WILLIAMS OBSTETRICS

Sixteenth Edition

Williams Obstetrics

Sixteenth Edition

JACK A. PRITCHARD, M.D.

Gillette Professor, Department of Obstetrics and Gynecology, University of Texas Southwestern Medical School, University of Texas Health Science Center at Dallas, and Director of Obstetrics, Parkland Memorial Hospital, Dallas, Texas

PAUL C. MACDONALD, M.D.

Professor, Department of Obstetrics and Gynecology and Biochemistry, University of Texas Southwestern Medical School, and Director of the Cecil H. and Ida Green Center for Reproductive Biology Sciences, University of Texas Health Science Center at Dallas, Texas

 APPLETON-CENTURY-CROFTS / New York

Prentice-Hall International, Inc., London
Prentice-Hall of Australia, Pty. Ltd., Sydney
Prentice-Hall of India Private Limited, New Delhi
Prentice-Hall of Japan, Inc., Tokyo
Prentice-Hall of Southeast Asia (Pte.) Ltd., Singapore
Whitehall Books Ltd., Wellington, New Zealand

Library of Congress Cataloging in Publication Data

Williams, John Whitridge, 1866–1931.
  Williams Obstetrics.

  Includes bibliographies and index.
  1. Obstetrics. I. Pritchard, Jack A., 1921–
II. MacDonald, Paul C., 1930–   III. Title.
IV. Title: Obstetrics.   [DNLM: 1. Obstetrics.
WQ100 P961w]
RG524.W7 1980   618.2   80–17633
ISBN 0–8385–9731–9

Text design: Alan Gold   Illustration Director: Tom Sims
Cover design: A Good Thing, Inc.   Production: John Morgan, Kathy Conyers

This edition of *Williams Obstetrics* is dedicated to Signe and Sue, whose love, loyalty, and devotion allowed us to pursue the careers that pleased us most—and whose patience, assistance, and criticism renewed our dedication to do so.

PREFACE

QUALITY of life for both the mother and the newborn rightfully has become our most important concern. Since the newborn faces the likelihood of 70 years or more of life, it is apparent that no greater service can be provided than ensuring that each newborn is well-born. Previously, medicine believed that cancer, heart disease, and stroke were the major problems facing our society. But since these maladies afflict the aged primarily, it is obvious that an untimely birth and birth-associated maladies are the problems that should have the highest priorities in medicine. Happily, we have entered an era in which the fetus can be rightfully considered and treated as our second patient. In this edition we have sought to do just that. Fetal diagnosis and therapy have now emerged as legitimate tools the obstetrician must possess. Moreover, the number of tools the obstetrician can employ to address the needs of the fetus increases each year. We are of the view that it is the most exciting of times to be an obstetrician. Who would have dreamed—even a few years ago—that we could serve the fetus as physician? Or, that the well-being and growth of the fetus could be monitored accurately and that the status of fetal health could be addressed? It is an exciting time, and we welcome you to join in this exciting adventure, Maternal-Fetal Medicine.

The revisions, and especially the additions, to this the sixteenth edition are almost too numerous to mention. One hundred of the figures represent either new drawings or extensive revisions of previous drawings. Nearly 200 pages have been added over and above deletions from the last edition. A few examples of the more extensive revisions are cited: Knowledge of the endocrinology of the placenta is now so great as to warrant a separate chapter, The Placental Hormones and Their Precursors (Chapter 7). Included in this new chapter are exciting discoveries concerned with the biogenesis of the major pregnancy hormone progesterone and a detailed description of the role of the fetal adrenal as a critical source of hormones and prehormones. Morphologic and Functional Development of the Fetus (Chapter 8) has been revised appreciably in keeping with the more definitive knowledge of fetal physiology that has become available recently. Technics to Evaluate Fetal Health (Chapter 14) has been revised and extended to reflect the value, and in a minority of instances, the lack of value, of specific procedures that may be applied to identify the status of the fetus. The unquestionable merit of sonography is emphasized, including 35 sonograms which serve to demonstrate its application in a variety of important pregnancy conditions. Physiology of Labor (Chapter 15) has been rewritten to include especially very recent biochemical observations concerned with the roles of glycerophospholipids, arachidonic acid, and prostaglandins in the initiation of labor. Diseases and Abnormalities of The Placenta and Fetal Membranes (Chapter 23) provides very recently acquired knowledge of the seemingly bizarre genetics that characterizes a true hydatidiform mole.

Pregnancy Complicated By Multiple Fetuses (Chapter 26) considers especially the marked reduction in perinatal mortality that has been accomplished in very recent years, at least in some institutions. Presented in Chapter 27, Hypertensive Disorders of Pregnancy, are intriguing concepts concerning the pathophysiology of pregnancy-induced hypertension and affirmation of the value of certain regimens of treatment. In Chapter 30, Dystocia Caused By Abnormalities In Presentation, Position, or Development of The Fetus, the question of delivery of the fetus who presents as a breech is carefully considered in light of recent experiences recorded by others as well as our own. Family Planning (Chapter 40) has been updated and the merits of some recommendations made previously which appeared to differ from general practice are affirmed. Cesarean Section and Cesarean Hysterectomy (Chapter 43) provides recent information concerning trends in delivery by cesarean birth as well as specific rates for some major institutions.

The magnitude of effort that was expended on this major revision required the participation of a large number of people to whom we are indeed grateful. Included among the many individuals in Dallas are Dr. Norman Gant, Chairman of the Department, and Dr. F. Gary Cunningham, Dr. Rigoberto Santos, Dr. Peggy J. Whalley, and all of our other faculty colleagues in the Department of Obstetrics and Gynecology, University of Texas Southwestern Medical School, who not only provided considerable information that we have incorporated into this edition, but who also performed many of our tasks within the department during the time of the revision.

Special praise and thanks must be given to Anita Lignoul who, with her monstrous machine, typed almost all of the manuscript, while improving its quality as she did so; to Tom Sims for his elegant art work in which he reaffirmed the adage, "A picture is worth a thousand words"; to Juanita Epperson for administrative leadership which allowed all of the many participants to provide excellent support; and last, but certainly not least, to Signe Pritchard who for at least 24 hours every day throughout the whole period of revision was concerned directly or indirectly with the myriad tasks essential to a successful outcome.

To Richard Lampert and John Morgan of Appleton-Century-Crofts, we are grateful for their excellent support, cooperation, effective persuasion, and the tolerance which they demonstrated during the preparation of this, the sixteenth edition.

CONTENTS

Colorplates

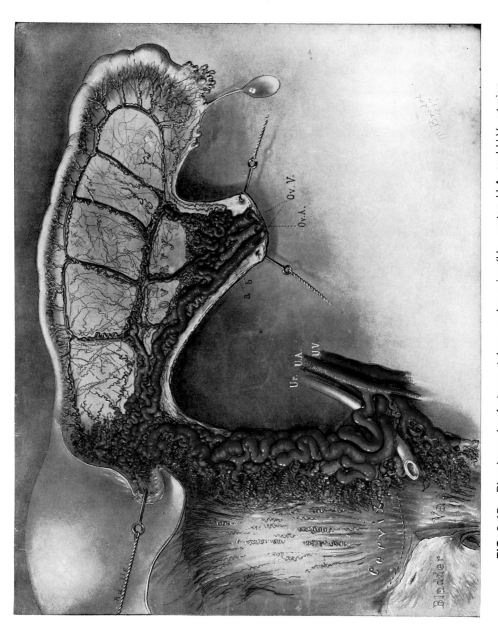

FIG. 2-15. Blood supply of uterus, tubes, and ovaries (Ur., ureter; U.A. and U.V., uterine artery and vein; Ov. A. and Ov. V., ovarian artery and vein).

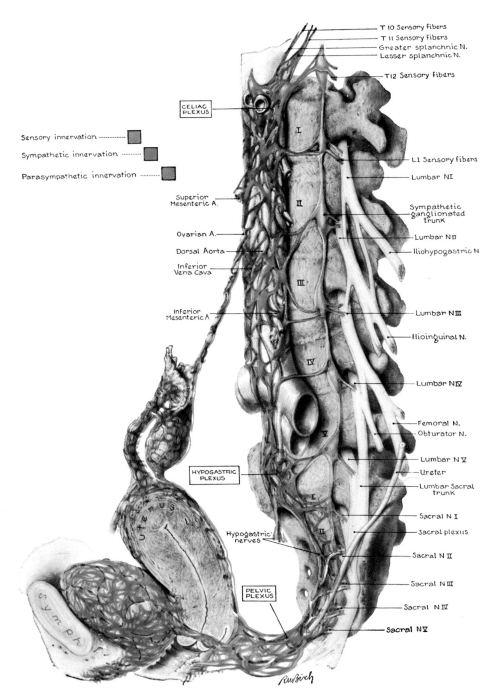

T 10 Sensory fibers
T 11 Sensory fibers
Greater splanchnic N.
Lesser splanchnic N.
T12 Sensory fibers

CELIAC
PLEXUS

L1 Sensory fibers

Lumbar N I

Sensory innervation
Sympathetic innervation
Parasympathetic innervation

Superior
Mesenteric A.

Sympathetic
ganglionated
trunk

Lumbar N II

Ovarian A.
Dorsal Aorta
Inferior
Vena Cava

Iliohypogastric N

Inferior
Mesenteric A

Lumbar N III

Ilioinguinal N.

Lumbar N IV

Femoral N.
Obturator N.

Lumbar N V

HYPOGASTRIC
PLEXUS

Ureter
Lumbar Sacral
trunk

Uterus

Sacral N I
Sacral plexus

Hypogastric
nerves

Sacral N II

Sacral N III

PELVIC
PLEXUS

Sacral N IV

Symph

Sacral N V

FIG. 2-16. Nerve supply of the uterus (Symph, symphysis pubis).

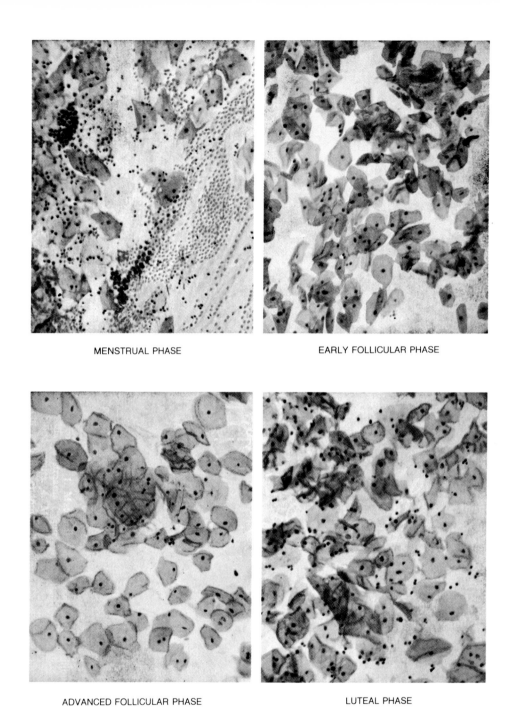

MENSTRUAL PHASE

EARLY FOLLICULAR PHASE

ADVANCED FOLLICULAR PHASE

LUTEAL PHASE

FIG. 4-13. Vaginal smears in normal menstrual cycle stained with OG6-EA36. Acidophilic cells red; basophilic cells blue-green. Photomicrographs colored by H. Murayama. (From Papanicolaou, Traut, and Marchetti. *The Epithelia of Woman's Reproductive Organs*. New York, Commonwealth Fund, 1948)

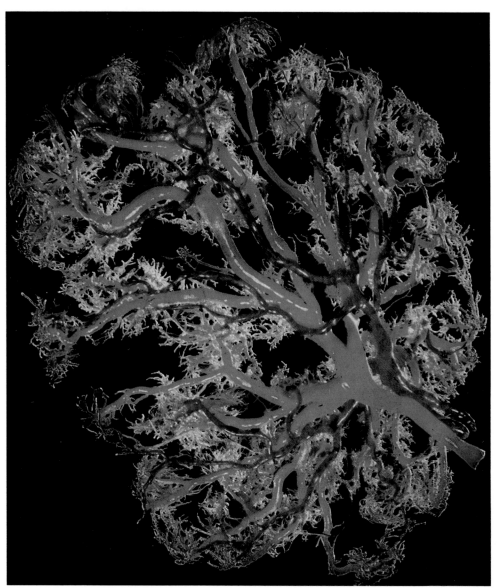

FIG. 6-19. Specimen of term human placenta obtained by corrosion. Fetal circulation viewed from the fetal side. (Prepared by Rudolph Skarda; courtesy of Abbott Laboratories)

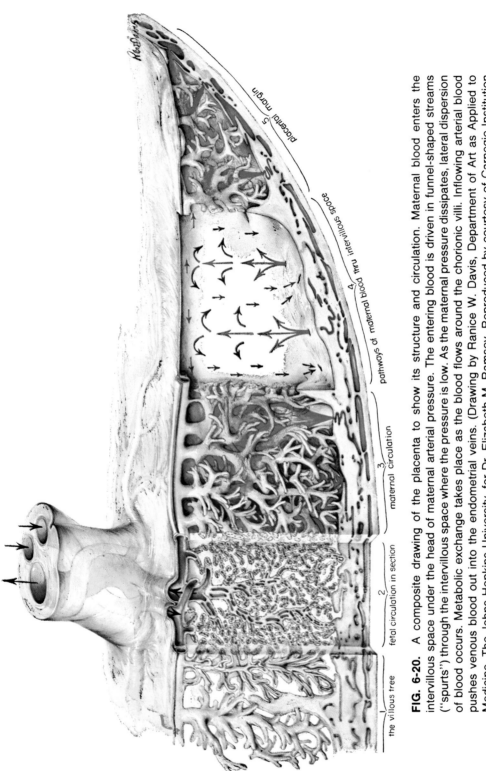

FIG. 6-20. A composite drawing of the placenta to show its structure and circulation. Maternal blood enters the intervillous space under the head of maternal arterial pressure. The entering blood is driven in funnel-shaped streams ("spurts") through the intervillous space where the pressure is low. As the maternal pressure dissipates, lateral dispersion of blood occurs. Metabolic exchange takes place as the blood flows around the chorionic villi. Inflowing arterial blood pushes venous blood out into the endometrial veins. (Drawing by Ranice W. Davis, Department of Art as Applied to Medicine, The Johns Hopkins University, for Dr. Elizabeth M. Ramsey. Reproduced by courtesy of Carnegie Institution of Washington.)

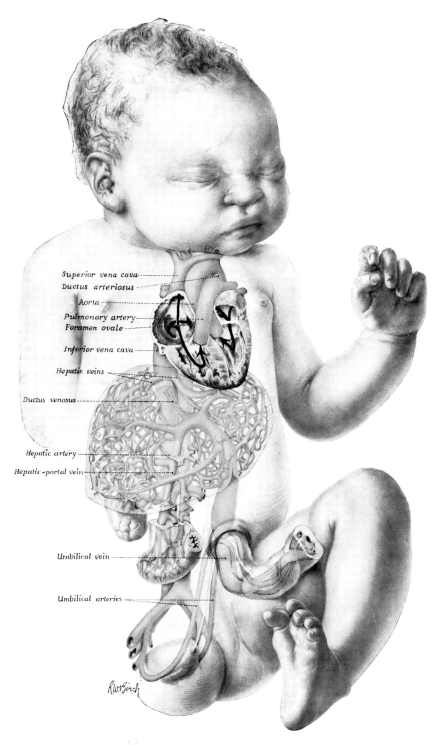

Superior vena cava

Ductus arteriosus

Aorta

Pulmonary artery

Foramen ovale

Inferior vena cava

Hepatic veins

Ductus venosus

Hepatic artery

Hepatic-portal vein

Umbilical vein

Umbilical arteries

R.W.Birch

FIG. 8-10. Cardiovascular system of fetus.

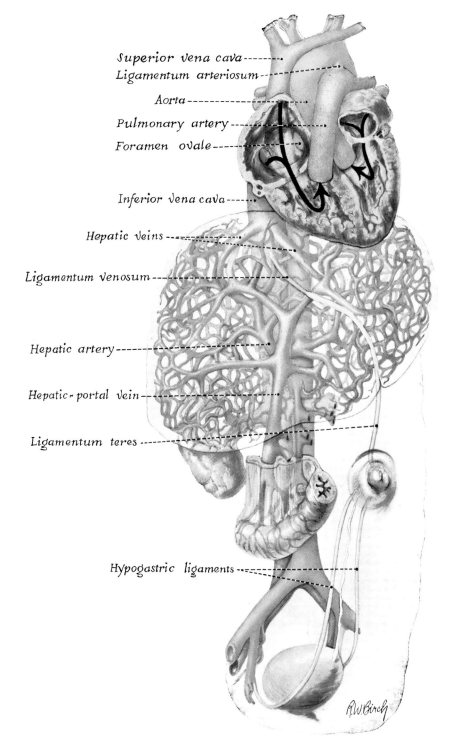

Superior vena cava

Ligamentum arteriosum

Aorta

Pulmonary artery

Foramen ovale

Inferior vena cava

Hepatic veins

Ligamentum venosum

Hepatic artery

Hepatic-portal vein

Ligamentum teres

Hypogastric ligaments

FIG. 8-11. Cardiovascular system of infant after birth.

WILLIAMS OBSTETRICS

Sixteenth Edition

1

Obstetrics in Broad Perspective

Obstetrics* is the branch of medicine that deals with parturition, its antecedents, and its sequels. It is concerned principally, therefore, with the phenomena and management of pregnancy, labor, and the puerperium, in both normal and abnormal circumstances.

In a broader sense, obstetrics is concerned with reproduction of a society. Appropriate obstetric care promotes health and well-being, both physical and mental, among younger people and their offspring and helps them develop healthy attitudes toward sex, family life, and the place of the family in society. Obstetrics is concerned with all the physiologic, psychologic, and social factors that profoundly influence both the quantity and the quality of human reproduction. The problems of population growth are the natural heritage of obstetrics. The vital statistics of the nation, published monthly by the National Center for Health Statistics, attest to society's concern with the charge of this specialty.

The word *obstetrics* is derived from the Latin term *obstetrix*, meaning midwife. The ety-

mology of obstetrix, however, is obscure. Most dictionaries connect it with the verb *obstare*, which means *to stand by* or *in front of*. The rationale of this derivation is that the midwife stood by or in front of the parturient. This etymology has long been attacked by some etymologists who believed that the word was originally *adstetrix* and that the *ad* had been changed to *ob*. In that case, obstetrix would mean *the woman assisting the parturient*. The fact that on certain inscriptions *obstetrix* is also spelled *opstetrix* has led to the conjecture that it was derived from *ops (aid)* and *stare*, meaning *the woman rendering aid*. According to Temkin,† the most likely interpretation is that obstetrix meant *the woman who stood by the parturient*. Whether it alluded merely to the midwife's standing in front of or near the parturient or whether it carried the additional connotation of rendering aid is not clear.

The term *obstetrics* is of relatively recent usage. The Oxford English Dictionary gives the earliest example from a book published in 1819, indicating that in 1828 it was necessary to apologize for the use of the word *obstetrician*. Kindred terms, however, are much older. For example, *obstetricate* occurs

* Oxford English Dictionary. Oxford at the Clarendon Press, 1933. The statements about the history of the term *obstetrics*, as well as the definition of obstetrics as stated in the first sentence of this chapter, were obtained chiefly from this source.

† Previous communication. Dr. Owsei Temkin, Associate Professor of the History of Medicine, Johns Hopkins University School of Medicine, graciously devoted time to a study of the etymology of the word *obstetrics*, and the comments cited were entirely his.

in English works published as early as 1623; *obstetricatory,* in 1640; *obstetricious,* in 1645; and *obstetrical,* in 1775. These terms were often used figuratively. As an example of such usage, the adjective *obstetric* appears in Pope's *Dunciad* (1742) in the famous couplet:

There all the Learn'd shall at the labour stand,

and Douglas lend his soft, obstetric hand.

The much older term *midwifery* was used instead of *obstetrics* until the latter part of the nineteenth century in both the United States and Great Britain. It is derived from the Middle English *mid,* meaning *with,* and *wif,* meaning wife in the sense of a *woman.* The term *midwife* was used as early as 1303, and *midwifery,* in 1483. In England today, the term *midwifery* carries the same connotation as obstetrics, and the two words are used synonymously.

Aims of Obstetrics. The transcendent objective of obstetrics is that every pregnancy be wanted and culminate in a healthy mother and a healthy baby. Obstetrics strives to minimize the number of women and infants who die as a result of the reproductive process or who are left physically, intellectually, or emotionally injured therefrom. Obstetrics is concerned further with the number and spacing of children so that both mother and offspring, indeed all the family, may enjoy optimal physical and emotional well-being. Finally, obstetrics strives to analyze and influence the social factors that impinge on reproductive efficiency.

Vital Statistics. To aid in the reduction of the number of mothers and infants who die as the result of pregnancy and labor, it is important to know how many such deaths occur in this country each year and in what circumstances. To try to help evaluate these data correctly, a variety of events concerned with pregnancy outcomes have been defined by various agencies:

Birth. This is the complete expulsion or extraction from the mother of a fetus irrespective of whether or not the umbilical cord has been cut or the placenta is attached. Fetuses weighing less than 500 g usually are not considered as births, but rather as abortions, for purposes of perinatal statistics. In the absence of a birth weight, a body length of 25 cm, crown to heel, is usually equated with 500 g. Twenty weeks gestation age is commonly considered to be equivalent to 500 g fetal weight; however, a 500 g fetus is more likely to be 22 weeks gestational age.

Birth Rate. The number of births per 1000 population is the birth rate, or crude birth rate.

Fertility Rate. This important term refers to the number of live births per 1000 female population aged 15 through 44 years.

Live Birth. Whenever the infant at or sometime after birth breathes spontaneously or shows any other sign of life such as heart beat or definite spontaneous movement of voluntary muscles, a live birth is recorded.

Stillbirth. None of the above signs of life are present at or after birth.

Neonatal Death. Early neonatal death refers to death of a live-born infant during the first 7 days of life. Late neonatal death refers to death after 7 but before 29 days of life.

Stillbirth Rate. The number of stillborn infants per 1000 infants born.

Fetal Death Rate. This term is synonymous with stillbirth rate.

Neonatal Mortality Rate. The number of neonatal deaths per 1000 live births.

Perinatal Mortality Rate. This rate is defined as the number of stillbirths plus neonatal deaths per 1000 total births.

Low Birth Weight. If the first weight obtained after birth is less than 2500 g, low birth weight is identified.

Term Infant. An infant born any time after 37 completed weeks of gestation through 41 completed weeks of gestation (260 to 287 days) has been defined by some to be a term infant. Such a definition implies that birth at any time within this period is optimal whereas birth before or afterward is not. Such an implication is not warranted. Some infants born between 37 and

38 weeks are at risk of functional prematurity, for example, the development of respiratory distress in the newborn infant of a diabetic mother (see Chap. 28, p. 743). Moreover, any risk to the fetus that might be imposed by remaining in utero until 42 weeks rather than 41 weeks does not appear to be appreciable. Consequently, there is no good reason for distorting the range for term birth to 3 weeks below the mean of 40 weeks but only 1 week beyond the mean. Therefore, it is our opinion that a term infant is better defined as one who is born no earlier than 38 completed weeks but no later than 42 completed weeks of gestation (see Chap. 37, p. 925).

Preterm or Premature Infant.   An infant born before 37 completed weeks has been so classified, although born before 38 completed weeks would seem more appropriate for reasons stated above.

Postterm Infant.   An infant born anytime after the beginning of the 42nd week has been classified by some as being postterm.

Abortus.   A fetus or embryo removed or expelled from the uterus during the first half of gestation (20 weeks or less), or weighing less than 500 g, or measuring less than 25 cm is also referred to as an abortus.

Direct Maternal Death.   Death of the mother resulting from obstetric complications of the pregnancy state, labor, or puerperium, and from interventions, omissions, incorrect treatment, or a chain of events resulting from any of the above is considered a direct maternal death. (Example: exsanguination from rupture of uterus.)

Indirect Maternal Death.   An obstetric death not directly due to obstetric causes but resulting from previously existing disease, or a disease that developed during pregnancy, labor, or the puerperium, but which was aggravated by the maternal physiologic adaptation to pregnancy, is classified as an indirect maternal death. (Example: mitral stenosis.)

Nonmaternal Death.   Death of the mother resulting from accidental or incidental causes in no way related to the pregnancy may be classified as a nonmaternal death. (Example: death from an airplane crash.)

Maternal Death Rate or Mortality.   The number of maternal deaths that occur as the result of the reproductive process per 100,000 live births. (Note: this rate is calculated per *one hundred thousand* live births and not per *one thousand.*)

The Birth Rate and Fertility Rate. One index of the need for obstetric personnel and facilities is the number of births each year. Additional indices are the birth rate and the fertility rate. From these data, particularly the fertility rate, the expected number of births in future years can be estimated.

In 1979, there were 3.47 million live births in the United States. This is 9 percent less than the number in 1970 but 8 percent more than 1975 when a nadir for that decade was achieved. The fertility rate was 68.0 in 1979 and 66.7 in 1975. Thus, the reason for more births in 1979 compared to 1975 was an increase in the number of women between 15 and 44 years of age as well as a slight increase in their fertility.

Maternal Mortality.   Maternal deaths per 100,000 live births have decreased remarkably in the past half century. There were only 320 maternal deaths in the United States reported in 1978, or 9.9 per 100,000 live births. By way of comparison, there were 12,544 maternal deaths, or 582.1 per 100,000 live births in 1935! Values for intervening years are presented in Table 1-1.

The nearly three-fold difference in maternal mortality rates that exists between white and black women appears to result primarily from social and economic factors, such as a relative lack of skilled personnel and appropriate facilities at delivery, lack of antepartum care, lack of family planning services, faulty health education, dietary deficiencies, and poor hygiene. As these unfavorable social and economic conditions are improved, the racial difference in the maternal death rates will doubtless decrease.

The maternal mortality rate varies also

with the age of the mother. In all races, the remarkable increase in mortality with advancing age can be explained only on the basis of an intrinsic maternal factor. The increasing frequency of hypertension with advancing years and the greater tendency to uterine hemorrhage contribute significantly to the elevation of the mortality rate. Advanced age and high parity act independently to increase the risk of childbearing, but their effects are usually additive. In the actual analysis of cases, it is difficult to dissociate these two factors.

COMMON CAUSES OF MATERNAL MORTALITY.   Hemorrhage, hypertension that is either induced or aggravated by pregnancy, and infection still account for half the maternal deaths in the United States. The causes of obstetric hemorrhage are multiple: postpartum hemorrhage, bleeding in association with abortion, bleeding from rupture of the fallopian tube (ectopic pregnancy), bleeding as the result of abnormal placental location or separation (placenta previa and abruptio placentae), and bleeding from rupture of the uterus. Hypertension induced or aggravated by pregnancy, occurring in about 6 or 7 percent of gravid women, is accompanied commonly by edema and proteinuria (preeclamp-

sia), and in some severe cases by convulsions and coma (eclampsia). Puerperal infection of the genital tract usually originates as metritis, which sometimes undergoes extension to cause peritonitis, thrombophlebitis, bacteremia, and distant foci of infection. Details of the origin, prevention, and treatment of these conditions form a considerable portion of the subject matter of obstetrics.

REASONS FOR DECLINE IN MATERNAL MORTALITY RATE.   Many factors and agencies are responsible for the dramatic fall in the maternal death rate in this country over the past 30 years. Obviously, there has been a general improvement in medical practice. The widespread use of blood transfusion and antibiotics and the maintenance of fluid, electrolyte, and acid–base balance in the serious complications of pregnancy and labor have materially changed obstetric practice. Equally important is the development of widespread obstetric training and continuing educational programs, which have provided more and better qualified specialists.

Obstetrics is unique in that no other branch of medicine is subject to such careful public scrutiny. Not only are births a matter of public record, but maternal and perinatal deaths are examined by municipal, state, and

TABLE 1-1.
MATERNAL MORTALITY IN THE UNITED STATES 1935–1978

MATERNAL DEATHS		RATE PER 100,000 LIVE BIRTHS		
Year	(No.)	Total	White	Other
1935	12,544	582.1	530.6	945.7
1940	8,876	376.0	319.8	773.5
1945	5,668	207.2	172.1	454.8
1950	2,960	83.3	61.1	221.6
1955	1,901	47.0	32.8	130.3
1960	1,579	37.1	26.0	97.9
1965	1,189	31.6	21.0	83.7
1970	803	21.5	14.4	55.9
1975	403	12.8	9.1	29.0
1976	390	12.3	9.0	26.5
1978*	320	9.9	—	—

* Provisional
From Facts of Life and Death, United States Department of Health, Education and Welfare, 1978, Publication No. 79–1222 and Monthly Vital Statistics Report, United States Department of Health, Education and Welfare, 27(13):8, 1979.

national health authorities. In many areas, local medical or obstetric and gynecologic societies also examine such deaths, and mortality conferences are frequently conducted as part of the continuing medical education of the obstetrician.

The *sine qua non* of good work in any field is well-trained personnel, but they could not have achieved the excellent results had there not been a great expansion in facilities for good obstetric care. Despite increased facilities, there remain areas in the United States where obstetric services are woefully inadequate, particularly in rural areas and in some of our large inner cities.

From the viewpoint of safer care during labor, the outstanding advance of the past 40 years has been the great increase in the proportion of hospital deliveries. As recently as 1940, only three out of five white births took place in hospitals; this figure now exceeds 99 percent. Hospital births not only mean better facilities but imply care by individuals specially trained in obstetrics and perinatology.

Perinatal Mortality. The sum of stillbirths and neonatal deaths is the perinatal mortality. The perinatal death rate has fallen by nearly 50 percent in the past 25 years (Table 1-2). Currently, there are about 180 perinatal deaths for every maternal death. With the current very low incidence of maternal deaths, perinatal loss rates not only are a better index of the level of obstetric care, but also give a valid indication of an equally important datum, the infant morbidity. To some extent, the total perinatal loss is correlated with the age and parity of the mother. The rates tend to be highest for the first born of very young women and births of the order of six and over.

FACTORS AFFECTING THE STILLBIRTH RATE. Nearly one-half of perinatal deaths are stillbirths. Stillbirths tend to decline as the quality of care during and throughout pregnancy improves. With improvement in prenatal care and proper hospitalization, some of these deaths need not occur. In too large a proportion of deaths in utero, unfortunately, there may be no obvious explanation.

NEONATAL DEATHS. In 1977, for the first time in the United States, there were fewer neonatal deaths than fetal deaths (stillbirths). Nearly half of the neonatal deaths occur in the first day of life. The number of deaths during those 24 hours exceeds that from the second month to the completion of the first year. The causes of this huge wastage during the neonatal period are numerous, but the most important is low birth weight usually as the consequence of delivery long before term. The proportion of infants of low birth weight differs among ethnic

TABLE 1-2.
PERINATAL MORTALITY IN THE UNITED STATES 1950–1977

YEAR	PERINATAL		FETAL		NEONATAL	
	Number	Ratio	Number	Ratio	Number	Ratio*
1950	141,117	39.7	68,262	19.2	72,855	20.5
1955	146,504	36.2	69,153	17.1	77,351	19.1
1960	148,213	34.8	68,480	16.1	79,733	18.7
1965	127,278	33.9	60,859	16.2	66,419	17.7
1970	109,240	29.3	52,961	14.2	56,279	15.1
1975	70,212	22.3	33,796	10.7	36,416	11.6
1977	65,913	19.6	33,053	9.8	32,860	9.9

From Facts of Life and Death, United States Department of Health, Education, and Welfare, 1978, Publication No. 79–1222.
* Deaths per 1,000 live births; neonatal deaths up to 28 days.

groups, ranging from about 60 per 1000 for white mothers to approximately 120 per 1000 births for black mothers. The interracial difference in the rates of low birth weight accounts for the major difference in neonatal mortality between these two groups. Social and environmental factors probably weigh more heavily than race, however, in the cause of this difference. As well as deaths, low birth weight has contributed appreciably to infant morbidity and for a large fraction of the neurologic and intellectual deficits that are tragic individually and costly to society. Why some women go into labor prematurely is one of the greatest unsolved problems of obstetrics.

The second most common cause of neonatal death is injury to the central nervous system. Here the word *injury* is used in its broad sense to indicate both cerebral injury resulting from hypoxia in utero and traumatic injury to the brain during labor and delivery. Some of these deaths could be prevented by more judicious management of labor. Another important cause of neonatal death is congenital malformation.

The Birth Certificate. Statutes in all 50 states and the District of Columbia require that a birth certificate be completed for every birth and submitted promptly to the local registrar. After the birth has been duly registered, notification is sent to the parents of the child and a complete report is forwarded to the National Center for Health Statistics in Washington.

There are many reasons why the complete and accurate registration of births is essential. Certification of the facts of birth is needed as evidence of age, citizenship, and family relationships. Moreover, the data they provide are of immeasurable importance to all agencies (social, public health, demographic, or obstetric) dealing with human reproduction. For instance, the data presented in the foregoing paragraphs were culled almost entirely from information published by the National Center for Health on the basis of birth certificates; they represent, furthermore, only a small fraction of the information obtainable from that source. A birth certificate, such as

that shown in Figure 1-1, provides even more data of direct obstetric importance. *Hence, the prompt and accurate completion of this certificate after each birth is not only a legal duty but a contribution to the broad field of obstetric knowledge.*

Obstetrics and Other Branches of Medicine. Obstetrics is a multifaceted subject, with close and numerous relations to other branches of medicine. It is so intimately related to the kindred subject of gynecology that obstetrics and gynecology are generally regarded as one specialty. Gynecology deals with the physiology and the pathology of the female reproductive organs in the nonpregnant state, whereas obstetrics deals with the pregnant state and its sequels. Correct differential diagnosis in either obstetrics or gynecology entails an intimate acquaintance with the clinical syndromes met in both; in addition, the methods of examination and many operative technics are common to both disciplines. It is therefore obligatory that every obstetrician have extensive experience in gynecology, and vice versa.

The scope of intrauterine diagnosis and treatment has broadened remarkably (see Chap. 14 and elsewhere). This, as well as the concern of obstetrics with the newborn infant, has brought the subject into close relation with pediatrics and given rise to the concept of perinatology. The boundaries between obstetrics and neonatology are not sharp, but rather overlap to the benefit of the fetus and infant. Even in metropolitan centers, inconvenient hours of birth often impose on the obstetrician the management of the newborn during the most critical hour of life. The obstetrician must possess expertise, therefore, in the management of the infant at this time as well as before birth.

Since pregnant and nonpregnant women are subject to the same diseases, the obstetrician commonly encounters and therefore must be knowledgeable about a variety of diseases in pregnant women. As emphasized in Chapter 28, the clinical picture presented by some of these disorders is altered greatly during pregnancy and the immediate puer-

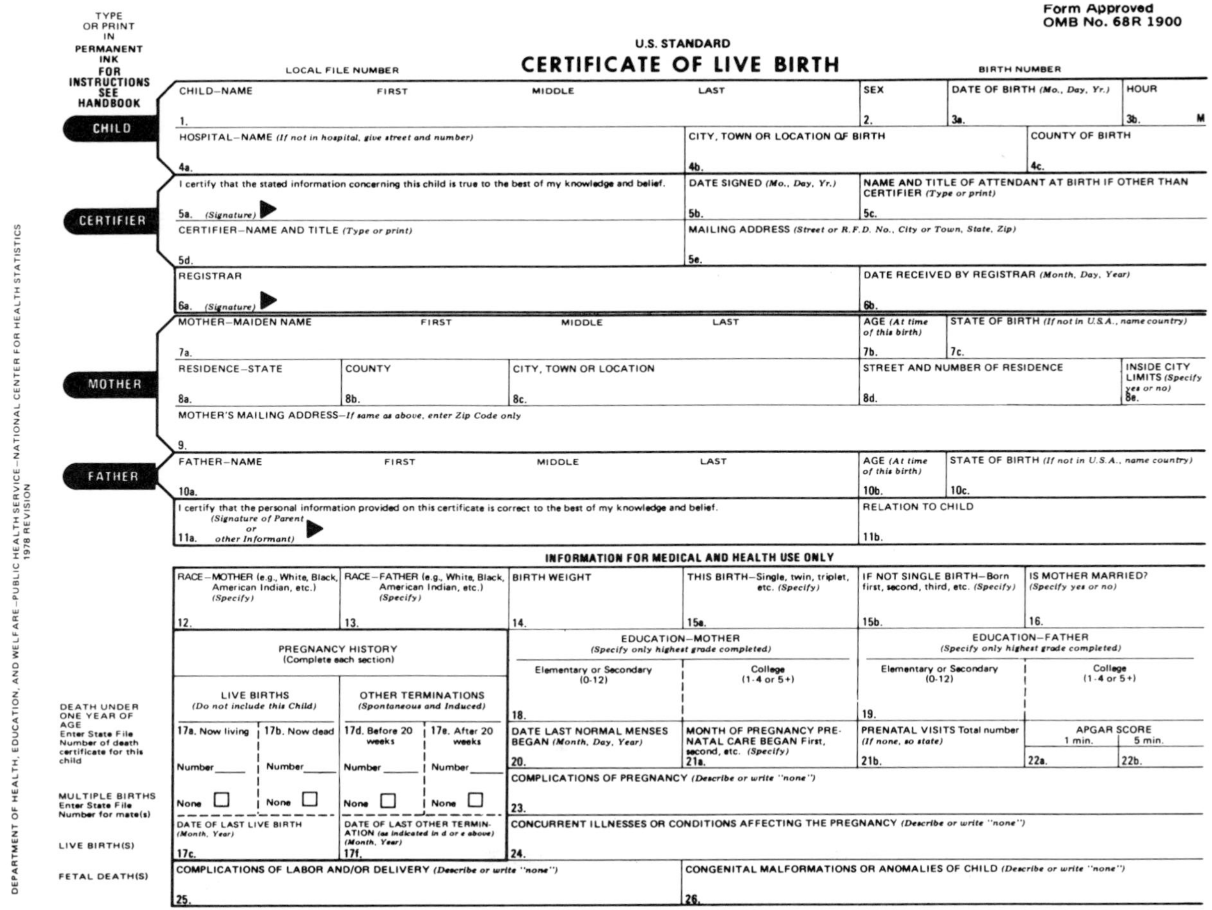

Form Approved
OMB No. 68R 1900

TYPE OR PRINT IN PERMANENT INK
FOR INSTRUCTIONS SEE HANDBOOK

U.S. STANDARD
CERTIFICATE OF LIVE BIRTH

LOCAL FILE NUMBER
BIRTH NUMBER

CHILD
CHILD–NAME FIRST MIDDLE LAST 1.
SEX 2.
DATE OF BIRTH (Mo., Day, Yr.) 3a.
HOUR 3b. M
HOSPITAL–NAME (If not in hospital, give street and number) 4a.
CITY, TOWN OR LOCATION OF BIRTH 4b.
COUNTY OF BIRTH 4c.

CERTIFIER
I certify that the stated information concerning this child is true to the best of my knowledge and belief.
5a. (Signature)
DATE SIGNED (Mo., Day, Yr.) 5b.
NAME AND TITLE OF ATTENDANT AT BIRTH IF OTHER THAN CERTIFIER (Type or print) 5c.
CERTIFIER–NAME AND TITLE (Type or print) 5d.
MAILING ADDRESS (Street or R.F.D. No., City or Town, State, Zip) 5e.
REGISTRAR 6a. (Signature)
DATE RECEIVED BY REGISTRAR (Month, Day, Year) 6b.

MOTHER
MOTHER–MAIDEN NAME FIRST MIDDLE LAST 7a.
AGE (At time of this birth) 7b.
STATE OF BIRTH (If not in U.S.A., name country) 7c.
RESIDENCE–STATE 8a.
COUNTY 8b.
CITY, TOWN OR LOCATION 8c.
STREET AND NUMBER OF RESIDENCE 8d.
INSIDE CITY LIMITS (Specify yes or no) 8e.
MOTHER'S MAILING ADDRESS–If same as above, enter Zip Code only 9.

FATHER
FATHER–NAME FIRST MIDDLE LAST 10a.
AGE (At time of this birth) 10b.
STATE OF BIRTH (If not in U.S.A., name country) 10c.
I certify that the personal information provided on this certificate is correct to the best of my knowledge and belief.
11a. (Signature of Parent or other Informant)
RELATION TO CHILD 11b.

INFORMATION FOR MEDICAL AND HEALTH USE ONLY

RACE–MOTHER (e.g., White, Black, American Indian, etc.) (Specify) 12.
RACE–FATHER (e.g., White, Black, American Indian, etc.) (Specify) 13.
BIRTH WEIGHT 14.
THIS BIRTH–Single, twin, triplet, etc. (Specify) 15a.
IF NOT SINGLE BIRTH–Born first, second, third, etc. (Specify) 15b.
IS MOTHER MARRIED? (Specify yes or no) 16.

PREGNANCY HISTORY (Complete each section)
LIVE BIRTHS (Do not include this Child)
17a. Now living Number ___ None ☐
17b. Now dead Number ___ None ☐
DATE OF LAST LIVE BIRTH (Month, Year) 17c.
OTHER TERMINATIONS (Spontaneous and Induced)
17d. Before 20 weeks Number ___ None ☐
17e. After 20 weeks Number ___ None ☐
DATE OF LAST OTHER TERMINATION (as indicated in d or e above) (Month, Year) 17f.

EDUCATION–MOTHER (Specify only highest grade completed)
Elementary or Secondary (0-12) College (1-4 or 5+) 18.
EDUCATION–FATHER (Specify only highest grade completed)
Elementary or Secondary (0-12) College (1-4 or 5+) 19.
DATE LAST NORMAL MENSES BEGAN (Month, Day, Year) 20.
MONTH OF PREGNANCY PRENATAL CARE BEGAN First, second, etc. (Specify) 21a.
PRENATAL VISITS Total number (If none, so state) 21b.
APGAR SCORE 1 min. 22a. 5 min. 22b.
COMPLICATIONS OF PREGNANCY (Describe or write "none") 23.
CONCURRENT ILLNESSES OR CONDITIONS AFFECTING THE PREGNANCY (Describe or write "none") 24.
COMPLICATIONS OF LABOR AND/OR DELIVERY (Describe or write "none") 25.
CONGENITAL MALFORMATIONS OR ANOMALIES OF CHILD (Describe or write "none") 26.

DEATH UNDER ONE YEAR OF AGE Enter State File Number of death certificate for this child
MULTIPLE BIRTHS Enter State File Number for mate(s)
LIVE BIRTH(S)
FETAL DEATH(S)

DEPARTMENT OF HEALTH, EDUCATION, AND WELFARE–PUBLIC HEALTH SERVICE–NATIONAL CENTER FOR HEALTH STATISTICS
1978 REVISION

FIG. 1-1. United States standard birth certificate contains data for statistical information and confidential data to be used only for medical statistical purposes.

perium; conversely, these diseases affect the course of gestation.

Obstetrics is intimately related to the preclinical sciences. The study of spontaneous abortion, for example, depends on knowledge of anomalies in the development of the early embryo and trophoblast. Abortion may also involve hormonal defects, which condition would link the subjects of obstetrics and endocrinology; or abortion may result from chromosomal defects, and such a condition would forge a link to cytogenetics. The concept of Rh isoimmunization has shown how immunologic factors may interfere with the successful outcome of pregnancy, but in turn, by appropriate immunotherapy, be successfully prevented. Obstetrics and general pathology meet most closely in the rapidly developing field of perinatal pathology. Other important relations of obstetrics to preclinical sciences include: microbiology, in the study of maternal and fetal infections; biochemistry and physiology, in relation to myriad events including labor; and pharmacology, in the action and metabolism of drugs in the mother and in the fetus and newborn infant. The numerous applications of the preclinical sciences to problems of human reproduction are evidenced in the relatively short but remarkable history of the National Institute of Child Health and Human Development.

Obstetrics is related also to certain fields that are not strictly medical. Since nutritional requirements are altered by pregnancy, obstetrics requires knowledge of the science of nutrition. In studies of fetal malformations, genetics is obviously of prime importance. Since the mother–child relationship is the basis of the family unit, the obstetrician is continually dealing with psychologic and sociologic problems. Economics play a prominent role in obstetrics since health care may be quite expensive, and especially so when those who provide it have little concern for costs. In addition, obstetrics has important legal aspects, especially in regard to the increasing number of malpractice suits.

Obstetrics, the Mother, and Her Family. In spite of the remarkable record of safety for the hospitalized expectant mother and her fetus-infant that has been achieved in recent years (Tables 1-1 and 1-2), there has evolved a small but quite vocal group of dissidents made up of former parturients, their partners, and those who would attempt to provide care during home delivery. Hopefully, those complaints about hospitalization for which there are real bases can be resolved short of sacrificing the safety that hospitalization for delivery can provide the mother and especially her fetus-infant.

There is no question but that some individuals who collaborate in the effort to provide optimal in-hospital care for the mother and the fetus-infant have not necessarily been as considerate of the pregnant mother and her family as they should have been. The expectant mother has been commonly treated as if she were seriously ill, even when she was quite healthy. All too often she has been forced to conform to a common pathway of care which stripped her of most of her individuality and much of her dignity. Niceties of surroundings have not been provided; instead, hospital austerity has prevailed. Hospital administrators have tended not to seek her business claiming they lost money on obstetrics. In recent years, obstetricians, for many good reasons, have worked mostly in groups and as a consequence, about the time of delivery, the ultimate event in the minds of the mother and her family, there may have been either a "changing of the obstetrical guard" or the obstetrician created the appearance of wanting to hurry the labor and delivery since he or she would soon be "going off." The same picture has been presented by the nurses and other personnel intimately involved in providing care for the mother and fetus-infant. Too often the expectant mother has felt that her fate and the fate of her baby were dependent not so much on skilled personnel but upon an electrical black box that appeared to possess some great power that prevailed above all other. Fortunately, appropriate applications of medical science do not require that excellent care be a dehumanizing ordeal. Excellent obstetric care and the many benefits that accrue can be provided in a hospital setting that, at the same time, is enjoyed by the mother and family, and is acceptable economically to all parties involved.

The Future. Although the recent decline in maternal mortality rate has been enormous, the millennium is neither here nor close by. If the nonwhite mortality rate were reduced to the level of that of the white by providing equal care, and if the white deaths considered preventable by many mortality studies were prevented, approximately two-thirds of these mothers' lives could be saved each year. Maternal mortality affects most seriously the socially and economically deprived. Many of these deaths result from sheer lack of adequate facilities, including lack of properly distributed units for antepartum care, lack of suitable hospital arrangements, and lack of readily available blood. Others are caused by errors of management by the obstetric personnel. Errors of omission include failure to provide antepartum care, failure to follow the woman and fetus carefully throughout labor and the early puerperium, and failure to obtain appropriate consultation. Among errors of commission, traumatic delivery looms large.

These several deficiencies in maternity care must obviously by corrected first if maternal and perinatal mortality rates are to be brought to the irreducible minimum. They can and doubtless will be lowered to that level by the same methods that have proved efficacious in the past: more and better trained personnel and equipped facilities available to all pregnant women and their fetuses.

The concept of the right of every child to be physically, mentally, and emotionally "well-born" is fundamental to human dignity. If obstetrics is to play a role in its realization, the specialty must maintain and even extend its role in the control of population. The right to be "well-born" in its broadest sense is simply incompatible with unrestricted fertility. Yet our knowledge of the forces operative in the fluctuation and control of population growth is still rudimentary. This concept of obstetrics as a social as well as a biologic science impels us to accept a responsibility unprecedented in American medicine.

2

The Anatomy of the Female Reproductive Tract

The organs of reproduction of women are classified as external and internal. The external organs and the vagina serve for copulation; the internal organs provide for development and birth of the fetus.

EXTERNAL GENERATIVE ORGANS

The *pudenda,* or the external organs of generation, are commonly designated the *vulva,* which includes all structures visible externally from the pubis to the perineum: the mons pubis, the labia majora and labia minora, the clitoris, hymen, vestibule, urethral opening, and various glandular and vascular structures (Fig. 2-1).

Mons Pubis. The mons pubis, or mons veneris, is the fat-filled cushion over the anterior surface of the symphysis pubis. After puberty, the skin of the mons pubis is covered by curly hair, forming the *escutcheon.* The distribution of pubic hair generally differs in the two sexes. In women, it occupies a triangular area, the base of which is formed by the upper margin of the symphysis, and a few hairs extend downward over the outer surface of the labia majora. In men, the escutcheon is not so well circumscribed, the hairs extending upward toward the umbilicus and downward over the inner surface of the thighs. Although considered a secondary sexual characteristic, the escutcheon of women occasionally resembles that of men.

Labia Majora. Extending downward and backward from the mons pubis there are two rounded folds of adipose tissue covered with skin, the labia majora. These structures vary in appearance, according to the amount of fat contained within them. The labia majora are homologous with the scrotum of men. The round ligaments terminate at their upper borders. The labia majora are less prominent after repeated childbearing, and in old age they usually shrivel. Ordinarily these structures are 7 to 8 cm in length, 2 to 3 cm in width, and 1 to 1.5 cm in thickness, and are somewhat tapered at their lower extremities. In children and nulliparous women the labia majora usually lie in close apposition, completely concealing the underlying parts, whereas in multiparous women they may gape widely (Fig. 2-1). The labia majora

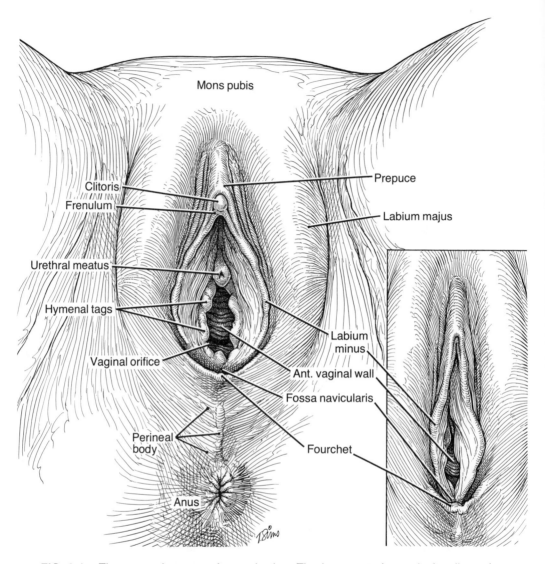

FIG. 2-1. The external organs of reproduction. The lower anterior vaginal wall can be seen through the gaping labia. The vaginal orifice is usually closed or nearly so (inset) except in some women of high parity.

are continuous directly with the mons pubis above and merge into the perineum posteriorly, where they join medially to form the *posterior commissure.*

Before puberty, the outer surface of each labium majus resembles the adjacent skin, but is covered with hair after puberty. In nulliparous women, the inner surface is moist, resembling a mucous membrane, whereas in multiparous women the inner surface be-comes more skinlike, but is not covered with hair. The labia majora are richly supplied with sebaceous glands. Beneath the skin, there is a layer of dense connective tissue, which is rich in elastic fibers and adipose tissue but is nearly free of muscular elements. Unlike the squamous epithelium of the vagina and cervix, parts of the vulvar skin contain many epithelial appendages. Beneath the skin there is a mass of fat, which provides the bulk of the volume of the labium; this adipose tissue is supplied with a plexus of veins which, as the result of external injury, may rupture to create a hematoma.

Labia Minora. Upon separating the labia majora, two flat reddish folds are visible. These structures are the labia minora, or nymphae, which meet at the upper extremity of the vulva. The labia minora vary greatly in size and shape. In nulliparous women, the labia minora are usually hidden, whereas in multiparous women the labia minora project beyond the labia majora.

Each labium minus consists of a thin fold of tissue which, when protected, presents a moist, reddish appearance, similar to that of a mucous membrane. However, these structures are covered by stratified squamous epithelium, into which numerous papillae project. The labia minora do not contain hair follicles but do contain many sebaceous follicles and occasionally a few sweat glands. The interior of the labial folds is made up of connective tissue, which contains many vessels and some smooth muscular fibers, as in typical erectile structures. These structures are extremely sensitive and abundantly supplied with several varieties of nerve endings.

The labia minora converge anteriorly where each divides into two lamellae, the lower two of which fuse to form the *frenulum of the clitoris,* and the upper pair merges into the *prepuce.* Posteriorly, the labia minora approach the midline as low ridges that fuse to form the *fourchet* in nulliparous women, but in multiparas they usually pass almost imperceptibly into the labia majora.

Clitoris. The clitoris, a homologue of the penis, is a small, cylindric, erectile body situated at the anterior extremity of the vulva and projects between the branched extremities of the labia minora, which form the prepuce and frenulum. The clitoris consists of a glans, a body (corpus), and two crura. The glans is made up of spindle-shaped cells, and the body contains two corpora cavernosa, in the walls of which are smooth muscle fibers. The long narrow crura arise from the inferior

surface of the ischiopubic rami and fuse just below the middle of the pubic arch to form the body of the clitoris.

The clitoris rarely exceeds 2 cm in length, even in a state of erection. It is sharply bent by traction exerted by the labia minora. As a result, the free end of the clitoris points downward and inward toward the vaginal opening. The glans, which rarely exceeds 0.5 cm in diameter, is covered by stratified epithelium which is richly supplied with nerve endings and is, therefore, extremely sensitive. The vessels of the highly erectile clitoris are connected with the vestibular bulbs. The clitoris is a major erogenous organ.

Krantz (1958) studied the abundant nerve supply of the external genitalia. The labia majora, as well as the labia minora and clitoris, contain a delicate network of free nerve endings, with the fibers terminating in small knoblike thickenings in or adjacent to the cells. These nerve endings are encountered more frequently in the papillae than elsewhere. Tactile discs also are found in abundance in these areas. The genital corpuscles, which are considered the main mediators of erotic sensation, vary considerably. They are sparsely and randomly distributed in the labia majora deep in the corium, but the labia minora contain a great number of the corpuscles, particularly in the prepuce and skin overlying the glans clitoridis.

Vestibule. The vestibule is the almond-shaped area that is enclosed by the labia minora laterally and extends from the clitoris to the fourchet anteroposteriorly. It is the remnant of the urogenital sinus of the embryo and is perforated usually by six openings: the urethra, the vagina, the ducts of Bartholin's glands, and, at times, the ducts of the paraurethral glands, also called Skene's ducts and glands (Fig. 2-2). The posterior portion of the vestibule between the fourchet and the vaginal opening is called the *fossa navicularis.* It is rarely observed except in nulliparous women, since it is usually obliterated as the result of childbirth.

Related to the vestibule are the *major vestibular glands,* or *Bartholin's glands* (Fig. 2-2).

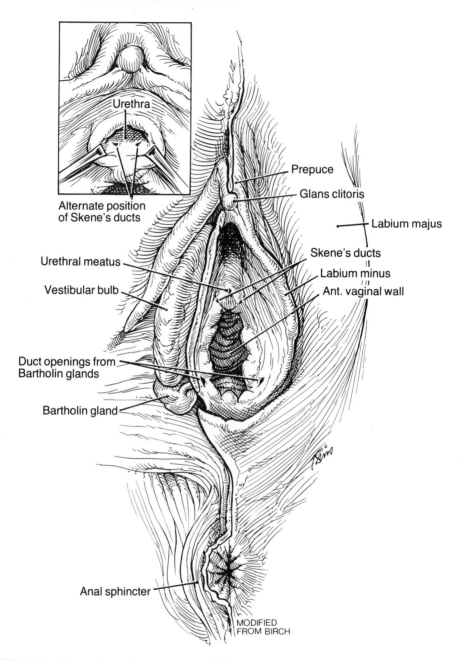

FIG. 2-2. The urethra, the openings of Skene's ducts, and the Bartholin glands and duct openings.

These are a pair of small compound glands, about 0.5 to 1 cm in diameter; one is situated beneath the vestibule on either side of the vaginal opening. The Bartholin glands lie under the constrictor muscle of the vagina and sometimes are found partially covered by the vestibular bulbs. The gland ducts are 1.5 to 2 cm long and open on the sides of the vestibule just outside the lateral margin of the vaginal orifice. Their small lumina ordinarily admit only the finest probe. During sexual excitement mucoid material is secreted by these glands. The ducts sometimes harbor gonococci, or other bacteria, which may gain access to the gland, causing suppuration and a Bartholin gland abscess.

Urethral Opening. The lower two-thirds of the urethra lies immediately above the anterior vaginal wall and terminates externally in the urethral meatus. The urinary meatus is in the midline of the vestibule, 1 to 1.5 cm below the pubic arch, and a short distance above the vaginal opening. It is usually puckered. Its orifice appears as a vertical slit, which can be distended to 4 or 5 mm in diameter. The *paraurethral ducts* open usually on the vestibule on either side of the urethra, but occasionally on the posterior wall of the urethra just inside the meatus (Fig. 2-2). These are of small caliber, about 0.5 mm in diameter, and of varying length. In the United States, they are generally known as *Skene's ducts.*

Vestibular Bulbs. Lying beneath the mucous membrane of the vestibule on either side are the vestibular bulbs, which are almond-shaped aggregations of veins, 3 to 4 cm long, 1 to 2 cm wide, and 0.5 to 1 cm thick. These bulbs lie in close apposition to the ischiopubic rami and are covered partially by the ischiocavernosus and constrictor vaginae muscles. The lower terminations of the vestibular bulbs are usually about the middle of the vaginal opening and anteriorly they extend upward toward the clitoris.

Embryologically, the vestibular bulbs correspond to the corpus spongiosum of the penis. During parturition, they are usually pushed up beneath the pubic arch; but since their posterior ends partially encircle the vagina, they are subject to injury and rupture, which may give rise to a hematoma of the vulva or to profuse hemorrhage.

Vaginal Opening and Hymen. The vaginal opening occupies the lower portion of the vestibule and varies considerably in size and shape. In virgins, it is most often entirely hidden by the overlapping labia minora, and when exposed, it usually appears almost completely closed by the membranous hymen.

The hymen presents marked differences in shape and consistency. It is comprised mainly of connective tissue, both elastic and collagenous. Both surfaces are covered by stratified squamous epithelium. Connective tissue papillae are more numerous on the vaginal surface and at the free edge. According to Mahran and Saleh (1964), there are no glandular or muscular elements in the hymen and it is not richly supplied with nerve fibers.

In the newborn, the hymen is very vascular and redundant; during pregnancy, the epithelium is thick and rich in glycogen; after menopause the epithelium thins, and focal cornification may appear. In adult virgins, the hymen is a membrane of varying thickness that surrounds the vaginal opening more or less completely and the aperture varies in size from that of a pinpoint to a caliber that admits the tip of one or even two fingers. The hymenal opening is usually crescentic or circular, but occasionally may be cribriform, septate, or fimbriated. Since the fimbriated variety may be mistaken for a ruptured hymen, it is wise to exercise caution in making definite statements regarding "rupture" of the hymen.

As a rule, during the first coitus, the hymen tears at several points, usually in its posterior portion. The edges of the tears soon cicatrize, and the hymen becomes permanently divided into two or more portions, separated by narrow slits extending down to its base. The extent to which rupture occurs varies with the structure of the hymen and the degree to which it is distended. Although it is commonly believed that rupture of the hymen is accompanied by bleeding, such does not occur in all cases. However, occasionally there may be profuse bleeding. Rarely, the membrane may be very resistant and require surgical incision before coitus can be accomplished.

The changes in the hymen brought about by coitus are occasionally of medico-legal importance, especially in cases of alleged rape, in which the physician is called upon to examine the victim and testify concerning the physical findings. In virgins who are examined a few hours after the sexual attack, the finding of fresh tears, abrasions, or bleeding points on the hymen constitute corroborative evidence of recent intercourse. The absence of such findings is of no significance, however, since the hymen may not be torn despite repeated coitus. In fact, many cases of pregnancy in women with unruptured hymens have been reported.

The changes produced in the hymen by childbirth, as a rule, are readily recognized. After the puerperium, the remnants of the hymen form several cicatrized nodules of varying size, the *myrtiform caruncles.*

An *imperforate hymen,* a rare lesion, occludes the vaginal orifice completely, causing retention of the menstrual discharge.

Vagina.   The vagina is a musculomembranous tube extending from the vulva to the uterus and is interposed between the bladder and the rectum (Fig. 2-3). The vagina constitutes the excretory duct of the uterus, through which uterine secretions and menstrual flow escape; it is the female organ of copulation; and, finally, it is part of the birth canal at delivery. The upper portion of the human vagina is believed to arise from the müllerian ducts and the lower portion from the urogenital sinus. Anteriorly, the vagina is in contact with the bladder and urethra,

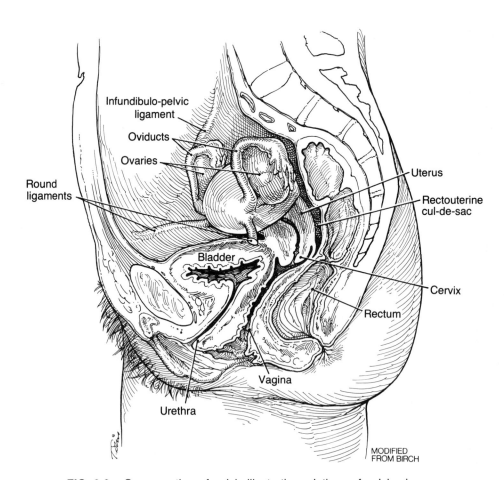

FIG. 2-3.   Cross section of pelvis illustrating relations of pelvic viscera.

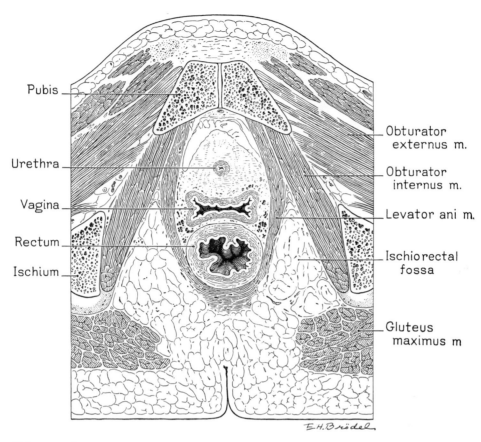

Pubis

Urethra

Vagina

Rectum

Ischium

Obturator externus m.

Obturator internus m.

Levator ani m.

Ischiorectal fossa

Gluteus maximus m

E.H.Brödel

FIG. 2-4.   Cross section through pelvis showing **H**-shaped lumen of vagina (m. = muscle).

from which it is separated by connective tissue which is often referred to as the vesicovaginal septum. Posteriorly, between the lower portion of the vagina and the rectum, there is similar tissue forming the rectovaginal septum. Usually the upper one-fourth of the vagina is separated from the rectum by the rectouterine pouch, or cul-de-sac of Douglas.

Normally, the anterior and posterior walls of the vagina lie in contact with only a slight space intervening between their lateral margins. Thus, when not distended, the vaginal canal is H-shaped on transverse section (Fig. 2-4). The vagina is capable of marked distension, as is evident during childbirth.

The upper end of the vagina is a blind vault into which the lower portion of the uterine cervix projects. The vaginal vault is subdivided into the anterior, posterior, and two lateral fornices. Since the vagina is attached higher up on the posterior wall than on the anterior wall of the cervix, the posterior fornix is considerably deeper than the anterior. The lateral fornices are intermediate in depth. The fornices are of considerable clinical importance since the internal pelvic organs usually can be palpated through their thin walls. Moreover, the posterior fornix usually provides ready surgical access to the peritoneal cavity. The vagina varies in length. The anterior and posterior vaginal walls commonly measure 6 to 8 cm and 7 to 10 cm in length, respectively.

Projecting into the vaginal lumen from the midlines of both the anterior and posterior walls are prominent longitudinal ridges. In nulliparous women, numerous transverse

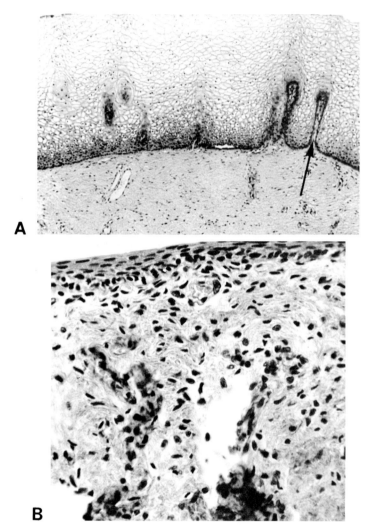

FIG. 2-5. **A.** Adult vagina showing noncornified, thick, stratified squamous epithelium. Epithelial appendages are absent. **Arrow** indicates a papilla. **B.** Thin vaginal epithelium of a prepubertal girl.

ridges, or *rugae,* extend outward from, and almost at right angles to, the longitudinal vaginal ridges. The rugae gradually fade away as they approach the lateral walls. They form a corrugated surface, which is not present before menarche and gradually becomes obliterated after repeated childbirth and after menopause. In elderly multiparas, the vaginal walls are often smooth. The mucosa of the vagina (Fig. 2-5) is composed of noncornified stratified squamous epithelium. Beneath the epithelium there is a thin fibromuscular coat; usually, an inner circular layer and an outer longitudinal layer of smooth muscle can be identified. Overlying the mucosa and muscularis there is a thin layer of connective tissue, rich in blood vessels, and occasional small lymphoid nodules. The mucosa and muscularis are attached very loosely to the underlying connective tissue, and are easily dissected off at operation. Some argument remains as to whether this connective tissue sometimes referred to as perivaginal endopelvic fascia, is a definite fascial plane in the strict anatomic sense.

Glands are normally not present in the vagina. In parous women, fragments of stratified epithelium, that sometimes give rise to cysts, are occasionally embedded in the vaginal connective tissue. These vaginal inclusion cysts are not glands but remnants of mucosal tags that were buried during the repair of vaginal tears after delivery. Other cysts lined by columnar or cuboidal epithelium may be found; these are derived from embryonic remnants.

From early infancy until after the menopause, the cells of the superficial layer of the vaginal mucosa contain considerable glycogen. Examination of exfoliated cells from the vagina permits identification of the various stages of the ovarian cycle (see Fig. 2-5).

In nonpregnant women, the vagina is kept moist by a small amount of secretion from the uterus. During pregnancy, there is copious vaginal secretion, which normally consists of a curdlike product of exfoliated epithelium and bacteria, which is markedly acidic. Bacilli are the predominant bacteria of the vagina during pregnancy, although cocci are also found. The acidic reaction is attributable to lactic acid, which arises from the breakdown of glycogen in the mucosa by Lactobacilli. The pH of the vaginal secretion varies with ovarian activity. Before puberty, it ranges between 6.8 and 7.2, whereas in adult women it is well below this, ranging between 4.0 and 5.0.

The vagina has an abundant vascular supply. The upper third is supplied by the cervicovaginal branches of the uterine arteries, the middle third by the inferior vesical arteries, and the lower third by the middle hemorrhoidal and internal pudendal arteries. Immediately surrounding the vagina there is an extensive venous plexus, the vessels from which follow the course of the arteries and empty eventually into the hypogastric veins. For the most part, the lymphatics from the lower third of the vagina along with those of the vulva empty into the inguinal lymph nodes, those from the middle third into the hypogastric nodes, and those from the upper third into the iliac nodes. The human vagina, according to Krantz (1958), is devoid of any special nerve endings (genital corpuscles), but occasionally free nerve endings are found in the papillae.

The Perineum. The many structures that make up the perineum are illustrated in Figure 2-6. Most of the support of the perineum is provided by the pelvic and urogenital diaphragms. The *pelvic diaphragm* consists of the levator ani muscles plus the coccygeus muscles posteriorly, and their fascial coverings. The levator ani muscles form a broad muscular sling that originates from the posterior surface of the superior rami of the pubis, from the inner surface of the ischial spine, and between these two sites, from the obturator fascia. The muscle fibers insert in the following locations: around the vagina and rectum to form efficient functional sphincters for each, into a raphe in the midline between the vagina and rectum, into a midline raphe below the rectum, and into the coccyx. The *urogenital diaphragm* is located external to the pelvic diaphragm, in the triangular area between the ischial tuberosities and symphysis pubis. The urogenital diaphragm consists of the deep transverse perineal muscles, the constrictor of the urethra, and internal and external fascial coverings.

PERINEAL BODY. The median raphe of the levator ani, between the anus and the vagina, is reinforced by the central tendon of the perineum, on which the bulbocavernosus muscles, the superficial transverse perineal muscles, and the external anal sphincter converge. These structures, which contribute to the perineal body and provide much support for the perineum, are often lacerated during delivery unless an adequate episiotomy is made at an appropriate time (Chap. 17, p. 430).

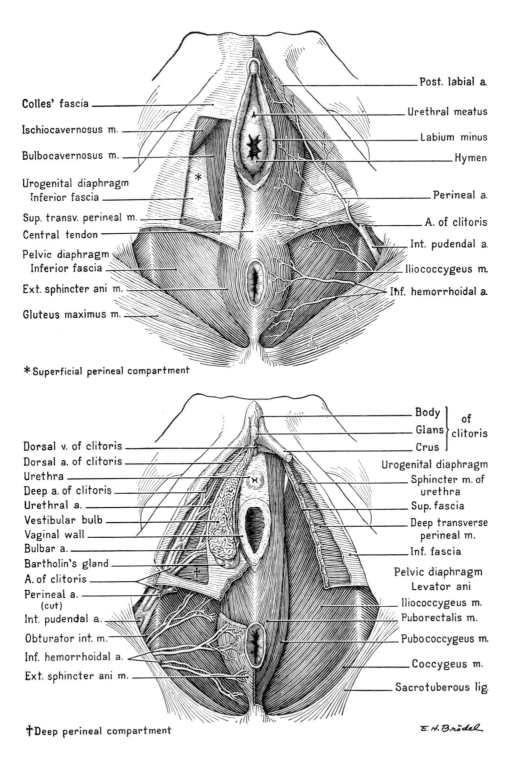

Post. labial a.

Colles' fascia

Ischiocavernosus m.

Bulbocavernosus m.

Urogenital diaphragm
  Inferior fascia

Sup. transv. perineal m.

Central tendon

Pelvic diaphragm
  Inferior fascia

Ext. sphincter ani m.

Gluteus maximus m.

Urethral meatus

Labium minus

Hymen

Perineal a.

A. of clitoris

Int. pudendal a.

Iliococcygeus m.

Inf. hemorrhoidal a.

*Superficial perineal compartment

Dorsal v. of clitoris
Dorsal a. of clitoris
Urethra
Deep a. of clitoris
Urethral a.
Vestibular bulb
Vaginal wall
Bulbar a.
Bartholin's gland
A. of clitoris
Perineal a.
  (cut)
Int. pudendal a.
Obturator int. m.
Inf. hemorrhoidal a.
Ext. sphincter ani m.

Body ⎫
Glans ⎬ of clitoris
Crus ⎭

Urogenital diaphragm
Sphincter m. of urethra
Sup. fascia
Deep transverse perineal m.
Inf. fascia
Pelvic diaphragm
Levator ani
Iliococcygeus m.
Puborectalis m.
Pubococcygeus m.
Coccygeus m.
Sacrotuberous lig.

†Deep perineal compartment

E. H. Brödel

FIG. 2-6. The perineum. The more superficial components are illustrated above and the deeper structures below (m. = muscle; a. = artery; lig. = ligament; Int. = internal; Ext. = external; Inf. = inferior).

INTERNAL GENERATIVE ORGANS

Uterus. The uterus is a muscular organ partially covered by peritoneum, or serosa. Its cavity is lined by the endometrium. During pregnancy, the uterus serves for reception, retention, and nutrition of the conceptus, which it expels during labor.

ANATOMIC RELATIONSHIPS. The uterus of the nonpregnant woman is situated in the pelvic cavity between the bladder anteriorly and the rectum posteriorly, and its inferior portion, the cervix, projects into the vagina. Almost the entire posterior wall of the uterus is covered by serosa, or peritoneum, the lower portion of which forms the anterior boundary of the *rectouterine cul-de-sac,* or pouch of Douglas. Only the upper portion of the anterior wall of the uterus is so covered (Fig. 2-7). The lower portion is united to the posterior wall of the bladder by a well-defined layer of normally loose connective tissue (Figs. 2-3, 2-8).

SIZE AND SHAPE. The uterus resembles a flattened pear in shape (Figs. 2-7, 2-8) and consists of two major but unequal parts: an upper triangular portion, the *body,* or *corpus,* and a lower, cylindric or fusiform portion, the *cervix.* The anterior surface of the body of the uterus is almost flat, whereas the posterior surface is distinctly convex. The oviducts, or fallopian tubes, emerge from the *cornua* of the uterus at the junction of the superior and lateral margins. The convex upper segment between the points of insertion of the fallopian tubes is called the *fundus uteri.* The lateral margins extend from the cornua on either side to the pelvic floor. Laterally, the portion of the uterus below the insertion of the fallopian tubes is not covered directly by peritoneum but receives the attachments of the broad ligaments.

There are marked variations in size and shape of the uterus, depending on age and parity. Before puberty, the organ varies from 2.5 to 3.5 cm in length. The uterus of nulliparous women measures from 6 to 8 cm in length as compared with 9 to 10 cm in multiparous women (Fig. 2-8). Uteri of nonparous and parous women also differ considerably in weight, the former normally weighing from 50 to 70 g, and the latter 80 g or some-

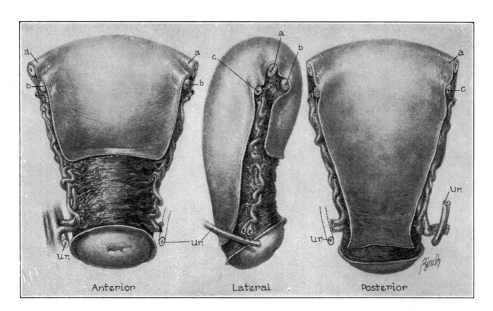

FIG. 2-7. Anterior, right lateral, and posterior views of the uterus of an adult woman; a, oviduct; b, round ligament; c, ovarian ligament; Ur., ureter.

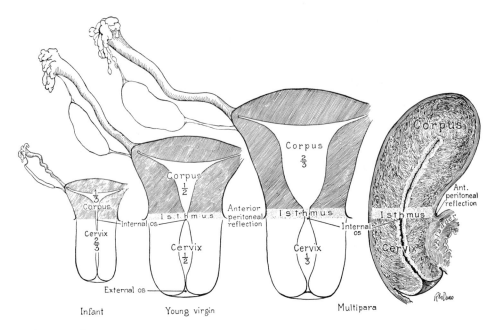

FIG. 2-8. The comparative size of prepubertal, adult nonparous, and multiparous uteri, frontal and sagittal sections.

what more (Langlois, 1970). The relation between the length of the body of the uterus and that of the cervix likewise varies widely. In the young child, the body of the uterus is only half as long as the cervix; in nulliparous women, the two are about equal length; in multiparous women the cervix is only a little more than one-third of the total length of the organ (Fig. 2-8).

The great bulk of the body of the uterus, but not the cervix, consists of muscle. The inner surface of the anterior and posterior walls of the uterus lie almost in contact, the cavity between them forming a mere slit (Fig. 2-9). The cervical canal is fusiform and contains a small opening at each end, the *internal os* and the *external os.* On frontal section, the cavity of the body of the uterus is triangular, whereas that of the cervix retains its fusiform shape. After childbearing, the triangular appearance of the uterine cavity is less pronounced, the margins then having become concave instead of convex. After menopause, the uterus decreases in size, with atrophy of myometrium and endometrium.

The *isthmus* (Fig. 2-8) is of special obstetric significance because in pregnancy it is essen-

tial to the formation of the lower uterine segment (see Chap. 15, p. 377).

UTERINE CERVIX. The cervix is the specialized portion of the uterus below the isthmus. Anteriorly, the upper boundary of the cervix, the internal os, corresponds approxi-

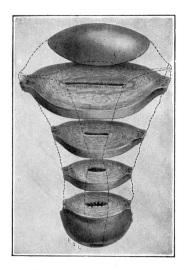

FIG. 2-9. Reconstruction of uterus showing shape of its cavity.

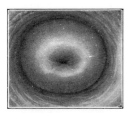

FIG. 2-10.   Nonparous cervical external os.

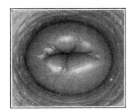

FIG. 2-11.   Parous cervical external os.

mately to the level at which the peritoneum is reflected upon the bladder.

The cervix is divided by the attachment of the vagina into vaginal and supravaginal portions. The supravaginal segment is covered on its posterior surface by peritoneum. Laterally it is attached to the cardinal ligaments and anteriorly it is separated from the overlying bladder by loose connective tissue. The vaginal portion of the cervix, or *portio vaginalis,* has the external os at its lower extremity.

The external os of the cervix may vary greatly in appearance. Before childbirth, it is a small, regular, oval opening. After childbirth, the orifice is converted into a transverse slit that divides the cervix into the so-called anterior and posterior lips. When the cervix has been torn deeply during labor it may become irregular, nodular, or stellate. These changes are sufficiently characteristic to permit the examiner to ascertain with some certainty whether the woman has borne children (Figs. 2-10, 2-11).

Basically the cervix is composed of connective tissue with occasional smooth muscle fibers, many vessels, and elastic tissue. The transition from the primarily collagenous tissue of the cervix to the primarily muscular tissue of the body of the uterus, although generally abrupt, may be gradual, extending over as much as 10 mm. The results of studies by Danforth, Buckingham, and Roddick (1960) are suggestive that the physical properties of the cervix are determined by the state of the connective tissue, and that during pregnancy and labor the remarkable ability of the cervix to dilate results from dissociation of collagen. Buckingham and co-workers (1965) were able to quantify the proportion of muscle to collagen in the human cervix. In the normal cervix, muscle formed an average of about 10 percent, whereas in "incompetent" cervices, the proportion of muscle appeared to be much greater.

Characteristically the mucosa of the cervical canal, although embryologically a direct continuation of endometrium, has differentiated in such a way that sections through the canal resemble a honeycomb. The mucosa is composed of a single layer of very high columnar epithelium which rests upon a thin basement membrane. The oval nuclei are situated near the base of the columnar cells, the upper portions of which look rather clear because of their mucoid content. These cells are abundantly supplied with cilia.

The numerous cervical glands extend from the surface of the endocervical mucosa directly into the subjacent connective tissue, since there is no submucosa as such, and furnish the thick, tenacious secretion of the cervical canal. If the ducts of the cervical glands are occluded, retention cysts may form, which are a few millimeters in diameter, the so-called *nabothian follicles* or *nabothian cysts.*

Normally, the squamous epithelium of the vaginal portion of the cervix and the columnar epithelium of the cervical canal form a sharp line of division very near the external os, the squamo-columnar junction. In response to inflammation or trauma, however, the stratified epithelium may gradually extend up the cervical canal and line the lower third or occasionally lower half of the canal. This change is more marked in multiparas, in whom the lips of the cervix are often everted. Uncommonly, the two varieties of epithelium abut on the vaginal portion outside the external os, as in *congenital ectropion.*

The cyclic changes in the cervical mucosa

are dependent upon the varying hormonal patterns of the menstrual cycle; as discussed on page 86.

BODY OF UTERUS. The wall of the uterine body is made up of three layers: serosal, muscular, and mucosal. The serosal layer is formed by the peritoneum covering the uterus, to which it is firmly adherent except just above the bladder and at the margins, where it is deflected to the broad ligaments.

ENDOMETRIUM. The innermost, or mucosal layer, which lines the uterine cavity in the nonpregnant state, is the *endometrium*. It is a thin, pink, velvetlike membrane, which on close examination is seen to be perforated by a large number of minute openings, the mouths of the uterine glands. Because of the constant cyclic changes that occur during the reproductive period of life, the endometrium normally varies greatly in thickness, measuring from 0.5 mm to as much as 5 mm. The endometrium consists of surface epithelium, glands, and interglandular tissue in which there are numerous blood vessels.

The histologic appearance of the normal endometrium is shown in Figures 2-2 to 2-5 of Chapter 4; ultrastructural features are illustrated in Figures 4-7 and 4-8 of that chapter. Since the uterus has no submucosa, the endometrium is attached directly to the underlying myometrium along a somewhat irregular boundary.

The epithelium of the endometrial surface is composed of a single layer of closely packed, high columnar, ciliated cells. During much of the endometrial cycle the oval nuclei are situated in the lower portions of the cells but not so near the base as in the endocervix.

Cilia have been demonstrated in the endometria of many mammals. The ciliated cells occur in discrete patches, whereas secretory activity appears to be limited to nonciliated cells. The ciliary current in both the tubes and the uterus is in the same direction, extending downward from the fimbriated end of the tubes toward the external os.

The tubular *uterine glands* are invaginations of the epithelium, which, in the resting state,

resemble the fingers of a glove. The glands extend through the entire thickness of the endometrium to the myometrium, which they occasionally penetrate for a short distance. Histologically, they resemble the epithelium of the surface and are lined by a single layer of columnar, partially ciliated epithelium that rests upon a thin basement membrane. The glands secrete a thin alkaline fluid that serves to keep the uterine cavity moist (see Chap. 4, Figs. 4-7 to 4-8).

In the classic monograph of Hitschmann and Adler published in 1908, it was reported that the endometrium undergoes constant, hormonally controlled, changes during each ovarian cycle. These three fundamental phases—*menstrual, proliferative (follicular),* and *secretory (luteal)*—are discussed in detail in Chapter 4 in the section on menstruation. In brief, immediately after menstruation the normal endometrium is quite thin, with the tubular glands well separated. Thereafter the endometrium rapidly increases in thickness and, before the next menstrual period, usually contains many convoluted or sacculated glands. After the menopause, the endometrium undergoes atrophy: the epithelium flattens, the glands gradually disappear, and the interglandular tissue becomes more fibrous.

The connective tissue of the endometrium, between the surface epithelium and the myometrium, is a mesenchymal stroma. Immediately after menstruation, the stroma consists of closely packed oval and spindle-shaped nuclei, around which there is very little cytoplasm. When separated by edema, the cells appear stellate, with branching cytoplasmic processes that form anastomoses. The cells are packed more closely around the glands and blood vessels than elsewhere. Several days before menstruation, the stromal cells usually become larger and more vesicular, resembling decidual cells, and, at the same time, there is a diffuse leukocytic infiltration.

The vascular architecture of the endometrium is of great importance in the phenomena of menstruation and pregnancy. Arterial blood is carried to the uterus by the uterine and ovarian arteries. As the arterial branches penetrate the uterine wall obliquely inward

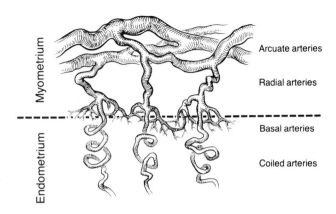

FIG. 2-12. Stereographic representation of myometrial and endometrial arteries in the macaque. Above are shown parts of myometrial arcuate arteries from which myometrial radial arteries course toward the endometrium. There are found larger endometrial coiled arteries and smaller endometrial basal arteries. (From Okkels and Engle. *Acta Pathol Microbiol Scand* 15:150, 1938)

reaching its middle third, they ramify in a plane parallel to the surface and are named the *arcuate arteries.* Radial branches extend from the arcuate arteries at right angles toward the endometrium. The endometrial arteries consist of *coiled,* or *spiral arteries,* which are a continuation of the radial arteries, and *basal arteries,* which branch from the radial arteries at a sharp angle, as illustrated in Figure 2-12. The coiled arteries supply most of the midportion and all of the superficial third of the endometrium. Their walls have been shown to react sensitively to hormonal influences, especially by vasoconstriction, and thus they probably play an important part in the mechanism of menstruation as described in Chapter 4 (p. 80). The straight basal endometrial arteries are smaller in both caliber and length than are the coiled vessels. They extend only into the basal layer of the endometrium, or at most a short distance into the middle layer, and are not under hormonal influence.

MYOMETRIUM. The major portion of the uterus, the myometrium, consists of bundles of smooth muscle which are united by connective tissue that contains many elastic fibers. According to Schwalm and Dubrauszky (1966), muscle fibers progressively diminish caudally to the extent that the cervix contains only about 10 percent muscle. The inner uterine wall of the body contains relatively more muscle than do the outer layers, and the anterior and posterior walls contain more than do the lateral walls. During preg-

nancy, the myometrium of the body of the uterus increases greatly but there is no significant change in the muscle content of the cervix. Anatomic changes in the myometrium during pregnancy are detailed in Chapter 9.

LIGAMENTS OF THE UTERUS. Extending from either side of the uterus are the broad, round, and uterosacral ligaments. The *broad ligaments* consist of two winglike structures that extend from the lateral margins of the uterus to the pelvic walls and divide the pelvic cavity into anterior and posterior compartments. Each broad ligament consists of a fold of peritoneum that encloses various structures and presents superior, lateral, inferior, and median margins. The inner two-thirds of the superior margin form the *mesosalpinx,* to which is attached the oviduct. The outer third of the superior margin of the broad ligament, extending from the fimbriated end of the oviduct to the pelvic wall, forms the *infundibulopelvic ligament* (suspensory ligament of the ovary), through which the ovarian vessels traverse.

The *parovarium,* which can be found in the scant loose connective tissue within the broad ligament in the vicinity of the mesosalpinx, consists of a number of narrow vertical tubules lined by ciliated epithelium. These tubules connect at their upper ends with a longitudinal duct that extends just below the oviduct to the lateral margin of the uterus, where it ordinarily ends blindly near the internal os, but, infrequently it may extend lateral to the vagina down to the level of the

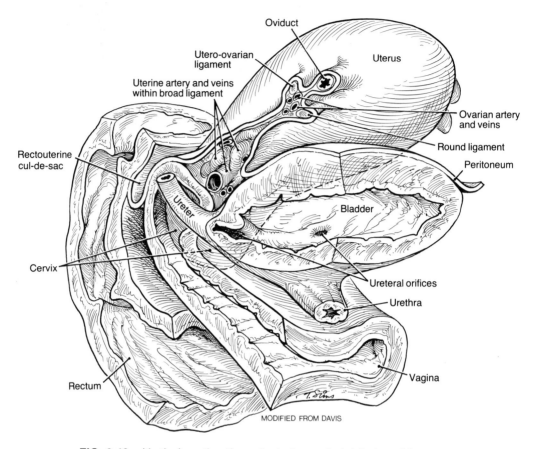

FIG. 2-13. Vertical section through uterine end of right broad ligament.

hymen. This canal, the remnant of the wolf-fian (mesonephric) duct in women, is called *Gartner's duct.* The parovarium, a remnant of the wolffian body, is homologous with the caput epididymidis in men. Its cranial portion is the *epoophoron,* or organ of Rosenmüller. Its caudal portion, or *paroophoron,* is a vestigial group of mesonephric tubules in or around the broad ligament. It is homologous with the paradidymis of men. The paroophoron usually disappears in the adult but occasionally forms macroscopic cysts.

At the lateral margin of each broad ligament, the peritoneum is reflected onto the side of the pelvis. The base of the broad ligament, which is quite thick, is continuous with the connective tissue of the pelvic floor. Its densest portion—referred to as the *cardinal ligament,* the transverse cervical ligament, or Mackenrodt's ligament—is composed of con-

nective tissue that is firmly united medially to the supravaginal portion of the cervix. The base of the broad ligament encloses the uterine vessels and the lower ureter.

A vertical section through the uterine end of the broad ligament is triangular, with the uterine vessels in its broad base (Fig. 2-13). In its lower part it is widely attached to the connective tissues adjacent to the cervix, the *parametrium.* The upper part consists of three folds which in turn nearly cover the oviduct, the utero-ovarian ligament, and the round ligament.

The *round ligaments* extend on either side from the lateral portion of the uterus arising somewhat below and anterior to the origin of the oviducts. Each round ligament lies in a fold of peritoneum continuous with the broad ligament and extends outward and downward to the inguinal canal, through which it passes, to terminate in the upper portion of the labium majus. In nonpregnant women, the round ligament varies from 3 to 5 mm in diameter, and is composed of smooth muscle cells, which are continuous directly with those of the uterine wall, and a certain amount of connective tissue. The round ligament corresponds to the gubernaculum testis of men. During pregnancy the round ligaments undergo considerable hypertrophy and increase appreciably in both length and diameter.

Each *uterosacral ligament* extends from its attachment posterolaterally to the supravaginal portion of the cervix to encircle the rectum, and insert into the fascia over the second and third sacral vertebrae. The uterosacral ligaments are composed of connective tissue and some smooth muscle covered by peritoneum. These ligaments form the lateral boundaries of the rectouterine cul-de-sac, or pouch of Douglas, and aid in retaining the body of the uterus in its usual anterior position by exerting traction posteriorly upon the cervix.

POSITION. When the nonpregnant woman is standing upright, the body of the uterus most often is almost horizontal and is flexed somewhat anteriorly with the fundus resting upon the bladder, whereas the cervix is directed backward toward the tip of the sacrum with the external os approximately at the level of the ischial spines. The position of the body of the uterus is altered according to the degree of distension of the bladder and rectum.

The normal uterus is a partially mobile organ. The cervix is anchored, but the body of the uterus is free to move in the anteroposterior plane. Therefore, posture and gravity influence the position of the uterus.

BLOOD VESSELS. The vascular supply of the uterus is derived principally from the uterine and ovarian arteries. The uterine artery, a main branch of the hypogastric artery (Fig. 2-14.A–G), after descending for a short distance, enters the base of the broad ligament and makes its way medially to the side of the uterus. In so doing, it crosses over the ureter, as described below. Immediately adjacent to the supravaginal portion of the cervix, the uterine artery divides into two main branches. The smaller cervicovaginal artery supplies the lower portion of the cervix and the upper portion of the vagina. The main branch turns abruptly upward and extends as a highly convoluted vessel along the margin of the uterus, giving off a branch of considerable size to the upper portion of the cervix and numerous other branches that penetrate the body of the uterus. Just before reaching the oviduct it divides into three terminal branches: fundal, tubal, and ovarian. The ovarian branch of the uterine artery anastomoses with the terminal branch of the ovarian artery; the tubal branch, making its way through the mesosalpinx, supplies part of the blood to the oviduct; the fundal branch is distributed to the uppermost portion of the uterus.

About 2 cm lateral to the cervix the uterine artery crosses over the ureter, as shown in Figures 2-7, 2-14, and 2-15. (For Figure 2-15, see colorplate.) The proximity of the uterine artery and uterine veins to the ureter at this point is of great surgical significance, because during hysterectomy the ureter may be injured or ligated in the process of clamping and tying the uterine vessels.

The *ovarian artery,* a direct branch of the aorta, enters the broad ligament through the infundibulopelvic ligament. On reaching the ovarian hilum, it divides into a number of smaller branches that enter the ovary, whereas its main stem traverses the entire length of the broad ligament very near the mesosalpinx and makes its way to the upper portion of the lateral margin of the uterus where it anastomoses with the ovarian branch of the uterine artery. There are numerous additional communications among the arteries on both sides of the uterus.

When the uterus is contracted, the lumina of the abundant veins are collapsed, but in injected specimens the greater part of the uterine wall appears to be composed of dilated venous sinuses. On either side, the arcuate veins unite to form the *uterine vein,* which

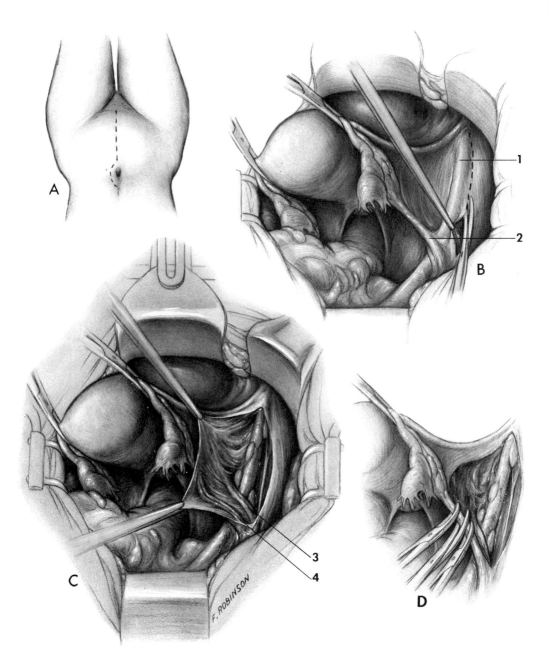

FIG. 2-14 (A-D). Illustrated are the pelvic viscera as seen through a long midline incision made in the lower abdomen **(A). B.** Retractors have been placed to spread the abdominal incision. The small intestine and omentum that overlie the pelvic contents have been displaced from the operative field. The oviducts, utero-ovarian ligaments, and round ligaments have been clamped bilaterally at their origin immediately adjacent to the uterus. Peritoneum just lateral to the right external iliac artery (1) is incised and the right infundibulo-pelvic ligament (2) is tensed by pulling the uterus to the left. **C.** The right broad ligament has been opened laterally. The right ureter (3) is now visible as it crosses the iliac vessels at the pelvic brim and courses medially and downward towards the cervix and bladder. The right ovarian artery and vein (4) are visible after dissection of the infundibulopelvic ligament. **D.** The ovarian vessels have been clamped and are being severed. (From Nelson JH Jr: Atlas of Radical Pelvic Surgery 2nd ed. p 131, 1977, Appleton) *(Continued)*

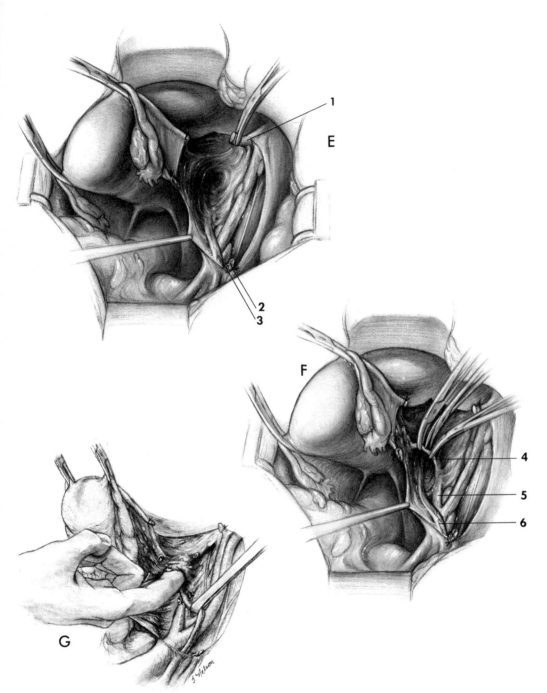

FIG. 2-14 (Cont.). **E.** The round ligament (1) and the ovarian vessels (2) have been ligated and severed. More of the ureter is visible (3). **F.** The origin of the right uterine artery (4) from the right hypogastric artery (5) is illustrated. Note the ureter (6) coursing beneath the uterine artery (4) just lateral to the junction of the cervix and body of the uterus. **G.** The operator's finger is in the paracervical ureteral tunnel through the right cardinal ligament just lateral to the supravaginal portion of the cervix. The ureter is being retracted laterally. (From Nelson JH Jr: Atlas of Radical Pelvic Surgery 2nd ed. p 133, 1977, Appleton)

empties into the hypogastric vein and thence into the common iliac vein.

Some of the blood from the upper part of the uterus and blood from the ovary and upper part of the broad ligament is collected by several veins that, within the broad ligament, form the large *pampiniform plexus,* the vessels from which terminate in the ovarian vein. The right ovarian vein empties into the vena cava, whereas the left ovarian vein empties into the left renal vein.

LYMPHATICS. The endometrium is abundantly supplied with lymphatics, but true lymphatic vessels are confined largely to its basal layer. The lymphatics of the underlying myometrium increase toward the serosal surface and form an abundant lymphatic plexus just beneath it, especially on the posterior wall of the uterus and, to a lesser extent, anteriorly.

The lymphatics from the various portions of the uterus drain into several sets of lymph nodes. Those from the cervix terminate mainly in the hypogastric nodes, which are situated near the bifurcation of the common iliac vessels between the external iliac and hypogastric arteries. The lymphatics from the body of the uterus are distributed to two groups of nodes. One set of vessels drains into the hypogastric nodes. The other set, after joining certain lymphatics from the ovarian region, terminates in the periaortic lymph nodes.

INNERVATION. The nerve supply is derived principally from the sympathetic nervous system, but also partly from the cerebrospinal and parasympathetic systems. (Fig. 2-16, see colorplate.) The parasympathetic system is represented on either side by the pelvic nerve, which consists of a few fibers derived from the second, third, and fourth sacral nerves; it loses its identity in the cervical ganglion of Frankenhäuser. The sympathetic system enters the pelvis through the hypogastric plexus which arises from the aortic plexus just below the promontory of the sacrum. After descending on either side, it also enters the uterovaginal plexus of Frankenhäuser, which consists of ganglia of varying size, but particularly of a large ganglionic plate situated on either side of the cervix just above the posterior fornix and in front of the rectum.

Branches from these plexuses supply the uterus, bladder, and upper part of the vagina and comprise both myelinated and nonmyelinated fibers. Some of these fibers terminate freely between the muscular fibers, whereas others accompany the arteries into the endometrium.

Both the sympathetic and parasympathetic nerves contain motor and a few sensory fibers. The sympathetic fibers cause muscular contraction and vasoconstriction, whereas the parasympathetics inhibit contraction and lead to vasodilatation. Since the Frankenhäuser plexus is derived from both sources, it has certain functions of both components of the autonomic nervous system.

The eleventh and twelfth thoracic nerve roots carry sensory fibers from the uterus, transmitting the painful stimuli of uterine contractions to the central nervous system. The sensory nerves from the cervix and upper part of the birth canal pass through the pelvic nerves to the second, third, and fourth sacral nerves, whereas those from the lower portion of the birth canal pass primarily through the pudendal nerve (Chap. 18).

Oviducts. The oviducts, or fallopian tubes, extend from the uterine cornua to the ovaries and provide access for the ova to the uterine cavity. The oviducts vary from 8 to 14 cm in length, are covered by peritoneum, and have a lumen lined by mucous membrane. Each fallopian tube is divided into an *interstitial portion, isthmus, ampulla,* and *infundibulum.* The interstitial portion is included within the muscular wall of the uterus. Its course is roughly obliquely upward and outward from the uterine cavity. The isthmus, or the narrow portion of the tube adjoining the uterus, gradually passes into the wider lateral portion, or *ampulla.* The *infundibulum,* or fimbriated extremity, is the

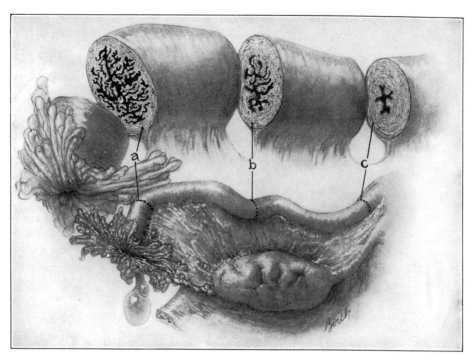

FIG. 2-17. The oviduct in cross section showing the gross structure of the epithelium in several portions: a, infundibulum; b, ampulla; c, isthmus.

funnel-shaped opening of the distal end of the fallopian tube (Fig. 2-17). The oviduct varies considerably in thickness, the narrowest portion of the isthmus measuring from 2 to 3 mm in diameter and the widest portion of the ampulla from 5 to 8 mm. The oviduct is surrounded completely by peritoneum except where the mesosalpinx is attached.

The fimbriated extremity of the infundibulum opens into the abdominal cavity. One projection, the *fimbria ovarica,* which is considerably longer than the other fimbriae, forms a shallow gutter which approaches or reaches the ovary.

The musculature of the fallopian tube is arranged, in general, in two layers, an inner circular and an outer longitudinal layer. In the distal portion of the oviduct, the two layers become less distinct and, near the fimbriated extremity, are replaced by an interlacing network of muscular fibers. The tubal musculature undergoes rhythmic contractions constantly, the rate of which varies with the

phases of the menstrual cycle. The contractions reach greatest frequency and intensity during transport of ova and are slowest and weakest during pregnancy.

The tube is lined by a mucous membrane, the epithelium of which is composed of a single layer of columnar cells, some ciliated and some secretory. The ciliated cells are most abundant at the fimbriated extremity; elsewhere, they form discrete patches. There are differences in the proportions of these two types of cells in different phases of the ovarian cycle. Since there is no submucosa, the epithelium is in close contact with the underlying muscle. The tubal mucosa undergoes cyclic changes histologically similar to, but much less striking than, those in the endometrium. The postmenstrual phase is characterized by a low epithelium that rapidly increases in height. During the follicular phase, the cells are taller, the ciliated elements are broad with nuclei near the margin, and the nonciliated cells are narrow with nu-

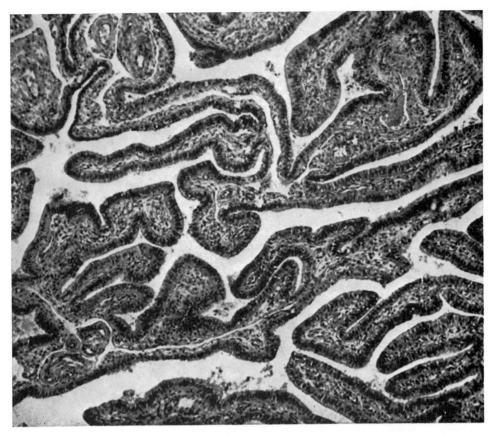

FIG. 2-18. Section through oviduct near fimbriated extremity, showing the complexity of the rugae.

clei nearer the base. During the luteal phase, the secretory cells enlarge, project beyond the ciliated cells, and extrude their nuclei. During the menstrual phase, these changes become even more marked. Changes in the fallopian tubes during late pregnancy and the puerperium include a low mucosa, plugging of the capillaries with leukocytes, and a decidual reaction.

The mucosa of the oviducts is arranged in longitudinal folds which become more complicated toward the fimbriated end. Consequently, the appearance of the lumen varies from one portion of the tube to another. On cross sections through the uterine portion, four simple folds are found, forming a figure that resembles a Maltese cross. The isthmus is more complex. In the ampulla, the lumen is almost completely occupied by the arborescent mucosa, which consists of very compli-

cated folds (Fig. 2-18).

The current produced by the tubal cilia is directed toward the uterine cavity. Indeed, minute foreign bodies introduced into the abdominal cavities of animals eventually appear in the vagina after making their way through the tubes and the cavity of the uterus. Tubal peristalsis is probably an important factor in transport of the ovum.

The tubes are richly supplied with elastic tissue, blood vessels, and lymphatics. Sympathetic innervation to the tube is extensive, in contrast to parasympathetic innervation. The role of these nerves in tubal function is poorly understood (Hodgson and Eddy, 1975).

Diverticula may extend occasionally from the lumen of the tube for a variable distance into its muscular wall and reach almost to its serosa. These diverticula may play a role in the development of ectopic pregnancy (Chap. 22).

Pertinent gross anatomic, histologic, and ultrastructural information about the human oviduct was well summarized by Woodruff and Pauerstein (1969).

EMBRYOLOGIC DEVELOPMENT OF THE UTERUS AND OVIDUCTS. The uterus and the tubes arise from the müllerian ducts, which first appear near the upper pole of the urogenital ridge in the 5th week of development in embryos 10 to 11 mm long. This ridge consists of the mesonephros, the gonad, and their ducts. The first indication of the müllerian duct is a thickening of the celomic epithelium at the level of the fourth thoracic segment. The thickening becomes the fimbriated extremity (infundibulum) of the fallopian tube, invaginating and growing caudally to form a slender tube at the lateral edge of the urogenital ridge. In the sixth week, the growing tips of the two müllerian ducts approach each other in the midline, reaching the sinus a week later (embryos of 30 mm). At that time, the two müllerian ducts have begun to fuse at the level of the inguinal crest, or gubernaculum (primordium of the round ligament), to form a single canal. The upper ends of the müllerian ducts thus produce the oviducts with the fused part giving rise to the uterus. The uterine lumen is completed from the fundus to the vagina during the third month. According to Koff (1933), the vaginal canal is not patent throughout its length until the sixth month.

The Ovaries. The ovaries are almond-shaped organs, the functions of which are the development and extrusion of ova and the elaboration of steroidal hormones. They vary considerably in size. During the childbearing period, they measure from 2.5 to 5 cm in length, 1.5 to 3 cm in breadth, and 0.6 to 1.5 cm in thickness. After menopause, they diminish markedly in size.

Normally, the ovaries are situated in the upper part of the pelvic cavity, resting in a slight depression on the lateral wall of the pelvis between the divergent external iliac and hypogastric vessels—the ovarian fossa of Waldeyer. When the woman is standing, the long axes of the ovaries are almost vertical, but became horizontal when she is supine. Their position, however, is subject to marked variation, and it is rare to find both ovaries at exactly the same level.

The lateral surface of the ovary is in contact with the ovarian fossa whereas the medial surface faces the uterus. The margin of the ovary that is attached to the mesovarium is more or less straight and is designated as the hilum, whereas the free margin is convex and is directed backward and inward toward the rectum.

The ovary is attached to the broad ligament by the *mesovarium.* The *utero-ovarian ligament* extends from the lateral and posterior portion of the uterus, just beneath the tubal insertion, to the uterine, or lower pole, of the ovary. It is usually several centimeters long and 3 to 4 mm in diameter. It is covered by peritoneum and is made up of muscle and connective tissue fibers continuous with those of the uterus. The *infundibulopelvic* or *suspensory ligament of the ovary* extends from the upper, or tubal, pole to the pelvic wall (Fig. 2-14.B). Through it course the ovarian vessels and nerves.

The exterior surface of the ovary varies in appearance with age. In young women, the organ presents a smooth, dull white surface through which glisten several small, clear follicles. As the woman grows older, the ovary becomes more corrugated and in elderly women its exterior may be markedly convoluted.

The general structure of the ovary can be studied best in cross sections, in which two portions may be distinguished, the *cortex* and the *medulla.* The cortex, or outer layer, varies in thickness with age, thinning with advancing years. It is in this layer that the ova and graafian follicles are located. The cortex of the ovary is composed of spindle-shaped connective tissue cells and fibers, among which are scattered primordial and graafian follicles in various stages of development. The follicles become less numerous as the woman grows older. The outermost portion of the cortex, which is dull and whitish, is designated the *tunica albuginea.* On its surface is a single layer of cuboidal epithelium, the germinal epithelium of Waldeyer.

The medulla, or central portion, of the ovary is composed of loose connective tissue, which is continuous with that of the mesovarium. The medulla contains a large number of arteries and veins and a small number of smooth muscle fibers continuous with those in the suspensory ligament. The muscle may function in movements of the ovary.

Both sympathetic and parasympathetic nerves supply the ovaries. The sympathetic nerves are derived in great part from the ovarian plexus, which accompanies the ovarian vessels; a few are derived from the plexus surrounding the ovarian branch of the uterine artery. The ovary is richly supplied with nonmyelinated nerve fibers, which for the most part accompany the blood vessels. These are merely vascular nerves, whereas others form wreaths around normal and atretic follicles, giving off many minute branches that have been traced up to, but not through the membrana granulosa.

DEVELOPMENT OF THE OVARY. The developmental changes in the human urogenital system have been followed from the third week after conception to maturity. At first, the changes are the same in both sexes. The earliest sign of a gonad appears on the ventral surface of the embryonic kidney between the eighth thoracic and fourth lumbar segments at about four weeks. As illustrated in Figure 2-19A, the coelomic epithelium has thickened, and clumps of cells bud off into the underlying mesenchyme. This circumscribed area of the coelomic epithelium is often called the *germinal epithelium.* At the fourth week, however, the region contains many large ameboid cells that have migrated into the body of the embryo from the yolk sac, where they have been recognized as early as the third week. These *primordial germ cells* are distinguished by their large size and certain morphologic and cytochemical features. They react strongly in tests for alkaline phosphatase (McKay, Robinson, and Hertig,

1949), and are recognizable even after repeated divisions. Primordial germ cells have been studied in many animals. If these cells are destroyed before they have begun to migrate or if they are prevented from reaching the genital area, a "gonad" lacking germ cells will develop.

When the primordial germ cells reach the genital area, some enter the germinal epithelium and others mingle with the groups of cells which proliferate from it or lie in the mesenchyme. Rapid division of all these types of cells results in development of a prominent *genital ridge* by the end of the fifth week. It projects into the body cavity medial to a fold that contains the mesonephric (wolffian) and the müllerian ducts (Fig. 2-19.B). Since the growth of the gonad is most rapid at the surface, it enlarges centrifugally. By the seventh week (Fig. 2-19.C), it has separated from the mesonephros except at the narrow central zone, the future hilum, where the blood vessels enter. At that time the sexes can be distinguished, since the testis can be recognized by well-defined radiating strands of cells (sex cords). They are separated from the germinal epithelium by mesenchyme that becomes the tunica albuginea. The sex cords, consisting of large germ cells and smaller epithelioid cells derived from the germinal epithelium, develop into the seminiferous tubules and tubuli recti. The rete, probably derived from mesonephric elements, establishes connection with the mesonephric tubules that develop into the epididymis. The mesonephric duct becomes the vas deferens.

In the female, the germinal epithelium continues to proliferate for a much longer period. The groups of cells thus formed lie at first in the region of the hilum. As connective tissue develops between them, they appear as sex cords. They give rise to the medullary cords and persist for variable periods (Forbes, 1942). By the third month, medulla and cortex are defined as illustrated in Figure 2-19D. The bulk of the organ consists of cortex, a mass of crowded germ and epithelioid cells that show some signs of grouping, but there are no distinct cords as in the testis. Strands of cells extend from the germinal ep-

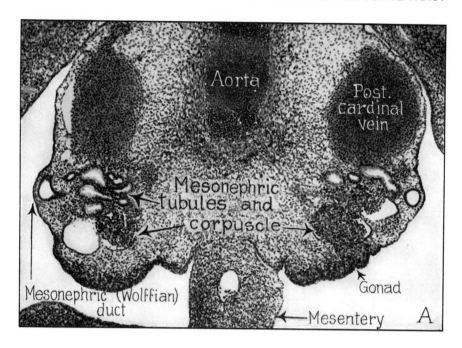

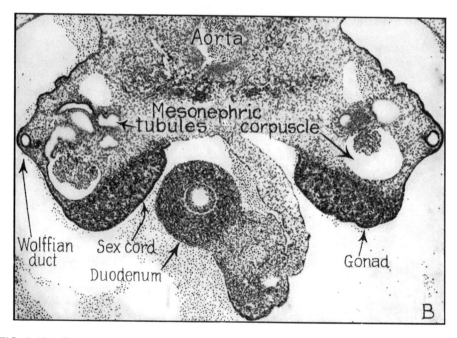

FIG. 2-19. Photomicrographs of sections of human embryos showing relations of gonads and metanophros. **A.** 11-mm embryo from fifth week after ovulation taken at level of arm bud. (Carnegie Collection No. 8773.) **B.** 14.2-mm embryo of 5 weeks from same level as **A.** Active proliferation has thickened gonad, which is still spread out on surface of mesonephros. On left, renal corpuscle opens into tubule. (Carnegie Collection No. 6520.) *(Continued)*

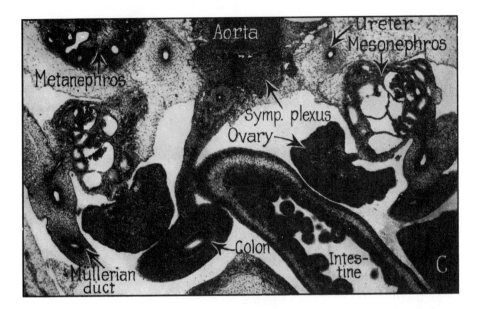

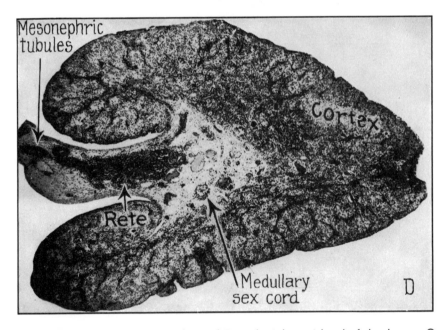

FIG. 2-19 (Cont.).   **C.** 31.5-mm embryo of 7 weeks taken at level of duodenum. Ovary has separated from mesonephros and appears homogeneous in structure. At right, a collecting tubule enters wolffian duct. (Carnegie Collection No. 6573.) **D.** 5½ month fetus, median section of ovary. Mesonephric tubules now included in mesovarium. Large mass of rete ovarii tubules, sex cords, and blood vessels in medulla. Cortex with nests of oocytes in stages of synapsis.

ithelium into the cortical mass, and mitoses are numerous. The rapid succession of mitoses soon reduces the size of the germ cells to the extent that they are no longer clearly differentiated from their neighbors. They are then called *oogonia*. Some of them in the medullary region are soon distinguished by a series of peculiar nuclear changes. Large masses of nuclear chromatin appear, very different from the chromosomes of the oogonial divisions. This change marks the beginning of *synapsis*, which involves interactions between pairs of chromosomes derived originally from father and mother. Various stages of synapsis can soon be seen throughout the cortex. Since similar changes occur in adjacent cells, groups (or "nests") appear. During one stage of synapsis, the chromatin is massed at one side of the nucleus, and the cytoplasm becomes highly fluid. Unless the preservation is prompt and perfect, these cells appear to be degenerating. Such artifacts have been misinterpreted frequently as evidence of widespread degeneration among oogonia.

By the fourth month, some germ cells, again in the medullary region, having passed through synapsis, have begun to enlarge. These are called *primary oocytes* (Fig. 2-20) at the beginning of the phase of growth that continues until they reach maturity. During this period of growth, many oocytes undergo degeneration, both before and after birth. The primary oocytes soon become surrounded by a single layer of flattened *follicle* cells (see Chap. 3, Fig. 3-1) derived originally from the germinal epithelium. They are then called *primordial follicles* and are seen first in the medulla and later in the cortex. Some begin to grow even before birth, and some are believed to persist in the cortex almost unchanged until the menopause.

By eight months of gestation, the ovary has become a long, narrow, lobulated structure attached to the body wall along the line of the hilum by the *mesovarium,* in which lies

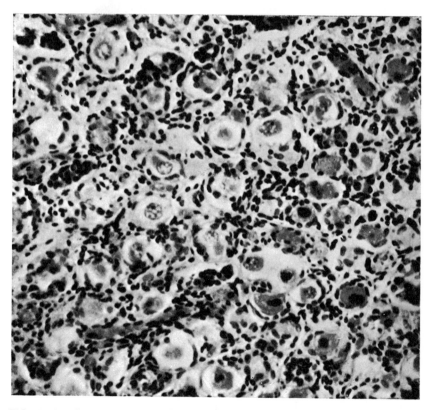

FIG. 2-20. Ovary of newborn girl. Numerous primordial follicles are shown.

the *epoophoron*. The germinal epithelium at that stage has been separated for the most part from the cortex by a band of connective tissue (tunica albuginea), which is absent in many small areas where strands of cells, usually referred to as cords of Pflüger, are in contact with the germinal epithelium. Among them are cells believed by many to be oogonia that have come to resemble the other epithelial cells as a result of repeated mitoses. The underlying cortex has two distinct zones. Superficially, there are nests of germ cells in synapsis, interspersed with Pflüger cords and strands of connective tissue. In the deeper zone, there are many groups of germ cells in synapsis, as well as primary oocytes, prospective follicle cells, and a few primordial follicles. In addition there are numerous scattered degenerating cells, although this zone is well vascularized. Such cellular degeneration is present regularly at certain stages in various rapidly growing regions of normal embryos.

At term, the various types of ovarian cells may still be found. In some cases, there are vesicular follicles in the medulla, which are all doomed to early degeneration.

MICROSCOPIC STRUCTURE OF OVARY. From the first stages of its development until after the menopause, the ovary undergoes constant change. The number of oocytes at onset of puberty has been variously estimated at 200,000 to 400,000 (see Chap. 5, p. 97). The duration of the period of atresia for a given follicle is unknown, although such data are essential to resolution of the question of neogenesis of ova in the adult. Since only one ovum is ordinarily cast off during a menstrual cycle, it is evident that a few hundred ova suffice for reproduction. The mode by which the others disappear is discussed in the section dealing with the corpus luteum and follicular atresia (see Chap. 3, p. 47).

Mossman and co-workers (1964), in an attempt to clarify the terminology of glandular elements in adult human ovaries, distinguished interstitial, thecal, and luteal cells. The interstitial glandular elements are formed from cells of the theca interna of de-

generating or atretic follicles; the thecal glandular cells are formed from the theca interna of ripening follicles; and the true luteal cells are derived from granulosal cells of ovulated follicles and from undifferentiated stroma surrounding them.

The huge store of primordial follicles at birth is gradually exhausted during the period of sexual maturity. Block (1952) found a gradual decline from a mean of 439,000 oocytes in girls under 15 years to a mean of 34,000 in women over the age of 36. Öhler (1951) and others have refuted the concept of continued oogenesis after birth in higher mammals, including man.

In the young girl, the greater portion of the ovary is composed of the cortex, which is filled with large numbers of closely packed primordial follicles. Those nearest the central portion of the ovary are at the most advanced stages of development. In young women, the cortex is relatively thinner but still contains a large number of primordial follicles separated by bands of connective tissue cells with spindle-shaped or oval nuclei. Each primordial follicle consists of an oocyte and its surrounding single layer of epithelial cells, which are small and flattened, spindle-shaped, and somewhat sharply differentiated from the still smaller spindly cells of the surrounding stroma (Fig. 2-20).

The oocyte is a single, large, roundish cell with a clear cytoplasm and a relatively big nucleus near the center. There are one large and several smaller nucleoli, and numerous masses of chromatin. The diameter of the smallest oocytes in the adult average 0.033 mm, and that of the nuclei, 0.020 mm.

REFERENCES

Block E: Quantitative morphological investigation of the follicular system in women. Acta Anat 14:108, 1952

Buckingham JC, Buethe RA Jr, Danforth DN: Collagen-muscle ratio in clinically normal and clinically incompetent cervices. Am J Obstet Gynecol 91:232, 1965

Danforth, DN, Buckingham JC, Roddick JW Jr: Connective tissue changes incident to cervical effacement. Am J Obstet Gynecol 80:939, 1960

Forbes TR: On the fate of the medullary cords of the human ovary. Contrib Embryol 30:9, 1942

Hitschmann F, Adler L: The structure of the endometrium of the sexually mature woman. Mschr Geburtsh Gynaek 27:1, 1908

Hodgson BJ, Eddy CA: The autonomic nervous system and its relationship to tubal ovum transport—a reappraisal. Gynecol Invest 6:162, 1975

Koff AK: Development of the vagina in the human fetus. Contrib Embryol 24:59, 1933

Krantz KE: Innervation of the human vulva and vagina. Obstet Gynecol 13:382, 1958

Langlois PL: The size of the normal uterus. J Reprod Med 4:220, 1970

Mahran M, Saleh AM: The miscroscopic anatomy of the hymen. Anat Rec 149:313, 1964

McKay DG, Robinson D, Hertig AT: Histochemical observations on granulosa cell tumors, thecomas and fibromas of the ovary. Am J Obstet Gynecol 58:625, 1949

Mossman HW, Koering MJ, Ferry D Jr: Cyclic changes in interstitial gland tissue of the human ovary. Am J Anat 115:235, 1964

Öhler I: Contribution to the knowledge of the ovarian epithelium and its relationship to oogenesis. Acta Anat 12:1, 1951

Schwalm H, Dubrauszky V: The structure of the musculature of the human uterus-muscles and connective tissue. Am J Obstet Gynecol 94:391, 1966

Woodruff JD, Pauerstein CJ: The Fallopian Tube. Baltimore, Williams and Wilkins, 1969

3

The Ovarian Cycle and Its Hormones

The obstetrician-gynecologist commonly assumes the role of endocrinologist, but as such has a significant advantage over his internist colleagues who deal with endocrine abnormalities in men. This is so because a detailed knowledge of the physiologic events of the ovarian cycle and the clinical manifestations of abnormalities thereof are sensitive guides to the endocrine milieu in young women. Specifically, the occurrence of spontaneous, predictable menses at reasonable intervals is strong evidence for the occurrence of ovulation. Moreover, if such menses are associated with some degree of discomfort, which may vary from only a prodroma of impending menstruation to severe dysmenorrhea, the likelihood of cyclic ovulation is even more assured. We do not subscribe to the thesis that regular, predictable menses may occur in anovulatory women (excepting those that are artificially produced by exogenous steroid compounds). For these reasons an equation can be formulated: cyclic, predictable, spontaneous menses = ovulation. Moreover, ovulation = normal sex hormone production. For women who are ovulatory, therefore, it can be assumed confidently that the production of pituitary gonadotropins, both follicle-stimulating hormone (FSH) and

luteinizing hormone (LH), as well as estrogens, androgens, and progesterone, are appropriate. Such a history is of more value than many hundreds of dollars worth of endocrine tests. For this reason, a thorough and carefully obtained menstrual history has both potential and real value. Consider the woman, for example, who has the regular, cyclic, predictable onset of menstruation, but sustains abnormal bleeding thereafter. Such a woman will almost invariably have some organic disease of the uterus to account for the abnormal bleeding. At the same time, excepting in women over 40 years of age, the occurrence of unpredictable uterine bleeding, i.e., unpredictable in onset, amount, and duration of bleeding, usually painless, is most often the result of chronic anovulation or undiagnosed pregnancy rather than organic uterine disease.

For these reasons, as well as the requirement of ovulation for pregnancy, this chapter and the next are devoted to a consideration of the closely integrated and synchronized phenomena that normally involve the ovary and endometrium of the nonpregnant woman during each ovarian cycle of her reproductive years. Teleologically, the purpose of the ovarian cycle is to provide an ovum for fertili-

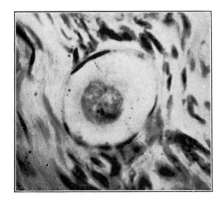

FIG. 3-1. Primordial follicle from adult ovary.

zation, whereas that of the endometrial cycle is to furnish a suitable site in which a fertilized ovum can implant and develop. Since the endometrial changes are regulated by the ovarian hormones, the two cycles are intimately related.

While both the ovarian and menstrual cycles are customarily considered to extend from the first day of one menstrual period to the day preceding the first day of the next, it is likely that the succeeding ovarian cycle, in the context of follicular maturation preparatory to the next ovulation, begins prior to the preceding menstruation. The typical human ovarian cycle is said to be 28 days, although 29 days is more usual, and variations are common and normal (see Chap. 4, p. 89).

Development of the Follicle.

Throughout the reproductive years, and in childhood to a lesser degree, certain primordial follicles undergo growth and development (Fig. 3-1). As the oocyte increases in size, the surrounding follicular cells become cuboidal, with nuclei that appear to be arranged in several layers (Figs. 3-2 and 3-3). The growth of the follicle soon becomes eccentric and the oocyte comes to lie at one side of the ball of follicular cells. Fluid accumulates between the cells to form a vesicle, with the ovum at one side (Fig. 3-4). While the follicle is still very small, a clear mucoid band, the *zona pellucida,* appears about the ovum (Fig. 3-5 and 3-6). The zona pellucida envelops the ovum and probably persists until after the fertilized ovum has reached the uterus.

MATURE GRAAFIAN FOLLICLE. The mature follicle is known as a *graafian follicle,*

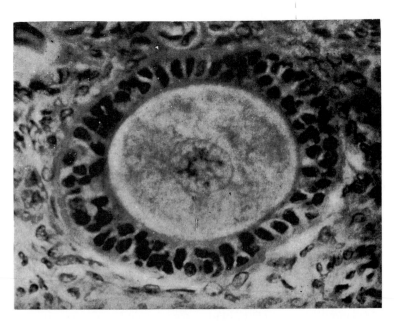

FIG. 3-2. Developing follicle.

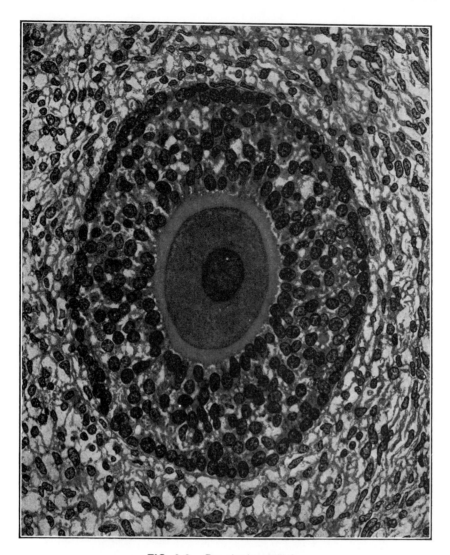

FIG. 3-3. Developing follicle.

after de Graaf, the Dutch anatomist, who described it in 1677. The follicular cells, or granulosa cells, that immediately surround the ovum constitute the *cumulus oophorus* or *discus proligerus,* which projects into the now abundant follicular fluid of the antrum. As the graafian follicle grows, the stromal cells surrounding it enlarge and the capillary net about them becomes closer, forming the theca interna, which is a cellular site of synthesis of estradiol-17β (Fig. 3-7). The cells of the theca interna develop lipid droplets; after ovulation these cells persist immediately adjacent to the enlarged follicular cells that are then called the granulosa lutein cells. The results of measurements of ova in sections of a well-preserved ovary are indicative that although the ovum grows slowly during the development of the graafian follicle, the volume of the ovum increases about 40-fold before complete maturity. The nucleus, however, increases only about 3-fold during this period. The large increase in cytoplasm includes the accumulation of nutrients such as yolk granules.

There is no reliable evidence that ova are formed normally in the human after birth. It has been estimated that there are 600,000 oogonia in the ovaries of female fetuses at 2 months gestation; 6,000,000 at 5 months

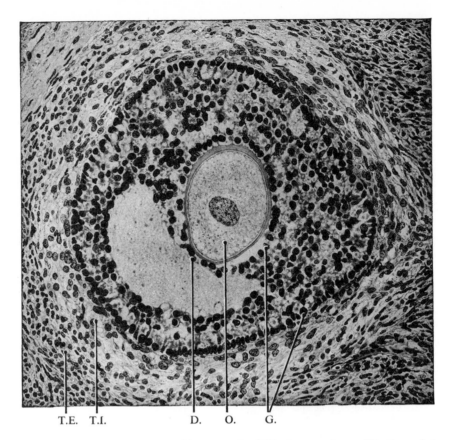

T.E. T.I.   D.   O.   G.

FIG. 3-4. Graafian follicle approaching maturity. T.E., theca externa; T.I., theca interna; D., discus proligerus (cumulus oophorus); O, ovum; G., granulosa cell layer.

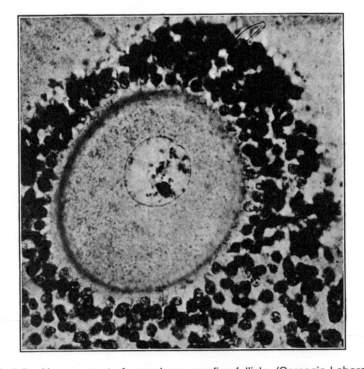

FIG. 3-5. Human oocyte from a large graafian follicle. (Carnegie Laboratory)

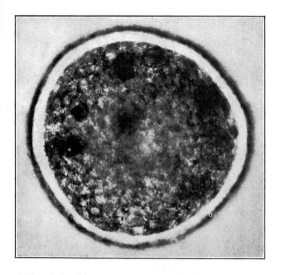

FIG. 3-6. Human ovum washed from tube. Fresh specimen, surrounded by semitransparent zona pellucida, consists largely of lipoid masses. Ovum measured 0.136 mm in the living state. (Carnegie Collection No. 6289, Dr. WH Lewis)

gestation. Degeneration occurs thereafter and 2,000,000 are found at birth, but only 300,000 in prepubertal girls (Baker, 1972). Before puberty, mature graafian follicles are found only in the deeper portions of the cortex. Later, however, mature follicles also develop in the superficial portions of the ovary. During each cycle, one follicle makes its way to the surface, where it appears as a transparent vesicle that may vary from a few to 10 or 12 mm in diameter. As the follicle approaches the surface of the ovary, its walls become thinner and more abundantly supplied with vessels (Fig. 3-8), except in its most prominent projecting portion, which appears almost bloodless and this site is designated the *stigma,* the spot where rupture of the follicle is to occur.

From outside inward, the mature graafian follicle consists of (1) a layer of specialized connective tissue, the theca folliculi; (2) an

Follicular fluid   Granulosa

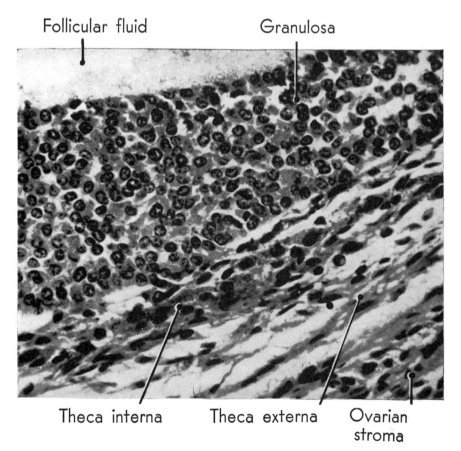

Theca interna   Theca externa   Ovarian stroma

FIG. 3-7. Section through the wall of a mature graafian follicle.

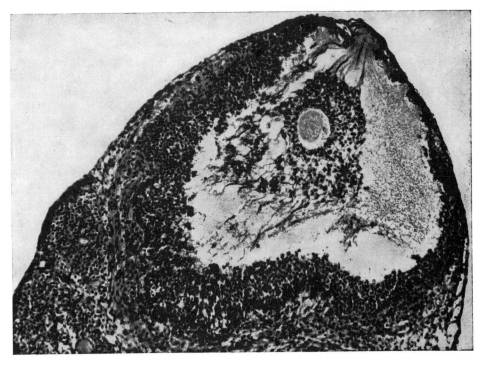

FIG. 3-8. Rat ovary just prior to ovulation. (Courtesy of Dr. Richard J. Blandau)

epithelial lining, the membrana granulosa; (3) the ovum; and (4) the liquor folliculi. The theca folliculi is comprised of an outer theca externa and an inner theca interna. The theca externa consists of ordinary ovarian stroma arranged concentrically about the follicle, but the connective tissue cells of the theca interna are greatly modified.

Almost as soon as the primordial follicle begins to develop, mitotic figures appear in the surrounding stroma, considerable multiplication of cells occurs, and the cells become distinctly larger than those of the surrounding connective tissue. As the follicle increases in size, these cells, the *theca lutein cells,* accumulate lipid and a yellowish pigment and appear granular. Simultaneously, there is a striking increase in the vascularity and in the number of lymphatic spaces of the theca.

The theca cells, before ovulation, are separated from the granulosa cells by a highly polymerized membrane. It is possible that luteinizing hormone may depolymerize this membrane at about the time of ovulation and allow vascularization of the granulosa cells to take place.

The epithelial lining of the follicle, or membrana granulosa, consists of several layers of small polygonal or cuboid cells containing round, darkly staining nuclei; the larger the follicle, the fewer the number of layers. At one point, the membrana granulosa is much thicker than elsewhere, forming a mound in which the ovum is included, the cumulus oophorus (discus proligerus).

The follicle is filled with a clear, proteinaceous fluid, the *liquor folliculi,* or follicular fluid. The granulosa cells do not take up the usual fat stains until the stage of preovulatory swelling, a period of rapid growth that commences about 24 hours before ovulation and is apparently related to the onset of, or preparation for, the secretion of progesterone.

MATURATION OF OVUM. As the human ovum approaches maturity, if it is brightly illuminated on a dark background, it is barely visible to the naked eye. According to Hartman (1929) and Allen and co-workers (1930), the average diameter of the mature human ovum in the fresh state is 0.133 mm.

If the nearly mature ovum is examined in the follicular fluid or in physiologic saline, the following structures may be distinguished in and about it: (1) a surrounding corona radiata; (2) a zona pellucida; (3) a perivitelline space; (4) a small clear zone of protoplasm; (5) a broad, finely granulated zone of protoplasm; (6) a central, deutoplasmic zone; (7) the nucleus, or germinal vesicle, with its germinal spot; and, if appropriately stained, (8) many small spheroid mitochondria. The ovum can rotate freely within the zona pellucida although its outer vitelline membrane appears closely applied to it. After fertilization, shrinkage of the ovum results in its complete separation from the zona pellucida as it floats in the perivitelline fluid. During growth, the oocyte accumulates deutoplasm (yolk granules). Before ovulation, the ovum is transparent with a faint yellowish tinge in the living state. There are also larger lipoid granules, which in preserved material appear to surround the nucleus (germinal vesicle). Numerous mitochondria are distributed through the cytoplasm. The spherical nucleus is located near the center of the oocyte. It has a large nucleolus and sparsely distributed chromatin. Shortly before ovulation, the nucleus migrates toward the periphery, and meiosis is reinitiated. At the completion of the first and second meiotic divisions, the number of chromosomes in the oocyte is halved, and two polar bodies are formed: the first before ovulation and the second after penetration of the oocyte by the sperm. Both polar bodies are extruded into the perivitelline space.

The mechanisms controlling meiosis and, consequently, the formation of polar bodies remain unknown. After oogonia have stopped undergoing mitosis (sometime during gestation but usually before the 7th month), they become primary oocytes. Characteristically, such cells have entered prophase of the first meiotic division. The primary oocytes continue through various stages of prophase (leptotene, zygotene, pachytene) until arrested in diplotene. By 6 months of age, all oocytes have either reached diplotene or else have become atretic. These primary oocytes remain in diplotene until shortly before ovulation unless they also undergo atresia. The factors responsible for arresting oocytes in diplotene are undefined; however, at the time of arrest, oocytes are encircled by a layer of follicle cells. The hypothesis has evolved that the follicle inhibits meiosis in some way. The theory of a follicular source of inhibition is supported by the fact that meiosis is reinitiated under one of two conditions: (1) after gonadotropic stimulation or (2) after removal from the follicle and culture in vitro in the absence of gonadotropins. The nature of the inhibitor has been postulated variously as a lack of oxygen, as steroids and currently as a protein. In accordance with the inhibition theory, gonadotropins overcome the inhibition by direct action on the oocyte or by indirect action through the follicle cells. There may be more than one inhibitor, since smaller oocytes will only mature to metaphase I in vitro, and oocytes progress only as far as metaphase II unless fertilization occurs. Another possibility exists, according to Baker (1972), that the so-called inhibition is really a stage in development, and the resumption of meiosis is dependent on the proper interaction among gonadotropins, follicle cells, and oocytes.

Ovarian follicles develop throughout childhood and occasionally attain considerable size, but do not normally rupture at this time, instead undergoing atresia in situ. Even in adults, many follicles that reach a diameter of 5 mm or more undergo atresia. Usually only one of a group of enlarging follicles continues to grow and to produce a normal mature egg that is extruded at ovulation. The mechanisms that normally limits maturation and ovulation to only one of the enlarging follicles, has not been defined and continues to constitute one of the major enigmas of ovarian physiology.

Ovulation. As the graafian follicle grows to a size of 10 to 12 mm in diameter, in response to the humoral mechanism described subsequently and schematically demonstrated on page 61, it gradually reaches the surface of the ovary and finally protrudes above it. Necrobiosis of the overlying tissues, rather than pressure within the follicle, is the principal factor causing follicular rupture. The cells at the exposed tip of the follicle float away at the site of the pale stigma so that the region becomes transparent. The thinnest clear area then bursts, and the follicular liquid and the ovum surrounded by the zona pellucida and corona radiata are extruded at the time of ovulation. The actual rupture of the follicle is not explosive. The discharge of the ovum with its zona pellucida and attached follicular cells takes not more than 2 to 3 minutes, and in the rabbit at least, it is expedited by the separation, just before rupture, of the ovum with the surrounding granulosa cells (corona radiata) from the follicular wall as the result of accumulation of fluid in the cumulus; hence, the ovum floats freely in the liquor. Recently, Strickland and Beers (1979) have demonstrated that granulosa cells produce plasminogen activator. The extracellular level of this enzyme activity is correlated closely with ovulation and is modulated by gonadotropins, cyclic nucleotides, and prostaglandins. Further, by the action of this enzyme on plasminogen, which is present in follicular fluid, the protease, plasmin, is generated, a proteolytic enzyme which Beers (1975) has shown can weaken the follicle wall.

Excellent motion pictures of the process of ovulation in the rat have been obtained by Richard Blandau and others. In Figures 3-8 and 3-9, two frames are illustrated. The follicle is shown just before ovulation and the expulsion of the ovum. In the first, the stigma is clearly visible, whereas in the second the actual expulsion of the ovum is shown.

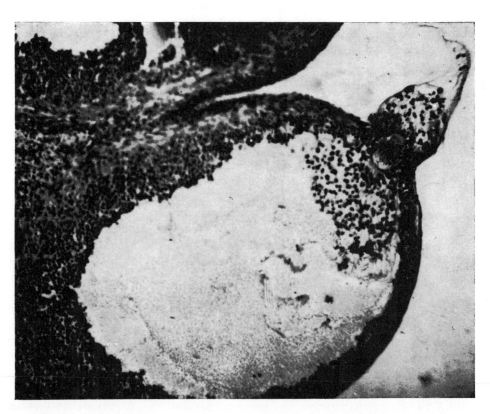

FIG. 3-9. Moment of ovulation in the rat. (Courtesy of Dr. Richard J. Blandau)

TIME OF OVULATION. The exact time of ovulation within the cycle is of the utmost importance for several reasons. First, since the life span of both the spermatozoa and the unfertilized ovum are limited, fertilization must take place within hours after ovulation if conception is to occur in that cycle. In infertile couples, detection of the time of ovulation and appropriate adjustment of the time of coitus are important steps in therapy. Second, to avoid conception, coitus could be limited to that part of the cycle several days from the time of ovulation, or the "safe period." Ovulation usually marks approximately the midpoint of both the ovarian and menstrual cycles. The period from the first day of menstrual bleeding to ovulation is designated the *preovulatory* or follicular phase of the cycle. The follicular phase encompasses roughly the first half of the ovarian cycle; the *postovulatory phase* is known as the luteal phase.

Various methods have been employed to attempt to determine the time of ovulation in women, the most dependable of which is the direct recovery of the ovum from the fallopian tube at operation. Allen and colleagues (1930) recovered mature unfertilized ova from the fallopian tube on the 12th, 15th and 16th days of the cycle, and concluded that ovulation occurs approximately on day 14 of a 28-day cycle. Other indirect methods for ascertaining the time of ovulation are the examination of fertilized ova and

evaluation of the changes that have taken place at the site of the ruptured follicle. By employing these technics it has been demonstrated that, although ovulation frequently occurs between the 12th and 16th days of the cycle, there is considerable variation. It is not uncommon for ovulation to take place at any time between the 8th and 20th days, as shown in Figure 3-10. The time of ovulation bears a closer temporal relation to the onset of the next menstrual period than to the previous menses, usually occurring approximately 14 days before the first day of the succeeding menstrual bleeding.

SIGNS AND SYMPTOMS OF OVULATION. On or about the day of ovulation, perhaps 25 percent of women experience lower abdominal discomfort on the involved side. This so-called *Mittelschmerz* is believed to result from peritoneal irritation by follicular fluid or blood escaping from the ruptured follicle. The symptom rarely occurs during every cycle.

A useful means of detecting ovulation is the shift in basal body temperature from a relatively constant lower level during the follicular or preovulatory phase to a higher level early in the luteal or postovulatory phase, as shown in Figure 3-11. Most likely ovulation occurs just before or during the shift in temperature. The increase in the basal body temperature is caused by the thermogenic action of progesterone. A similar ther-

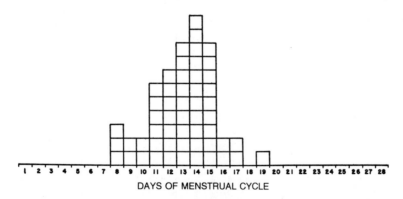

DAYS OF MENSTRUAL CYCLE

FIG. 3-10. Day of ovulation in 54 women calculated from the apparent age of the corpus luteum. Each block represents an observation of one woman.

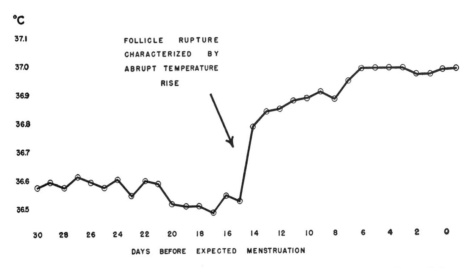

FIG. 3-11. Basal temperature shift characteristic of rupture of follicle. (From Palmer. *Obstet Gynecol Survey* 4:1, 1949)

mal response can be induced by injecting progesterone into a castrated subject. The rise in basal body temperature, therefore, may provide evidence for the development of a corpus luteum and the secretion of progesterone. Extensive luteinization of the granulosa, however, may occur in a follicle that still contains an ovum (luteinized follicle or entrapped ovum). Such an event is believed to be a cause of a short luteal phase and infertility.

OTHER TESTS FOR OVULATION. During the follicular phase, the cervical mucus increases in amount. Near the time of ovulation, the appearance of the cervical mucus changes from opaque to clear. At this time, the viscosity decreases considerably and the mucus can be drawn into long threads with considerable elastic recoil (*Spinnbarkeit*). Also at this time, when the cervical mucus is spread on a glass slide and allowed to dry, it undergoes marked arborization, or "ferning," because of its content of sodium chloride (see Chap. 4, Fig. 4-11, and p. 86). These changes in cervical mucus become maximal at about the time of ovulation. Unfortunately, these cyclic changes in cervical mucus offer no proof of ovulation, but in normal circum-

stances simply herald the augmented secretion of estrogen unopposed by progesterone. Similar changes in cervical mucus may be induced in castrated women by the administration of appropriate doses of estrogen. After ovulation, the changes in the mucus regress; the arborization of dried mucus is lost and a beaded, or "cellular," pattern develops.

As discussed in Chapter 4, there are numerous characteristic morphologic changes that take place in the endometrium after the formation of the corpus luteum and the secretion of progesterone. Since ovulation is nearly always associated with these changes, the demonstration of a well-developed secretory endometrium is strong evidence that ovulation has occurred during that cycle.

Increased plasma levels of progesterone in a nonpregnant woman is additional evidence that luteinization of a follicle and very likely ovulation have taken place. Convenient, rapid, and inexpensive methods of measuring the progesterone in serum by protein displacement or radioimmunoassay technics are now readily available. These tests, though not absolute for establishing that ovulation has occurred, are extremely valuable in reaching this presumptive conclusion.

Generally, plasma progesterone measurements have replaced the more tedious measurement of urinary pregnanediol as a reflection of progesterone secretion.

Many other tests, ranging from detection of altered symptoms or physical findings to biochemical or biophysical changes, have been proposed for detecting ovulation. Most of these have been reviewed by Speck (1959). There is still, however, no accurate test that can be conducted readily by women to warn them of impending ovulation. The striking increase in LH secretion that gives rise to the preovulatory LH surge is the most predictable endocrine event that precedes ovulation. It is conceivable that this "surge" could be monitored by sensitive and specific immunoassay techniques in order to predict more precisely that ovulation was imminent provided the time to complete the test were sufficiently short. Such a technic would have obvious utility in problems of infertility, but as yet undefined advantages in the prevention of pregnancy.

Corpus Luteum. The corpus luteum normally forms in the ovary at the site of the ruptured follicle immediately after ovulation. It is colored by a golden pigment, from which it derives its name, which means "yellow body." Microscopically, it has been observed that the corpus luteum undergoes four stages: proliferation, vascularization, maturity, and regression.

When the mature graafian follicle ruptures, the ovum, follicular liquid, and a considerable portion of the surrounding granulosa are discharged. The collapsed walls of the empty follicle form convolutions about the blood-filled cavity (Fig. 3-12). The remaining granulosa cells appear polyhedral, with round, vesicular nuclei and frothy cytoplasm. There are many large lacunae that contain extravasated blood but, initially, no blood vessels. The theca interna is invaginated, and its vascular channels are greatly dilated. Endothelial sprouts from these vessels penetrate the granulosa and the hemorrhagic cavity of the ruptured follicle. Hertig

(1964) described the K cells (Fig. 3-13) which can be recognized in the mature graafian follicle as stellate cells with deeply eosinophilic, homogenous cytoplasm. During the proliferative stage, strands of K cells, having migrated from the theca, extend into the membrana granulosa to as far as the central coagulum.

In the stage of vascularization that soon follows ovulation, the blood-filled cavity of the ruptured follicle undergoes rapid organization. Grossly, the central coagulum appears pale gray, with only a few hemorrhagic foci. Microscopically, there are fibroblasts but no capillaries within the coagulum. Elsewhere in the granulosa layer, dilated capillaries are conspicuous. As the stage of vascularization of the corpus luteum progresses to maturity, there is peripheral vacuolation in the luteinized cells originating from granulosa, a finding that is suggestive of physiologic activity. The theca interna cells are also vacuolated; when stained for lipid, many more coarse droplets are found than in the granulosa lutein cells. The K cells continue to constitute a prominent portion of the corpus luteum cell mass at that stage and also contain lipid, as well as a high concentration of alkaline phosphatase. The mature corpus luteum is usually 1 to 3 cm in diameter but occasionally may occupy a third or more of the entire ovary. At this stage, the corpus luteum characteristically is bright yellow.

Regressive changes occur in the corpus luteum, occasionally as early as the 23rd day of the cycle. These changes become progressively more marked up to the onset of menstruation until the central coagulum has been obliterated by connective tissues and blood pigment has been removed by leukocytes. There is no further capillary proliferation; the nuclei of the granulosa lutein cells become pale, and peripheral vacuolization of the cytoplasm decreases as coarse lipid droplets accumulate. The theca cells can be seen only in widely separated clumps. The K cells develop hyperchromatic nuclei, and the cellular outlines almost disappear. There is progressive loss of lipid-staining material

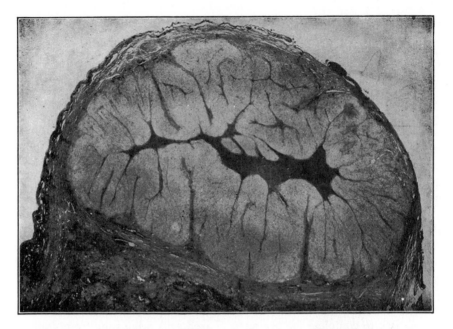

FIG. 3-12. Corpus luteum of pregnancy (Low power; see also Fig. 3-14).

"K" cell   Theca lutein   Lutein cells

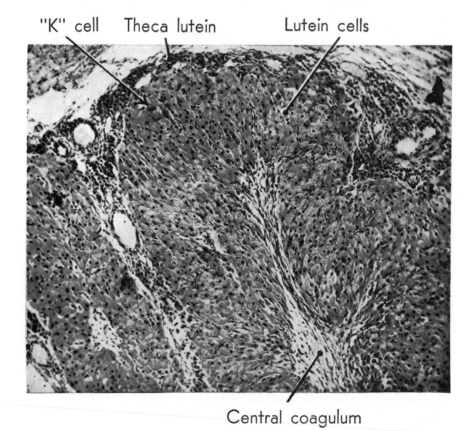

Central coagulum

FIG. 3-13. Section through the wall of a mature corpus luteum of menstruation.

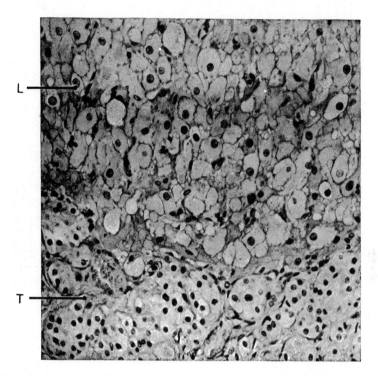

FIG. 3-14. Corpus luteum of pregnancy (High power; L, lutein cells; T, theca lutein cells).

throughout the entire corpus luteum. Before menstruation, complete regression of the corpus luteum takes place. If fertilization does not take place, the corpus luteum is destined to be a *corpus luteum of menstruation.* If fertilization does take place, a *corpus luteum of pregnancy* is initiated, presumably by the action of hCG, and the degenerative changes are postponed (Fig. 3-14).

ULTRASTRUCTURE.   Adams and Hertig (1969) described the ultrastructure of human corpora lutea obtained approximately 2, 3, 5, 11, and 15 days after ovulation. The day 5 (ovarian cycle day 19) corpus luteum, compared with younger, differentiating and older, regressing specimens, had ultrastructural characteristics that were consistent with maximal secretion of progesterone. The day 5 luteal cell contained a peripheral mass of agranular endoplasmic reticulum, which merged with a large paranuclear Golgi area. Parallel cisternae of granular endoplasmic reticulum were found in the periphery. Lipid droplets and mitochondria with tubular cris-

tae were numerous in the physiologically active cells, the complex plasma membranes which suggested specialized activities.

Corpus Luteum of Pregnancy. The duration and the function of the corpus luteum of pregnancy have been the subjects of much speculation and investigation. The scientific validity of hormonal therapy in the prevention of early abortion after surgical removal of the corpus luteum is dependent on an understanding of the function of this structure.

Hertig (1964) enumerated the morphologic criteria of a very early corpus luteum of pregnancy, these included increased congestion; a surge of hyperplasia from the 23rd to 28th day after the last period, presumably resulting, at least in part, from the stimulus of chorionic gonadotropin; an increasing number of K cells; and the absence of atrophic, ischemic, or regressive changes similar to those that appear when menstruation is imminent. The degenerative changes in the corpus luteum are delayed for a variable length of time but take place most frequently at about 6 months of gestation, although normal-appearing corpora lutea have been found at term.

ULTRASTRUCTURE.   Adams and Hertig (1969) compared the ultrastructure of human corpora lutea obtained during the 6th, 10th, 16th, and 35th weeks of pregnancy to those obtained during the menstrual cycle. In pregnancy, the luteal cell appears more highly compartmentalized, with a peripheral mass of endoplasmic reticulum and a central area in which mitochondria and Golgi complexes are concentrated. The area rich in mitochondria and Golgi complexes extends to the cell surface where microvilli are found that face a vascular space. Certain luteal cells with irregular nuclear membranes contain vesicular aggregates within the peripheral nucleoplasm or the perinuclear cytoplasm. These nuclear vesicular aggregates and certain spherical bodies may reflect prolonged endocrine stimulation and secretory exhaustion, which ultimately produce electron-dense cells with pyknotic nuclei.

Crisp and co-authors (1970), in an ultrastructure study, compared the granulosa and theca lutein cells of human corpora lutea. In early pregnancy, granulosa lutein cells were distinguished from theca lutein cells on the basis of their more homogeneous, electron-lucent matrix, enlarged pleomorphic mitochondria, abundant endoplasmic reticulum, and several other important ultrastructural features. They found, furthermore, that granulosa lutein cells of early pregnancy may be distinguished from those of the progestational phase of the menstrual cycle by their better developed endoplasmic reticulum, large spherical mitochondria, more numerous membrane-bound granules, and greater numbers of intercellular canaliculi. They suggested that these differences are caused by the action of chorionic gonadotropin during early gestation. On the basis of morphologic specializations, it seems likely that the corpus luteum may secrete, in addition to steroids, a proteinaceous product, i.e., relaxin.

FUNCTION IN PREGNANCY.   In the human, the corpus luteum is necessary for maintenance of pregnancy for only a short time after implantation. Among other species, the need for corpus luteum to maintain pregnancy is highly variable. Numerous human pregnancies have succeeded despite early ablation of the corpus luteum. Pratt (1927) reported continuation of pregnancy after such an operation performed as early as the 20th day after the last menstrual period, or about the time of implantation. In a review of cases in which the corpus luteum had been removed early in pregnancy, Hall (1955) reported a rate of abortion of a little over 20 percent. He believed that rate was not higher than expected following any abdominal surgery in the first trimester. In a well-designed study, Tulsky and Koff (1957) removed the corpora lutea from 14 women on whom they intended to perform sterilization and therapeutic abortion. Spontaneous abortion occurred in only two. In the remainder, the pregnancies were terminated by dilatation and curettage; 10 of the 14 women continued to excrete normal quantities of pregnanediol until the conceptus was removed.

The degenerative changes in the corpus luteum of an infertile cycle are delayed by the administration of chorionic gonadotropin. The corpus luteum, of course, secretes progesterone, but soon after implantation the human placenta apparently produces enough progesterone to maintain pregnancy. The corpus luteum, though necessary for implantation in the human, is not required for pregnancy beyond the earliest stages.

Inevitably, however, the clinician must face certain therapeutic choices when obliged to remove the corpus luteum in early pregnancy from a woman who wishes to continue that pregnancy. Our choice is the utilization of a parenteral progestin, 17α-hydroxyprogesterone caproate (Delalutin, 150 mg) when the corpus luteum is removed prior to 10 weeks gestation. We choose hydroxyprogesterone caproate because it has a predictable duration of action, does not virilize a female fetus, and can be given intramuscu-

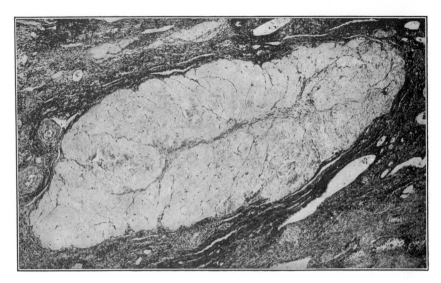

FIG. 3-15.   Corpus albicans.

larly. Beyond 8 weeks gestation, we administer the progestin only at the time of surgery, if at all. Between 6 and 8 weeks, there may be some merit in a second injection 1 week after surgery.

Corpora Albicantia.   In the absence of pregnancy, degenerated lutein cells are rapidly resorbed, and, in a short time, the corpus luteum is replaced by newly formed connective tissue closely resembling that of the surrounding ovarian stroma. The structures formed, called corpora albicantia, appear on cut-section to be dull and white, somewhat like scar tissue. They are, however, gradually invaded by the surrounding stroma and are broken up into increasingly small hyaline masses, which eventually are completely resorbed. Ultimately, the site of the original follicle is indicated only by an area of slightly thickened connective tissue. In older women, this process may be slower and less complete. In women near the age of menopause, it is not uncommon to find their ovaries to be almost filled by scars of various sizes (Fig. 3-15).

Atretic Follicles.   Theca lutein cells are admixed somewhat with granulosa lutein cells, but for the most part the two cell types are distinctive in appearance. The granulosa lutein cells are larger, more highly vacuolated, and are provided with a smaller nucleus; the theca lutein cells are somewhat smaller, more deeply stained, and have a relatively larger nucleus. The theca lutein cells play a prominent part in the life history of follicles that degenerate without rupture. This process, *follicular atresia,* is particularly pronounced during pregnancy. In such circumstances, after the follicle has attained a certain size, the ovum undergoes cytolysis, while the membrana granulosa degenerates and is cast off into the liquor folliculi and eventually resorbed. While these changes are in progress, the theca lutein cells proliferate to form about the follicle a tunic many layers thick which frequently becomes yellowish. Eventually, as the follicular fluid disappears, the walls of the follicle collapse and the theca cells surrounding it undergo fatty and hyaline change. Finally, an irregular hyaline body results that cannot be distinguished from a similar structure derived from a corpus luteum.

Atresia is the fate of the vast majority of follicles that develop beyond the primordial stage; the process begins during intrauterine life and continues until after the menopause.

Corpora lutea, however, always develop only from the comparatively few follicles that rupture after reaching maturity. Possibly one of the functions of the corpus luteum is obliteration of the spaces left by the ruptured follicles without the formation of cicatricial tissue, thus preventing conversion of the entire organ to scar tissue.

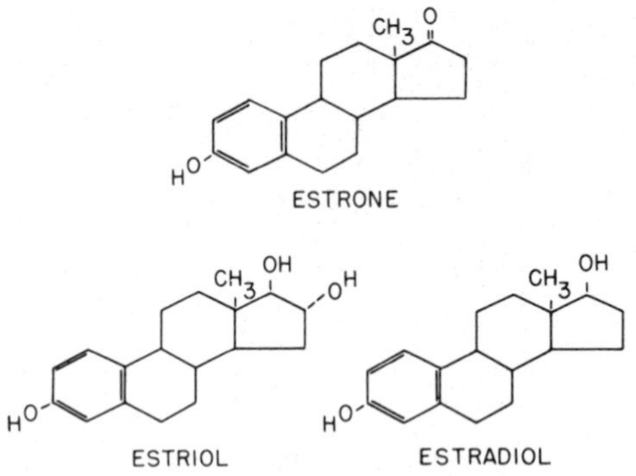

THE OVARIAN HORMONES

Estrogens

Discovery. In 1900, Knauer, in a classic study, demonstrated that ovarian transplants prevented atrophy of the uterus in ovariectomized rabbits. Twelve years later, Adler (1912) extracted a substance from ovaries that caused estrus in the guinea pig, and in 1917, Stockard and Papanicolaou described cyclic variations in the vaginal smear of the guinea pig. This bioassay enabled Allen and Doisy, in 1923, to isolate a potent estrogen from follicular fluid of the sow's ovary. In 1927, Aschheim and Zondek found that urine in pregnancy was rich in estrogenic substances. With a ready source of crude material and a satisfactory method of bioassay, the way was paved for final chemical identification. Within the next 2 years, Doisy (1929) and Butenandt (1929) almost simultaneously announced the crystallization from urine of an estrogenic substance later designated as *estrone* (Fig. 3-16). In 1930, Browne, working in Collip's laboratory, isolated the estrogenic steroid *estriol* from placental tissue (Fig. 3-16). It was not until 1936, however, that MacCorquodale and his associates, working in Doisy's laboratory, crystallized *estradiol-17β* (Fig. 3-16), the most potent growth-promoting factor of these three estrogenic substances.

Terminology. In 1936, the Council on Pharmacy and Chemistry of the American Medical Association adopted *estrogen* as the collective term for all substances capable of

FIG. 3-16. Structural formulas of the three important estrogens.

producing the typical changes of estrus: enlargement of the uterus, "cornification" of the vagina, and mating behavior in immature animals or in oophorectomized adult animals. The chemical names of the common estrogens in the human are estradiol-17β, estrone, and estriol.

Chemistry of the Estrogens. The parent hydrocarbon of the naturally occurring estrogens, estrane, possesses an 18-carbon skeleton and differs from the parent compound of the C_{19}-steroid series in that the angular methyl group at position 10 is absent. All the estrogens that have been isolated from human sources possess this structure, and, in addition, ring A is characteristically aromatic, as in estratriene (Fig. 3-17). The hydroxyl group at position 3 of the estrogens is therefore phenolic, that is, weakly acidic. The phenolic structure accounts for the solubility of these compounds in alkali and provides the basis for their separation from neutral steroids, such as the 17-ketosteroids.

The biosynthesis and metabolism of the classic estrogens—estradiol-17β, estrone, and estriol—have been studied extensively; however, a large number of additional metabolites have been isolated and characterized from human urine and various other sources. By the technic of isotope dilution in vivo, it has been shown that most of these metabolites are derived from the classic estrogens,

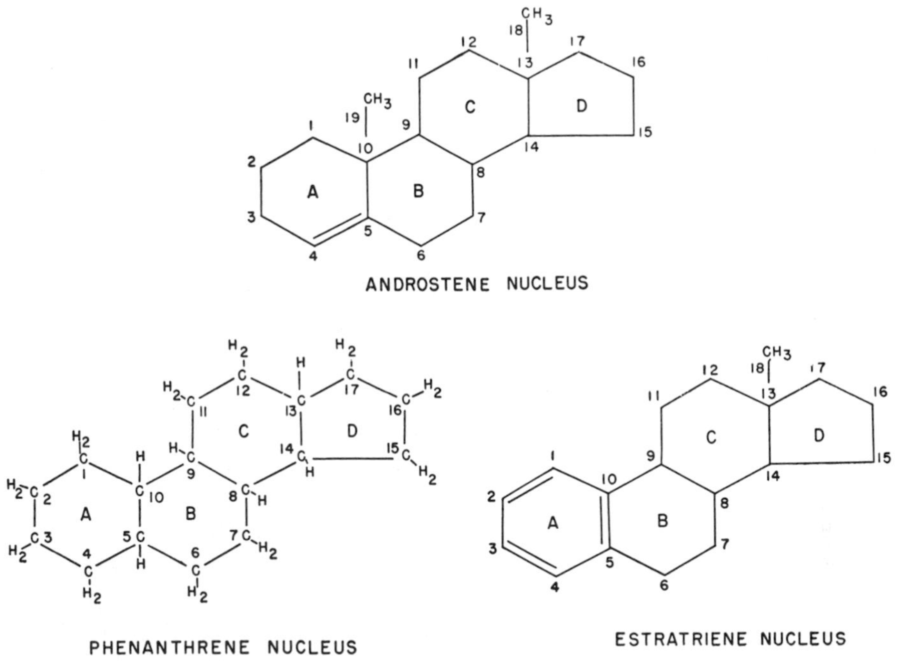

ANDROSTENE NUCLEUS

PHENANTHRENE NUCLEUS

ESTRATRIENE NUCLEUS

FIG. 3-17. Theoretical structural nuclei from which the estrogens and androgens are derived.

estradiol-17β and estrone. The biologic role, if any, of these compounds, however, is at present unknown.

The estrogens in urine occur mostly in conjugated forms, linked to either glucuronic or sulfuric acid, or both; while in blood, the unconjugated forms and the sulfates are found. The estrogen in highest concentration in blood in nonpregnant subjects is estrone sulfate.

Catechol Estrogens. The major metabolites of the naturally produced estrogens, estrone, and estradiol-17β are the catechol estrogens. The catechol estrogens are so called because they possess a hydroxyl function at the C-2 position of the A-ring. The two hydroxyl groups ortho to one another in an aromatic ring is a structural feature common to the catecholamines—dopamine, epinepherine, and norepinepherine. Because of this structural similarity to the catecholamines, it is suspected that the catechol estrogens may modulate the metabolism or action

of catecholamines. Impetus for this postulate was gained from the observation that the catechol estrogens have a much greater affinity for the enzyme, catechol-O-methyltransferase than do the catecholamines. Catechol-O-methyltransferase catalyzes the conversion of the catecholamines to inactive methyl ether (metanephrine) metabolites.

Sources of Estrogens. The results of the histochemical investigations of Dempsey and Bassett (1943) and of McKay and Robinson (1947) were indicative that the thecal cells elaborate estradiol-17β. Additional experimental data gathered from implantation of granulosal or thecal cells into castrated animals were suggestive that endocrine activity was associated only with the transplanted thecal cells. Furthermore, ovarian irradiation that resulted in destruction of the granulosa and proliferation of the theca allowed a persistence of estrogenic activity. Observations of experimentally produced ovarian tumors were indicative that the thecal component of the granulosa cell tumor, rather than the granulosa component, secreted estrogens. However, the conversion of C_{19}-steroids to estrogens, an enzymatic process referred to as aromatization, can be demonstrated in isolated granulosa cells in vitro. Presently, the relative contribution of each of the cellular elements of the follicle to total estradiol-17β production by the ovary is not known, nor is it known if such contributions may be profoundly different in the follicular and luteal phases of the ovarian cycle. The theca cells are considered to be the principal site of formation of estrogens in the developing follicle, but the granulosa cells of the corpus luteum are enzymatically competent to produce estrogens and may serve as a quantitatively significant source during the luteal phase of the ovarian cycle.

In addition, estrogens in the plasma and urine of nonpregnant women are derived from yet another source. The existence of an extraglandular source of estrogen is now established. This extraglandular estrogen is derived from the conversion of plasma androstenedione to estrone (MacDonald et al., 1967). Indeed, extraglandular estrogen production constitutes the principal mechanism for estrogen formation in prepubertal children and in postmenopausal women. Moreover, in young adult men, estrogen is derived largely from extraglandular sources from the conversion of plasma androstenedione and plasma testosterone. A small amount of estradiol-17β is secreted directly by the testes in normal men. In young women, extraglandular estrogen is principally the result of the formation of estrone, in many extraglandular sites, from the aromatization of plasma androstenedione. The plasma prehormone, androstenedione, originates by direct secretion from both the adrenal cortex and the ovaries. In young women, approximately 3 to 4 mg of androstenedione enter the blood each day from these two sources of direct secretion. Approximately 1.5 percent of this androstenedione is converted, in extraglandular sites, to the product hormone, estrone. Thus, in young women, the extraglandular estrogen production rate amounts to 40 to 60 μg of estrone per day. In certain anovulatory women, with excessive production of androstenedione (usually of ovarian origin) the extraglandular formation of estrone may be increased as a result of the increasing availability of the plasma substrate. Indeed, in such women, extraglandular estrone may be the principal source of estrogen formation. In normal ovulatory women, however, the fluctuating secretion of estradiol-17β by the ovary is additive to the extraglandular estrogen production, and total estrogen production in such women is the sum of its formation from these two sources.

Biosynthetic Pathways of the Formation of Estrogen in the Ovary. Through the work of numerous investigators, many of the steps involved in ovarian biosynthesis of estrogens have been elucidated. These steps are illustrated in Figure 3-18, in which several noteworthy features of this biosynthetic system are shown.

First, incubation of ovarian tissue with simple precursors such as acetate or cholesterol results in formation of estrogen (Ryan and Smith, 1959). Unlike the placenta, therefore (see Chap. 7), the ovary does not require circulating C_{19}-steroid precursors for the biosynthesis of estrogens, but rather has the capacity for estrogen synthesis de novo.

Second, several investigators have demonstrated that at least two separate pathways for the synthesis of estradiol-17β may be operative in the human ovary. One proceeds via Δ-4-androstenedione and testosterone in the biosynthesis of estradiol-17β; the other proceeds via Δ^5-3 β-hydroxysteroid intermediates, namely pregnenolone, 17 α-hydroxypregnenolone and dehydroisoandrosterone in the synthesis of estradiol-17β. Ryan (1959) speculated that the two pathways may have a cellular separation in the ovary. It is possible that the Δ^5-3 β-hydroxy pathway is preferred in the theca cells, whereas the Δ^4-3 ketone pathway may be utilized principally in corpus luteum, which is known to be a rich source of 3 β-hydroxysteroid dehydrogenase, the enzyme that catalyzes the con-

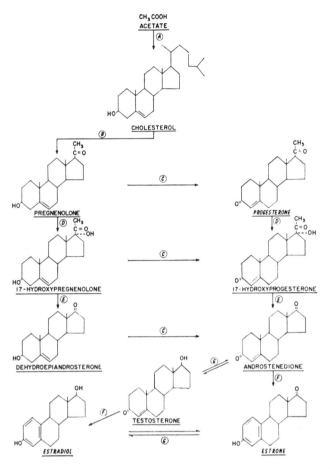

FIG. 3-18. Pathway of steroid biosynthesis in the ovary. **A.** formation of sterol from acetate. **B.** cleavage of cholesterol side chain—converts C_{27} to C_{21} compound. **C.** 3β-hydroxysteroid dehydrogenase and Δ^4-Δ^5-isomerase reaction. **D.** 17α-hydroxylation. **E.** cleavage of side chain—converts C_{21} to C_{19} compounds. **F.** aromatizing reaction. **G.** 17β-hydroxysteroid dehydrogenase (reversible). (From Smith and Ryan. *Am J Obstet Gynecol* 84:141, 1962)

version of Δ^5-3 β-hydroxysteroids to the Δ^4-3-ketone moiety. It is quite possible, of course, that the synthetic capacities of the two cellular types differ quantitatively rather than qualitatively, so that an absolute division of enzymatic capacities is not demonstrable by in vitro technics. It must be recalled that androstenedione is the precursor of estrogen biosynthesis via either pathway.

Third, as stated, both proposed pathways of ovarian estrogen synthesis proceed through "androgenic" intermediates, dehydroisoandrosterone, Δ^4-androstenedione, and testosterone. Thus, not only is the enzymatic potential of the ovary to produce androgen established, but the secretion of androgens, including testosterone, during the normal cycle has been demonstrated.

Nature of the Ovarian Secretion of Estrogen. Estimations of the daily "production rate" of estrogen in menstruating women have been made. This rate is a measure of the total daily production of estrogen, that is, the amount of estrogen produced from all sources. Although the production rate does not measure directly ovarian secretion, it does measure the total estrogen produced both by ovarian secretion (estradiol-17β) and by extraglandular formation (estrone) from plasma androstenedione. The daily production rates of estradiol-17β have been calculated from the amount of dilution by endogenously produced hormone of an intravenously administered tracer dose of isotope-labeled estradiol-17β. The extent to which endogenous hormone dilutes the administered tracer is estimated by measuring the specific activity of a urinary metabolite, estradiol-17β glucuronoside. Employing this experimental design, Goering and Herrmann (1964) found that the production rate of estradiol-17β during the immediate premenstrual and postmenstrual phases of the cycle was about 50 μg per 24 hours, but rose to 150 to 300 μg per 24 hours at the time of ovulation. These results are in good agreement with estimates made by indirect technics. From studies in plasma, it appears that the estradiol-17β secretory rate may reach upward to 400 to 600 μg per 24 hours just prior to the LH surge at midcycle. Levels this high are not measured by urinary technics, since these methods compute the "average" daily production over the 3- to 5-day period of urine collections.

These isotope studies as well as those involving direct sampling of ovarian venous blood have also provided results that are supportive of the view that the principal ovarian estrogenic secretory product is estradiol-17β, which, in turn, is the precursor of multiple urinary estrogenic metabolites. Fishman and co-workers (1960) demonstrated that estradiol-17β introduced into the circulation is quickly converted to estrone. Although intravenously administered estrone is also converted to estradiol-17β, this transformation proceeds at a much slower rate. Gurpide and associates (1963) found that more than 90 percent of intravenously administered isotope-labeled estradiol-17β was metabolized via estrone, whereas 50 percent of intravenously administered radioactive estrone was metabolized via estradiol-17β. The conversion of plasma estradiol-17β to plasma estrone and of plasma estrone to plasma estradiol-17β, however, is considerably less than

90 and 50 percent, respectively. Namely, only 15 percent of estradiol-17β appears in plasma as estrone, whereas only 5 percent of estrone appears in plasma as estradiol-17β. The reason for the differences as measured by urinary and plasma methods is that there is further metabolism of the product in the tissue sites of conversion prior to reentry of the product into plasma. Estradiol-17β, for example, may be converted in a tissue site to estrone, but the estrone formed may be further metabolized irreversibly, e.g., to estrone glucuronoside, prior to reentry into blood.

Estrogens in Biologic Fluids. The estrogens circulating in blood are principally sulfuric acid conjugates, whereas the metabolites found in urine are principally glucuronic acid conjugates. Only a small fraction of the total amount of estrogens produced is excreted in the urine. (The combined concentration of estradiol-17β, estrone, and estriol in 24 hours of urine equals about 15 percent of the estradiol-17β and estrone daily production rate.) Substantial amounts of estrogens have been identified in the feces.

Frank and associates (1932) first noted the tendency toward a biphasic curve of estrogen excretion in urine, with one peak at or near the time of ovulation and a second peak during the midluteal phase. During the 4 or 5 days before the next menstrual period, the excretion of estrogens declines rapidly. A similar pattern has been identified for the levels of estrogens in plasma, as shown in Figure 3-19.

Actions of the Estrogens. Estradiol-17β may be regarded as a growth hormone with selective affinity for tissues derived from the müllerian ducts, namely, the fallopian tubes, the endometrium, the myometrium, the cervix, and the vagina. Jensen and Jacobson (1962), as well as others, have shown that while only a small amount of a physiologic dose of estradiol-17β can be found in a growth-responsive tissue, the tissues derived from müllerian ducts have a much greater capacity to "incorporate and retain

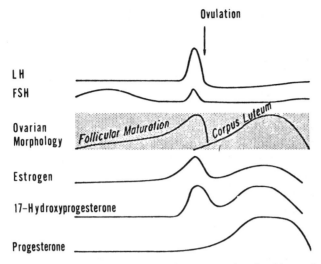

FIG. 3-19. Changes in plasma of the various hormones involved in ovulation in women. LH, luteinizing hormone; FSH, follicle-stimulating hormone. (From Strott, Yoshimi, Ross, Lipsett. *J Clin Endocrinol Metab* 29:1166, 1969)

estradiol-17β (but not estrone) for a prolonged period of time" than do other tissues, such as liver, kidney, and skeletal muscle.

The developmental role, if any, of estrogens in sexual differentiation remains to be ascertained. Jost (1953) and others have shown that the male sex hormone, testosterone, is necessary for the development of the wolffian ducts into the male internal genitalia as well as the differentiation of the genital tubercle into the male external genitalia. Moreover, yet another fetal testicular secretory product—likely a macromolecule (estimated molecular weight = 15,000 daltons) and seemingly of seminiferous tubule origin—causes regression of the müllerian ducts, hence the name *müllerian duct regression factor* or substance. It has been assumed, by inference, that the female sex hormone is unnecessary in the embryo for the proper development of the müllerian ducts, although this has, by no means, been satisfactorily demonstrated. It is likely, however, that in the absence of the testis the müllerian ducts and the genital tubercle differentiate along female lines, no positive stimulus being necessary.

At puberty, the effects of estrogens are seen in the development of the adult female habitus. Vaginal cornification occurs and the uterus attains the adult size and configuration. The ratio of the size of the body of the uterus to that of the cervix changes from 1 to 1 to the adult ratio of 2 to 1. In addition to producing these end-organ responses, estrogens also influence the actions of other endocrine glands and their hormones.

EFFECTS ON UTERUS. It has been demonstrated convincingly that estrogens act on the uterus via at least two mechanisms. One of these is through a system that involves a cytosolic receptor in uterine tissue which provides for the concentration of estradiol-17β in the cytosol and the subsequent translocation to the nucleus of the receptor–estrogen complex. After a conformational change, the complex apparently elicits DNA transcription with a resultant messenger RNA response and ultimately protein synthesis. Additionally, Szego and Davis (1969) have shown that estradiol-17β will evoke, within 15 seconds of administration, an increase in the uterine concentration of cyclic AMP, the so-called second messenger, apparently resulting from an interaction of trophic hormone and inner cell membrane adenyl-cyclase system. No doubt many other metabolic effects of estrogens at other sites within the uterine cell will be defined ultimately.

The spiral arteries respond to the growth stimulus of estrogens even more actively than does the rest of the endometrium; as a result, their tips progressively approach the epithelial surface. In addition, estrogens affect the activity of the cervical epithelium in such a way that the cervical mucus increases in quantity and pH, attains a clear fluid state, and is more readily penetrated by spermatozoa. Microscopically, the dried mucus is characterized by the formation of a "fern," as discussed on page 86.

EFFECTS ON VAGINA. Estrogens produce thickening of the vaginal epithelium. In castrated women, estrogens cause a change in the vaginal epithelium from a structure two or three cells thick to a membrane densely packed with compressed cells.

EFFECTS ON FALLOPIAN TUBES. Estrogens stimulate growth of the fallopian tubes and appear to influence the activity of the tubal musculature. In experimental animals, tubal contractions become maximal at estrus. The dependence of these contractions on estrogens is indicated by their disappearance after ovariectomy and their restoration by the administration of estrogens.

EFFECTS ON BREASTS. The administration of estrogens to the immature or ovariectomized animal in which the mammary glands are rudimentary or atrophic causes an extension of the ducts comparable to that seen in the sexually mature, nulliparous animal. The type of growth varies in different species. In the human and in the monkey, partial lobule-alveolar growth is induced, as well as ductal development. In other animals, the action of estrogens is solely on the ducts, the action of progesterone being necessary for the proliferation of the lobule-alveolar system.

EFFECTS ON OTHER ENDOCRINE ORGANS. Estrogens suppress the secretion of follicle-stimulating hormone (FSH) by the pituitary, as demonstrated by Frank and Salmon (1935), who showed that the elevated urinary FSH titer found in menopausal or ovariectomized women could be lowered by the administration of estrogens. The actual pituitary content of FSH was lowered after estrogen administration, a finding that is indicative that the effect was not just the result of secretory suppression and increased glandular storage. In women, there is evidence that estrogens can trigger the release of luteinizing hormone (LH), which, in turn, brings about ovulation in a mature ovarian follicle.

EFFECTS ON OVARY. Bradbury (1961) demonstrated that there is direct action of estrogenic hormones on ovarian tissue itself. Estradiol-17β, by a local effect, stimulates the growth of the ovarian follicle even in the absence of FSH and thereby potentiates the response to gonadotropins. This action of an estrogen on the follicle likely accounts for the almost exponential rise in estradiol-17β secretion and concentration in blood just prior to the LH "surge."

EFFECTS ON SKELETAL SYSTEM. Estrogens promote linear growth of bone and epiphyseal closure in immature animals, including the human.

Progesterone

During the postovulatory phase of the ovarian cycle, progesterone is secreted by the corpus luteum.

Prenant, in 1898, first suggested that the corpus luteum was an organ of internal secretion. Fraenkel, in 1910, demonstrated that the corpus luteum in the rabbit was necessary for the maintenance of pregnancy. In the same year, Bouin and Ancl (1910) described the histology of the progestational endometrium, providing the foundation upon which Corner and Allen (1929) established their classic method of bioassay of progesterone, which enabled them, in 1928, to isolate from sows' ovaries the hormone that they named "progestin" to indicate its specific role in gestation. Somewhat later, when Butenandt characterized progesterone as a steroid, he suggested that the chemical nature be indicated in the nomenclature by the suffix "sterone." The term *progesterone* thus arose from the combination of the two words.

Butenandt (1930) described a urinary steroid excreted in large amounts during pregnancy; pregnanediol. The significance of the compound, however, was not recognized until 1937, when Venning demonstrated a correlation between the excretion of pregnanediol in the urine and the presence of endogenous or exogenous progesterone. She demonstrated that pregnanediol, excreted as sodium pregnanediol glucuronoside, was a metabolite of progesterone. Previously, only minute amounts of progesterone had been isolated directly from the corpus luteum or from the blood of the ovarian vein. No metabolites of progesterone had been identified, and, therefore, no means of monitoring the secretion of progesterone were available.

Definition. Progesterone is a specific, biologically active steroid which produces progestational changes in the uterus of suitably estrogen-prepared immature or ovariectomized animals.

Chemistry of Progesterone. Progesterone, the principal hormone secreted by the corpus luteum, is a derivative of the 21-carbon skeleton, pregnane. In addition to the 2-carbon side chain at carbon 17, progesterone has a ketone group at carbon-20 and a Δ^4-3-ketone configuration in ring A, a characteristic of several hormonally active steroids. Progesterone and two compounds closely related structurally, 20α- and 20β-dihydroprogesterone have been isolated from the corpus luteum and ovarian vein blood, the placenta, and the adrenal. Progesterone is found in peripheral venous blood, but little is found in the urine or feces.

Metabolism of Progesterone. In the human, the major urinary metabolite of pro-

gesterone is pregnanediol. Dorfman, Ross, and Shipley (1948) found pregnanolone in the urine after administration of progesterone; the "allo" forms of both pregnanolone and pregnanediol are also recoverable in much smaller amounts. The liver has been identified as a major site of conversion of progesterone to these compounds.

From the results of a number of studies, however, it has been shown that progesterone is a preferred substrate for the ubiquitous but metabolically important enzyme, 5α-reductase. Progesterone, acting as a preferred substrate, serves as a competitive inhibitor for the 5α-reductase system (Massa and Martini, 1971). The enzyme catalyzes the conversion of testosterone to dihydrostestosterone, a compound which, in turn, modulates androgenic effects in certain end-organs. Moreover, from the results of some studies, it appears possible that progesterone may exert its definitive biologic action through its conversion to 5α-dihydroprogesterone in some tissues. Recently, it has been shown that there are considerable amounts of 5α-dihydroprogesterone in the blood of normally pregnant women (Milewich et al., 1975). The exact source of this compound and the biologic significance of this finding are not yet clear.

Employing histologic studies, Jones, Wade, and Goldberg (1952) showed that the glandular cells that are rich in glycogen are low in alkaline phosphatase, an enzyme that decreases greatly when large amounts of progesterone are given. They also found that progesterone blocks the formation of high-energy phosphate in hepatic mitochondria of the rat, favoring production of glycogen.

Progesterone and Metabolites in Blood and Urine. Progestational activity in the blood of ovulating women reaches a maximum about 1 week after ovulation. About 65 percent of injected progesterone can be recovered as metabolites in the excreta, with 20 percent in the urine, and 45 percent in the bile or feces. In the urine, half is excreted as pregnanediol, 10 to 20 percent as pregnanolone, and a small amount as other metabolites. The material in the bile is apparently from 50 to 60 percent pregnane-diol, 30 to 40 percent pregnanolone, and about 10 percent unidentifiable, more polar (i.e., water soluble) material. In women with normal ovarian cycles, the peak excretion of pregnanediol occurs on the 20th and 21st days. Excretion of pregnanediol usually declines and may be almost absent 2 days before menstruation.

These findings correlate well with those of the progesterone assays of the corpus luteum of menstruation conducted by Hoffman (1948), who found the first measurable progesterone was found on the 14th day of the cycle. The levels increased to maximal values by the 16th day and remained elevated until the 24th day of the cycle, after which there was a gradual decline until menstruation. The rate of secretion of progesterone by the mid-luteal phase corpus luteum has been estimated to be 25–30 mg per day, the highest rate of steroid secretion per unit weight of tissue of any endocrine organ.

Actions of Progesterone. The more profound effects of progesterone recognized thus far include the following: conversion of proliferative endometrium to secretory endometrium and then to decidua; inhibition of the contractility of smooth muscle, especially in the uterus; stimulation of natriuresis and, in turn, increased aldosterone production; and stimulation of the respiratory center and an increased respiratory rate. More recently, it has been shown by several investigators that small amounts of progesterone given to castrated or postmenopausal women who had been given an estrogen leads to a sudden and transient rise in circulating luteinizing hormone.

EFFECTS ON ENDOMETRIUM. A major function of progesterone is the preparation of the endometrium for blastocyst implantation and maintenance of pregnancy. The classic progestational changes in the endometrium were described by Hitschmann and Adler (1908) and were detailed later by Noyes, Hertig, and Rock (1950). In the properly estrogen-primed endometrium, progesterone produces manifold evidences of se-cretory activity. The tubular endometrial glands characteristic of the preovulatory phase are converted into tortuous structures. Subnuclear vacuoles in the epithelial cells are the first histologic evidence of progesterone effect on endometrial gland secretion. These vacuoles increase in size and migrate toward the luminal margin of the cell, finally allowing secretion to pour into the lumens of the glands. If these same glandular epithelial cells are suitably stained, glycogen can be demonstrated at about the time vacuolization first appears. Thereafter, glycogen steadily increases in amount until shortly before menstruation; the alkaline phosphatase activity, however, appears to reach its maximum around the time of ovulation. The stroma becomes edematous, and the constituent cells undergo hypertrophy with an increased amount of cytoplasm. If stimulation persists, the stromal cells form sheets of decidual cells. These characteristic histologic, cytochemical, and ultrastructural changes are discussed further in Chapter 4 (Fig. 4-1–4-5 and p. 76).

The normal menstrual flow occurs from the progestational endometrium. The amount of progesterone necessary to produce these typical endometrial effects is influenced by the previous estrogenic stimulation as well as the duration of the stimulation by progesterone and the continuity of the dosage. Progesterone, 10 mg given intramuscularly daily for 7 days, produces minimal secretory glandular changes. The level for vascular response, however, seems to be lower than that for the glandular reaction, since half this dose may produce withdrawal bleeding in the absence of any glandular progestational effect. To prevent menstruation, in the presence of a regressing corpus luteum, it is necessary to give large amounts of progesterone, 100 to 250 mg daily in divided doses. With these amounts of progesterone, menstruation can be delayed for 10 to 14 days or longer.

MAINTENANCE OF PREGNANCY. The progestational endometrium, with the deposition of glycogen that occurs under the influence of progesterone, furnishes proper nutritive conditions for the nidation and support of the fertilized ovum. If, because of a deficiency of progesterone, the endometrial bed degenerates, products of conception implanted therein are aborted. In many animals, e.g., the rat and mouse, the presence of the corpus luteum seems to be necessary throughout pregnancy, since its removal at any stage leads to abortion. As classically described by Corner and Allen (1929), ovariectomy in the pregnant rabbit or destruction of all the corpora lutea before the last few days of its gestational period regularly causes abortion. By administering an extract of sow's corpora lutea they were able to maintain pregnancy to term (31 days, approximately) in rabbits ovariectomized shortly after mating.

The ability of women to carry pregnancy to completion in the absence of the corpus luteum in no way indicates that progesterone per se is unnecessary. The placenta, which normally produces progesterone and estrogens in large quantities throughout much of pregnancy, is able to synthesize these hormones even at a very early stage in gestation in sufficient quantities to maintain gestation.

EFFECTS ON UTERINE MOTILITY. Knaus (1926) concluded that, in rabbits, progesterone acts on both endometrium and myometrium. He demonstrated decreased spontaneous uterine activity and complete inhibition of the response to the oxytocic hormone in the postovulatory phase of the ovarian cycle during the time of transportation, implantation, and early development of the fertilized ovum. He found that progesterone also inhibited spontaneous contractility and the response to posterior pituitary extracts in the human uterus. Csapo (1954) found, using isolated muscle, that progesterone decreased the electrochemical gradient and, depending upon the extent of its domination, could inhibit myometrial functions in the presence of a complete actomyosin and adenosine triphosphate system. The decrease of the electrochemical gradient makes the muscle insensitive to oxytocin, epinephrine, acetylcholine, and histamine.

EFFECTS ON FALLOPIAN TUBES. From histologic studies, it was shown that, to a degree, the tubal mucosa undergoes cyclic changes. During the luteal phase, it undergoes changes that are indicative of secretory activity. This interpretation is substantiated by Joël's observation (1939) that the content of glycogen and ascorbic acid in the human tubal mucosa reaches its height during the luteal phase. This has been demonstrated in the rabbit by Westman and co-workers (1931) and by Caffier (1938). Cyclic variations in the activity of the tubal musculature have also been ascribed to progesterone. There are rhythmic contractions, the amplitude of which is greatest at the height of the follicular phase and least during the luteal phase of the cycle; the relative quiescence in the latter phase, attributed to the action of progesterone, may play an important part in transport of the fertilized ovum to the uterine cavity. A very specific action of progesterone on the chick oviduct, the elaboration of avidin, has been demonstrated by the elegant studies of O'Malley and co-workers (1970).

EFFECTS ON CERVIX. The cervix produces different types of mucus during various phases of the cycle. After ovulation, the secretions are scanty, viscid, full of leukocytes, impermeable to spermatozoa, and do not form a fern pattern. These characteristics presumably are the effect primarily of progesterone counteracting estrogen.

EFFECTS ON OVULATION. Hertz, Meyer, and Spielman (1937) showed that progesterone caused the copulatory response in the guinea pig. In women, however, progesterone is produced after ovulation.

EFFECTS ON BREASTS. Progesterone is largely responsible for the acinar and lobular development during the luteal phase of the menstrual cycle, following the action of estrogens on the ductal epithelium. Progesterone plus estrogens, by dual action, are capable of bringing about complete mammary development, estrogens acting chiefly on the ductal system and progesterone on the lobular alveolar apparatus. Progesterone apparently also inhibits the action of prolactin in α-lactalbumin synthesis. This apparently explains in part the enigma of the failure of lactation during pregnancy when prolactin levels are greater than those found in puerperal women. Upon delivery of the placenta and the removal of the source of the massive progesterone production, the inhibitory effect on the breast of progesterone is removed and lactation can proceed under the influence of prolactin.

EFFECTS ON OTHER ENDOCRINE SYSTEMS. Progesterone will not suppress the pituitary production of FSH according to Greep and Jones (1950), and is ineffective in the relief of menopausal vasomotor symptoms. Salhanick and associates (1952) thought that progesterone might suppress the secretion of luteinizing hormone, but this point is still debated.

THERMOGENIC EFFECTS. The induction of an increase in the basal body temperature by progesterone has been used to identify luteal function.

Synthetic Progestogens. Several synthetic steroid compounds with various degrees of progesteronelike activities are used in clinical medicine, especially combined with estrogens, as oral contraceptives (see Chap. 40, p. 1012).

Androgens

The human ovary is enzymatically capable of synthesizing dehydroisoandrosterone, androstenedione, and testosterone. Evidence obtained by isolation of steroids from incubations of ovarian tissue, analysis of ovarian venous blood, and measurements of secretory rates before and after adrenal suppression, is indicative that the normal ovary secretes dehydroisoandrosterone, androstenedione and testosterone. Androstenedione levels in blood from the ovarian vein increase sharply in the late follicular phase, decrease slightly during the early luteal phase, and then rise again (Baird et al., 1974). In normal ovula-

tory women, plasma androstenedione originates from both adrenal and ovarian secretion. Dehydroisoandrosterone and its sulfate ester are derived principally from adrenal secretion. Testosterone, on the other hand, is derived primarily from the extraglandular conversion of androstenedione to testosterone, with a lesser amount of testosterone arising by direct ovarian secretion. During the premenopausal years, women produce approximately 300 μg of testosterone per day, one-half to two-thirds of which is derived from the extraglandular conversion of the plasma prehormone, androstenedione. Thus, androstenedione represents a plasma prehormone for conversion at extraglandular sites not only to estrogen but to the biologically important androgen, testosterone, as well.

RELAXIN

Relaxin is a polypeptide that has been identified in many mammalian species. Its exact function is poorly understood; its effects vary from one species to another. The main source of the hormone is probably the ovary, but in many animals it may be produced by the placenta as well. Relaxin is said to cause softening of the cervix in several mammals. On that basis, its use in slowly progressing human labors was suggested. Even if relaxin produces cervical softening, however, it does not overcome the main problem of dysfunctional labor. The production of relaxin by the corpus luteum of pregnancy is considered further in Chapter 9.

PITUITARY GONADOTROPIC HORMONES

The importance of the pituitary gland in the sexual cycle was first appreciated from the results of studies conducted by Philip Smith (1927) in hypophysectomized animals. Fluhmann, in 1929, contributed to our early clinical understanding of gonadotropin secretion when he discovered large amounts of pituitary gonadotropin in the blood of postmenopausal women. In 1931, Fevold, Hisaw, and Leonard succeeded in demonstrating that this pituitary gonadotropic fraction actually contained two active components, FSH and LH. In 1939, the Evans Laboratory in Berkeley, California, and the Squibb Biological Research Laboratory, directed by Van Dyke, almost simultaneously described the chemical separation and identification of these substances. These findings made possible experiments with relatively pure hormones and provided for further elucidation of the physiologic activity of the pituitary gonadotropins.

The next major contribution in the control of the ovarian cycle by the pituitary hormones came from Harris (1952), who appreciated the importance of the hypophysial portal system, a series of blood vessels along the pituitary stalk communicating with the hypothalamic centers. Wislocki (1938) showed that the blood flow in this system was principally from the hypothalamus to the anterior pituitary gland rather than in the reverse direction. The results of other studies are indicative that changes in the hypothalamus are responsible for the onset of puberty, rather than maturation of the ovary or the pituitary, both of which are capable of adult function at birth if properly stimulated. Some of the complexities of the neurohumoral control of anterior pituitary function, originally emphasized by Harris, are discussed below.

Follicle Stimulating Hormone. FSH, when administered to hypophysectomized immature female rats, causes growth of the follicle, development of the antrum, and increased ovarian weight. FSH is essential for the production of estrogen by the ovary. The metabolic fate of FSH is largely unknown. It appears to be partly excreted in the urine in much the same form in which it is secreted by the pituitary.

Although FSH was one of the first gonadotropic hormones to be identified, it was one of the last to be isolated in a pure preparation.

It is a readily water soluble glycoprotein. The isoelectric point of the hormone isolated from pituitary of swine is pH 4.8. The carbohydrate fraction of the protein includes mannose and hexosamine.

FSH usually is detectable in the blood and urine of children, but it begins to increase at about 11 years of age. Just prior to puberty the gonadotropins are found to increase principally at night, primarily during sleep. During the normal menstrual cycle, before ovulation, the FSH levels remain relatively constant or change only slightly until just prior to ovulation, when the levels rise somewhat. By the time of ovulation, any previous increase in the FSH level has receded to nearly base line levels. During the remainder of the ovarian cycle, FSH levels remain low and rise again very slightly just prior to menstruation (Figs. 3-19, 3-20). The modest rise in plasma FSH just before ovulation coincides with an increase in luteinizing hormone, i.e., the LH surge, that is much greater in magnitude than is that of FSH.

After the menopause, when the secretion of estrogens by the ovary is negligible or absent, the level of FSH in plasma and the amount excreted in the urine are very much increased. Administration of an estrogen lowers markedly but does not abolish completely the secretion of FSH by the pituitary.

Luteinizing Hormone. LH is also referred to as interstitial cell-stimulating hormone. LH restores the interstitial cells in the ovary of a hypophysectomized mature female rat and stimulates testicular interstitial cells to secrete androgen in the hypophysectomized mature male rat.

An electrophoretically pure preparation was obtained from pituitary glands of sheep and swine in 1939; the fractions obtained from the two sources have slightly different chemical characteristics. LH, like FSH, is a highly water-soluble glycoprotein.

According to Yussman and Taymor (1970), the LH levels in plasma rise sharply 12 to 24 hours before the estimated time of ovulation and reach a peak about 8 hours later. These investigators also noted that FSH

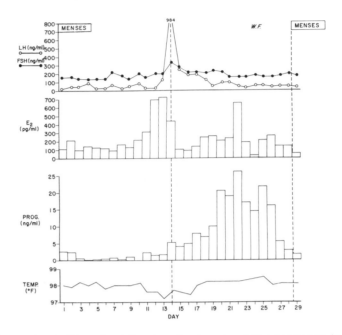

FIG. 3-20. Plasma levels throughout the menstrual cycle of the hormones involved in ovulation. LH, luteinizing hormone; FSH, follicle-stimulating hormone; E₂, estradiol; Prog., progesterone; Temp., basal body temperature; ng, nanogram; pg, picogram. (From Vande Wiele et al. *Recent Prog Horm Res* 126:63, 1970)

follows a similar but less marked pattern of response. Plasma progesterone levels were noted by them to increase after the rise in LH. Therefore, even though progesterone in small doses has been demonstrated to trigger LH release, the evidence is that in the normal menstrual cycle, significant amounts of circulating progesterone are not present until after the LH surge.

Estradiol-17β will trigger the release of LH. Moreover, estradiol-17β in plasma has been found to reach a peak level at or probably just before the time of increased LH release. Vande Wiele and associates (1970) treated mature rats with an antibody to estradiol-17β and thereby successfully blocked the commonly recognized end-organ responses to estrogen and also prevented LH release and ovulation. Treatment with stilbestrol, however, which is not inhibited by antibodies to estradiol-17β, restored ovulation. The results obtained by Vande Wiele et al. with antiestradiol were in sharp contrast to those obtained with antibodies to progesterone. Al-

though progesterone antibodies blocked the recognized end-organ response to progesterone, these antibodies did not prevent the discharge of LH or ovulation. Thus, a rise in circulating estrogen appears to be the important stimulus for the preovulatory LH surge.

Luteotropic Hormones. Even in the rat there does not appear to be a single luteotropic hormone. Instead, luteinizing hormone, follicle-stimulating hormone, and estrogens as well as prolactin all appear to be required for normal function of the corpus luteum.

Vande Wiele and associates (1970) studied corpus luteum function in women who previously had undergone hypophysectomy. Ovulation and corpus luteum formation were induced by giving repeated injections of FSH and then LH (Fig. 3-21). In one woman, the dosage of LH, all given in one day, was sufficient to stimulate the normal LH surge that occurs just before ovulation. There were increases initially in estrogens and progester-

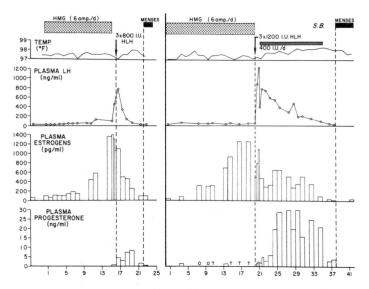

FIG. 3-21. Induction of ovulation in a woman without a pituitary by giving human menopausal gonadotropin (HMG) for 14 days followed by human luteinizing hormone (HLH). LH, luteinizing hormone; FSH, follicle-stimulating hormone; ng, nanogram; pg, picogram. (From Vande Wiele et al. *Recent Prog Horm Res* 126:63, 1970)

one in the plasma but these were not sustained. Within 5 days, the levels of estrogens and progesterone became very low; and on the sixth day after injecting the LH, the patient menstruated. These results were duplicated in other women who received LH for only 1 day. The studies were then repeated, but the injection of LH was continued daily. Progesterone and estrogens were detectable in the plasma until the onset of menstruation 17 days after LH treatment was commenced. Vande Wiele and associates (1970) were not able to prolong the life of the corpus luteum by giving LH and thereby delay the onset of menstruation much beyond the normal time of about 14 to 15 days. One woman conceived during the course of these studies. She subsequently gave birth to quintuplets who survived. These investigators concluded that LH is essential to maintain the normal life span of the corpus luteum, but that the life span of the corpus luteum cannot be prolonged for more than a few days by LH.

Luteolytic factors, the activities of which depend in some way on the presence of a uterus, have been suggested on the basis of the results of experiments in several species, including sheep, sow, and guinea pig. No proof of a uterine luteolytic factor in women has yet been provided, however.

Prolactin. There is no evidence from results of experiments in women that prolactin serves as a luteotropic hormone. Indeed, from measurements of prolactin by radioimmunoassay during the course of the menstrual cycle there is no clear-cut pattern of prolactin concentration that can be related to the events of the ovarian cycle. There is episodic secretion of prolactin, and increased plasma concentrations of prolactin have been observed in women during sleep. Interestingly, thyrotropin-releasing hormone (TRH) has been shown to cause a significant increase in the secretion of prolactin in the human. This finding may in part explain the previously inexplicable occurrence of galactorrhea in hypothyroid women and the occurrence of galactorrhea together with sexual precocity in hypothyroid girls. The physiologic role or roles of prolactin in the human are yet to be defined. Historically as well as phylogenetically, prolactin occupies a crucial role in many species in salt and water metabolism, lipid metabolism, renal function, and glucose metabolism, and prolactin influences significantly the kinetics of a host of important enzyme reactions. Nonetheless, the importance of prolactin in human health and disease, excepting for lactation, remains largely undefined.

In addition to the possible role of TRH in eliciting prolactin secretion by the pituitary, direct and indirect evidence has been obtained for the existence of a prolactin-inhibitory factor (PIF) of hypothalamic origin. Moreover, a close relationship between the apparent activity of prolactin inhibitory factor and that of luteinizing hormone releasing-factor (LHRH) have been described. Thus, with increasing activity of LHRH and PIF, the net result is an increase in gonadotropins and a decrease in prolactin secretion. Conversely, with decreasing LHRH and decreasing PIF, the net result is a decrease in gonadotropin and an increase in prolactin secretion. This combination of events is commonly observed in clinical medicine and results in the common triad of amenorrhea, estrogen deficiency, and galactorrhea. This state is commonly induced by a number of drugs that either inhibit the synthesis of catecholamines, e.g., dopamine, or deplete the brain concentration of such agents, e.g., certain tranquilizers and reserpine. Presently there is considerable evidence which is supportive of the view that *dopamine* is PIF.

NEUROHUMORAL CONTROL

Anterior pituitary function is under neurohumoral control. Humoral agents, now called releasing factors or hormones, are liberated from nerve endings of the hypothalamic tracts into the capillaries that empty into the portal vessels in the median eminence. The releasing factors are then carried through the hypophysial-portal circulation to the anterior pituitary (Porter, 1973).

During the past decade, considerable evidence has accumulated for the existence of distinct releasing factors for each of the hormones secreted by the anterior pituitary. The

releasing factors all appear to be peptides of quite low molecular weight. Two of them, TRH and LHRH, have been identified and synthesized. In addition there are factors (hormones) originating in the hypothalamus that inhibit the secretion of anterior pituitary hormones; e.g., PIF (dopamine) inhibits the secretion of prolactin, and somatostatin inhibits the secretion of growth hormone.

During the past decade, our view of the control of pituitary hormone release and subsequent ovarian response has altered materially. For a time, the possibility was considered that the anterior pituitary was principally under the control of the brain through a series of events that led to the production of hypophysiotrophic substances that traversed the long portal vessels and were conveyed in the blood to the sinusoids of the anterior pituitary. In turn, it was envisioned that the activity of the ovary, principally through the secretion of estradiol-17β, influenced brain function in this regard, and thus the ovarian follicle was considered to control, in part, its own fate. The massive increase in concentration of estradiol-17β, for example, at midovarian cycle precedes and is believed to elicit the midcycle LH surge. Thus, the ovary could signal the brain that a follicle was mature enough to respond to a significant increase in LH, the result being ovulation. While this formulation of the sequence of events still has considerable merit, it is now clear that the interaction between the ovary, brain, and pituitary is considerably more complex. Porter and associates (1976), for example, have shown that there is not a direct relationship between the concentration of LRF in the portal blood and the rate of secretion of LH by the pituitary. The LH to LHRH molecular secretory ratio in diestrous female rats was found to be 53 whereas the LH to LHRH molecular secretory ratio in castrated females was 1300. Thus, it is apparent that either a considerable increase in gain is effected with increasing LHRH secretion or the hormones elaborated by the ovaries significantly influence pituitary responsiveness, or both. In this regard Yen and others (1972, 1974) have demonstrated that LH response to administered LHRH women is augmented considerably by endogenous or exogenously administered estrogens.

REFERENCES

Adams EC, Hertig AT: Studies on the human corpus luteum: I. Observations on the ultrastructure of development and regression of the luteal cells during the menstrual cycle. J Cell Biol 41:696, 1969

Adams EC, Hertig AT: Studies on the human corpus luteum: II. Observations on the ultrastructure of luteal cells during pregnancy. J Cell Biol 41:716, 1969

Adler L: (Physiology and pathology of ovarian function). Arch Gynaekol 95:349, 1912

Allen E, Doisy EA: An ovarian hormone: a preliminary report on its localization, extraction, and partial purification, and action on test animals. JAMA 81:819, 1923

Allen E, Pratt JP, Newell QU, Bland LJ: Human tubal ova: related early corpora lutea and uterine tubes. Contrib Embryol 22:45, 1930

Aschheim S, Zondek B: (Anterior pituitary hormone and ovarian hormone in the urine of pregnant women). Klin Wochenchr 6:248, 1927

Baird DT, Burger PE, Heavon-Jones GD, Scaramuzzi RJ: The site of secretion of androstenedione in non-pregnant women. J Endocrinol 63:201, 1974

Baker, TG: Oogenesis and ovulation. In Austin CR, Short RV (eds): Reproduction in Mammals: I. Germ Cells and Fertilization. Cambridge, Cambridge University Press, 1972

Beers WH: Follicular plasminogen and plasminogen activator and the effect of plasmin on ovarian follicle wall. Cell 6:379, 1975

Blandau R: Personal communication.

Bouin P, Ancel P: (Research on the function of the corpus luteum). J Physiol Pathol Gen 12:1, 1910

Bradbury J: Direct action of estrogen on the ovary of the immature rat. Endocrinology 68:115, 1961

Browne JSL: Further observations on ovary stimulating hormones of placenta. Cited by Collip JB, Can Med Assoc J 22:761, 1930

Butenandt A: (On "Progynon," a crystallized female sexual hormone). Naturwissenschaften 17:879, 1929

Butenandt A: (On pregnanediol, a new steroid derivative from pregnant urine). Ber Chem Ges 63:659, 1930

Caffier P: (On the hormonal influence of the human tubal mucosa and its therapeutic utilization). Zeutralbl Gynaekol 62:1024, 1938

Corner GW, Allen WM: Physiology of the corpus luteum: II. Production of a special uterine reaction (progestational proliferation) by extracts of the corpus luteum. Am J Physiol 88:326, 1929

Crisp TM, Dessouky DA, Denys FR: The fine structure of the human corpus luteum of early pregnancy and during the progestational phase of the menstrual cycle. Am J Anat 127:37, 1970

Csapo AI: The molecular basis of myometrial function and its disorders. In La Prophylaxie en Gynecologie et Obstetrique, Congres International de Gynecologie et Obstetrique. Geneva, Georg, 1954, p 693

de Graaf R: De Mulierum organis generationi inservientibus. Lugd, Batav, 1677, p 161

Dempsey EW, Bassett DL: Observations on the fluorescence, birefringence and histochemistry of the rat ovary during the reproductive cycle. Endocrinology 33:384, 1943

Doisy EA, Veler CD, Thayer S: Folliculin from urine of pregnant women. Am J Physiol 90:329, 1929

Dorfman RI, Ross E, Shipley RA: Metabolism of the steroid hormones: the metabolism of progesterone and ethynyl testosterone. Endocrinology 42:77, 1948

Fevold HL, Hisaw FL, Leonard SL: The gonad-stimulating and the luteinizing hormones of the anterior lobe of the hypophysis. Am J Physiol 97:291, 1931

Fishman J, Bradlow HL, Gallagher TF: Oxidative metabolism of estradiol. J Biol Chem 235:3104, 1960

Fluhmann CF: Anterior pituitary hormone in blood of women with ovarian deficiency. JAMA 93:672, 1929

Frank RT, Goldberger MA: The female sex hormone. JAMA 86:1686, 1926

Frank RT, Salmon UJ: Effect of administration of estrogenic factor upon hypophyseal hyperactivity in the menopause. Proc Soc Exp Biol Med 33:311, 1935

Frank RT, Goldberger MA, Spielman F: Utilization and excretion of female sex hormone. Proc Soc Exp Biol Med 29:1229, 1932

Fraenkel L: (New experiments on the function of the corpus luteum). Arch Gynaekol 91:705, 1910

Goering RW, Herrmann WL: Estrogen secretion rate studies in normal women. Clin Res 12:115, 197, 1964

Greep RO, Jones IC: Recent Progress in Hormone Research, vol 5. New York, Academic, 1950

Gurpide E, Hausknecht R, Vande Wiele RL, Lieberman S: Abstract, 45th Meeting, Endocrinological Society, 1963

Hall RE: Removal of the corpus luteum in early pregnancy: a review of the literature and report of 2 cases. Bull Sloane Hosp Women 1:49, 1955

Harris GW: Hypothalamic control of the anterior pituitary gland. CIBA Found Colloq Endocrinol 4:105, 1952

Harris GW: Ovulation. Am J Obstet Gynecol 105:659, 1969

Hartman CG: How large is the mammalian egg? Q Rev Biol 4:581, 1929

Hertig AT: Gestational hyperplasia of endometrium: a morphologic correlation of ova, endometrium, and corpora lutea during early pregnancy. Lab Invest 13:1153, 1964

Hertz R, Meyer RK, Spielman MA: Specificity of progesterone in inducing sexual receptivity in ovariectomized guinea pig. Endocrinology 21:533, 1973

Hitschmann F, Adler L: (The structure of the endometrium of sexually mature women with special reference to menstruation). Monatsschr Geburtshilfe Gynaekol 27:1, 1908

Hoffman F: (On the content of progesterone in the ovary and blood during the cycle). Geburtshilfe Frauenheilkd 8:723, 1948

Jensen EV, Jacobson HI: Basic guides to the mechanism of estrogen action. Recent Prog Horm Res 18:387, 1962

Joël K: The glycogen content of the fallopian tubes during the menstrual cycle and during pregnancy. J Obstet Gynaecol Br Emp 46:721, 1939

Jones HW, Wade R, Goldberg B: Phosphate liberation by endometrium in the presence of adenosinetriphosphate. Am J Obstet Gynecol 64:1118, 1952

Jost A: Problems of fetal endocrinology. Recent Prog Horm Res 8:379, 1953

Knauer E: (Ovarian transplantation). Arch Gynaekol 60:322, 1900

Knaus H: The action of pituitary extract upon the pregnant uterus of the rabbit. J Physiol 61:383, 1926

MacCorquodale DW, Thayer SA, Doisy EA: The isolation of the principal estrogenic substance of liquor folliculi. J Biol Chem 115:435, 1936

MacDonald PC, Rombaut RP, Siiteri PK: Plasma precursors of estrogen. I. Extent of conversion of plasma Δ^4 androstenedione to estrone in normal males and nonpregnant normal, castrate and adrenalectomized females: J Clin Endocrinol Metab 27:1103, 1967

McKay DG, Robinson D: Observations on fluorescence, birefringence and histochemistry of human ovary during menstrual cycle. Endocrinology 41:378, 1947

Massa R, Martini L: Interference with the 5 α-reductase system. A new approach for developing anti-androgens. Gynecol Invest 2:253, 1971

Milewich L, Gomez-Sanchez C, Madden JD, MacDonald PC: Isolation and characterization of 5 α-pregnane-3, 20-dione and progesterone in peripheral blood of pregnant women. Measurement throughout pregnancy. Gynecol Invest 6:291, 1975

Noyes RW, Hertig AT, Rock J: Dating the endometrial biopsy. Fertil Steril 1:3, 1950

Porter JC, Ben-Jonathan N, Oliver C, Eskay RL, Winters AJ: The interrelationship of the CSF, hypophysial portal vessels, and the hypothalamus and their role in the regulation of anterior pituitary function. In Anand Kumar TC (ed): Neuroendocrine Regulation of Fertility, Basel, Karger, 1976

Porter JC, Mical RS, Ben-Jonathan N, Ondo JG: Neurovascular regulation of the anterior hypophysis. Horm Res 29:161, 1973

Pratt JP: Corpus luteum in its relation to menstruation and pregnancy. Endocrinology 11:195, 1927

Prenant A: (On the morphologic importance of the corpus luteum, and its physiologic and possible therapeutic action). Rev Med Liest 30:385, 1898

Ryan KJ: Biological aromatization of steroids. J Biol Chem 234:268, 1959

Ryan KJ: Synthesis of hormones in the ovary. In Grady HG, Smith DE (eds): The Ovary. Baltimore, Williams & Wilkins, 1963, p 69

Ryan KJ, Smith OW: Biogenesis of estrogens by the human ovary: I. Conversion of acetate-1-ΔC^{14} to estrone and estradiol. J Biol Chem 234:268, 1959

Salhanick HA, Hisaw FL, Zarrow MX: The action of estrogen and progesterone on the gonadotrophin content of the pituitary of the monkey. J Clin Endocrinol Metab 12:310, 1952

Smith OW, Ryan KJ: Estrogen in the human ovary. Am J Obstet Gynecol 84:141, 1962

Smith PE: The disabilities caused by hypophysectomy and their repair. JAMA 88:158, 1927

Speck G: The determination of the time of ovulation. Obstet Gynecol Survey 14:798, 1959

Stockard CR, Papanicolaou GN: The existence

of a typical oestrous cycle in the guinea pig, with a study of its histological and physiological changes. Am J Anat 22:225, 1917

Strickland S., Beers WH: Studies of the enzymatic basis and hormonal control of ovulation. In Midgley AR, Sadler WA (eds): Ovarian Follicular Development. New York, Raven Press, 1979

Strott CA, Yoshimi T, Ross GT, Lipsett MB: Ovarian physiology: Relationship between plasma LH and steroidogenesis by the follicle and corpus luteum; effect on HCG. J Clin Endocrinol Metab 29:1157, 1969

Szego CM, Davis JS: Inhibition of estrogen-induced cyclic AMP elevation in rat uterus: II. By glucocorticoids. Life Sci 8:1109, 1969

Tulsky AS, Koff AK: Some observations on the role of the corpus luteum in early human pregnancy. Fertil Steril 8:118, 1957

Vande Wiele RL, Bogumil J, Dyrenfurth I, Ferin M, Jewelewicz R, Warren M, Rizkallah T, Mikhail G. Mechanisms regulating the menstrual cycle in women. Recent Prog Horm Res 126:63, 1970

Venning EH, Browne JSL: Urinary excretion of sodium pregnanediol glucuronidate in the menstrual cycle. (An excretion product of progesterone). Am J Physiol 119, 417, 1937

Westman A, Jorpes E, Widström G: (Investigation of the mucosal cycle in the uterine tube, its hormonal regulation and the significance of the tubal secretion for vitality of the fertilized eggs). Acta Obstet Gynecol Scand 11:279, 1931

Wislocki GB: The vascular supply of the hypophysis cerebri of the rhesus monkey and man. Proc A Res Nerv Ment Dis 17:48, 1938

Yen SSC, Vandenberg G, Rebar R, Thara Y: Variation of pituitary responsiveness to synthetic LRF during different phases of the menstrual cycle. J Clin Endocrinol Metab 35:931, 1972

Yen SSC, Vandenberg G, Siler TM: Modulation of pituitary responsiveness to LRF by estrogen. J Clin Endocrinol Metab 39:170, 1974

Yussman MA, Taymor ML: Serum levels of follicle stimulating hormone and luteinizing hormone and of plasma progesterone related to ovulation by corpus luteum biopsy. J Clin Endocrinol 30:396, 1970

4

The Endometrium and Menstruation:
Unique Properties

The human endometrium is a remarkable tissue. During a woman's life, the endometrium normally is shed and regenerated no less than 400 times. The lifetime cumulative menstrual blood loss normally associated with endometrial shedding is 20 liters or more, an amount of blood containing at least three times the total body iron content of the average adult woman.

This unique tissue, the endometrium, has become a model for investigations concerned with elucidation of the mechanism of action of steroid hormones and other agents, e.g., the prostaglandins. The accessibility of human endometrial tissue, together with recently developed technics that allow the separation of endometrial glandular epithelium from stroma, have rightfully attracted endocrinologists and molecular biologists who seek to define the nature of hormone action on target tissues.

Estrogen Action. Estradiol-17β promotes growth of the endometrium in a manner that now stands as a model for hormone mechanism of action. Estradiol-17β, biologically the most potent of the naturally occurring estrogens, enters the endometrial cell

apparently by simple diffusion. In the cell, the hormone becomes associated with a cytosolic macromolecule characterized by a high affinity for estradiol-17β. The receptor-estradiol-17β complex is translocated to the nucleus of the cell where it becomes associated with the chromatin of the cell's nucleus. The result is a transcriptional event with synthesis of messenger RNA and subsequent protein synthesis. Among the proteins synthesized are macromolecules with high affinity for progesterone, i.e., progesterone receptors, as well as additional receptor molecules for estradiol-17β. Thus, the action of estradiol-17β on the endometrium is one that provides both for the perpetuation of the cellular milieu in which estrogen acts and for the initiation of the action of progesterone.

Progesterone Action. This hormone also enters the endometrial cell by diffusion and becomes associated with receptors with high affinity for progesterone. The concentration of progesterone receptors is dependent, however, on previous estrogen action. The progesterone-receptor complex is also translocated to the nucleus, but its action there is strikingly different from that of the estradiol-17β-receptor complex. The progesterone-receptor complex brings about a decrease in the production of estradiol-17β receptor molecules, an action which eventually negates the action of estrogen. Progesterone also brings about an increase in the activity of the enzyme estradiol-17β dehydrogenase, the enzyme that catalyzes the interconversion of estradiol-17β and estrone. Tseng and co-workers (1974) have shown that the reaction kinetics of estradiol-17β dehydrogenase favor the formation of estrone, a biologically weaker estrogen than estradiol-17β. Thus, progesterone may attenuate estrogen action by (1) reducing the rate of synthesis of estrogen receptors and (2) by bringing about a reduction in the intracellular level of estradiol-17β.

These important studies have also provided tools for the investigator to identify markers of estrogen and progesterone action—tools believed to be important in the identification of hormone responsive tumors. A marker of estrogen action is the presence of progesterone receptors. Horwitz and colleagues (1975) have pioneered the delineation of estrogen-responsive breast cancer by showing that tumors which possess progesterone receptors are affected by endocrine ablation procedures. The presence of estradiol-17β dehydrogenase activity is indicative of progesterone action, and the existence of this enzyme in endometrial carcinoma tissue may signal responsiveness therapeutically of such tumors to progesterone and related progestational agents.

Decidua. The human decidua, the specialized endometrium of pregnancy produced by prolonged stimulation by progesterone and estrogen, is a tissue of great interest to immunologists as well. The special relationship that exists between endometrium-decidua and invading trophoblast, seemingly defies the laws of transplant immunology. The success of this unique autograft is not only a curiosity but an event that many investigators believe harbors the solution to the future of successful transplantation surgery and perhaps the control of neoplasia as well.

The mysteries of the human decidua continue to increase. Convincing evidence has been presented by Riddick and co-workers (1979) and Golander and co-workers (1978) for example, which is supportive of the view that the decidua is a source of the enormous amounts of prolactin found in the amnionic fluid during human pregnancy. Levels of prolactin of 10,000 ng/ml of amniotic fluid are found during the 20th to 24th week of pregnancy compared to levels of 150 ng/ml in plasma of term pregnant women (Tyson et al., 1972). Thus the human endometrium not only occupies a unique role in the physiology of womanhood but constitutes a marvelous model system for study by endocrinologists, molecular biologists, immunologists, oncologists, and lipid biochemists.

THE ENDOMETRIAL CYCLE

The histologic changes in the endometrium during the menstrual cycle are summarized in Figure 4-1, from Noyes, Hertig, and Rock (1950). So characteristic are these alterations that an experienced pathologist can "date" an endometrium accurately from its microscopic appearance.

In response to the endocrine changes that occur during each ovulatory ovarian cycle, there are morphologic changes in the endometrium that evolve with such precise regularity that the histologic features of the endometrium can be used to date the ovarian cycle. The endocrine changes during the ovarian cycle, as described in the preceding chapter and on page 84, is summarized as follows: (1) During the preovulatory, or follicular phase of the ovarian cycle, estradiol-17β is secreted by the chosen follicle in increasing quantity. (2) During the postovulatory, or luteal, phase of the cycle, progesterone, in addition to estradiol-17β, is secreted by the corpus luteum. (3) During the premenstrual phase the corpus luteum regresses and both estradiol-17β and progesterone secretion diminishes. Consequent upon these phases of the ovarian cycle are the four main stages

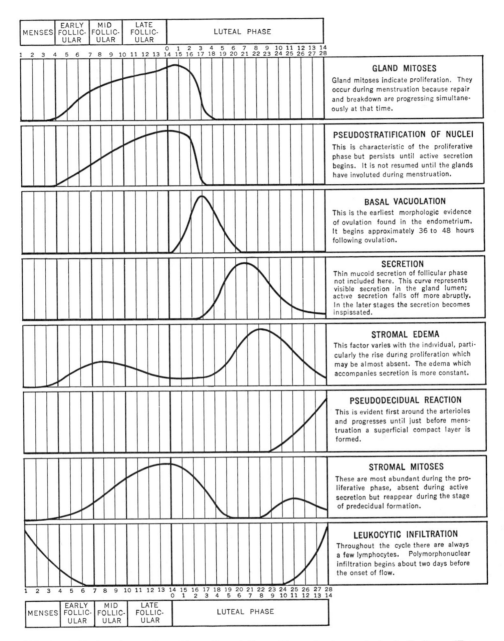

FIG. 4-1. Dating the endometrium. Correlation of important morphologic findings. (From Noyes, Hertig, Rock. *Fertil Steril* 1:3, 1950)

of the endometrial cycle: (1) postmenstrual reorganization and *proliferation* in response to stimulation by estradiol-17β (2) abundant glandular *secretion,* resulting from the combined action of progesterone and the estrogen; (3) *premenstrual ischemia* and involution; and (4) *menstruation* with collapse and des-

quamation of all but the deep layers of the endometrium, as the consequence of withdrawal of both estradiol-17β and progesterone. The follicular, preovulatory, or proliferative phase, and the postovulatory, luteal, or secretory phase are customarily divided into early and late stages. The normal secretory

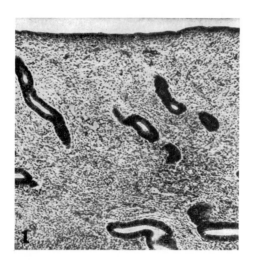

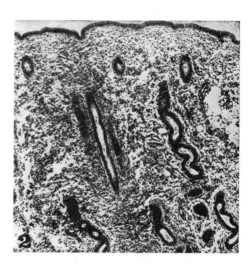

FIG. 2. Early proliferative endometrium. Shortly after menstruation. Glands are short and relatively straight and narrow. Stroma is moderately dense.

FIG. 3. Late proliferative endometrium. Endometrium is thicker than in Figure 2. Glands are more tortuous with higher epithelium. Stroma is more edematous.

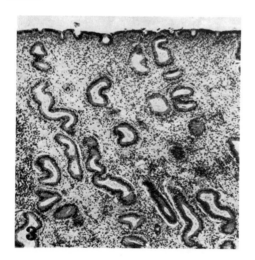

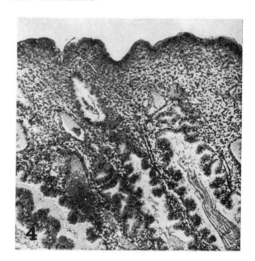

FIG. 4. Early secretory endometrium. About 3 days after ovulation. Subnuclear secretory vacuoles are evident in epithelium. Total thickness of endometrium is not significantly greater than in Figure 3.

FIG. 5. Late secretory endometrium. Several days before menstruation. Glands are tortuous, serrated, and exhausted of secretion. Early predecidual change of superficial stroma.

FIGS. 4-2–4-5. Histologic changes during the endometrial cycle. (Courtesy of Dr. Ralph M. Wynn)

phase may be subdivided rather finely, according to histologic criteria, from shortly after ovulation until the onset of menstruation.

Early Proliferative Phase. The histologic appearance of an early proliferative stage of the endometrial cycle is depicted in Figure 4-2. The endometrium is thin, usually less than 2 mm in depth. The glands are narrow tubular structures that pursue almost a straight course from the surface toward the basal layer. The glandular epithelium is low columnar, and the nuclei are round and basal. In the deeper part of the endometrium, the cells of the stroma are rather densely packed and their nuclei are deep-staining and small. In the superficial reorganizing layer, the stromal cells are more loosely packed, and the nuclei are more nearly round, more vesicular, and larger than in the deeper layers. Mitotic figures, especially in the glands, are present by Day 5 and mitotic activity is evident until 2 to 3 days after ovulation. Although the blood vessels are numerous and prominent, there is no extravasated blood or lymphocytic infiltration at this stage.

Late Proliferative Phase. As shown in Figure 4-3, the endometrium becomes thicker, as a result of both hyperplasia and increase in stromal ground substance. The loose stroma is especially prominent superficially, and the glands are widely separated compared with those of the deeper zone, where they are crowded and tortuous and the stroma is denser. This zoning becomes more pronounced in the secretory phase. Gradually, the glandular epithelium becomes taller and pseudostratified toward the time of ovulation. After ovulation, there is often a variable but transient increase in the density of the stroma.

Early Secretory Phase. Following ovulation, there are regularly occurring morphologic events that allow the endometrium to be dated quite precisely. The total thickness of the endometrium may decrease slightly because of loss of fluid. During the secretory stage, three zones become well defined: the basal zone or layer adjacent to the myometrium; the compact zone or layer immediately beneath the endometrial surface; and the spongy zone or layer between the compact and basal layers. Actually, the basal layer undergoes little if any histologic alteration during the menstrual cycle, but mitoses are found in the glands. The spongy middle layer comprises a lacy labyrinth with little stroma between the tortuous and serrated glands, and is the most characteristic feature of the luteal phase. In the compact superficial layer, the glands are more nearly straight and are narrower, but their lumens often are filled with secretion. Edema of the abundant stroma is an important factor in the thickening of the endometrium, but there is also an increase in dry weight. The secretory endometrium commonly attains a thickness of 4 to 5 mm (Fig. 4-4).

Late Secretory Phase. This stage represents the culmination of the histologic changes of the endometrial cycle. The endometrium now is extremely vascular, succulent, rich in glycogen, and ideal for the implantation and growth of the fertilized ovum. The stromal cells, particularly those around the blood vessels, undergo hypertrophic changes similar to, but less extensive than, those of the true decidua in pregnancy (p. 122). At the time of the cycle corresponding to implantation, i.e., about a week after ovulation, the endometrium is 5 to 6 mm thick and the secretory changes preparatory to nidation of the fertilized ovum are maximal (Fig. 4-5).

A further characteristic of the secretory phase is the striking development of the spiral, or coiled, arteries, which become much more tortuous (Fig. 2-12, p. 25). They branch in the compact layer, and the arterioles break up into capillaries within this zone. During the first week of the menstrual cycle, the arterioles extend only about halfway through the endometrium. Since the arterioles lengthen more rapidly than the endometrium thickens, their distal ends reach progressively closer to the surface of the endometrium. Mitoses are common in their walls. This unequal growth results in a disproportion between the length of the arterioles and the thickness of the endometrium, and, for this reason, the vessels become increasingly coiled.

Premenstrual Phase.   This phase of the cycle occupies the 2 or 3 days before menstruation and corresponds to the regression of the corpus luteum and, in turn, lack of secretion of progesterone and estrogen. The chief histologic characteristic of the premenstrual phase is infiltration of the stroma by polymorphonuclear or mononuclear leukocytes, producing a pseudoinflammatory appearance. At the same time, in the superficial zone, the reticular framework of the stroma disintegrates. As a result of the loss of tissue fluid and secretion, the thickness of the endometrium often decreases appreciably during the 2 days before menstruation (Fig. 4-1). In the process of reduction, the glands and arteries collapse.

Endometrial Ischemia.   In a classic study, Markee (1940) described the vascular changes that occur before menstruation, as observed in intraocular transplants of endometrium in the rhesus monkey. He found that as the result of the compression of the endometrium, the coiling of the arterioles increases markedly. Although the coils are fairly regular earlier in the cycle, just before menstruation they become quite irregular.

Markee furthermore demonstrated two entirely different vascular phenomena in endometrial transplants for the few days preceding menstrual bleeding. Beginning 1 to 5 days before the onset of menstruation, there is a period of slowed circulation, or relative stasis, during which vasodilatation may occur. There follows a period of vasoconstriction beginning 4 to 24 hours before the extravasation of any blood. The period of stasis is extremely variable, ranging from less than 24 hours to 4 days. It was Markee's opinion that the slowing of the circulation leading to stasis is caused by the increased resistance to blood flow offered by the coiled arteries. As more coils are added, the blood flow becomes in-

creasingly slower. Another explanation, however, must be invoked for the bleeding during anovulatory cycles and for bleeding following the withdrawal of estrogens, in which circumstances the arteries may be quite simple or relatively uncoiled. In such cases, there may be a more direct mechanism involving arteriolar vasoconstriction.

Thus, it is envisioned by most authorities that vasoconstriction of the arterioles and coiled arteries precedes the onset of menstrual bleeding by 4 to 24 hours, corresponding to the premenstrual ischemic phase. After the constriction has begun, the superficial half to two-thirds of the endometrium receive an inadequate supply of blood during the remainder of that menstrual cycle; the anemic appearance of the functional zone may be striking. When, after a period of constriction, an individual coiled artery relaxes, hemorrhage occurs from that artery or its branches. Then, in sequence, these constricted arteries relax and bleed, the succession of small hemorrhages from individual arterioles or capillaries continuing for a variable period of time. Although this sequence of vasoconstriction, relaxation, and hemorrhage appears to be well established, the mechanism that actually brings about the escape of blood from the vessels remains an enigma. It is entirely possible that the damage to the walls of the vessels during the period of vasoconstriction results in their rupture when the constricted segment relaxes and the blood flow is resumed.

The Role of Prostaglandins in Menstruation.   The prostaglandins, a unique class of tissue hormones, are synthesized in the cells in which they exert their action or in nearby cells. Thus, this group of substances are tissue rather than humoral hormones. These substances are degraded rapidly in the tissues of origin and in more remote sites, such as the lungs. Most of the prostaglandins or prostaglandinlike substances are synthesized from an essential fatty acid, namely arachidonic acid. Most often, however, arachidonic acid is found in tissues in an esterified form, usually in the *sn*-2 position of glycerophospholipids. The enzyme, phospholipase A_2, catalyzes the hydrolysis of the *sn*-2 fatty acid ester of glycerophospholipids to effect the release of free arachidonic acid. The rate of release of free arachidonic acid is believed to be the rate-limiting step in the formation of prostaglandins. Both endometrium and decidua are richly endowed with prostaglandin synthetase activity. It has been shown that the decidua is also enriched with arachidonic acid. The possible role of prostaglandin synthesis by the decidua in the initiation of parturition is discussed in Chapter 15 (p. 372).

A role for prostaglandins in the initiation of menstruation is also envisioned (Casey et al., 1980). The administration of prostaglandin $F_{2\alpha}$ ($PGF_{2\alpha}$) will bring about menstruation in nonpregnant women. It has been proposed that this action of prostaglandins is mediated by the induction of vasoconstriction of the endometrial arterioles. Menstrual blood contains large amounts of prostaglandins and prostaglandin administration gives rise to symptoms that mimic the dysmenorrhea commonly associated with normal ovulatory menses, i.e., menses triggered by progesterone withdrawal.

Prostaglandin 15-hydroxydehydrogenase (PGDH), the enzyme which catalyzes the first reaction in the degradation of prostaglan-

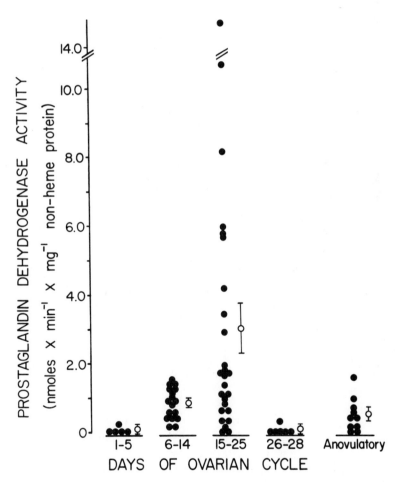

FIG. 4-6. 15-Hydroxyprostaglandin dehydrogenase activity in the cytosolic fraction of human endometrial tissue. The open circles and bars denote means ±S.E.M. for PGDH activity in each group. Number of samples (n): days 1–5, n = 5; days 6–14, n = 17; days 15–25, n = 26; days 26–27, n = 6; anovulatory, n = 10. (From Casey et al. Submitted to Prostaglandins, 1980)

dins, is found in endometrium principally in the cells of the glandular epithelium (Casey et al., 1980). The specific activity of this enzyme is highest in endometrium tissue during the luteal phase of the cycle whereas it is barely detectable or absent on Days 26 to 28 just before the onset of menses and Days 1 to 5 of the menstrual cycle (Fig. 4-6). Thus, the activity of the enzyme, PGDH, appears to follow the level of progesterone. It has been hypothesized that the fall in activity of PGDH during progesterone withdrawal, and, in turn, the reduced rate of degradation of prostaglandins, may serve to enhance the level of prostaglandins in the endometrium.

Menstrual Phase. Menstrual bleeding may be either arterial or venous, with the former predominating. It appears at the outset to result from rhexis of a coiled artery with consequent formation of a hematoma, but occasionally it takes place by leakage through the vessel. When a hematoma forms, the superficial endometrium becomes distended and ruptures. Subsequently, fissures develop in the adjacent functional layers, and bloody fragments of tissue of various sizes become detached. Although autolysis occurs, as a rule, fragments of tissue can be identified in the vagina and in the menstrual discharge. Hemorrhage stops when the coiled artery re-

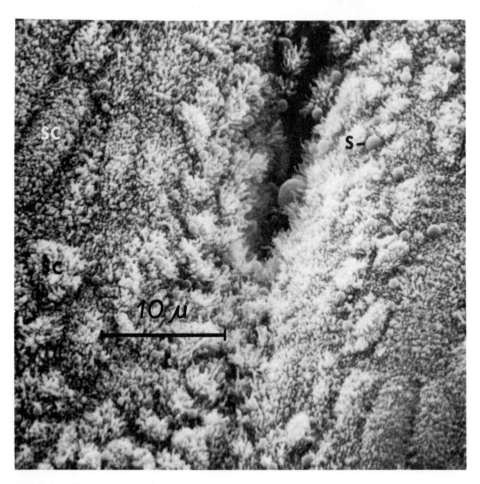

FIG. 4-7. Gland ostium and surrounding endometrium in proliferative phase seen by scanning electron microscopy. Many secretory droplets are seen on cell surfaces. Microvilli are prominent on secretory cells (SC) and individual cell margins are identified. (From White and Buchsbaum. *Gynecol Oncol* 1:330, 1973)

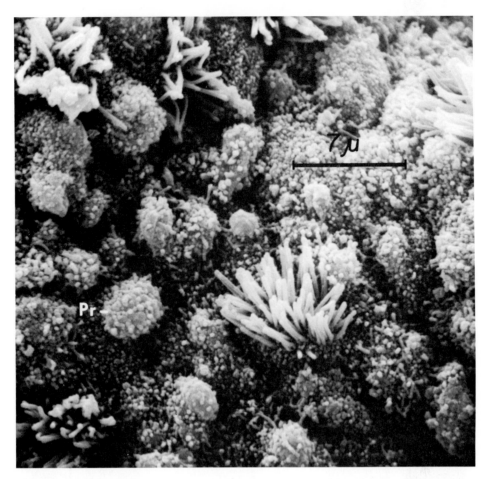

FIG. 4-8.   Cellular detail of secretory phase endometrium on day 24 of the cycle, demonstrated by scanning electron microscopy. Microvilli are prominent and cellular protuberances (Pr) are evident. (From White and Buchsbaum. *Gynecol Oncol* 1:330, 1973)

turns to a state of constriction. The changes accompanying partial necrosis seal off the tip of the vessel, and, in the superficial portion, often only the endothelium remains. The endometrial surface is restored, according to Markee (1940), by growth of the flanges, or collars, forming the everted free ends of the uterine glands. These flanges increase in diameter very rapidly, and the continuity of the epithelium is effected by the fusion of the edges of these sheets of thin migrating cells.

Among the more thorough studies of menstruation are those of McLennan and Rydell (1965) who believed that loss of endometrial tissue may be less extensive than previous investigators had suggested. In their opinion, regeneration of the uterine surface occurs from residual spongy layer rather than from the most basal elements.

Ultrastructure.   According to the findings of the ultrastructural studies of Wynn and associates (1967) and White and Buchsbaum (1973), in the endometrium there is cytoplasmic secretion into the glandular lumens throughout the menstrual cycle (Figs. 4-7 and 4-8). The terms *secretory* and *proliferative,* therefore, reflect less accurately the histologic pattern than do *preovulatory* (follicular) and *postovulatory* (luteal).

TABLE 4-1.

CORRELATION OF THE OVARIAN AND ENDOMETRIAL CYCLES (IDEAL 28-DAY CYCLE)

PHASE	MENSTRUAL	EARLY FOLLICULAR	ADVANCED FOLLICULAR	OVULATION	EARLY LUTEAL	ADVANCED LUTEAL	PREMEN-STRUAL
Days	1–3 to 5	4 to 6–8	9 to 12–16	12–16	15–19	20–25	26–32
Ovary	Involution of corpus luteum	Growth and maturation of graafian follicle		Ovulation	Active corpus luteum		Involution of corpus luteum
Estrogen	Diminution	Progressive increase		High concentration	Secondary rise		Decreasing
Progesterone	——— Absent ———			Appearing	——— Rising ———		Decreasing
Endometrium	Menstrual desquamation and involution	Reorganization and proliferation	Further growth and watery secretion	—	Active secretion and glandular dilatation	Accumulation of secretion and edema	Regressive
Pituitary secretion							
FSH	Fairly constant until just before ovulation			Moderate increase just before	——Rapid decrease to previous levels——		
LH	———— Same as above ————			Marked increase just before	————Same as above————		

The Endometrial Cycle in Retrospect.
The correlation of the ovarian cycle and its
hormones with the endometrial cycle and the
action of the pituitary gonadotropic hormones is summarized in Table 4-1 and in
Figures 4-9 and 4-10. Although the cycle is
divided into phases for descriptive purposes
and for convenience in diagnosis, the changes
are continuous throughout an ovulatory cycle. Furthermore, there is considerable individual variation in both the activity of the
endocrine glands and in the response of the
target organ, the uterus. Secretory changes
closely resembling those of the luteal phase
may appear occasionally before ovulation. Although the postovulatory phase of the cycle
is generally very close to 14 days in length,
the normal follicular phase may vary from
1 to 3 weeks. Finally, whereas the bleeding
at the end of a typical ovulatory menstrual
cycle is preceded by endometrial ischemia,
bleeding, on occasion, may appear at the expected time even without prior ovulation,
formation of a corpus luteum, or secretion
of progesterone. The histologic features of
anovulatory cycles are reproduced in the
bleeding endometria of patients after abrupt
withdrawal of estrogens. Anovulatory cycles
sometimes occur in otherwise apparently normal women, but the incidence is difficult to
ascertain because adequate observations of
the ovaries are rarely possible. It appears that
in some such cycles a follicle enlarges but
becomes cystic and degenerates. In others,
no follicles grow beyond a few millimeters
throughout an entire cycle. Withdrawal of
progesterone, therefore, is not essential for
cyclic uterine bleeding. *It is rare, however, for
women with persistent anovulation to menstruate
regularly unless they are using oral contraceptives.*

At about 27 to 35 days after the last menstrual period, there may be bleeding around
the site of implantation of the fertilized ovum,
resulting in slight vaginal bleeding that is
sometimes mistaken for a menstrual period.
According to Hartman (1932), this "placental sign" of bleeding always occurs during
pregnancy in the rhesus monkey.

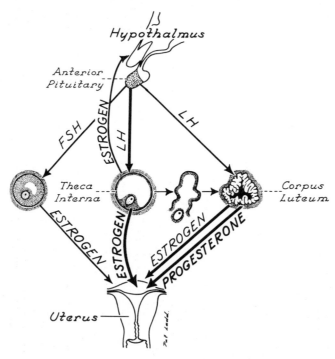

FIG. 4-9. Hormonal relationships of the hypothalamus, pituitary, ovaries, and endometrium
in the menstrual cycle.

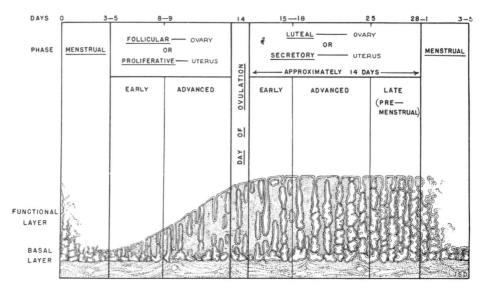

FIG. 4-10. Cyclic changes in thickness and in form of glands and arteries of endometrium and their relation to ovarian cycle.

CERVICAL, VAGINAL, AND TUBAL CYCLES

Cervix. Cyclic changes occur in the endocervical glands, especially during the follicular phase of the cycle. During the early follicular phase, the glands are only slightly tortuous and the secretory cells are not very tall. Secretion of mucus is meager. The late follicular phase is characterized by pronounced tortuosity of the glands, deep invagination, tumescence of the epithelium, high columnar cells, and abundant secretion. The connective tissue acquires a looser texture and better vascularization. Ovulation is followed by regression of these changes.

The secretory activity of the endocervical glands becomes maximal about the time of ovulation and is the result of estrogenic stimulation. Only at that time, in most women, is the cervical mucus of such a quality as to permit passage of the spermatozoa. The property of the cervical mucus that permits it to be drawn out in long strands is termed *Spinnbarkeit,* which is maximal at the time of ovulation. The synchronization of the height of secretory activity in the cervical and endometrial cycles is precise and purposeful.

In the cervix, where the mucus facilitates passage of the spermatozoa, it occurs when the ovum is just ready to be fertilized, a period of probably not more than about 15 hours. In the endometrium, where the purpose of the highly developed secretory activity seems to be to provide a site favorable for nidation of the fertilized ovum, the changes are maximal about 6 days later, when the fertilized ovum is ready to implant.

The "Fern Pattern." If cervical mucus is aspirated, spread on a glass slide, allowed to dry for about 10 minutes, and examined microscopically, characteristic patterns can be discerned, depending on the stage of the menstrual cycle and the presence or absence of pregnancy. From about the 7th day of the menstrual cycle to about the 18th day, a fern-like pattern is seen (Fig. 4-11); it is sometimes called "arborization" or the "palm leaf pattern." After approximately the 21st day, this fern pattern has disappeared and is replaced by a quite different, beaded or cellular picture (Fig. 4-12). This beaded pattern is usually encountered also in pregnancy.

The crystallization of the mucus, which is necessary for the production of the fern, or

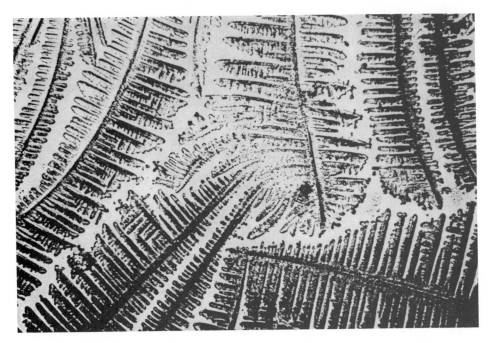

FIG. 4-11. Typical "fern arborization" pattern in cervical smears at midcycle in normal menstruating women. Note fullness and regular branching.

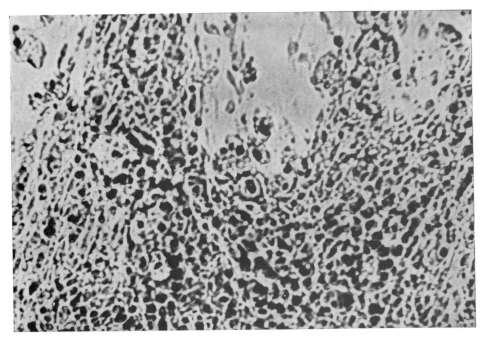

FIG. 4-12. A smear of cervical mucus from a pregnant patient at 8 months. The beaded pattern is evident. (Courtesy of Dr. J.C. Ullery)

arborized pattern, is dependent upon the concentration of electrolytes, mainly sodium chloride, in the secretion. In general, a 1 percent concentration of sodium chloride is required for the full development of a fern pattern; below that concentration either a beaded pattern or atypical, incomplete arborization is seen.

The concentration of sodium chloride, and, in turn, presence or absence of the fern pattern, is determined by hormonal action. Whereas the cervical mucus is relatively rich in sodium chloride when estrogen but not progesterone is being produced, the secretion of progesterone even without a reduction in the secretion of estrogen promptly lowers the sodium chloride content of the mucus, either cervical or nasal, to a level at which ferning will not occur in a dried specimen. During pregnancy, progesterone usually exerts a similar effect, even though the amount of estrogen produced is enormous compared with that of a normal menstrual cycle.

Vagina. Because of the constant desquamation of the vaginal epithelium, the cellular content of the vaginal fluid is reflective to some degree of the changes in the epithelium of the surface of the vagina. The human vaginal epithelium, under estrogenic stimulation, is characterized by cyclic changes during which the greatest development is reached at the end of the follicular phase. As shown in Figure 4-13 (see color plate), this stage is characterized by enlargement, flattening, and spreading of these cells and by relative leukopenia, whereas in the smear taken in the luteal phase there is an increase in the number of basophilic cells and leukocytes, as well as irregular grouping.

CLINICAL ASPECTS OF MENSTRUATION

Menstruation is the normal periodic, physiologic discharge of blood, mucus, and cellular debris from the uterine mucosa, occurring

at more or less regular intervals from puberty to menopause except during periods of pregnancy and lactation.

The Menarche and Puberty. The age at which menstruation begins (menarche) has declined steadily until recent years (Fig. 4-14). This decline has ceased in the United States. The average time at which menstruation begins is now between the 12th and 13th year but in a small minority of apparently normal girls its onset may occur as early as the 10th or as late as the 16th year. The menarche refers specifically to the onset of the first menstruation, whereas puberty is a broader term, referring to the entire transitional stage between childhood and maturity. The menarche, hence, is just one sign of puberty.

The Menopause and Climacteric. Menopause is the cessation of menses which occurs, on the average, at 47 years of age. There are wide variations in the age at which menopause occurs, however. About one-half of all women cease menstruating between 45 and 50, about one-quarter stop before 45, and another one-quarter continue to menstruate until past 50. The term climacteric is de-

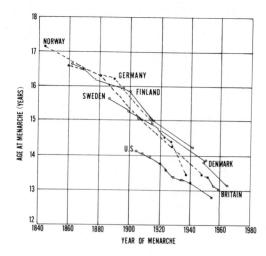

FIG. 4-14. The steady decline of the age of menarche in the United States and other countries. (From Tanner. *Sci. Am* 218:21, 1968)

rived from the Greek word meaning "rung of a ladder" and bears the same relation to the menopause as the term *puberty* bears to menarche. The climacteric refers to the critical period in a woman's life known to the laity as the "change of life."

Interval and Duration. Although the *modal interval* at which menstruation occurs is 28 days, there is considerable variation among women in general as well as in the cycles of any individual woman. Marked irregularity in the length of the menstrual cycle does not necessarily mean sterility. Arey (1939), who analyzed 12 different studies comprising about 20,000 calendar records from 1500 women and girls, reached the conclusion that there is no evidence of perfect regularity. In a study by Gunn, Jenkin, and Gunn (1937) of 479 normal British women, the typical difference between the shortest and longest cycle was 8 or 9 days. In 30 percent, it was more than 13 days but in no case was it fewer than 2 days. Arey found that in an average adult woman one-third of her cycles departed by more than 2 days from the mean length of her cycle. Arey's analysis of 5322 cycles in 485 normal white women indicated an average interval of 28.4 days; his figure for the average cycle in pubertal girls was longer, 33.9 days. Chiazze and associates (1968) analyzed the length of 30,655 menstrual cycles of 2316 women. The mean for all cycles was 29.1 days. For cycles rang-

ing from 15 to 45 days, the average length was 28.1 days. The degree of irregularity was such that only 13 percent of the women had cycles that varied in length by less than 6 days. Haman (1942) surveyed 2460 cycles in 150 housewives attending a clinic where special attention was directed to recording accurately the length of the menstrual cycles. Haman's data and that of Arey for white women, superimposed in the distribution curves shown in Figure 4-15, are almost identical.

Duration and Amount. The duration of menstrual flow is also variable; the usual duration is 4 to 6 days, but lengths between 2 and 8 days may be considered physiologic. In any individual woman, however, the duration of the flow is usually fairly similar from cycle to cycle.

The menstrual discharge consists of shed fragments of endometrium mixed with a variable quantity of blood. Usually the blood is liquid, but if the rate of flow is excessive, clots of varying size may appear. Considerable attention has been directed to the usual state of incoagulability of menstrual blood. The most logical explanation for its incoagulability is that the blood, having already undergone coagulation as it was shed, was promptly liquefied by fibrinolytic activity. Endometrial tissue possesses not only potent thromboplastic properties, which promptly initiate clotting, but also a potent activator

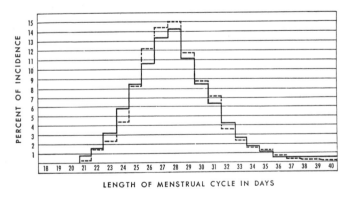

FIG. 4-15. Duration of menstrual cycle based on distribution data of Arey (continuous line) and Haman (broken line). (Courtesy of Eli Lilly and Co.)

of plasminogen to plasmin, which effects prompt lysis of fibrin clot.

At one time the toxic properties of the menstrual discharge attracted considerable interest. The discharge undoubtedly contains toxic proteins and peptides (Smith and Smith, 1940), arising most likely both from proteolytic activity inherent in the mixture of blood and endometrium and also from bacterial contamination (Zondek, 1953).

The average amount of blood lost by normal women during a menstrual period has been measured by several groups of investigators who found it to range from about 25 to 60 ml (Baldwin et al., 1961; Barker and Fowler, 1936; Hallberg et al., 1966; Hytten et al., 1964; Millis, 1951). With a normal hemoglobin concentration of 14 g per dl and a hemoglobin iron content of 3.4 mg per g, these volumes of blood contain from 12 to 29 mg of iron and represent a loss equivalent to 0.4 to 1.0 mg of iron for every day of the cycle, or about 150 to 400 mg per year. Finch (1959) has measured the rate of decrease in the specific activity of the miscible iron of the body for a period of years after the injection of Fe^{55} to ascertain the rate of loss of iron from the body. Women who menstruated lost on the average 0.6 mg of iron per day more than did men and postmenopausal women. Since the amount of iron that is absorbed from the usual diet is quite limited, this "negligible" iron loss is important because it contributes to the low iron stores found in a majority of women (Hallberg et al., 1968; Scott and Pritchard, 1967).

Changes in Body Weight. It has been reported frequently that about 30 percent of women gain 1 to 3 pounds shortly before the onset of menstruation, which they lose promptly as menstruation begins. Although only a minority of women manifest gains, there has been a tendency to regard the increase in weight as a normal characteristic of the cycle, reflecting the influence of steroid hormones. Actually, the average gain is insignificant, perhaps a quarter of a pound, as shown in a statistical study of this question by Chesley and Hellman (1957) and by Go-

lub and associates (1965). It would appear, therefore, that the concept of appreciable premenstrual weight gain as a physiologic phenomenon is not valid. Preece and co-workers (1975) identified no consistent change in total body water during the menstrual cycle.

REFERENCES

Arey LB, The degree of normal menstrual irregularity: an analysis of 20,000 calendar records from 1,500 individuals. Am J Obstet Gynecol 37:12, 1939

Baldwin RM, Whalley PJ, Pritchard JA: Measurements of menstrual blood loss. Am J Obstet Gynecol 81:739, 1961

Barker AP, Fowler WM: The blood loss during normal menstruation. Am J Obstet Gynecol 31:979, 1936

Casey ML, Hemsell DL, MacDonald PC, Johnston JM: NAD+-dependent 15-hydroxyprostaglandin dehydrogenase activity in human endometrium. Prostaglandins, 19:122, 1980

Chesley LC, Hellman LM: Variations in body weight and salivary sodium in the menstrual cycle. Am J Obstet Gynecol 74:582, 1957

Chiazze L, Brayer FT, Macisco JJ, Parker MP, Duffy BJ: The length and variability of the human menstrual cycle. JAMA 203:377, 1968

Finch CA: Body iron exchange in man. J Clin Invest 38:392, 1959

Golander A, Hurley T, Barret J, Hizi A, Handwerger S: Prolactin synthesis by human chorion decidual tissue. A possible source of prolactin in the amniotic fluid. Science 202:311, 1978

Golub LJ, Menduke H, Conly SS Jr: Weight changes in college women during the menstrual cycle. Am J Obstet Gynecol 91:89, 1965

Gunn DL, Jenkin PM, Gunn AL: Menstrual periodicity; statistical observations on a large sample of normal cases. J Obstet Gynaecol Br Emp 44:839, 1937

Hallberg L, Hogdahl A-M, Nilsson L, Rybo G: Menstrual blood loss, a population study: variation at different ages and attempts to define normality. Acta Obstet Gynecol Scand 45:320, 1966

Hallberg L, Hallgren J, Hollender A, Hogdahl AM, Tibblin G: Occurrence of iron deficiency anemia in Sweden. Symp Swedish Nutri Found 6:19, 1968

Haman JO: The length of the menstrual cycle: a study of 150 normal women. Am J Obstet Gynecol 43:870, 1942

Hartman CG: Studies in the reproduction of the monkey *Macaca (Pithecus) rhesus* with special reference to menstruation and pregnancy. Contrib Embryol 23:1, 1932

Horwitz KB, McGuire WL, Pearson OH, Segaloff A: Predicting response to endocrine therapy in human breast cancer: a hypothesis. Science 189:726, 1975

Hytten FE, Cheyne GA, Klopper AI: Iron loss at menstruation. J Obstet Gynaecol Br Commw 71:255, 1964

Markee JE: Menstruation in intraocular endometrial transplants in the rhesus monkey. Contrib Embryol 28:219, 1940

McLennan CE, Rydell AH: Extent of endometrial shedding during normal menstruation. Obstet Gynecol 26:605, 1965

Millis J: The iron losses of healthy women during consecutive menstrual cycles. Med J Aust 2:874, 1951

Noyes RW, Hertig AT, Rock J: Dating the endometrial biopsy. Fertil Steril 1:3, 1950

Preece PE, Richards AR, Owen GM, Hughes LE: Mastalgia and total body water. Br Med J 4:498, 1975

Riddick DH, Luciano AA, Kusmik WF, Maslar IA: Evidence for a nonpituitary source of amniotic fluid prolactin. Fertil Steril 31:35, 1979

Scott DE, Pritchard JA: Iron deficiency in healthy young college women. JAMA 199:897, 1967

Smith OW, Smith GV: Menstrual discharge of women: I. Its toxicity in rats. Proc Soc Exp Biol Med 44:100, 1940

Tseng L, Gurpide E: Estradiol and 20 α-dihydroprogesterone dehydrogenase activities in human endometrium during the menstrual cycle. Endocrinology 94:419, 1974

Tyson JE, Hwang P, Guyda H, Friesen HG: Studies of prolactin secretion in human pregnancy. Am J Obstet Gynecol 113:14, 1972

White AJ, Buchsbaum HJ: Scanning electron microscopy of the human endometrium. Gynecol Oncol 1:330, 1973

Wynn RM, Harris JA: Ultrastructural cyclic changes in the human endometrium: I. Normal preovulatory phase. Fertil Steril 18:632, 1967

Wynn RM, Woolley RS: Ultrastructural cyclic changes in the human endometrium: II. Normal postovulatory phase. Fertil Steril 18:721, 1967

Zondek B: Does menstrual blood contain a specific toxin? Am J Obstet Gynecol 65:1065, 1953

5

Gametogenesis and Development of the Ovum

GAMETOGENESIS

Primitive germ cells are present in the human embryo by the end of the third week of development. Both *oogenesis,* in the course of which mature ova are formed from primitive oogonia, and *spermatogenesis,* which results in the production of spermatids, share the basic biologic feature of maturation, or reduction, division. Such special cellular division, known as *meiosis,* is limited to germ cells. Meiosis is characterized by a long and unusual prophase, and involves a process that provides for the exchange of genic material between homologous chromosomes and eventually for reduction of the *diploid* number of chromosomes to the *haploid* number. In man, the 46 chromosomes, comprising 44 autosomes and 2 sex chromosomes, are halved during a meiotic division, with the result that each mature gamete contains 22 autosomes and 1 sex chromosome. The diploid number is not restored until union of the egg and sperm during fertilization (Fig. 5-1). *Spermatogenesis,* comprising the final changes leading to production of mature male gametes, involves alterations in the shape of the spermatids and their transformation to spermatozoa. The fact that the mature germ cells are derived directly from primitive cells that may have migrated from the yolk sac to the developing gonads as early as the 5th week of embryonic life underlies the concept of *continuity of the germ plasm.* It explains, moreover, how some germ cells, reaching maturity at a very late date, as in the case of human ova, may have remained dormant for as long as 40 years.

Meiosis. All primitive germ cells, *oogonia* and *spermatogonia,* contain the diploid number of 46 chromosomes. When these stem cells divide to produce primary oocytes and spermatocytes, each chromosome undergoes replication by splitting longitudinally to form a double-stranded structure. During this typical *mitosis,* one strand of each chromosome enters each daughter cell, which thus obtains the identical chromosomal components of the parent cell (Fig. 5-2).

However, when the primary oocytes and spermatocytes continue their maturation to form secondary oocytes and spermatocytes, respectively, the ensuing meiotic division is quite different, in that each of the newly formed cells receives only 23, or the haploid number of chromosomes. The basic differ-

NORMAL GAMETOGENESIS

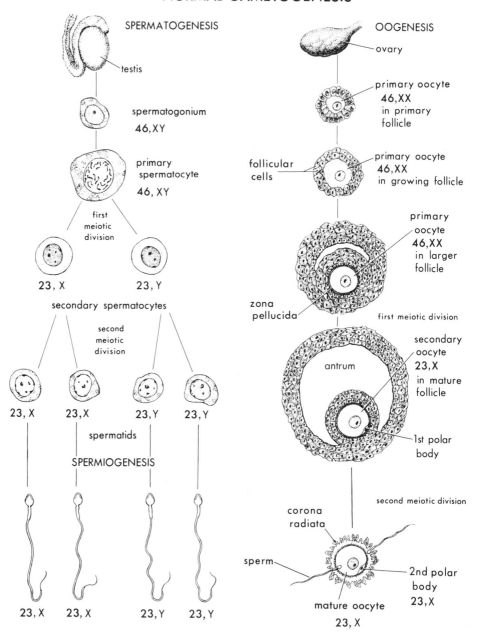

FIG. 5-1. Drawings comparing spermatogenesis and oogenesis. The chromosome complement of the germ cells is shown at each stage. The number designates the total number of chromosomes, including the sex chromosome(s) shown after the comma. Note that (1) following the two meiotic divisions, the diploid number of chromosomes, 46, is reduced to the haploid number, 23; (2) *four sperms* form from one primary spermatocyte, whereas only *one* mature oocyte (ovum) results from maturation of a primary oocyte; and (3) the cytoplasm is conserved during oogenesis to form one large cell, the mature oocyte (ovum). (From Moore. *The Developing Human.* Philadelphia, Saunders, 1977)

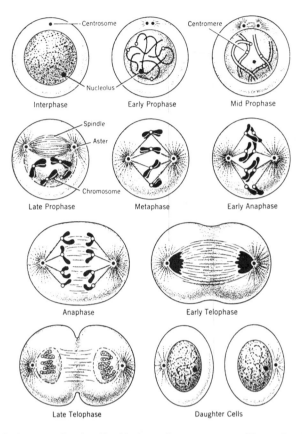

FIG. 5-2. Mitosis in an animal cell with four chromosomes. (From Gardner. *Principles of Genetics.* Courtesy of Wiley)

ence between meiosis and ordinary mitosis is the prolonged meiotic prophase, during which there is preliminary pairing of homologous chromosomes before division. During the *leptotene* stage of meiotic prophase, the 46 chromosomes appear as single slender threads (Fig. 5-3); in the next, or *zygotene,* stage, the homologous chromosomes are aligned parallel to each other in *synapsis,* with the formation of 23 bivalent components. Each chromosome then divides longitudinally, except at the *centromere,* and the ensuing *pachytene* stage is comprised of *tetrads* of four chromatids, the shape of which is dependent on the position of the centromere. At this point, the chromatids break and recombine with strands from the homologous chromosome to effect an exchange of genic material. During the next, or *diplotene,* stage, the homologus strands separate. During the meta-

phase of the first meiotic division, the bivalents (two chromatids making up each chromosome) become oriented on the spindle; when the cell divides, the members of each pair moved toward opposite poles into the daughter cells, which then contain the haploid number of chromosomes, still double-stranded except at the centromere. *The individual chromosomes now are no longer genetically identical with the parent cell.* Each secondary oocyte will thus receive 22 autosomes and an X chromosome, and each secondary spermatocyte will receive 22 autosomes and either an X or a Y chromosome.

At the second meiotic division the *diad* splits at the centromere to form two *monads,* one of which passes into each daughter cell, probably having already undergone a typical mitotic longitudinal replication. The mature ovum (22 + X), if fertilized by a spermato-

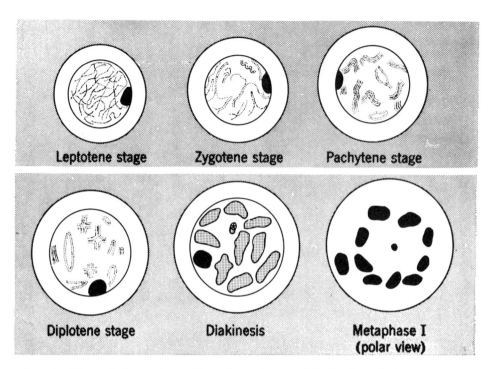

FIG. 5-3.   The meiotic prophase, illustrating pairing and duplication of chromosomes in the zygotene and pachytene stages, respectively. (From Gardner. *Principles of Genetics.* Courtesy of Wiley)

cyte containing 22 + Y chromosomes, will produce a male zygote (44 + XY), if fertilized by an X-containing spermatocyte, the result will be a female (44 + 2X).

Biochemistry of Cellular Division. The helical structure of DNA (deoxyribonucleic acid) is shown in Figure 5-4. During mitotic interphase, synthesis of DNA occurs simultaneously with the duplication of the chromosomes. The results of autoradiographic studies of the incorporation of tritiated thymidine into chromosomes are indicative that duplication is accomplished by separation of the two original DNA subunits of each chromosome and by subsequent synthesis of two new subunits. At the following cellular division, each chromatid receives one original and one new subunit.

Oogenesis.   In the sections of Chapters 2 and 3 dealing with the embryology of the ovary, the derivation of the primitive germ

cells from the yolk sac and the histogenesis of the granulosal and thecal elements are described. Pinkerton and colleagues (1961) were able to trace the development of the human ovum by employing histochemical

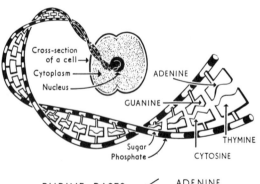

PURINE BASES < ADENINE / GUANINE

PYRIMIDINE BASES < CYTOSINE / THYMINE

FIG. 5-4.   The double helix of the DNA molecule.

technics depending mainly upon the high content of alkaline phosphatase characteristic of the germ cells. In the first phase (migration), the germ cells reach the medial slope of the mesonephric ridge, where the gonads arise, divide rapidly, and become oogonia; in the second phase (division), the germ cells divide mitotically at a rate that is maximal during the 8th to 20th week, gradually slowing, and finally ceasing at birth; in the third phase (maturation), the cells enter the prophase of the first meiotic division, acquiring a ring of granulosa cells and becoming definitive oocytes within the primary follicles.

It is well to remember that all oocytes are derived from the primitive germ cells. Blandau and co-workers (1963) have recorded cinematographically in the mouse the ameboid migration of primitive germ cells from the yolk sac to the germinal ridges. The primitive oogonia, furthermore, continue localized movements within the developing ovary even after reaching the pachytene stage of meiosis.

There is no evidence of *neogenesis* of human ova. Of the total number of primary oocytes at birth, estimated to be about 2,000,000, and at puberty to be 400,000 to 500,000 (Baker, 1963), only 400 to 500 will actually be ovulated; the majority degenerate in situ. After puberty several oocytes may begin to enlarge during each cycle, but ordinarily only one reaches full maturity.

The primary oocytes increase in size, while proliferating cuboidal follicular cells form increasingly thick coverings around them (Fig. 5-5). The follicular cells, furthermore, deposit on the surface of the oocyte an acellular glycoprotein mantle, which gradually thickens to form the *zona pellucida*. Irregular fluid-filled spaces between the follicular cells then coalesce to form an antrum. The radially elongated follicular cells surrounding the zona pellucida form the *corona radiata*. A solid mass of follicular cells surrounding the ovum in the side of a developing vesicular ovarian follicle is the *cumulus oophorus (discus proligerus)* (Fig. 5-6). As the follicle nears maturity, the cumulus projects farther into the antrum,

as a consequence the oocyte appears to be supported by a column of follicular cells. At this stage, the follicle varies from 6 to 12 mm in diameter and lies immediately beneath the surface of the ovary.

The oocyte finally completes the first meiotic division, which it began before birth, during the final stage of transformation of the primordial follicle into the mature graafian follicle. The important result is the formation of two daughter cells, each with 23 chromosomes but of greatly unequal size. One receives almost all the cytoplasm of the mother cell to become a secondary oocyte; the other, the first polar body, receives very

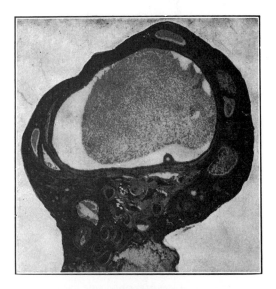

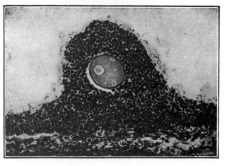

FIG. 5-5. Transverse section of macaque ovary showing ovum in almost fully grown 5-mm follicle. Top, × 10. Bottom, same ovum × 100. (Macaque No. 100, collection of Dr. GW Corner)

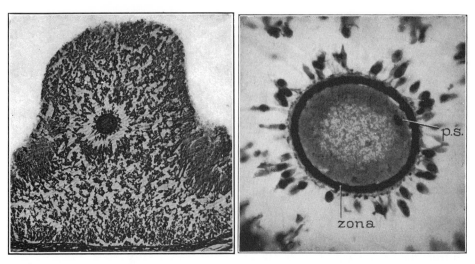

FIG. 5-6. Ovum in mature 7-mm follicle. Left, × 50. Note loosening of cells of cumulus oophorus. Right, same ovum × 358, containing first polar spindle, p.s., and surrounded by corona radiata. (Macaque No. 109, collection of Dr. GW Corner)

little cytoplasm. The polar body lies between the zona pellucida and the vitelline membrane of the secondary oocyte. In studies of tubal ova, Hertig and Rock (1944) found that the first polar body is cast off while still in the ovary. A second division consummates in the formation of the second polar body at the moment the sperm penetrates the egg.

One of the most interesting, but unsolved riddles in this field, is the mechanism(s) that prevents all ova but one from undergoing simultaneous maturation and ovulation during the first cycle. The factors normally responsible for allowing only one ovum normally to reach maturity each month are considered in Chapter 3 (p. 47).

In women, the second maturation division is completed only if the ovum is fertilized. Failing penetration by a spermatozoon within a few hours of ovulation, the ovum begins to degenerate; however, it is probably capable of being fertilized successfully for 15 to 18 hours (Blandau, 1975). Although it is not certain that the first polar body always undergoes subsequent division, fertilized ova have been found accompanied by three polar bodies. During maturation, the diameter of the human ovum increases from 19 μ in the origi-

nal oocyte to 135 μ in the fully mature ovum, a sevenfold increase.

Spermatogenesis. In the male embryo, as previously described in the female, the primordial germ cells enter the developing gonad during the 5th week but locate in the medulla rather than in the cortex as in the ovary. There the germ cells are incorporated into irregularly shaped primitive sex cords composed of cells derived from the surface epithelium.

At birth, the sex cords are solid, only later developing a lumen to become the seminiferous tubules. Two kinds of cells are found in the sex cords; the larger type, located along the basement membrane, contain a pale-staining nucleus with one or more nucleoli and probably represents the primordial germ cell; the other type, also found along the basement membrane, is much smaller and contain coarsely granuated nuclei; these cells cease to proliferate at birth and become sustentacular (Sertoli) cells.

The nuclear changes that ensue during spermatogenesis are analogous to those in oogenesis. Each primary spermatocyte enters the long prophase of the first meiotic division.

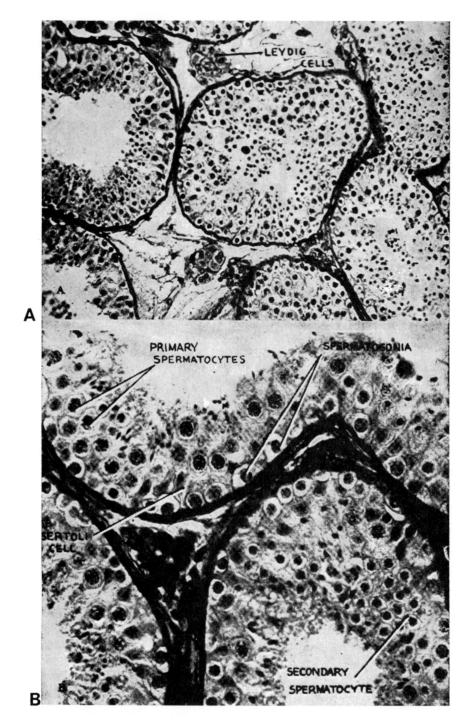

FIG. 5-7. Sections of normal human testes. **A.** testis of man aged 26, showing Leydig cells. **B.** testis of man aged 34 with sperm count 120 million per ml, showing stages of spermatogenesis. (From Nelson. In Greep (ed): *Histology.* Courtesy of Blakiston)

Upon completion of the first reduction division, secondary spermatocytes are formed, each containing the haploid number of chromosomes; but unlike the products of the first meiotic division of the ovum, the secondary spermatocytes receive equal shares of cytoplasm from the parent cell. Almost immediately after formation, the secondary spermatocytes begin the second meotic division, which results in the production of four spermatids. Theoretically, each primary spermatocyte, after two meiotic divisions, gives rise to four spermatids, which are analogous chromosomally to the mature ovum and second polar body, and which develop subsequently into spermatozoa (Figs. 5-1 and 5-7).

Immediately after they are formed, the spermatids undergo extensive changes in shape to become spermatozoa. The newly formed spermatid has a spherical nucleus, a

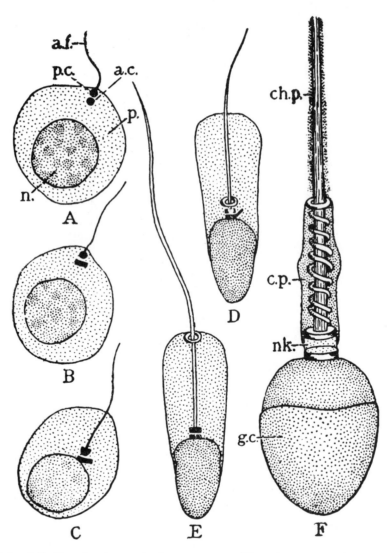

FIG. 5-8. A-F. The development of spermatozoa (Meves): a.c., anterior centrosome; a.f., axial filament; c.p., connecting pieces; ch.p., chief piece; g.c., galea capitis; n, nucleus; nk, neck; p, protoplasm; p.c., posterior centrosome. (From Greep (ed): *Histology*. Courtesy of Blakiston)

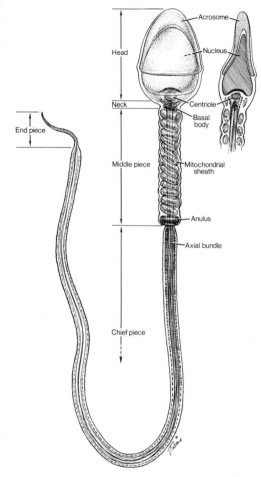

FIG. 5-9. Ultramicroscopic structure of human spermatozoön.

prominent Golgi zone, and many mitochondria. An initial change in the Golgi is the appearance of the dense *acrosomic granule,* which later forms a thin membrane over the surface of the nucleus, the head cap. The centrioles migrate to the pole of the nucleus opposite the head cap and form the flagellum, while the nucleus itself becomes condensed and slightly flattened and elongated. At the same time, mitochondria move toward the flagellum to form a collar around the axial filament. Distally, the mitochondrial collar is limited by an annular structure, and together with the centriole, the collar and ring form the middle piece of the spermatozoon. The cytoplasm and the Golgi material not incorporated into the spermatozoa are cast off. Though only slightly motile when they first enter the seminiferous tubules, the spermatozoa become fully motile in the epididymis (Figs. 5-8 and 5-9).

TRANSPORT OF OVA AND SPERMATOZOA

Tubal Transport. In women, the ovaries normally lie free in the peritoneal cavity except for the supporting mesovarium and ovarian ligament. About the time of ovulation, however, the fimbriae of the oviduct, as the consequence of appropriate hormonal and neural regulation, very likely completely cover the site of ovulation. Ovulation is not an explosive phenomenon; instead, as the stigma is digested by proteolytic enzymes, there is a gentle outpouring of the contents of follicle, including the egg surrounded by the cumulus oophorus. The cumulus cells appear to be important for pickup and transport of the egg by the oviduct. In the oviduct of the monkey, ciliary action is the prominent force in the movement of the ovum in the tube, whereas peristalis appears to be so in the rabbit (Blandau, 1975). The relative contribution of each of these mechanisms in women is not known. Since fertilization in mammals usually occurs in the ampulla, whatever the roles of the tubal cilia and peristalsis may be, an adequate theory must explain how ova are moved down and spermatozoa moved up the fallopian tube.

Migration of the Ovum. In most mammals, the fertilized ovum requires 3 to 3½ days for transit through the oviduct, reaching the cavity of the human uterus about 3 to 4 days after ovulation. In women, the ovum may wander across the pelvis to be picked up by the opposite tube *(external migration)* or, theoretically, may cross inside the uterus and migrate up the opposite tube *(internal migration).* Presumptive clinical evidence of migration of the ovum includes a successful intrauterine pregnancy in women who have only one tube and the contralateral ovary. It is likely that the entire subject of migration of the ovum in women has received more attention than it deserves. In their normal anatomic relations, as observed at laparotomy, both tubes usually hang freely, with their fimbriated extremities posterior to the uterus and rather closely approximated. In view of the known motility of the fallopian tubes, it is entirely reasonable that the ovum may be picked up directly by the opposite tube, without recourse to complicated mechanisms of internal or external migration.

Transport of Spermatozoa. During human coitus, an average ejaculate of 2 to 5 ml containing an average of 70 million sperm per milliliter is deposited in the vagina. Of these 100 million spermatozoa, or more, of which between 80 and 90 percent are normal forms, perhaps 15 to 50 actually reach the site of fertilization. For successful fertilization, of course, only one spermatozoa must meet, in the upper portion of the fallopian tube, the single mature ovum released during each normal ovulatory cycle.

Sperm reach the site of fertilization in the ampulla of the oviduct in perhaps 1 to 1½ hours after ejaculation, which is much faster than can be explained by their flagellar action. Blandau (1975) believes that the spermatozoa must make their own way through the mucus that fills the cervical canal. The first spermatozoa appear to burrow through the mucus by chemical as well as mechanical means; the leaders very likely depolymerize the cervical mucus by releasing proteases contained in the acrosome, and thereby render the mucus more easily penetrable by spermatozoa that follow and successfully enter the uterine cavity. The uterine cavity in vivo may well be nearly obliterated except for canals that extend from the internal os of the cervix to the uterotubal junctions. As the consequences of such canals, sperm are directed to the oviduct. In much of the oviduct, including the lower portion, there is dual ciliary action in opposite directions; one set of cilia move material down, for example, the ovum, while an adjacent set propels material up, especially sperm.

FERTILIZATION

As soon as the sperm penetrates the zona pellucida and touches the vitelline membrane, a second polar body is formed and the female pronucleus, as well as the male pronucleus, are evident in the ovum. Ordinarily, the penetration of the zona pellucida and vitelline membrane by one sperm inhibits entry by other sperm, but, at times, more than one do enter. The mechanism by which the sperm penetrates the tough zona pellucida is unknown but probably involves enzymatic action. Materials other than genic material contained in the sperm degenerate within the ovum.

Zona Pellucida. Dickmann and Noyes (1961) found that the zona pellucida in the rat is shed from the blastocyst during the 5th day after fertilization. The shedding, moreover, appears unrelated to a specific uterine environment, but rather is an intrinsic manifestation of growth and maturation of the blastocyst. The zona is clearly not necessary for implantation; on the contrary, its removal is a prerequisite for implantation, at least in the laboratory rodents studied thus far.

Abnormal Sexual Differentiation. Since there are two chromosomally different kinds of spermatozoa in mammals, the male gamete determines the sex of the offspring. In birds, on the other hand, the ovum or the female parent determines chromosomal sex. Although heredity is the principal determinant of sex in mammals, environment factors must also be operative, as evidenced by the various intersexes and, in the opossum, for example, the phenomenon of sexual transformation. In general, in mammals a Y chromosome will lead to male sexual differentiation, even in the presence of more than one X chromosome.

Abnormalities of sexual development may result from meiotic *nondisjunction* of the monads and diads of the sex chromosomes of either parent during diakinesis, the final stage of prophase. Thus, instead of producing two cells with one X each, a primary oocyte may give rise to one cell with two X chromosomes, and one with none. Similarly, a primary spermatocyte may give rise to two cells, with XY and O chromosomal complements, respectively. If then, a normal mature oocyte (X) is fertilized by a spermatozoon with no sex chromosome, an individual with 45 chromosomes and an XO karyotype results. Clinically, such a person represents a variety of gonadal dysgenesis, *Turner syndrome,* who is *chromatin-negative* and sterile. By analogy, nondisjunction of the homologous X chromosomes may result in an XX mature oocyte, which, if fertilized by a normal Y-bearing spermatozoon, produces an XXY individual. Such a person, representing a common type of *Klinefelter syndrome,* will have 47 chromosomes and *chromatin-positive* cells. Cases of Klinefelter syndrome with more than 47 chromosomes, for example, the XXXY karyotypes, may be explained either on the basis of nondisjunction of the gametes of both parents, or on the statistically much more likely basis of nondisjunction of the female gamete during both the first and second meiotic divisions.

Chromosomal mosaicism, however, requires a different explanation. An XXX/XO mosaic, for example, might result from mitotic nondisjunction, with the shift of an X from one strain to another, but an XXX/XX chromosomal pattern is more difficult to explain. Nondisjunction or translocation of an *autosome* (a chromosome other than an X or a Y), furthermore, may result in other clinically significant genetic abnormalities, such as Down syndrome (mongolism), which typically is characterized by 47 chromosomes, or an autosomal trisomy, involving chromosome 21.

Aging of Gametes.   The increased incidence of the trisomy 21 variety of Down syndrome late in reproductive life is well established. It may be related to an increased tendency toward nondisjunction in ova that remained dormant in the ovary for 40 years or more. Although the incidence of this syndrome in the population as a whole is only 3 per 2000 live births, the incidence rises to about 1 in 100 in women by age 40.

Tesh and Glover (1969) noted that aging of the male gametes also exerted deleterious effects on the embryo and fetus. They reported that aging of rabbit sperm in the male reproductive tract led to loss of fertilizing capacity. Moreover, if such sperm fertilized eggs, an increase in embryonic anomalies resulted.

Vickers (1969) observed that delayed fertilization also led to an increase in chromosomal anomalies of the embryo. In mice in which fertilization was delayed (7 to 13 hours), triploidy, for example, was increased ninefold. Vickers postulated that the chromosomal aberrations may have resulted from errors in meiosis, fertilization, or cleavage.

DEVELOPMENT OF FERTILIZED OVUM

Cleavage of the Ovum.   After fertilization, the mature ovum becomes a zygote, which then undergoes segmentation, or cleavage, into blastomeres. With the accumulation of fluid between the blastomeres, the blastocyst is formed. Although it is not strictly correct to refer to segmenting zygotes as ova, the earliest stages of human development have traditionally been so designated. The blastocyst, or "ovum," then implants in the endometrium, while the fetal membranes and germ layers of the embryo are formed. Although the distinction between embryo and fetus is essentially arbitrary, it is customary to refer to the human conceptus from fertilization through the first 8 weeks of development as an *embryo,* and from 8 weeks after ovulation until term as a *fetus.* During the embryonic period, the major organ systems are formed, and during fetal life histogenesis, or differentiation of the tissues, proceeds.

The first typical mitotic division of the segmentation nucleus of the zygote results in the formation of two blastomeres. A photomicrograph of the living segmenting monkey's ovum (Fig. 5-10) shows the blastomeres and polar bodies suspended in the perivitelline fluid and surrounded by the zona pellucida. The human ovum (Fig. 5-11) undergoes similar changes.

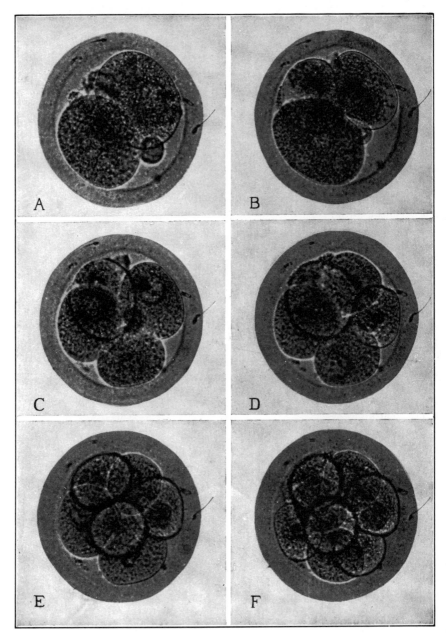

FIG. 5-10. Photomicrographs (× 300) of living monkey fertilized ovum showing its cleavage divisions. The fertilized ovum was washed out of the tube and cultivated in plasma; its growth changes were recorded cinematographically. The illustrations are enlargements from single frames of the film. **A.** two-cell stage, 29 hours and 30 minutes after ovulation. **B.** three-cell stage, 36 hours and 4 minutes after ovulation. **C.** four-cell stage, 37 hours and 35 minutes after ovulation. **D.** five-cell stage, 48 hours and 39 minutes after ovulation. **E.** six-cell stage, 49 hours exactly after ovulation. **F.** eight-cell stage, 48 hours and 48 minutes after ovulation. These cleavages normally occur as the ovum passes down the fallopian tube. Note the spermatozoon in the zona pellucida. (After Lewis and Hartman. *Contrib Embryol* 24:187, 1933)

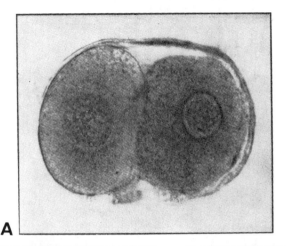

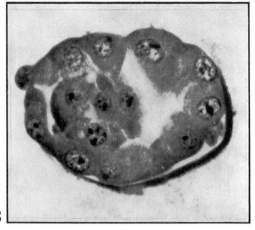

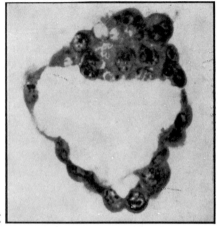

FIG. 5-11. Human preimplantation stages. **A.** two-celled stage. Intact fertilized ovum surrounded by zona pellucida, photographed after fixation. Washed from fallopian tube about 1½ days after conception. Nuclei shimmer through granular cytoplasm. Polar body in perivitelline space. (Carnegie Collection No. 8698. × 500.) **B.** 58-celled blastula with intact zona pellucida found in uterine cavity 3 to 4 days after conception. Thin section showing outer (probably trophoblastic) and inner (embryo-forming) cells and beginning segmentation cavity. (Carnegie Collection No. 8794. × 600.) **C.** 107-celled blastocyst found free in uterine cavity about 5 days after conception. A shell of trophoblastic cells enveloping fluid-filled blastocele, and inner mass consisting of embryo-forming cells. (Carnegie Collection No. 8663. × 600.) (From Hertig, Rock, Adams, Mulligan. *Contrib Embryol* 35:199, 1954)

During its 3 days within the fallopian tube, the fertilized ovum undergoes slow cleavage, as indicated by the recovery from the uterine cavity of human ova with only 12 blastomeres. As the blastomeres continue to divide, a solid mulberrylike ball of cells, the *morula,* is produced. The gradual accumulation of fluid within the morula results in formation of the blastocyst, at one pole of which is a compact mass of cells, the *inner cell mass,* destined to produce the embryo (Figs. 5-12 and 5-13); the outer layer of cells is the *trophoblast,* which provides nourishment to the ovum.

The Early Human Ovum.   Much of our knowledge of the earliest stages of human development is derived from the material ob-

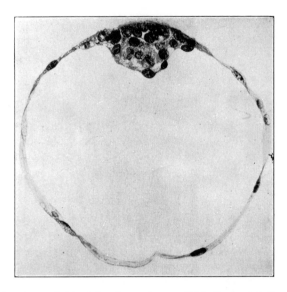

FIG. 5-12. Section through blastula of monkey. × 300. Post-ovulation age 9 days. The delicate trophoblast forms the outer wall of the segmentation cavity; the embryo develops from the inner cell mass at the pole uppermost in this figure. (C 522, Carnegie Collection), (retouched photomicrograph)

tained by Hertig and Rock (1944) and prepared by Heuser (1945) with unsurpassed histologic skill. The earliest human ovum available for study was the pronuclear form discovered by Noyes and co-workers (1964; Fig. 5-14). In the normal two-celled egg flushed from the fallopian tube (Fig. 5-11), Hertig and Rock (1944) found the blastomeres and a polar body free in the perivitelline fluid and surrounded by a thick zona pellucida (cf. monkey's ovum, Fig. 5-10.A). They provisionally considered as abnormal the four cleavage stages with 5, 8, 9, and 11 to 12 blastomeres that they found in the uterine cavity, but recovered morphologically normal stages comprising 12 and 58 cells. The normal ova, still surrounded by a zona pellucida, measured 0.150 and 0.154 mm, respectively, in the fresh state. In the 58-cell morula (Fig. 5-11.B), the outer cells can be distinguished, presumably destined to produce the trophoblast, and the inner cells that form the

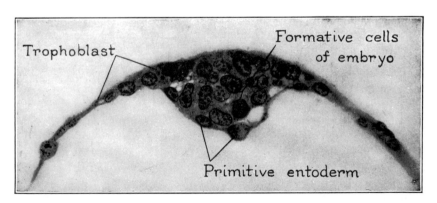

FIG. 5-13. Section through embryonic area of monkey. × 500 (retouched photomicrograph)

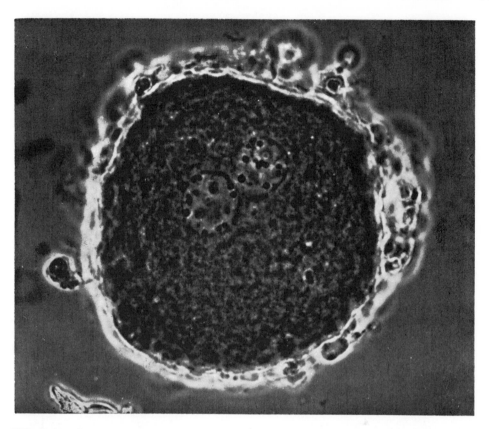

FIG. 5-14. Pronuclear egg after fixation and staining. Note two pronuclei. Absence of zona pellucida is an artifact of processing. Phase contrast. (Courtesy of Dr. Zeev Dickmann and Dr. Robert W Noyes)

embryo. The next stage that Hertig and Rock (1945) obtained was a 107-cell blastocyst (blastodermic vesicle), which was no larger than the earlier cleavage stages, despite the accumulated fluid (Fig. 5-11.C). It measured 0.153 × 0.155 mm in diameter before fixation and after the disappearance of the zona pellucida. The eight formative (embryo-producing) cells were surrounded by 99 trophoblastic cells. The "ovum," now a blastocyst, was ready to implant.

Implantation. Before implantation, the zona pellucida disappears and the blastocyst adheres to the endometrial surface. After erosion of the epithelium, the blastocyst sinks into the endometrium. From the findings of Hertig and Rock it is apparent that in the woman the pole of the blastocyst at which the inner cell mass is located enters first.

One of the earliest implantation sites discovered by Hertig and Rock (1944, 1945) is shown in Figure 5-15. It measured only 0.36 × 0.31 mm, its discovery remaining a remarkable achievement. The blastocyst shown in Figure 5-15 was in the process of entering the endometrium, with its thin outer wall still within the uterine cavity. An ovum at a similar stage, with dimensions of 0.45 × 0.30 × 1.125 mm, is shown in Figure 5-16. It appears to have flattened out in penetrating the uterine epithelium, in the fashion of the blastocyst of the rhesus monkey. The enlargement and multiplication of the trophoblastic cells in contact with the endometrium are alone responsible for the increase in size of the implanted blastocyst as compared with the free one. The hole in the uterine epithelium created by the ovum as it implants is indicative of the size of the zygote

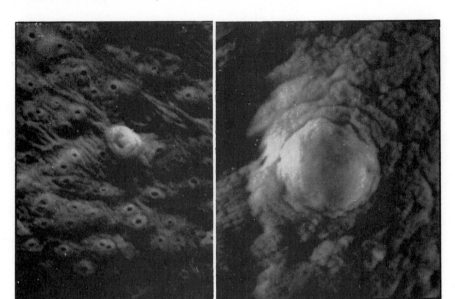

FIG. 5-15. Low- and high-power photographs of surface of view on an early human implantation obtained on day 22 of cycle, less than 8 days after conception. Site was slightly elevated and measured 0.36 by 0.31 mm. Mouths of uterine glands appear as dark spots surrounded by halos. (Carnegie Collection No. 8225)

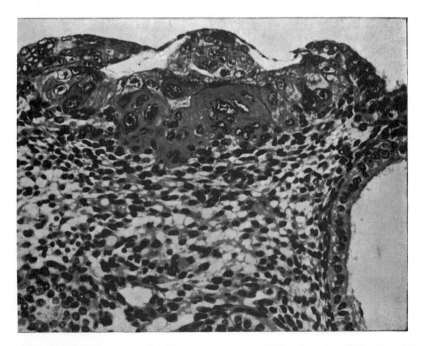

FIG. 5-16. Young human ovum (about 7½ days). × 300. (Carnegie Collection No. Mu-8020.) Implantation is still shallow so that the characteristics of the collapsed blastocyst wall continue in evidence. Ovum is well anchored to the endometrium, by its trophoblast, however. The embryo is the small globular mass situated between the blastocyst wall above and the proliferating trophoblast underneath it. (From Hertig and Rock. *Am J Obstet Gynecol* 47:149, 1944)

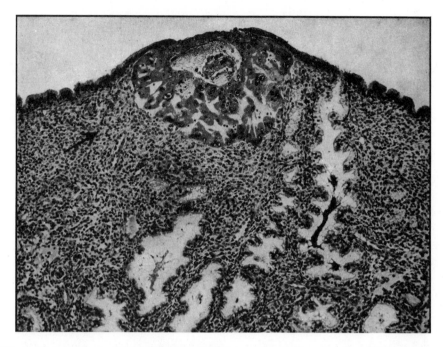

FIG. 5-17. A thin section of ovum obtained on 25th day of cycle, 9½ days or less after conception. Area still exposed to uterine lumen, 0.38 × 0.26 mm bordered as in Figure 5-20. Synctiotrophoblast, a complex network filling enlarged implantation site. Within cytotrophoblastic shell, two-layered embryo and amnion-forming cells. Arrow is pointed to zone of enlarged stromal cells. (Carnegie Collection No. 8004.) Photomicrograph × 100. (From Hertig and Rock. *Contrib Embryol* 31:65, 1945)

at the onset of erosion of the surface. The defect is bounded by a zone of maternal epithelium that shriveled as the trophoblast spread out beneath it (Fig. 5-17). When correction was made for the additional shrinkage resulting from preparation of the histologic sections, the diameter of the ovum at the moment of implantation was estimated as 0.23 mm. According to Hertig and Rock (1945), the smaller human zygote implants at about 6 days after fertilization.

MECHANISM OF IMPLANTATION. Although little is known of the fundamental nature of implantation in man, some information based on studies of lower species is available. As the blastocyst contacts the endometrium, syncytiotrophoblast differentiates from cytotrophoblast. Development of syncytiotrophoblast undoubtedly is a major factor in the successful invasion of the endometrium. In women, a full decidual response

is not elicited until the trophoblast has eroded the superficial uterine epithelium.

Whereas in women the free blastocystic period is 4 to 6 days, in some species there is a "developmental diapause," or delayed implantation, in which the blastocysts may remain unattached for much longer intervals (6 months or more in the pine marten).

Free blastocysts recovered from the uterus of the cow and the sheep and kept frozen in liquid nitrogen for up to 3 weeks have been then implanted successfully in recipient animals to produce normal offspring. Human ova have been fertilized in vitro and successful implantation and successful pregnancies have been reported (Steptoe and Edwards, 1978).

A thoughtful review of the subject of "external human fertilization" has been provided by Grobstein (1979).

Development of Ovum After Implantation. At 7½ days, the stage shown in Figure

5-16, the wall of the blastocyst facing the uterine lumen consists of a single layer of flattened cells, whereas the thicker opposite wall comprises two zones—the trophoblast and the embryo-forming inner cell mass. The maternal tissues in contact with the trophoblast show definite signs of injury, and the decidua immediately adjacent appears condensed, perhaps as a result of withdrawal of water by the invading trophoblast. Within the trophoblast, two subdivisions are distinguishable, the *cytotrophoblast,* comprising individual cells with relatively pale-staining cytoplasm, and the *syncytiotrophoblast,* in which dark-staining nuclei are irregularly distributed within a common basophilic cytoplasm.

In the trophoblast, mitotic figures are confined to the cellular elements. As early as 7½ days, the inner cell mass, now the *embryonic disc,* has already differentiated into a thick plate of primitive ectoderm and an underlying layer of endoderm. Between the embryonic disc and the trophoblast appear some small cells that soon enclose a space that will become the amnionic cavity.

In the next stage of the Hertig and Rock series, the 9½-day ovum (Fig. 5-17), the increase in size is mainly a result of development of the syncytium, which comprises a complex network of protoplasmic strands, enclosing irregular fluid-filled spaces, the *lacunae,* which later become confluent. The

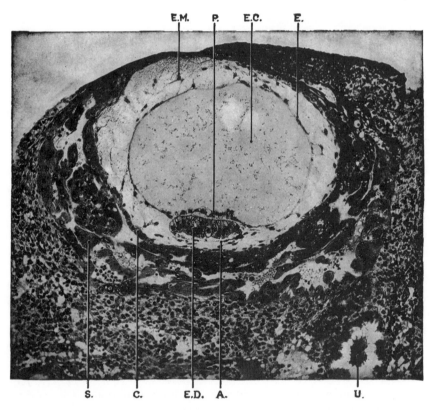

FIG. 5-18. Human fertilized ovum of previllous stage. × 120. (Carnegie Collection No. 7700). Free cells are delaminating from inner surface of trophoblast around its entire circumference, forming amnion adjacent to germ disc. E.D., embryonic disc; P., primitive entoderm; A., amnion; E., exocelomic membrane; E.C., exocelomic cavity; C., cytotrophoblast; S., syncytium; E.M., extraembryonic mesoblast. U., uterine gland. Removed on the twenty-ninth day after the onset of the last menstrual period. Its age is estimated as about 12 days. (From Hertig and Rock. *Contrib Embryol* 31:65, 1945)

embryonic disc now consists of a "dorsal" ectoderm, made up of tall columnar cells, and a "ventral" endoderm, formed of somewhat irregular cells. The remainder of the blastocyst is occupied by a proteinaceous coagulum, limited externally by a layer of flattened cells (the *exocelomic,* or *Heuser's, membrane*) of uncertain origin. The amnionic cavity dorsal to the embryonic disc is now well defined. With regard to the amnion, it seems reasonable that at least the epithelium is delaminated from the trophoblast. There is no convincing evidence that the inner cell mass produces any of the extraembryonic mesoderm.

As the embryo enlarges, more maternal tissue is destroyed and the walls of its capillaries are eroded, with the result that maternal blood enters the lacunae. With deeper burrowing of the ovum into the endometrium, the trophoblastic strands branch to form the solid primitive villi traversing the lacunae. Located originally over the entire surface of the ovum, the villi later disappear except over the most deeply implanted portion, the future placental site. The mesenchyme first appears as isolated cells within the cavity of the ovum. When the cavity is completely lined with mesoderm, it is termed the *chorionic vesicle,* and its membrane, now called the *chorion,* is composed of trophoblasts and mesenchyme.

The 12-day embryo shown in Figure 5-18 has reached a diameter of almost 1 mm. The mesenchymal cells within the cavity are most numerous about the embryo, where they eventually condense to form the *body stalk,* which serves to join the embryo to the nutrient chorion and later develops into the umbilical cord. The site of entry of the blastocyst into the endometrium is then covered by regenerated epithelium. The defect itself is plugged by fibrin and cellular debris. The syncytiotrophoblast of the chorionic shell is permeated by a system of intercommunicating channels or trophoblastic lacunae contain-

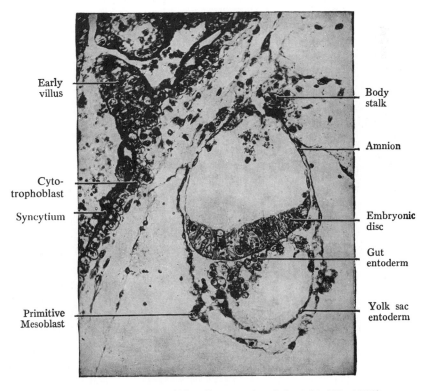

FIG. 5-19. Embryo. × 180. (After Brewer. *Am J Anat* 61:429, 1938)

ing maternal blood. At the same time, in the surrounding endometrial stroma there develops a decidual reaction, characterized by enlargement of the connective tissue cells and storage of glycogen therein. The amnionic cavity is then lined by ectoderm, apparently contiguous with that of the embryonic disc. At this stage, the endoderm probably delaminates from the inferior surface of the embryonic disc and soon spreads peripherally beyond the disc to line the blastocele. The process results in the formation of the yolk sac. The remainder of the blastocyst is filled with primary mesoderm, consisting of sparse mesenchymal cells in a loose matrix. The mesoderm, according to one school of thought, arises from the trophoblast, but its precise mode of origin in man remains to be elucidated.

The Germ Layers.   In Figures 5-19 and 5-20, the amnion and yolk sac with both epithelial and mesenchymal components can be seen. The body stalk, representing the future caudal end of the embryo, can also be recog-

nized at this stage. Cellular proliferation in the embryonic disc marks the beginning of a thickening in the midline that clearly indicates the embryonic axis and is called the *primitive streak.* Cells spread out laterally from the primitive streak between ectoderm and endoderm to form the mesoderm. These three germ layers then give rise to the various organs of the body. From the *ectoderm* are derived the entire nervous system, central and peripheral, and the epidermis with such derivatives as the crystalline lens and the hair. The *endoderm* develops into the lining of the gastrointestinal tract, from pharynx to rectum, and such derivative organs as the liver, pancreas, and thyroid. The dermis, the skeleton, the connective tissues, the vascular and urogenital systems, and most skeletal and smooth muscle arise from the *mesoderm.* The cavity that later divides the somatic and visceral sheets of intraembryonic mesoderm is the *celom.*

Formation of the Somites.   During the third week postfertilization (5th week gesta-

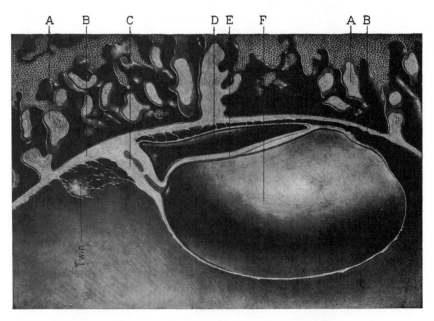

FIG. 5-20. Median view of wax reconstruction of Mateer fertilized ovum, showing the amnionic cavity and its relations to chorionic membrane and yolk sac. × 50. A. chorionic villi, B. chorionic membrane; C. body stalk with allantois; D. flattened amniotic cavity; E. embryonic area; F. yolk sac. (After Streeter. *Contrib Embryol* 9:389, 1920)

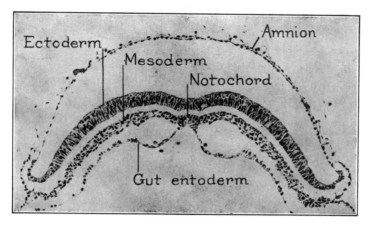

FIG. 5-21. Photomicrograph of transverse section through presomite human embryo. × 125. (No. 5960 Carnegie Collection.) (From Heuser, Hertig, and Rock. *Contrib Embryol* 31:85, 1945)

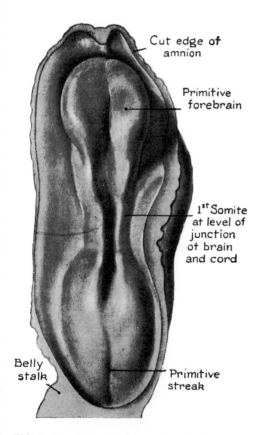

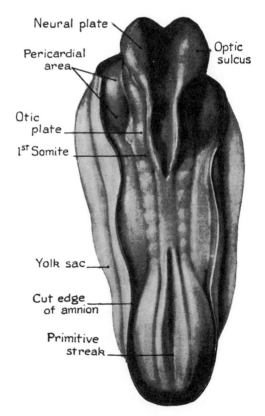

FIG. 5-22. Human embryo at beginning of segmentation. × 67. Dorsal view of model showing open neural groove. (Carnegie Collection No. 1878. Drawing by Didusch after Ingalls. *Contrib Embryol* 11:61, 1920. From Streeter. *Sci Monthly* 32:495, 1931)

FIG. 5-23. Seven-somite human embryo. × 45. Estimated (Streeter) 21 days after ovulation. Note closure of neural tube in middle region. (Carnegie Collection No. 4216. Drawing by Didusch after Payne. *Contrib Embryol* 16:115, 1925. From Streeter. *Sci Monthly* 32:495, 1931)

tional age), the primitive streak becomes a prominent structure, leading to recognition of cephalic and caudal ends of the embryo. As cells proliferate rapidly and spread laterally from the primitive streak, a midline *primitive groove* develops. Simultaneously, the yolk sac enlarges, with the result that the embryonic disc is spread out upon it. In Figure 5-20 there is shown a well-defined body stalk, into which a narrow endodermal diverticulum, the allantois, has extended. In many mammals, the allantois develops into a large sac that vascularizes the chorion. A forward extension of the primitive streak, the *notochord* (Fig. 5-21), constitutes the primordial supporting structure of vertebrates and remains as a continuous column of cells throughout embryonic life. Remnants of the notochord persist in the adult as the nucleus pulposus of the intervertebral discs.

Since differentiation of structure proceeds from cephalic to caudal ends in a sequence characteristic of all vertebrate embryos, most of the substance of the early embryo will enter into formation of the head, the subsequent development of the primitive streak providing material for the rest of the body. In Figure 5-22, the thickened ectoderm that forms the neural plate is shown. Soon there develops a *neural groove* (Fig. 5-23), as neural folds arise on either side. Connecting the cavity of the future neural tube with the future lumen of the gut is the *neurenteric canal*. As the neural folds develop, the underlying lateral mesoderm is divided into discrete blocks, the *somites* (Figs. 5-22–5-24), which give rise to the skeletal and connective tissues, the muscles, and the dermis. The first three or four somites enter into formation of the occipital region of the head. The primordium of the heart already has appeared beneath the pharynx as it is separated from the yolk sac by a fold that also lifts the cephalic end of the embryo above the level of the yolk sac. In Figure 5-25 (A–E) the elevation of the neural folds is shown as is the closure of these folds to form a tube, which is wider from the outset in the region of the fourth pair of somites. Although the head remains relatively enormous during the embryonic period, the rest of the body takes form after the 4th week, and the head becomes smaller in proportion. By the 7th week, after fertilization, the neck can be recognized, the tail filament has disappeared, and the embryo can be identified as human. From the eighth week after fertilization, changes in the shape of the human fetus are less striking. Some of the principal features are outlined in Chapter 8.

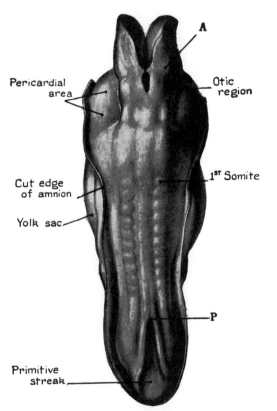

Pericardial area

Otic region

Cut edge of amnion

Yolk sac

1ˢᵗ Somite

A

P

Primitive streak

FIG. 5-24. Ten-somite human embryo. × 25. A and P mark superior and inferior limits of neural tube closure. (Carnegie Collection No. 5074. Drawing by Didusch after Corner. *Contrib Embryol* 20:81, 1929. From Streeter. *Sci Monthly* 32:495, 1931)

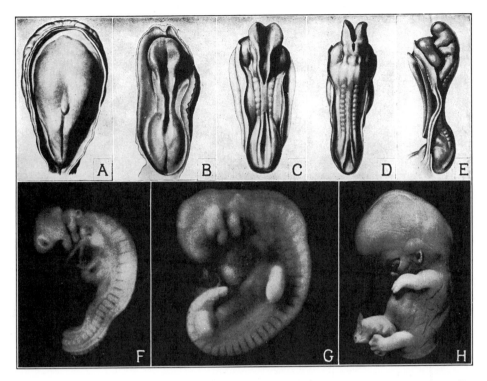

FIG. 5-25. Human embryogenesis. (Carnegie Collection.) A. Heuser, × 30, 19 days. B. Ingalls, × 28. C. Payne, × 23. D. Corner, × 23. E. Atwell, × 15.5, 21 to 22 days. F. × 12, fourth week. G. × 8.5, fifth week. H. × 2.5, eighth week. (From Streeter. *Sci Monthly* 32:495, 1931)

REFERENCES

Baker TG: A quantitative and cytological study of germ cells in human ovaries. Proc R Soc (Biol) 158:417, 1963

Blandau R: Personal communication, 1975

Blandau RJ, White BJ, Rumery RE: Observations on the movements of the living primordial germ cells in the mouse. Fertil Steril 14:482, 1963

Brewer JI: A normal human ovum in a stage preceding the primitive streak. Am J Anat 61:429, 1938

Dickman Z, Noyes RW: Zona pellucida at the time of implantation. Fertil Steril 12:310, 1961

Grobstein C: External human fertilization. Sci Am 240:57, 1979

Hertig AT, Rock J: On the development of the early human ovum with special reference to the trophoblast of the previllous stage: a description of 7 normal and 5 pathologic human ova. Am J Obstet Gynecol 47:149, 1944

Hertig AT, Rock J: Two human ova in the previllous stage, having a developmental age of about 7 and 9 days respectively. Contrib Embryol 31:65, 1945

Hertig AT, Rock J, Adams EC, Mulligan WJ: On the preimplantation stages of the human ovum. Contrib Embryol 35:199, 1954

Heuser C, Hertig AT, Rock J: Two human embryos showing early stages of the definitive yolk sac. Contrib Embryol 31:85, 1945

Noyes RW, Dickmann Z, Clewe TH, Bonney WA: Pronuclear ovum from a patient using an intrauterine contraceptive device. Science 147:744, 1964

Pinkerton JHM, McKay DG, Adams EC, Hertig AT: Development of the human ovary: study using histochemical technics. Obstet Gynecol 18:152, 1961

Steptoe PC, Edwards RG: Birth after the reimplantation of human embryo (letter). Lancet 2:366, 1978

Streeter GL: A human embryo (Mateer) of the presomite period. Contrib Embryol 9:389, 1920

Tesh JM, Glover TD: Aging of rabbit spermatozoa in the male tract and its effect on fertility. J Reprod Fertil 20:287, 1969

Vickers AD: Delayed fertilization and chromosomal anomalies in mouse embryos. J Reprod Fertil 20:69, 1969

6

The Placenta and Fetal Membranes

Scientific interest in the placenta derives not only from its enormous diversity of form and function but also from the unique metabolic, endocrine, and immunologic properties of its trophoblasts.

DEVELOPMENT OF THE HUMAN PLACENTA

Early Trophoblasts. In the discussion of the earliest stages of human placentation (see Chap. 5), the wall of the primitive blastodermic vesicle was described as consisting of a single layer of ectoderm. As early as 72 hours after fertilization, Hertig (1962) observed that the 58-cell blastula had differentiated into 5 embryo-producing cells and 53 cells destined to form trophoblasts. Although trophoblasts have not been identified before nidation of the ovum, both cellular and syncytial trophoblast are apparent in the earliest implanted blastocyst of the monkey. Indeed, some evidence has been presented that is suggestive that the elaboration of human chorionic gonadotropin (hCG) may precede implantation. Soon after implantation, the

trophoblasts proliferate rapidly and invade the surrounding decidua. In their invasive and cytolytic behavior, their histologically characteristic cytoplasmic vacuolization, and in ultrastructure, the early trophoblasts resemble choriocarcinoma (see Chap. 23, p. 568). As invasion of the endometrium proceeds, maternal blood vessels are tapped and cytoplasmic vacuoles coalesce to form larger lacunae (Fig. 6-1) that are soon filled with maternal blood. As the lucunae join, a complicated labyrinth is formed which is partitioned by solid trophoblastic columns. The trophoblast-lined labyrinthine channels and the solid cellular columns form the intervillous space and primary villous stalks, respectively. Much of our knowledge of the formation of the intervillous space of both men and the macaque is based on the findings of the classic studies of Wislocki and Streeter (1938).

Chorionic Villi. Villi may be easily distinguished first in the human placenta on about the 12th day after fertilization. When the solid trophoblast is invaded by a mesenchymal core, presumably derived from cytotrophoblast, secondary villi are formed. After

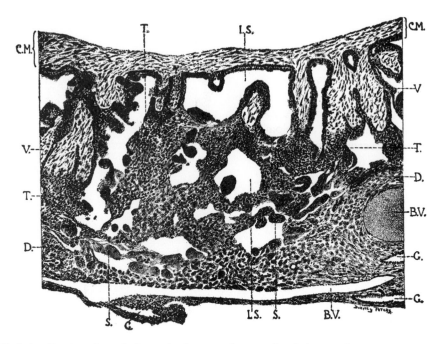

FIG. 6-1. Section through 3 weeks human placenta (ovulation age), showing chorion, decidua, and intervillous spaces. B.V., maternal blood vessel; C.M., chorionic membrane; D., decidua; G., uterine gland; I.S., intervillous space; S., syncytium; T., trophoblast; V., villus.

angiogenesis occurs in situ from the mesenchymal cores, the resulting villi are termed tertiary. Maternal venous sinuses are tapped early, but until the 14th or 15th day after fertilization, maternal arterial blood does not enter the intervillous space. By about the 17th day, both fetal and maternal blood vessels are functional and a placental circulation is established. The fetal circulation is completed when the blood vessels of the embryo are connected with chorionic blood vessels that are likely formed in situ from cytotrophoblast. Some villi, in which absence of angiogenesis results in a lack of circulation, may distend with fluid and form vesicles. A striking exaggeration of this process is present in the development of hydatidiform mole (see Chap. 23, p. 558).

Proliferation of cellular trophoblast at the tips of the villi produces the cytotrophoblastic cell columns, which are not invaded by mesenchyme but are anchored to the decidua at the basal plate. Thus, the floor of the intervillous space consists of cytotrophoblast from the cell columns, peripheral syncytium of the trophoblastic shell, and decidua of the basal plate. The chorionic plate, consisting of the two trophoblasts externally and fibrous mesoderm internally, forms the roof of the intervillous space.

Between the 18th and 19th days of development, the blastocyst (including the chorionic shell) measures 6 × 2.5 mm in diameter. At this time, the embryo is in the primitive-streak stage with a maximal length of 0.6 to 0.7 mm. The trophoblastic shell is thick, with villi formed of cytotrophoblastic projections, a central core of chorionic mesoderm in which blood vessels are developing, and an external covering of syncytiotrophoblast, or syncytium. The blastocyst lies buried in the decidua and is separated from the myometrium by the decidua basalis and from the uterine epithelium by the decidua capsularis. The embryo itself is trilaminar, and its endoderm is continuous with the lining of the yolk sac. An intermediate layer of intraembryonic mesoderm can be traced and found to be contiguous with the extraembryonic mesoderm, which later forms part of the walls of the amnion and yolk sac and connects the embryonic structures to the chorionic mesoderm by the body stalk, or abdominal pedicle, the forerunner of the umbilical cord. At this stage, the secondary or definitive yolk sac is completely lined by endoderm. External to the yolk sac the fluid-filled exocelomic cavity is found, the early formation of which prevents approximation of the yolk sac and trophoblasts in man, and hence precludes formation of a choriovitelline placenta.

By about three weeks after fertilization, the relations of chorion to decidua are clearly evident in the human embryo. The chorionic membrane consists of an inner connective tissue layer and an outer epithelium from which rudimentary villi project. The connective tissue consists of spindly cells with protoplasmic processes within a loose intercellular matrix. The trophoblast differentiates into cuboidal or nearly round cells with clear cytoplasm and light-staining vesicular nuclei (cytotrophoblast or Langhans cells) and an outer syncytium containing irregularly scattered, dark-staining nuclei within a coarsely granulated cytoplasm (syncytiotrophoblast).

In early pregnancy, the villi are distributed over the entire periphery of the chorionic membrane; grossly, an ovum dislodged from the endometrium at this stage of development appears shaggy (Fig. 6-2). The villi in contact with the decidua basalis proliferate to form the leafy chorion, or *chorion frondosum*, the fetal component of the placenta, whereas those in contact with the decidua capsularis cease to grow and undergo almost complete degeneration. The greater part of the chorion, thus denuded of villi, is designated the smooth, or bald, chorion or the *chorion laeve*. It is formed, according to Hertig (1962), as the result of a combination of direct pressure and interference with its vascular supply. The chorion laeve is more nearly opaque generally than the amnion even though rarely exceeding 1 mm in thickness. The chorion laeve contains ghost villi and, clinging to its surface, a few shreds of decidua. Until near the end of the third month, the chorion laeve remains separated from the

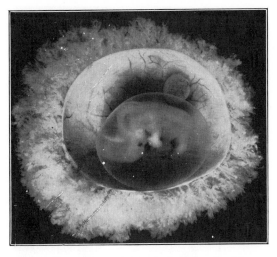

FIG. 6-2. Human chorionic vesicle. Ovulatory age, 40 days. (Carnegie Collection No. 8537)

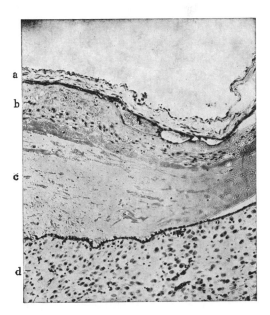

FIG. 6-3. Unfused decidua vera and capsularis. Section through uterus at 10 weeks gestation, showing that the decidua vera and capsularis have not yet fused. a, amnion chorionic membrane; b, degenerating decidua capsularis; c, uterine cavity; d, decidua vera.

amnion by the exocelomic cavity. Thereafter the amnion and chorion are in intimate contact (Fig. 6-3). *In the human, the chorion laeve and amnion form an avascular amniochorion which, nevertheless, is an important site of transfer and metabolic activity.*

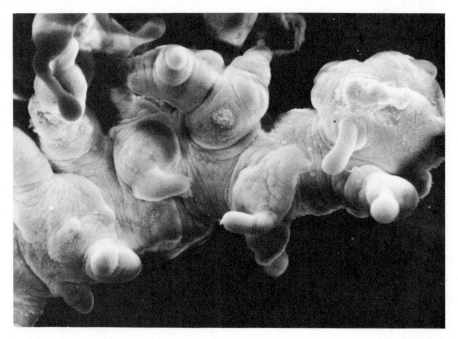

FIG. 6-4. Scanning electron micrograph of the placental villi at 10 to 14 weeks gestation. Note the larger stem villi and the small syncytial sprouts at various stages of formation. Furrows or creases on the surface are also evident, especially at the bases of larger villi. (× 289) (From King and Menton. *Am J Obstet Gynecol* 122:824, 1975)

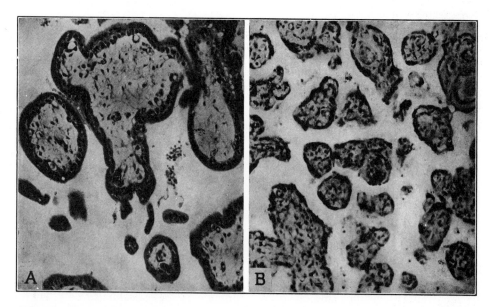

FIG. 6-5. Comparison of chorionic villi in early and late pregnancy. **A.** 2 months gestation. Note inner Langhans' cells and outer syncytial layer. **B.** Term placenta. Syncytial layer is obvious, but Langhans' cells are difficult to recognize at low magnification in light micrographs.

Placental Cotyledons.   Certain villi of the chorion frondosum extend from the chorionic plate to the decidua and serve as anchoring villi. Most villi, however, arboresce and end freely in the intervillous space without reaching the decidua (Fig. 6-4). As the placenta matures, the short, thick, early stem villi branch repeatedly, forming progressively finer subdivisions and greater numbers of increasingly small villi (Fig. 6-5). Each of the main stem villi and its ramifications constitutes a placental cotyledon.

Placental Septa.   The origin and exact composition of the placental septa continue to stimulate controversy. They appear to consist of decidual tissue in which trophoblastic elements are encased and thus are very likely of dual origin, i.e., fetal and maternal.

Especially recommended for an elegant pictorial description of human placentation is Boyd and Hamilton's extensively illustrated treatise, *The Human Placenta* (1970).

Placental Size and Weight.   The steady increase in size and weight of the placenta throughout pregnancy is shown in Table 6-1. The data obtained from weighing the placenta vary considerably, depending upon how the placenta is prepared. If membranes and most of the cord are left attached and adherent maternal blood clot is not removed, the weight is increased by nearly 50 percent (Thomson et al., 1969). Crawford (1959) suggested that the total number of cotyledons

remains the same throughout gestation, but individual cotyledons continue to grow until term, although less actively in the final weeks.

Placental Aging.   As the villi continue to branch and the terminal ramifications become more numerous and smaller, the volume and prominence of cytotrophoblast (Langhans cells) in the villi decrease, although cytotrophoblast remains obvious in the placental floor. As the syncytium thins and forms knots, the vessels become more prominent and lie closer to the surface. The stroma of the villi also exhibits changes associated with aging. In placentas of early pregnancy, the branching connective tissue cells are separated by an abundant loose intercellular matrix; later the stroma becomes denser, and the cells more spindly and more closely packed. Another change in the stroma involves the so-called *Hofbauer cells,* still of somewhat uncertain nature, origin, and significance. These are nearly round cells with vesicular, often eccentric nuclei and very granular or vacuolated cytoplasm. These cells are characterized, histochemically, by intracytoplasmic lipid and are readily distinguished from plasma cells.

As the placenta grows and ages, certain of the accompanying histologic changes are suggestive of an increase in the efficiency of transport to meet the metabolic requirements of the growing fetus. Such changes involve a decrease in thickness of the syncytium, partial disappearance of Langhans cells, decrease

TABLE 6-1.
GROWTH OF THE PLACENTA

DURATION (DAYS)	DIAMETER (cm)	VOLUME (ml)	SURFACE (cm²)	WEIGHT (g)	FETAL WEIGHT PLACENTAL WEIGHT	FETAL WEIGHT PLACENTAL SURFACE
105–135	10.0	115	62	120	2/50	4/83
135–165	12.0	235	167	245	3/22	4/73
165–195	14.0	230	145	245	4/17	7/01
195–225	15.0	349	199	365	4/84	9/19
225–240	16.0	394	219	407	6/67	12/80
240–296	18.0	430	243	464	7/29	13/98

Data from Snoeck: *Le Placenta Humain.* Masson et Cie; and from Crawford: *Br J Obstet Gynaec* 66:885, 1959.

in the stroma, and an increase in the number of capillaries and their approximation to the syncytial surface. By 4 months, the apparent continuity of the cytotrophoblast is broken, and the syncytium forms knots on the more numerous, smaller villi. At term, the villous covering may be focally reduced to a thin layer of syncytium with minimal connective tissue with fetal capillaries that apparently abut the trophoblast. The villous stroma, Hofbauer cells, and Langhans cells are markedly reduced, and the villi appear filled with thin-walled capillaries. Other changes, however, appear to decrease the efficiency for placental exchange, as, for example, the thickening of basement membranes of endothelium and trophoblast, obliteration of certain vessels, deposition of fibrin on the surface of the villi, and deposits of fibrin in the basal and chorionic plates and elsewhere in the intervillous space.

THE DECIDUA

Decidual Reaction. The decidua is the endometrium of the pregnant uterus, and is so named because much of it is shed following parturition. The decidual reaction encompasses the changes that begin in response to progesterone following ovulation and prepare the endometrium for implantation and nutrition of the blastocyst. In human pregnancy, the decidual reaction is not completed until several days after nidation. It first commences around maternal blood vessels, spreading in waves throughout the mucosa of the uterus. During development of the decidua, the endometrial stromal cells enlarge and form polygonal or round *decidual cells.* The nuclei become round and vesicular, and the cytoplasm becomes clear, slightly basophilic, and surrounded by a translucent membrane.

During pregnancy, the decidua thickens,

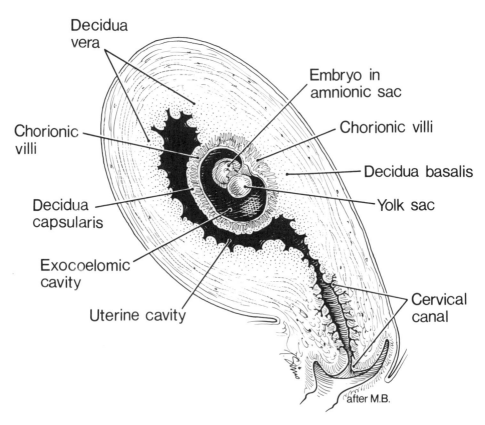

FIG. 6-6. Chorion frondosum and chorion laeve of early pregnancy. Three portions of the decidua (basalis, capsularis, and parietalis, or vera) are also illustrated.

eventually attaining a depth of 5 to 10 mm. With a magnifying glass, furrows and numerous small openings, representing the mouths of uterine glands, can be detected. The portion of the decidua directly beneath the site of implantation forms the *decidua basalis;* that overlying the developing ovum and separating it from the rest of the uterine cavity is the *decidua capsularis* (Figs. 6-6, 6-7). The remainder of the uterus is lined by *decidua vera,* or *decidua parietalis.*

There is a space between the decidua capsularis and the decidua vera since the gestational sac does not fill the entire uterine cavity during the early months of pregnancy. By the fourth month, the growing sac fills the uterine cavity; and with fusion of the capsularis and vera, the uterine cavity is obliterated. The decidua capsularis is most prominent about the second month of pregnancy, consisting of decidual cells covered by a single layer of flattened epithelial cells without traces of glands; internally, it contacts the chorion laeve.

The decidua vera and the decidua basalis each are composed of three layers (Fig. 6-8): a surface, or compact zone *(zona compacta);* a middle portion, or spongy zone *(zona spongiosa)* with glands and numerous small blood vessels; and a basal zone *(zona basalis).* The

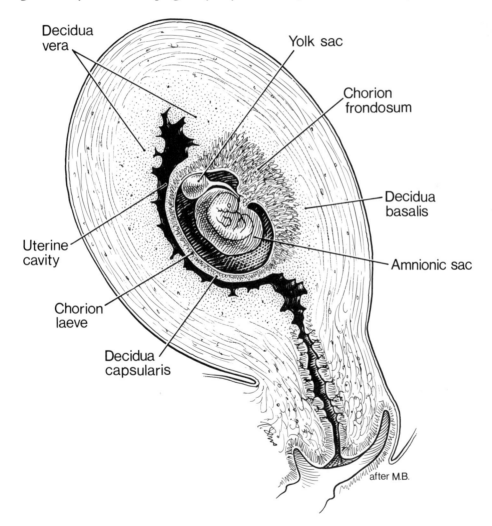

FIG. 6-7. More advanced stage of pregnancy, showing atrophic chorion laeve and chorion frondosum (chorionic villi) proliferating into decidua basalis.

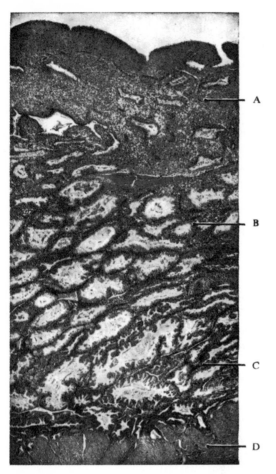

FIG. 6-8. Early decidua vera (parietalis). **A,** compact layer (see Fig. 6-9); **B,** spongy layer; **C,** uterine glands just above the basal layer; **D,** myometrium. (Compare with Figs. 2 through 5 in Chap. 4)

compacta and the spongiosa together form the functional zone *(zona functionalis).* The basal zone remains after delivery and gives rise to new endometrium. As pregnancy advances, the glandular epithelium of the decidua vera changes from a cylindric to a cuboid or flattened form, at times even resembling endothelium. After the fourth month, because of uterine distension, the decidua vera gradually thins from its maximal height of 1 cm in the first trimester to only 1 or 2 mm at term.

HISTOLOGY. The compact layer of the decidua consists of large, closely packed, epithelioid, polygonal, lightly staining cells with round, vesicular nuclei (Fig. 6-9). Many stromal cells appear stellate, particularly when the decidua is edematous, with long protoplasmic processes that anastomose with those of adjacent cells. Numerous small round cells containing very little cytoplasm are scattered among typical decidual cells, especially early in pregnancy. Formerly considered to be lymphocytes, these cells are now regarded as precursors of new decidual elements. In the early months of pregnancy, ducts of uterine glands are found in the decidua compacta, but these become less obvious in late pregnancy.

The spongy layer of the decidua consists of large distended glands, often exhibiting marked hyperplasia but separated by minimal stroma. At first, the glands are lined by typical cylindric uterine epithelium with abundant secretory activity. Presumably the glandular secretion contributes to the nourishment of the ovum during its histotrophic phase, before the establishment of a placental circulation. The epithelium gradually becomes cuboidal or even flattened, later degenerating and sloughing to a great extent into the lumens of the glands. The interglandular stroma of the spongy zone undergoes little change during pregnancy.

From the basal zone of the decidua vera (not to be confused with decidua basalis) some of the endometrium regenerates during the puerperium (see Chap. 19, p. 458). In comparing the decidua vera at four months gestation with the nonpregnant, early proliferative endometrium (see Fig. 4-1), it is clear that during decidual transformation of the endometrial stroma, there is marked hypertrophy but only slight hyperplasia.

The decidua basalis enters into the formation of the *basal plate* of the placenta and differs, histologically, from the decidua vera in two respects (Fig. 6-10). First, the spongy zone of the decidua basalis consists mainly of arteries and widely dilated veins; by term, the glands have virtually disappeared. Second, the decidua basalis is invaded extensively by trophoblastic giant cells which first

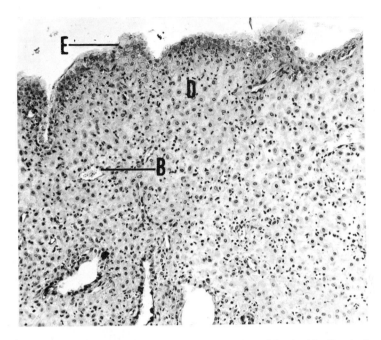

FIG. 6-9. Decidua vera (parietalis) showing epithelium (E), decidualized stromal cells (D), and blood vessel (B). (Courtesy of Dr. Ralph M. Wynn)

appear as early as the time of implantation. The number and depth of penetration of the giant cells vary greatly. Although generally confined to the decidua, they may penetrate the myometrium. In such circumstances, their number and invasiveness may be so extensive as to be suggestive of choriocarcinoma to the inexperienced observer.

Aging of the Decidua. Where invading trophoblast meets the decidua, there is a zone of fibrinoid degeneration, *Nitabuch's layer.* Whenever the decidua is defective, as in placenta accreta (see Chap. 34, p. 883), Nitabuch's layer is usually absent. There is also an inconstant deposition of fibrin, *Rohr's stria,* at the bottom of the intervillous space and surrounding the fastening villi. McCombs and Craig (1964) found that decidual necrosis is a normal phenomenon in the first and probably the second trimester. The presence of necrotic decidua obtained through curettage following spontaneous abortion in the first trimester should not, therefore, be inter-

preted necessarily as either a cause or an effect of the abortion.

Histochemistry and Ultrastructure. In their elegant studies of placental histochemistry, Wislocki and Dempsey (1948, 1955) found difficulty in distinguishing, with conventional stains, trophoblast from decidua in the basal plate. However, they observed differences in the distribution of RNA and mitochondria and characteristic "capsules" surrounding individual decidual cells. Wynn's electron microscopic findings (1967) of the human basal plate demonstrated that this complex region of the placenta comprises intimately related fetal and maternal cells. Well-preserved trophoblastic and endometrial cells are rarely in direct contact, however, but remain separated by degenerating tissue and fibrinoid. The giant cells in the region are derived from the syncytium or arise from differentiation of cytotrophoblast in situ. These syncytial masses may be hormonally active late in pregnancy. Moe (1969) confirmed these findings by showing that there is no intimate contact between apparently viable cytotrophoblast and decidua. The immunologic implications of these cellular relations are discussed subsequently.

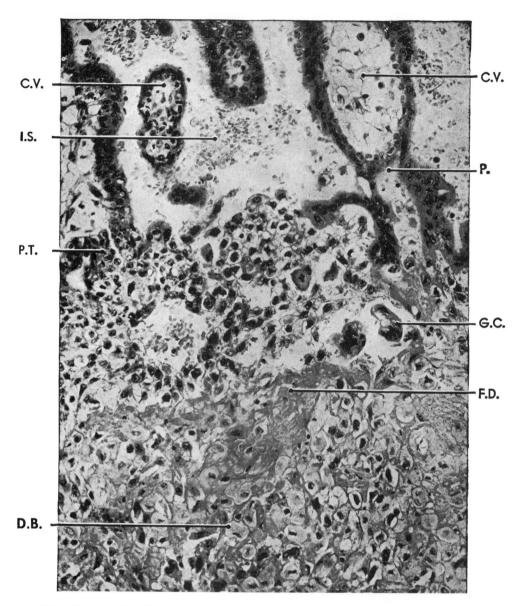

FIG. 6-10. Section through junction of chorion and decidua basalis. Fourth month of gestation. C.V., chorionic villi; D.B., decidua basalis; F.D., fibrinoid degeneration; G. C., giant cell; I.S., intervillous space containing maternal blood; P., fastening villus; P.T., proliferating trophoblast.

BIOLOGY OF THE TROPHOBLAST

Origin of the Syncytiotrophoblast. Of all placental components, the trophoblast is the most variable in structure, function, and development. Its invasiveness provides for attachment of the blastocyst to the uterus; its role in nutrition of the conceptus is reflected in its name; and its function as an endocrine organ is requisite to the maintenance of pregnancy. Morphologically, the trophoblast may be cellular or syncytial and it may appear as uninuclear cells or multinuclear giant cells. The true syncytial character of the human syncytiotrophoblast (syncytium) has been confirmed by electron microscopy. The mechanism of growth of the syncytium, however, has remained a mystery, in view of the discrepancy between increase in the number of nuclei in the syncytiotrophoblast and only equivocal evidence of intrinsic nuclear replication. Mitotic figures are completely absent from the syncytium, being confined to the cytotrophoblast. To distinguish amitotic nuclear proliferation within the syncytium from cytotrophoblastic origin of the syncytiotrophoblast, Galton (1962) employed microspectrophotometry, based on the Feulgen method for measuring DNA. He noted a diploid, unimodal distribution of DNA in the syncytium at a time of rapid placental growth, whereas a high proportion of cytotrophoblastic nuclei contained DNA in excess of the diploid amount, reflecting synthesis of DNA in interphase nuclei preparatory to division (see Chap. 5).

Galton concluded that the rapid accumulation of nuclei in the syncytiotrophoblast is explained by cellular proliferation within the cytotrophoblast, followed by coalescence of daughter cells in the syncytium.

Further evidence was provided by Richart (1961), who noted the early incorporation of tritiated thymidine in the cytotrophoblast

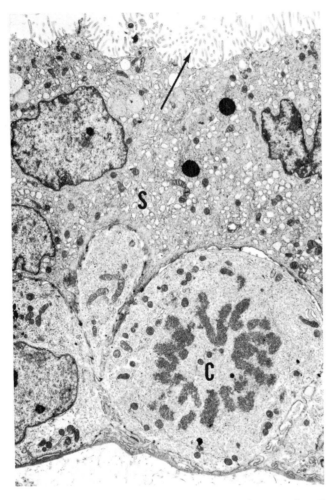

FIG. 6-11. Electron micrograph of human placenta at 6 weeks gestation. Note prominent border of microvilli (arrow), syncytium (S), and mitotic figure in cytotrophoblast (C). (Courtesy of Dr. Ralph M. Wynn)

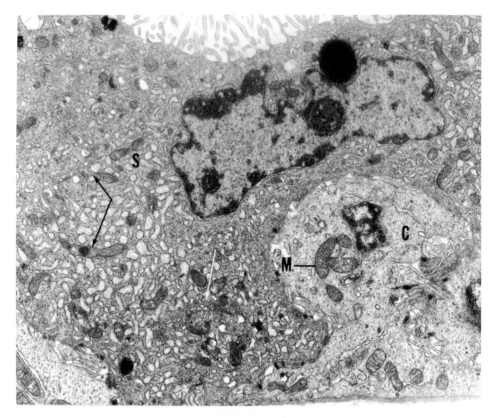

FIG. 6-12. First-trimester human placenta, showing well-differentiated syncytiotrophoblast (S) with numerous mitochondria (black arrows) and Golgi complexes *(white arrow).* Cytotrophoblast (C) has large mitochondria (M) but few other organelles. (Courtesy of Dr. Ralph M. Wynn)

but not in the syncytium. Midgley and co-workers (1963) subsequently extended the idea and found that although tritiated thymidine appeared at first only in the nuclei of the cytotrophoblast, the label could be detected 22 hours later in the syncytiotrophoblast, indicating that the syncytium is derived from cytotrophoblast and is itself a mitotic end stage.

Ultrastructure. From the electron microscope studies of Wislocki and Dempsey (1955) the basic data were provided upon which the functional interpretation of placental fine structure is based. The prominent microvilli of the syncytial surface, corresponding to the so-called brush border of light microscopy, and their associated pinocytotic vacuoles and vesicles are related to the ab-

sorptive and secretory functions of the placenta. The Langhans cells, which persist to term although often compressed against the trophoblastic basal lamina, retain their ultrastructural simplicity. They possess few specialized organelles, with abundant free ribosomes but scant ergastoplasm. Desmosomes connect individual Langhans cells with one another and with the syncytium, from which complete plasma membranes are absent. The syncytium is, ultrastructurally, relatively complex, containing abundant endoplasmic reticulum, Golgi bodies, and mitochondria, as well as numerous secretory droplets, lipid granules, and highly convoluted plasma membranes. The electron density of the syncytial nuclei is related to the high content of deoxyribonucleoprotein, and the abundant ribosomes and granular endoplasmic reticulum of the syncytial cytoplasm are correlated with a high content of the ribonucleoprotein and deep basophilia. As the syncytium matures, the fine struc-

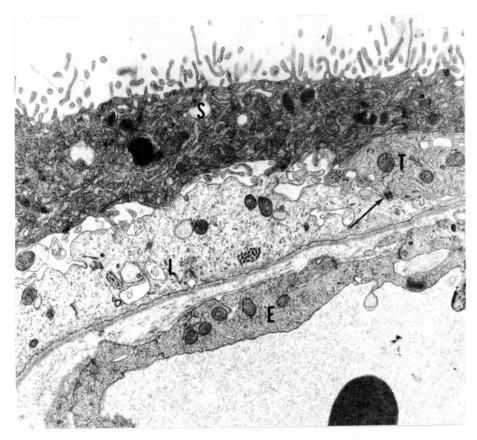

FIG. 6-13. Term human placenta, showing electron-dense syncytium (S), Langhans' cells (L), transitional cytotrophoblast (T), and capillary endothelium (E). Arrow points to desmosome. (Courtesy of Dr. Ralph M. Wynn)

tural changes reflect functional maturation. Early syncytiotrophoblast often exhibits a microvesicular endoplasmic reticulum; later, at the height of active synthesis of proteins, flattened ergastoplasmic channels assume prominence; and still later, associated with storage and transport of proteins, there appear dilated cisternae of endoplasmic reticulum, the largest of which are visible with the light microscope. Secretory granules, at least those thought to be glycoproteins and osmiophilic lipid granules correspond to PAS-positive and sudanophilic droplets, respectively (Figs. 6-11–6-13).

As the placenta matures, the collagen-rich stromal connective tissue decreases, as do the numbers of fibroblasts and Hofbauer cells. The human placental membrane may be reduced, anatomically, to a thin covering of trophoblast, capillary endothelium, and trophoblastic and endothelial basement membranes separated by mere wisps of connective tissue. Although at term, there is focal villous degeneration, morphologic evidence of activity in all layers persists. Since not only the trophoblast but the endothelium and even the basal laminas may show evidence of pinocytosis and other metabolic activity, it is hardly reasonable to equate the number of layers in the histologic "barrier" with the functional efficience of the placenta. Reduction of the number of layers may result in more rapid transplacental passage of substances to which the laws governing simple diffusion apply, but metabolites regulated by "carrier systems" are not proportionally affected. As for pinocytosis, a virtually continuous system of vesicles and vacuoles may be found extending from the syncytial surface to the capillary endothelium. Boyd and co-workers (1968) described a direct connection of some of these vacuoles with the perinuclear space, which receives tubular communications with the endoplasmic reticulum. The term *barrier* as applied to placental physiology should therefore be replaced by the more accurate term, *placental membrane.* The number of layers, furthermore, is a poor index of the true approximation of the circulations, since in the six-layered epitheliochorial placenta of the pig, for example (p. 142), the indentation of both fetal and maternal epithelium by the respective capillaries results in a rather close vascular relation. Comparative ultrastructure has thus posed an apparently insurmountable obstacle to the acceptance of the Grosser classification (p. 141) as a basis for comparative functional placentology.

Localization of Placental Hormones. That the syncytium is a source of placental steroids has not been questioned seriously since Wislocki's histochemical localization in the syncytiotrophoblast of sudanophilic droplets, which he associated with estrogen and progesterone. Thiede and Choate (1963) localized chorionic gonadotropin by immunofluorescent technics to the syncytium. A much smaller amount appeared in the amnion, but no specific fluorescence was detected in the cytotrophoblast. In combined ultrastructural and immunofluorescent studies, Pierce and Midgley (1963), working with human choriocarcinoma, likewise detected the chorionic gonadotropin in the syncytium but not in the cytotrophoblast. Sciarra and co-workers (1963) noted the protein hormone placental lactogen to be in the syncytium but not in the Langhans cells (p. 149). Wynn and Davies (1965) demonstrated by electron microscopy that only the syncytium contained the subcellular organelles required for synthesis of proteins, particularly abundant endoplasmic reticulum, and well developed Golgi complexes, whereas the cytotrophoblast was, ultrastructurally, simple.

CIRCULATION IN THE MATURE PLACENTA

Since the placenta functionally represents a rather intimate presentation of the fetal capillary bed to maternal blood, its gross anatomy primarily concerns vascular relations. The human placenta at term is a discoid organ measuring approximately 15 to 20 cm in diameter and 2 to 3 cm in thickness. It weighs approximately 500 g and generally is located in the uterus anteriorly or posteriorly near the fundus. The fetal side is covered by transparent amnion beneath which the fetal vessels course, with the arteries passing over the veins. A section through the placenta in situ (Figs. 6-14–6-16) includes amnion, chorion, chorionic villi and intervillous spaces, decidual plate, and myometrium. The maternal surface of the placenta (Fig. 6-17) is divided into irregular lobes by furrows produced by septa, which consist of fibrous tissue with sparse vessels confined mainly to their bases. The broadbased septa ordinarily do not reach the chorionic plate, thus providing only incomplete partitions.

Fetal Circulation.   Fetal blood flows to the placenta through the two umbilical arteries, which carry deoxygenated, or "venous," blood. The vessels branch repeatedly beneath the amnion and again within the dividing villi, forming capillary networks in the terminal divisions (Figs. 6-18, 6-19; see Colorplate for Fig. 6-19). Blood with a significantly higher oxygen content returns to the fetus from the placenta through the single umbilical vein (see Chap. 8, p. 183).

Maternal Circulation.   Only relatively recently has the mechanism of the maternal placental circulation been explained in physiologic terms. Insofar as fetal homeostasis is dependent on efficient placental circulation, the extensive efforts of investigators to elucidate the factors regulating the flow of blood into and from the intervillous space have led to important practical applications in obstetrics. An adequate theory must explain how blood may actually leave the maternal circulation, flow into an amorphous space lined by trophoblastic syncytium rather than capillary endothelium, and return through maternal veins without producing arteriovenous-like shunts that would prevent the blood from remaining in contact with the villi long enough for adequate exchange.

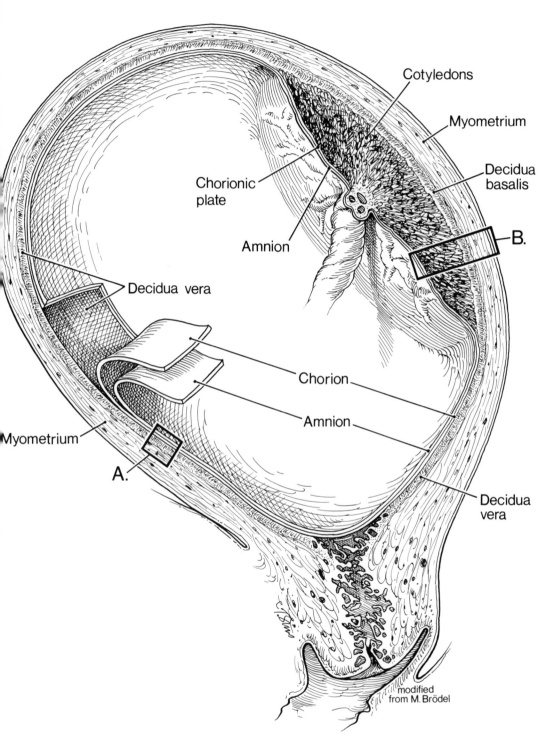

FIG. 6-14. A pregnant uterus showing normal placenta in situ. **A.** Location of section shown in Figure 6-15. **B.** Location of section shown in Figure 6-16.

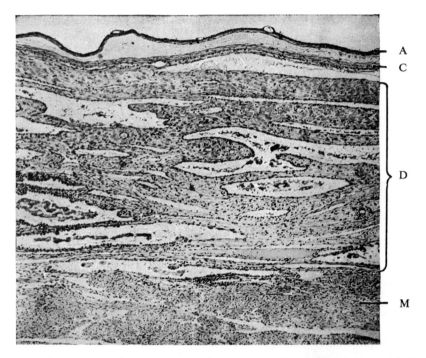

FIG. 6-15. Section of fetal membranes and uterus opposite placental site at **A** in Figure 6-14. A, amnion; C, chorion; D, decidua parietalis; M, myometrium.

It was not until the objective studies of Ramsey and her co-workers that a "physiologic" mechanism of placental circulation, consistent with both experimental and clinical findings, was available (Fig. 6-20; see Colorplate). Discarding the crude corrosion technics of her predecessors, Ramsey and co-workers, by careful, slow injections of radiocontrast material under low pressure that avoided disruption of the circulation, proved that the venous exits as well as the arterial entrances are scattered at random over the entire base of the placenta. The maternal blood entering through the basal plate is driven by the head of maternal arterial pressure high up toward the chorionic plate before lateral dispersion occurs. After bathing the chorionic villi, the blood drains through venous orifices in the basal plate and enters the maternal placental veins. The maternal blood thus traverses the placenta randomly without preformed channels, propelled by the maternal arterial pressure. The spiral arteries are generously per-pendicular and the veins parallel to the uterine wall, an arrangement that facilitates closure of the veins during a uterine contraction and prevents squeezing of essential maternal blood from the intervillous space. According to Brosens and Dixon (1963), there are about 120 spiral arterial entries into the intervillous space of the human placenta at term, discharging blood in spurts that displace the adjacent villi, as described by Borell and co-workers (1958).

Ramsey and Harris (1966) compared the uteroplacental vasculature and circulation of the rhesus monkey with those of women. The most significant morphologic variation is the greater dilatation of human uteroplacental arteries. In the woman, particularly in early pregnancy, there may be multiple openings from a single arterial stem into the intervillous space. The force of the spurts is eventually dissipated with the creation of a small lake of blood roughly 5 mm in diameter about halfway toward the chorionic plate.

The closeness of the villi slows the flow of blood, providing adequate time for exchange.

Ramsey's concept is supported by numerous arteriographic studies that clearly show the spiral arterial spurts associated with the "lakes" and by many pressure studies, which demonstrate the closure of uteroplacental veins at the beginning of uterine contractions. Corroboration has been provided by results of cineradioangiography, which shows how, in the macaque, debouching streams from the spiral arteries connect with and develop into the small lakes, which then disperse in a general effusion of blood throughout the intervillous space (Fig. 6-21).

In Ramsey's motion pictures, the effect of myometrial contractions upon placental circulation is shown unequivocally to involve diminution of arterial inflow and cessation of venous drainage. Continued observation of the contrast medium by televised fluoroscopy indicates that myometrial contractions cause a slight delay in appearance of the contrast medium in the veins of the uterine wall when injection occurs during a strong contraction. The pressure in the intervillous space may be decreased to the point at which blood cannot be expressed against the prevailing myometrial pressure. Ramsey has provided further evidence of independent activity of the spiral arterioles, as indicated by the appearance of spurts in different locations even when injections are performed under conditions of minimal myometrial pressure. Not all endometrial spiral arteries are continuously patent, nor do they all necessarily discharge blood into the intervillous space simultaneously.

In summary, Ramsey's concept holds that the maternal blood enters the intervillous space in spurts produced by the maternal blood pressure. The vis a tergo forces blood in discrete streams toward the chorionic plate until the head of pressure is reduced. Lateral spread then occurs. Continuing influx of arterial blood exerts pressure on the contents of the intervillous space, pushing the blood toward exits in the basal plate, from which it is drained through uterine and other pelvic veins. During uterine contractions, both inflow and outflow are curtailed, although the volume of blood in the intervillous space is maintained, thus providing for continual, though reduced, exchange.

Freese (1968) added support to older anatomic studies that showed that in both the

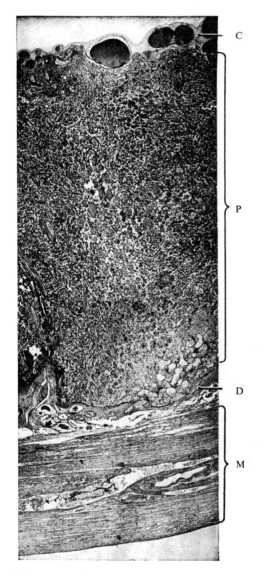

FIG. 6-16. Section of placenta and uterus through **B** in Figure 6-14. C, chorionic plate with fetal blood vessels; P, placental villi; D, decidua basalis; M, myometrium.

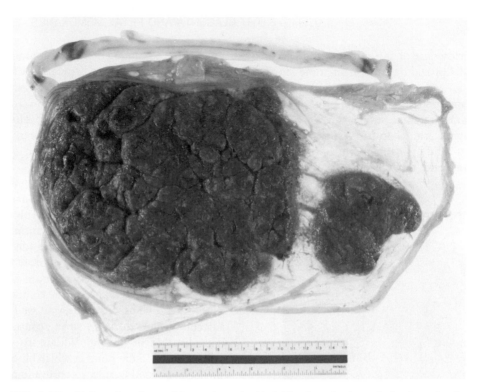

FIG. 6-17. Maternal surface of term placenta. Variably discrete, irregularly shaped adjacent lobes are evident plus a large separate (succenturiate) lobe.

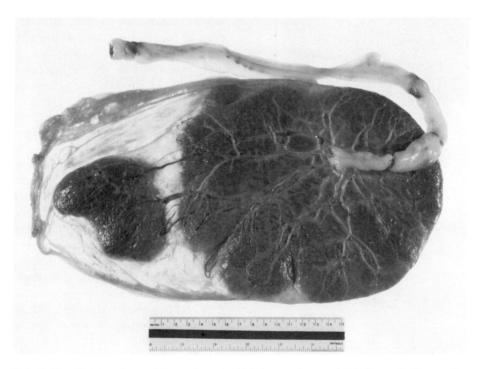

FIG. 6-18. Fetal surface of term placenta. Fetal vessels are visible beneath the amnion overlying the placenta. The fetal vessels extend to the adjacent separate (succenturiate) lobe.

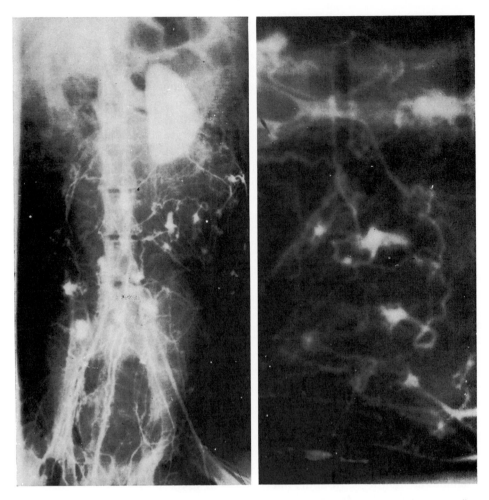

FIG. 6-21. *Left.* Radiogram 6 seconds after injection of a radiopaque contrast medium into the right femoral artery of a monkeys on day 111 of pregnancy. The primary placenta is below on the left; the secondary placenta is above on the right. *Right.* High magnification of an artery at the center of the secondary placenta in the same monkey. (Courtesy of Dr. Elizabeth M. Ramsey)

rhesus monkey and man, each placental coty-ledon is supplied by one spiral artery, which is located beneath a central empty space. He believed that this relatively hollow central portion of the cotyledon, which he called the intracotyledonary space, is the preferential site of entry of blood. Wigglesworth (1969) suggested that the structure of the fetal coty-ledon may determine, in part, the pattern of maternal blood flow through the placenta and that fetal cotyledons develop around the spi-ral artery. Variations in structure of the villi in this region imply that growth occurs

around the center of the cotyledon since villi there are less mature. The intervillous space thus has arterial, capillary, and venous zones. In this connection, Reynolds and co-workers (1968) showed that the blood pressure was highest around the central cavity of the cotyl-edon, the gradient diminishing radially and toward the subchorial lake. They postulated that Braxton-Hicks contractions (p. 265) en-hance the movement of blood from the cen-ter of the cotyledon through the intervillous space.

Bleker and associates (1975) identified by

serial sonography in normally laboring women, that the length, thickness, and surface of the placenta increased during uterine contractions. They attributed these changes to distension of the intervillous spaces by blood as the consequence of relatively greater impairment of venous outflow compared to arterial inflow. During contractions, therefore, a somewhat larger volume of blood is available for exchange even though the rate of flow is decreased.

Prostaglandins or prostaglandin-like substances very likely have an autoregulatory role in placental hemodynamics. Speroff (1975), for example, reported a rise in E prostaglandins and an increase in uterine blood flow in response to angiotensin II in pregnant monkeys while indomethacin had the opposite effect.

The principal factors regulating the flow of blood in the intervillous space are thus shown to include arterial blood pressure; intrauterine pressure; the pattern of uterine contraction, including the contour of the individual contraction wave; and factors acting specifically upon the arteriolar walls. The lack of homogeneity of blood throughout the intervillous space has been emphasized by Fuchs and co-workers (1963), who measured blood samples thought to be from the intervillous space and found considerable variations in the P_{O_2}, P_{CO_2}, pH, and standard bicarbonate. The values of some samples resembled arterial and others uterine venous blood. They stressed, however, the difficulty of ascertaining the precise source of blood obtained by transuterine puncture of the placenta.

Studies of the human placental circulation provide no evidence of counter-current flow, a system by which fetal blood of low oxygen content as it enters the villous capillaries would flow first close to maternal blood of low oxygen content and then move in close proximity to progressively more oxygenated maternal blood. In the hemochorial villous placenta of man, strict countercurrent flow is precluded by the random distribution of villi, in the capillaries of which the direction of fetal-to-maternal flow can bear no fixed relationship.

Harris and Ramsey (1966) published a summary of their anatomic studies of the uteroplacental vasculature. They noted that cytotrophoblastic elements are confined initially to the terminal portions of the uteroplacental arteries but later extend proximally. By the 16th week, cytotrophoblasts are found in many of the arteries of the inner layer of myometrium. Intra-arterial accumulation of trophoblast ultimately may stop circulation through some of these vessels. The number of arterial openings into the intervillous space gradually is reduced by cytotrophoblast and by breaching of the walls of the more proximal parts of the arteries by deeply penetrating trophoblast. Brosens and co-workers (1967) found that the cytotrophoblast not only breaches the maternal spiral vessels but also plays a major role in their progressive conversion to large tortuous channels by replacement of the normal muscular and elastic tissue of the wall by fibrous tissue and fibrinoid. After the 30th week, a prominent venous plexus separates the decidua basalis from the myometrium, thus providing a plane of cleavage for separation of the placenta.

PLACENTAL IMMUNOLOGY

The placenta appears to defy the laws of transplantation immunology. Today it is still enigmatic that the mother tolerates the fetal graft in light of the now well-established antigenic competence of both the trophoblast and the fetus. Indeed, there is suggestive evidence to support the view that the greater the genetic disparity between mother and fetus, the better the pregnancy, at least in terms of placental and fetal weight.

Breaks in the Placental "Barrier." The failure of the placenta to maintain absolute integrity of the fetal and maternal circulations is documented by numerous studies of the passage of cells between mother and fetus in both directions, and best exemplified clinically by the occurrence of erythroblastosis fetalis (see Chap. 38, p. 968). Typically a few fetal blood cells are found in the mother's blood; rarely, the fetus may exsanguinate into the maternal circulation (see Chap. 23, p. 574). Leukocytes from the fetus may replicate in the mother; leukocytes bearing a Y chromosome have been identified in women for up to five years after giving birth to a son (Ciaranfi et al., 1977). Desai and Creger (1963) labeled maternal leukocytes and platelets with atabrine and found that they crossed the placenta from mother to fetus. Lymphocytes passing into the fetus create the possibility of *chimerism,* the subject of a review by Benirschke (1970). If the maternal cells then colonize, a "graft-versus-host" reaction or autoimmune process may result.

Cells of fetal origin other than constituents of the blood have also been identified in the maternal circulation. Cells morphologically identical with trophoblast have been identified in the uterine venous blood (Douglas et al., 1959) as well as in cord blood (Salvaggio et al., 1960). The immunologic significance of continuous release of fetal elements into the maternal circulation remains to be explained.

Immunologic Considerations. Except in parthenogenesis, or in situations in which both parents are genetically identical, the fetus and his trophoblast confront the mother with foreign antigens. A fertilized egg transplanted to a recipient's uterus may, furthermore, result in a pregnancy with immunologic characteristics of a homograft. Interspecific hybrids, analogous to heterografts, represent even more flagrant violations of the laws of immunology. Attempts to explain the survival of the "homograft" have occupied the attention of several of the world's outstanding biologists. An explanation based on antigenic immaturity of the fetus must be discarded in light of Billingham's demonstration (1964) that transplantation antigens appear very early in life. A second explanation, based on diminished immunologic reactivity of the mother during pregnancy, provides only an ancillary factor in the prevention of the development of maternal isoimmunization during pregnancy in a few species. If the uterus were an immunologically privileged site, as in a third explana-

tion, advanced ectopic pregnancies could never occur. Since transplantation immunity can be evoked and expressed in the uterus as elsewhere, the survival of the homograft must be related to a peculiarity of the fetus and placenta rather than of the uterus. A fourth explanation involves a physiologic barrier between fetus and mother. Lanman and colleagues (1962) provided indirect support for the last hypothesis in their experiments in which fertilized rabbit's ova were transferred to a recipient's uterus. Neither prior exposure of the foster mother to skin grafts from the parents nor reexposure to homografts from these donors at the time of egg transfer or at midpregnancy adversely affected the pregnancy.

Kobayashi and co-workers (1979) have reported a dose-dependent suppression of the bidirectional mixed lymphocyte reaction by progesterone in concentrations comparable to those of the placenta. Therefore, they suggest a role for progesterone at its site of production in immunoregulation during pregnancy. Siiteri and co-workers (1977) previously demonstrated that the rejection of grafted hamster skin is delayed by the presence of progesterone.

One reasonable explanation for the survival of the homograft appears to be a fairly complete anatomic separation of maternal and fetal circulations. Comparative electron microscopy of the placenta has supported the concept of the prime role of the trophoblast in maintaining the "immunologic barrier." In all placentas examined with the electron microscope, at least one layer of trophoblast has been shown to persist essentially throughout gestation.

The suggestion by Kirby and co-workers (1964) that deposition of fibrinoid was a general phenomenon of mammalian placentation rekindled interest in these amorphous deposits. (We have used the term *fibrinoid* in the restricted conventional sense of the histopathologist to refer to a group of substances recognized with the light microscope.) Although fibrinoids are not demonstrable in all mammalian placentas, a submicroscopic glycocalyx may be found with the electron microscope to coat most trophoblastic plasma membranes. It is still not clear whether these polysaccharide barriers serve as mechanical barriers to the passage of transplantation antigens from fetus to mother, or to provide for local shields from maternal lymphocytes.

Maternal lymphocyte function is altered during pregnancy, as reflected by a reduction in phytohemagglutinin-induced transformation (Finn et al., 1972; Purtilo et al., 1972). It has been suggested by Finn (1975) that lymphocytes possess individual-specific surface repellent molecules and that these can cross the placenta and coat maternal lymphocytes, thus preventing them from attacking fetal cells. It has also been suggested that various secretory products of the trophoblast, e.g., hCG and progesterone, may confer immunologic privilege to the trophoblast.

Finn and associates (1977) provided an attractive explanation for the tolerance of the fetus and placenta by the mother. They demonstrated maternal and fetal lymphocytes to be tolerant of each other in the bidirectional mixed lymphocyte reaction. They believed the tolerance between maternal and fetal cells to be largely due to a genetic mechanism since the bidirectional mixed lymphocyte reaction between parents and older children was also reduced when compared with that between randomly selected controls. Tolerance between maternal and fetal cells was not demonstrated in an undirectional mixed lymphocyte reaction, which suggested that the tolerance requires viability of both cell populations. They have postulated that the mother has two allelic surface markers, one of which must pass to the cells of the fetus, and thus there is a common marker on maternal and fetal cells. These markers are mutually repellent and keep the cell surfaces sufficiently separated to prevent contact between major HLA antigens and thereby prevent an immunologic reaction.

THE AMNION

The human amnion either develops by delamination from the cytotrophoblast about the seventh or eighth day of development of the normal ovum or it develops essentially as an extension of the fetal ectoderm. Initially a minute vesicle (see Fig. 5-18), the amnion develops into a small sac that covers the dorsal surface of the embryo. As the amnion enlarges, it gradually engulfs the growing embryo, which prolapses into its cavity. Distension of the amnionic sac eventually brings it into contact with the interior of the chorion; apposition of the mesoblasts of chorion and amnion near the end of the first trimester results in obliteration of the extraembryonic celom. The amnion and chorion, though slightly adherent, are never intimately connected and usually can be separated easily, even at term.

The normal amnion is 0.02 to 0.5 mm in thickness. The epithelium normally consists of a single layer of nonciliated, cuboid cells. According to Bourne (1962), there are five layers, comprising, from within outward, epithelium, basement membrane, the compact layer, the fibroblastic layer, and the spongy layer. Electron microscopic studies of amnion by Wynn and French (1968) and by Hoyes (1968) have not, however, confirmed such sharply defined layers (Fig. 6-22).

Bourne (1962) was unable to find blood vessels or nerves in the amnion at any stage of development and, despite the occurrence of suggestive spaces in the fibroblastic and spongy layers, could not identify distinct lymphatic channels.

At term, small rounded plaques are often found on the amnion, particularly near the attachment of the umbilical cord. These *amnionic caruncles* consist of stratified squamous epithelium that histologically resembles skin (see Chap. 23, p. 577).

Fetal Membranes and Steroid Hormone Metabolism. Studies directed toward a definition of the role of the fetal membranes in the initiation of parturition were initiated by MacDonald and co-workers (1974). Among the early findings was the clear demonstration that both the amnion and chorion laeve possesses extensive enzymatic capabilities for steroid hormone metabolism including 5α-reductase, 3β-hydroxy steroid

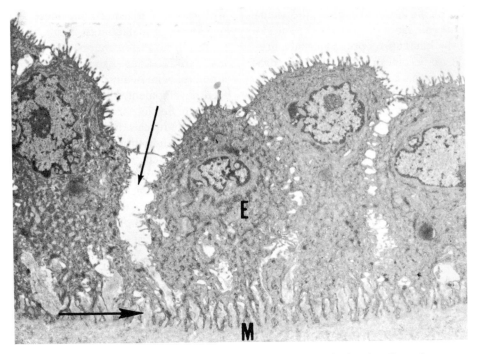

FIG. 6-22. Electron micrograph of human amnion at term obtained at time of cesarean section. Epithelium (E) and mesenchyme (M) are shown. Thin arrow indicates intercellular space. Thick arrow points to specializations of basal plasma membranes. (Courtesy of Dr. Ralph M. Wynn)

dehydrogenase, Δ^{5-4}-isomerase, 20α-steroid oxidoreductase, 17α-dehydrogenase and other enzyme activities.

The fetal membranes are rich in glycerophospholipids containing arachidonic acid, the obligate precursor of prostaglandins E_2 and $F_{2\alpha}$. The fetal membranes also have phospholipase A_2, an enzyme that catalyzes the hydrolysis of glycerophospholipids to yield arachidonic acid, an essential and likely the rate-limiting step in prostaglandin biosynthesis (see Chap. 15, p. 371).

Amnionic Fluid. The normally clear fluid that collects within the amnionic cavity increases in quantity as pregnancy advances until near term, when it normally decreases. An average volume of somewhat less than 1000 ml is found at term, although the volume may vary widely from a few milliliters to many liters in abnormal conditions (oligohydramnios and polyhydramnios, or hy-

dramnios). The origin, composition, and function of the amnionic fluid are discussed further in Chapter 8 (p. 206).

UMBILICAL CORD AND RELATED STRUCTURES

Development of the Cord and Related Structures. The yolk sac and the umbilical vesicle into which it develops are quite prominent at the beginning of pregnancy. At first the embryo is a flattened disc interposed between amnion and yolk sac. Since the dorsal surface grows faster than the ventral surface, in association with the elongation of the neural tube, the embryo bulges into the amnionic sac and the dorsal part of the yolk sac is incorporated into the body of the embryo to form the gut. The allantois projects into the base of the body stalk from the caudal wall of the yolk sac or, later, from the anterior wall of the hindgut. As pregnancy advances, the yolk sac becomes smaller and its pedicle relatively longer. By about the middle of the third month, the expanding amnion obliterates the exocelom, fuses with the chorion laeve, and covers the bulging placental disc and the lateral surface of the body stalk, which is then called the umbilical cord, or funis. Remnants of the exocelom in the anterior portion of the cord may contain loops of intestine, which continue to develop outside the embryo. Although the loops are later withdrawn, the apex of the midgut loop retains its connection with an attenuated vitelline duct that terminates in a crumpled, highly vascular sac 3 to 5 cm in diameter lying on the surface of the placenta between amnion and chorion or in the membranes just beyond the placental margin, where occasionally it may be identified at term.

In an electron microscopic study of the human yolk sac, Hoyes (1969) confirmed that its endoderm is the origin of fetal blood cells. The epithelium of the yolk sac has ultrastructural features that are usually associated with those of a tissue that serves as a site of transfer of metabolites.

The three vessels in the cord at term normally are two arteries and one vein. The right umbilical vein usually disappears early during fetal development, leaving only the original left vein. Section of any portion of the cord frequently reveals, near the center, the small duct of the umbilical vesicle, lined by a single layer of flattened or cuboid epithelial cells. In sections just beyond the umbilicus, but never at the maternal end of the cord, another duct representing the allantoic remnant occasionally is found. The intra-abdominal portion of the duct of the umbilical vesicle, which extends from umbilicus to intestine, usually atrophies and disappears, but occasionally it remains patent, forming Meckel's diverticulum. The most common vascular anomaly in man is the absence of one umbilical artery. This subject is discussed further in Chapter 23 (p. 573).

Structure and Function of the Cord. The umbilical cord, or funis, extends from the fetal umbilicus to the fetal surface of the placenta. Its exterior is dull white,

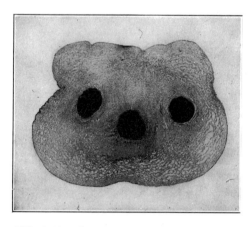

FIG. 6-23. Cross section of umbilical cord fixed after blood vessels had been emptied. The umbilical vein, carrying oxygenated blood to the fetus, is in the center; on either side are the two umbilical arteries carrying deoxygenated blood from the fetus to the placenta. (From Reynolds. *Am J Obstet Gynecol* 68:69, 1954)

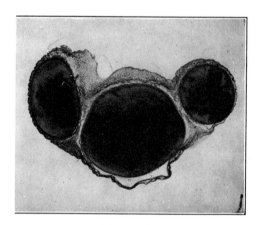

FIG. 6-24. Cross section of same umbilical cord shown in Figure 6-23, but through a segment from which the blood vessels had not been emptied. This photograph probably represents more accurately the conditions in utero. (From Reynolds. *Am J Obstet Gynecol* 68:69, 1954)

moist, and covered by amnion, through which the three umbilical vessels may be seen. Its diameter is 1 to 2.5 cm, with an average length of 55 cm and a usual range of 30 to 100 cm. Folding and tortuosity of the vessels, which are longer than the cord itself, frequently create nodulations on the surface, or *false knots,* which are essentially varices. The matrix of the cord consists of Wharton's Jelly (Figs. 6-23, 6-24). After fixation, the umbilical vessels appear empty, but Figure 6-24 is more accurately representative of the situation in vivo, when the vessels are not emptied of blood. The two arteries are smaller in diameter than the vein. When fixed in its normally distended state, the umbilical artery exhibits transverse intimal *folds of Hoboken* across part of its lumen (Chacko, Reynolds, 1954). The mesoderm of the cord, which is of allantoic origin, fuses with that of the amnion.

The egress of blood from the umbilical vein is via two routes, the ductus venosus, which empties directly into the inferior vena cava, and numerous smaller openings into the fetal hepatic circulation and thence into the inferior vena cava by the hepatic vein (Fig. 8-10 Colorplate). The blood takes the path of least resistance through these alternate routes. Resistance in the ductus venous is controlled by a sphincter, which is situated at the origin of the ductus at the umbilical recess and innervated by a branch of the vagus nerve.

Ellison and co-workers (1970) studied the innervation of the umbilical cord of the rat by means of localization of acetylcholinesterase and catecholamines. Cholinesterase-positive nerves were confined to periarterial plexus while adrenergic nerves were entirely absent from the cord. By these technics, certain nerves could be traced to the placenta but not into it. Although several recent investigators, relying on histochemical methods, have reported nerves in placenta and amnion, ultrastructural confirmation is lacking. The question of innervation of the placenta and membranes thus remains open. Humoral stimuli, however, may well be transmitted across the placenta.

COMPARATIVE ANATOMY

Types of Placentation. The debt of all comparative placentologists to George B. Wislocki, late Professor of Anatomy at Harvard University, and Harland W. Mossman, Professor Emeritus of Anatomy at the University of Wisconsin, can scarcely be overemphasized, as amply demonstrated by reference to the writings of Amoroso, Enders, Wimsatt, Wynn, and others. In this brief discussion only generalizations are outlined, insofar as they focus attention on fundamental problems in human placentology.

CHORIOALLANTOICPLACENTATION. Since the chorioallantoic placenta is the principal organ of fetomaternal exchange in most higher mammals, including man, it has been subjected to numerous attempts at classification. In dealing with biologic variation, however, overclassification reflects gaps in detailed knowledge rather than scholarly perfection. The well-known scheme of Grosser (1927) in which placentas are classified according to the number of layers separating fetal and maternal blood, has proved progressively less useful in proportion to the increasing knowledge of placental structure and function. In Grosser's original classification the minimal placental "barrier" comprised the three fetal components (trophoblast, connective tissue, and endothelium), forming a *hemochorial* placenta, in which trophoblast was directly exposed to maternal blood. The persistence of maternal endothelium added a fourth layer to form an *endotheliochorial* placenta. If, in addition, endometrial connective tissue remains, a *syndesmochorial* placenta results. When the epithelium of the endometrium enters into formation of a six-layered placenta, an epitheliochorial condition obtains (Fig. 6-25).

The inadequacies of the Grosser classification involve its failure to account for anatomic variations within the placenta, changes accompanying placental aging, and accessory placental organs. Its basic deficiency, however, was the implication that a reduction in the number of layers in the placental "barrier" was equivalent to increased placental efficiency. Whereas the transfer of substances that cross the placenta by simple diffusion may be influenced directly by the thickness of the barrier, the Grosser scheme failed to consider the physiologic activity of the highly complex placental membrane, particularly with respect to active transport of metabolites.

Although attempts to modify the Grosser classi-

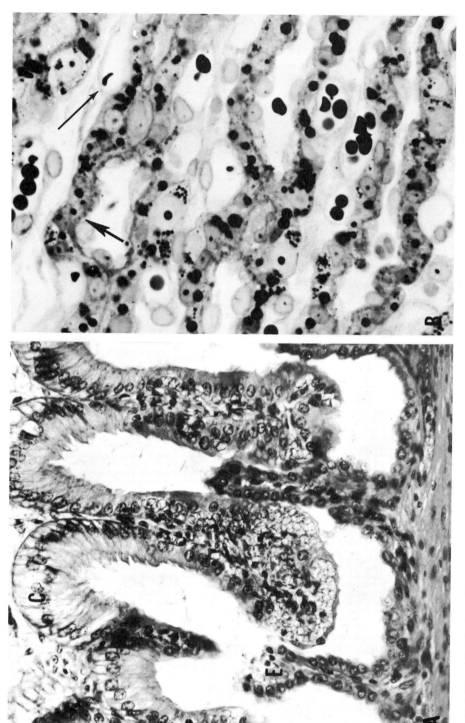

FIG. 6-25. Histologic variation in placental membranes. **A.** Epitheliochorial (six-layered placenta of pig, showing chorionic epithelium (trophoblast) (C) and endometrium (E). The separation of layers is an artifact. (Courtesy of Dr. Harland W. Mossman) **B.** Endotheliochorial (four-layered) placenta of cat, showing maternal (thick arrow) and fetal (thin arrow) vessels. The designation, *vasochorial,* is more appropriate to this placenta. (Courtesy of Dr. Ralph M. Wynn)

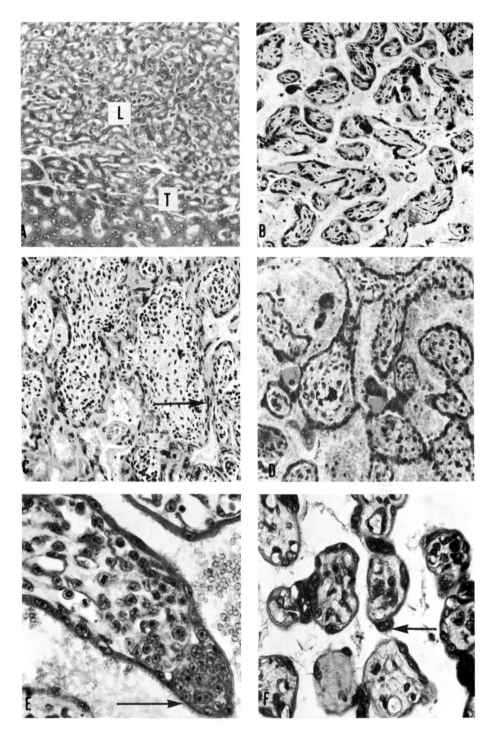

FIG. 6-26. Histologic variants of the hemochorial placenta. **A.** Completely labyrinthine placenta of guinea pig, showing syncytiotrophoblastic lamellae (L) and trophospongium (T). **B.** Villous placenta of rhesus monkey, showing free villi resembling those of human placenta. **C.** Pseudolabyrinth of placenta of New World squirrel monkey, showing trophoblastic trabecula (arrow). **D.** Semivillous placenta of spotted hyena, showing resemblance to that of platyrrhine monkey. This placenta may be partially endotheliochorial. **E.** Villus of nine-banded armadillo, showing cytotrophoblastic (arrow) restricted to tip. **F.** Term human placenta, showing completely free villi with syncytial "knot" (arrow). (Courtesy of Dr. Ralph M. Wynn)

fication have been generally unsuccessful, the introduction of the term *vasochorial* by Wislocki represents an improvement, inasmuch as the occurrence of entirely unsupported endothelium, as implied in the term *endotheliochorial*, is most unlikely. In the lamellae of the cat's "vasochorial" placenta, furthermore, decidualike cells persist, in an almost syndesmochorial relation. Rigid classifications, moreover, neglect the transitions between various histologic types within the same placenta and the fundamental differences in origin and function of numerous placental specializations that appear superficially homologous. In the "hematoma" of the typical carnivore's placenta, for example, stagnant blood extravasates between the chorion and the endometrial surface. Such a structure is *histotrophic*, a term used to describe nutrition obtained for the trophoblast from sources other than circulating blood, such as glandular secretions and extravasated blood. In contrast, the hemochorial placenta of man is representative of a true *hemotrophic* condition in that nutrition is derived from the circulating blood. The two conditions, though superficially similar histologically, are basically different in origin and function.

Mossman (1937) originally described placentas allegedly more intimate than the hemochorial types and postulated that even the trophoblast may disappear focally to produce hemoendothelial placentas. The results of comparative electron microscopic studies, however, consistently have demonstrated at least one layer of trophoblast in all placentas studied thus far (Enders, 1965; Mossman, 1967). Enders suggested a most useful classification of hemochorial placentas based on the number of complete layers of trophoblast. The placentas of man and the guinea pig, for example, are *hemomonochorial;* that of the rabbit is *hemodichorial;* and that of the mouse is *hemotrichorial.*

Additional factors of importance in the classification of chorioallantoic placentas are gross shape and presence or absence of true decidua. In general, placentas may be grossly divided into diffuse, cotyledonary, zonary, and discoid types. The definitive shape usually is determined by the initial distribution of villi over the chorionic surface, although occasionally it is derived secondarily. In the pig and horse, the distribution of villi over almost the entire chorionic surface produces a diffuse placenta. In the ruminants (sheep, cow, deer, and antelope), the villi are restricted to separate tufts of cotyledons, widely scattered over the chorion to form a cotyledonary, or multiplex, placenta. In most carnivores, the Sirenia, and the Tu-bulidentata (aardvark), the grouping of villi in bands around the equator of the chorioallantoic sac results in a zonary placenta. In anthropoids, rodents, bats, and most insectivores, the placenta consists of a single disc, as in man, or a double disc, as in certain monkeys and primitive tree shrews. The definitive shape of the human placenta is a result of the disappearance of villi from all but a circumscribed locus on the chorion. Finally, placentas may be classified as deciduate (man, guinea pig), adeciduate (ungulates), or contrade-ciduate allegedly (some insectivores).

THE HEMOCHORIAL VILLOUS PLACENTA. Hemochorial placentas, which are of special interest because they include the human placenta, comprise both labyrinthine and villous forms. In the hemochorial labyrinth, the trophoblast forms lamellae between blood-filled spaces. The villous condition results from the initial rupture by the trophoblast of the maternal vessels, with escape of blood to form large sinusoids and trabeculae across the blood-filled spaces. In studies employing both light and electron microscopy, Wynn and Davies (1965) and Enders (1965) demonstrated the villous condition in a variety of taxonomically unrelated animals, such as the scaly-tailed squirrel, the armadillo, and a variety of primates including man. They confirmed, furthermore, the presence of transitions from villous to labyrinthine forms, seen particularly well in the New World monkeys. In the human placenta the villi are almost entirely free; the apparent intervillous connections are formed not by syncytiotrophoblast, as Stieve (1942) believed, but rather by fibrinous adhesions resulting from the organization of minute hematomas. The breakdown of syncytium in the placentas of certain New World monkeys, for example, converts the trabeculae in these areas to villi, and the labyrinthine to the villous condition (Fig. 6-26).

REFERENCES

Benirschke K: Spontaneous chimerism in mammals: a critical review. In Current Topics in Pathology. Berlin, Springer-Verlag, 1970, p 1

Billingham RE: Transplantation immunity and the maternal-fetal relation. New Engl J Med 270:667, 720, 1964

Bleker OP, Kloosterman GJ, Mieras DJ, Oosting J, Salle HJA: Intervillous space during uterine contractions in human subjects: an ultrasonic study. Am J Obstet Gynecol 123:697, 1975

Borell U, Fernström I, Westman A: (An arteriographic study of the placental circulation). Geburtshilfe Frauenheilkd 18:1 1958

Bourne GL: The Human Amnion and Chorion. Chicago, Year Book, 1962

Boyd JD, Hamilton WJ: The Human Placenta. Cambridge, England, Heffer, 1970

Boyd JD, Boyd CAR, Hamilton WJ: Observations on the vacuolar structure of the human syncytiotrophoblast. Z Zellforsch Mikrosk Anat 88:57, 1968

Brosens I, Dixon HG: The anatomy of the maternal side of the placenta. Br J Obstet Gynaecol 73:357, 1963

Brosens I, Robertson WB, Dixon HB: The physiological response of the vessels of the placental bed to normal pregnancy. J Pathol Bact 98:569, 1967

Chacko AW, Reynolds SRM: Architecture of distended and nondistended human umbilical cord tissues, with special references to the arteries and veins. Contrib Embryol 35:135, 1954

Ciaranfi A, Curchod A, Odartchenko N: Survie de lymphocytes foetaux dans de sang maternel post-partum. Schweiz Med Wschr 107:134, 1977

Crawford JM: A study of human placental growth with observations on the placenta in erythroblastosis foetalis. Br J Obstet Gynaecol 66:885, 1959

Desai RG, Creger WP: Maternofetal passage of leukocytes and platelets in man. Blood 21:665, 1963

Douglas GW, Thomas L, Carr M, Cullen NM, Morris R: Trophoblast in the circulating blood during pregnancy. Am J Obstet Gynecol 78:960, 1959

Ellison JP, Hibbs RG, Ferguson MA, Mahan M, Blasini EJ: The innervation of the umbilical cord. Anat Red 166:302, 1970

Enders AC: A comparative study of the fine structure of the trophoblast in several hemochorial placentas. Am J Anat 166:29, 1965

Finn R: Survival of the genetically incompatible fetal allograft. Lancet 1:835, 1975

Finn R, St. Hill CA, Govan AJ, Ralfs IG, Gurney FJ, Denye V: Immunological responses in pregnancy and survival of fetal homograft. Br Med J 3:150, 1972

Finn R, Davis JC, St. Hill CA, Hipkin LJ: Fetomaternal bidirectional mixed lymphocyte reaction and survival of fetal allograft. Lancet

21:200, 1977

Freese UE: The uteroplacental vascular relationship in the human. Am J Obstet Gynecol 101:8, 1968

Fuchs F, Spackman T, Assali NS: Complexity and nonhomogencity of the intervillous space. Am J Obstet Gynecol 86:226, 1963

Galton M: DNA content of placental nuclei. J Cell Biol 13:183, 1962

Grosser O: Frühentwicklung, Einautbildung and Placentation des Menschen und der Saugetiere, Dt. Frauenheilke, Vol 5, Bergmann 1927

Harris JWS, Ramsey EM: The morphology of human uteroplacental vasculature. Contrib Embryol 38:43, 1966

Hertig AT: The placenta: some new knowledge about an old organ. Obstet Gynecol 20:859, 1962

Hoyes AD: Fine structure of human amniotic epithelium in early pregnancy. Br J Obstet Gynaecol 75:949, 1968

Hoyes AD: The human foetal yolk sac: An ultrastructural study of four specimens. Z Zellforsch 99:469, 1969

Kirby DRS, Billington WD, Bradbury S, Goldstein DJ: Antigen barrier of the mouse placenta. Nature (London) 204:548, 1964

Kobayashi H, Mori T, Suzuki A, Nishimura T, Nishimoto H, Harada M: Suppression of mixed lymphocyte reaction by progesterone and estradiol-17β. Am J Obstet Gynecol 134:255, 1979

Lanman JT, Dinerstein J, Fikrig S: Homograft immunity in pregnancy: lack of harm to fetus from sensitization of mother. Ann NY Acad Sci 99:706, 1962

MacDonald PC, Schultz FM, Duenhoelter JH, Gant NF, Jimenez JM, Pritchard JA, Porter JC, Johnson JM: Initiation of human parturition: I. Mechanism of action of arachidonic acid. Obstet Gynecol 44:629, 1974

McCombs HL, Craig JM: Decidual necrosis in normal pregnancy. Obstet Gynecol 24:436, 1964

Midgley AR Jr, Pierce GB Jr, Deneau GA, Gosling JRS: Morphogenesis of syncytiotrophoblast in vivo: an autoradiographic demonstration. Science 141:349, 1963

Moe N: The deposits of fibrin and fibrin-like materials in the basal plate of the normal human placenta. Acta Pathol Microbiol Scand 75:1, 1969

Mossman HW: Comparative morphogenesis of the fetal membranes and accessory uterine structures. Contrib Embryol 26:129, 1937

Mossman HW: Comparative biology of the placenta and fetal membranes. In Wynn RM (ed): Fetal Homeostasis. New York, New York Academy of Sciences, 1967, Vol 2, p 13

Pierce GB Jr, Midgley AR Jr: The origin and function of human syncytiotrophoblastic giant cells. Am J Pathol 43:153, 1963

Purtilo DT, Hallgren H, Yunis EJ: Depressed maternal lymphocyte response to phytohaemagglutinin in human pregnancy. Lancet 1:769, 1972

Ramsey EM, Davis RW: A composite drawing of the placenta to show its structure and circulation. Anat Rec 145:366, 1963

Ramsey EN, Harris JWS: Comparison of uteroplacental vasculature and circulation in the rhesus monkey and man. Contrib Embryol 38:59, 1966

Reynolds SRM, Freese UE, Bieniarz J, Caldeyro-Barcia R, Mendez-Bauer C, Escarcena L: Multiple simultaneous intervillous space pressures recorded in several regions of the hemochorial placenta in relation to functional anatomy of the fetal cotyledon. Am J Obstet Gynecol 102:1128, 1968

Richart RM: Studies of placental morphogenesis: I. Radioautographic studies of human placenta utilizing tritiated thymidine. Proc Soc Exp Biol Med 106:829, 1961

Salvaggio AT, Nigogosyan G, Mack HC: Detection of trophoblasts in cord blood and fetal circulation. Am J Obstet Gynecol 80:1013, 1960

Sciarra JJ, Kaplan SL, Grumbach MM: Localization of anti-human growth hormone serum within the human placenta: evidence for a human chorionic-growth-hormone-Prolactin. Nature (London) 199:1005, 1963

Siiteri PK, Febres F, Clemens LE, Jeffry Chang R, Gondos B, Sites D: Progesterone and maintenance of pregnancy: Is progesterone nature's immunosuppressant? Ann NY Acad Sci 286:384, 1977

Speroff L: An autoregulatory role for prostaglandins in placental hemodynamics: their possible influence on blood pressure in pregnancy. J Reprod Med 15:181, 1975

Stieve H: (The intervillous space of the human placenta in the fourth and fifth months and at the end of pregnancy). Arch Gynaekol 174:452, 1942

Thiede HA, Choate JW: Chorionic gonadotropin localization in the human placenta by immunofluorescent staining: II. Demonstration of HCG in the trophoblast and amnion epithelium of immature and mature placentas. Obstet Gynecol 22:433, 1963

Thomson AM, Billewicz WZ, Hytten FE: The weight of the placenta in relation to birthweight. Br J Obstet Gynaecol 76:865, 1969

Wislocki GB, Dempsey EW: The chemical histology of human placenta and decidua with reference to mucoproteins, glycogen, lipids and acid phosphatase. Am J Anat 83:1, 1948

Wislocki GB, Denpsey EW: Electron microscopy of the human placenta. Anat Rec 123:133, 1955

Wislocki GB, Streeter GL: On the placentation of the macaque (Macaca mulatta), from the time of implantation until the formation of the definitive placenta. Contrib Embryol 27:1, 1938

Wynn RM: Comparative electron microscopy of the placental junctional zone. Obstet Gynecol 29:644, 1967

Wynn RM: Fetomaternal cellular relations in the human basal plate: an ultrastructural study of the placenta. Am J Obstet Gynecol 97:832, 1967

Wynn RM, Davies J: Comparative electron microscopy of the hemochorial villous placenta. Am J Obstet Gynecol 91:533, 1965

Wynn RM, French GL: Comparative ultrastructure of the mammalian amnion. Obstet Gynecol 31:759, 1968

7

The Placental Hormones
and Their Precursors

The human placenta produces, in abundance, the protein hormones *chorionic gonadotropin* (hCG) and *placental lactogen* (hPL) as well as the steroid hormones *progesterone* and *estrogens*. Some evidence has accumulated that trophoblast also synthesizes a *thyroid-stimulating hormone*. The human placenta may form a *corticotropin* (chorionic ACTH), although the existence of chorionic ACTH has not been proven. The trophoblast also can synthesize certain hormones that are similar immunologically, at least, to some of the hypothalamic-releasing hormones that act on the pituitary.

CHORIONIC GONADOTROPIN

Human chorionic gonadotropin (hCG) is believed to be produced principally by syncytiotrophoblast rather than cytotrophoblast, as pointed out in Chapter 6, page 130. The most apparent function of hCG in women is to maintain the corpus luteum during early pregnancy, but a role for hCG in the initiation of testosterone secretion by the fetal testes is probable and, a role in the maintenance

of cholesterol side chain-cleavage in the placenta must be considered. Moreover, a role for hCG in the provision of immunologic privilege to the trophoblast has been suggested.

In the human ovary, appropriately primed by FSH (follicle-stimulating hormone), hCG induces ovulation and is sometimes so used as an LH (luteinizing hormone) surrogate in the treatment of infertility due to anovulation and hypogonadotropic hypogonadism.

The original demonstration of the "pregnancy hormone" in urine by Ascheim and Zondek in 1927 formed the basis for consideration of the placenta as an endocrine organ. Not until 1938, however, when Gey, Jones, and Hellman demonstrated the production of hCG by trophoblastic cells maintained in tissue culture, was the placental source of the hormone verified. The hormone was finally crystallized in 1948 by Claesson and co-workers.

The methods for assaying hCG are of considerable clinical importance, since these assays form the basis for the majority of tests for pregnancy. Unfortunately, neither the immunoassays nor bioassays commonly employed for pregnancy testing are absolutely

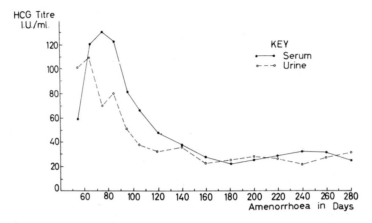

FIG. 7-1. Mean levels of serum and urine chorionic gonadotropin in 600 normally pregnant women; the technic of hemagglutination-inhibition was used. (From Teoh. *J Obstet Gynaecol Br Comm* 74:77, 1967)

specific for hCG. More recently, it was demonstrated that the hCG molecule is comprised of two specific peptide chains. The peptide chain designated as the α-chain of hCG is very similar, chemically and immunologically, to the α-chain of pituitary FSH (follicle-stimulating hormone), LH (luteinizing hormone), and thyrotropin. The similarity of the immunologic determinants in the α-chains, but not β-chains, of these various hormones accounts for their cross reactivity when immunoassay procedures are employed. Moreover, the apparent hCG activity in biologic fluids at times differed appreciably, depending upon whether immunoassay or bioassay was employed. Wide and Hobson (1967), and also Bridson and associates (1970), demonstrated that hCG synthesized in vitro by cloned choriocarcinoma cells yielded values twice as great by immunoassay as by bioassay. They suggested that the reduction in biologically active material compared with that found employing urinary hCG was the result of alterations in the hormone molecule after it was secreted by the trophoblast. Moreover, such cells may secrete the α-chain or β-chain

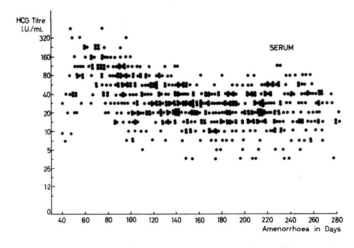

FIG. 7-2. Individual serum chorionic gonadotropin levels used to construct the curve in Figure 7-1. Note the scale along the ordinate of the graph is logarithmic. (From Teoh. *J Obstet Gynaecol Br Comm* 74:75, 1967.)

of hCG; the separate chains are biologically inactive but are recognized by antibodies. Some of the technics in current use for detecting chorionic gonadotropin are considered further in Chapter 10, page 265.

The rate of excretion of chorionic gonadotropin into the maternal urine during pregnancy gradually increases, attaining peak levels between the 60th and 70th days of gestation. Thereafter, the titer begins to fall, although more slowly than it rose, reaching a lower level between the 100th and 130th days, which is maintained throughout the remainder of pregnancy. The levels of hCG in the serum closely parallel those in the urine, rising rapidly from approximately 1 IU per ml by six weeks after the commencement of the last menstrual period to an average value of about 100 IU per ml between the 60th and 80th days after the last menstrual period (Fig. 7-1). Although most curves constructed from mean values for chorionic gonadotropin in serum or urine are quite similar, such curves do not emphasize the considerable variations in the levels of this hormone among individual women at the same duration of gestation, as demonstrated by the data presented in Figure 7-2.

Significantly higher titers of hCG are likely to be found in pregnancies with multiple fetuses, in pregnancies with a single erythroblastic fetus resulting from maternal isoimmunization, and especially in women with hydatidiform mole and choriocarcinoma. Interestingly, many nontrophoblastic tumors produce hCG, and Yoshimoto and co-workers (1979) have demonstrated that many normal tissues also secrete hCG, in small amounts. Borkowski and Muquardt (1979) found that hCG could be detected, albeit in very small amounts, in the blood of 12 of 16 blood donors who were believed to be normal men.

HUMAN PLACENTAL LACTOGEN

Human placental lactogen (hPL) is detectable in the trophoblast as early as the third week after ovulation. It was described first by Ito

and Higashi in 1961. Josimovich and MacLaren isolated the hormone in 1962 and characterized it as a polypeptide found in extracts of human placenta and retroplacental blood. Since hPL has both potent lactogenic activity and an immunochemical resemblance to human growth hormone, it was first called *human placental lactogen* or chorionic growth hormone. Later, this substance was referred to as chorionic somatomammotropin. More recently, most authors have employed the original terminology, human placental lactogen. This protein consists of a single polypeptide chain with a molecular weight of about 20,000 daltons (Li et al., 1968). Placental lactogen contains 184 amino acid residues, compared to 188 in human growth hormone; the amino acid sequence in each hormone is also quite similar. Grumbach and Kaplan (1964) found, by immunofluorescence studies, that this hormone, like hCG was concentrated in the syncytiotrophoblast.

Placental lactogen can be detected in the serum of pregnant women as early as the 6th week of gestation (or 4 weeks after fertilization). Its concentration rises steadily during the first and second trimesters and the concentration in maternal blood is approximately proportional to placental mass. The concentration of hPL in maternal serum, as measured by radioimmunoassay, reaches higher levels in late pregnancy than those of any other known protein hormone. These high levels, coupled with a very short half-life in the circulation, attest to a rate of production of hPL by the placenta of considerable magnitude, which has been estimated to be 1 to 2 g per day. Practically no hPL is found in the fetal circulation or in the urine of the mother or newborn; the concentration of the hormone in amnionic fluid is somewhat lower than that in the maternal plasma. Since hPL is secreted primarily into the maternal circulation with only very small amounts found in cord blood, it appears that the role of the hormone in pregnancy is mediated through maternal rather than fetal tissues.

Placental lactogen participates, directly or indirectly, in a number of profound metabolic actions. These include lipolysis and elevation of circulating free fatty acids, thereby providing a source of energy for maternal metabolism and fetal nutrition, and the inhibition of both the uptake of glucose and of gluconeogenesis in the mother, thereby sparing both glucose and protein (see Chap. 9, p. 231). The antiinsulin action of hPL leads normally to increased maternal levels of insulin, which favor protein synthesis and, in turn, ensures a mobilizable source of amino acids for transport to the fetus. However, the presence of the hormone does not appear to be required for a successful pregnancy outcome. Nielsen and associates (1979) have described a pregnancy in which no hPL could be identified in either maternal serum or the placenta when analyzed by several technics in a number of laboratories.

Spellacy and Buhi (1969) could not detect hPL in the early postpartum period and also noted a deficient output of pituitary growth hormone at this time. They suggested that this relative lack of insulin antagonists is associated with low fasting levels of blood glucose during this period.

Differing from hCG, the level of hPL in neoplastic trophoblastic disease is low compared to that of a normal pregnancy. However, hPL production is not restricted to the trophoblast. The hormone has been detected by direct radioimmunoassay in sera from men and women with various malignancies other than those originating in trophoblast or gonad, including bronchogenic carcinoma, hepatoma, lymphoma, and pheochromocytoma (Weintraub and Rosen, 1970).

Possible indications in clinical obstetrics for assaying hPL are considered especially in Chapter 14, page 348. A clear utility of the measurement of hPL in highrisk pregnancy has not been established.

CHORIONIC THYROTROPIN AND ADRENOCORTICOTROPIN

There is convincing evidence that the placenta produces a chorionic thyrotropin (hCT) but there is little or no evidence that this substance has significant biologic activity in

human pregnancy. The neoplastic trophoblast of hydatidiform mole and choriocarcinoma may produce a family of chorionic thyrotropins, but the increased thyroid-stimulating activity in women with neoplastic trophoblastic disease has been attributed by some chiefly to the thyroid-stimulating properties of hCG. An ACTH-like protein has also been isolated from placental tissue but sufficient evidence has not accrued yet to support the proposition that this compound is undoubtedly of placental origin or that it is chemically distinct from pituitary ACTH. There are several lines of evidence, however, which are supportive of the likelihood that ACTH is produced in chorionic tissue. Odagiri and colleagues (1979) found that ACTH, lipotropin, and β-endorphin, which are presumably derived from the same precursor molecule, are all found in placental extracts. This was an important observation since lipotropin and β-endorphin are not believed to be present normally in the circulation. Moreover, Liotta and colleagues (1977) found that ACTH may be produced by dispersed placental cells.

OTHER HORMONES

The placenta contains an appreciable amount of immunoreactive *luteinizing hormone releasing hormone* (LHRH) according to Siler-Khodr and Khodr (1978). Interestingly, these investigators also demonstrated that immunoreactive LHRH was present in the cytotrophoblast but not in the syncitiotrophoblast. Moreover, Gibbons and co-workers (1975) and Khodr and Siler-Khodr (1980) have demonstrated that the human placenta can synthesize in vitro both LHRH and *thyrotropin-releasing hormone* (TRH). The role of these releasing hormones, if indeed they arise in chorionic tissue, cannot be resolved presently. It is interesting to speculate that the finding of these substances in placental tissue is indicative that there may be a hierarchy of control of formation of chorionic trophic agents such as hCG, and chorionic thyrotropin and ACTH.

ESTROGENS

Mechanism of Estrogen Formation in Pregnancy.
The mechanism of estrogen formation in normal pregnant women differs from that in nonpregnant women. In summary:

1. The placenta is the site of origin of estrogens during human pregnancy.
2. The placenta synthesizes estrogens from externally supplied precursor hormones transported in the maternal and fetal plasma.
3. The disproportionately elevated urinary estriol levels in pregnancy result from the synthesis of estriol in the placenta, principally from the utilization of 16-hydroxy-dehydroisoandrosterone sulfate most of which arises in the fetus.

During normal human pregnancy, a hyperestrogenic state of continually increasing proportions exists that terminates abruptly after expulsion of the products of conception. The amount of estrogens produced by the normal pregnant woman near term in one day may exceed the total amount of estrogens produced by a nonpregnant, ovulatory woman in three years. Moreover, during the course of a normal pregnancy the gravid woman produces more estrogen than an ovulatory woman produces in 150 years.

There is little doubt that the site of origin of the increased amounts of estrogens is the placenta. As early as the seventh week of gestation, more than 50 percent of estrogens entering the maternal circulation are of placental origin (Siiteri and MacDonald 1965). Indeed, Diczfalusy and Borell (1961) demonstrated that urinary estrogens do not decrease following bilateral oophorectomy performed on the 78th day of pregnancy. Similar results were obtained in several studies of urinary estrogen excretion by pregnant women after surgical removal of the corpus luteum. Thus, it is evident that the ovary is not a quantitatively important source of estrogens after the first few weeks of human pregnancy.

The mechanism of estrogen formation in normal pregnant women is quite different from that in nonpregnant women. As pointed out in Chapter 3, the principal estrogen secreted by the ovary in nonpregnant women is estradiol-17β, while that of extraglandular origin is estrone, and from these two estrogens the multiple urinary estrogenic metabolites are derived. In nonpregnant women, the ratio of the concentrations of urinary estriol to that of estrone plus estradiol-17β is approximately one. During pregnancy, however, this ratio increases to ten or more near term (Brown, 1956). This disproportionate increase in estriol formation during human pregnancy results from the placental formation of estriol from 16α-hydroxydehydroisoandrosterone sulfate rather than from an alteration in the fractional conversion of estrone and estradiol-17β to estriol in mother or fetus.

The biosynthetic pathways of estrogen formation in the placenta differ considerably from those in other endocrine organs. From the results of in vitro studies, it is clear that estrogens of ovarian origin arise de novo, i.e., from acetate or cholesterol (Fig. 3-18, p. 59); however it has not been possible to demonstrate that acetate or cholesterol or even progesterone can serve as a precursor of estrogens synthesized by the placenta. The placenta appears to lack steroid 17α-hydroxylase activity, and consequently is incapable of converting C_{21}-steroids to C_{19}-steroids. Thus, progesterone is not metabolized further in the placenta. Ryan (1959), in classic experiments, demonstrated that placental tissue possessed exceptionally high capacity to convert certain C_{19}-steroids to estrone and estradiol-17β. Dehydroisoandrosterone, androstenedione, and testosterone were converted efficiently to estrone, estradiol-17β, or both, by placental preparations in vitro. These findings led to an investigation of the role of C_{19}-steroids in maternal or fetal blood as precursors for the placental biosynthesis of estrogens.

Amoroso (1960) concluded that the placenta, might, through its abundant enzymatic activity, bring about the conversion of inactive materials derived from elsewhere in the body. Support for this deduction was provided by Frandsen and Stakemann (1961) who found that women pregnant with an anencephalic fetus excreted in the urine approximately one-tenth the amount of estrogens that women pregnant with a normal fetus did at the same stage of gestation. Pointing to the characteristic absence of the fetal zone of the adrenal cortex in anencephalic fetuses, Frandsen and Stakemann postulated that the fetal adrenal was the site of origin of a substance that serves as the precursor of placental estrogen.

PLASMA-BORNE PRECURSORS. The first proof that the placenta utilizes plasma-borne precursors was provided by the demonstration that radiolabeled dehydroisoandrosterone sulfate, introduced into the maternal plasma, was converted efficiently to estrogens by the placenta (Baulieu and Dray, 1963; Siiteri and MacDonald, 1963). It was also shown that other C_{19}-steroids, namely, dehydroisoandrosterone, androstenedione, and testosterone, introduced into the maternal circulation were also converted to estrogens. The abundance of dehydroisoandrosterone sulfate in the plasma, however, and its much longer half-life uniquely qualify it as the principal circulating precursor of placental estrone and estradiol-17β. The arrival of dehydroisoandrosterone at the site of conversion as the sulfate does not preclude its utilization in the synthesis of estrogen, since the placenta normally is a rich source of sulfatase (Pulkkinen, 1961; Warren and Timberlake, 1962). By infusing isotope-labeled dehydroisoandrosterone sulfate into pregnant women, it was shown that as early as the seventh week of gestation there is readily demonstrable conversion of circulating maternal dehydroisoandrosterone sulfate to estradiol-17β. By the 30th week of pregnancy, 25 percent or more of dehydroisoandrosterone sulfate in the maternal plasma is converted to estradiol-17β by the placenta. Additionally, maternal dehydroisoandrosterone sulfate is converted ultimately to estriol

via an estrone-estradiol-17β independent pathway (MacDonald and Siiteri, 1964) to be described below. The utilization of circulating maternal dehydroisoandrosterone sulfate for placental estrogen biosynthesis undoubtedly accounts, in part, for the decrease in the concentration of dehydroisoandrosterone sulfate in the plasma of pregnant women (Migeon et al., 1955), as well as the decrease of the 11-deoxy-17-ketosteroids excreted in the urine as pregnancy advances.

In extensive studies of the metabolism of maternal plasma dehydroisoandrosterone sulfate during the course of human gestation, Gant and co-workers (1971) found that there was a striking increase in the rate of clearance of dehydroisoandrosterone sulfate from the plasma of normally pregnant women at term compared to the clearance in men and nonpregnant women. Whereas the metabolic clearance rate of dehydroisoandrosterone sulfate in nonpregnant individuals is 6 to 8 liters per 24 hours, the rate of clearance of this substance from maternal plasma of gravidas at term is increased by 10- to 20-fold. Since the maternal adrenal production rate of dehydroisoandrosterone sulfate is not significantly changed during the course of human pregnancy, the concentration in plasma will decrease with increasing rates of clearance.

The increase in clearance of dehydroisoandrosterone sulfate from the plasma of pregnant women appears to be attributable principally to two processes: (1) its removal through conversion to estradiol-17β by the trophoblasts, and (2) an increased rate of metabolism attributable to increased 16α-hydroxylation of dehydroisoandrosterone sulfate in the maternal compartment. Approximately 30 percent of dehydroisoandrosterone sulfate in the plasma of pregnant women is converted to 16α-hydroxydehydroisoandrosterone sulfate. While the extent of these conversions are high, the maternal adrenal does not produce significantly increased quantities of dehydroisoandrosterone sulfate during pregnancy; therefore, the fetal adrenal constitutes the principal source of placental estriol precursor.

PLACENTAL CLEARANCE OF DEHYDRO-ISOANDROSTERONE SULFATE. Utilizing the principle of determining the total rate of clearance of dehydroisoandrosterone sulfate and simultaneously measuring the fraction of that clearance which is uniquely the consequence of trophoblastic utilization for the formation of estradiol-17β, Gant and co-workers (1971) developed a technique for measuring the placental clearance rate of dehydroisoandrosterone sulfate through estradiol-17β formation. In normally pregnant, ambulatory women near term the placental clearance of maternal plasma dehydroisoandrosterone sulfate to estradiol-17β is approximately 25 ml per minute. On the other hand, in women whose pregnancies are complicated by pregnancy-induced hypertension, the placental clearance is markedly reduced. Employing this technique to monitor placental function, Gant and associates (1976) showed that there was a consistent decrease in placental clearance in both normal and hypertensive subjects following sodium depletion either from the ingestion of low salt diets or the administration of diuretics. Moreover, the metabolic clearance rates of dehydroisoandrosterone sulfate in young primigravid subjects who were ostensibly normal but identified as being at high risk for the development of pregnancy-induced hypertension (i.e., the onset of angiotensin II pressor sensitivity early in pregnancy), were found to have higher metabolic clearance rates of dehydroisoandrosterone sulfate than did young primigravid women who remained normal (see Chap. 27, p. 670). The results of these studies, together with those of others who found increased plasma renin levels early in pregnancy, as well as increased concentrations of estriol in women who later developed pregnancy-induced hypertension compared to those who remained normotensive, are suggestive that preeclampsia is preceded by a state of hyperplacentosis (Robertson et al., 1971).

As pregnancy advances, however, the utilization of *maternal* plasma dehydroisoandrosterone sulfate accounts for only a fraction of the estrogens produced by the placenta. The observation by Frandsen and Stakemann (1961) of lower excretion of estrogens in women pregnant with an anencephalic fetus, in whom characteristically the fetal zone of the adrenal cortex is absent, together with the finding of high levels of dehydroisoandrosterone sulfate in the cord blood of normal infants (Colás et al., 1964), were suggestive of the likelihood that precursors secreted by the fetal adrenal contributed to the synthesis of placental estrogens. Confirmation of this hypothesis was provided by the experiments of Bolté and co-workers (1964), who demonstrated that dehydroisoandrosterone sulfate introduced into the umbilical artery and perfused through the placenta in situ was converted to estrone and estradiol-17β.

While dehydroisoandrosterone sulfate circulating in both fetal and maternal plasma is utilized in the production of estrone and estradiol-17β by the placenta, an explanation was still required for the inordinately large amount of estriol found in the urine of pregnant women. The estriol present in the urine of pregnant women cannot be accounted for on the basis of metabolism of estrone and estradiol-17β. In this regard, it is important to recall that Pearlman and co-workers (1957), and Fishman and associates (1961), demonstrated that the metabolism of estradiol-17β in the pregnant woman was not significantly different from that found in non-pregnant women. Moreover, it has been impossible to demonstrate conversion of more than trace amounts of estradiol-17β to estriol in the placenta, indicating that the critical step of 16α-hydroxylation is not efficiently performed by placental tissue. Consequently, several other explanations were offered to account for the formation of estriol in pregnancy.

One of the several hypothesis held that placental estrone and estradiol-17β were circulated to the fetus and therein converted to estriol, which thereafter reentered the maternal circulation (Fishman et al., 1961; Gurpide et al., 1962). Another explanation, advanced by Bolté and co-workers (1964), held that placental estrone was converted to 16α-hydroxy-estrone by the fetus, circulated back to the placenta where reduction to estriol occurred. A third explanation required the production of a 16α-hydroxy C_{19}-steroid in the fetus or mother as a circulating precursor for placental biosynthesis of estriol. Although all three explanations are supported by data, quantitatively, the third mechanism is the most important. Ryan (1959) demonstrated that 16α-hydroxylated C_{19}-steroids such as 16α-hydroxydehydroisoandrosterone, 16α-hydroxy-Δ^4-androstenedione, and 16α-hydroxytestosterone were efficiently converted to estriol by preparations of placental tissue. In addition, large amounts of 16α-hydroxydehydroisoandrosterone sulfate are found in umbilical cord blood (Colás et al., 1964). Finally, the conversion of radiolabeled 16α-hydroxydehydroisoandrosterone and 16α-hydroxydehydroisoandrosterone sulfate, introduced into the maternal circulation, to radiolabeled estriol was demonstrated (Siiteri and MacDonald, 1964; Madden et al., 1978).

Thus, the adrenal cortices of both mother and fetus are the sites of origin of precursors of placental estrogens. In the absence of the fetal zone of the adrenal cortex, as in anencephaly, the rate of formation of placental estrogens (especially estriol) is severely limited due to the lack of precursor formation in the fetus. Verification of the diminished levels of precursors in cord blood of anencephalic monsters was provided by the finding of low levels of dehydroisoandrosterone sulfate in cord blood of such newborns (Nichols, 1958). In addition, it was shown that the total production of estrogens can be accounted for by the placental utilization of maternal plasma dehydroisoandrosterone sulfate in women 33 to 40 weeks pregnant with an anencephalic fetus (MacDonald and Siiteri, 1965). Furthermore, in such pregnancies, the production of estrogens can be increased by the administration of ACTH, which stimulates the rate of dehydroisoandrosterone sulfate secretion by the maternal adrenal. Finally, placental production of estrogens can be decreased by the administration of a potent glucocorticosteroid, which suppresses ACTH se-

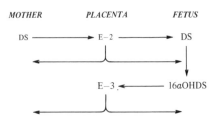

FIG. 7-3. Estrogen biosynthesis during human pregnancy. (From Worley et al. *Semin Perinat* 2:15, 1978)

cretion and thus decreases the rate of secretion of dehydroisoandrosterone sulfate from the maternal adrenal cortex (MacDonald and Siiteri, 1965).

Women with Addison's disease have decreased excretion of estrogens during pregnancy (Baulieu et al., 1956), although the decrease is principally in the urinary estrone and estradiol-17β fractions, since the fetal contribution to the synthesis of estriol, particularly in the latter part of pregnancy, is of paramount importance. Figure 7-3 is a schematic representation of the pathways of estrogen formation by the placenta.

The Fetal Adrenal. The fetal adrenal cortex assumes a major role in the biosynthesis of estrogen by the placenta. Indeed, the human fetal adrenal is a unique organ. Comparatively, the fetal adrenal is the largest organ of the fetus. Moreover, it is a unique structure in other ways. More than 85 percent of the fetal adrenal gland is composed normally of a fetal zone that is not present in the adult adrenal. At term, the weight of the fetal adrenals approximates the weight of the adrenals of the adult.

While measurements of fetal adrenal secretory activity have not been possible, it can be computed that in some fetuses the adrenals must produce 100 to 200 mg of steroids per day. Considering that the normal production of steroids by the adrenals of the nonstressed, resting, adult rarely exceeds 15 to 20 mg per day, it is apparent that the fetal adrenal is a truly remarkable endocrine organ.

Immediately after birth, the fetal adrenal cortex undergoes rapid involution and the weight of the adrenals decreases strikingly

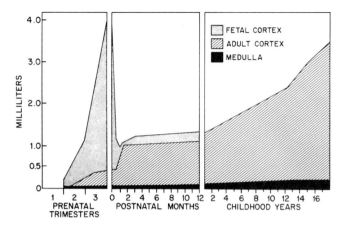

FIG. 7-4. Size of the adrenal gland and its component parts in utero, during infancy, and during childhood. (Adapted from Bethune. *The Adrenal Cortex, A Scope Monograph.* Kalamazoo, Mich., Upjohn Co, 1974)

during the first few months of life. The size attained by the fetal adrenal just prior to delivery is not achieved again until late in adolescent life (Fig. 7-4). Based on the importance of the fetal adrenal in the biogenesis of placental estrogen precursors and the potential importance of the fetal adrenal secretions in the initiation of labor and in fetal lung maturation, considerable interest and investigative efforts have been directed toward an elucidation of the factors which control the secretory activity and growth of the fetal adrenal cortex.

EARLY DEVELOPMENT. Early in embryonic life, the fetal adrenal is composed of cells that resemble the fetal zone of the adrenal cortex; these cells rapidly appear and proliferate prior to the time that vascularization of the pituitary by the hypothalamus is complete. This is suggestive that the early development of the fetal adrenal is under trophic influences which do not conform to those of the adult. Either ACTH is secreted by the fetal pituitary in the absence of hypothalamic-corticotropin-releasing factor, or ACTH arises from sources other than the fetal pituitary, e.g., chorionic ACTH synthesized by trophoblast. ACTH of maternal origin does not cross the placenta. Even in the anencephalic fetus, the fetal adrenal apparently con-

tinues to grow normally until approximately 20 weeks gestation. At this time, a progressive decrease in fetal adrenal size usually occurs in the anencephalic fetus. In the normal fetus, however, the adrenal continues to grow, and during the last 5–6 weeks of gestation an explosive rate of growth of the fetal adrenal is observed. The results of a variety of studies are suggestive that the rate of fetal adrenal growth and steroid secretion are not controlled by a single trophic stimulus but rather by a multiplicity of influences, which acting in concert, result in the peculiar development, growth rate, and steroid synthesis characteristic of the human fetal adrenal. First, there is a relative deficit in the expression of the enzyme complex 3β-hydroxysteroid dehydrogenase, $\Delta^{5,4}$-isomerase in the fetal adrenal. The absence of effective expression of this enzyme attenuates the conversion of pregnenolone to progesterone, an obligatory step in cortisol synthesis, and it also precludes the conversion of dehydroisoandrosterone to androstenedione. Serra and associates (1971) demonstrated, however, that the lack of expression of this enzyme is not because of an absence of the enzyme but rather may be the consequence of inhibition of its expression through the high levels of progesterone, and possibly estrogen as described by Bongiovanni and associates

(1967). In any event, the failure of expression of the 3β-hydroxysteroid dehydrogenase enzyme activity will decrease the capacity for cortisol biosynthesis from cholesterol and pregnenolone. This set of events sets the stage for the potential of a cycle that can be envisioned to act to control the activity and growth of the fetal adrenal.

The early growth of the fetal adrenal, prior to the development of vascular control of the pituitary by the hypothalamus, may be the consequence of the elaboration of chorionic ACTH (p. 150). The results of several studies are now suggestive that in early pregnancy an ACTH-like substance is elaborated from the placenta. If this were true, the production of chorionic ACTH would reach a nadir at about 120 to 140 days of gestation. At this time, vascularization of the pituitary via the long hypophyseal-portal vessels has been completed, and theoretically, at least, corticotropin-releasing factor from the fetal brain could now influence the release of ACTH by the fetal anterior pituitary. In the absence of adequate pituitary production of ACTH (e.g., in the anencephalic fetus), it is conceivable that the adrenal would begin to undergo involution at about 20 weeks gestation. It appears that ACTH alone, however, does not produce the total physiologic response observed in fetal adrenal growth and steroid secretion since it has been demonstrated that there is a continuing decrease in the concentration of ACTH in fetal plasma as human pregnancy advances (Winters et al., 1974).

For the reasons just cited, a second trophic agent is envisioned that will work cooperatively with ACTH to stimulate the fetal adrenal cortex in its rate of growth and steroid secretion. Many investigators have sought to identify the "second trophic stimulus" of the fetal adrenal. Every compound known to be secreted by the pituitary and each of the peptide hormones of the placenta have been considered candidates for this role. The results of recent investigations, however, are consistent with the view that an alternative explanation may be more appropriate to account for stimulation of growth and steroid excretion by the fetal adrenal.

CHOLESTEROL AS A STEROID PRECURSOR. As pointed out above, the output of steroids from the fetal adrenal is enormous. Indeed, fetal adrenal steroid hormone production requires the utilization of an amount of cholesterol equivalent to one-fourth of the daily cholesterol turnover of the adult. If the relative size of the fetus is taken into account, it can be computed that the rate of turnover of the cholesterol pool in the fetus must be six times that of the adult just to accommodate the needs of the fetal adrenal for steroidogenesis. From this analysis we believe that the more cogent question is, "What is the source of fetal adrenal steroid precursor?" rather than, "What is the alternate adrenocorticotrophic agent?" Others have proposed that progesterone and pregnenolone produced by the placenta may serve as precursors for fetal adrenal cortisol and dehydroisoandrosterone sulfate biosynthesis, respectively. The role of fetal plasma progesterone in the biosynthesis of adrenal cortisol remains to be defined. Progesterone may act on the one hand to restrict the de novo synthesis of cortisol by inhibiting the adrenal enzyme, 3β-hydroxysteroid dehydrogenase. Fetal plasma progesterone, on the other hand, may be converted to cortisol in the fetal adrenal cortex. The conversion of isotope-labeled progesterone introduced into the fetal circulation to isotope-labeled cortisol has been demonstrated. The relative importance, however, of this pathway of cortisol formation compared to that of de novo synthesis to total fetal cortisol production is unknown. It is clear, however, that the utilization of pregnenolone in the fetal circulation cannot account for more than a tiny fraction of the enormous quantity of dehydroisoandrosterone sulfate secreted by the fetal adrenals near term.

We come then to what we now consider to be a most important issue concerning fetal adrenal steroidogenesis, namely, "What is the source of cholesterol utilized in fetal adrenal steroidogenesis?" Several investigations have demonstrated that fetal adrenal tissue, in vitro, can synthesize steroid hormones. From these findings, it is clear that the fetal adrenal can also synthesize cholesterol from two carbon fragments, viz., acetate. The rate of cholesterol synthesis by fetal adrenal tissue, however, is such that this source of cholesterol can account for only a small fraction of the steroids produced by the fetal adrenals at term. Thus, the fetal adrenal must assimilate cholesterol from the fetal circulation in order to meet the demands for steroidogenesis. Circulating cholesterol and cholesterol esters are present in the form of lipoproteins. Lipoproteins are designated according to their density as determined by ultracentrifugation, e.g., very low-density lipoprotein (VLDL), low-density lipoprotein (LDL), and high-density lipoprotein (HDL). In studies employing human fibroblasts in culture, Goldstein and Brown (1974) demonstrated the presence of a specific plasma membrane receptor with high affinity for LDL. Following binding of LDL to the plasma membrane receptor, LDL is internalized by an adsorptive endocytotic process. The internalized endocytotic vesicle fuses with lysosomes and the hydrolytic enzymes of the lysosomes catalyze the hydrolysis of the protein component of LDL, which give rise to amino acids, and the hydrolysis of the cholesterol esters of LDL, which give rise to cholesterol and fatty acids.

In recent studies Goldstein and Brown, 1974; Anderson and associates, 1976; and Faust and colleagues, 1977 have shown that most nonhepatic tissues possess plasma membrane receptors for LDL. Simpson and coworkers (1979) conducted experiments designed to ascertain if human fetal adrenals utilize circulating lipoproteins as a source of cholesterol for steroidogenesis. Employing explants of human fetal adrenal tissue maintained in organ culture, they found that the presence of lipoprotein caused a marked stimulation of steroidogenesis by ACTH-treated fetal adrenal tissue. HDL was much less effective than LDL, whereas VLDL was devoid of stimulatory activity. Carr and associates (1979) also evaluated the relative contribution of cholesterol synthesized de novo and that of cholesterol derived from the uptake of LDL to fetal adrenal steroidogenesis. First, they found that the activity of the rate-limiting enzyme in de novo cholesterol synthesis in the fetal adrenal, 3-hydroxy-3-methyl glutaryl coenzyme A (HMG Co A) reductase, was sufficient to account for only a fraction of the cholesterol required for fetal adrenal steroidogenesis. Second, they demonstrated that if LDL were removed from the medium of fetal adrenal explants in organ culture, the rate of steroidogenesis decreased even in the presence of ACTH. Thus, the fetal adrenal is highly dependent upon circulating lipopro-

TABLE 7-1.

CONCENTRATIONS OF DEHYDROISOANDROSTERONE SULFATE (DHAS) AND LIPOPROTEINS IN UMBILICAL CORD PLASMA*

NEWBORN CLASSIFICATION	NUMBER OF SAMPLES	DHAS (ng/ml)	LIPOPROTEINS (MG CHOLESTEROL/DL)		
			LDL	HDL	VLDL
Normal	26	2012 ± 125†	31.1 ± 1.2	24.2 ± 1.0	2.3 ± 0.3
Mild pregnancy-induced hypertension	5	1838 ± 315	29.5 ± 3.9	27.6 ± 3.9	4.4 ± 1.9
Severe pregnancy-induced hypertension or chronic hypertension	9	1321 ± 205‡	48.6 ± 4.1§	22.4 ± 3.0	3.9 ± 1.3
Anencephaly	3	337 ± 70§	88.2 ± 6.3§	27.3 ± 8.2	Undetectable

* Expressed as lipoprotein-cholesterol levels.   ‡ P < 0.01—When compared to normal.
† All data presented as mean ± Standard error.   § P < 0.001—When compared to normal.
LDL = Low Density Lipoproteins; HDL = High Density Lipoproteins; VLDL = Very Low Density Lipoproteins.
From Parker and coworkers, in press, *Science:* 1980.

teins as a source of cholesterol for steroido-genesis. Indeed, alterations in lipoprotein cholesterol levels in cord plasma appear to be highly dependent upon the status of fetal adrenal steroid biosynthesis before birth (Table 7-1). Therefore, an important question to be addressed is the source of circulating cholesterol in the human fetus. Pitkin and co-workers (1972), from the results obtained in studies of subhuman primates, and in the study of one human pregnancy, concluded that no more than 20 percent of fetal choles-terol could be attributed to transfer from the mother. A model of cholesterol metabolism in the fetal adrenal proposed by Simpson and colleagues is presented in Figure 7-5. The low level of LDL-cholesterol in the plasma of the fetus is likely due to its rapid utilization by the fetal adrenal for steroidogenesis. As illustrated in Table 7-1, the levels of LDL-cholesterol are high in umbilical cord plasma of the anencephalic newborn in whom the adrenal is atrophic. Moreover, there is a higher level of LDL in infants of women with hypertension in whom estriol is low. More-over, there is an inverse correlation between the cord plasma levels of LDL and dehydro-isoandrosterone sulfate.

FETAL PROLACTIN AS TROPHIC STIMU-LUS. Thus, in addition to ACTH, the cho-lesterol contained in plasma lipoprotein, es-pecially LDL, appears to occupy a crucial role

in fetal adrenal steroidogenesis. Nonetheless, the likelihood that yet another trophic stimu-lus for the fetal adrenal exists is still attrac-tive. The unique pattern of fetal adrenal secre-tion, i.e., the secretion of large amounts of dehydroisoandrosterone sulfate and small amounts of cortisol is reminiscent of the ste-roid secretory patterns observed in women with virilizing adrenal adenomas.

In yet another pathophysiologic state, hy-perprolactinemia due to pituitary microade-nomas, high plasma levels of dehydroisoan-drosterone sulfate and normal levels of cortisol are observed commonly. Impor-tantly, when such women were treated with bromocriptine, dehydroisoandrosterone sul-fate levels in plasma dropped appreciably. Thus, the second hormone that appears most likely to serve a role in fetal adrenal steroido-genesis is fetal pituitary prolactin. In support of this view, it has been demonstrated that while ACTH levels in plasma decline throughout the course of gestation in the fe-tus, increasing concentrations of prolactin are observed. Indeed, the concentrations of pro-lactin during the last five weeks of pregnancy increase and are maintained at a high level during the time of maximum fetal adrenal growth (Winters et al., 1975).

Prolactin will cause cholesterol storage in some endocrine glands. ACTH, on the other hand, promotes the cleavage of the choles-terol side chain to give rise to pregnenolone.

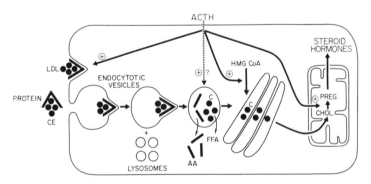

FIG. 7-5. Model proposed to describe the metabolism of low-density lipoprotein (LDL) by human fetal adrenal tissue: CE = cholesteryl esters; AA = amino acids; FFA = free fatty acids; CHOL = cholesterol; Preg = pregnenolone; HMG-CoA = 3-hydroxy-3 methyl-glutaryl coenzyme A reductase. (Courtesy of Dr. Evan R Simpson)

These two events working in concert in the face of a relative deficit in the expression of the enzyme 3β-hydroxysteroid dehydrogenase would favor the production of dehydroisoandrosterone or its sulfate by the fetal adrenal. As discussed previously, dehydroisoandrosterone sulfate of fetal adrenal origin serves, ultimately, as the principal precursor for placental estrogen production. The estrogen thus produced could serve to perpetuate the cyclicity of the dualistic trophic stimulus of the fetal adrenal. The increasing production of estrogen favors the release of prolactin by the pituitary. Most investigators, including ourselves, however, have been unable to show a direct stimulatory effect of prolactin on fetal adrenal tissue. Therefore, it appears that if prolactin has a role in fetal adrenal growth and steroidogenesis, it must be indirect, e.g., in lipoprotein synthesis or in fetal adrenal steroid sulfotransferase stimulation.

POSTNATAL CHANGES. Following birth, there is a precipitous fall in the concentration of prolactin in the newborn and a concomitant decrease in the size and in the rate of secretion of steroids by the adrenal of the newborn child.

MEASUREMENT OF URINARY OR PLASMA ESTRIOL DURING PREGNANCY AS A TEST OF FETAL WELL-BEING

Rationale. With the discovery that urine of pregnant women contained large amounts of estrogens that originated in the placenta (Aschheim and Zondek, 1927), measurements of the urinary excretion of the metabolites of these hormones have been performed in an attempt to provide an index of "placental function." Since the principal estrogen in the urine during pregnancy is estriol, most investigators have concentrated on developing reliable methods for its measurement. The discovery that the fetus plays an important role in contributing precursors for the synthesis of estriol strengthened the

possibility that abnormal pregnancies may be recognized by abnormal rates of urinary excretion of estriol.

It has long been known that fetal death is accompanied by a marked reduction in the levels of urinary estrogens. Moreover, Cassmer (1959) demonstrated that ligation of the umbilical cord with the fetus and placenta left in situ was followed by an abrupt and striking decrease in production of placental estrogens. These findings were subject to at least two interpretations, both of which are probably valid in part.

The first explanation was that maintenance of the fetal circulation is essential to the functional endocrine integrity of the placenta. This explanation was substantiated by the fact that in Cassmer's preparation the placental production of estrogens was maintained at "preligation" levels by perfusion of the placenta in situ through the fetal vessels with maternal blood after disconnecting the fetus. Further substantiation of this explanation is afforded by the demonstration that fetal death may be associated with a considerable reduction in the placental utilization of dehydroisoandrosterone sulfate circulating in the maternal plasma (Siiteri and MacDonald, 1963).

A second explanation of the marked decrease in urinary estrogens following fetal death is that there is an elimination of one source of precursors of placental estrogens: the fetus. The quantitative importance of fetal precursors of placental estriol in normal pregnancy is demonstrated amply by the low levels of urinary estriol found in pregnancies with an anancephalic fetus.

Levels of estriol in the urine of pregnant women, therefore, may be influenced not only by the biosynthetic integrity of the placenta, but also by the availability of precursors of placental estrogens, and probably by other factors as yet unknown. The clinical usefulness of these measurements as corroborative evidence of fetal death is well established, but whether a clinically useful index of placental function or evaluation of the condition of the fetus is provided by estimations of urinary estriol remains to be proved. *The clinical value of these tests can be established only by proof of increased infant salvage resulting directly from therapeutic regimens predicated upon the results of estriol measurements.* The development of this aspect of obstetric endocrinology is discussed thoroughly by Frandsen and Stakemann (1963), who reviewed the development of methods for measuring urinary estriol and described reliable procedures developed in their laboratories for the estimation of urinary estriol throughout normal human pregnancy. The range of variation in amounts of urinary estriol excreted among different normal pregnant women is great as illustrated in Figure 7-6. With reliable urine collections and accurate chemical methods, however, Frandsen found that the day-to-day variation of estriol excretion by the same woman was relatively small, four-fifths of his subjects having less than 20 percent day-to-day variation during the last 30 weeks of pregnancy.

The interpretation of "abnormal" levels of urinary estriol associated with possibly or definitely abnormal pregnancies must be made with caution and with appreciation of the following factors:

1. The wide range of normal values for excretion rates of estriol severely restricts the significance of a single measurement that falls in the "normal range" (Fig. 7-6).
2. In view of the difficulties of accurately ascertaining both duration of gestation and completeness of the collection of urine, and of eliminating technical error, a *single measurement considerably outside the "normal range" must be verified.*
3. Restriction of the supply of placental precursors of estriol, as in anencephaly or during the administraion of potent glucocorticosteroids to the mother, will result in decreased production of placental estriol, independent of placental function.
4. Factors apparently unrelated to the fetoplacental unit may be associated with decreased urinary estriol. For example, Taylor and colleagues (1963) found low levels of urinary estriol in women with acute pyelonephritis who subsequently recovered and delivered a healthy infant. Moreover, low levels of estriol are found during the ingestion of certain drugs, including certain antibiotics and even aspirin (Castellanos et al., 1975).
5. Low levels of urinary estriol have been observed that resulted from a placental deficiency of sulfatase activity (France and Liggins, 1969), a situation that would preclude the utilization of the sulfurylated precursors, dehydroisoandrosterone sulfate or 16α-hydroxydehydroisoandrosterone sulfate, for placental estrogen biosynthesis. The infants (all males to date) of these pregnancies are apparently normal but labor may not occur at term and is seemingly difficult to induce.

For these reasons, there is general agreement that a single measurement of the level of urinary estriol may not reflect reliably or accurately the status of the fetoplacental unit. Repeated measurements to confirm the results or to identify a pattern are therefore essential.

High rates of excretion of estriol occur in women with multiple fetuses and in some sensitized Rh-negative women carrying an erythroblastotic fetus (Greene and Touchstone, 1963; Taylor et al., 1963). It is also theoretically possible that women pregnant with a fetus affected by congenital adrenal hyperplasia will have elevated levels of urinary estriol as a result of the increased production of C_{19}-steroids by the affected fetal adrenal cortex.

Plasma Estriol.   In addition to the utilization of urinary estriol levels to monitor high-risk pregnancies, plasma estriol has been similarly employed for the same purpose. Generally, the results of plasma estriol measurements by a variety of techniques, as well as total plasma estrogens, have correlated well with the results of urinary estrogen determination. The advantage of utilization of plasma estriol is the ease of collection of plasma compared to 24-hour urine collections, and the avoidance of technical difficulties both in the collection and in the processing of urine.

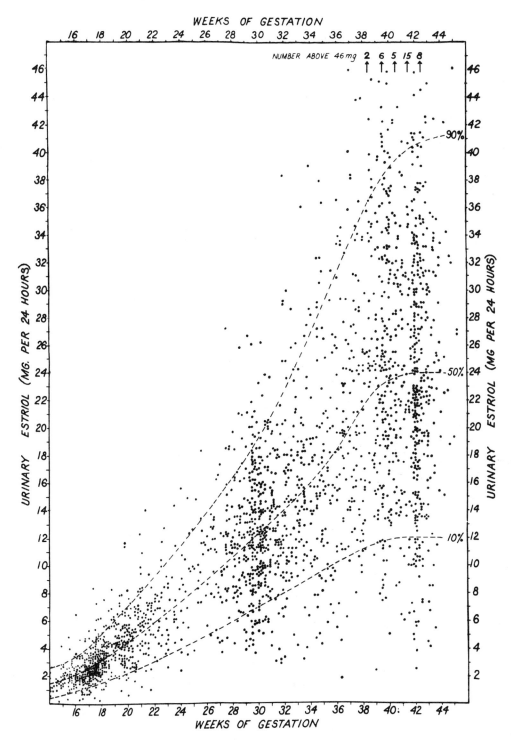

FIG. 7-6. Urinary estriol values from 14 weeks gestation showing tenth, fiftieth, and ninetieth percentiles. (From Beischer et al. *Am J Obstet Gynecol* 103:483, 1969)

Estetrol. Some interest has been focused on the possible merits of the measurement of plasma or urinary estetrol to monitor fetal well-being. Estetrol is 15α-hydroxy estriol. This compound has several features that make it unique as a metabolite of fetal metabolic function. First, it is derived principally from estriol, which itself is attributable primarily to production from fetal precursors, and, moreover, estetrol is produced almost exclusively in the fetus. The 15α-hydroxylation capability resident in the fetus and requisite for formation of estetrol is not demonstrable in the maternal compartment. Thus, estetrol represents a compound whose production relies principally upon fetal precursors and upon fetal metabolism for its finite and final formation. However, to date, the results reported are not supportive of the view that the measurement of estetrol has an advantage over that of estriol determinations in the monitoring of high-risk pregnancy.

Clinical Utility. One of the greatest problems in obstetric management today is the proper timing of delivery when complications threaten the life and well-being of the fetus. The difficult but common problem is to choose between prematurity and the high fetal risk of continued intrauterine existence. In such situations, notably diabetes, pregnancy-induced or chronic hypertension, poor previous obstetric history, fetal growth retardation, suspected postmaturity and others the need for an accurate index of fetal well-being is urgent. The results of future studies may substantiate the value of measurements of urinary or plasma estriol (or estetrol) as a guide to obstetric management in these difficult situations. Barnes (1965) emphasized that there is little evidence that therapy based on levels of urinary estriol increased the rate of infant salvage beyond that accomplished by sound clinical judgment alone. Moreover, the results of the only prospective, controlled study reported to date were suggestive that the measurement of estriol has little or no clinical utility in reducing perinatal mortality or morbidity (Duenhoelter et al., 1976). Specifi-

cally, the results of this study were supportive of the proposition that expert clinical management offers the greatest potential to date for the reduction of perinatal mortality and morbidity and that the measurement of hormones produced by the placenta offers no unique insight into a complicated pregnancy in which the fetus is at high risk.

For these reasons, we do not employ estriol measurements in the management of pregnancies in which the fetus is considered to be at risk. In a recent study of pregnancies complicated by mild chronic hypertension, Arias and Zamora (1979) also found that estriol measurements were of no utility in the management of such complicated pregnancies. Similarly, Schneider and associates (1978) concluded that 24-hour urinary estriol excretion measured 3 times per week were of no value in management of postterm pregnancies.

Other investigators who do employ estriol measurements in obstetric management generally agree that the level of estriol does not always reflect accurately the well-being of the fetus. Hagerman (1979), for example, has written, "It seems likely that the greatest value of the test (plasma estriol) resides in the predictive value of a negative result, which can provide a modest degree of reassurance that the status of the infant is satisfactory. No laboratory test is perfect, and this one is less informative than some. Nevertheless, it is probably as good as, or better than, many other tests used in this area of clinical medicine. The overall classification of correct results with an efficiency of 59 percent is satisfactory. The false-negative rate is disappointingly high." His comments serve to emphasize the need for better tests rather than the perpetuation of some of those that have been commonly used in recent years even though they are, in fact, of little predictive value.

PROGESTERONE

Site of Production. The production of progesterone is accomplished by the placental

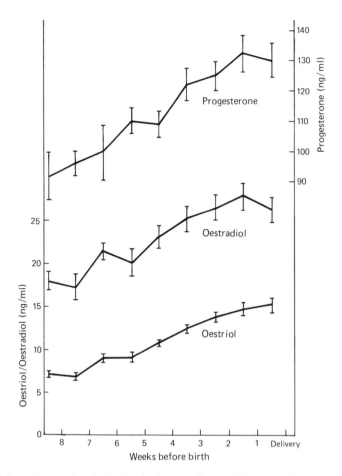

FIG. 7-7. Mean plasma levels (±standard error of mean) for progesterone, unconjugated estradiol-17β, and unconjugated estriol in 33 normal pregnant women during the last 9 weeks before delivery. (From Tungsubutra and France. *Aust NZ J Obstet Gynaecol*, 18:97, 1978)

utilization of maternal lipoprotein cholesteryl esters. Although much more progesterone than estrogen is produced during normal human pregnancy, relatively much less was known about its biosynthesis until very recently. The placenta produces large amounts of progesterone during pregnancy, and as documented in the review of Diczfalusy and Troen (1961), a relatively small fraction of the total production of progesterone takes place in the ovary after the first few weeks of gestation. Surgical removal of the corpus luteum or even bilateral oophorectomy performed during the seventh to tenth weeks of gestation does not result in a decrease in the rate of urinary excretion of pregnanediol, the principal metabolite of progesterone. During normal human pregnancy there is a gradual increase in the levels of plasma progesterone as well as those of estradiol-17β and estriol, as shown in Figure 7-7.

Production Rate.   Isotope dilution technics for the measurement of endogenous rates of hormonal secretion were first applied to the study of progesterone secretion in pregnancy. The results of these studies, performed by Pearlman in 1957, were indicative that the daily production of progesterone in late pregnancy was about 250 mg. The results of studies in which other methods have been employed are in agreement with that figure.

Source of Cholesterol Precursor for Progesterone Biosynthesis.

The biosynthetic origin of placental progesterone was an enigma until very recently. Solomon and colleagues (1954) demonstrated that in vitro perfusion of the placenta with radiolabeled cholesterol resulted in the formation of radiolabeled progesterone. In addition, incubation of Δ^5-pregnenolone with placental tissue preparations also resulted in the formation of progesterone; and an exceedingly great capacity of the placenta to convert Δ^5-pregnenolone to progesterone has been demonstrated by in situ placental perfusion studies conducted in Diczfalusy's laboratories.

While the placenta produces a prodigious amount of progesterone, this organ has a very limited capacity for the biosynthesis of cholesterol. The rate of incorporation of radiolabeled acetate into cholesterol by placental tissue procedes very slowly and the activity of the rate-limiting enzyme in cholesterol biosynthesis, viz., 3-hydroxy-3 methylglutaryl coenzyme A (HMG-Co A) reductase, in placental tissue microsomes is limited.

By in vivo studies, Bloch (1945) and Werbin and co-workers (1957) demonstrated that after the intravenous administration of isotope-labeled cholesterol to pregnant women the specific activity of urinary pregnanediol was similar to that of plasma cholesterol. Hellig and associates (1970) also demonstrated that maternal plasma cholesterol was the principal precursor (up to 90 percent) of progesterone biosynthesis in human pregnancy.

Role of Lipoprotein Cholesterol.

In studies similar to those described employing fetal adrenal tissue, Simpson and associates (1979) have shown that the placenta preferentially utilizes lipoprotein cholesterol for progesterone biosynthesis. Thus, production of placental progesterone, like that of placental estrogens, occurs through the utilization of circulating precursors; but unlike estriol, which is formed principally from the utilization of fetal adrenal precursors, placental progesterone biosynthesis procedes through the utilization of a maternal precursor which is taken up in the form of lipoprotein cholesterol.

These findings not only provide new insights into the biochemical mechanisms of placental progesterone formation, but may also provide clues to other aspects of maternal-placental-fetal physiology:

First, the rate of progesterone secretion may be largely dependent on the number of low-density lipoprotein receptors on the plasma membrane of the trophoblasts and primarily independent of uteroplacental blood flow. This obtains for several reasons:

1. Cholesterol side-chain cleavage by placental mitochondria is continually in a highly activated state. Some investigators have taken this to mean that the placenta is under constant trophic stimulation and that hCG may be the trophic substance. Indeed, a hierarchy of control of placental hormone production was suggested from the finding of immunoreactive LHRH in placental tissue (Siler-Khodr and Khodr, 1978).
2. De novo cholesterol synthesis by the placenta is very limited.
3. The fetus contributes little or no precursors for placental progesterone biosynthesis.
4. Maternal levels of LDL-cholesterol should never be rate-limiting in the placental assimilation of cholesterol from the maternal circulation.

Second, the metabolism of LDL by the trophoblasts will result in the hydrolysis of LDL protein and cholesteryl esters. The hydrolysis of the protein of LDL gives rise to amino acids, many of which are essential amino acids. The hydrolysis of cholesterol esters gives rise to cholesterol, which is utilized for progesterone biosynthesis, and to fatty acids. The principal fatty acid of LDL cholesteryl esters is linoleic acid, an essential fatty acid. It seems reasonable to speculate, therefore, that the metabolism of LDL by the trophoblasts constitutes a means of obtaining cholesterol for placental progesterone biosynthesis and a mechanism for sequestering essential fatty acids and amino acids for transport to the fetus. Interestingly, Simpson and Burkhardt (1979) also found that progesterone, in concentrations similar to those found in placental tissue, inhibits the activity of the enzyme that catalyzes the esterification of cholesterol. It can be envisioned that this physiologic event will serve to ensure a supply of cholesterol for progesterone biosynthesis by preventing the sequestration of cholesterol into an inappropriate storage form, viz, cholesteryl esters, and to protect essential fatty acids from reesterification with cholesterol.

The intimate relationships that exist between the fetus and placenta in the production of estrogen cannot be demonstrated in the case of progesterone. Fetal death, ligation of the umbilical cord in situ, and anencephaly are all associated with very low maternal urinary excretion of estrogens, but a concomitant decrease in excretion of pregnanediol to anywhere near the same extent does not occur in these situations.

REFERENCES

Anderson RGN, Goldstein JL, Brown MS: Localization of low-density lipoprotein receptors on plasma membranes of normal human fibroblasts and their absence in cells from a familial hypercholesterolemia homozygote. Proc Natl Acad Sci USA 73:2434, 1976

Amoroso EC: Comparative aspects of the hormonal functions. In Villee CA (ed): The Placenta and Fetal Membranes. Baltimore, Williams and Wilkins, 1960, p 3

Arias F, Zamora J: Antihypertensive treatment and pregnancy outcome in patients with mild chronic hypertension. Obstet Gynecol 53:489, 1978

Ascheim S, Zondek B: (Anterior pituitary hormone and ovarian hormone in the urine of pregnant women). Klin Wochensehr 6:248, 1927

Barnes AC: Discussion of paper by JW Greene. Am J Obstet Gynecol 91:688, 1965

Baulieu EE, Bricaire H, Jayle MF: Lack of secretion of 17-hydroxycorticosteroids in a pregnant woman with Addison's disease. J Clin Endocrinol 16:690, 1956

Baulieu EE, Dray F: Conversion of H³ dehydroisoandrosterone (3β-hydroxy-Δ⁵-androsten-17-one) sulfate to H³-estrogens in normal pregnant women. J Clin Endocrinol 23:1298, 1963

Beischer NA, Brown JB, Smith MA, Townsend L: Studies in prolonged pregnancy. II. Clinical Results and Urinary Excretion in Prolonged Pregnancy. Am J Obstet Gynecol 103:483, 1969

Bloch K: The biological conversion of cholesterol to pregnanediol. J Biol Chem 157:661, 1945

Bolté E, Mancuso S, Eriksson G, Wiqvist N, Diczfalusy E: Studies on the aromatisation of neutral steroids in pregnant women: 1. Aromatisation of C-19 steroids by placentas perfused in situ. Acta Endocrinol 35:535, 1964a

Bolté E, Mancuso S, Eriksson G, Wiqvist N, Diczfalusy E: Studies on the aromatisation of neutral steroids in pregnant women: 2. Aromatisation of dehydroisoandrosterone and of its sulphate administered simultaneously into a uterine artery. Acta Endocrinol 45:560, 1964b

Bolté E, Mancuso S, Eriksson G, Wiqvist N, Diczfalusy E: Studies on the aromatisation of neutral steroids in pregnant women: 3. Over-all aromatization of dehydroisoandrosterone sulfate circulating in the foetal and maternal compartments. Acta Endocrinol 45:576, 1964c

Bongiovanni AM, Eberlein WR, Goldman AS, New M: Disorders of adrenal steroid biogenesis. Recent Progr Horm Res 23:375, 1967

Borkowski A, Maquardt C: Human chorionic gonadotropin in the plasma of normal, nonpregnant subjects. N Engl J Med 301:298, 1979

Bridson WE, Ross GT, Kohler PO: Immunologic and biologic activity of chorionic gonadotropin synthesized by cloned choriocarcinoma cells in tissue culture. Clin Res 18:356, 1970

Brown JB: Urinary excretion of oestrogens during pregnancy, lactation, and the reestablishment of menstruation. Lancet 1:704, 1956

Carr BR, Parker CR Jr, Milewich L, Porter JC, MacDonald PC, Simpson ER: Effect of various lipoproteins on steroidogenesis by human fetal adrenal (HFA) tissue. 26th Annual Meeting Society of Gynecological Investigation, 1979, p 141

Cassmer O: Hormone production of the isolated human placenta. Acta Endocrinol 32(Suppl): 45, 1959

Castellanos JM, Aranda M, Cararach J, Cararach V: Effect of aspirin on oestriol excretion in pregnancy. Lancet 1:859, 1975

Claesson L, Högberg B, Rosenberg T, Westman A: Crystalline human chorionic gonadotrophin and its biological action. Acta Endocrinol 1:1, 1948

Colás A, Heinrichs WL, Tatum HJ: Pettenkofer chromogens in the maternal and fetal circulations: detection of 3β, 16α-dihydroxyandrost-5-en-17-one in umbilical cord blood. Steroids 3:417, 1964

Diczfalusy E, Borell U: Influence of oophorectomy on steroid excretion in early pregnancy. J Clin Endocrinol 21:1119, 1961

Diczfalusy E, Troen P: Endocrine functions of the human placenta. Vit Horm 19:229, 1961

Duenhoelter JH, Whalley PJ, MacDonald PC: An analysis of the utility of plasma immunorectine estrogen measurements in determining delivery time of gravidas with a fetus considered at high risk. Am J Obstet Gynecol 125:889, 1976

Faust JR, Goldstein JL, Brown MS: Receptor-mediated uptake of low density lipoprotein and utilization of its cholesterol for steroid synthesis in cultured mouse adrenal cells. J Biol Chem 252:4861, 1977

Fishman J, Brown JB, Hellman L, Zumoff B, Gallagher TF, Estrogen metabolism in normal and pregnant woman. J Biol Chem 237:1489, 1961

France JT, Liggins GC: Placental sulfatase deficiency. J Clin Endocrinol 29:138, 1969.

Frandsen VA, Stakemann G: The site of production of oestrogenic hormones in human pregnancy: hormone excretion in pregnancy with anencephalic foetus. Acta Endocrinol 38:383, 1961

Frandsen VA, Stakemann G: The urinary excretion of oestriol during the early months of pregnancy. Acta Endocrinol 44:196, 1963

Gant NF, Hutchinson HT, Siiteri PK, MacDonald PC: Study of the metabolic clearance rate of dehydroisoandrosterone sulfate in pregnancy. Am J Obstet Gynecol 111:4:555, 1971

Gant NF, Madden JD, Siiteri PK, MacDonald PC: The metabolic clearance rate of dehydro-isoandrosterone sulfate. IV. Acute effects of induced hypertension, hypotension, and naturesis in normal and hypertensive pregnancies. Am J Obstet Gynecol 124:143, 1976

Gey GO, Jones GES, Hellman LM: The production of a gonadotrophic substance (prolan) by placental cells in tissue culture. Science 88:306, 1938

Gibbons JM, Mitnick M, Chieffo V: In vitro biosynthesis of TSH- and LH-releasing factors by human placenta. Am J Obstet Gynecol 121:127, 1975

Goldstein JL, Brown MS: Binding and degradation of low density lipoproteins by cultured human fibroblasts. J Biol Chem 249:5153, 1974

Greene, JW, Touchstone JC: Urinary estriol as an index of placental function. Am J Obstet Gynecol 85:1, 1963

Grumbach MM, Kaplan SL: On placental origin and purification of chorionic growth hormone-prolactin and its immunoassay in pregnancy. Trans NY Acad Sci 27:167, 1964

Gurpide E, Angers M, Vande Wiele R, Lieberman S: Determination of secretory rates of estrogens in pregnant and nonpregnant women from the specific activities of urinary metabolites. J Clin Endocrinol 22:935, 1962

Hagerman DD: Clinical use of plasma total estriol measurements late in pregnancy. J Reproduct Med 23:179, 1979

Hellig HD, Gattereau D, Lefevre Y, Bolté E: Steroid production from plasma cholesterol: I. Conversion of plasma cholesterol to placental progesterone in humans. J Clin Endocrinol 30:624, 1970

Ito Y, Higashi K: Studies on prolactin-like substance in human placenta. II: Endocrinol Jap 8:279, 1961

Josimovich JB, MacLaren JA: Presence in human placenta and term serum of highly lactogenic substance immunologically related in pituitary growth hormone. Endocrinology 71:209, 1962

Khodr GS, Siler-Khodr TM: Placental luteinizing hormone-releasing factor and its synthesis. Science 207:315, 1980

Li CH, Grumbach MM, Kaplan SL, Josimovich JB, Friesen H, Cati KG: Human chorionic somatomammotropin (HCS), proposed terminology for designation of a placental hormone. Experientia 24:1288, 1968

Liotta A, Osathanondh R, Ryan KJ, Krieger DT: Presence of Corticotropin in human placenta: Demonstration of in vitro synthesis. Endocrinology 101:1552, 1977

MacDonald PC, Siiteri PK: Utilization of circulating dehydroisoandrosterone sulfate for estrogen synthesis during human pregnancy (abstract). Clin Res 12:67, 1964

MacDonald PC, Siiteri PK: The conversion of isotope-labeled dehydroisoandrosterone and dehydroisoandrosterone sulfate to estrogen in normal and abnormal pregnancy. In Paulsen CA (ed): Estrogen Assays in Clinical Medicine. Seattle, University of Washington Press, 1965, p 251

MacDonald PC, Siiteri PK: Origin of estrogen in women pregnant with an anencephalic fetus. J Clin Invest 44:465, 1965

Madden JD, Gant NF, MacDonald PC: Studies of the kinetics of conversion of maternal plasma dehydroisoandrosterone sulfate to 16α-hydroxydehydroisoandrosterone sulfate, estradiol and estriol. Am J Obstet Gynecol 132:392, 1978

Migeon CJ, Keller AR, Holmstrom EG: Dehydroisoandrosterone, androsterone and 17-hydroxycorticosteroid levels in maternal and cord plasma in cases of vaginal delivery. Bull Johns Hopkins Hosp 97:415, 1955

Nichols J, Lescure OL, Migeon CJ: Levels of 17-hydroxycorticosteroids and 17-ketosteroids in maternal and cord plasma in term anencephaly. J Clin Endocrinol 18:444, 1958

Nielsen PV, Pedersen H, Kampmann E-M: Absence of human placental lactogen in an otherwise uneventful pregnancy. Am J Obstet Gynecol 135:322, 1979

Odagiri E, Sherrill BJ, Mount CD, Nicholson WE, Orth DN: Human placental immunoreactive corticotropin, lipotropin, and β-endorphin. Evidence for a common precursor. Proc Natl Acad Sci USA 16:2027, 1979

Parker RC Jr, Simpson ER, Bilheimer DW, Leveno KJ, Carr BR, MacDonald PC: Inverse relation between low-density lipoprotein-cholesterol and dehydroisoandrosterone sulfate in human fetal plasma. Science 208:512, 1980

Pearlman WH: (16-³H) Progesterone metabolism in advanced pregnancy and in oophorectomized-hysterectomized women. Biochem J 67:1, 1957

Pitkin RM, Connor WE, Lin DS: Cholesterol metabolism and placental transfer in the pregnant rhesus monkey. J Clin Invest 51:2584, 1972

Pulkkinen MO: Arylsulphatase and the hydrolysis of some steroid sulphates in developing organism and placenta. Acta Physiol Scand 52, Suppl 180, 1961

Robertson JIS, Weir RJ, Düsterdieck GO, Fraser R, Tree M: Renin angiotensin and aldosterone in human pregnancy and the menstrual cycle. Scot Med J 16:183, 1971

Ryan KJ: Metabolism of C-16-oxygenated steroids by human placenta: The formation of estriol. J Biol Chem 234:2006, 1959

Schneider JM, Olson RW, Curet LB: Screening for fetal and neonatal risk in the postdate pregnancy. Am J Obstet Gynecol 131:473, 1978

Serra GB, Perez-Palacios G, Jaffe RB: Enhancement of 3β-hydroxysteroid dehydrogenase-isomerase in the human fetal adrenal by removal of the soluble cell fraction. Biochem Biophys Acta 244:186, 1971

Siler-Khodr TM, Khodr GS: Content of luteinizing hormone-releasing factor. Am J Obstet Gynecol 130:216, 1978

Siiteri PK, MacDonald PC: The utilization of circulating dehydroisoandrosterone sulfate for estrogen synthesis during human pregnancy. Steroids 2:713, 1963

Siiteri PK, MacDonald PC: The biogenesis of urinary estriol during human pregnancy (abstract). Clin Res 12:44, 1964

Siiteri PK, MacDonald PC: Estrogen biosynthesis during human pregnancy. Federation Proceedings 24:384, 1965

Simpson ER, Burkhart M: ACYL COA: Cholesterol ACYL. Transferase activity in human placental microsomes: Inhibition by progesterone. Arch Biochem Biophy, in press, 1980

Simpson ER, Carr BR: Metabolism of serum lipoproteins by the human fetal adrenal. Proceedings of the 61st Annual Meeting of the Endocrine Society, 1979, p 218

Simpson ER, Carr BR, Parker CR, Milewich L, Porter JC, MacDonald PC: The role of serum lipoproteins in steroidogenesis by the human fetal adrenal cortex. J Clin Endocrinol Metab, 1979, in press

Solomon S, Lentz AL, VandeWiele RL, Lieberman S: Pregnenolone an intermediate in the biogenesis of progesterone and the adrenal hormones. Proc Am Chem Soc abstract 29C, 1954

Spellacy WN, Buhi WC: Pituitary growth hormone and placental lactogen levels measured in normal term pregnancy and at the early and late postpartum periods. Am J Obstet Gynecol 105:888, 1969

Taylor ES, Hassner A, Bruns PD, Drose VE: Urinary estriol excretion of pregnant patients with pyelonephritis and Rh isoimmunization. Am J Obstet Gynecol 85:10, 1963

Warren JC, Timberlake CE: Steroid sulfatase in the human placenta. J Clin Endocrinol 22:1148, 1962

Weintraub D, Rosen SW: Ectopic production of human chorionic somatomammotropin (HCS) in patients with cancer. Clin Res 18:375, 1970

Werbin H, Plotz EJ, LeRoy GV, David ME: Cholesterol: a precursor of estrone in vivo. J Am Chem Soc 79:1012, 1957

Wide L, Hobson B: Immunological and biological activity of human chorionic gonadotropin in urine and serum of pregnant women and women with a hydatidiform mole. Acta Endocrinol 54:105, 1967

Winters AJ, Colston C, MacDonald PC, Porter JC: Fetal plasma prolactin levels. J Clin Endocrinol Metab 41:626, 1975

Winters AJ, Oliver C, Colston C, MacDonald PC, Porter JC: Plasma ACTH levels in the human fetus and neonate as related to age and parturition. J Clin Endocr Metab 39:269, 1974

Worley RJ, Everett RB, Madden JD, MacDonald PC, and Gant NF: Fetal Considerations. Metabolic clearance rate of maternal plasma dehydroisoandrosterone sulfate. Seminars in Perinatology, 2:15, 1978

Yoshimoto Y, Wolfsen AR, Hirose F, Odell WD: Human chorionic gonadotropin-like material: Presence in normal human tissues. Am J Obstet Gynecol 134:729, 1979

8

The Morphologic and Functional Development of the Fetus

Since World War II, and especially in the last two decades, knowledge of fetal development, function and environment has increased remarkably. As an important consequence, the fetus has acquired the status of a patient who should be given the same care by the physician that we have long given the pregnant woman. Investigations of human life in utero have been and will continue to be among the most rewarding in all of biology, and they are of great clinical importance. This chapter considers the development of the normal fetus. Technics for identifying fetal well-being, or fetal health, are emphasized in Chapter 14. Anomalies, injuries, and diseases that affect the fetus and newborn infant are considered in Chapters 37, 38, and 39.

The Fetus at Various Times in Pregnancy. The different terms commonly used to indicate the duration of pregnancy and fetal age are somewhat confusing. *Menstrual age* or *gestational age* commences on the first day of the last menstrual period at a time before conception, or about 2 weeks before ovulation and fertilization, or nearly 3 weeks before implantation of the fertilized ovum. About 280 days, or 40 weeks, elapse, on the

average, between the first day of the last menstrual period and delivery of the infant; 280 days correspond to 9⅓ calendar months, or 10 units of 28 days each. The unit of 28 days has been referred to commonly but imprecisely as a lunar month of pregnancy; the time from one new moon to the next is actually 29½ days.

It is the usual practice for the obstetrician to calculate the gestational age on the basis of menstrual age. Embryologists, however, cite events in days or weeks from the time of ovulation *(ovulation age)* or conception *(conception age)*, the latter two being nearly identical. Occasionally, it is of some value to divide the period of gestation into three units of three calendar months each, or three *trimesters,* since some important obstetric events may be categorized conveniently by trimesters. The possibility of spontaneous abortion, for example, is limited principally to the first trimester of pregnancy, whereas the likelihood of survival of the prematurely born infant is confined, with few exceptions, to pregnancies that reach the third trimester.

The following short description of various periods of development of the ovum and embryo is included. For a more detailed description, based on Streeter's (1920) timetables of human development ("Horizons"), the reader is referred to the text by Hamilton and Mossman (1972).

THE OVUM. During the first 2 weeks after ovulation, the products of conception usually are designated as the ovum, even though the ovum has been fertilized. The successive phases of development during this period are as follows: (1) ovulation, (2) fertilization of the ovum, (3) formation of free blastocyst (the events of the first week after ovulation are illustrated diagramatically in Figure 8-1), and (4) implantation of blastocyst, which starts at the end of the first week after ovulation. Primitive chorionic villi begin to form after implantation. It is conventional to refer to the products of conception after the development of chorionic villi not as a fertilized ovum but as an embryo. The early stages of preplacental development are

discussed in Chapter 5, and the formation of the placenta in Chapter 6.

THE EMBRYO. The beginning of the embryonic period is taken as the beginning of the 3rd week after ovulation, or the 5th week after the onset of the last menstrual period, and coincides in time with the expected time of menstruation. Most pregnancy tests in clinical use are usually positive by this time (see Chap. 10, p. 265). The embryonic disc is well-defined and the body stalk is diferentiated. At this stage, the chorionic sac measures approximately 1 cm in diameter (Figs. 8-2 and 8-3). The chorionic villi at this time are distributed equally around the circumference of the chorionic sac. There is a true intervillous space containing maternal blood and villous cores with angioblastic chorionic mesoderm.

By the end of the 4th week *after ovulation,* the chorionic sac measures 2 to 3 cm in diam-

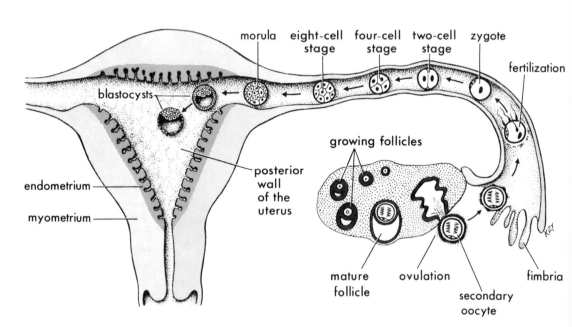

FIG. 8-1. Diagrammatic summary of the ovarian cycle, fertilization, and human development during the first week. Developmental stage 1 begins with fertilization and ends when the zygote forms. Stage 2 (days 2 to 3) comprises the early stages of cleavage (from 2 to about 16 cells or the morula). Stage 3 (days 4 to 5) consists of the free unattached blastocyst. Stage 4 (days 5 to 6) is represented by the blastocyst attaching to the center of the posterior wall of the uterus, the usual site of implantation. (From Moore. *The Developing Human,* 2nd ed. Philadelphia, Saunders, 1977)

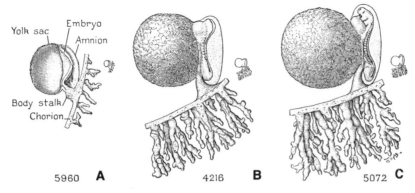

FIG. 8-2. Early human embryos. Only the chorion adjacent to the body stalk is shown. Small outline to right of each embryo gives its actual size. Ovulation ages: **A.** Carnegie collection (presomite), 19 days. **B.** (7 somites), 21 days. **C.** (17 somites), 22 days. (After drawings and models in the Carnegie Institution)

eter, and the embryo about 4 to 5 mm in length (Fig. 8-4). The heart and pericardium are very prominent because of the dilatation of the chambers of the heart. Arm and leg buds are present, and the amnion is beginning to ensheath the body stalk, which becomes the umbilical cord.

At the end of the 6th week from the time of ovulation, or about 8 weeks after the onset of the last menstrual period, the embryo measures 22 to 24 mm in length, and the head is quite large compared with the trunk. Fingers and toes are present, and the external ears form definitive elevations on either side of the head.

The end of the embryonic period and the beginning of the fetal period are arbitrarily considered by most embryologists to occur 8 weeks after ovulation, or 10 weeks after the last menstrual period. At this time, the embryo measures nearly 4 cm. Few, if any, new major structures are formed thereafter; development during the fetal period consists of growth and maturation of structures formed during the embryonic period.

3 LUNAR MONTHS. By the end of the 12th week by menstrual age, or 10 weeks since ovulation, the crown-rump length of the fetus is 6 to 7 cm in length (Fig. 8-5.

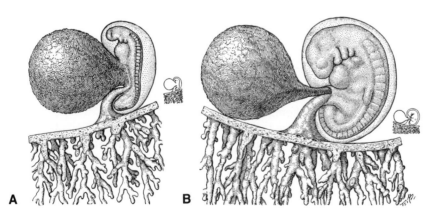

FIG. 8-3. Early human embryos. Small outline to right of each embryo gives its actual size. Ovulation ages: **A.** 22 days. **B.** 23 days. (After drawings and models in the Carnegie Institution)

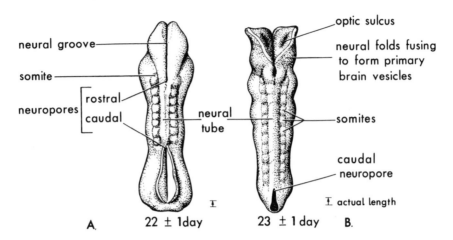

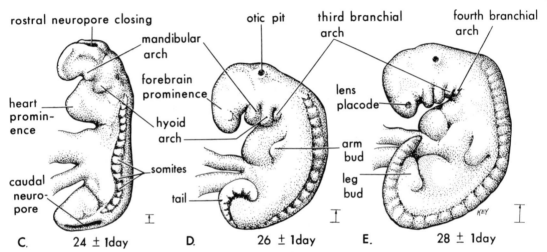

FIG. 8-4. Three to four-week embryos. **A** and **B.** dorsal views of embryos during stage 10 of development (about 22 to 23 days) showing 8 and 12 somites, respectively. **C, D,** and **E.** lateral views of embryos during stages 11, 12, and 13 of development (24 to 28 days) showing 16, 27, and 33 somites, respectively. (From Moore. *The Developing Human,* 2nd ed. Philadelphia, Saunders, 1977)

A and B), and the uterus usually is just palpable above the symphysis pubis. Centers of ossification have appeared in most bones; the fingers and toes have become differentiated and are provided with nails; scattered rudiments of hair appear; the external genitalia are beginning to show definite signs of male or female sex. A fetus born at this time may make spontaneous movements if still within the amnionic sac or if immersed in warm saline.

4 **LUNAR MONTHS.** By the end of the 16th week by menstrual age, the crown-rump length of the fetus is 12 cm, and it weighs about 110 g. By careful examination of the external genital organs the sex of the fetus can be determined.

5 **LUNAR MONTHS.** The end of the 5th lunar month, or the end of the 20th week, is the midpoint of pregnancy if gestation is calculated from the time of the last normal menstrual period. The fetus now weighs somewhat more than 300 g. The skin has become less transparent, and a downy lanugo covers its entire body, while some scalp hair is evident.

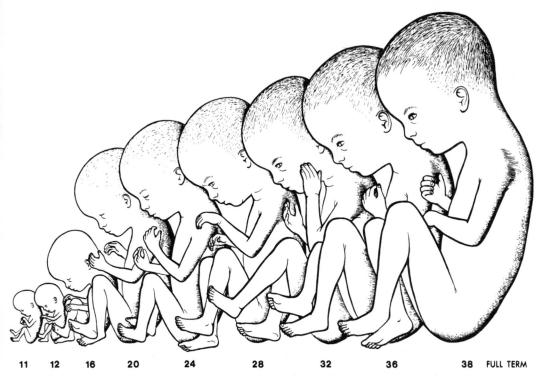

FIG. 8-5. A. The embryonic period ends at the end of the 8th week after fertilization; by this time, the beginnings of all essential structures are present. The fetal period, extending from the 9th week until birth, is characterized by growth and elaboration of structures. Sex is clearly distinguishable by 12 weeks. The above 11- to 38-week fetuses (13- to 40-week menstrual age) are about half actual size. (From Moore. *The Developing Human,* 2nd ed. Philadelphia, Saunders, 1977)

6 LUNAR MONTHS. By the end of the 24th week, the fetus now weighs about 630 g. The skin is characteristically wrinkled, and fat is being deposited beneath it. The head is comparatively quite large; eyebrows and eyelashes are usually recognizable. A fetus born at this period will attempt to breathe but practically always dies shortly after birth.

7 LUNAR MONTHS. By the end of the 28th week after the onset of the last menstrual period, the fetus has attained a crown-rump length of about 25 cm and weighs about 1100 g. The thin skin is red and covered with vernix caseosa. The pupillary membrane has just disappeared from the eyes. An infant born at this period moves his limbs quite energetically and cries weakly. The infant, with expert care, may survive.

8 LUNAR MONTHS. At the end of the 8th lunar month, or 32 weeks, the fetus has attained a crown-rump length of about 28 cm and a weight of about 1800 g. The surface of the skin is still red and wrinkled. Infants born at this period usually survive with proper care.

9 LUNAR MONTHS. At the end of 36 weeks the average crown-rump length of the fetus is about 32 cm long and weighs about 2500 g. Because of the deposition of subcutaneous fat, the body has become more rotund and the face has lost its previous wrinkled appearance. Infants born at this time have an excellent chance of survival if given proper care.

10 LUNAR MONTHS. Term is reached at 10 lunar months, or 40 weeks after the last menstrual period. At this time the fetus

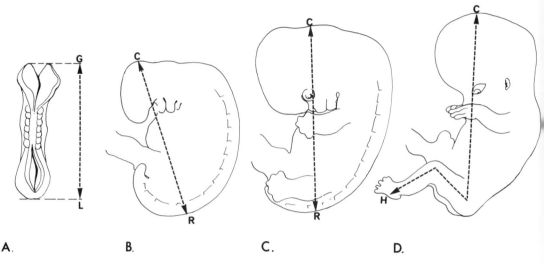

A.   B.   C.   D.

FIG. 8-5. B. Sketches showing methods of measuring the length of embryos. **A.** Greatest length. **B** and **C.** Crown-rump length. **D.** Crown-heel length. (From Moore. *The Developing Human,* 2nd ed. Philadelphia, Saunders, 1977)

is fully developed, with the characteristic features of the newborn infant to be described here. The average crown-rump length of the fetus at term is about 36 cm, and weighs approximately 3400 g with the variations to be discussed subsequently.

Length of Fetus. Because of the variability in the length of the legs and the difficulty of maintaining them in extension, measurement of the sitting height (crown to rump) is more accurate than that of the standing height (Fig. 8-5.B). The average sitting height and weight of the fetus at the end of the various lunar months were ascertained by Streeter (1920) from 704 specimens and still are similar to those found more recently as shown in Table 8-1. Such values are approximate, and generally the length is a more accurate criterion of the age of a fetus than is the weight.

Haase (1875) suggested that for clinical purposes the length in cm of the fetus measured from crown to heel may be approximated during the first 5 months by squaring the number of the lunar month to which the pregnancy has advanced and, in the second half of pregnancy, by multiplying the month by 5.

Weight of the Newborn. The average term infant at birth weighs about 3000 to 3600 g. depending upon race, economic status, size of the parents, and parity of the mother, with boys roughly 100 g (3 ounces) heavier than girls. The observations of Gruenwald (1967) and other investigators established that during the second half of pregnancy the fetal weight increases linearly with time until about the 37th week of gestation, and then it slows in rate variably. Gruenwald emphasized that the principal determinants of the extent to which fetal growth late in pregnancy departs from the previously linear pattern are related in large part to the socioeconomic status of the mothers. In general, the greater the socioeconomic deprivation, the slower the rate of growth late in pregnancy.

Birth weights over 5000 g occur occasionally, but most tales of huge babies vastly exceeding this figure are based on hearsay and inaccurate measurements at best. Presumably, the largest baby recorded in the literature is that described by Belcher (1916), a stillborn female weighing 11,340 g (25 pounds). In spite of these exceptional cases of macrosomia, extreme skepticism is justified in accepting reports concerning phenomenally heavy children. Term infants, however, frequently weigh

TABLE 8-1.
CRITERIA FOR ESTIMATING AGE DURING THE FETAL PERIOD

AGE (WEEKS)		CR LENGTH (mm)*	FOOT LENGTH (mm)*	FETAL WEIGHT (g)†	MAIN EXTERNAL CHARACTERISTICS
Menstrual	Fertilization				
11	9	50	7	8	Eyes closing or closed. Head more rounded. External genitalia still not distinguishable as male or female. Intestines are in the umbilical cord.
12	10	61	9	14	Intestine in abdomen. Early fingernail development.
14	12	87	14	45	Sex distinguishable externally. Well-defined neck.
16	14	120	20	110	Head erect. Lower limbs well developed.
18	16	140	27	200	Ears stand out from head.
20	18	160	33	320	Vernix caseosa present. Early toenail development.
22	20	190	39	460	Head and body (lanugo) hair visible.
24	22	210	45	630	Skin wrinkled and red.
26	24	230	50	820	Fingernails present. Lean body.
28	26	250	55	1000	Eyes partially open. Eyelashes present.
30	28	270	59	1300	Eyes open. Good head of hair. Skin slightly wrinkled.
32	30	280	63	1700	Toenails present. Body filing out. Testes descending.
34	32	300	68	2100	Fingernails reach finger tips. Skin pink and smooth.
38	36	340	79	2900	Body usually plump. Lanugo hairs almost absent. Toenails reach toe tips.
40	38	360	83	3400	Prominent chest; breasts protrude. Testes in scrotum or palpable in inguinal canals. Fingernails extend beyond finger tips.

From Moore: The Developing Human, 2nd ed. Philadelphia, Saunders, 1977.
* These measurements are averages and so may not apply to specific cases; dimensional variations increase with age. The method for taking CR (crown-rump) measurements is illustrated in Figure 8-5.B.
† These weights refer to fetuses that have been fixed for about two weeks in 10 percent formalin. Fresh specimens usually weigh about 5 percent less.

less than 3200 g and sometimes as little as 2250 g (5 pounds) or even less. In the past, it was customary, when the birth weight was 2500 g or less, to classify the infant as premature even though in some instances the low birth weight was not the consequence of prematurity but rather intrauterine growth retardation.

The many factors intimately involved in fetal growth are considered further in this chapter in the sections on placental transfer and fetal nutrition (pp. 177, 203), as well as in Chapters 13 and 37.

Fetal Head. Obstetrically, the head of the fetus is a most important part, since an essential feature of labor is an adaptation between the fetal head and the maternal bony pelvis. Only a comparatively small part of the head of the fetus at term is represented by the face; the rest is composed of the firm skull, which is made up of two frontal, two parietal, and two temporal bones, along with the upper portion of the occipital bone and the wings of the sphenoid. These bones are not united rigidly but are separated by membranous spaces, the *sutures* (Fig. 8-6). The most important sutures are the *frontal*, between the two frontal bones; the *sagittal*, between the two parietal bones; the two *coronal*, between the frontal and parietal bones; and the two *lambdoid*, between the posterior margins of the parietal bones and upper margin of the occipital bone. With vertex presentations, all the sutures are palpable during labor, except the *temporal* sutures, which are situated on either side between the inferior margin of the parietal and the upper margin of the temporal bones, covered by soft parts, and cannot be felt in the living child.

Where several sutures meet an irregular space forms, which is enclosed by a membrane and designated a *fontanel* (Fig. 8-6). Four such structures are usually distinguished, namely the greater, the lesser, and the two temporal fontanels. The *greater, or anterior, fontanel* is a lozenge-shaped space situated at the junction of the sagittal and the coronal sutures. The *lesser, or posterior, fontanel* is represented by a small triangular area at the intersection of the sagittal and lambdoid sutures. Both may be felt readily during labor, and their recognition gives important information concerning the presentation and position of the fetus. The *temporal, or casserian,* fontanels, situated at the junction of the lambdoid and temporal sutures, have no diagnostic significance.

It is customary to measure certain critical *diameters* and *circumferences* of the infant's head. The diameters most frequently used and their average lengths are

1. The *occipitofrontal* (11.5 cm), which follows a line extending from a point just above the root of the nose to the most prominent portion of the occipital bone.
2. The *biparietal* (9.5 cm), the greatest transverse diameter of the head, which extends from one parietal boss to the other.
3. The *bitemporal* (8.0 cm), the greatest distance between the two temporal sutures.
4. The *occipitomental* (12.5 cm), from the chin to the most prominent portion of the occiput.

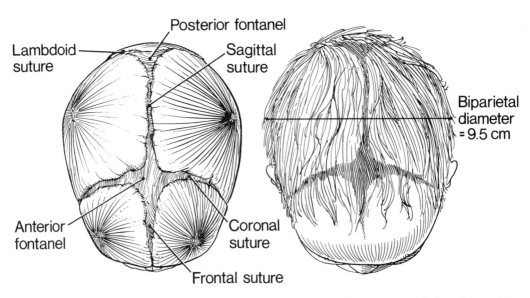

FIG. 8-6. Fetal head at term showing various fontanels, sutures, and diameter.

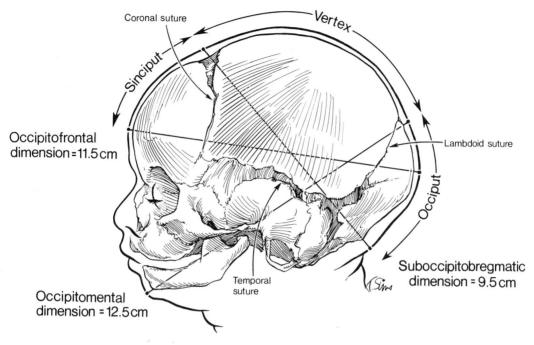

FIG. 8-7.   Diameters of the fetal head at term.

5. The *suboccipitobregmatic* (9.5 cm), which follows a line drawn from the middle of the large fontanel to the undersurface of the occipital bone just where it joins the neck (Figs. 8-6 and 8-7).

The greatest circumference of the head, which corresponds to the plane of the occipitofrontal diameter, averages 34.5 cm, and the smallest circumference, corresponding to the plane of the suboccipitobregmatic diameter, is 32 cm. As a rule, white infants have larger heads than do nonwhite infants, boys somewhat larger than girls, and the infants of multiparas larger heads than those of nulliparas.

Because of the widely varying mobility at the sutures between the bones of the skull, fetal heads differ appreciably in their ability to adapt to the maternal pelvis by *molding.* The bones of one fetus may be soft and readily molded, whereas those of another are firmly ossified, only slightly mobile, and therefore incapable of significant reduction in size.

Fetal Brain.   As pregnancy advances the fetal brain changes remarkably in appearance, as well as in function (Fig. 8-8). Therefore, it is possible to identify fetal age rather precisely from the external appearance of the brain (Dolman, 1977).

PLACENTAL TRANSFER

General Concepts.   A major function of the placenta is to transfer oxygen and a great variety of nutrients from the mother to the fetus and, conversely, to convey carbon dioxide and other metabolic wastes from fetus to mother. To appreciate the complexity of the placenta as an organ of transfer, it is necessary only to reflect on the fact that the placenta, and to a limited extent the attached membranes, supply all material for fetal growth and energy production while removing all products of fetal catabolism.

There are no continuous direct communi-

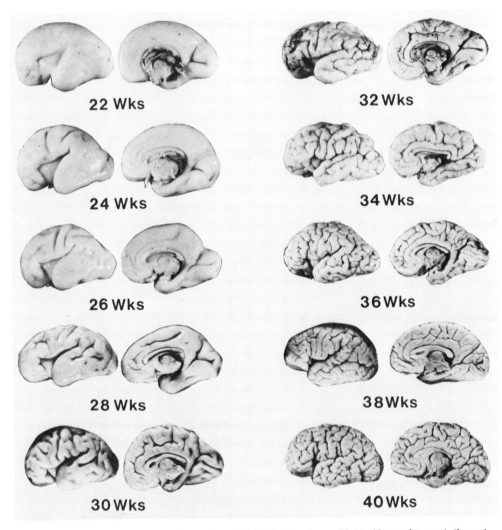

22 Wks   32 Wks

24 Wks   34 Wks

26 Wks   36 Wks

28 Wks   38 Wks

30 Wks   40 Wks

FIG. 8-8. Characteristic configuration of fetal brains from 22 to 40 weeks gestation at two-week intervals. (From Dolman. *Arch Pathol Lab Med* 101:193, 1977)

cations between the fetal blood in the vessels of the chorionic villi and the maternal blood in the intervillous space. Throughout most of pregnancy, nearly all the erythrocytes in the fetal circulation can be shown, by their resistance to acid elution, to be rich in fetal hemoglobin, whereas only rarely does an erythrocyte in the maternal circulation display this property. The one exception to this generalization regarding the independence of the circulations is the development of occasional breaks in the chorionic villi, permitting the escape of varying numbers of fetal erythrocytes into the maternal circulation (see

Chap. 6, p. 136). This leakage is the clinically significant mechanism by which some Rh-negative women become sensitized by the erythrocytes of their Rh-positive fetus (see Chap. 38, p. 961). These occasional leaks, however, do not controvert the basic principle that no *gross* intermingling of the macromolecular constituents of the two circulations occurs. The transfer of substances from mother to fetus and from fetus to mother, therefore, depends primarily on mechanisms that permit the transport of such substances through the intact chorionic villus.

At least nine variables determine the effectiveness of the human placenta as an organ of transfer.

1. The concentration in the maternal plasma of the substance under consideration and in some instances the extent to which it is bound to another compound.
2. The rate of maternal blood flow through the intervillous space.
3. The area available for exchange across the villous epithelium.
4. In case the substance is transferred by diffusion, the physical properties of the tissue barrier interposed between blood in the intervillous space and blood in the fetal capillaries.
5. For any substance actively transported, the capacity of the biochemical machinery of the placenta for effecting active transfer.
6. The amount of the substance metabolized by the placenta during transfer.
7. The area for exchange across the fetal capillaries in the placenta.
8. The concentration in the fetal blood of the substance, exclusive of any that is bound.
9. The rate of fetal blood flow through the villous capillaries.

Unfortunately, in human pregnancy many of these processes, including blood flow, cannot be measured accurately in either the mother or the fetus. In recent years, however, technics have been developed for doing so in experimental animals.

The Intervillous Space. The intervillous space functions as the depot from which materials are transferred, either passively or actively, through the chorionic epithelium to the fetal vessels, and where substances from the fetus enter the maternal circulation. Since this process of transfer supplies the fetus with oxygen as well as nutriment and provides for elimination of metabolic waste products in addition, the chorionic villi and the intervillous space, together, function for the fetus as a lung, gastrointestinal tract, and kidney.

The circulation of maternal blood within the intervillous space has been considered in detail in Chapter 6. The residual volume of the intervillous space of the delivered term placenta measures about 140 ml; however, the normal volume of the intervillous space before delivery is probably twice this value (Aherne and Dunnill, 1966). Uteroplacental blood flow near term has been estimated to be about 600 ml per minute, with most of the blood apparently going through the intervillous space. Although much more remains to be learned about the hemodynamics of the intervillous space even in normal pregnancy, on the basis of a variety of animal studies, as well as clinical observations made in women, the following conclusions can be drawn: uterine contractions reduce blood flow through the intervillous space, the degree of reduction depending in large part upon the intensity of the contraction. Blood pressure within the intervillous space is significantly less than uterine arterial pressure but somewhat greater than uterine venous pressure. Uterine venous pressure, in turn, varies depending upon several factors, including posture. When the mother is supine, for example, pressure in the lower part of the inferior vena cava is elevated; consequently, in this circumstance, pressure in the uterine and ovarian veins and, in turn, the intervillous space, is elevated. An even greater increase in intervillous pressure is likely when the mother stands.

The hydrostatic pressure in the capillaries of the chorionic villi is probably not appreciably different from that in the intervillous space. During normal labor, the rise in fetal blood pressure must parallel the pressure in the amnionic fluid and the intervillous space. Otherwise, the capillaries in the chorionic villi would collapse and fetal blood flow through the placenta would cease.

Chorionic Villus. Substances that pass from the maternal blood to the fetal blood must traverse trophoblast, stroma, and fetal capillary wall. These layers have a minimal aggregate thickness of 3 to 6 μ, according to Wislocki (1955). Although the histologic "barrier" separates the maternal and fetal circulations, it does not behave uniformly like a simple physical barrier, because throughout pregnancy it either actively or passively permits, facilitates, and adjusts the amount and rate of transfer of a wide range of substances to the fetus. Certain histologic alterations in the villus with advancing pregnancy appear to enhance placental permeability. As the prominence of Langhans cells, or cytotrophoblast, decreases, the villous epithelium consists predominantly of syncytiotrophoblast. The walls of the villous capillaries likewise become thinner, and the relative number of fetal vessels increases in relation to the villous connective tissue.

Several attempts have been made to estimate the total surface area of chorionic villi in the human placenta at term. The planimetric measurements made by Aherne and Dunnill (1966) of the villous surface area of the placenta were demonstrative of a close correlation with fetal weight. According to their findings, the total surface area at term is approximately 10 square meters.

Transfer by Diffusion. Most substances with a molecular weight less than 500 daltons can diffuse readily through the placental tissue interposed between the maternal and fetal circulations. Molecular weight clearly has a bearing on the rate of transfer by diffusion; all other things equal, the smaller the molecule, the more rapid is the rate. Diffusion, however, is by no means the only mechanism of transfer of compounds with a low molecular weight. The placenta actually facilitates the transfer of a variety of such compounds, especially those which are in low concentration in maternal plasma but are essential for the rapid growth of the fetus.

Simple diffusion appears to be the mechanism involved in the transfer of oxygen, carbon dioxide, and water, and most but not all electrolytes. Anesthetic gases also pass through the placenta rapidly and do so apparently by simple diffusion.

Insulin, steroid hormones from the adrenal, and hormones from the thyroid cross the placenta but at very slow rates. The hormones synthesized by the placenta enter both the maternal and fetal circulations but not necessarily to the same degree. For example, the concentrations of chorionic gonadotropin and placental lactogen are appreciably lower in fetal plasma than in maternal plasma. Substances of very high molecular weight do not usually traverse the placenta, but there are pronounced exceptions, such as immune gamma globulin G with a molecular weight of about 160,000 daltons.

TRANSFER OF OXYGEN AND CARBON DIOXIDE. Normal values for oxygen, carbon dioxide, and pH in maternal and fetal blood, as compiled by Longo (1972), are presented in Table 8-2. Because of the continuous passage of oxygen from the maternal blood in the intervillous space to the fetus, the oxygen saturation of this blood resembles that in the maternal capillaries, and is less than that of the mother's arterial blood. The average oxygen saturation of intervillous space blood is estimated to be 65 to 75 percent, with a partial pressure (PO_2) of about 30 to 35 mm Hg. The oxygen saturation of the umbilical vein blood is similar, but with an oxygen partial pressure somewhat lower. In the estimations reported for the PO_2 of blood from the intervillous space, inconsistently high or low figures are often encountered, suggesting that, if the needle is actually in the intervillous space, this blood is not thoroughly mixed. If the needle or electrode were to be at a point where it is bathed by a jet of arterial blood into the intervillous space,the estimate of oxygen saturation becomes falsely high, whereas the reverse obtains if the needle or electrode is placed at a location where the circulation is relatively sluggish or is mistakenly placed in an adjacent uterine vein. The collection of umbilical venous or arterial blood at delivery that is truly representative of the oxygenation in utero is fraught with even greater errors.

Despite the relatively low PO_2, normally the fetus does not suffer from lack of oxygen. The human fetus probably behaves like the lamb fetus and, therefore, has a cardiac out-

TABLE 8-2.
NORMAL VALUES FOR OXYGEN, CARBON DIOXIDE, AND pH
IN HUMAN MATERNAL AND FETAL BLOOD

	UTERINE		UMBILICAL	
	Artery	Vein	Vein	Artery
PO_2 (mm Hg)	95	40	27	15
O_2Hb (percent saturation)	98	76	68	30
O_2 content (ml per dl)	15.8	12.2	14.5	6.4
Hemoglobin (g per dl)	12.0	12.0	16.0	16.0
O_2 capacity (ml O_2 per dl)	16.1	16.1	21.4	21.4
PCO_2 (mm Hg)	32	40	43	48
CO_2 content (mM per liter)	19.6	21.8	25.2	26.3
HCO_3^- (mM per liter)	18.8	20.7	24.0	25.0
pH	7.40	7.34	7.38	7.35

put considerably greater per unit of body weight than does the adult. The high cardiac output and, late in pregnancy, the increased oxygen-carrying capacity of fetal blood as the consequence of a higher hemoglobin concentration compensate effectively for the low oxygen tension. Both of these mechanisms are considered further in this chapter under "Fetal Circulation" and under "Fetal Blood." Additional evidence that the fetus does not normally experience lack of oxygen is supplied by measurement of the lactic acid content of fetal blood, which is only slightly higher than that of the mother.

Assali and co-workers (1968, 1974) were able to raise the PO_2 in the umbilical vein of the lamb fetus by 10 mm Hg when the mother breathed 100 percent oxygen at atmospheric pressure. They detected no fall in uteroplacental or umbilical blood flow in response to 100 percent oxygen. When the ewe breathed hyperbaric oxygen that raised the maternal arterial PO_2 to 1300 mm Hg, uteroplacental blood flow did not change and umbilical flow decreased only slightly, although the PO_2 in umbilical blood rose to nearly 600 mm Hg (Fig. 8-9). With normally functioning maternal and fetal circulations, therefore, oxygen can be delivered across the placenta,

at least to the fetus of the sheep, under increased tension and without remarkably restricting umbilical blood flow. Employing the usual equipment for providing oxygen to the mother, the increase is modest, however.

There are no precise measurements of the ability of the human fetus to withstand severe hypoxia. Myers (1970) has measured the tolerance of the brain of the monkey fetus to hypoxia induced by cord compression with complete cessation of flow. The rates at which bradycardia, hypotension, and acidosis developed varied with gestational age, so that the more mature the fetus, the more rapid the rate of deterioration.

In general, the transfer of carbon dioxide from the fetus to the mother obeys the same laws as those described for oxygen, although carbon dioxide traverses the chorionic villus more rapidly than does oxygen. Near term, the partial pressure of carbon dioxide in the umbilical arteries is estimated to average about 48 mm Hg, or about 5 mm or so more than in the maternal blood in the intervillous space. For several reasons, fetal blood has somewhat less affinity for carbon dioxide than does the blood of the mother, thereby favoring the transfer of carbon dioxide from the fetus to the mother.

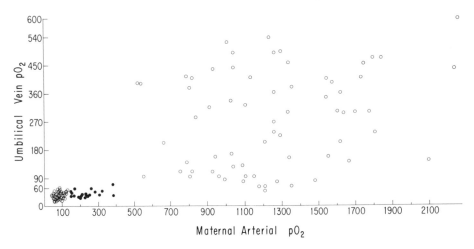

FIG. 8-9. Changes in umbilical vein blood Po₂ during progressively increasing maternal blood Po₂. Note that when the maternal blood Po₂ was raised to about 300 mmHg by ventilating the maternal lungs with 100 percent oxygen *(black dots)*, umbilical vein blood Po₂ remained below 60 mmHg. This illustrates the boundary imposed on fetal oxygenation. Only when the maternal blood Po₂ was increased by hyperbaric oxygenation *(open circles)* did the fetal blood Po₂ increase to high levels. (From Assali. In Gluck (ed): *Modern Perinatal Medicine*. Chicago, Year Book, 1974)

Selective Transfer. Although diffusion is an important method of placental transfer, the chorionic villus exhibits enormous selectivity in transfer, maintaining different concentrations of a variety of metabolites on the two sides of the villus. One example of this selectivity is in the transfer of the two isomers of histidine, as demonstrated by Page (1957). D-Histidine, the unnatural isomer, traverses the placenta more slowly, coming to equilibrium with the fetal blood within 3 or 4 hours. If only passive transfer by simple diffusion were involved, L-histidine, the natural isomer, would be expected to behave similarly, but in the case of this isomer, equilibrium is attained within a few minutes. The concentrations of a number of substances that are not synthesized by the fetus are several times higher in fetal than in maternal blood. Ascorbic acid is a good example of this phenomenon. This crystalline substance of relatively low molecular weight chemically resembles the pentose and hexose sugars and might be expected to traverse the placenta by simple diffusion. The concentration of ascorbic acid, however, is regularly 2 to 4 times higher in fetal plasma than in maternal plasma (Braestrup, 1937; Manahan and Eastman, 1938). The unidirectional transfer of iron across the placenta provides another example of the unique capabilities of the human placenta for transport. Typically, the mineral is present in the plasma at a lower concentration in the mother than in the fetus, and, at the same time, the iron-binding capacity of the plasma is much greater in the mother than in the fetus. Nonetheless, iron is transported actively from maternal to fetal plasma, and in the human fetus the amount transferred appears to be independent of maternal iron status (Pritchard, unpublished).

Intrauterine infections caused by viruses, bacteria, and protozoa are occasionally encountered. Many viruses, including those responsible for rubella, chickenpox, measles, mumps, smallpox, vaccinia, poliomyelitis, cytomegalic inclusion disease, coxsackie virus disease, and western equine encephalitis, may cross the placenta and infect the fetus. *Treponema pallidum, Toxoplasma, Plasmodium* species, and *Mycobacterium tuberculosis* may similarly produce intrauterine infection. With protozoal and bacterial, but not necessarily viral, infections, there is almost always histologic evidence of involvement of the placenta.

PHYSIOLOGY OF FETUS

Fetal Circulation. Since practically all materials needed for growth and maintenance are brought to the fetus from the placenta by the umbilical vein, the fetal circulation must differ fundamentally from that of the adult (Figs. 8-10 and 8-11; see Colorplate). The single umbilical vein in the umbilical cord carries oxygenated, nutriment-bearing blood from the placenta to the fetus. The umbilical vein enters the fetus through the umbilical ring and ascends along the anterior abdominal wall to the liver. The vein then divides, with some branches carrying blood to the hepatic veins primarily of the left side of the liver, while others deliver umbilical vein blood to the intrahepatic portal circulation. The major "branch" of the umbilical vein, the *ductus venosus,* traverses the liver to enter directly the inferior vena cava. The blood flowing to the fetal heart from the inferior vena cava, therefore, consists of an admixture of "arterial" blood that passes through the ductus venosus and less well oxygenated blood that collects from most of the veins below the level of the diaphragm. As a consequence, the oxygen content of blood delivered to the heart from the inferior vena cava is decreased with respect to that which leaves the placenta, but it is greater than that from the superior vena cava.

As emphasized by Dawes (1962), the *foramen ovale* opens directly off the inferior vena cava so that blood from the inferior vena cava is, for the most part, immediately deflected by the *crista dividens* through the foramen ovale into the left atrium. Little or none of the less well oxygenated blood from the superior vena cava normally passes through the foramen ovale. The preferential flow of blood from the inferior vena cava through the foramen ovale to the left atrium bypasses the right ventricle and pulmonary circulation and permits delivery to the left ventricle of more highly oxygenated blood than if complete admixture had occurred in the right atrium. The more highly oxygenated blood that passes through the foramen ovale and is ejected from the left ventricle perfuses two vital organs, the heart and the brain. The blood that is typically venous in character, coming from the superior vena cava and ejected from the right ventricle into the pulmonary trunk, is, for the most part, shunted through the *ductus arteriosus* into the descending aorta. Only about one-third of the blood goes through the lungs.

The lamb fetus has been studied intensively by several groups of investigators who believe that the circulatory function of the mature lamb fetus is similar in many respects to that of the mature human fetus. Before birth, in man and in sheep, both ventricles of the fetal heart, as the consequence of the shunts just described, work in parallel rather than in series. Attempts to measure cardiac output in the lamb fetus have yielded somewhat variable results. Assali (1974) and associates (1968) have ascertained a mean value of about 225 ml per kg per minute but with considerable individual variation; Paton and co-workers (1973) found very similar values in baboon fetuses. Such a high fetal cardiac output, which per unit of weight is about three times that of an adult at rest, would compensate for the low oxygen content of fetal blood. The high cardiac output is accomplished in part by the fast heart rate of the fetus.

Before birth and expansion of the lungs, the high pulmonary vascular resistance accounts for the high pressure and the low blood flow in the fetal pulmonary circuit. At the same time, resistance to flow through the ductus arteriosus and the umbilicoplacental circulation is low, probably accounting for the overall low fetal systemic vascular resistance. It is estimated that in the fetal lamb about one-half the combined output of the two ventricles goes to the placenta. Rudolph and Heymann (1968), by injecting isotopically labeled plastic microspheres into the fetal lamb circulation at various sites, determined the distribution of cardiac output during the last third of gestation to be roughly as follows: placenta, 41 percent; carcass, 35 percent; brain, 5 percent; heart, 5 percent; gastrointestinal tract, 5 percent; lungs, 4 percent; kidneys, 2 percent; spleen, 2 percent; liver (hepatic artery only), 2 percent.

After birth, the umbilical vessels, the ductus arteriosus, the foramen ovale, and the ductus venosus normally constrict or collapse and consequently the hemodynamics of the fetal circulation undergo pronounced changes. According to Assali (1974) and associates (1968), clamping of the umbilical cord and expansion of the fetal lungs, either through spontaneous breathing or artificial respiration, promptly induce a variety of hemodynamic changes in sheep. The systemic arterial pressure initially falls slightly, apparently the result of the reversal in the direction of blood flow in the ductus arteriosus, but it soon recovers and then rises above the control value. They concluded that several factors played a role in regulating the flow of blood through the ductus arteriosus, including the difference in pressure between the pulmonary artery and aorta and especially the oxygen tension of the blood passing through the ductus arteriosus. They were able to influence flow through the ductus arteriosus by altering the PO_2 of the blood. When the lungs were ventilated with oxygen and the PO_2 rose above 55 mm Hg, ductus flow dropped, but ventilation with nitrogen, initially at least, returned ductus flow to the original pattern.

The effects from variations in oxygen tension of blood flowing through the ductus arteriosus are thought to be mediated through the actions of prostaglandins on the ductus. Prostaglandins E_1 and E_2 dilate the constricted ductus arteriosus and are intimately involved in maintaining normal patency in utero. Inhibitors of prostaglandin synthetase,

when given to the mother, may lead to premature closure of the ductus arteriosus (see Chap. 37, p. 936).

With expansion of the lungs, pressures in the right ventricle and pulmonary arteries fall because of the marked decrease in pulmonary vascular resistance. Theoretically, at least, an increase in the left atrial pressure above that of the right atrium would close the foramen ovale. There is some disagreement, however, as to when closure actually occurs. The experiments of Barclay and co-workers (1939) indicate that functional closure of the foramen ovale occurs within several minutes of birth. Arey (1946), however, states that anatomic fusion of the two septa of the foramen ovale is not completed until about 1 year after birth, and that in 25 percent of cases perfect closure is never attained. When the foramen ovale remains functionally patent, circulatory disturbances of variable gravity result.

The more distal portions of the hypogastric arteries, which course from the level of the bladder along the abdominal wall to the umbilical ring and into the cord as umbilical arteries, undergo atrophy and obliteration within 3 to 4 days after birth, to become the *umbilical ligaments;* intraabdominal remnants of the umbilical vein form the *ligamentum teres.*

Fetal Blood. Hematopoiesis is demonstrable first in the yolk sac of the very early embryo. The next major site of erythropoiesis is the liver and finally the bone marrow. The contributions made by each site throughout the growth and development of the embryo and fetus are demonstrated graphically in Figure 8-12. The first erythrocytes formed are nucleated, but as fetal development progresses, more and more of the circulating erythrocytes are nonnucleated. As the fetus grows, not only does the volume of blood in the common circulation of the fetus and placenta increase but the hemoglobin concentration rises as well. As shown by the studies of Walker and Turnbull (1953), the hemoglobin of fetal blood rises to the

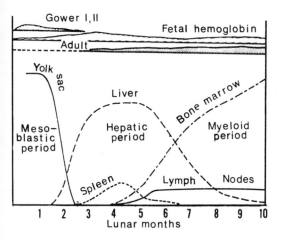

FIG. 8-12. Sites of hematopoiesis and kinds of hemoglobin synthesized at various stages of fetal development. (From Brown. *Biology of Gestation, Vol. II. The Fetus and Neonate.* New York, Academic, 1968, p 361)

adult male level of about 15.0 g per dl at midpregnancy, and at term it is somewhat higher. Fetal blood at or near term is characterized, therefore, by a hemoglobin concentration that is high by maternal standards. The reticulocyte count falls from a very high level in the very young fetus to about 5 percent at term. Pearson (1966), using a variety of technics, found the life span of erythrocytes from more mature fetuses to be approximately two-thirds that of erythrocytes of normal adults, but erythrocytes of less mature fetuses have an even shorter life span. These data are supportive of the concept that fetal erythrocytes are "stress erythrocytes." The erythrocytes of the fetus differ metabolically from those of the adult; several enzymes, for example, have appreciably different activities. The fetus is capable of making erythropoietin in increased amounts when severely anemic and of excreting it into the amnionic fluid (Finne, 1966).

Precise measurements of the volume of blood contained in the human fetoplacental circulation are lacking. However, Usher, Shepard, and Lind (1963) have carefully measured the volume of blood of term normal infants very soon after birth and noted

an average of 78 ml per kg when immediate cord-clamping was carried out. Gruenwald (1967) found the volume of blood of fetal origin contained in the placenta after prompt cord-clamping to average 45 ml per kg of fetus. These combined results are suggestive that the fetoplacental blood volume at term is approximately 125 ml per kg of fetus. Pritchard and co-workers (unpublished observations) have measured the volumes of blood in infants with erythroblastosis fetalis as well as their placenta and cord immediately after delivery. The "fetoplacental" blood volume in these circumstances was very close to 120 ml per kg of infant weight.

In the embryo and fetus, the globin moiety of much of the hemoglobin differs from that of the normal adult. In the embryo, three major forms of hemoglobin may be found (Pearson, 1966). The most primitive forms are Gower-1 and Gower-2. The globin moiety of Gower-1 consists of four ϵ-peptide chains per molecule of protein, whereas in Gower-2 there are two α- and two ϵ-chains. All normal hemoglobins elaborated after Gower-1 contain a pair of α-chains, but the other pair of peptide chains differs for each kind of hemoglobin. Hemoglobin F (so-called fetal hemoglobin or alkaline resistant hemoglobin) contains a pair of α-peptide chains and a pair of γ-chains per molecule of hemoglobin. Actually, two varieties of γ-chains have been identified in hemoglobin F, their ratios changing steadily as the fetus and infant mature (Huisman et al., 1970). As shown in Figure 8-12, hemoglobin A, the fourth hemoglobin to be formed by the fetus and the major hemoglobin formed after birth in normal persons, is present after the 11th week of gestation in progressively greater amounts as the fetus matures (Pataryas and Stamatoyannopoulos, 1972). The globin of hemoglobin A is made up of a pair of α-chains and a pair of β-chains. Hemoglobin A_2, the globin of which contains a pair of α-chains and a pair of σ-chains, is present in very small concentrations in the mature fetus but increases after birth. Thus, as growth proceeds, there is a shift not only

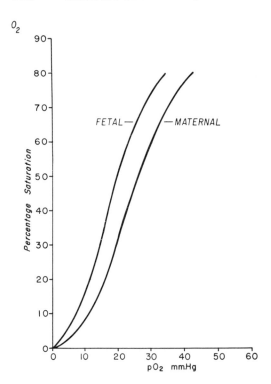

FIG. 8-13. Oxygen dissociation curves of fetal and maternal human bloods prepared at pH 7.40. (Courtesy of Dr. André Hellegers)

in the amounts but also in the kinds of globin synthesized by the embryo and fetus.

As demonstrated in Figure 8-13, at any given oxygen tension and at identical pH, fetal erythrocytes that contain mostly hemoglobin F bind more oxygen than do erythrocytes containing nearly all hemoglobin A. The major reason for this difference is that hemoglobin A binds 2, 3 diphosphoglycerate more avidly than does hemoglobin F (De Verdier and Garby, 1969) and diphosphoglycerate so bound lowers the affinity of the hemoglobin molecule for oxygen. The increased oxygen affinity of the fetal erythrocyte compared to that of the maternal erythrocyte, in which the diphosphoglycerate level is increased compared to the nonpregnant state, facilitates transfer of oxygen from mother to fetus (see Chap. 9, 234).

Since fetal erythrocytes formed late in pregnancy contain less hemoglobin F and more hemoglobin A than do the cells formed

earlier, the content of hemoglobin F of the fetal erythrocytes falls somewhat during the latter weeks of pregnancy. At term, about three-fourths of the total hemoglobin normally is hemoglobin F. During the first 6 to 12 months after delivery, the proportion of hemoglobin F continues to fall, eventually to reach the low level found in erythrocytes of normal adults (Schulman and Smith, 1953).

Evidence of a physiologic role for erythropoietin in fetal erythropoiesis has been provided by Zanjani and co-workers (1974). The injection of antierythropoietin into the sheep fetoplacental circulation was followed by a fall in reticulocytes and incorporation of radioiron into erythrocytes; moreover, induction of anemia in the fetus resulted in elevated levels of erythropoietin-like material. In utero the fetal liver, rather than the kidney, appears to be an important source of erythropoietin. After birth, erythropoietin normally may not be detectable for up to 3 months.

The kinds and numbers of leukocytes in the fetus are highly variable, depending upon the degree of maturity and the impact of labor.

The concentrations of several coagulation factors at birth are appreciably below the levels that develop within a few weeks after birth (Sell and Corrigan, 1973). The factors that are low in cord blood are II, VII, IX, X, XI, XII, XIII and fibrinogen. Without prophylactic vitamin K, vitamin K-dependent coagulation factors usually decrease even further during the first few days after birth and may lead to hemorrhage in the newborn infant (see Chap. 38, p. 976). Platelet counts in cord blood are in the normal range for nonpregnant adults, while fibrinogen levels are somewhat less than in nonpregnant adults. For reasons unknown, the time for conversion of fibrinogen in plasma to fibrin clot when thrombin is added (thrombin time) is somewhat prolonged compared with that of older children and adults. Measurements of factor VIII coagulant activity have proved to be of value in accurately making or excluding the diagnosis of hemophilia in male infants (Kasper et al., 1964). Functional factor XIII (fibrin-stabilizing factor) levels in plasma are significantly reduced compared to those in normal adults (Henriksson et al., 1974). Nielsen (1969) described the finding of low levels of plasminogen and somewhat increased fibrinolytic activity in cord plasma compared to that in maternal plasma.

The mean total plasma protein and plasma albumin concentrations in maternal and cord blood are similar. For example, Foley and associates (1978) identified maternal and cord total plasma proteins to average 6.5 g/dl and 5.9 g/dl respectively with maternal and cord plasma albumin levels of 3.6 g/dl and 3.7 g/dl respectively.

Near term, the immunoglobulin IgG is present in approximately the same concentrations in cord and maternal sera but IgA and IgM are considerably lower in cord serum. Although IgA and IgM of maternal origin are effectively excluded from the fetus, IgG crosses the placenta with considerable efficiency (Gitlin et al., 1972). All four major subclasses of human IgG appear to cross the placenta from mother to fetus but whether by the same or different transport systems is not clear (Gitlin, 1974). Increased amounts of IgM are found in the fetus only after the fetal immune mechanism has been provoked into antibody response by an infection in the fetus.

The viscosities of maternal and cord bloods are similar (Foley and associates, 1978). The increase in viscosity imposed by the higher hematocrit of cord blood is offset by the lower levels of fibrinogen and IgM in the cord plasma.

Urinary System.   Two primitive urinary systems, the pronephros and the mesonephros, precede the development of the metanephros. Embryologic failure of either of the first two may result in anomalous development of the definitive urinary system.

By the end of the first trimester, the nephrons have some capacity for excretion through glomerular filtration, although the kidneys are functionally immature throughout fetal life. The ability to concentrate and

to modify the pH of urine is quite limited even in the mature fetus. Fetal urine is hypotonic with respect to fetal plasma because of low concentrations of electrolytes. In the lamb fetus, and most likely in the human fetus, the fraction of the cardiac output perfusing the kidneys is low and renal vascular resistance is high, compared with these values later in life (Assali et al., 1968; Rudolph and Heymann, 1968). In the lamb fetus, urine flow varies considerably in response to stress. Transient marked fetal polyuria postoperatively that dissipates apparently with recovery of fetal well-being has been noted by Gresham and co-workers (1972).

Urine is usually found in the bladder even in small fetuses. Wladimiroff and Campbell (1974) estimated urine production for human fetuses using an ultrasonic method to determine bladder volumes. They report a mean production of 10 ml per hour at 30 weeks, with an increase at term to 27 ml, or 650 ml per day. Maternally-administered diuretic (furosemide) increases fetal urine formation.

After obstruction of the urethra, the bladder, ureters, and renal pelves may become quite dilated; the bladder may become sufficiently distended that dystocia results. The kidneys in these circumstances seem capable of excreting urine until back pressure ultimately destroys the renal parenchyma. Kidneys are not essential for survival in utero, but are important in the control of the composition and volume of amnionic fluid (see Chap. 23, p. 581). Abnormalities that cause chronic anuria most often are accompanied by oligohydramnios.

RESPIRATORY SYSTEM

Maturation of Fetal Lung.   The biochemical maturation of the fetal lung is of considerable concern to the obstetrician. This obtains since functional immaturity of the lung at birth leads to the development of the respiratory distress syndrome. Kiedel and Gluck (1975), as well as Farrell and Avery

(1975), have recounted succinctly the history of the clinical identification of respiratory distress syndrome. The signs and symptoms of this disorder were described in 1903 by Hocheim who observed a nebulous lining in the lungs of two infants who died shortly after birth. His observation led to the utilization of the descriptive phrase, "hyaline membrane disease," which is employed to describe the pathologic features of the respiratory distress syndrome. In 1929, von Neergard compared the pressure-volume curves of lungs distended with air with those of lungs distended with a gum arabic solution, and from the results of these studies he concluded that the forces that promote deflation or collapse of air-containing lung result principally from surface tension at the air-tissue interface of the alveolus. Clements (1957) demonstrated a surface tension-lowering material in saline extracts of lung lavage material. Subsequently it was demonstrated that the surface-active components of the alveoli is attributable to a lipoprotein, *surfactant*. Klaus and associates (1961) demonstrated that the principal surface-active component of surfactant was a specific lecithin, dipalmitoylphosphatidylcholine, in which the palmitoyl radical is present in both the sn-1 and sn-2 positions of the glycerophospholipid. Avery and Mead (1959) were the first to point out that the respiratory distress is caused by a deficiency in lung surfactant biosynthesis. Subsequently, several investigators have shown that augmented surfactant synthesis appears in fetal lungs according to a developmental timetable.

The recognition of the importance of surfactant in the prevention of respiratory distress syndrome led many investigators to study the composition of surfactant (Fig. 8-14). There are several unique features which characterize the phospholipid composition of this complex lipoprotein. Approximately 80 percent of the phospholipids are comprised of phosphatidylcholines (lecithins); and, importantly, a single phosphatidylcholine, i.e., dipalmitoylphosphatidylcholine, accounts for nearly 50 percent of the glycerophospholipids of surfactant. Surfactant also has an unusually high content of phosphatidylglycerol,

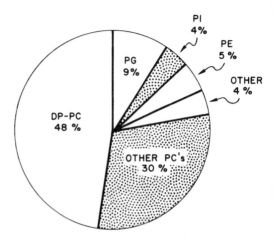

FIG. 8-14. Glycerophospholipid composition of pulmonary surfactant: DP-PC = dipalmitoylphosphatidylcholine, PC = phosphatidylcholine, PG = phosphatidylglycerol, PI = phosphatidylinositol, and PE = phosphatidylethanolamine. (From Johnston et al. In *Enzymes of Lipid Metabolism.* New York, Plenum, 1978, 328)

9 to 15 percent, an amount much greater than that found in any other mammalian tissue (White, 1973). Importantly, phosphatidylglycerol is the second most surface-active component of surfactant, but more than that, phosphatidylglycerol appears to confer a certain stability to the surfactant moiety over and above that which can be attributed to its surface-active properties alone. This as yet ill-defined action of phosphatidylglycerol is believed to be important in the prevention of the respiratory distress syndrome since infants born before the phosphatidylglycerol content of their surfactant has risen are at increased risk of respiratory distress even though the dipalmitoylphosphatidylcholine content of their surfactant is high.

In an elegant series of studies, Gluck and associates (1967, 1970, 1971, 1972, 1974) demonstrated that an increasing concentration of dipalmitoylphosphatidylcholine (lecithin) in amnionic fluid, relative to that of sphingomyelin (the lecithin to sphingomyelin, or L/S, ratio), constitutes an index of fetal lung maturation. These studies succeeded because of the ingenious idea of measuring the concentration of sphingomyelin as a reference for general phospholipid synthesis by the lung, whereas the measurement of acetone-precipitable phosphatidylcholine (disaturated lecithin) was a specific index of surfactant synthesis. More recently, Hallman and co-workers (1976) observed that identification of phosphatidylglycerol in amnionic fluid is also an indicator of lung maturation. From these diverse observations, it is apparent that augmented synthesis of surfactant and specifically that of dipalmitoylphosphatidylcholine and phosphatidylglycerol are required in the preparation of the fetal lung for the transition from a water–alveolar interface to an air–alveolar interface, events which must take place in order to prevent alveolar collapse on expiration. Thus, the regulation of the rate of synthesis of dipalmitoylphosphatidylcholine and phosphatidylglycerol becomes of signal importance. The biosynthetic pathways involved in the formation of the glycerophospholipids of surfactant are illustrated in Figure 8-15.

The biosynthesis of phosphatidylcholine and phosphatidylglycerol involves several common reactions. The glycerol backbone for both phosphatidylcholine and phosphatidylglycerol synthesis is provided by either glycerol-3-phosphate or dihydroxyacetone phosphate, or both. It is noteworthy that glycerol-3-phosphate originates from glycerol in tissues containing glycerolkinase activity and from glucose through glycolysis. Glycerol-3-phosphate is acylated in a stepwise fashion, a process which gives rise to phosphatidic acids containing two of a variety of fatty acids. The acyl donor to the glycerol backbone is fatty acid-coenzyme A (CoA). Generally, phosphatidic acids contain a saturated fatty acid in the sn-1 position and an unsaturated fatty acid in the sn-2 position. In the biosynthesis of phosphatidic acids by lung tissue, there is no evidence for preferential incorporation of palmitoyl-CoA in the sn-2 position. It is important to note that phosphatidic acid is a substrate common to the formation of the two principal surface-active glycerophospholipids, i.e., dipalmitoylphosphatidylcholine and phosphatidylglycerol. Thus, the metabolism of phosphatidic acids constitutes a critical branch point in the regulation of the biosynthesis of the surface-active glycerophospholipids of surfactant.

First, let us consider the biosynthesis of dipalmitoylphosphatidylcholine. Phosphatidic acids are hydrolyzed through the action of the enzyme phosphatidate phosphohydrolase (PAPase), to yield sn-1,2-diglycerides. The sn-1,2-diglycerides serve as co-substrates with cytidine diphosphate (CDP)-choline in the formation of phospha-

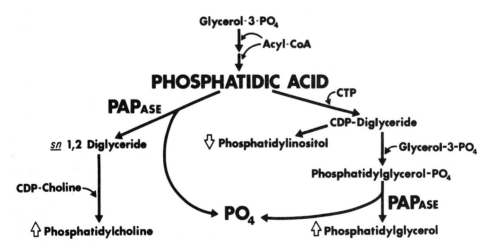

FIG. 8-15.   The pathways for the biosynthesis of phosphatidylcholine, phosphatidylglycerol, and phosphatidylinositol (See text for abbreviations). (Courtesy of Dr. John M. Johnston)

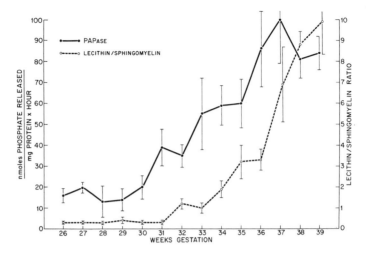

FIG. 8-16. Specific activity of PAPase in human amnionic fluid as a function of fetal gestational age, and the relationship of PAPase specific activity to the L/S ratio. (From Jimenez and Johnston. *Pediatr Res* 10:767, 1976)

tidylcholines. This latter reaction is catalyzed by the enzyme choline phosphotransferase (CPTase). In this reaction the co-substrate, CDP-choline, is formed through the action of choline kinase which gives rise to phosphorylcholine. Phosphorylcholine, in turn, is converted to CDP-choline through the action of cytidine triphosphate (CTP) phosphocholine cytidylyltransferase. Most of the resultant phosphatidylcholines contain a saturated fatty acid, commonly palmitic acid, in the sn-1 position, whereas an unsaturated fatty acid is commonly present in the sn-2 position. Obviously, some molecular rearrangement of such phosphatidylcholines must occur in order to produce dipalmitoylphosphatidylcholine. Two separate mechanisms have been proposed to account for the enrichment of phosphatidylcholines with palmitic acid in the sn-2 position. Both mechanisms require the action of the enzyme, phospholipase A_2. The action of phospholipase A_2 results in the deacylation of glycerophospholipids at the sn-2 position. One product of this reaction is sn-1-palmitoyllysophosphatidylcholine. This lysophosphatidylcholine may be acylated with palmitoyl-CoA through the action of acyltransferase, resulting in the product, dipalmitoylphosphatidylcholine (Lands, 1958). It is interesting that this pathway was first demonstrated in lung tissue. Alternatively, the remodeling of phosphatidylcholine can come about as the result of the transfer of the acyl moiety from the sn-1 position of an sn-1-palmitoyllysophosphatidylcholine to the sn-2

position of a second sn-1-palmitoyllysophosphatidylcholine. Through this pathway, dipalmitoylphosphatidylcholine can also be formed. This latter mechanism for remodeling phosphatidylcholine originally was demonstrated in liver tissue (Marinetti, 1958), but has also been demonstrated in lung tissue (van den Bosch et al., 1965).

Much effort has been directed toward defining the mechanisms that give rise to augmented surfactant biosynthesis during fetal lung maturation. A number of investigators working in the laboratories of Dr. John M. Johnston have accumulated considerable evidence in support of the view that the enzyme PAPase occupies a regulatory role in the biosynthesis of the glycerophospholipids of surfactant (Delahunty et al., 1979; Douglas et al., 1976; Herbert et al., 1978; Jimenez et al., 1974, 1975, 1976; Johnston et al., 1978; Rosenfeld et al., 1979; Schultz et al., 1974; Spitzer et al., 1975). The specific activity of PAPase in fetal rabbit lung tissue increases strikingly just prior to the accumulation of dipalmitoylphosphatidylcholine. In view of this striking increase in the specific activity of PAPase in fetal rabbit lung just prior to the lecithin "surge," Johnston, Jimenez and colleagues investigated the PAPase activity in human amnionic fluid as a function of gestational age. They found that PAPase was present in amnionic fluid and that the specific activity of this enzyme began to increase at about 29 to 32 weeks of gestation (Fig. 8-16). Moreover, the increase in PAPase activity preceded or was concomitant with the increase in the L/S ratio.

These investigators also demonstrated that the specific activity of PAPase in the nasopharyngeal fluid was greater than that of amnionic fluid, a finding that is indicative that PAPase in amnionic fluid arises in fetal lung tissue. Thus, PAPase is translocated from the type II pneumonocytes into the alveolar space and thence into the bronchi and is swept into the amnionic fluid by fetal thoracic movements. It appears that PAPase and surfactant are secreted by the type II pneumocytes as a closely associated unit, viz, the lamellar body, by a process that involves the microtubule system (Fig. 8-17. A, B, and C).

Johnston and associates (1978) also found that the hydrolysis of phosphatidylglycerol phosphate to give rise to phosphatidylglycerol was catalyzed by PAPase, and that the enzyme previously presumed to be PGPase (Fig. 8-15) was in fact PAPase. Thus, the increase in activity of PAPase in fetal lung is envisioned to bring about a series of events that regulate the rate of surfactant formation in developing lungs.

1. PAPase catalyzes the hydrolysis of phosphatidic acids to give rise to diglycerides, the cosubstrate for phosphatidylcholine formation.
2. Diglycerides, in increased concentrations, bring about an activation of the enzyme CTP-phosphocholine citidylyltransferase, which catalyzes the reaction giving rise to CDP-choline, the other cosubstrate for phosphatidylcholine biosynthesis.
3. PAPase is the enzyme that brings about the hydrolysis of phosphatidylglycerophosphate to give rise to phosphatidylglycerol.

The control of phosphatidylglycerol synthesis warrants careful investigation since Gluck and co-workers have shown that increased concentrations of phosphatidylglycerol together with decreased concentrations of phosphatidylinositol in surfactant also herald lung maturation. Furthermore, it has been shown that phosphatidylglycerol also acts to increase the activity of the lung tissue enzyme, CTP:phosphocholine cytidylyltransferase, an enzyme necessary for phosphatidylcholine biosynthesis. Moreover, some infants who are born of diabetic mothers develop respiratory distress syndrome despite high concentrations of phosphatidylcholine in their amnionic fluid. These infants are characterized by having in their surfactant low levels of phosphatidylglycerol and high levels of phosphatidylinositol. Thus, an understanding of the regulation of formation of phosphatidylglycerol becomes of crucial importance in a consideration of fetal lung maturation. Presently the control of phosphatidylinositol and phosphatidylglycerol biosynthesis is incompletely understood. It seems likely that the decrease in concentration of phosphatidylinositol with a concomitant increase in phosphatidylglycerol in surfactant with lung maturation is brought about by a change in the flux of CDP-diglycerides through the pathways involved in the synthesis of these acidic glycerophospholipids (Bleasdale et al., 1979) (Fig. 8-15). In any event, it is known that with fetal lung maturation there is first a "surge" in phosphatidylcholine synthesis which is followed in time by an in-

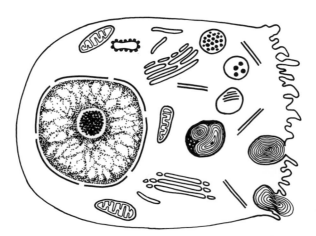

FIG. 8-17. A. Proposed mechanism for the origin and secretion of lamellar bodies by the type II pneumocyte. (Courtesy of Dr. J. Snyder and Dr. John M. Johnston)

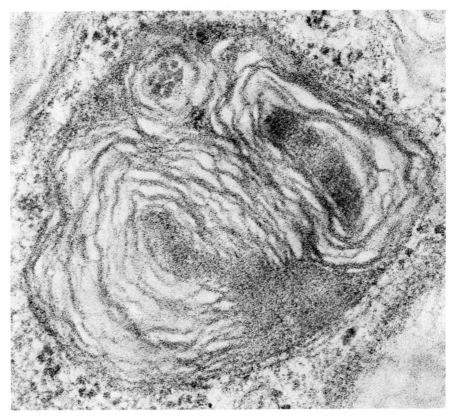

FIG. 8-17. B. Transmission electron micrograph of fused human fetal lung lamellar bodies. (Courtesy of Dr. J. Snyder and Dr. John M. Johnston)

crease in phosphatidylglycerol and a concomitant decrease in phosphatidylinositol in surfactant.

Hormonal Regulation of Surfactant Formation in Human Fetal Lung. Although it is of signal importance to elucidate the biochemical events involved in the synthesis and release of surfactant, it is equally important to define the mechanisms involved in the control of the synthesis and release of surfactant. Many substances have been proposed as being important in these processes. However, the interest of most investigators who have directed their attention to this question has centered on a few agents. Of these, the most intensively investigated compounds are cortisol and other glucocorticosteroids.

CORTISOL AND FETAL LUNG MATURATION. The basis for suspecting that the glucocorticosteroids stimulate surfactant secretion was provided by Liggins (1969). He observed that the lungs of prematurely delivered lambs which had received glucocorticosteroids prior to birth appeared to have accelerated lung maturation. Since that time, many investigators have suggested that fetal cortisol is the natural trigger for augmented surfactant synthesis. It has been observed that the administration of glucocorticosteroids to the fetus resulted in increased incorporation of radiolabeled choline into phosphatidylcholine in fetal rabbit lungs (Barrett et al., 1975; Farrell and Zachman, 1973) and fetal rat lungs (Russell et al., 1974). The inclusion of glucocorticosteroids in the medium of human fetal lung explants (Erelund et al., 1975) and rabbit mixed lung cells grown in tissue culture (Smith and Torday, 1975) resulted in increased incorporation of radiolabeled choline into phosphatidylcholine. The admin-

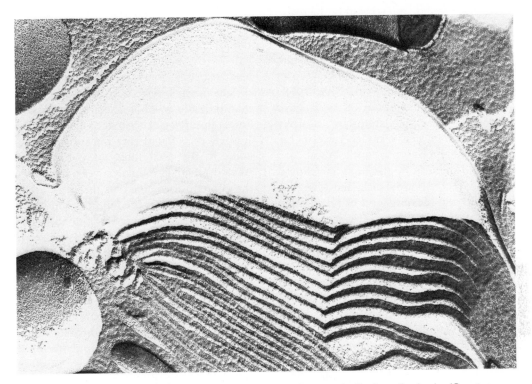

FIG. 8-17. C. Freeze-fracture scanning electron micrograph of a lamellar body. (Courtesy of Dr. R. C. Reynolds and Dr. John M. Johnston)

istration of glucocorticosteroids to fetuses has been found to increase the specific activity of lung CPTase (Farrell and Zachman, 1973) glycerolphosphate phosphatidyltransferase (Rooney et al., 1977), lipoprotein lipase (Hamosh et al., 1977), and PAPase (Brehier et al., 1978). On the other hand, the increase in the specific activity of CPTase and glycerophosphate phosphatidyltransferase following glucocorticosteroid administration was not observed in the rabbit by Rooney and co-workers (1975) or by Brehier and colleagues (1977). Glucocorticosteroid receptors have been demonstrated in cytosolic and nuclear fractions prepared from fetal lung tissues (Ballard and Ballard, 1972; Giannopoulus, 1973).

There is evidence to support the view that glucocorticosteroids, when administered in large doses to the mother at certain critical times during gestation, increase the rate of maturation of the human fetal lung as indicated by a reduced incidence of respiratory distress syndrome in newborns of such glucocorticosteroid-treated mothers compared to those whose mothers were not so treated (Liggins and Howie, 1972). The precise role of glucocorticosteroids in fetal lung maturation has not been fully defined, however, and from the evidence available it cannot be concluded that cortisol is the single physiologic regulator of the activities of enzymes involved in surfactant formation in most species, including man. There is little doubt that the administration of glucocorticosteroids to pregnant women during the 29th to 33rd week of gestation is associated with a reduced incidence of respiratory distress in their prematurely born infants, but there are various conclusions regarding the mechanism(s) by which such treatment is effective. Some investigators have found that the lecithin (phosphatidylcholine)-to-sphingomyelin ratio in amnionic fluid increases after glucocorticosteroid treatment of the mother (Spellacy et al., 1973; Zuspan et al., 1977); yet, Liggins and Howie found no consistent increase. Some investigators have found in amnionic fluid a temporal relationship between the levels of cortisol and increasing lecithin-to-sphingomyelin ratios (Fencl et al., 1975; Tan et al., 1976); but we (Milewich et al., 1978) and others (Sivakoumaran et al., 1975) have not found such a relationship. Murphy (1975) found a significant correlation between the level of cortisol in umbilical cord plasma and the lecithin-to-sphingomyelin ratio in amnionic fluid; Sybulski and Manghan (1976) did not. Murphy found a relationship between the levels of cortisol in cord plasma and the subsequent development of respiratory distress syndrome in these newborns; Hauth and associates (1978) did not.

It should be pointed out that the failure to find a correlation between the levels of cortisol in umbilical cord plasma and in amnionic fluid with alterations in the L/S ratio in the amnionic fluid and with the subsequent development of respiratory distress syndrome should be viewed with caution. This obtains since it is likely that the metabolic clearance rate of plasma cortisol in the fetus increases as a function of the size of the fetus and in its vascular volume. Thus, the levels of fetal plasma cortisol may remain relatively constant during the latter few weeks of gestation while the rate of cortisol secretion by the fetal adrenal may be rising appreciably. If this were the case, then static measurements of fetal plasma cortisol at one point in time, i.e., at the time of birth, would not be reflective of the rate of secretion of cortisol by the fetal adrenal cortex. At the same time, the level of cortisol in amnionic fluid may not necessarily reflect the rate of cortisol secretion by the fetal adrenal. This obtains since cortisone arising in the maternal compartment can be converted to cortisol by the human fetal membranes (Murphy, 1977). Moreover, alterations in the rate of excretion of cortisol and cortisol sulfate by the developing fetal kidneys, together with increasing clearance of substances in amnionic fluid through increased fetal "breathing" and fetal swallowing as gestation advances, as well as transport from the amnionic fluid to the maternal compartment, are factors likely to give rise to significant alterations in the levels of cortisol in amnionic fluid independent of the rate of secretion of cortisol by the fetal adrenal cortex. Nonetheless, Johnson and colleagues (1978) found that the administration of glucocorticosteroids to pregnant subhuman primates was not associated with an increase in surfactant content in the fetal lungs. Rather, they found that the principal alteration in the fetal lungs of corticosteroid-treated pregnant monkeys was a decrease in the content of collagenous tissue.

Thus, in view of the failure to find a consistent relationship between glucocorticosteroid administration and an increase in activity of an enzyme involved in surfactant synthesis, the failure to find consistently a response in phosphatidylcholine formation (as indicated by an increased L/S ratio) after the administration of glucocorticosteroids to pregnant women, the failure to demonstrate consistently a temporal relationship between increased cortisol (as indicated by cortisol levels in amnionic fluid or in umbilical cord plasma) and increased surfactant formation, some investigators have been led to the conclusion that cortisol may not be the only trigger for augmented surfactant formation in the maturing human fetal lung (Hauth et al., 1978). This conclusion is strengthened by the well known clinical observation that the respiratory distress syndrome is not observed in many human neonates whose capacity to secrete cortisol is limited. Such infants include those who have anencephaly, adrenal hypoplasia, and congenital adrenal hyperplasia. It may be that cortisol is one of several hormones that act cooperatively to effect fetal lung maturation. For example, cortisol is believed to stabilize the ribosomal-endoplasmic reticulum complex of mammary tissue such that this organ can respond to prolactin and insulin and secrete milk (Oka and Topper, 1971).

PROLACTIN AND FETAL LUNG MATURATION. Winters and colleagues (1975) found that prolactin levels in fetal plasma increased strikingly during the last few weeks of human pregnancy. Hauth and co-workers (1978) found that the rise in fetal prolactin levels was temporally related to the increase in the L/S ratio in amnionic fluid (Fig. 8-18). They also noted that a role for prolactin can be envisioned by recalling that prolactin has a profound effect on the gills of fish, the phylogenetic homologue of lung (Lam, 1969) and that there are certain metabolic similarities between the maturing human lung and the prolactin-stimulated mammary gland. These two tissues share a common and almost unique lipid biosynthetic capability, i.e., an extraordinary capacity to incorporate palmitic acid into the *sn*-2 position of the glycerophospholipids of surfactant and the *sn*-2 position of triglycerides of milk (Breckenridge et al., 1969). Prolactin increases the capacity of mammary tissue maintained in culture to synthesize fatty acids (Hollowes et al., 1973) and other milk constituents such as casein and lactose (Turkington et al., 1973). Type II cell tumors of the lung and presumably nontumorous type II pneumocytes have a large capacity to synthesize palmitic acid when compared to the other cells of the lung (Voelker et al., 1976). Prolactin administration to fetal rabbits has been shown to increase the phosphatidylcholine concentration in fetal lungs (Hamosh and Hamosh, 1977). Interestingly, the action of prolactin

in mammary tissue is dependent upon pretreatment of such tissue with glucocorticosteroids and insulin.

On the other hand, it should be pointed out that Ballard and colleagues (1978) were unable to induce increased phosphatidylcholine content in the lung tissue of rabbit fetuses by prolactin treatment. Specifically, they did not find an increase in phosphatidylcholine concentration following the injection of prolactin into fetal rabbits of similar magnitude to that found by Hamosh and Hamosh (1977). Moreover, Ballard and associates administered prolactin to sheep fetuses and again were unable to find an increase in the phosphatidylcholine content of the tracheal fluid of such treated sheep fetuses. However, it should be noted that the lecithin content of tracheal fluid in the sheep fetus does not rise during glucocorticosteroid treatment. It has been reported recently that the newborn of a woman treated with bromocriptine did not suffer from respiratory distress syndrome (Bigazzi et al., 1979). This finding is important, since the levels of prolactin in the mother and in the newborn of this bromocriptine-treated woman were quite low. On the other hand, the level of prolactin in amnionic fluid of this subject was not reduced.

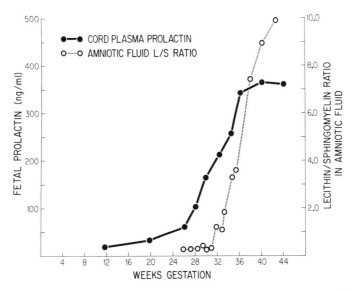

FIG. 8-18. Temporal relationship between fetal plasma prolactin concentrations and the amniotic fluid L/S ratio. (From Hauth et al. *Obstet Gynecol* 51:81, 1978)

TABLE 8-3.

THE INCIDENCE OF RESPIRATORY DISTRESS AND CORD
PLASMA PROLACTIN LEVELS IN VARIOUS GESTATIONAL
AGE GROUPS

GESTATIONAL AGE AT DELIVERY (WKS)	INCIDENCE OF RESPIRATORY DISTRESS SYNDROME				
	Newborn Cord Plasma Prolactin				
	(<200 ng/ml)		(≥200 ng/ml)		
	Incidence	Percent	Incidence	Percent	P*
≤26	4/4	100	0/0		—
26.5–29	12/14	86	0/0		—
29.5–33	20/25	80	0/10	0	<.001
33.5–36	7/25	28	2/43	5	<0.01
≥36.5	1/20	5	2/50	4	0.642

* Computed from the exact probability test of Fisher
From Hauth et al.: Obstet Gynecol 51:81, 1978.

Johnson and associates (1979) have recently proposed that prolactin in amnionic fluid, inspired into the fetal alveoli during fetal thoracic movements, may serve an important role in the maturation of fetal lungs. Thus, as in the case of cortisol, one cannot conclude that prolactin, either of fetal pituitary or amnionic fluid origin, is the sole stimulant for the biochemical maturation of the fetal lung.

Nonetheless, it has been found that the concentration of prolactin in umbilical cord plasma and the incidence of respiratory distress syndrome were inversely correlated (Table 8-3). In the study by Hauth and co-workers (1978) it was found that in those infants in whom the prolactin concentration in cord plasma was equal to or greater than 200 ng per ml, respiratory distress occurred uncommonly, 0 percent in infants delivered from 29.5 to 33 weeks of gestation and 5 percent in infants delivered from 33.5 to 36 weeks of gestation. When the prolactin level in cord plasma was less than 200 ng per ml, respiratory distress occurred often, 80 percent in infants delivered from 29.5 to 33 weeks, and 28 percent in those delivered from 33.5 to 36 weeks. All infants delivered from 25 to 29 weeks of gestation had prolactin levels less than 200 ng per ml; and among

these infants, the incidence of respiratory distress was 89 percent. Smith and co-workers (1978) have also measured cord plasma prolactin levels in 58 newborns ranging from 27 weeks gestation to term. They found that the incidence of respiratory distress was markedly increased in those infants in whom the cord plasma prolactin levels were less than 140 ng per ml, as compared to those in whom the prolactin levels were greater than 140 ng per ml. Gluckman and associates (1978) have also found that infants who develop respiratory distress had lower prolactin plasma concentrations at the time of birth than did those infants who did not develop respiratory distress. Similar findings have been reported recently by Grosso and colleagues (1979).

It can be argued that augmented surfactant biosynthesis and prolactin secretion are independent events in fetal lung maturation. However, the presence of prolactin receptors in fetal lung tissue (Josimovich et al., 1977) and the demonstrated participation of prolactin in lipid biosynthesis by the fetal lung and by mammary tissue are supportive of the view that prolactin has a role in the process of augmented surfactant formation. Additional support for this proposed action of prolactin in the biochemical maturation of the fetal lung is provided by the finding that the incidence of respiratory distress in premature infants born of heroin addicts is markedly decreased (Glass et al., 1971). Opiates, for example, morphine, are potent stimuli for prolactin secretion (Tolis et al., 1975). These several lines of evidence taken together have led some investigators to the conclusion that increased prolactin secretion and augmented synthesis of surfactant by the human fetus during the last trimester of gestation may be causally related, and that prolactin and cortisol may act in concert to bring about augmented surfactant synthesis.

ESTROGENS AND FETAL LUNG MATURATION.   It is of interest that many of the tissues that contain prolactin receptors also have receptors for estrogens. In fact, it appears that estrogens, directly or indirectly, regulate the number of prolactin receptors in the liver and mammary gland (Gelato et al., 1975; Kelly et al., 1975; Posner et al., 1975). Many of the actions of prolactin and estrogens appear to be interrelated, especially with regard to lipid metabolism and growth. Estrogens are anabolic steroids that have been shown to regulate lipoprotein synthesis in the liver (Luskey et al., 1974) and lipid metabolism in the rat uterus (Chan et al., 1976). Increased lipid synthesis is one of the earliest and most dramatic responses of the rat uterus to estrogenic hormones (Aizawa et al., 1961). Spooner and Gorski (1972) showed that estrogens enhanced both fatty acid synthesis and the incorporation of choline into phospholipids of the rat uterus. Dickey and Robertson (1969) reported that decreased maternal and neonatal urinary estrogens were found in instances where respiratory distress subsequently developed. Pasqualini and associates (1976), studying guinea pig fetuses, demonstrated a high concentration of estradiol-17β receptors in lung tissue cytosol as well as nuclear binding of the steroid. Moreover, the number of estrogen receptors in the lung of the guinea pig fetus increased with gestational age (Sumida et al., 1977). Mendleson and associates

(1980) have demonstrated estrogen binding in cytosolic fractions prepared from rat and human fetal lung tissues. Moreover, in a recent study, Khosla and Rooney (1979) found that when pregnant rabbits were injected with estradiol-17β, fetal lung surfactant content was increased.

THYROXINE AND FETAL LUNG MATURATION.   A role for thyroxine in the rate of surfactant synthesis has been proposed by a number of investigators. Thyroxine administration to rabbit fetuses of 24 to 25 days gestation is associated with accelerated maturation of the fetal lung and an early appearance of osmiophilic lamellar inclusions within the type II pneumonocytes (Rooney et al., 1974; Wu et al., 1971, 1973). Smith and Torday (1974) found that thyroxine treatment was associated with an increased incorporation of choline into phosphatidylcholine in cultured cells prepared from rabbit fetuses of 28 days gestation. On the other hand, Rooney and co-workers found no effect of thyroxine treatment on the activities of lysophosphatidic acid acyltransferase, CPTase CDP-diglyceride:inositol phosphatidyltransferase, glycerolphosphate phosphatidyltransferase, acyltransferase, or fatty acid biosynthesis. Mason and associates (1973), in a study of the effect of thyroxine treatment on the concentration of dipalmitoylphosphatidylcholine in lungs of hyperthyroid and in euthyroid rats, found that thyroxine had little effect on the concentration of dipalmitoylphosphatidylcholine. Thus, the role of thyroxine, if any, in the biochemical maturation of the fetal lung type II pneumonocyte is unclear.

CONCLUSION.   Presently, it seems reasonable to conclude that the hormonal stimulation of surfactant synthesis in the type II pneumonocytes of developing fetal lung is brought about by a complex interaction of several hormones. It is well established that pretreatment of breast tissue with estrogens followed by cortisol, prolactin, and insulin treatment is essential for lactation. Perhaps a similar sequence of events leads to surfactant formation in maturing fetal lungs.

Respiration. Within a very few minutes after birth, the respiratory system must be able to provide oxygen as well as eliminate carbon dioxide if the neonate is to survive. Development of air ducts and alveoli, pulmonary vasculature, muscles of respiration, and coordination of their activities through the central nervous system to a degree that allows the fetus to survive, at least for a time, can be demonstrated by the end of the second trimester of pregnancy. The majority of fetuses born before this time, however, succumb immediately or during the next few days from respiratory insufficiency, as pointed out in Chapter 38 (p. 957).

Movements of the fetal chest wall have been detected by sophisticated ultrasonic technics as early as 11 weeks gestation (Boddy et al., 1975). From the beginning of the 4th month, the fetus is capable of respiratory movement sufficiently intense to move amnionic fluid in and out of the respiratory tract. In the roentgenogram in Figure 8-19, obtained 26 hours after injection of Thorotrast into the amnionic sac, the contrast medium in the lungs of the very immature fetus is clearly demonstrated. From this and similar studies by Davis and Potter (1946) it was shown that the longer the exposure in utero after a single injection of Thorotrast, the greater the apparent concentration in the lungs.

Duenhoelter and Pritchard (1976, 1977) demonstrated in both the human and the rhesus fetus that chromium-labeled erythrocytes and other labeled particles injected into the amnionic sac accumulated in the lungs as well as the gastrointestinal tract (Fig. 8-20). They interpreted their findings to mean that throughout the last two trimesters progressively larger volumes of amnionic fluid are normally inspired and presumably for the most part expired by the fetus. The pressure changes with some inspirations demonstrated by Martin and co-workers (1974) in the rhesus fetus are sufficient to account for such movement.

Boddy and Dawes (1975) identified fetal breathing movement in the normal human fetus that are episodic and irregular; their

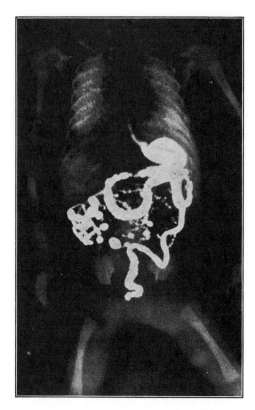

FIG. 8-19. X-ray of 115-g fetus in which Thorotrast is present in the lungs, esophagus, stomach, and entire intestinal tract following injection of Thorotrast into the amnionic cavity 26 hours before delivery. It demonstrates not only intrauterine respiration of the fetus but also active swallowing of amniotic fluid by the fetus. (From Davis and Potter. *JAMA* 131:1194, 1946)

frequency ranged typically from 30 to 70 per minute. Asphyxia was followed by cessation of normal breathing movements and the initiation of gasping respiratory efforts.

VAGITUS UTERI. Crying in utero is a rare phenomenon. Following rupture of the membranes air may gain access to the amnionic cavity and be inspired by the fetus. Thiery and associates (1973) described three cases in which fetal crying was heard during vaginal examination, amnioscopy, or application of a clip electrode to the fetus. Hiccuping in utero is a much more common phenomenon.

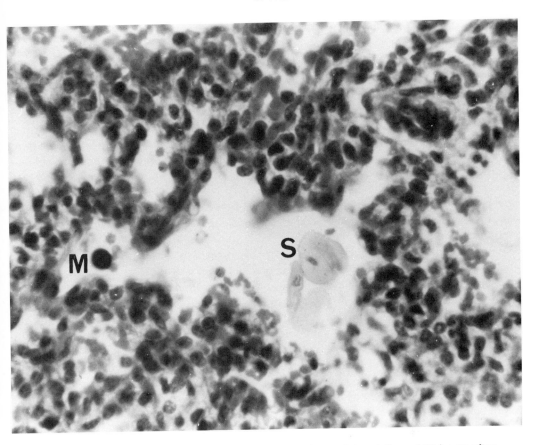

FIG. 8-20. Photomicrograph of lung of a near-term rhesus fetus delivered 24 hours after labeling the amnionic fluid with radiostrontium-labeled microspheres as well as chromium-labeled erythrocytes. Contained in the alveolus immediately adjacent to the dense microsphere (M) are labeled erythrocytes that were also inhaled, as were fetal squamous cells, or squames (S). From the amount of chromium within the lungs, it was calculated that at least 62 ml of amnionic fluid was inhaled in 24 hours by a fetus that weighed 281 g. (From Duenhoelter and Pritchard. *Am J Obstet Gynecol* 125:306, 1976)

Digestive System. As early as the 11th week of gestation, the small intestine demonstrates peristalsis and is capable of transporting glucose actively (Koldovsky et al., 1965). By the 4th month, gastrointestinal function is sufficiently developed to allow the fetus to swallow amnionic fluid, absorb much of the water from it, and, as shown in Figure 8-19, propel unabsorbed matter as far as the lower colon. Hydrochloric acid and some of the digestive enzymes characteristic of the gastrointestinal tract of the adult are demonstrable in the early fetus but in very small amounts, compared with those in postnatal life.

Fetal swallowing at various stages of pregnancy has been measured by introducing a small volume of maternal erythrocytes labeled with isotopic chromium into the amnionic sac and subsequently measuring the chromium that accumulated in the gastrointestinal tract either directly in fetuses that succumbed from immaturity after delivery or in the meconium and feces passed after birth by more mature fetuses (Pritchard, 1965, 1966). Term-size fetuses were thought to swallow relatively large volumes of amnionic fluid; in one study, the amount appeared to average nearly 450 ml of amnionic fluid per 24 hours. Gitlin and associates (1972) found that the rate of clearing of radiolabeled albumin from amnionic fluid, presumably by swallowing, was very similar to this value. More recent studies indicate, however, that the volumes of amnionic fluid swallowed directly by the fetus are probably somewhat less than what has been reported. More likely some of the label in the amnionic fluid was removed by inhalation and the inspired label, in turn, was either absorbed across the lung or was propelled from the lung by ciliary movement into the pharynx from which it was swallowed (Duenhoelter and Pritchard, unpublished). In either event the apparent volume of fluid swallowed would be somewhat greater than that actually swallowed.

Fetal swallowing appears to have little effect on amnionic fluid volume early in pregnancy, since the volume swallowed is small compared with the total volume of amnionic fluid present. Late in pregnancy, however, the volume of amnionic fluid surrounding the fetus appears to be regulated to some degree by fetal swallowing, and when swallowing is inhibited, hydramnios is common (see Chap. 23, p. 578).

The act of swallowing may enhance growth and development of the alimentary canal and condition the fetus for alimentation after birth, although anencephalic fetuses, which usually swallow little amnionic fluid, have gastrointestinal tracts that appear normal. In the latter part of pregnancy, swallowing serves to remove some of the insoluble debris that is normally shed into the amnionic sac and sometimes abnormally excreted into it. The undigested portions of the swallowed debris can be identified in meconium collected at birth. The amnionic fluid swallowed probably contributes little to the caloric requirements of the fetus but may contribute essential nutrients. Gitlin (1974) demonstrated that late in pregnancy about 0.8 g of soluble protein, approximately one-half albumin, appears to be ingested by the fetus each day.

Meconium consists not only of undigested debris from swallowed amnionic fluid, but to a larger degree, of various products of secretion, excretion, and desquamation by the gastrointestinal tract. The dark greenish-black appearance is caused by pigments, especially biliverdin. Hypoxia has been implicated in the evacuation of meconium from the large bowel into the amnionic fluid. Small-bowel obstruction may lead to vomiting in utero (Shrand, 1972). Indeed fetuses who suffer from congenital chloride diarrhea may have diarrhea *in utero* which leads to hydramnios and premature delivery (Holmberg et al., 1977).

Liver and Pancreas. Hepatic function in the fetus differs in several ways from that of the adult. Many enzymes of the fetal liver are present in considerably reduced amounts compared with those in later life. The liver has a very limited capacity for converting free *bilirubin* to bilirubin diglucuronoside (see Chap. 38, p. 972). The more immature the fetus, the more deficient is the system for conjugating bilirubin.

As mentioned in the discussion of fetal blood, the life span of the erythrocyte of the fetus is shorter than that of the normal adult; as the result, relatively more bilirubin is produced. Only a small fraction of the bilirubin is conjugated by the fetal liver and excreted through the biliary tract into the intestine where, for the most part, it is oxidized to biliverdin. Studies of the fate of bilirubin in the fetus have been conducted in the monkey and the dog by Bashore and associates (1969) and by Bernstein and co-workers (1969), who demonstrated that radiolabeled unconjugated bilirubin is cleared promptly from the fetal circulation by the placenta to be conjugated by the maternal liver and excreted through the maternal biliary tract. The transfer of the unconjugated bilirubin across the placenta, however, is bidirectional. This observation is supported by the rarely encountered case of fetal hyperbilirubinemia as the consequence of high levels of unconjugated bilirubin in maternal plasma. Conjugated bilirubin is not exchanged to any significant degree between mother and fetus.

Glycogen appears in low concentration in the fetal liver during the second trimester of pregnancy, but near term there is a rapid and marked increase in normal fetuses to levels 2 to 3 times those in adult liver. After delivery, the glycogen content falls precipitously.

The exocrine function of the fetal pancreas appears to be limited but not necessarily absent. For example, radioiodine-labeled human albumin injected into the amnionic sac and swallowed by the fetus is absorbed from the fetal intestine. It is not absorbed as undigested protein, however, since the iodine is excreted promptly in the maternal urine when pretreatment with iodide has been provided to enhance the clearance of the digested radiolabeled iodine (Pritchard, 1965).

Insulin-containing granules can be identified in the fetal pancreas by nine weeks gestation, and plasma *insulin* is detectable at 12 weeks (Adam, 1969). The fetal pancreas responds to hyperglycemia by increasing plasma insulin (Obershain et al., 1970). Although the precise role played by insulin of fetal origin is not clear, fetal growth must be determined to a considerable extent by the amounts of basic nutrients from the mother and, through the action of insulin, the anabolism of these materials by the fetus. Insulin levels are not only high in serum from infants of diabetic mothers but also in other large-for-gestational-age infants, whereas they are low in infants who are small for gestational age (Brinsmead, Liggins, 1979). Proof that insulin of fetal origin helps meet the needs of the diabetic mother is lacking.

Glucagon has been identified in the pancreas at 8 weeks gestation. Induced hypoglycemia and infused alanine increase glucagon levels in the rhesus mother, yet similar stimuli to the fetus do not. Within 12 hours of birth, however, the infant is capable of responding (Chez et al., 1975). Moreover, fetal alpha cells of the pancreas are capable of responding to L-dopa (Epstein et al., 1977). Therefore, the alpha cell nonresponsiveness to hypoglycemia and to infused alanine was the consequence of failure of release of glucagon rather than inadequate production of the hormone.

Other Endocrine Glands. Before the end of the first trimester, the fetal pituitary is able to synthesize and store pituitary hormones. Growth hormone, corticotropin (ACTH), prolactin, luteinizing hormone, and follicle-stimulating hormone have been identified in the pituitary of the human fetus by 10 weeks gestation. Moreover, the fetal pituitary is responsive to hypophysiotropic hormones and is capable of secreting these hormones from early in gestation (Grumbach and Kaplan, 1974).

Winters and co-workers (1974) have shown that by the 12th week ACTH levels are high in fetal plasma and remain so until late in pregnancy, when they decrease significantly. As gestation advances, however, *prolactin* in fetal plasma rises remarkably, to levels on the average 6 times greater at 35 to 42 weeks gestation than at 16 to 19 weeks.

The levels of pituitary *growth hormone* are rather high in cord blood, although the hormone's role in fetal growth and development is not clear. Decapitation in utero does not appreciably impair the growth of the rest of the animal fetus, as shown by Bearn (1967) as well as others. Furthermore, human anencephalic fetuses with little pituitary tissue are not remarkably different in weight from normal fetuses.

The pituitary-thyroid system is capable of function by the end of the first trimester (Table 8-4). However, until midpregnancy secretion of thyroid-stimulating hormone and thyroid hormones is low. There is considerable increase after this time (Fisher, 1975). Probably very little *thyrotropin* crosses the placenta from mother to fetus, whereas the pathologic long-acting thyroid stimulators LATS and LATS Protector do so (see Chap. 28 p. 749).

The human placenta actively concentrates iodide on the fetal side, and throughout the second and third trimesters of pregnancy the fetal thyroid concentrates iodide more avidly than does the maternal thyroid. Therefore, the hazard to the fetus of administering to the mother either radioiodide or appreciable amounts of ordinary iodide is obvious.

Most evidence is indicative that thyroid hormones of maternal origin cross the placenta to a very *limited* degree, with triiodothyronine crossing more readily than thyroxin. The fetus is dependent upon hormone pro-

TABLE 8-4.
PHASES OF THYROID MATURATION IN THE HUMAN FETUS
AND NEWBORN INFANT

PHASE	EVENTS	GESTATIONAL AGE
I	Embryogenesis of pituitary-thyroid axis	2–12 weeks
II	Hypothalamic maturation	10–35 weeks
III	Development of neuroendocrine control	20 weeks to 4 weeks after birth
IV	Maturation of peripheral monodeiodination systems	30 weeks to 4 weeks after birth

From Fisher: Ross Conference on Obstetrical Decisions and Neonatal Outcome, San Diego, May, 1979.

duced by the fetal thyroid gland. From the fact that athyreotic cretins generally have euthyroid mothers it can be implied that a normal rate of maternal thyroid secretion cannot compensate for inadequate fetal glandular synthesis.

Immediately after birth there are major changes in thyroid function and metabolism. Atmospheric cooling evokes sudden and marked increase in thyrotropin secretion which, in turn, causes a progressive increase in serum thyroxine levels maximal 24 to 36 hours after birth. There are nearly simultaneous elevations of serum triiodothyronine levels.

There is good evidence that the fetal parathyroids elaborate *parathormone* by the end of the first trimester, and the glands appear to respond in utero to regulatory stimuli. Newborn infants of mothers with hyperparathyroidism, for example, may suffer hypocalcemic tetany.

Lack of *antidiuretic hormone* production by the fetus has been suggested to account for the lack of urine-concentrating ability in the newborn infant. However, several investigators have found that the levels of arginine vasopressin in umbilical cord plasma are strikingly increased compared to the levels found in maternal plasma.

The *adrenal* of the human fetus is very much larger in relation to total body size than is that of the adult; the bulk of the enlargement is made up of the central or so-called fetal zone of the adrenal cortex. The normally hypertrophied fetal zone involutes rapidly after birth. The fetal zone is scant to absent in rare instances where the fetal pituitary is missing. The function of the fetal adrenal and the control of fetal adrenal steroidogenesis are discussed in detail in Chapter 7 (p. 154).

The fetal adrenal synthesizes *aldosterone.* In one study, aldosterone levels in cord plasma near term exceeded those in maternal plasma, as did renin and renin substrate (Katz et al., 1974). The renal tubules of the newborn, and presumably the fetus, appear relatively insensitive to aldosterone (Kaplan, 1972).

Catecholamines are present in the adrenal medulla from very early in fetal life.

Siiteri and Wilson (1974) have demonstrated synthesis of *testosterone* by the fetal testis from progesterone and pregnenolone by 10 weeks gestation. The capacity for steroidogenesis by the ovary is limited before the development of primary and graafian follicles in the second half of gestation (Grumbach and Kaplan, 1974).

Components of the fetoplacental endocrine system very likely play a prominent role in the initiation of spontaneous labor, as discussed in Chapter 15.

Nervous System and Sensory Organs. Synaptic function is developed sufficiently by the eighth week of gestation to demonstrate flexion of neck and trunk (Temiras et al., 1968). If the fetus is removed from the uterus during the 10th week, spontaneous movements may be observed, although movements in utero usually are not felt by the mother until several weeks later. At 10 weeks, local stimuli may evoke squinting, opening the mouth, incomplete finger closure, and plantar flexion of the toes. Complete finger closure is achieved during the fourth lunar month. Swallowing and respiration are also evident during the fourth lunar month, as demonstrated in Figure 8-19, but the ability to suck is not present until the 6th month.

During the third trimester of pregnancy, integration of nervous and muscular function proceeds rapidly, so that the majority of fetuses delivered after the thirty-second week of gestation survive.

By the 7th lunar month, the eye is sensitive to light, but perception of form and color is not complete until long after birth.

The internal, middle, and external components of the ear are well developed by midpregnancy. The fetus apparently hears some sounds in utero as early as the 24th to 26th week of gestation (Westin, 1968).

Taste buds are evident histologically in the third lunar month; by the seventh month of gestation, the fetus is responsive to variations in the taste of ingested substances.

Immunology. Infections in utero have provided an opportunity to examine some of the mechanisms for immune response by the human fetus. The opinion that the fetus is immunologically incompetent is no longer tenable. Indeed, morphologic evidence of immunologic competence in the human fetus has been reported as early as 13 weeks gestational age by Altshuler (1974), who described infection of the placenta and fetus by cytomegalovirus with characteristic severe imflammatory cell proliferation as well as virus inclusions. Moreover, synthesis by fetal organs of components of complement late in the first trimester has been demonstrated by Kohler (1973). All components of human complement are produced at an early stage of fetal development. In cord blood at or near term, the average level for most components of complement are about one-half the values for adults (Adinolfi, 1977).

In the absence of a direct antigenic stimulus in the fetus, such as infection, the immunoglobulins in the fetus consist almost totally of species of immune globulin G (IgG) synthesized by the mother and subsequently transferred across the placenta by both diffusion and active transport, as described on page 180 of this chapter. Therefore, the antibodies in the fetus and the newborn infant most often reflect the immunologic experiences of the mother.

Differing from many animals, the human newborn infant does not acquire much in the way of passive immunity from the absorption of humoral antibodies ingested in colostrum. Nonetheless, IgA ingested in colostrum may provide protection against enteric infections, since the antibody resists digestion and is effective on mucosal surfaces. The same is possibly true for IgA ingested with amnionic fluid before delivery.

In the adult, production of immune globulin M (IgM) in response to antigen is superseded in a week or so predominantly by production of IgG. In contrast, the IgM response remains the dominant one for weeks to months in the fetus and newborn. IgM serum levels in umbilical cord blood and identification of specific antibodies may be of aid in the diagnosis of intrauterine infection.

The transfer of some IgG antibodies from mother to fetus is harmful rather than protective to the fetus. The classic clinical example of antibodies of maternal origin that are dangerous to the fetus is hemolytic disease of the fetus and newborn resulting from Rh isoimmunization. In this disease, maternal antibody to fetal erythrocyte antigen crosses to the placenta to destroy the fetal erythrocytes (see Chap. 38, p. 961).

Nutrition of the Fetus. During the first 2 months of pregnancy, the embryo consists almost entirely of water; in later months, relatively more solids are added. The amounts of water, fat, nitrogen, and certain minerals in the fetus at successive weeks of pregnancy are shown in Table 8-5, adapted from Widdowson (1968). Because of the small amount of yolk in the human ovum, growth of the fetus from the very early stage of develop-

TABLE 8-5.

TOTAL AMOUNTS OF FAT, NITROGEN, AND MINERALS IN THE BODY OF THE DEVELOPING FETUS

BODY WEIGHT (g)	APPROXIMATE FETAL AGE (weeks)	WATER (g)	FAT (g)	N (g)	Ca (g)	P (g)	Mg (g)	Na (mEq)	K (mEq)	Cl (mEq)	Fe (mg)	Cu (mg)	Zn (mg)
30	13	27	0.2	0.4	0.09	0.09	0.003	3.6	1.4	2.4	—	—	—
100	15	89	0.5	1.0	0.3	0.2	0.01	9	2.6	7	5.1	—	—
200	17	177	1.0	2.8	0.7	0.6	0.03	20	7.9	14	10	0.7	2.6
500	23	440	3.0	7.0	2.2	1.5	0.10	49	22	33	28	2.4	9.4
1000	26	860	10	14	6.0	3.4	0.22	90	41	66	64	3.5	16
1500	31	1270	35	25	10	5.6	0.35	125	60	96	100	5.6	25
2000	33	1620	100	37	15	8.2	0.46	160	84	120	160	8.0	35
2500	35	1940	185	49	20	11	0.58	200	110	130	220	10	43
3000	38	2180	360	55	25	14	0.70	240	130	150	260	12	50
3500	40	2400	560	62	30	17	0.78	280	150	160	280	14	53

From Widdowson: In Assali (ed): Biology of Gestation, Vol. II, The Fetus and Neonate. New York, Academic, 1968.

ment depends on nutrition obtained from the mother. During the first few days after implantation, the nutrition of the fertilized ovum is derived directly from the interstitial fluid of the endometrium and from the surrounding maternal tissue, which has undergone proteolysis as the result of trophoblastic invasion. Within the next week, the forerunners of the intervillous space arise, comprising at first simply lacunae filled with maternal blood. During the 3rd week after ovulation, blood vessels appear in the chorionic villi. During the 4th week after ovulation, a cardiovascular system has formed, and thereby a true circulation, both within the embryo and between the embryo and the chorionic villi.

Ultimately, the maternal diet is the source of the nutrients supplied to the fetus. The mother eats varying amounts and kinds of food several times a day. In turn, the food is digested, its constituents are absorbed, and, for the most part, they are immediately stored. The storage forms are then made available continuously in an orderly way to meet the demands for energy, tissue repair, and new growth, including pregnancy. Three major storage depots, namely, the liver, muscle, and adipose tissue, and the storage hormone, insulin, are involved intimately in the metabolism of the nutrients absorbed from the maternal gut. Insulin is released from the maternal islands of Langerhans in response to various materials liberated from food during digestion and absorption. The secretion of insulin is sustained by rising levels of blood glucose and amino acids. The net effect is to store glucose as glycogen primarily in the liver and muscle, to retain some amino acids as protein, and to store the excess as fat.

During the fasting state, glucose is released from glycogen, but glycogen stores are not large in the mother and cannot in themselves provide an adequate amount of glucose to meet the requirements of the mother and fetus for energy and growth. The cleavage of stored triglycerides in adipose tissue, however, can provide the mother with energy in the form of free fatty acids. The process of lipolysis is activated directly or indirectly by a number of hormones, including glucagon, norepinephrine, placental lactogen, glucocorticoids, and thyroxine. Neutral fat does not cross the placenta but glycerol does. The extent of transport of free fatty acids is not known, although Szabo and associates (1969) noted the active transfer of palmitic acid from the maternal to the fetal side of the human placenta perfused in vitro. Portman and co-workers (1969), furthermore, demonstrated rapid transfer of palmitic and linoleic acids from mother to fetus in subhuman primates. Glucose and the naturally occurring forms of amino acids, of course, readily cross the placenta to the fetus. It appears that glucose transfer across the placenta is carrier-mediated, or "facilitated" although this is not an established fact (Hay, 1979). The fetus is not exposed to a constant supply of glucose since even in normal pregnant women the maternal plasma level may vary by up to 75 percent. Granted the fetus is quite dependent on his mother ultimately for nutrition, but he is not a passive parasite. He can actively participate through appropriate humoral and metabolic interaction in providing for his own nutrition.

The placenta is known to concentrate a large number of amino acids intracellularly from maternal plasma (Lemons, 1979). The actual uptake of amino acids by the placenta occurs by diffusion and by active transport. Presumably, fetal uptake of amino acids is dependent to an appreciable extent upon this concentrating capacity of the placenta. Essential amino acids for the fetus include methionine, cystine, histidine, isoleucine, leucine, lysine, phenylalanine, threonine, tryptophan, and valine (Lemons, 1979).

Since glucose is a major nutrient for growth and energy in the fetus, it would seem advantageous during pregnancy, as emphasized by Freinkel (1969), for the operational mechanisms to be those that minimize glucose utilization by the mother and thereby make the limited maternal supply available to the fetus. One metabolic action of placental lactogen, a hormone normally present in abundance in the mother but not the fetus, is to block the utilization of glucose by the mother while promoting the mobilization and utilization of free fatty acids. Placental lactogen does not appear to be absolutely required for a normal pregnancy outcome, however. Neilsen and co-workers (1979) have described an otherwise normal pregnancy in which *no* placental lactogen could be identified by a variety of technics applied in several laboratories.

For obvious reasons, a great deal of investigative effort continues to be focused on maternal nutrition and its effect on the growth and development of the fetus. Fetal size is not just a function of fetal age. For example, in maternal diabetes mellitus without significant maternal vascular disease, the fetus is much larger typically than normal, but if severe maternal vascular disease further complicates the diabetes, the fetus may be appreciably smaller than normal (see Chap. 28, p. 745). Page (1970), in an interesting theoretical discussion of fetal growth, analyzed the factors known to control the delivery of a primary nutrient, glucose, to the fetus. Since maternal hyperglycemia leads to increased transfer of glucose across the placenta, he suggested that hyperglycemia and hyperinsulinemia in the fetus together accelerate fetal growth. Brinsmead and Liggins (1979) have observed insulin levels to be higher in cord plasma from large-for-gestational-age infants and lower when infants were small for gestational age.

Factors leading to growth retardation in the human fetus, are complex. Growth retardation might result from insufficient concentration of a nutrient in the maternal arterial plasma, inadequate uterine blood flow and placental perfusion, reduced functional surface area of the chorionic villi, impairment of placental transport mechanisms, inadequate vascularity of the chorionic villi, or insufficient umbilical blood flow to transfer the nutrient in appropriate amounts from the placenta to the fetus. Maternal dietary deficiencies among species in which the weight of the fetus is relatively large compared with the mother's weight, and in which the duration of gestation is short, commonly cause fetal growth retardation. In women, however, in whom fetal size is slight compared with that of the mother and the duration of

gestation is long, it has been difficult to demonstrate a clear-cut correlation between maternal nutritional deficiency and fetal growth retardation (see Chap. 13, p. 309). It is possible that subtle but nonetheless deleterious changes in the human fetus may be induced by faulty maternal nutrition, be it either undernutrition or the ingestion of excessive amounts of nutrients, including protein (Stein et al., 1978).

AMNIONIC FLUID

The fluid filling the amnionic sac serves several important functions. It provides a medium in which the fetus can readily move, cushions him against possible injury, helps him maintain an even temperature, and provides, when appropriately tested, useful information concerning the health and maturity of the fetus (see Chap. 14). If the presenting part of the fetus is not closely applied to the lower uterine segment during labor, the hydrostatic action of the amnionic fluid may be important in dilating the cervical canal.

By the 12th day after fertilization of the ovum, a cleft enclosed by primitive amnion has formed adjacent to the embryonic plate. Rapid enlargement of the cleft and fusion of the surrounding amnion first with the body stalk, and later with the chorion, create the amnionic sac, which fills with an essentially colorless fluid. The amnionic fluid increases rapidly to an average volume of 50 ml at 12 weeks gestation and to 400 ml at midpregnancy; it reaches a maximum of about a liter at 36 to 38 weeks gestation. The volume then decreases as term approaches, and if the pregnancy is prolonged, amnionic fluid may become relatively scant. There are rather marked individual differences in amnionic fluid volume, however, as reported by Fuchs (1966) and as the data of Gillibrand (1969), plotted in Figure 8-21, clearly show. The physician performing amniocentesis for diagnostic purposes soon appreciates the considerable variability in the volume of amnionic fluid present at the same time in different

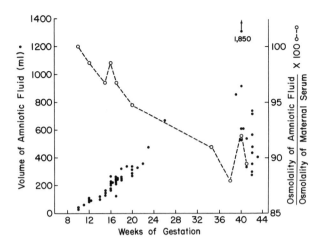

FIG. 8-21. Amnionic fluid volume, black dots and osmolality, open circles. The first and second trimesters are characterized by a rather orderly increase in volume, but at term the volume is quite variable. The osmolality decreases in approximately linear fashion as pregnancy advances. (From Gillibrand. *Br J Obstet Gynaecol* 76:527,893, 1969)

pregnancies as well as at different times in the same pregnancy.

The composition and volume of amnionic fluid change as pregnancy advances. In the first half of pregnancy, the fluid has essentially the same composition as maternal plasma except for a much lower protein concentration, and it is nearly devoid of particulate matter. As gestation advances, phospholipids, primarily from the lung, accumulate in the fluid and variable amounts of particulate matter in the form of desquamated fetal cells, lanugo and scalp hair, and vernix caseosa are shed into the fluid. The concentrations of various solutes also change significantly and, as a consequence, the osmolality decreases on the average about 20 to 30 mOsm, or about 10 percent, as shown in Figure 8-21.

Ions and small molecules move rapidly into and out of amnionic fluid but at rates that are specific for each substance. In contradistinction to bulk movement of amnionic fluid, as with swallowing, this process involves simply molecular or ionic trade across a membrane without necessarily inducing changes in volume or concentration (Plentl, 1968).

There is no single mechanism that will account for all the variations in composition and volume of amnionic fluid that have been observed during the course of a normal pregnancy. One relatively simple explanation is that amnionic fluid in early pregnancy is a product primarily of the amnionic membrane covering the placenta and cord. It is likely that fluid also passes across the fetal skin at this time (Lind et al., 1972). As the pregnancy advances, the surface of the amnion expands and the volume of fluid increases, but from about the 4th month the fetus is capable of modifying amnionic fluid composition and volume by urinating and swallowing progressively larger amounts of fluid. At the same time, movement of fluid into and out of the respiratory tract is likely to modify further the volume and composition of amnionic fluid.

Changes in osmolality are indicative that as gestation advances, the fetal urine makes an increasingly important contribution to the amnionic fluid. Fetal urine is quite hypotonic compared with maternal or fetal plasma, because of the lower electrolyte concentration in the urine, but it contains more urea, creatinine, and uric acid than does plasma. These observations have been made repeatedly on amnionic fluid and urine obtained at the time of delivery and have been shown to exist in utero as early as the 24th week of pregnancy. Mandelbaum and Evans (1969) examined urine obtained inadvertently from the fetal bladder in utero at the time of attempted intrauterine transfusion and compared the concentrations of several of the constituents of the urine with those of amnionic fluid. Even at 24 weeks gestation, the urea and creatinine concentrations were two to three times higher in the urine, whereas the concentrations of sodium, potassium, and chloride were only about one-third to one-fifth as great as those in the amnionic fluid. The admixture of sizable volumes of fetal urine with the amnionic fluid, therefore, would logically be expected to lower the osmolality, as demonstrated in Figure 8-21, and, at the same time, raise the concentration of urea, creatinine, and uric acid. Indeed, late in pregnancy, amnionic fluid normally differs from plasma in precisely these ways.

The fetus undoubtedly swallows amnionic fluid during much of pregnancy. Often, but not always, a great excess of amnionic fluid (hydramnios) develops whenever fetal swallowing is greatly impaired (see Chap. 23, p. 578). A classic example of a lesion in which fetal swallowing cannot take place and thereby leads to hydramnios is fetal esophageal atresia. Conversely, when urination in utero cannot take place, as in instances of renal agenesis or atresia of the urethra, the volume of amnionic fluid surrounding the fetus typically is extremely limited (oligohydramnios).

Although lack of fetal swallowing with continuous production of normal amounts of fluid by the amnion and by the fetal kidneys may lead to hydramnios, this mechanism is certainly not the sole cause of hydramnios. Progressive hydramnios has been observed in instances in which a normal fetus was known to ingest relatively large amounts of amnionic fluid, and in which maternal diseases known to predispose to hydramnios, such as diabetes, were not identified (Pritchard, 1966). Presumably, in these instances, increased production by the amnion or, unlikely, intense fetal polyuria, or even both, cause the increase in amnionic fluid volume. Whether the respiratory tract is involved at times in the development of hydramnios is not clear.

SEX OF THE FETUS

Sex Ratio. The accepted secondary sex ratio, that is, the sex ratio of human fetuses reaching viability, is approximately 106 males to 100 females. This figure has been obtained by the examination of term and premature infants. Many attempts have been made to establish a sex ratio for fetuses of earlier gestational age. In general, such studies have been misleading, for as Wilson (1926) showed, external genitals are an unreliable index of sex before the 50-mm stage.

Since, theoretically, there should be as many Y-bearing as X-bearing sperm, the primary sex ratio, or the ratio at the time of fertilization, should be 1 to 1. If so, the secondary sex ratio of 106 to 100 is suggestive that more females than males are lost during the early months of pregnancy. Establishment of the primary sex ratio in man is at present impracticable, for it requires the recovery and assignment of zygotes that fail to cleave and blastocysts that fail to implant. The results of Carr's studies (1963), nevertheless, are suggestive that the primary sex ratio in the human may be unity.

Sex Differentiation. One of the greatest responsibilities of the obstetrician is the assignment of sex to the newborn. An incorrect assignment of sex portends grave psychological and social problems for the baby and family. Yet we are of the view that sex assignment can be made correctly even with newborns with genital ambiguity. In order to address this issue together with that of making a definitive diagnosis in genitalia, the mechanisms of normal and abnormal sex differentiation should be considered. It is clear that male differentiation is directed by the testis. *In the absence of the testis, female differentiation ensues irrespective of the genetic sex.* For example, Jost (1973) found that if castration of the rabbit fetus were accomplished before differentiation of the genital anlagen, all newborns were phenotypic females with female external genitalia and müllerian ducts, which developed into upper vagina, uterus, and fallopian tubes. On the other hand, if castration of the fetus before differentiation of the genital anlagen were followed by implantation of a testis on one side, all fetuses were male phenotypes; the external genitalia of such fetuses was masculinized and on the side of the testicular implant there was wolffian duct development to form a vas deferens, epididymis, and seminal vesicles. Moreover, on the side of the testicular implant the müllerian structures, i.e., uterine horn and fallopian tube, were not present. On the other hand, the müllerian duct did develop on the side not containing a testis graft. Jost also found that following castration of the fetus at the sexually indifferent stage and implantation of a testosterone pellet, the external genitalia masculinized as did the wolffian duct, but that the müllerian duct, i.e., uterine horn and fallopian tube, did not regress. These fundamental observations, together with those of Wilson and collaborators (1970) form the basic framework of our understanding of the mechanisms of sex differentiation. Wilson and Gloyna, 1970, demonstrated that in most androgen responsive tissues, the androgen, testosterone, is converted to a 5 α-dihydrotestosterone by the action of the enzyme, 5 α-reductase. In these tissues, androgen action is expressed by this 5 α-reduced metabolite. The 5 α-dihydrotestosterone is bound to a cytosolic binding protein and the steroid-receptor protein complex is translocated to the nucleus to become associated with chromatin. Thus, in the genital tubercle and urogenital sinus, testosterone acts only after conversion to 5 α-dihydrotestosterone. There is a notable exception, however, to this generalization for testosterone action. Wilson and Lasnitzki (1971) demonstrated that testosterone acts on the wolffian duct of the embryo before 5 α-reductase activity is present in this tissue.

Based on these observations, the biochemical basis of sex differentiation can be formulated as illustrated diagramatically in Figure 8-22 and summarized below:

1. Genetic sex is established at the time of fertilization of the ovum.
2. Gonadal sex is determined by the action of a locus on the Y chromosome that codes for a plasma membrane antigen called the H-Y antigen. Such action brings about differentiation of the primitive gonad as a testis.
3. The fetal testis elaborates a proteinaceous substance called müllerian duct regression factor that brings about the regression of the müllerian duct: failure of development of uterus, fallopian tube, and upper vagina. Müllerian duct regression factor is produced by the Sertoli cells of the seminiferous tubules. It is important to recall that the seminiferous tubules appear in the

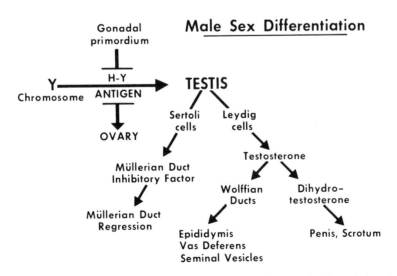

FIG. 8-22. Scheme of male sex differentiation. (From Grumbach. In *Genetic Mechanisms of Sexual Development.* New York, Academic, 1979)

fetal gonad before the Leydig cells, the cellular site of origin of testosterone. Therefore, müllerian duct regression is initiated before virilization by testosterone commences. Importantly, müllerian duct regression factor acts locally, i.e., near the site of formation; therefore, if a testis were absent on one side, the müllerian duct on that side would persist.

4. The fetal testis, under the influence of chorionic gonadotropin initially and thence pituitary LH, secretes testosterone which acts directly on the wolffian duct to effect the development of the vas deferens, epididymis, and seminal vesicles. Testosterone, of fetal testicular origin, enters the blood, reaches the genital tubercle and urogenital sinus, and, in these tissues, testosterone is converted to 5 α-dihydrotestosterone that brings about the androgenic action that leads to virilization of the external genitalia.

The development of ambiguous genitalia is brought about invariably by abnormal androgen representation in utero. This means, simply, too much androgen for an embryo or fetus destined to be female, or too little androgen representation for a fetus destined to be male. In the case of the fetus destined to be male, inadequate androgen representation may be caused by deficient fetal testicular secretion of testosterone or by a deficiency in responsiveness to testosterone or 5 α-dihydrotestosterone in tissues that nominally respond to androgens.

Based on these premises we believe that all abnormalities of sexual differentiation can be placed in one of three general categories:

Category 1. Female pseudohermaphroditism

Category 2. Male pseudohermaphroditism

Category 3. Dysgenetic gonads and true hermaphroditism

Category 1. Considered here are abnormalities that conform to the following guidelines: (1) müllerian duct regression factor *not* produced; (2) androgen exposure, variable; (3) karyotype-46,XX; (4) ovaries present. Category 1 is also

referred to as female pseudohermaphroditism. This obtains since all subjects in this category were destined to be female by virtue of genetic and gonadal sex. Thus, the only abnormality that can occur is androgen excess. Since müllerian duct regression factor was not produced, each subject in this category will have uterus, fallopian tubes, and upper vagina. If such embryos are exposed to a small androgen excess reasonably late in embryologic development, the only abnormality may be slight clitoral hypertrophy, with an otherwise normal female phenotype. With somewhat greater androgen excess, clitoral hypertrophy and posterior labial fusion may develop. With progressively increasing androgen excess somewhat earlier in embryologic development, there is greater virilization. This process of virilization can proceed through the formation of labioscrotal folds, the development of a urogenital sinus (in which the vagina empties into the posterior urethra) and even to the development of a penile urethra, the "empty scrotum" syndrome. The cause of female pseudohermaphroditism is excessive androgen. The androgen excess most commonly arises from the fetal adrenal by virtue of excess secretion of androgen in instances of enzymatic defects in the pathway to cortisol formation, i.e., congenital adrenal hyperplasia. With inadequate cortisol synthesis, it is presumed that ACTH secretion is elevated. Excessive stimulation of the adrenals leads to excessive secretion of cortisol precursors and their metabolites, which include androgens, principally androstenedione, which can be converted to testosterone in extraglandular tissues. Another cause of female pseudohermaphroditism is fetal androgen excess due to excessive androgen arising in the maternal compartment. The excess androgen in the mother may arise by secretion from maternal ovaries, hyperreactio lutealis, or tumors of the maternal ovary, e.g., luteomas or arrhenoblastomas, hilar cell tumors, etc. Commonly, however, the female fetus of a pregnant woman with an androgen-secreting tumor does not virilize. During much of pregnancy, the female fetus is protected from androgen excess in the mother because of the extraordinary capacity of the trophoblast to convert C_{19}-steroids (androgens) to estrogens. Certain drugs given to pregnant women will bring about virilization of their female fetus. Most commonly, such drugs are synthetic progestins. It is not altogether clear how progestins cause virilization of the female fetus. On the one hand, some of these compounds, especially the 19-nortestosterone group, may act on fetal tissues as androgens. On the other hand, these agents may act to inhibit aromatization in the placenta and thus allow the transfer to the fetus of androgens that escaped aromatization. In summary, all subjects of Category 1 can be normal females, including fertility, if the proper diagnosis is made and appropriate therapy initiated.

Category 2. Subjects with ambiguous genitalia, whose abnormalities conform to the following guidelines are considered here: (1) müllerian duct regression factor produced; (2) androgen representation, variable; (3) karyotype-46,XY; (4) testes, or no gonads, present. Category 2 is also referred to as male pseudohermaphroditism. This obtains since all subjects in this category were destined to be male by virtue of genetic sex. Thus, the only abnormality that can occur is inadequate virilization.

Diminished masculinization can arise by virtue of deficient production of testosterone by the fetal testis or by deficient responsiveness of genital tissues to normal quantities of androgen. Since müllerian duct regression factor was produced in these subjects during embryologic life, there is no uterus, fallopian tubes, or upper vagina. Deficient testosterone production may occur if there is an enzymatic defect in the testis involving one of the enzymes in the pathway to testosterone formation. There are five enzymatic steps in the conversion of cholesterol to testosterone. Defects in each of these enzymatic steps have been described.

If the testis regresses during embryologic life, there will be deficient testosterone production. Such an occurrence has been referred to as embryologic testicular regression (Edman et al., 1977).

Deficiencies in androgen responsiveness may be due to inadequate or abnormal androgen receptor macromolecules in the cytosol of androgen responsive tissues, or both, or may be due to failure of conversion of testosterone to 5 α-dihydrotestosterone in such tissues due to absence of 5 α-reductase enzyme activity. The most extreme form of the androgen resistance disorders is that of testicular feminization. In this disorder, there appears to be virtually no tissue responsiveness to androgen. Such subjects have a female phenotype with short, blind ending vagina, no uterus or fallopian tubes, and no wolffian duct structures. At the expected time of puberty testosterone levels rise to values similar to or greater than those found in normal adult men. Nonetheless, virilization does not occur and even sexual hair, i.e., pubic and axillary hair, does not develop because of the androgen resistance. Presumably because of androgen resistance at the level of brain and pituitary, LH levels are elevated in these women. As a consequence there is increased testicular secretion of estrogen compared to normal men (MacDonald et al., 1979). In the absence of androgen responsiveness, feminization, i.e., breast development, ensues. In the disorder called incomplete testicular feminization, there appears to be slight androgen responsiveness. In such subjects, there is modest clitoral hypertrophy at birth and at the expected time of puberty virilization does not occur but pubic and axillary hair do develop. These women also develop feminine breasts, presumably through the same endocrine mechanisms as in women with the complete form of testicular feminization (Madden et al., 1975).

A third syndrome of androgen resistance has been referred to as familial male pseudohermaphroditism, Type I (Walsh et al., 1974). This entity is commonly referred to as Reifenstein syndrome but constitutes a spectrum of abnormalities of genital virilization varying from a phenotype similar to that of women with incomplete testicular feminization to a male phenotype with only a bifid scrotum, sterility and gynecomastia. In these subjects, androgen resistance was also established by the demonstration of diminished 5 α-dihydrotestosterone binding capacity in fibroblasts grown in culture from genital skin biopsies.

The fourth form of androgen resistance is caused by a deficiency, in androgen responsive tissues, of the enzyme activity, 5 α-reductase. Since androgen action in the genital tubercle and urogenital sinus is mediated by 5 α-dihydrotestosterone, persons with 5 α-reductase deficiency have female external genitalia (modest clitoral hypertrophy). However, since androgen action in the wolffian duct of the embryo is mediated by testosterone per se, such persons have a well developed epididymis, seminal vesicles, vas deferens, and the ejaculatory ducts empty into the vagina.

A composite photograph of the genitalia of subjects with each of the four types of androgen resistance is shown in Figure 8-23.

Enzymatic defects in testicular testosterone biosynthesis give rise to decreased rates of fetal testosterone secretion. Incomplete masculinization of the external genitalia is the consequence. The phenotype of such newborns is variable in the degree of ambiguity since the degree of enzyme deficit varies.

The phenotype of subjects with embryologic testicular regression is dependent upon the time

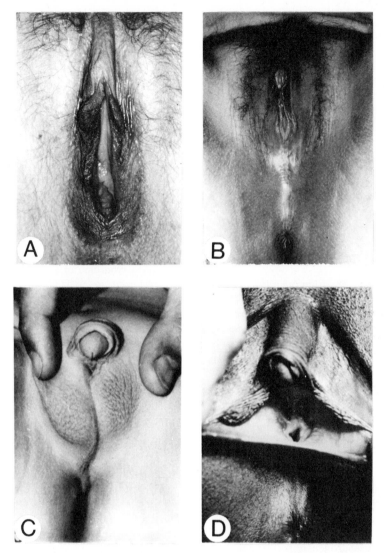

FIG. 8-23. External genitalia of representative patients with male pseudo-hermaphroditism due to androgen resistance. **A.** Testicular feminization. **B.** Incomplete testicular feminization. **C.** Familial male pseudohermaphroditism, Type I (Reinfenstein syndrome). **D.** 5-Reductase deficiency. (From Wilson and MacDonald. In *Metabolic Basis of Inherited Disease*. New York, McGraw-Hill, 1978)

in embryologic life that the fetal testis regressed. The time course of gonadal development and sexual differentiation is illustrated in Figure 8-24.

Edman and associates (1977) analyzed the phenotypes of reported cases of agonadism in 46, XY persons, and in three cases of their own. They compared these findings with those that would be expected to occur if the testis regressed at various stages of development according to embryo-

logic findings of the time course of sex differentiation (Jirasek, 1967, 1970, 1971). They found that a spectrum of phenotypes (cases *a-i,* Fig. 8-24) had been described which ranged from normal female phenotype with absent uterus, fallopian tubes and upper vagina, to normal male phenotype with anorchia. Since müllerian regression commences before virilization is initiated in embryonic life, such a spectrum of phenotypes was to be ex-

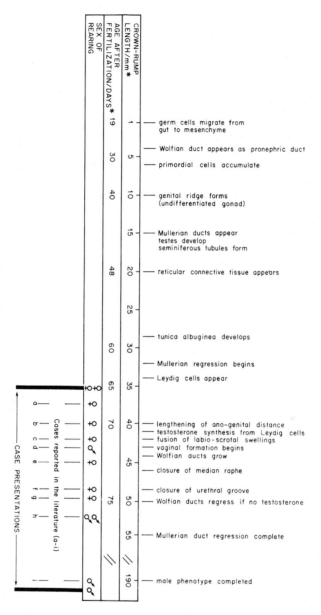

FIG. 8-24. The temporal relations of the sequence of morphologic changes that occur during male embryogenesis, and a comparison of this sequence to the phenotypes reported in subjects with embroyologic testicular regression. (From Edman et al. *Obstet Gynecol* 49:208, 1977)

pected if testicular regression were to occur at various times during sexual differentiation.

Category 3. This category of our classification of subjects with ambiguous genitalia encompasses those in whom the following guidelines are met:

(1) müllerian duct regression factor not produced; (2) androgen production, varied; (3) karyotype, varied and commonly abnormal; (4) gonads, neither ovaries nor testis (but rarely both). All of these subjects are characterized by having a uterus,

fallopian tubes and upper vagina. The majority of subjects in Category 3 have dysgenetic gonads. With the typical case of gonadal dysgenesis (e.g., those with Turner syndrome) there is a female phenotype and at the time of expected puberty sexual infantilism persists. Some persons with gonadal dysgenesis have ambiguous genitalia, a finding that is indicative that an abnormal gonad produced androgen, albeit in small amounts, during embryonic development. Generally, such subjects have mixed gonadal dysgenesis, i.e., a dysgenetic gonad on one side and an abnormal testis or ontogenetic tumor on the other side. Most subjects with true hermaphroditism fall into Category 3. True hermaphrodites are those persons with both ovarian and testicular tissue, specifically those who have in their gonads the germ cells, ova and sperm, of both sexes.

PRELIMINARY DIAGNOSIS. A preliminary diagnosis of the etiology of genital ambiguity can be made at the time of birth of an affected child. By rectal examination of the newborn, the experienced examiner can ascertain whether the child has a uterus. If the uterus is present, the diagnosis must be female pseudohermaphroditism, testicular or gonadal dysgenesis, or true hermaphroditism. A family history of congenital adrenal hyperplasia is helpful. If the uterus is not present, the diagnosis is male pseudohermaphroditism. Androgen resistance and enzymatic defects in testicular testosterone biosynthesis are familial.

SEX ASSIGNMENT. The critical decision of sex assignment by the obstetrician, in our view, is an easy decision to make. In our judgment, any newborn with ambiguity of the genitalia, and with the urethra opening onto the perineum, should be designated as female. This conclusion is reached on the basis of the following considerations: (1) All persons in Category 1 of our classification (i.e., female pseudohermaphroditism) can be normal, fertile women. (2) The subjects in Category 2 of this classification either cannot produce testosterone or are refractory to its action. Moreover, all of the subjects of Category 2 are infertile. (3) Reconstruction of the penis in such a manner that a sexually

functional organ is produced is difficult, if not presently impossible.

REFERENCES

Adam PAJ, Teramo K, Raiha N, Gitlin D, Schwartz R: Human fetal insulin metabolism early in gestation: response to acute elevation of the fetal glucose concentration and placental transfer of human insulin-I-131. Diabetes 18:409, 1969

Adinolfi M: Human complement: Onset and site of synthesis during fetal life. Am J Dis Child 131:1015, 1977

Aherne W, Dunnill MS: Morphometry of the human placenta. Br Med Bull 22:1, 1966

Aizawa Y, Mueller GC: The effect *in vivo* and *in vitro* of estrogens on lipid synthesis in the rat uterus. J Biol Chem 236:381, 1961

Altshuler G: Immunologic competence of the immature human fetus. Obstet Gynecol 43:811, 1974

Arey LB: Developmental Anatomy: A Textbook and Laboratory Manual of Embryology, 5th ed. Philadelphia, Saunders, 1946

Assali NS: In Gluck L (ed): Modern Perinatal Medicine. Chicago, Year Book, 1974

Assali NS, Morris JA: Maternal and fetal circulations and their interrelationships. Obstet Gynecol Survey 19:923, 1964

Assali NS, Bekey GA, Morrison LW: Fetal and neonatal circulation. In Assali NS (ed): Biology of Gestation, Vol II. The Fetus and Neonate. New York, Academic, 1968

Assali NS, Kirschbaum TH, Dilts PV: Effects of hyperbaric oxygen on uteroplacental and fetal circulation. Circ Res 22:573, 1968

Avery ME, Mead J: Surface properties in relation to atelectasis and hyaline membrane disease. Am J Dis Child 97:517, 1959

Ballard PL, Ballard RA: Glucocorticoid receptors and the role of glucocorticoids in fetal lung development. Proc Natl Acad Sci USA 69:2668, 1972

Ballard PL, Gluckman PD, Brehier A, Kitterman JA, Kaplan SL, Rudolph AM, Grumbach MM: Failure to detect an effect of prolactin on pulmonary surfactant and adrenal steroids in fetal sheep and rabbits. J Clin Invest 62:879, 1978

Barclay AE, Barcroft J, Barron DH, Franklin KJ: Radiographic demonstration of circulation through heart in adult and in foetus, and identification of ductus arteriosus. Br J Radiol 12:505, 1939

Barrett CT, Sevanian A, Kaplan SA: Cyclic AMP (cAMP) and surfactant production: New means for enhancing lung maturation in the fetus. Pediatr Res 9:394, 1975

Bashore RA, Smith F, Schenker S: Placental transfer and disposition of bilirubin in the pregnant monkey. Am J Obstet Gynecol 103:950, 1969

Bearn JG: Role of fetal pituitary and adrenal glands in the development of the fetal thymus of the rabbit. Endocrinology 80:979, 1967

Belcher DP: A child weighing 25 pounds at birth. JAMA 67:950, 1916

Bernstein RB, Novy MJ, Piasecki GJ, Lester R, Jackson BT: Bilirubin metabolism in the fetus. J Clin Invest 48:1678, 1969

Bigazzi M, Ronga R, Lancranjan I, Ferraro S, Branconi F, Buzzoni P, Martorana G, Scarselli GF, Del Pozo E: A pregnancy in an acromegalic woman during bromocriptine treatment: Effects on growth hormone and prolactin in the maternal, fetal, and amniotic compartments. J Clin Endocrinol Metab 48:9, 1979

Bleasdale JE, Wallis P, MacDonald PC, Johnston JM: Characterization of the forward and reverse reactions catalyzed by CDP-diacylglycerol: Inositol transferase in rabbit lung tissue. Biochim Biophys Acta 575:135, 1979

Boddy K, Dawes GS: Fetal breathing. Brit Med Bull 31:3, 1975

Braestrup PW: Studies of latent scurvy in infants: II. Content of ascorbic (cevitamic) acid in the blood serum of women in labor and in children at birth. Acta Paediat 19 (Suppl 1):328, 1937

Breckenridge WC, Makai L, Kuksis A: Triglyceride structure of human milk fat. Can J Biochem 47:761, 1969

Brehier A, Benson BJ, Williams MC, Mason RJ, Ballard PL: Corticosteroid induction of phosphatidic acid phosphatase in fetal rabbit lung. Biochem Biophys Res Commun 77:886, 1977

Brinsmead MW, Liggins GC: Somatomedin-like activity, prolactin, growth hormone and insulin in human cord blood. Aust NZ Obstet Gynaec 19:129, 1979

Brown A: Biology of Gestation, Vol. II. The Fetus and Neonate. New York, Academic, 1968

Carr D: Chromosome studies in abortuses and stillborn infants. Lancet 2:603, 1963

Chan L, Jackson RL, O'Malley BW: Synthesis of very low density lipoproteins in the cockerel. Effects of estrogen. J Clin Invest 58:368, 1976

Chez RA, Mintz DH, Reynolds WA, Hutchinson DL: Maternal-fetal plasma glucose relationships in late monkey pregnancy. Am J Obstet Gynecol 121:938, 1975

Clements, JA: Surface tension of lung extracts. Proc Soc Exper Biol Med 95:170, 1957

Davis ME, Potter EL: Intrauterine respiration of the human fetus. JAMA 131:1194, 1946

Dawes GS: The umbilical circulation. Am J Obstet Gynecol 84:1634, 1962

Delahunty TJ, Spitzer HL, Jimenez JM, Johnston JM: Phosphatidate phosphohydrolase activity in porcine pulmonary surfactant. Am Rev Resp Dis 119:75, 1979

De Verdier CH, Garby L: Low binding of 2, 3-diphosphoglycerate to hemoglobin F. Scand J Clin Lab Invest 23:149, 1969

Dickey RP, Robertson AF: Newborn estrogen excretion. Am J Obstet Gynecol 104:551, 1969

Dolman CL: Characteristic configuration of fetal brains from 22 to 40 weeks gestation at two week intervals. Arch Pathol Lab Med 101:193, 1977

Douglas WHJ, Delvecchio PJ, Steiniger GE, Teel RW, Spitzer HL, Johnston JM: Organotypic cultures of diploid type II alveolar pneumonocytes: phosphatidic acid phosphohydrolase (PAPase) activity, Intern Congr Cell Biol (Abs) 70:8ba, 1976

Duenhoelter JH, Pritchard JA: Unpublished observations

Duenhoelter JH, Pritchard JA: Fetal respiration: quantitative measurements of amnionic fluid inspired near term by human and rhesus fetuses. Am J Obstet Gynecol 125:306, 1976

Duenhoelter JH, Pritchard JA: Fetal respiration. A review. Am J Obstet Gynecol 129:326, 1977

Edman CD, Winters AJ, Porter JC, Wilson J, MacDonald PC: Embryonic testicular regression. A clinical spectrum of XY agonadal individuals. Obstet Gynecol 49:208, 1977

Ekelund L, Arvidson G, Åstedt B: Cortisol induced accumulation of phospholipids in organ culture of human fetal lung. Scand J Clin Lab Invest 35:419, 1975

Epstein M, Chez RA, Oakes GK, Mintz DH: Fetal pancreatic glucagon responses in glucose-intolerant nonhuman primate pregnancy. Am J Obstet Gynecol 127:268, 1977

Farrell PM, Avery ME: Hyaline membrane disease. Am Rev Resp Dis 111:657, 1975

Farrell PM, Zachman RD: Induction of choline phosphotransferase and lecithin synthesis in the fetal lung by corticosteroids. Science 179:297, 1973

Fencl MD, Montserrat deM, Tulchinsky D: Total cortisol in amniotic fluid and fetal lung maturation. N Engl J Med 292:133, 1975

Finnne PH: Antenatal diagnosis of the anemia in erythroblastosis. Acta Paediatr Scand 55:609, 1966

Fisher DA: Fetal thyroid hormone metabolism. Contemporary Ob/Gyn 3:47, 1975

Foley ME, Isherwood DM, McNicol GP: Viscosity, haematocrit, fibrinogen and plasma proteins in maternal and cord blood. Br J Obstet Gynaecol 85:500, 1978

Freinkel N: Homeostatic factors in fetal carbohydrate metabolism. In Wynn RM (ed): Fetal Homeostasis. Vol. IV. New York, Appleton, 1969

Fuchs F: Volume of amniotic fluid at various stages of pregnancy. Clin Obstet Gynecol 9:449, 1966

Gelato M, Marshall S, Boudreau M, Bruni J, Campbell GA, Meit J: Effects of thyroid and ovaries on prolactin binding activity in rat liver. Endocrinology 96:1292, 1975

Giannopoulus G: Glucocorticoid receptors in lung. I. Specific binding of glucocorticoids to cytoplasmic components of rabbit fetal lung. J Biol Chem 248:3876, 1973

Gillibrand PN: Changes in amniotic fluid volume with advancing pregnancy. J Obstet Gynaecol Br Commonw 76:527, 1969

Gitlin D: Protein transport across the placenta and protein turnover between amnionic fluid, maternal and fetal circulation. In Moghissi and Hafez (eds): The Placenta. Springfield, Ill., Thomas, 1974

Gitlin D, Kumate J, Morales C, Noriega L, Arevalo N: The turnover of amniotic fluid protein in the human conceptus. Am J Obstet Gynecol 113:632, 1972

Glass L, Rajegowda BK, Evans HE: Absence of respiratory distress syndrome in premature infants of heroin-addicted mothers. Lancet 2:685, 1971

Gluck L, Kulovich MV, Borer RC: The interpretation and significance of the lecithin-sphingomyelin ratio in amniotic fluid. Am J Obstet Gynecol 120:142, 1974

Gluck L, Landowne RA, Kulovich MV: Biochemical development of surface activity in mammalian lung: III. Structural changes in lung lecithin during development of the rabbit fetus and newborn. Pediatr Res 4:352, 1970

Gluck L, Kulovich MV, Borer RC, Brenner PH, Anderson GG, Spellacy WN: Diagnosis of the respiratory distress syndrome by amniocentesis. Am J Obstet Gynecol 109:440, 1971

Gluck L, Motoyama EK, Smits HL, Kulovich MV: The biochemical development of surface activity in mammalian lung. I. The surface-active phospholipids; the separation and distribution of surface-active lecithin in the lung of the developing rabbit fetus. Pediatr Res 1:237, 1967

Gluck L, Kulovich MV, Eidelman AI, Cordero L, Khazin AF: Biochemical development of surface activity in mammalian lung: IV. Pulmonary lecithin synthesis in the human fetus and newborn and etiology of the respiratory distress syndrome. Pediatr Res 6:81, 1972

Gluckman PD, Ballard PL, Kaplan SL, Liggins GC, Grumbach MM: Prolactin in umbilical cord blood and the respiratory distress syndrome. J Ped 93:1011, 1978

Gresham EL, Rankin JHG, Makowski EL, et al.: Fetal renal function in unstressed pregnancies. J Clin Invest 51:149, 1972

Grosso DS, MacDonald CP, Thomasson JE, Christian CD: Newborn serum prolactin (PRL) levels: Relationship to respiratory distress syndrome (RDS) and pre-eclampsia. Presented before Society for Gynecologic Investigation, San Diego, Calif, March 21, 1979

Gruenwald P: Growth of the human foetus. In McLaren A (ed): Advances in Reproductive Physiology. New York, Academic, 1967

Grumbach MM, Kaplan SL: Fetal pituitary hormones and the maturation of central nervous system regulation of anterior pituitary function. In Gluck L (ed): Modern Perinatal Medicine. Chicago, Year Book, 1974

Haase W: Maternity annual report for 1875. Charite Annalen 2:669, 1875

Hallman M, Kulovich MV, Kirkpatrick E, Sugarman RG, Gluck L: Phosphatidylinositol and phosphatidylglycerol in amniotic fluid: Indices of lung maturity. Am J Obstet Gynecol 125:613, 1976

Hamilton WJ, Mossman HW: Human Embryology, 4th ed. Baltimore, Williams & Wilkins, 1972

Hamosh M, Hamosh P: The effect of prolactin on the lecithin content of fetal rabbit lung. J Clin Invest 59:1002, 1977

Hauth JC, Parker CR, MacDonald PC, Porter JC,

Johnston JM: Role of fetal prolactin in lung maturation. Obstet Gynecol 51:81, 1978

Hay WW Jr: Fetal glucose metabolism. Semin Perinatol 3:157, 1979

Henriksson P, Hedner V, Nilsson IM, Boehm J, Robertson B, Lorand L: Fibrin-stabilization factor XIII in the fetus and the newborn infant. Pediatr Res 8:789, 1974

Herbert WNP, Johnston JM, MacDonald PC, Jimenez JM: Fetal lung maturation: Human amniotic fluid phosphatidate phosphohydrolase activity through normal gestation and its relation to the lecithin/sphingomyelin ratio. Am J Obstet Gynecol 132:373, 1978

Hocheim H: Cited by Kiedel W and Gluck L in Scarpelli (ed): Pulmonary Physiology of the Fetus, Newborn, and Child. Philadelphia, Lea & Febiger, 1975

Hollowes RC, Wang DY, Lewis DJ: The stimulation by prolactin and growth hormone of fatty acid synthesis in explants from rat mammary glands. J Endocrinol 57:265, 1973

Holmberg C, Perheentupa J, Launiala K, Hallman N: Congenital chloride diarrhoea. Archives of Disease in Childhood 52:255, 1977

Huisman THJ, Schroeder WA, Brown AK: Changes in the nature of human fetal hemoglobin during the first year of life. Presented before Society for Pediatric Research, Atlantic City, N.J., May 1, 1970

Jimenez JM, Johnston JM: Fetal lung maturation: IV. The release of phosphatidic acid phosphohydrolase and phospholipids into the human amniotic fluid. Pediatr Res 10:767, 1976

Jimenez JM, Schultz FM, Johnston JM: Fetal lung maturation. III. Amniotic fluid phosphatidic acid phosphohydrolase (PAPase) and its relation to the lecithin/sphingomyelin ratio. Am J Obstet Gynecol 46:588, 1975

Jimenez JM, Schultz FM, MacDonald PC, Johnston JM: Fetal lung maturation: II. Phosphatidic acid phosphohydrolase in human amniotic fluid. Gynecol Invest 5:245, 1974

Jirasek JE: The relationship between the structure of the testis and differentiation of the external genitalia and phenotype in man. In Wolstenholm, O'Conner (eds): Ciba Foundation Colloquia on Endocrinology. Endocrinology of the Testis. Boston, Little, Brown, 1967

Jirasek JE: The relationship between differentiation of the testicle, genital ducts and external genitalia in fetal and postnatal life. In Rosenberg, Paulsen (eds): The Human Testis: Advances in Experimental Medicine and Biology, Vol. 10. New York, Plenum Press, 1970

Jirasek JE: Development of the genital system in human embryos and fetuses. Development of the Genital System and Male Pseudohermaphroditism. Baltimore, Johns Hopkins Press, 1971

Johnson JWC, Mitzner W, London WJ, Palmer AE, Scott R, Kearney K: Glucocorticoids and the rhesus fetal lung. Am J Obstet Gynecol 130:905, 1978

Johnson JWC, Tyson JE, Mitzner W, London W, Palmer A, Andreassen B, Beck J: Prolactin and rhesus fetal lung characteristics. Presented before Society for Gynecologic Investigation, San Diego, Calif., March 21, 1979

Johnston JM, Porter JC, MacDonald PC: The biosynthesis and hormonal regulation of surfactant formation. In Gatt S, Freysz L, Mandel P (eds): Enzymes of Lipid Metabolism. New York, Plenum, 1978, p 327

Johnston JM, Reynolds G, Wylie MB, MacDonald PC: The phosphohydrolase activity in lamellar bodies and its relationship to phosphatidylglycerol and lung surfactant formation. Biochim Biophys Acta 531:65, 1978

Josimovich JB, Merisko K, Boccella L: Binding of prolactin by fetal rhesus cell membrane fractions. Endocrinology 100:557, 1977

Jost A, Vigier B, Prepin J: Studies on sex differentiation in mammals. Rec Prog Horm Res 29:1, 1973

Kaplan S: Disorders of the endocrine system. In Assali NS (ed): Pathophysiology of Gestation: III. Fetal and Neonatal Disorders. New York, Academic, 1972

Kasper CK, Hoag MS, Aggeler PM, Stone S: Blood clotting factors in pregnancy: Factor VIII concentrations in normal and AHF-deficient women. Obstet Gynecol 24:242, 1964

Katz FH, Beck P, Makowski EL: The renin-aldosterone system in mother and fetus at term. Am J Obstet Gynecol 118:51, 1974

Kelly PA, Posner BI, Friesen HG: Effects of hypophysectomy, ovariectomy, and cycloheximide on specific binding sites for lactogenic hormones in rat liver. Endocrinology 97:1408, 1975

Khosla SS, Rooney SA: Stimulation of fetal lung surfactant production by administration of 17β-estradiol to the maternal rabbit. Am J Obstet Gynecol 133:213, 1979

Kiedel W, Gluck L: In Scarpelli E (ed): Pulmonary physiology of the fetus, newborn, and child. Philadelphia, Lea and Febiger, 1975, p 96

Klaus MH, Clements JA, Havel RJ: Composition of surface-active material isolated from beef lung. Proc Natl Acad Sci USA 47:185, 1961

Kohler PF: Maturation of the human complement system. J Clin Invest 52:671, 1973

Koldovsky O, Heringova A, Jirsova U, Jirasek JE, Uher J: Transport of glucose against a concentration gradient in everted sacs of jejunum and ileum of human fetuses. Gastroenterology 48:185, 1965

Lam TJ: Effect of prolactin on loss of solutes via the head region of the early-winter marine threespine stickelback (gasterosteus aculeatus L., form tacherus) in fresh water. Can J Zool 47:865, 1969

Lands WE: Metabolism of glycerolipids: A comparison of lecithin and triglyceride synthesis. J Biol Chem 231:883, 1958

Lemons JA: Fetal-placental nitrogen metabolism. Semin Perinat 3:177, 1979

Liggins GC: Premature delivery of foetal lambs infused with glucocorticoids. J Endocrinol 45:515, 1969

Liggins GC, Howie MB: A controlled trial of antepartum glucocorticoid treatment of prevention of the respiratory distress syndrome in premature infants. Pediatrics 50:515, 1972

Lind T, Kendall A, Hytten FE: The role of the fetus in the formation of amniotic fluid. J Obstet Gynaecol Br Commonw 79:289, 1972

Longo L: In Assali NS (ed): Pathophysiology of Gestation, Vol II. New York, Academic, 1972

Luskey KL, Brown MS, Goldstein JL: Stimulation of the synthesis of very low density lipoproteins in rooster liver by estradiol. J Biol Chem 249:5939, 1974

MacDonald PC, Madden JD, Brenner PF, Wilson JD, Siiteri PK: Origin of estrogen in normal men and in women with testicular feminization. J Clin Endocrinol Metab 49:905, 1979

Madden JD, Walsh PC, MacDonald PC, Wilson JD: Clinical and endocrinological characterization of a patient with syndrome of incomplete testicular feminization. J Clin Endocrinol Metab 41:751, 1975

Manahan CP, Eastman NJ: The cevitamic acid content of fetal blood. Bull Hopkins Hosp 62:478, 1938

Mandelbaum B, Evans TN: Life in the amniotic fluid. Am J Obstet Gynecol 104:365, 1969

Marinetti GV, Erbland J, Witter RF, Petix J, Stotz E: Metabolic pathways of lipolecithin in a soluble rat-liver system. Biochim Biophys Acta 30:223, 1958

Martin CB, Murata Y, Petrie RH: Respiratory movements in fetal rhesus monkeys. Am J Obstet Gynecol 119:934, 1974

Mason RJ: Disaturated lecithin concentration of rabbit tissues. Am Rev Resp Dis 107:678, 1973

Mendelson CR, MacDonald PC, Johnston JM: Estrogen binding in human fetal lung cytosol. Endocrinology 106:368, 1980

Milewich L, Johnston JM, Bradfield DJ, Herbert WNP, MacDonald PC, Jimenez JM: The relationship of amniotic fluid dehydroisoandrosterone sulfate (DS) and cortisol (F) concentrations with lecithin to sphingomyelin (L/S) ratios during human gestation. Pediatr Res 12:397, 1978 (abstract)

Moore K L: The Developing Human, 2nd ed. Philadelphia, Saunders, 1977

Murphy BEP: Cortisol and cortisone levels in the cord blood at delivery of infants with and without the respiratory distress syndrome. Am J Obstet Gynecol 119:1112, 1975

Murphy BEP: Chorionic membrane as an extra-adrenal source of foetal cortisol in human amniotic fluid. Nature 266:179, 1977

Myers RE: Fetal brain tolerance to umbilical cord compression according to gestational age. Presented at the seventeenth annual meeting of the Society for Gynecologic Investigation, New Orleans. April 2, 1970

Nielsen NC: Coagulation and fibrinolysin in normal women immediately postpartum and in newborn infants. Acta Obstet Gynecol Scand 48:371,1969

Nielson PV, Pedersen H, Kampmann E-M: Absence of human placental lactogen in an otherwise uneventful pregnancy. Am J Obstet Gynecol 135:322, 1979

Obenshain SS, Adam PAJ, King KC, Teramo K, Raivio KO, Räihä N, Schwartz R: Human fetal insulin response to sustained maternal hyperglycemia N Engl J Med 283:566, 1970

Oka T, Topper YJ: Hormone-dependent accumulation of rough endoplasmic reticulum in mouse mammary epithelial cells in vitro. J Biol Chem 246:7701, 1971

Page EW: Transfer of materials across the human placenta. Am J Obstet Gynecol 74:705, 1957

Page EW: Problems of nutrition in the perinatal period. Report of the 60th Ross Conference on Pediatric Research, Columbus, Ohio, 1970

Page EW, Glendening MB, Margolis A, Harper HA: Transfer of D- and L-histidine across the human placenta. Am J Obstet Gynecol 73:589, 1957

Pasqualini JR, Sumida C, Gelly C: Cytosol and nuclear [³H]oestradiol binding in the foetal tissues of guinea pig. Acta Endocrinol 83:811, 1976

Pataryas HA, Stammatoyannopoulos G: Hemoglobins in human fetuses: evidence for adult hemoglobin production after the 11th gestational week. Blood 39:688, 1972

Paton JB, Fisher DE, DeLannoy CW, Behrman RE: Umbilical blood flow, cardiac output, and organ blood flow in the immature baboon fetus. Am J Obstet Gynecol 117:560, 1973

Pearson HA: Recent advances in hematology. J Pediatr 69:466, 1966

Plentl AA: Physiology of the placenta: III. Dynamics of amniotic fluid. In Assali NS (ed): Biology of Gestation, Vol I, The Maternal Organism. New York, Academic 1968

Portman OW, Behrman RE, Soltys P: Transfer of free fatty acids across the primate placenta. Am J Physiol 216:143, 1969

Posner BI, Kelly PA: Prolactin receptors in rat liver: Possible induction by prolactin. Science 188:57, 1975

Pritchard JA: Deglutition by normal and anencephalic fetuses. Obstet Gynecol 25:289, 1965

Pritchard JA: Fetal swallowing and amniotic fluid volume. Obstet Gynecol 28:606, 1966

Pritchard JA: Unpublished observations, 1975

Rooney SA, Gross I, Motoyama EK, Warshaw JB: Effects of cortisol and thyroxine on fatty acid and phospholipid biosynthesis in fetal rabbit lung. Physiologist 17:323, 1974

Rooney SA, Gross J, Gassenheimer LN, Motoyama EK: Stimulation of glycerolphosphate phosphatidyltransferase activity in fetal rabbit lung by cortisol administration. Biochim Biophys Acta 398:433, 1975

Rosenfeld CR, Andujo O, Johnston JM, Jimenez JM: Phosphatidate phosphohydrolase (PAPase) and phospholipids (PL) in tracheal (TF) and amniotic (AF) fluid during ovine gestation. Pediatr Res 13:363, 1979

Rudolph AM, Heymann MA: The fetal circulation. Ann Rev Med 19:195, 1968

Russell BJ, Nugent L, Chernick V: Effects of steroids on the enzymatic pathways of lecithin production in fetal rabbits. Biol Neonat 24:306, 1974

Schulman I, Smith CH: Fetal and adult hemoglobins in premature infants. Am J Dis Child 86:354, 1953

Schultz FM, Jimenez JM, MacDonald PC, Johnston JM: Fetal lung maturation. I. Phospha-

tidic acid phosphohydrolase in rabbit lung. Gynecol Invest 5:222, 1974

Sell EJ, Corrigan JJ Jr: Platelet counts, fibrinogen concentrations, and factor V and factor VIII levels in healthy infants according to gestational age. J Pediatr 82:1028, 1973

Shrand II: Vomiting in utero with intestinal atresia. Pediatrics 49:767, 1972

Siiteri PK, Wilson JD: Testosterone formation and metabolism during male sex differentiation in human embryo. J Clin Endocrinol 38:113, 1974

Sivakumaran T, Duncan ML, Effer SB, Younglai EV: Relationship between cortisol and lecithin/sphingomyelin ratios in human amniotic fluid. Am J Obstet Gynecol 122:291, 1975

Smith YF, Mullan DK, Hamosh M, Scanlon JW, Hamosh P: Prolactin and human lung maturation. Pediatr Res 12:569, 1978

Spellacy WN, Buhi WC, Riggall FC, Holsinger KL: Human amniotic fluid lecithin/sphingomyelin ratio changes with estrogen or glucocorticoid treatment. Am J Obstet Gynecol 115:216, 1973

Spitzer HL, Johnston JM: Characterization of phosphatidate phosphohydrolase activity associated with isolated lamellar bodies. Biochim Biophys Acta 531:275, 1978

Spitzer HL, Rice JM, MacDonald PC, Johnston JM: Phospholipid biosynthesis in lung lamellar bodies. Biochem Biophys Res Commun 66:17, 1975

Spooner PM, Gorski J: Early estrogen effects on lipid metabolism in the rat uterus. Endocrinology 91:1273, 1972

Stein Z, Susser M, Rush D: Prenatal nutrition and birth weight: Experiments and quasi-experiments in the past decade. J Reprod Med 21:287, 1978

Streeter GL: Weight, sitting height, head size, foot length, and menstrual age of the human embryo, Contrib Embryol 11:143, 1920

Sumida C, Gelly C, Nugyen BL, Pasqualini JR: Cytosol and nuclear ³H-estradiol receptors in fetal guinea pig kidney, lung and uterus during fetal development. Acta Endocrinol (Suppl 212) 85:36, 1977

Sybulski S, Manghan GB: Relationship between cortisol levels in umbilical cord plasma and development of the respiratory distress syndrome in premature newborn infants. Am J Obstet Gynecol 125:239, 1976

Szabo AJ, Grimaldi RD, Jung WF: Palmitate transport across perfused human placenta. Metabolism 18:406, 1969

Tan SY, Gewolb IH, Hobbins JC: Unconjugated cortisol in human amniotic fluid: Relationship to lecithin/sphingomyelin ratio. J Clin Endocrinol Metab 43:412, 1976

Temiras PS, Vernadakis A, Sherwood NM: Development and plasticity of the nervous system. In Assali NS (ed): Biology of Gestation, VII. The Fetus and Neonate. New York, Academic, 1968

Thiery M, Yo Le Sian A, Vrijens M, Janssens D: Vagitus uterinus. J Obstet Gynaecol Brit Commonw 80:183, 1973

Tolis G, Hickey J, Guyda H: Effects of morphine on serum growth hormone, cortisol, prolactin, and thyroid stimulating hormone in man. J Clin Endocrinol Metab 41:797, 1975

Turkington RW, Majumderi GC, Kadohama N: Hormone regulation of gene expression in mammary cells. Rec Prog Horm Res 29:417, 1973

Usher R, Shephard M, Lind J: The blood volume of the newborn infant and placental transfusion. Acta Paediatr 52:497, 1963

Van Den Bosch J, Bonte HA, vanDeenen LLM: On the anabolism of lipolecithin. Biochim Biophys Acta 98:648, 1965

Voelker DR, Ten-Ching L, Snyder F: Fatty acid biosynthesis and dietary regulation in pulmonary adenomas. Arch Biochem Biophys 176:753, 1976

Von Neergaad K: Neue auffassungen uber einen grundbegriff de Atemmechanik Die Retraktionskraft der Lunge Abhängig von der Oberfläch enspannung in den Alveolen. Z Ges Expt Med 66:373, 1929

Walker J, Turnbull EPN: Haemoglobin and red cells in the human foetus and their relation to the oxygen content of the blood in the vessels of the umbilical cord. Lancet 2:312, 1953

Walsh PC, Madden JD, Harrod MJ, Goldstein JL, MacDonald PC, Wilson JD: Familial incomplete male pseudohermaphroditism, Type 2. Decreased dihydrotestosterone formation in pseudovaginal perineoscrotal hypospades. N Engl J Med 291:944, 1974

White DA: In Ansell, GB, Dawson, RMC, Hawthorne, JN, (eds.); Form and Function of Phospholipids. Amsterdam, Elsevier, 1973, p. 441

Widdowson EM: Growth and composition of the fetus and newborn. In Assali NS (ed): Biology of Gestation, Vol II. The Fetus and Neonate. New York, Academic, 1968

Wilson JD, Gloyna RE; The intranuclear metabolism of testosterone in the accessory organs of reproduction. Recent Prog Horm Res 26:309, 1970

Wilson JD, Lasnitzki I. Dihydrotestosterone formation in fetal tissues of the rabbit and rat. Endocrinology 89:659, 1971.

Wilson JD, MacDonald PC: Male pseudohermaphroditism due to androgen resistance: testicular feminization and related syndromes. In Stanbury JB, Wyngaarden JD, Frederickson DS (eds): The Metabolic Basis of Inherited Disease. New York, McGraw-Hill, 1978

Wilson KM: Correlation of external genitalia and sex-glands in the human embryo. Contrib Embryol 18:23, 1926

Winters AJ, Colston C, MacDonald PC, Porter JC: Fetal plasma prolactin levels. J Clin Endocrinol Metab 41:626, 1975

Winters AJ, Oliver C, Colston C, MacDonald PC, Porter JC: Plasma ACTH levels in the human fetus and neonate as related to age and parturition. J Clin Endocrinol Metab 39:269, 1974

Wislocki GB: In Villee CA (ed): Gestation. Transactions of the First Conference. New York, The Josiah Macy, Jr. Foundation, 1955

Wladimiroff JW, Campbell S: Fetal urine-production rates in normal and complicated pregnancy. Lancet 1:151, 1974

Wu B, Kikkawa Y, Orzalesi MM, Motoyama EK, Kaibara M, Zigas CJ, Cook CD: The effect of thyroxine on the maturation of fetal rabbit lungs. Biol Neonat 22:161, 1973

Wu B, Kikkawa Y, Orzalesi MM, Motoyama EK, Kaibara M, Zigas CJ, Cook CD: Accelerated maturation of fetal rabbit lungs by thyroxine. Physiologist 14:253, 1971

Zanjani ED, Peterson EN, Gordon AS, Wasserman LR: Erythropoietin production in the fetus: role of the kidney and maternal anemia. J Lab Clin Med 83:281, 1974

Zuspan FR, Cordero L, Semchyshyn S: Effects of hydrocortisone on lecithin-sphingomyelin ratio. Am J Obstet Gynecol 128:571, 1977

9

Maternal Adaptation to Pregnancy

The duration of human pregnancy averages very close to 266 days (38 weeks) from the time of ovulation, or 280 days (40 weeks) from the first day of the last menstrual period (see Chap. 8, p. 169 and Chap. 13, p. 304). During this period, adaptive changes quite remarkable in number and degree are experienced by the pregnant woman.

UTERUS

Hypertrophy and Dilatation. One of the several unique features of the uterus is its remarkable capacity to increase in size in a few months and then to return essentially to its original state within a very few weeks. During normal intrauterine pregnancy, the almost solid uterus, with a cavity of 10ml or less, is transformed into a relatively thin-walled muscular container of sufficient capacity to accommodate the fetus, placenta, and amnionic fluid. The total volume of the contents of the uterus at term averages about 5 liters but may be as much as 10 liters or more, so that by the end of pregnancy the uterus has achieved a 500- to 1000-times greater capacity than in the nonpregnant state. A cor-

responding increase in weight occurs. The body of the uterus at term weighs approximately 1100 g, compared to about 70 g in the nonpregnant woman. During pregnancy, uterine enlargement involves stretching and marked hypertrophy of existing muscle cells, whereas the appearance of new muscle cells is limited. At the time of parturition, a single myometrial cell is about 500 μ in length and the nucleus is eccentrically placed in the thickest part of the cell. The cell is surrounded by an irregular array of collagen fibrils. The force of contraction is transmitted from the contractile proteins of the muscle cell to the surrounding connective tissue through the reticulum of collagen (Carsten, 1968). Accompanying the increase in size of the uterine muscle cells during pregnancy, there is an accumulation of fibrous tissue, particularly in the external muscular layer, together with a considerable increase in elastic tissue. The network thus formed adds materially to the strength of the uterine wall. There is, concomitantly, a great increase in the size and number of blood vessels and lymphatics in the uterus. The veins which drain at the placental site are transformed into the large uterine sinuses. Hypertrophy of the nerve supply of the uterus also takes place, exemplified by the increase in size of Frankenhäuser's cervical ganglion.

During the first few months of pregnancy, hypertrophy of the uterine wall is probably stimulated chiefly by the action of estrogen and perhaps that of progesterone. It is apparent that the early hypertrophy of the uterus is not the result of mechanical distension by the products of conception since similar uterine changes occur when the embryo is implanted in the fallopian tube or ovary. However, after the third month, the increase in uterine size is, in large part, due to the effect of pressure exerted by the expanding products of conception.

Rapid growth of tissues is correlated with increased synthesis of *polyamines.* The polyamines, spermidine and spermine and their immediate precursor, putrescine, are believed to play crucial roles in tissue growth and cell hypertrophy. (For review see Russell, Durie, 1978.) Russell, et al., (1978) have shown that polyamine levels in the urine of normally pregnant women are strikingly elevated and that the highest levels are attained at 13 to 14 weeks gestation (Fig. 9-1). It is interesting to speculate that the increased rate of synthesis of polyamines at this time in gestation is related to the hypertrophy

of the myometrium that occurs during this stage of pregnancy.

During the first few months of pregnancy, the uterine walls become considerably thicker than in the nonpregnant state, but as gestation advances the uterine wall gradually thins. At term, the walls of the uterine corpus are for the most part 1.5 cm or less in thickness. Early in pregnancy, the uterus loses the firmness and resistance characteristic of the nonpregnant organ. In the later months, the uterus is changed into a muscular sac with thin, soft, readily indentable walls, demonstrable by the ease with which the fetus usually can be palpated through the abdominal wall and by the readiness with which the uterine walls yield to the movements of the fetal extremities.

The enlargement of the uterus is not symmetrical, rather it is most marked in the fundus. The differential growth is readily apparent by observing the relative positions of the attachments of the fallopian tubes and ovarian ligaments. In the early months of pregnancy, these structures insert only slightly below the apex of the fundus, whereas in the later months, they are inserted slightly above the middle of the uterus. The position of the placenta also influences the extent of uterine hypertrophy, since the portion of the uterus surrounding the placental site enlarges more rapidly than does the myometrium distal to the site of placental implantation.

Arrangement of the Muscle Cells. The musculature of the pregnant uterus is arranged in three strata: an external hoodlike layer, which arches over the fundus and extends into the various ligaments; an internal layer, consisting of sphincterlike fibers around the orifices of the tubes and the internal os; and lying between the two, a dense network of muscle fibers perforated in all directions by blood vessels. The main portion of the uterine wall is formed by the middle layer, which consists of an interlacing network of muscle fibers between which extend the blood vessels. Each cell in this layer has a double curve, so that the interlacing of any two gives approximately the form of the figure 8. As a result of such an arrangement, when the cells contract after delivery they constrict the blood vessels and thus act as ligatures. The muscle cells composing the uterine wall

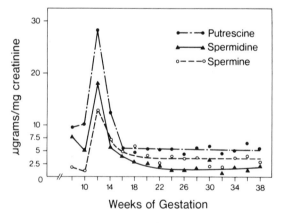

FIG. 9-1. Polyamines in the urine of women with normal pregnancies as a function of weeks of gestation. Each point is the mean value of results obtained in the urine of at least five separate women. (From Russell et al.: *Am J Obstet Gynecol* 132:649,1978)

in pregnancy, especially in its lower portion, over-lap one another like shingles on a roof. One end of each fiber arises beneath the serosa of the uterus and extends obliquely downward and inward toward the decidua, forming a large number of muscular lamellae which are interconnected by short muscular processes. When the tissue is slightly spread apart, it appears sievelike and, on closer examination, is found to comprise innumerable rhomboidal spaces.

Changes in Uterine Size, Shape, and Position.

As the uterus increases in size, it also undergoes important modifications in shape. For the first few weeks, its original pear shape is maintained, but as pregnancy advances the corpus and fundus soon assume a more globular form, becoming almost spherical by the third lunar month. Thereafter, the organ increases more rapidly in length than in width and assumes an ovoid shape.

By the end of the third lunar month (12 weeks), the uterus has become too large to remain wholly within the pelvis. Thereafter, as the uterus continues to enlarge, it contacts the anterior abdominal wall, displaces the intestines laterally and superiorly, and continues to rise, reaching ultimately almost to the liver. As the uterus rises, tension is exerted upon the broad ligaments, which partly unfold in their median and lower portions, and upon the round ligaments.

During pregnancy, the uterus is rather mobile. With the pregnant woman standing, the longitudinal axis of the uterus corresponds to an extension of the axis of the pelvic inlet. The abdominal wall supports the uterus and, unless the abdominal wall is quite relaxed, maintains this relation between the long axis of the uterus and the axis of the pelvic inlet. When the pregnant woman is supine, the uterus falls back to rest upon the vertebral column and the adjacent great vessels, especially the inferior vena cava and the aorta.

As the uterus rises out of the pelvis, it usually rotates somewhat to the right, thereby directing its left margin more anteriorly. This *dextrorotation* has been considered to result in large measure from the presence of the rectosigmoid in the left side of the pelvis. However, *levorotation* occurs occasionally, especially if there is a pelvic or low abdominal mass on the right side, for example, a transplanted kidney.

Changes in Contractility.

From the first trimester of pregnancy onward, the uterus undergoes irregular contractions, which normally are painless. In the second trimester such contractions may be detected by bimanual examination and, later by abdominal examination alone. The relaxed uterus transiently becomes firm and then returns to its original relaxed state. Since attention was first called to this phenomenon by Braxton Hicks, the contractions have been known by his name. Such contractions appear unpredictably and sporadically, are usually nonrhythmic, and their intensity, according to Alvarez and Caldeyro-Barcia (1950), is somewhat more than 8 cm of water. Until the last month of gestation, *Braxton Hicks contractions* are infrequent, but increase in frequency during the last week or two. At this time, the contractions may occur as often as every 10 to 20 minutes and may assume some degree of rhythmicity. Late in pregnancy these contractions may cause some discomfort and account for so-called false labor.

Uteroplacental Blood Flow.

The delivery of most substances essential for the growth and metabolism of the fetus and placenta, as well as the removal of most metabolic wastes, is dependent upon adequate perfusion of the placental intervillous space. Placental perfusion by maternal blood depends, in turn, upon blood flow to the uterus through the uterine and ovarian arteries. There is no question that there is a progressive increase in uteroplacental blood flow large in magnitude during pregnancy. The reported values, which average roughly 500 ml/per minute late in pregnancy, must be viewed as approximations because of inherent errors in the methods of measurement as well as the undoubtedly appreciable changes in uterine blood flow that likely are induced by various body positions (Kauppi-laetal, 1980).

Assali and associates (1953,1960), Metcalfe and co-workers (1955), and Blechner and associates (1975), employing the nitrous oxide method to estimate uteroplacental blood flow in human pregnancy, found that the total flow averages about 500 ml per minute at term. Browne and Veall (1953) arrived at approximately the same values, using the rate of disappearance of ^{24}Na.

Rekonen and co-workers (1976) attempted measurement of intervillous and myometrial blood flow in pregnant women in the supine position using intravenously injected ^{133}Xe. They obtained mean values for intervillous flow of 135 ml per minute per dl and myometrial flow of 7.7 ml per minute per 100 g. Thus for a placenta of 500 g and a uterus of 1000 g, uteroplacental blood flow estimated by this technic averaged 750 ml per minute. There was appreciable variation among individuals, although the reproducibility in the same individual was good.

Edman and colleagues (1979) have measured minimal placental intervillous blood flow from the placental clearance of maternal plasma androstenedione through 17 β-estradiol formation. These investigators found values of approximately 450 ml of blood per minute for placental intervillous flow at or near term.

Assali and co-workers (1968), and others, using electromagnetic flowmeters, studied the effects of spontaneous and oxytocin-induced labor on uteroplacental blood flow in sheep and dogs at term. They noted that uterine contractions, either spontaneous or induced, caused a decrease in uterine blood flow that was roughly proportional to the intensity of the contraction; a tetanic contraction caused a precipitous fall in uterine blood flow. Harbert and associates (1969) made similar observations in gravid monkeys, and the same pattern of change undoubtedly occurs during the myometrial contractions of human parturition.

Obviously, a great deal remains to be learned about the factors that control uterine blood flow and effective perfusion of the placenta, including not only the effects of maternal posture, physical activity, and emotional state, but also the impact of maternal diseases and, in turn, the effect of various treatments employed.

Changes in the Cervix. During pregnancy, pronounced softening and cyanosis of the cervix occurs, often demonstrable as early as a month after conception. These changes comprise two of the very earliest physical signs of pregnancy. The factors responsible for these changes are increased vascularity and edema of the entire cervix, together with hypertrophy and hyperplasia of the cervical glands.

As shown in Figures 9-2 and 9-3, the glands of the cervical mucosa undergo such marked proliferation that by the end of pregnancy they occupy approximately one-half of the entire mass of the cervix, rather than a small fraction, as in the nonpregnant state. Moreover, the septa separating the glandular spaces become progressively thinner, resulting in the formation of a structure resembling a honeycomb, the meshes of which are filled with tenacious mucus. Soon after conception a clot of very thick mucus obstructs the cervical canal. At the onset of labor, if not before, this so-called *mucous plug* is expelled. The glands near the external os proliferate beneath the stratified squamous epithelium of the portio vaginalis, giving the cervix the velvety consistency characteristic of pregnancy.

So-called *erosions of the cervix* are common during pregnancy. These lesions are customarily red and velvety in appearance and are covered by columnar epithelium, spreading from the external os to involve the portio vaginalis of the cervix to various degrees. The high frequency of cervical "erosions" in pregnancy is best explained on the basis that they are normal, representing an extension, or *eversion,* of the proliferating endocervical glands and the columnar endocervical epithelium. Although the term erosion implies an "eating out" or ulceration of the covering epithelium, the cause in pregnancy is rarely inflammatory.

During pregnancy, there is a change in

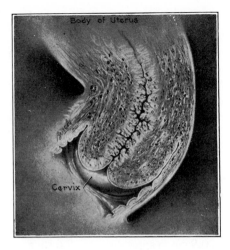

FIG. 9-2. Cervix in the nonpregnant woman.

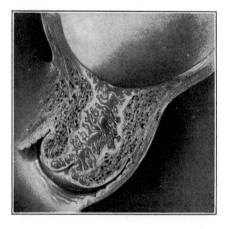

FIG. 9-3. Cervix in pregnancy. Note the elaboration of the mucosa into a honeycomblike structure, the meshes of which are filled with a tenacious mucus—the so-called mucous plug (drawn to approximately one-third the scale of cervix shown in Fig. 9-2).

the consistency of the cervical mucus. In the great majority of pregnant women, cervical mucus, spread and dried on a glass slide, is characterized by fragmentary crystallization, or "beading," typical of the effect of progesterone (see Chap. 4, p. 87). Arborization of the crystals, or "ferning," however, is not necessarily associated with a poor outcome of pregnancy (Salvatore, 1968). Chrétien (1978), employing scanning electron microp-

scopy, has studied the structural variations in cervical mucus during normal pregnancy.

During pregnancy, basal cells near the squamocolumnar junction of the cervix, histologically, are likely to be prominent in size, shape, and staining qualities. These changes are considered by most authorities to be estrogen-induced (Hellman et al., 1954).

Although the cervix contains a small amount of smooth muscle, its major component is connective tissue. The cervix undergoes profound changes during pregnancy, especially during labor, and these must involve its collagen-rich connective tissue. Danforth and Buckingham (1964) found an appreciable decrease in the hydroxyproline content of the cervix as pregnancy advances, as well as a marked decrease in the compactness and cohesiveness of the collagen fibers immediately after vaginal delivery. The mechanisms responsible for the orderly effacement and dilatation of the cervix are still poorly understood, but Liggins (1978) has shown that many of these changes can be induced in the cervix of the gravid sheep by the administration of prostaglandin.

OVARIES AND OVIDUCTS

Ovarian Function. Ovulation ceases during pregnancy and the maturation of new follicles is suspended. As a rule, only a single corpus luteum of pregnancy can be found in the ovaries of pregnant women. Yoshima and associates (1969) found that the level of plasma progesterone reached a nadir by the eighth week of pregnancy and then rose again. By contrast, maternal plasma 17 α-hydroxyprogesterone levels continued to decline to a level only somewhat higher than those found during the luteal phase. These observations are indicative that the corpus luteum of pregnancy most likely functions maximally during the first four weeks after ovulation and conception but thereafter contributes relatively little to progesterone production during the remainder of human pregnancy.

RELAXIN. This protein hormone is secreted by the corpus luteum during human pregnancy. It is detectable in serum by the time of the first missed menses and is believed to be secreted in a pattern similar to that of hCG. Thus the secretion of this corpus luteum hormone differs from that of the steroids of the corpus luteum. Whereas 17 α-hydroxyprogesterone and presumably progesterone secretion by the corpus luteum has declined to negligible rates by the seventh to eighth week of pregnancy, relaxin secretion continues throughout pregnancy. The role, if any, of relaxin in human pregnancy is unknown. Relaxin is not required for a successful pregnancy outcome since oophorectomy at or after eight weeks or so usually does not adversely affect the pregnancy. For a review of this subject, see Schwabe and associates (1978).

PREGNANCY LUTEOMA. In 1963, Sternberg described a solid ovarian tumor that developed during pregnancy that was composed of large acidophilic luteinized cells. The observations of Krause and Stembridge (1966), Garcia-Bunuel and co-workers (1975) and others, are suggestive that this luteoma of pregnancy represents an exaggeration of the luteinization reaction of the ovary of normal pregnancy and is not a true neoplasm. The luteoma regresses after delivery, and normal ovarian function returns even in those instances in which the luteoma is responsible, transiently, for maternal virilization. In the immediate puerperal state, the luteoma may be responsive to exogenously administered hCG.

Even though maternal virilization is prominent, the fetus may not be affected presumably because of the protective role of the placenta through its high capacity to convert androgens to estrogens. Verkauf and colleagues (1977) in one case found in cord blood dramatically lower levels of androgens and relatively higher levels of 17 β-estradiol and estriol in comparison to maternal blood.

OTHER CHANGES. A *decidual reaction* on and beneath the surface of the ovaries, similar to that found in the endometrial stroma, is common in pregnancy and is commonly observed at cesarean section. These elevated patches of tissue bleed easily and may, on first glance, resemble freshly torn adhesions. Similar decidual reactions are occasionally seen on the posterior uterine serosa and upon or within other pelvic or even extrapelvic abdominal organs.

By inspection of the ovarian veins at cesarean section, their enormous caliber is startling. By actual measurement, Hodgkinson (1953) found that the diameter of the ovarian vascular pedicle increased during pregnancy from 0.9 cm to approximately 2.6 cm at term.

Oviducts. The musculature of the fallopian tubes undergoes little hypertrophy during pregnancy. The epithelium of the tubal mucosa is flattened during gestation, compared to that of the nonpregnant state. Decidual cells may develop in the stroma of the endosalpinx, but a continuous decidual membrane is not formed.

VAGINA AND OUTLET

During pregnancy increased vascularity and hyperemia develops in the skin and muscles of the perineum and vulva and there is softening of the normally abundant connective tissue of these structures.

Increased vascularity prominently affects the vagina. The copious secretion and the characteristic violet color of the vagina during pregnancy (Chadwick's sign), similar to the changes that occur in the cervix during pregnancy, probably result chiefly from hyperemia. The vaginal walls undergo striking changes seemingly in preparation for the distension that occurs during labor, with a considerable increase in thickness of the mucosa, loosening of the connective tissue, and hypertrophy of the smooth-muscle cells to nearly the same extent as in the uterus. These changes effect such an increase in length of the vaginal walls that sometimes, in parous women, the lower portion of the anterior vaginal wall protrudes slightly through the vulvar opening. The papillae of the vaginal mucosa also undergo considerable hypertrophy, creating a fine hobnailed appearance.

Vaginal Secretion. The considerably increased cervical and vaginal secretion during pregnancy consists of a somewhat thick, white discharge. Its pH is acidic, varying from 3.5 to 6, the result of increased production of lactic acid from glycogen in the vaginal epithelium by the action of *Lactobacillus acidophilus.* The acidic pH probably serves to control the rate of multiplication of pathogenic bacteria in the vagina.

Vaginal Cytology. Early in pregnancy the vaginal epithelial cells are similar to those found during the luteal phase of the menstrual cycle (see Chap. 4, p. 88), but as pregnancy advances two patterns of response are seen:

1. Small intermediate cells, called navicular cells by Papanicolaou, are found in abundance in small, dense clusters. The ovoid navicular cells contain a vesicular, somewhat elongated nucleus.

2. Vesicular nuclei without cytoplasm, or so-called naked nuclei, are evident along with an abundance of *Lactobacillus,* a normal organism in the vagina. Evaluation of the epithelial cells, identified in scrapings from the lateral walls of the upper vagina, has been considered by some investigators, but certainly not all, to be of value in prognosticating the outcome of pregnancy (McLennan, McLennan, 1969; Meisels, 1968).

ABDOMINAL WALL AND SKIN

Striae Gravidarum. In the later months of pregnancy, reddish, slightly depressed streaks commonly develop in the skin of the abdomen and sometimes in the skin over the breasts and thighs. These striae gravidarum occur in about one-half of all pregnant women (Fig. 9-4). In multiparous women, in addition to the reddish striae of the present pregnancy, glistening, silvery lines that represent the cicatrices of previous striae are seen frequently.

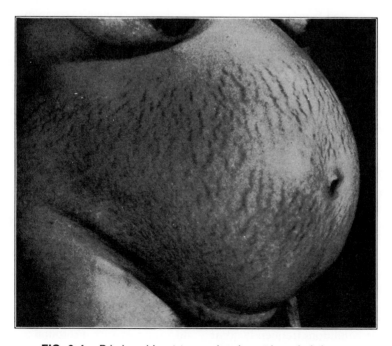

FIG. 9-4. Primigravida at term, showing striae of abdomen.

Diastasis Recti. Occasionally, the muscles of the abdominal walls do not withstand the tension to which they are subjected, and the rectus muscles separate in the midline, creating a diastasis recti of varying extent. If severe, a considerable portion of the anterior uterine wall is covered by only a layer of skin, attenuated fascia, and peritoneum. In extreme instances, herniation of the gravid uterus through the diastasis may be so great that the fundus of the uterus drops below the level of the pelvic inlet when the woman is standing.

Pigmentation. In many women, the midline of the abdominal skin becomes markedly pigmented, assuming a brownish-black color to form the *linea nigra.* Occasionally, irregular brownish patches of varying size appear on the face and neck, giving rise to *chloasma* or the *mask of pregnancy,* which, fortunately, usually disappears, or at least regresses considerably, after delivery. Oral contraceptives may cause chloasma in these same women. There is very little known of the nature of these pigmentary changes, although melanocyte-stimulating hormone, a polypeptide similar to ACTH, has been shown to be remarkably elevated from the end of the second month of pregnancy until term. Estrogen and progesterone, moreover, are reported to exert a melanocyte-stimulating effect (Diczfalusy, Troen, 1961).

Cutaneous Vascular Changes. Angiomas, called *vascular spiders,* develop in about two-thirds of white women and approximately 10 percent of black women during pregnancy (Bean and colleagues, 1949). These are minute, red elevations on the skin, particularly common on the face, neck, upper chest, and arms, with radicles branching out from a central body. The condition is often designated as nevus, angioma, or telangiectasis. *Palmar erythema* is also frequently encountered in pregnancy, having been observed by Bean and associates in about two-thirds of white women and one-third of black women. The two conditions frequently occur together but are of no clinical significance,

disappearing in most women shortly after the termination of pregnancy. The high incidence of vascular spiders and palmar erythema in pregnancy is most likely the consequence of the hyperestrogenemia of pregnancy.

BREASTS

During pregnancy, striking changes occur in the breasts. In the early weeks, the pregnant woman often experiences tenderness and tingling of the breasts. After the second month, the breasts increase in size and become nodular as a result of hypertrophy of the mammary alveoli. As the breasts increase in size, delicate veins become visible just beneath the skin (Figs. 9-5, 9-6). The changes in the nipples and areolae are even more characteristic. The nipples become considerably larger, more deeply pigmented, and more erectile. After the first few months, a thick, yellowish fluid, *colostrum,* often can be expressed from the nipples by gentle massage. At that time, the areolae become broader and more deeply pigmented. The depth of pigmentation varies with the woman's complexion. Scattered through the areolae are a number of small elevations, the so-called glands (follicles) of Montgomery, which are hypertrophic sebaceous glands. If the increase in size of the breasts is very extensive, striations similar to those observed in the abdomen may develop. Histologic and functional changes of the breasts induced by pregnancy and delivery are discussed further in Chapter 19 (p. 460).

METABOLIC CHANGES

In response to the rapidly growing fetus and placenta and their increasing demands, the pregnant woman undergoes metabolic changes that are numerous and intense. Certainly no other physiologic event in postnatal life induces such profound metabolic alterations.

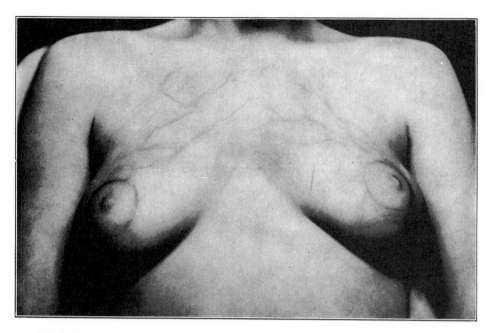

FIG. 9-5. Infrared photograph of nonlactating breasts in a nonpregnant woman.

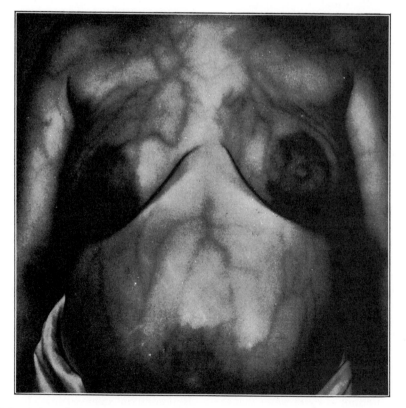

FIG. 9-6. Infrared photograph of gravida one month before term, showing accentuated venous pattern over breasts and abdomen.

Weight Gain. One of the most notable alterations in pregnancy is maternal weight gain. Most of the increase in weight is attributable to the weight of the products of conception (fetus, placenta, fetal membranes, and amnionic fluid) and to the hypertrophy of the uterus. A smaller fraction of the increase in maternal weight is the result of metabolic alterations, especially retention of water and deposition of fat and protein. In an exhaustive survey, Chesley (1944) found that the average total weight gain in pregnancy was 24 pounds (11 kg). During the first trimester, the average gain was only 2 pounds (1 kg), compared with about 11 pounds (5 kg) during each of the last two trimesters.

In the average pregnancy at term, the fetus weighs approximately 7½ pounds, the placenta and membranes 1½ pounds, the amnionic fluid 2 pounds, and the uterus 2½ pounds. Thus the uterus and its contents account for more than half of the weight gain in pregnancy. The breasts probably increase about 1 pound, and the blood volume is expanded by about 1500 ml, or 3½ pounds, leaving only about 6 pounds of the usual total weight gain not immediately explained. Retention of fluid, especially in tissues below the level of the uterus, and some deposition of fat account for the remaining 6 pounds.

Water Metabolism. Increased retention of water has long been regarded as a characteristic physiologic alteration of late pregnancy. Inasmuch as an exaggeration of this phenomenon, i.e., edema, is commonly associated with one of the principal complications of gestation, preeclampsia-eclampsia, water metabolism has long been of keen interest to obstetricians.

At term, the water content of the fetus, placenta, and amnionic fluid amounts to about 3.5 liters. Approximately 3.0 liters more water accumulates as a result of increases in the maternal blood volume and in the size of the uterus and the breasts. Thus, the minimum amount of extra water that the average woman could be expected to retain during normal pregnancy is about 6.5 liters.

Clearly demonstrable pitting edema of the ankles and legs occurs in a substantial proportion of pregnant women, especially at the end of the day, before retiring. This accumulation of fluid, which may amount to a liter or so, is caused by an increase in venous pressure below the level of the uterus because of the increased venous pressure in all body positions except lateral recumbent.

The amount of water to be mobilized and excreted by the mother after delivery will depend upon the amount retained during pregnancy, the degree of hydration or dehydration during labor, and the amount of blood lost at delivery. In normal primiparas without demonstrable edema before vaginal delivery, weight loss during the first 10 days after delivery averaged nearly 5 pounds (2 kg) (Dennis, Bytheway, 1965).

Protein Metabolism. The products of conception, as well as the uterus and maternal blood, are relatively rich in protein rather than fat or carbohydrate. Nonetheless, their protein content is rather small compared with the total body protein of the mother. At term, the fetus and placenta together weigh about 4 kg and contain approximately 500 g of protein, or about one-half of the total increase normally induced by pregnancy (Hytten, Leitch, 1971; Widdowson, 1968). Approximately 500 g more of protein is added to the uterus as contractile protein, to the breasts primarily in the glands, and to the maternal blood in the form of hemoglobin and plasma proteins. At the same time, the concentrations of several plasma proteins are altered by pregnancy. The albumin concentration decreases significantly (p. 248) while fibrinogen rises (p. 236). The concentrations of IgG, IgA, and IgM fall somewhat. (Amino et al., 1978).

Dietary protein requirements during pregnancy and lactation are discussed in Chapter 13, (p. 311).

Carbohydrate Metabolism. Pregnancy is potentially diabetogenic. Diabetes mellitus may be aggravated by pregnancy and clinical diabetes may appear in some women only during pregnancy. Consequently, considerable attention has been focused on the metabolism of carbohydrates and insulin in pregnant women. In healthy women, the fasting plasma glucose concentration falls somewhat during pregnancy (Fig. 9-7). The effect of normal pregnancy on *insulin* levels is disputed. Increased fasting levels of insulin have been reported by some investigators (Bleicher et al., 1964; Spellacy et al., 1963) while others have found them to be unchanged (Taylor et al., 1978), or even lower during pregnancy (Tyson et al., 1976).

Bleicher and associates (1964) presented the concept that the lower fasting glucose levels and the higher concentration of plasma free fatty acids found normally in pregnant women result from a state of "accelerated starvation" brought about by the "host–parasite" relation between mother and conceptus. During pregnancy, there are safeguards that

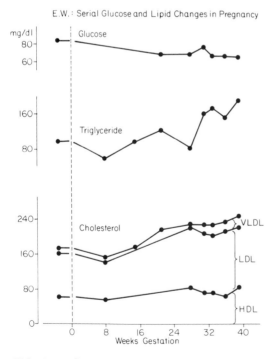

E.W.: Serial Glucose and Lipid Changes in Pregnancy

FIG. 9-7. Serial changes in concentrations of glucose and lipids during normal pregnancy. VLDL = very low-density lipoproteins; LDL = low-density lipoproteins; HDL = high-density lipoproteins. (From Knopp, RH: *Contemporary Ob/Gyn* 12:83, 1978)

spare utilization of glucose by maternal tissues while allowing "parasitization" of glucose and gluconeogenic precursors by the fetus to continue. The placenta is known to synthesize and secrete a growth-hormone-like substance, placental lactogen (p. 149). This hormone promotes lipolysis, bringing about an increase in plasma free fatty acids, and thereby provides alternative fuel substrates for the mother. The ability of placental lactogen to oppose the action of insulin leads to increased maternal requirements for insulin during pregnancy.

Estrogen, progesterone, and cortisol may also contribute to the diabetogenic predisposition apparent in pregnancy. Progesterone given to monkeys was shown by Beck (1969) to produce a marked increase in the plasma insulin response to intravenous glucose similar to that noted in human pregnancy. Moreover, Beck and Wells (1969) found that the potent synthetic estrogen, mestranol (ethinyl estradiol-3-methyl ether), caused not only an increased plasma insulin response to intravenous glucose but also a decreased sensitivity to the hypoglycemic action of exogenous insulin. Only the subjects with limited ability to increase insulin production demonstrated decreased glucose tolerance after mestranol treatment, however, presumably because of failure to compensate for insulin resistance induced by mestranol. Plasma cortisol levels are increased appreciably during pregnancy. Evidence is equivocal however that the level of free cortisol is greater in the pregnant than in the nonpregnant woman.

Insulinase activity has been found in the human placenta. It seems unlikely, however, that accelerated degradation of insulin by placental insulinase contributes appreciably to the diabetogenic state induced by pregnancy, since the rate of degradation of radiolabeled insulin in vivo does not appear to differ among pregnant and nonpregnant women (Burt, Davidson, 1974).

Intravenous glucose tolerance tests are commonly used by the clinician, but from the results of these tests one cannot demonstrate any distinct differences in the magnitude and duration of the induced hyperglycemia between normal pregnant and nonpregnant women. Employing oral glucose tolerance tests, the hyperglycemia induced may persist somewhat longer than in normal nonpregnant women, probably because of slower and therefore more prolonged absorption of glucose. However, this explanation may be an oversimplification of the problem. The hypoglycemic effect of tolbutamide is not nearly so great in normal pregnant women as it is in nonpregnant women even though insulin release is appreciably greater (Spellacy and associates, 1965). The decreased hypoglycemic effect of tolbutamide in pregnancy results, therefore, mainly from the increased peripheral resistance to insulin that is induced by pregnancy.

The frequent occurrence of *glucosuria* in healthy women during pregnancy results from increased glomerular filtration and less effective renal tubular reabsorption than in the nonpregnant state (Davison, Hytten, 1975).

Fat Metabolism.   Plasma lipids increase appreciably during the latter half of pregnancy. This increase involves total lipids, esterified and nonesterified cholesterol, phospholipids, neutral fat, lipoproteins, and free fatty acids. The magnitude of some of the changes is illustrated in Table 9-1 and Figure 9-7. Cholesterol, triglyceride, and lipoprotein levels decrease at different rates after delivery (Potter, Nestel, 1979).

In pregnant women, starvation induces much more intense ketonemia and ketonuria than it does in nonpregnant women. Women at midpregnancy who before abortion were starved experimentally for upward of four days, demonstrated remarkably increased levels of plasma free fatty acids, glycerol, and ketones as glucose fell more than one-third. Similar changes occurred in amnionic fluid (Kim, Felig, 1972).

Hytten and Thomson (1968) concluded that storage of fat takes place during early and midpregnancy, the fat being deposited mostly in central rather than peripheral sites. Later in pregnancy, as the nutritional demands of the fetus increase remarkably, storage of fat decreases. These workers cited some evidence that progesterone may act to reset a "lipostat" in the hypothalamus; at the end of pregnancy the lipostat returns to its previous nonpregnant level and the added fat is lost. Such a mechanism for energy storage, theoretically at least, might protect the mother and fetus during times of prolonged starvation or hard physical exertion. Otherwise, according to some current views, such deposition of fat might be undesirable.

Mineral Metabolism.   The requirements for iron during pregnancy are considerable, and often exceed the amounts available (p. 234). With respect to most other minerals, pregnancy induces little change in their metabolism other than their retention in amounts equivalent to those utilized for growth of fetal and, to a lesser extent, maternal tissues (see Chap. 8, p. 204; Chap. 13, p. 312). Copper and ceruloplasmin in the

TABLE 9-1.
CHANGES IN SERUM LIPIDS (FASTING) INDUCED BY PREGNANCY

	NONPREGNANT	37–40 WEEKS	% CHANGE
Serum total lipids (mg/dl)	711	1039	+46
Serum total cholesterol (mg/dl)	178	249	+40
Esterified cholesterol (%)	74	77	—
Serum phospholipids (mg/dl)	256	350	+37
Free fatty acids (μeq/liter)	768	1226	+60

Data from deAlvarez and associates: *Am J Obstet Gynecol* 82:1096, 1961; and from Burt: *Obstet Gynecol* 15:460, 1960.

plasma increase considerably early in pregnancy, because of the increases in estrogens, which will produce the same changes when administered to nonpregnant subjects (Russ, Raymunt, 1956).

During pregnancy, the calcium and magnesium levels are reduced very slightly, the reduction probably reflecting for the most part the lowered plasma protein concentration and the consequent decrease in the amount of each electrolyte that is bound to protein. Serum phosphorus levels are within the nonpregnant range.

Acid-Base Equilibrium and Blood Electrolytes. Normally, the pregnant woman hyperventilates, compared with the nonpregnant subject, and this causes a respiratory alkalosis by lowering the PCO_2 of the blood. A moderate reduction in plasma bicarbonate from about 26 mmoles to about 22 mmoles per liter effectively compensates for the respiratory alkalosis. As a result, there is only a minimal increase in blood pH (Sjöstedt, 1962). The concentration of some of the electrolytes and of total protein in the plasma is decreased slightly during pregnancy. The serum osmolality and the concentration of potassium and sodium are reduced about 3 percent.

HEMATOLOGIC CHANGES ASSOCIATED WITH NORMAL PREGNANCY

Blood Volume and Iron Metabolism. The maternal blood volume increases markedly during pregnancy. In a study of 50 normal women, the blood volumes at or very near term averaged about 45 percent above their nonpregnant levels (Pritchard, 1965). This increase is similar to that described by Caton and associates, (1949), by Dahlström and Ihrman (1960), and Ueland (1976).

The degree of expansion varies considerably; in some women there is only a modest increase and in others their blood volume nearly doubles. A fetus is not essential for the development of hypervolemia during pregnancy, for increases in blood volume identical with those found during normal pregnancy have been demonstrated in some women with hydatidiform mole (Pritchard, 1965).

The pregnancy-induced hypervolemia serves to meet the demands of the enlarged uterus with its greatly hypertrophied vascular system, to protect the mother and, in turn, the fetus against the deleterious effects of impaired venous return in the supine and erect positions, and to safeguard the mother against the adverse effects of blood loss associated with parturition.

The maternal blood volume starts to increase during the first trimester, expands most rapidly during the second trimester, and then rises at a much slower rate during the third trimester, attaining a plateau during the last several weeks of pregnancy. A significant decrease in maternal blood volume in late pregnancy was found in some earlier studies, but this finding has not been confirmed.

The increase in blood volume results from an increase in both plasma and erythrocytes. The usual pattern is that of an initial rise in the plasma volume, followed by an increase in the volume of circulating erythrocytes. Although more plasma than erythrocytes is usually added to the maternal circulation, the increase in the volume of circulating erythrocytes is considerable, averaging, in the 50 women previously mentioned, about 450 ml of erythrocytes, or an increase of about 33 percent. The importance of this increase in creating a demand for iron is discussed below. The increase in the volume of circulating erythrocytes in pregnancy is accomplished by accelerated production rather than by prolongation of the life span of the erythrocyte (Pritchard, Adams, 1960).

The mean age of circulating maternal red cells is lower during the latter half of pregnancy because the rate of red cell production exceeds that of destruction. For the same reason, the *mean cell volume* is increased since a red cell is largest when first released from the bone marrow and becomes progressively smaller with age. In normally pregnant women, the concentration of 2,3-diphosphoglycerate in red cells is increased and, consequently, their affinity for oxygen is decreased (Bille-Brahe, Rørth, 1979). The combination of lowered oxygen affinity of maternal red cells and lowered blood P_{CO_2} facilitates the transport of oxygen and carbon dioxide across the placenta.

Moderate erythroid hyperplasia is present in the bone marrow, and the reticulocyte count is elevated slightly during normal pregnancy. Manasc and Jepson (1969) found increased levels of erythropoietin in maternal plasma and urine during pregnancy. They concluded that a major stimulus to erythropoiesis during human pregnancy is increased production of erythropoietin. Jepson and Friesen (1968) reported that administration of placental lactogen, purified from human placenta, to polycythemic mice accelerated the incorporation of iron into their erythrocytes, an effect that was abolished by its incubation with antibody to placental lactogen but not with antisheep erythropoietin. The precise roles of these substances in augmenting erythropoiesis during pregnancy await further clarification.

CHANGES IN HEMATOCRIT. In spite of the augmented erythropoiesis, the concentrations of hemoglobin and erythrocytes, as well as the hematocrit, commonly decrease slightly during normal pregnancy. In Sturgeon's careful study (1959), for instance, in which iron was readily available to the mother for erythropoiesis, he found that the hemoglobin concentration at term averaged 12.1 g, as compared with a level of 13.3 g per dl for nonpregnant women. In a similar study, the hemoglobin concentration at term averaged 12.5 g, with a level below 11.0 g per dl in only 6 percent of the pregnant subjects (Pritchard, Hunt, 1958). In many more recent studies these results have been confirmed. A hemoglobin concentration much below 11.0 g per dl, especially late in pregnancy, is suggestive of an abnormal process, usually iron deficiency, rather than the physi-

TABLE 9-2.
MEASUREMENT OF HEMOGLOBIN IRON AND IRON STORES IN HEALTHY YOUNG WOMEN (NEVER PREGNANT AND NEVER EXPERIENCED ABNORMAL BLOOD LOSS)

	AVERAGE	RANGE
Age	23	21 to 26
Weight (kg)	60	49 to 72
Height (in)	65	60 to 68
HGB conc. (g/dl)	14.1	13.0 to 15.6
Serum iron conc. (μg/dl)	105	76 to 132
HGB mass (g)	443	358 to 492
HGB iron (mg)	1505	1210 to 1670
Iron stores* (mg)	347	150 to 629

From Pritchard and Mason: *JAMA* 190:897, 1964.
* Iron converted to hemoglobin in response to repeated phlebotomy.

ologic effect of the hypervolemia of pregnancy alone (see Chap. 28, p. 714).

IRON STORES. It has been stated commonly that the total body iron content averages about 4 g, or slightly more, in the adult. This value, however, applies to normal men. In healthy young women of average size, the body iron content is probably not much more than half that amount (Table 9-2). Commonly, iron stores of normal young women are only about 0.3 g (Pritchard, Mason, 1964; Scott, Pritchard, 1967). As in men, heme iron in myoglobin and enzymes, and transferrin-bound circulating iron, together total only a few hundred mg. The total iron content of normal adult women, therefore, is probably in the range of 2.0 to 2.5 g.

IRON REQUIREMENTS. The iron requirements of normal pregnancy total about 1 g (Fig. 9-8). About 300 mg are actively transferred to the fetus and placenta (Widdowson, Spray, 1951) and about 200 mg are lost through various normal routes of excretion. These are obligatory losses and occur even when the mother is iron deficient. The average increase in the total volume of circulating erythrocytes of about 450 ml during pregnancy, when iron is available, utilizes an-

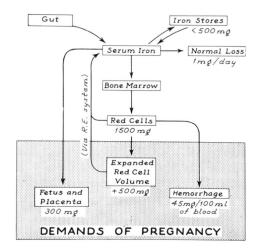

FIG. 9-8. The iron requirements of normal pregnancy. The 300 mg of iron transferred to the fetus are permanently lost from the mother. The 500 mg incorporated into maternal hemoglobin usually are not all lost; the amount recovered for storage depends upon the amount of blood lost at and after delivery.

other 500 mg of iron since 1 ml of normal erythrocytes contains 1.1 mg of iron. Practically all the iron for these purposes is utilized during the latter half of pregnancy. Therefore, the iron requirement becomes quite large during the second half of pregnancy, averaging 6 to 7 mg per day (Pritchard, Scott, 1970). Since this amount of iron is not available from body stores in most women, the desired increase in maternal erythrocyte volume and hemoglobin mass will not develop unless exogenous iron is made available in adequate amounts. In the absence of added exogenous iron, the hemoglobin concentration and hematocrit fall appreciably as the maternal blood volume increases. Hemoglobin production in the fetus, however, will not be impaired, since the placenta obtains iron from the mother in amounts sufficient for the fetus to establish normal hemoglobin levels even when the mother has severe iron-deficiency anemia.

The amounts of iron absorbed from diet, together with that mobilized from stores, is usually insufficient to meet the demands im-

posed by pregnancy, even though iron absorption from the gastrointestinal tract appears to be moderately increased during pregnancy (Hahn and associates, 1951). Supplemental iron therefore, is valuable, during the latter half of pregnancy, and for several weeks after delivery if the infant is to be breast-fed (See Chap. 13, p. 313).

Without supplemental iron, the maternal *plasma iron concentration* often decreases during pregnancy. Undoubtedly, in most instances, iron deficiency contributes significantly to the fall. The *plasma iron-binding capacity* (transferrin) increases during pregnancy even when iron deficiency has been eliminated by appropriate treatment (Sturgeon, 1959). Several investigators have found that the administration of estrogen to nonpregnant women produced an increase in plasma transferrin levels comparable to those of pregnancy.

BLOOD LOSS. Not all the iron added to the maternal circulation in the form of hemoglobin is lost from the mother. During usual delivery and through the next few days, nearly half of the erythrocytes added to the maternal circulation during pregnancy are lost by way of the placental implantation site, the placenta itself, the episiotomy wound and lacerations, and the modest amount in the lochia. On the average, an amount of maternal erythrocytes corresponding to about 600 ml of predelivery blood is lost during and after vaginal delivery of a single fetus (Newton, 1966; Pritchard, 1965; Ueland, 1976). The average blood loss associated with the vaginal delivery of twins, however, is about 1 liter, or nearly twice that lost with the delivery of a single fetus. When delivery is accomplished by cesarean section, the loss of erythrocytes from the maternal circulation is appreciably greater than in vaginal delivery of a single fetus. In elective repeat cesarean section, the average loss of erythrocytes and hemoglobin is nearly twice that in vaginal delivery, or the amount lost is that contained in nearly 1 liter of maternal blood before delivery (Pritchard, 1965, Ueland, 1976;

Wilcox et al., 1959). Therefore, depending upon the means of the delivery and the number of fetuses, on the average nearly one-half to two-thirds of the erythrocytes added to the maternal circulation during pregnancy will be lost. However, it is not rare for the quantity of erythrocytes lost to equal or exceed the added volume accumulated during pregnancy.

Generally, the pattern of change in maternal blood volume during labor, vaginal delivery, and the puerperium is as follows: (1) there is some hemoconcentration during labor, which varies with the degree of muscular activity and dehydration; (2) during and soon after delivery there is a further reduction in volume which closely parallels the amount of blood lost; (3) during the first few days of the puerperium there is little change or a slight increase in blood volume, especially if hemoconcentration during labor or blood loss at delivery was sizable; (4) by one week after delivery there is a further reduction in plasma volume to the extent that the maternal blood volume is only slightly greater than several months later (McLennan et al., 1959, Pritchard, 1965).

Following delivery, any excess circulating hemoglobin above the amount normally present in the nonpregnant state ultimately yields iron for storage. The mechanism by which this occurs is most likely not accelerated erythrocyte destruction during the late puerperium, but rather reduced production of new erythrocytes. A similar process occurs after a normal nonanemic person receives transfused cells, or when a normal person with polycythemia, induced by high altitude, returns to sea level. There is no evidence of an increased rate of erythrocyte destruction in normal puerperal women who have a moderate excess of erythrocytes after delivery.

Leukocytes. The blood leukocyte count varies considerably during normal pregnancy. (Efrati et al., 1964). Usually it ranges from 5000 to 12,000 per mm³, but during labor and the early puerperium it may become markedly elevated, attaining levels

of 25,000 or even more. The cause for the marked increase is not known, but the same response occurs during and after strenuous exercise. It probably represents the reappearance in the circulation of leukocytes previously shunted out of the active circulation (Wintrobe, 1961).

Beginning quite early in pregnancy, the activity of alkaline phosphatase in the leukocytes is increased. Elevated leukocyte phosphatase activity is not peculiar to pregnancy but occurs in a wide variety of conditions, including most inflammatory states. During pregnancy there is a neutrophilia which consists predominantly of mature forms. By close examination of smears of the peripheral blood, of pregnant women, one can find an occasional myelocyte.

Blood Coagulation. The levels of several blood coagulation factors are increased during pregnancy. Plasma fibrinogen (factor I) measured as thrombin-clottable protein in normal nonpregnant women, averages very close to 300 mg and ranges from about 200 to 400 mg per dl. During normal pregnancy, the concentration of fibrinogen increases about 50 percent, averaging about 450 mg late in pregnancy, with a range from approximately 300 to 600 mg per dl. The increase in the concentration of fibrinogen undoubtedly contributes greatly to the striking increase in the blood *sedimentation rate* in normal pregnancy. The increased sedimentation rate in pregnancy, therefore, has no diagnostic or prognostic value when employed for the usual clinical purpose, such as the assessment of the activity of rheumatic heart disease.

Other clotting factors, the activities of which are increased appreciably during normal pregnancy, are factor VII (proconvertin), factor VIII (antihemophiliac globulin), factor IX (plasma thromboplastin component or Christmas factor), and factor X (Stuart factor). Usually, the level of factor II (prothrombin) is increased only slightly, whereas those of factors XI (plasma thromboplastin antecedent) and XIII (fibrin-stabilizing factor) are decreased during pregnancy (Coopland et al.,

1969; Kasper et al., 1964; Talbert, Langdell, 1964). The Quick one-stage prothrombin time and the partial thromboplastin time are both shortened slightly as pregnancy progresses.

Although some investigators have described a moderate decrease in the number of platelets per unit volume (Pitkin, Witte, 1980), our experience has been that there is no remarkable change in their number, appearance, or function. The clotting times of whole blood in either plain glass tubes (wettable surface) or silicone-coated or plastic tubes (nonwettable surface) do not differ significantly in normal pregnant and nonpregnant women. Some, but not all, of the pregnancy-induced changes in the levels of coagulation factors can be induced in part by the administration of one of several of the estrogen plus progestin contraceptive tablets commonly used (Fletcher, Alkjaersig, 1969).

High molecular weight soluble fibrin-fibrinogen complexes circulate in normal pregnancy and lower levels of antithrombin III and an increased capacity for neutralizing heparin have been described. Some of these alterations in coagulation factors during normal pregnancy may be equated with a continuing low-grade process of intravascular coagulation, as emphasized by Bonnar (1978) who, employing electron microscopy, identified fibrin deposited in the intervillous space of the placenta and in the walls of the spiral arteries that supply blood to the intervillous space.

During normal pregnancy, the level of maternal plasminogen (profibrinolysin) in plasma increases considerably, a phenomenon that can be induced by estrogen treatment. Even so, fibrinolytic, or plasmin, activity, measured either as the time for clotted whole plasma to dissolve or as the time for the clotted euglobulin fraction from plasma to undergo lysis, is distinctly prolonged compared with that of the normal nonpregnant state. Astedt (1972) implicated the placenta in the reduced fibrinolytic activity that characterizes normal pregnancy, since delivery normally is immediately followed by a prompt increase in plasma fibrinolytic activity (Margulis and associates, 1954; Ratnoff and co-workers, 1954). At the same time, fibrin degradation products usually rise slightly after delivery (Woodfield and associates, 1968).

CARDIOVASCULAR SYSTEM

During pregnancy and the puerperium there are remarkable changes involving the heart and the circulation.

Heart. Typically, the resting pulse rate increases about 10 to 15 beats per minute during pregnancy. As the diaphragm is elevated progressively during pregnancy, the heart is displaced to the left and upward, while at the same time it is rotated somewhat on its long axis. As a result, the apex of the heart is moved somewhat laterally from its position in the normal pregnant state, and an increase in the size of the cardiac silhouette is found in roentgenograms (Fig. 9-9). The extent of these changes is influenced by the

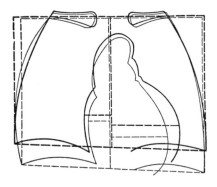

FIG. 9-9. Change in cardiac outline that occurs in pregnancy. The light lines represent the relations between the heart and thorax in the nonpregnant woman, and the heavy lines represent the conditions existing in pregnancy. These findings are based on teleoroentgenograms and represent the average findings in 33 women. (From Klafen and Palugyay: *Arch Gynaekol* 131:347, 1927)

size and position of the uterus, the strength of the abdominal muscles, and the configurations of the abdomen and thorax. Variability of these factors makes it difficult to precisely identify moderate degrees of cardiomegaly by physical examination or by simple roentgenographic studies. The physician must, therefore, be cautious in making a diagnosis of pathologic cardiomegaly during pregnancy.

In several studies using frontal and sagittal roentgenograms, the cardiac volume was found to increase normally by about 75 ml, or a little more than 10 percent, between early and late pregnancy (Ihrman, 1960). Such an increase in cardiac volume might involve slight hypertrophy, dilatation, or more likely, both. Katz and co-workers (1978) have studied left ventricular performance during pregnancy and the puerperium using echocardiography. Both left ventricular wall mass and end-diastolic dimensions were observed to increase during pregnancy as did heart rate, calculated stroke volume, and cardiac output. The changes in stroke volume were directly proportional to end-diastolic volume, implying, at least, that there is little change in the inotropic state of the myocardium during normal pregnancy and the puerperium.

During pregnancy some of the cardiac sounds may be altered to the extent that they would be considered abnormal in the absence of pregnancy. Cutforth and MacDonald (1966) obtained phonocardiograms at varying intervals during pregnancy in 50 normal women and documented the following changes:

Heart sounds: An exaggerated splitting of the first heart sound with increased loudness of both components; no definite changes in the aortic and pulmonary elements of the second sound; a loud, easily heard third sound.

Heart murmurs: A systolic murmur in 90 percent of pregnant women, intensified during inspiration in some or expiration in others, and disappearing very shortly after delivery; a soft diastolic murmur transiently in 19 percent; continuous murmurs arising apparently in breast vasculature in 10 percent.

The physician must be cautious when interpreting the significance of murmurs during pregnancy, especially systolic murmurs.

Normal pregnancy induces no characteristics changes in the *electrocardiogram* other than slight deviation of the electrical axis to the left as a result of the altered position of the heart.

Cardiac Output. During normal pregnancy, the arterial blood pressure and vascular resistance decrease while the blood volume, maternal weight, and basal metabolic rate increase. Each of these events would be expected to affect cardiac output with some leading to decreased output but others causing an increase. Many years ago, it was proposed, on the basis of relatively few observations, that maternal cardiac output rose progressively until about 32 to 34 weeks gestation but fell thereafter. This report had an unusually profound impact on clinical management of pregnant women with heart disease. It was generally taught that if pregnancy were tolerated until about the 34th week no further problems should be anticipated, because cardiac output and simultaneously cardiac work would fall at or before this time. The fact that such a conclusion, which was drawn from the limited laboratory observations, did not fit many clinical experiences went almost unnoticed.

From the results of more recent studies it has become clear that cardiac output *at rest,* when measured in the lateral recumbent position, increases appreciably during the first trimester and remains elevated during the second and third trimesters. Typically, cardiac output in late pregnancy is appreciably higher when the woman is in the lateral recumbent position than when she is supine, since in the supine position the large uterus and its contents often impede venous return to the heart (Kerr, 1965; Lees et al., 1968). Ueland and Hansen (1969), for example, found cardiac output to increase 1100 ml (22 percent) when the pregnant woman was moved from her back onto her side. In some individuals, the differences were much more striking.

Cardiac output in response to physical activity by the ambulatory woman must be greater late in pregnancy than it would be if she were not pregnant. Increase in mass alone demands such a response.

During the first stage of labor, maternal cardiac output increases moderately, and during the second stage of labor, with vigorous expulsive efforts, the cardiac output is appreciably greater. Most of the increase in cardiac output induced by pregnancy is lost very soon after delivery (Ueland, Metcalfe, 1975).

Circulation. The posture of the pregnant woman affects *arterial blood pressure.* Typically, blood pressure in the brachial artery is highest when the gravida is sitting, lowest when lying in the lateral recumbent position, and intermediate when supine, except for a few women who become quite hypotensive in the supine position. Usually, arterial blood pressure decreases to a nadir during the second trimester or early third trimester, and rises thereafter. Any sustained rise of 30 mm systolic or 15 mm diastolic under basal conditions, is indicative of an abnormality, most likely pregnancy-induced hypertension (see Chap. 27, p. 665).

The antecubital *venous pressure* remains unchanged during pregnancy, but in the supine position the femoral venous pressure rises steadily from 8 cm of water pressure early in pregnancy to 24 cm at term (Fig. 9-10). Employing radiolabeled tracers, Wright and co-workers (1950) and many others have demonstrated that blood flow in the legs is retarded during pregnancy except when the subjects were in the lateral recumbent position. This tendency toward stagnation of blood in the lower extremities during the latter part of pregnancy is attributable to the occlusion of the pelvic veins and inferior vena cava by pressure of the enlarged uterus. The elevated venous pressure returns to normal if the pregnant woman lies on her side and immediately after delivery of the infant by cesarean section (McLennan, 1943). From a clinical viewpoint, the retarded blood flow and increased venous pressure in the legs, which are demonstrable in the latter months of pregnancy, are of great importance. These alterations contribute to the dependent edema frequently experienced by women as they approach term and to the development of varicose veins in the legs and vulva, as well as hemorrhoids, during gestation.

OTHER CIRCULATORY EFFECTS FROM SUPINE POSITION. In the supine position, the large uterus of pregnancy rather consistently compresses the venous system that returns blood from the lower half of the body to the extent that cardiac filling may be re-

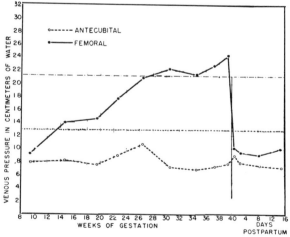

FIG. 9-10. Serial changes in antecubital and femoral venous blood pressure throughout normal pregnancy and early puerperium. These measurements were made on women in the supine position. (From McLennan: *Am J Obstet Gynecol* 45:568, 1943.)

duced and cardiac output decreased. Infrequently, this causes significant arterial hypotension sometimes referred to as the supine hypotensive syndrome (Howard et al., 1953). Moreover, Bieniarz and associates (1968) observed that in the supine position the large pregnant uterus may compress the aorta sufficiently to lower arterial blood pressure below the level of compression. They demonstrated that the usual sphygmomanometric measurement of blood pressures in the brachial artery does not provide a reliable estimate of the pressure in the uterine or other arteries that lie distal to the compression exerted on the aorta by the gravid uterus and its contents. When the pregnant woman is supine, uterine arterial pressure is significantly lower than that in the brachial artery. In the presence of systemic hypotension, as occurs with spinal anesthesia, the decrease in uterine arterial pressure is even more marked than in arteries above the level of compression of the aorta.

Blood Flow to Skin. Increased cutaneous blood flow in pregnancy serves to dissipate excess heat generated by the increased metabolism imposed by pregnancy (Burt, 1950, Spetz,1964).

RESPIRATORY TRACT

Anatomic Changes. The level of the diaphragm rises about 4 cm during pregnancy. The subcostal angle widens appreciably as the transverse diameter of the thoracic cage increases about 2 cm and its circumference about 6 cm but not to a degree sufficient to prevent a reduction in the residual volume of air in the lungs created by the elevated diaphragm. The idea that the elevated diaphragm was "splinted" during normal pregnancy has been disproved by the findings of fluoroscopic studies (Möbius, 1961). Diaphragmatic excursion is actually greater during pregnancy than when nonpregnant.

Pulmonary Function. At any stage of normal pregnancy, the amount of oxygen de-

livered by the increase in tidal volume described below clearly exceeds the oxygen need imposed by the pregnancy. Moreover, the amount of hemoglobin in the circulation and, in turn, the total oxygen-carrying capacity, increases appreciably during normal pregnancy, as does cardiac output. As the consequence, *maternal arteriovenous oxygen difference* is decreased during pregnancy.

The respiratory rate is changed little during pregnancy but the *tidal volume, minute ventilatory volume, and minute oxygen uptake* increase appreciably as pregnancy advances (Table 9-3). The *maximum breathing capacity* and *forced (or timed) vital capacity* are not altered appreciably. The *functional residual capacity* and the *residual volume* of air are decreased as the consequence of elevation of the diaphragm. *Lung compliance* is unaffected by pregnancy while *airway conductance* is increased and *total pulmonary resistance* is reduced. Gee and associates (1967) speculated that increased airway conductance from decreased bronchomotor tone may be effected by progesterone action.

The *closing volume*, i.e., the lung volume at which airways in the dependent parts of the lung begin to close during expiration, has been considered to be higher in pregnancy by some investigators but not by others (Baldwin and associates, 1977).

An increased awareness of a desire to breathe is common even early in pregnancy (Milne et al., 1978) and may be interpreted as dyspnea which, in turn, suggests pulmonary or cardiac abnormalities even though most often none exists. The increased tidal volume normally lowers slightly the blood Pco2 causing mild respiratory alkalosis, which is compensated for by a lowering of the bicarbonate concentration.

The increased respiratory effort and, in turn, the reduction in Pco2 during pregnancy most likely is induced in large part by progesterone and to a lesser degree estrogen. The site of action of the hormones appears to be central, i.e., a direct stimulatory effect on the respiratory center.

Although pulmonary function is not impaired by pregnancy, diseases of the respiratory tract may be more serious during gesta-

TABLE 9-3.
RESTING RESPIRATORY FUNCTION

FUNCTION	NOT PREGNANT	PREGNANT	CHANGE (%)
Respiratory rate	15	16	—
Tidal Volume (ml)	487	678	+39*
Minute ventilation (ml)	7270	10,340	+42*
Minute O$_2$ uptake	201	266	+32*
Vital capacity (ml)	3260	3310	+ 1
Maximum breathing capacity (predicted; %)	102	97	− 5
Inspiratory capacity (ml)	2625	2745	+ 5
Residual volume (ml)	965	770	−20*

From Cugell and associates: *Am Rev Tuberc* 67:568, 1953.
* Highly significant differences.

tion. Important factors are undoubtedly the increased oxygen requirements imposed by pregnancy and perhaps an increase in closing volume, especially when supine.

URINARY SYSTEM

Remarkable changes in both structure and function take place in the urinary tract during normal pregnancy.

Kidney. Apparently, the kidney increases slightly in size during pregnancy. Bailey and Rolleston (1971), for example, found that the kidney was 1.5 cm longer during the early puerperium than when measured 6 months later.

Glomerular filtration rate (GFR) and renal plasma flow (RPF) increase early in pregnancy, the former as much as 50 percent by the beginning of the second trimester, and the latter not quite so much (Chesley, 1963; Sims, 1963). The precise mechanism by which RPF and GFR are increased in pregnancy has not been identified. Placental lactogen may play a role, since it possesses many of the actions of pituitary growth hormone and the latter has been demonstrated experimentally to induce increases in both RPF and GFR. The elevated GFR has been found by

most investigators to persist to term (Fig. 9-11), whereas the RPF decreases during the third trimester toward values found in nonpregnant persons.

Most studies of renal function carried out during pregnancy have been performed while the subjects were supine, a position that late in pregnancy may produce marked systemic hemodynamic changes and which lead to alterations in several aspects of renal function, as described on page 239. Late in pregnancy, for instance, urinary flow and sodium excretion are affected significantly by posture, averaging less than half the rate of excretion in the supine position, compared to the lateral recumbent position (Chesley, Sloan, 1964, Hendricks, Barnes, 1955; Pritchard et al., 1955).

Whereas posture clearly affects sodium and water excretion in late pregnancy, its impact on GFR and RPF seems to be much more variable. Chesley and Sloan (1964), for example, found GFR and RPF to be reduced commonly when the pregnant woman was in the supine position, whereas Dunlop (1976) identified little or no reduction. Pritchard and associates (1955) detected decreases in GFR and RPF while supine compared to lateral recumbent in some, but not most, of the late pregnant women studied. Davison and Hytten (1974) have rightfully pointed out that an estimate of glomerular filtration rate is only valid for the conditions

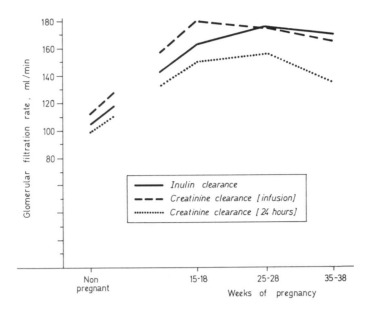

FIG. 9-11. Mean glomerular filtration rate measured in healthy women over a short period with infused inulin (Inulin clearance), simultaneously as creatinine clearance during the inulin infusion (Creatinine clearance [infusion]), and over 24 hours as endogenous creatinine clearance (Creatinine clearance [24 hours]). (From Davison and Hytten: *Br J Obstet Gynaecol* 81:588, 1974)

under which it is measured and that changes with posture represent the real life situation rather than artifact.

A possible cause of the changes in renal function in the supine position compared to the lateral recumbent is reduced venous return to the heart, which results from obstruction of the inferior vena cava and iliac veins by the large pregnant uterus, which could lead to reduction in cardiac output and, in turn, lowering of RPF and GFR. This sequence of events, however, does not appear to be essential to the mechanism that triggers sodium and water retention when supine. In a woman at term with a renal transplant in the right iliac fossa, a change to the supine from the lateral recumbent position had no obvious affect on water and sodium excretion or on GFR (Pritchard, unpublished).

Another possible mechanism to account for decreased sodium and water excretion in supine pregnant women is elevated ureteral pressure. Fulop and Brazeau (1970) induced increased tubular reabsorption of sodium and water in dogs by elevating ureteral pressure moderately. Pritchard and associates (1955) were not able to prevent such decreases in the supine position following the insertion of ureteral catheters well above the pelvic brim; however, increased intraureteric pressure may not have been completely prevented by this maneuver.

It has been suggested by some that the release of antidiuretic hormone (ADH) plays a role, but ADH is probably not essential, since postural changes have produced similar reductions in a pregnant woman with severe diabetes insipidus (Whalley et al., 1961).

LOSS OF NUTRIENTS. One unusual feature of the pregnancy-induced changes in renal excretion is the remarkably increased amounts of various nutrients in the urine. Amino acids and water-soluble vitamins are lost in the urine of pregnant women in much greater amounts than in the urine of nonpregnant women (Hytten, Leitch, 1971).

Tests of Renal Function. The results of several of the tests of renal function in general clinical use may be altered during normal pregnancy and therefore be quite misleading. During pregnancy the concentrations in plasma of creatinine and urea normally decrease as a consequence of the increased GFR. At times, the urea concentration may be so low as to suggest impaired hepatic synthesis, which sometimes occurs with severe liver disease.

Creatinine clearance is a most useful test of renal function in pregnancy (provided that complete urine collection is made over an accurately timed period preferably of at least several hours). *Urine concentration tests* may give results that are misleading. During the day, pregnant women tend to accumulate water in the form of dependent edema (see p. 230), and at night, while recumbent, they mobilize this fluid and excrete it via the kidneys. This reversal of the usual nonpregnant diurnal pattern of urinary flow causes nocturia and the nighttime excretion of urine more dilute than in the nonpregnant state. The failure of a pregnant woman to excrete a concentrated urine after withholding fluids for approximately 18 hours does not necessarily mean renal damage. The kidney, in fact, in these circumstances functions perfectly normally by excreting mobilized extracellular fluid of relatively low osmolality. *Dye excretion tests,* such as the timed measurement of the amount of injected phenosulfonphthalein (PSP) excreted in the urine, may also give results in pregnant women that are misleading. The dye may very well be excreted by the kidney but at low rates of urinary flow it is not collected and measured because of stagnation of urine in the considerably dilated renal pelves and ureters, which is described below.

URINALYSIS. *Glucosuria* during pregnancy is not necessarily abnormal. The appreciable increase in glomerular filtration, together with impaired tubular reabsorptive capacity for filtered glucose accounts in most cases for the glucosuria. Chesley (1963) calculated that for these reasons alone about one-sixth of all pregnant women should spill glucose in the urine. Even though glucosuria is common during pregnancy, the possibility of diabetes mellitus cannot be ignored. *Pro-*

teinuria does not occur normally during pregnancy except occasionally in slight amounts during or soon after vigorous labor. If not the result of contamination during collection, blood cells in the urine during pregnancy indicate disease somewhere in the urinary tract. Difficult labor and delivery, of course, can cause hematuria because of trauma to the lower urinary tract.

HYDRONEPHROSIS AND HYDRO-URETER. In pregnant women, after the uterus rises completely out of the pelvis, it rests upon the ureters, compressing them at the pelvic brim (Figs. 9-12, 9-13). Increased intraureteral tonus above the level of the pelvic brim compared with that of the pelvic portion of the ureter has been identified (Rubi, Sala, 1968). No such differences were demonstrable in nonpregnant women.

Typically, ureteral dilatation above the pelvic brim is more marked on the right side. Schulman and Herlinger (1975) found ureteral dilatation to be greater on the right side in 86 percent of pregnant women studied. The unequal degrees of dilatation may result from a cushioning provided the left ureter by the sigmoid colon and perhaps from greater compression of the right ureter as the consequence of dextrorotation of the uterus. Bellina and co-workers (1970) emphasized that the right ovarian vein complex, which is remarkably dilated during pregnancy, lies obliquely over the right ureter and may contribute significantly to right ureteral dilatation.

Another possible mechanism causing hydronephrosis and hydroureter is hormonal, presumably an effect of progesterone. Major support for this concept was provided by Van Wagenen (1939) who described in the monkey further dilatation of the ureters after removal of the fetus if the placenta remained in situ. However, the relatively abrupt onset of dilatation in women at midpregnancy, described by Schulman and Herlinger, is more consistent with ureteral compression from a translocated enlarging uterus than a humoral effect.

Elongation accompanies distension of the

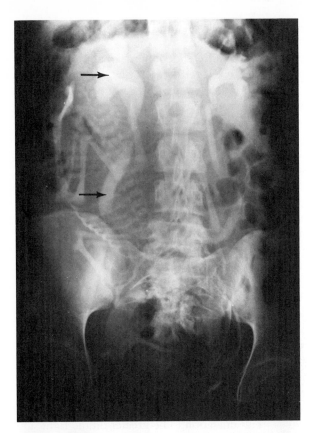

FIG. 9-12. Normal intravenous pyelogram at 36 weeks gestation. Pregnancy-induced hydronephrosis (upper arrow) and hydroureter (lower arrow) are more marked on the mother's right side. Elongation, dilatation, and peristalsis of the ureter create the appearance of discontinuity of the ureter.

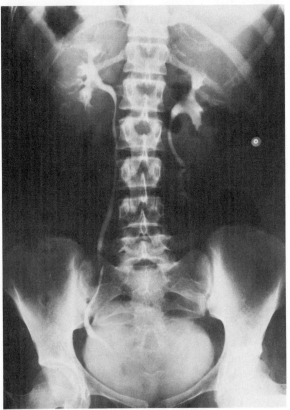

FIG. 9-13. Intravenous pyelogram one week postpartum on the same woman. There has been rapid resolution of much of the pregnancy-induced hydronephrosis and hydroureter evident in Figure 9–12.

ureter, which is frequently thrown into curves of varying size, the smaller of which may be sharply angulated, producing, at least theoretically, partial or complete obstruction. These so-called kinks are poorly named, since the term connotes obstruction. They are, in fact, in most cases, merely single or double curves, which, when viewed in the roentgenogram taken in the same plane as the curve, appear as more or less acute angulations of the ureter. Another exposure at right angles nearly always identifies them to be more gentle curves rather than kinks. The ureter, in both its abdominal and pelvic por-

tions, undergoes not only elongation but frequently lateral displacement by the pressure of the enlarged uterus.

Remarkable pregnancy-induced hydronephrosis with some degree of hydroureter has been demonstrated after transplant of a donor kidney to the iliac fossa (Fig. 9-14A, B). In this particular subject, the creatinine clearance increased from 75 ml per minute very early in pregnancy to 120 ml per minute during the third trimester.

After delivery, there is resolution so that by six to eight weeks the urinary tract has returned to pregestational dimensions. The

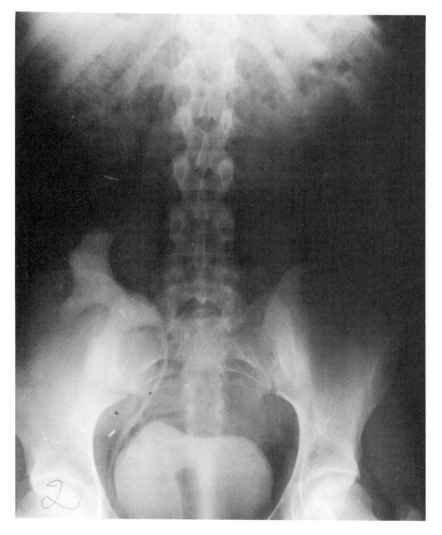

FIG. 9-14. A. Intravenous pyelogram of renal transplant: Before pregnancy.

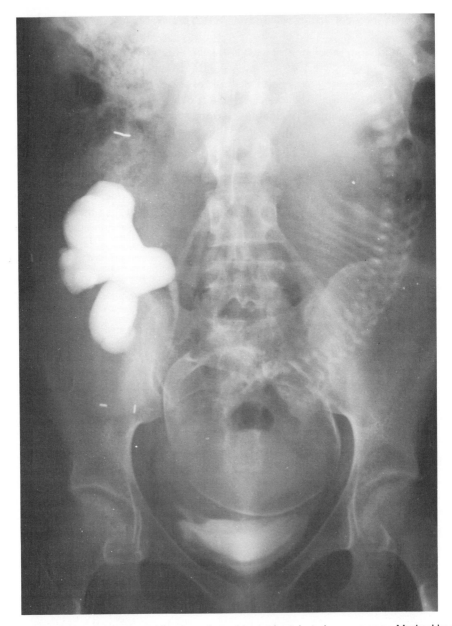

FIG. 9-14. B.   Intravenous pyelogram of renal transplant: Late in pregnancy. Marked levo-rotation of the uterus was identified at cesarean section.

stretching and dilatation do not continue long enough to impair permanently the elasticity of the ureter unless infection supervenes. These changes induced by pregnancy have been reviewed by Fainstat (1963) and by Schulman and Herlinger (1975).

Bladder.   There are few significant anatomic changes in the bladder before the fourth month of pregnancy. From that time onward, however, the increased size of the uterus, together with the hyperemia which affects all pelvic organs and the hyperplasia of the muscle and connective tissues, elevates the trigone and causes thickening of its posterior, or interureteric, margin. Continuation of this process to the end of pregnancy produces a marked deepening and widening of the trigone. The bladder mucosa undergoes no change other than an increase in the size and tortuosity of its blood vessels.

Toward the end of pregnancy, particularly in nulliparas in whom the presenting part often engages before the onset of labor, the entire base of the bladder is pushed forward and upward, converting the normal convex surface into a concavity, as viewed through the cystoscope. As a result, difficulties in diagnostic and therapeutic procedures are increased greatly. In addition, the pressure of the presenting part impairs the drainage of blood and lymph from the base of the bladder, often rendering the area edematous, easily traumatized, and probably more susceptible to infection.

Normally there is little residual urine in nulliparas, but occasionally it develops in multiparas with relaxed vaginal walls and cystoceles. Incompetence of the ureterovesical valve may supervene, with the consequent probability of vesicoureteral reflux of urine, as Lund and co-workers (1959) demonstrated, employing cinefluoroscopy.

GASTROINTESTINAL TRACT

As pregnancy progresses, the stomach and intestines are displaced by the enlarging uterus. As the result of the positional changes in these viscera, the physical findings in certain diseases are altered. The appendix, for instance, is usually displaced upward and somewhat laterally as the uterus enlarges, and at times it may reach the right flank (p. 761).

There are usually decreased tone and motility of the gastrointestinal tract, which lead to prolongation of the times of gastric emptying and intestinal transit. The large amounts of progesterone produced by the placenta contribute to the generalized relaxation of smooth muscle characteristic of pregnancy. During labor, especially after the administration of analgesic agents, *gastric-emptying time* typically is appreciably prolonged. A major danger of general anesthesia for delivery is regurgitation and aspiration of either food-laden or highly acidic gastric contents (see Chap. 18, p. 440).

Pyrosis (heartburn), common during preg-

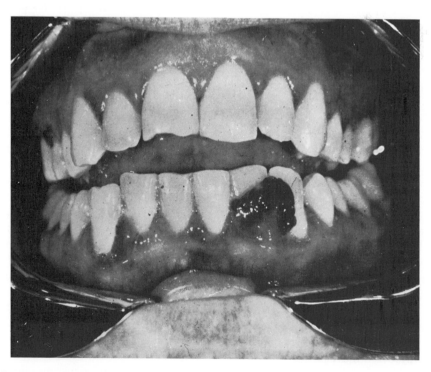

FIG. 9-15. Pregnancy epulis, a benign vascular lesion that may bleed vigorously if traumatized. After pregnancy, it usually regresses spontaneously. (Courtesy of Dr. Robert Walker)

nancy, is most likely caused by reflux of acidic secretions into the lower esophagus, the altered position of the stomach probably contributing to its frequent occurrence. Esophageal and gastric tone are altered by pregnancy with intraesophageal pressures being lower and intragastric pressures higher in pregnant women. At the same time, esophageal peristalsis has lower wave speed and lower amplitude (Ulmsten, Sundström, 1978). These changes favor gastroesophageal reflux.

The gums may become hyperemic and softened during pregnancy and may bleed when mildly traumatized, as with a toothbrush. A focal, highly vascular swelling of the gums, the so-called epulis of pregnancy (Fig. 9-15) develops occasionally but typically regresses spontaneously after delivery. There is no good evidence that pregnancy per se incites tooth decay.

Hemorrhoids are fairly common during pregnancy. They are caused in large measure by constipation and the elevated pressure in veins below the level of the enlarged uterus.

LIVER AND GALLBLADDER

Liver. Although the liver in some animals increases remarkably in size during pregnancy, there is no evidence of such an increase in human pregnancy (Combes, Adams, 1971). Moreover, by histologic evaluation of liver obtained by biopsy, including examination with the electron microscope, it has been demonstrated that no distinct changes in liver morphology occur in response to normal pregnancy (Adams, Ashworth, unpublished; Ingerslev, Teilum, 1946). The results of the very few measurements of hepatic blood flow during pregnancy are in conflict; there is perhaps a slight increase.

Some of the laboratory tests commonly used to evaluate hepatic function yield appreciably different results during normal pregnancy. Moreover, the changes induced by pregnancy often occur in the same direction as those found in patients with hepatic disease. Total *alkaline phosphatase* activity in serum approximately doubles during normal pregnancy and commonly reaches levels that would be considered abnormal in the nonpregnant woman. Much of the increase is attributable to alkaline phosphatase isozymes from the placenta, which are heat-stable up to 65C. Whether all of the increase is caused by enzymes of placental origin is not clear, since nonpregnant women given estrogen in amounts comparable with those found in pregnancy frequently have increased serum alkaline phosphatase activity in their blood. (Song, Kappas, 1968). Mendenhall (1970), as part of a study of the effects of pregnancy on several serum proteins, reconfirmed the presence of a decrease in *plasma albumin* concentration, showing it to average 3.0 g per dl late in pregnancy compared with 4.3 g in nonpregnant women. The reduction in serum albumin, combined with a slight increase in globulins that occurs normally during pregnancy, results in a decrease in the albumin to globulin ratio similar to that in certain hepatic diseases. Serum *cholinesterase* activity is reduced during normal pregnancy, as it is in certain liver diseases. The magnitude of the decrease is about the same as the decrease in the concentration of albumin, namely, i.e., 25 percent (Pritchard, 1955).

Leucine aminopeptidase activity is markedly elevated in serum from pregnant women; at term it reaches a level approximately three times the nonpregnant value. The increase in total serum leucine aminopeptidase activity during pregnancy results from the appearance of a pregnancy-specific enzyme (or enzymes) with distinct substrate specificities (Song, Kappas, 1968). The pregnancy-induced aminopeptidase has oxytocinase activity and has been called cystine aminopeptidase by Page and co-workers (1954). The site of origin of the enzymes for oxytocin is not clear.

Combes and associates (1963) demonstrated that the capacity of the liver for excreting sulfobromophthalein into bile is somewhat decreased during normal pregnancy, while, at the same time, the ability of the liver to extract and store sulfobromophtha-lein is increased. The administration of estrogens to nonpregnant women induces comparable changes (Mueller, Kappas, 1964). *Spider nevi and palmer erythema,* both of which occur in patients with liver disease, are commonly found in normal pregnant women, most probably as a result of the increased circulating estrogens during pregnancy, but they disappear soon after delivery (Bean et al., 1949).

Gallbladder.   Gallbladder function is altered during pregnancy. Potter (1936) noted at the time of cesarean section that quite often the gallbladder is distended but hypotonic; moreover, aspirated bile was quite thick. It is commonly accepted that pregnancy predisposes to formation of gallstones (p. 759).

ENDOCRINE GLANDS

Some of the most important endocrine changes of pregnancy have been discussed: the production of estrogens, progesterone, chorionic gonadotropin, placental lactogen, chorionic thyrotropin, and corticotropin (see Chap. 7, p. 147).

Pituitary.   The pituitary enlarges somewhat during pregnancy. Although there have been suggestions that it may increase in size sufficiently to compress the optic chiasma and reduce the visual fields, such visual changes during normal pregnancy are either absent or minimal. However, striking enlargement of microadenomas of the pituitary do occur during pregnancy. This complication is a much feared sequelae in women treated for infertility due to hyperprolactinemia-induced anovulation usually accompanied by galactorrhea. Enlargement of the pituitary during pregnancy likely results from the action of estrogen. The maternal pituitary gland is not essential for the maintenance of pregnancy (Kaplan, 1961). There now are a number of women who have undergone hypophysectomy, completed pregnancy successfully and

have undergone spontaneous labor while receiving glucocorticosteroids along with thyroid hormone and vasopressin. Extensive destruction of both the maternal and the fetal pituitary glands in monkeys during the second trimester does not interrupt gestation (Hutchinson and co-workers, 1962). In these hypophysectomized primates, marked adrenal atrophy did not occur, thus the placenta may be a source of an adrenal corticotropin in this species.

PITUITARY   GROWTH   HORMONE. Although placental lactogen (hPL) is abundant in the pregnant woman's blood, the level of pituitary growth hormone is decreased. After delivery, hPL rapidly disappears, but pituitary growth hormone remains quite low for some time (Spellacy, Buhi, 1969). The relative lack of these hormones, with the loss of their diabetogenic effect, may account in part for the usually abrupt and rather marked reduction in insulin requirements of women with diabetes mellitus during the early puerperium.

PROLACTIN.   During the course of human gestation, there is a marked increase in the levels of prolactin in the maternal plasma. In fact, the levels increase to such an extent that mean concentrations of 150 ng per ml, values 10 times greater than those in normal nonpregnant women, are observed at term (Friesen et al., 1972; Riggs et al., 1977). Paradoxically, following delivery, there is a decrease in plasma prolactin concentration even in the lactating mother. During early lactation, there are pulsatile bursts of secretion of prolactin apparently in response to suckling. The physiologic cause of the marked increase in prolactin prior to parturition is unknown. But, when the marked increase in secretion that occurs in the experimental animal under estrogen influence is considered, it is tempting to relate the increase in prolactin secretion during pregnancy to the increase in estrogens in the gravid woman. Moreover, it is likely that the action of prolactin in mediating lactalbumin synthesis is inhibited during the course of pregnancy by the steroid hormone, proges- terone. Thus, following delivery, with the re- moval of the inhibitory influence of proges- terone, lactation may proceed.

Prolactin is also found, throughout the course of gestation, in high concentration in the fetal plasma, attaining highest concentra- tions during the last five weeks of pregnancy (Winters et al., 1975). Considerable evi- dence has accrued which is supportive of the view that prolactin in fetal plasma is of fetal pituitary origin and not of maternal pituitary origin.

For reasons not yet clearly understood, the concentrations of prolactin in the amnionic fluid are highest early in gestation and, in fact, levels of 10,000 ng per ml can be ob- served in the amnionic fluid at 20 weeks ges- tation. Several groups of investigators have presented convincing evidence that the uterine decidua is one site of synthesis of at least a part of the prolactin in amnionic fluid. The levels of prolactin in amnionic fluid de- crease after about 24 weeks of gestation such that by term the concentrations are one-tenth those observed in early pregnancy (Friesen et al., 1972).

Thyroid. During pregnancy there is moderate enlargement of the thyroid caused by hyperplasia of the glandular tissue and in- creased vascularity. The basal metabolic rate increases progressively during normal preg- nancy by as much as 25 percent. Most of this increase in oxygen consumption, how- ever, is the result of the metabolic activity of the products of conception. As was shown by Sandiford and Wheeler (1924), if the body surface of the fetus is considered along with that of the mother, the predicted and the measured basal metabolic rates are quite similar.

THYROXINE.   Beginning as early as the second month of pregnancy, the concentra- tion of thyroid hormone, measured as pro- tein-bound iodine (PBI), butanol-extractable iodine (BEI), or *thyroxine,* rises sharply in the mother's plasma to a plateau, which is main- tained until after delivery. The plateau is

reached at levels from 9 to 16 μg per dl of thyroxine as compared with 5 to 12 μg in nonpregnant euthyroid women.

Such an elevation of circulating thyroid hormone incorrectly suggests an overtly hy- perthyroid state during pregnancy. During pregnancy, the *thyroxine-binding proteins* of plasma, principally an α-globulin, are consid- erably increased. Mulaisho and Utiger (1977) provide the following mean values for thyroid-binding globulin levels in plasma: 7.1 mg per dl in the first trimester, 9.0 in the second, and 8.9 in the third trimester, compared to values of 3.6 mg per dl for nor- mal nonpregnant women. Therefore, even though the total concentrations of thyroxine and triiodothyronine are elevated, the amounts of unbound, or effective, hormone are not appreciably higher (Osathanondh et al., 1976). The increase in circulating estro- gens during pregnancy presumably is the ma- jor cause of these changes in circulating hor- mones and binding capacity, for they can be reproduced by administering estrogen, in- cluding most oral contraceptives, to nonpreg- nant women. Although the normal early in- crease in thyroxine and thyroid-binding globulin and the decrease in triiodothyronine resin uptake are sometimes absent in women destined to abort, the abortion almost cer- tainly is not the result of failure of hormones and binding protein to increase, but rather is due to an abnormal conceptus.

During pregnancy, there is increased up- take of ingested radioiodide by the maternal thyroid gland, again suggesting a hyperthy- roid state. Aboul-Khair and associates (1964), however, claimed that although the clearance of inorganic iodine is increased by the thyroid gland during pregnancy, the abso- lute uptake is not increased. They concluded that the goiter of pregnancy simply reflects and compensates for the lower concentration of circulating iodide available for synthesis of thyroxine.

Hershman and Starnes (1969) as well as others, identified a thyrotropic substance ob- tained from human placenta but the role of chorionic thyrotropin, if any, in stimulating the thyroid is unclear. In women with hydatidiform moles, increased thyroid activity is likely due to the action of hCG which is known to have intrinsic thyroid stimulating activity.

RESIN UPTAKE OF TRIIODOTHYRO-NINE. In 1957, Hamolsky and associates reported that the in vitro uptake of radioactive triiodothyronine by erythrocytes was increased during incubation with serum from hyperthyroid subjects but was decreased if the serum came from hypothyroid subjects or pregnant women. Furthermore, the administration of estrogen lowered the uptake of triiodothyronine. The decreased uptake by erythrocytes, or by resin, both in pregnancy and following administration of estrogen, is clearly the result of increased binding of the triiodothyronine to thyroid binding proteins, especially α-globulin. The change in uptake is similar in time of appearance to that of thyroxine, but in the opposite direction. *Therefore, an elevated plasma thyroxine level and simultaneously a lowered uptake of triiodothyronine by resin are indicative of hyperestrogenemia, including that induced by pregnancy or by estrogen-containing oral contraceptives.* In Table 9-4, the pregnancy-induced changes, those found in hyperthyroidism, and those induced by administration of estrogen, are compared.

Thyroxine, thyroxine-binding capacity, and triiodothyronine resin uptake values in cord serum are less than those in maternal serum but greater than levels in nonpregnant adults (Russell et al., 1964).

Parathyroids. Increased plasma levels of parathyroid hormone are observed in pregnancy. Reitz and co-workers (1977), for example, identified the level of hormone during the third trimester to be about twice that of normal nonpregnant controls. In general, the level of ionized calcium in plasma is of major importance in the operation of a feedback mechanism regulating the secretion of the hormone, but during normal pregnancy, the level of ionized calcium is not appreciably different from the nonpregnant state (Pitkin, Gebhardt, 1977). Therefore, Reitz and co-workers suggest that during pregnancy a new "set point" exists between the levels of parathyroid hormone and ionized calcium.

Calcitonin, which originates in the parafollicular, or C cells of the thyroid, may protect the skeleton during calcium stress. During pregnancy and lactation calcitonin levels in plasma are appreciably higher than in nonpregnant women and are comparable to those of men and in women who are using estrogen-progestin contraceptives (Hillyard et al., 1978; Stevenson and co-workers, 1979).

Adrenal. In normal pregnancy, there is

TABLE 9-4.

COMPARISON OF EFFECTS OF PREGNANCY AND OF ESTROGEN ADMINISTRATION ON TESTS USED TO EVALUATE THYROID FUNCTION

TESTS	NORMAL PREGNANCY	ESTROGEN ADMINISTRATION	HYPER-THYROIDISM
Basal metabolic rate	Increased	Not increased	Increased
Total thyroxine	Increased	Increased	Increased
Thyroxine-binding globulin	Increased	Increased	Not increased
Free thyroxine	Not increased	Not increased	Increased
Total triiodothyronine	Increased	Increased	Increased
Free triiodothyronine	Not increased	Not increased	Increased
Radioiodine uptake (percent)	Increased	Not increased	Increased
Absolute iodine uptake	Not increased	Not increased	Increased
Triiodothyronine resin uptake	Decreased	Decreased	Increased
Serum cholesterol level	Increased	Variable	Decreased

probably very little morphologic change in the maternal adrenal.

CORTISOL. There is a considerable increase in the concentration of circulating cortisol, but much of it is bound by the cortisol-binding globulin, *transcortin*. The rate of secretion of cortisol by the maternal adrenal is not greater; probably it is even lower than it is in the nonpregnant state. However, the metabolic clearance rate of cortisol is lower during pregnancy, as indicated by the fact that in a pregnant woman, the half-life of intravenously injected radiolabeled cortisol is nearly twice as long as it is in nonpregnant women (Migeon et al., 1957). Administration of estrogen, including those in most oral contraceptives, causes changes in levels of cortisol and transcortin similar to those of pregnancy.

In early pregnancy, the levels of circulating corticotropin (ACTH) are strikingly reduced. As pregnancy progresses, the levels of ACTH and cortisol rise. This apparent paradox is not completely understood. It is believed to be due to alterations in cortisol metabolism induced by estrogen and progesterone, and perhaps due to a direct effect of progesterone on the brain by modulating corticotropin-releasing factor.

ALDOSTERONE. As early as the 15th week of normal pregnancy, the maternal adrenal secretes considerably increased amounts of aldosterone. By the third trimester, about 1 mg per day is secreted. If sodium intake is restricted, aldosterone secretion is even further elevated (Watanabe et al., 1963). At the same time, levels of renin and angiotensin substrate are normally increased especially during the latter half of pregnancy (Geelhoed, Vander, 1968; Massani et al., 1967). This gives rise to increased angiotensin II plasma levels which appear to account for the markedly elevated secretion of aldosterone. It has been suggested that the elevated secretion of aldosterone during normal pregnancy affords protection against the natriuretic effect of progesterone (Landau, Lugibihl, 1961). Progesterone administered

to nonpregnant women is associated with a prompt and marked increase in aldosterone excretion (Laidlaw et al., 1962).

DESOXYCORTICOSTERONE. There is a striking increase in the maternal plasma levels of desoxycorticosterone (DOC) during the last trimester of human pregnancy. Brown et al. (1972) and Nolten and associates (1978) found that in nonpregnant women and during the first two trimesters of pregnancy, the levels of plasma DOC are less than 10 ng per dL. During the last few weeks of pregnancy, DOC levels rise to 150 ng per dL or more (Fig. 9-16). The origin of these increased amounts of DOC are not clear. Interestingly, Nolten et al. found that the administration of a potent glucocorticosteroid, dexamethasone, to pregnant women to reduce ACTH secretion is not accompanied by a reduction in plasma DOC levels. Moreover, ACTH administration to pregnant women is not accompanied by an increase in plasma DOC concentration.

These findings, together with the finding of significant quantities of DOC in the fetal circulation and of DOC sulfate in the amnionic fluid, led these investigators to suggest that the increased levels of DOC in maternal plasma arise in the fetus. This may be true.

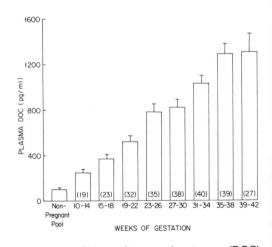

FIG. 9-16. Plasma deoxycorticosterone (DOC) in primigravid women. (From Parker and coworkers, 1980, submitted to *Am J Obstet Gynecol*)

Alternatively, it has been suggested (Winkel et al., 1979) that maternal plasma progesterone may serve as a precursor for DOC biosynthesis in the maternal compartment. These investigators demonstrated that [³H] progesterone administered to pregnant and nonpregnant persons is converted to [³H] DOC since [³H] tetrahydro DOC is found in the urine of such subjects. The extent of conversion of plasma progesterone to DOC (based on the ³H:¹⁴C ratio of urinary tetrahydro DOC following the intravenous infusion of [³H] progesterone and [¹⁴C] DOC) is approximately 1 percent. However, it is not yet clear whether the DOC derived from the conversion of plasma progesterone ever enters the circulation as DOC. It seems likely that this conversion occurs in the maternal liver. If this is true, it is possible that the DOC derived by conversion of progesterone in the hepatocyte is reduced to tetrahydro DOC before it leaves the liver cell. The fractional conversion of plasma progesterone to urinary tetrahydro DOC is similar in nonpregnant and pregnant humans. However, it is possible that as progesterone levels rise in the latter stages of pregnancy, a greater portion of DOC derived from progesterone may escape 5 β-reductase enzyme by progesterone itself. If this were true, there may be a threshold level of plasma progesterone that is reached before DOC, derived from progesterone conversion, has access to maternal plasma. Such an occurence could have profound physiologic and pathophysiologic consequences, in instances of large placental mass and high plasma progesterone levels, e.g., multiple pregnancy, hydatidiform mole, and with hydrops fetalis.

OTHER STEROIDS. As discussed in Chapter 7 (p. 152), the levels of *dehydroisoandrosterone sulfate* circulating in maternal blood and excreted in the urine are not increased during normal pregnancy, but rather decreased as a consequence of an increased rate of removal, through extensive 16 α-hydroxylation in the maternal liver and estrogen formation in the placenta.

The maternal plasma levels of *androstenedione* and *testosterone* are increased during pregnancy. This finding is not explained by alterations in the metabolic clearance rates of these androgens. On the one hand, maternal plasma androstendione and testosterone are converted to estradiol in the placenta, which increases the rate of clearance, but, on the other hand, there is an increased amount of testosterone-estradiol-binding globulin in plasma of pregnant women which retards the rate of testosterone clearance. Thus, there is an increased plasma production rate of maternal testosterone and androstenedione during human pregnancy. The source of this increased androgen production is unknown but it likely originates in the ovary. Interestingly, little or no testosterone in maternal plasma enters the fetal circulation as testosterone. Even when massive testosterone levels are found in the circulation of pregnant women with androgen-secreting tumors, the testosterone level in umbilical cord venous plasma is likely to be so low as to be undetectable. This finding is the result of the near complete conversion of testosterone to β-estradiol by the trophoblast (Hensleigh, Woodruff, 1978).

MUSCULOSKELETAL SYSTEM

Progressive *lordosis* is a characteristic feature of normal pregnancy. Compensating for the anterior position of the enlarging uterus, the lordosis shifts the center of gravity back over the lower extremities. There is increased mobility of the sacroiliac, sacrococcygeal, and the pubic joints during pregnancy, presumably as a result of hormonal changes. Their mobility may contribute to the alteration of maternal posture and, in turn, cause discomfort in the lower portion of the back, especially late in pregnancy. During the last trimester of pregnancy, aching, numbness, and weakness are occasionally experienced in the upper extremities, possibly as a result of the marked lordosis with anterior flexion of the neck and slumping of the shoulder girdle, which, in turn, produces traction on the ulnar and median nerves (Crisp, DeFrancesco, 1964).

PRECOCIOUS AND LATE PREGNANCY

The youngest mother whose history is authenticated is Lina Medina, who was delivered by cesarean section in Lima, Peru, on May 15, 1939. It was claimed that she was four years and eight months old, but a careful review of her birth records indicates that she may have been five years and eight months of age. In either event, it is a record.

Although true precocious puberty, as suffered by Lina Medina, is still very uncommon, the average age of menarche and ovulation is appreciably lower than it was several decades ago (see Chap. 4, p. 88). The mean age of menarche in the United States is now estimated to be 12.3 years.

As a consequence of earlier menarche, and perhaps of greater sexual freedom, most obstetric services have witnessed a marked increase in the number of extremely young pregnant women (Duenhoelter and co-workers, 1975).

Although it was predicted by some that long-term suppression of ovulation by oral contraceptives might result in continued ovulation for years after the usual time of menopause, there is no evidence to support the occurrence of such a phenomenon. Pregnancy after the age of 47 years is uncommon. In a careful review of the literature from 1860 to 1964 on this subject, Wharton (1964) cited 26 women over the age of 50 with normal pregnancy; the oldest was said to be 63. The paucity of reports of pregnancy in women of advanced age is probably an underestimate of the prevalence, but it nevertheless indicates the rarity of pregnancy in the sixth decade of life.

Horger and Smythe (1977) have reviewed the pregnancy experiences of 440 women whose ages ranged from 40 to 54 years. Pregnancy terminated in abortion in 22 percent, one-half of which were electively induced.

The perinatal mortality rate was 101 per 1000 (10.1 percent) and neonatal morbidity, including low birth weight, was increased. Hypertensive disorders were common. Abruptio placentae complicated 16 pregnancies (4.6 percent) and in five instances the infants were stillborn. Postpartum, one woman died from carcinoma of the pancreas.

REFERENCES

Aboul-Khair SA, Crooks J, Turnbull AC, Hytten FE: The physiological changes in thyroid function during pregnancy. Clin Sci 27:195, 1964

Adams RH, Ashworth CT: unpublished

Alvarez H, Caldeyro-Barcia R: Contractility of the human uterus recorded by new methods. Surg Gynecol Obstet 91:1, 1950

Amino N, Tanizawa O, Miyai K, Tanaka F, Hayashi C, Kawashima M, Ichihara K: Changes in serum immunoglobulins IgG, IgA, IgM, and IgE during pregnancy. Obstet Gynecol 52:415, 1978

Assali NS, Dilts PV, Plentl AA, Kirschbaum TH, Gross SJ: Physiology of the placenta. In Assali NS (ed): Biology of Gestation: The Maternal Organism, Vol I. New York, Academic, 1968

Assali NS, Douglass RA, Baird WW, Nicholson DB, Suyemoto R: Measurement of uterine blood flow and uterine metabolism: IV. Results in normal pregnancy. Am J Obstet Gynecol 66:248, 1953

Assali NS, Rauramo L, Peltonen T: Measurement of uterine blood flow and uterine metabolism: VIII. Uterine and fetal blood flow and oxygen consumption in early human pregnancy. Am J Obstet Gynecol 79:86, 1960

Åstedt B: Significance of placenta in depression of fibrinolytic activity during pregnancy. J Obstet Gynaecol Br Commonw 79:205, 1972

Bailey RR, Rolleston GL: Kidney length and ureteric dilatation in the puerperium. J Obstet Gynaecol Br Commonw 78:55, 1971

Baldwin GR, Moorthi DS, MacDonnell KF: New lung functions and pregnancy. Am J Obstet Gynecol 127:235, 1977

Bean WB, Cogswell R, Dexter M, Embick JF: Vascular changes of the skin in pregnancy-vascular spiders and palmar erythema. Surg Gynecol Obstet 88:739, 1949

Beck P: Effects of gonadal hormones and contraceptive steroids on glucose and insulin metabolism. In Salhanick HA, Kipnis DM, Vande Wiele RL (eds): Metabolic Effects of Gonadal Hormones and Contraceptive Steroids. New York, Plenum, 1969

Beck P, Wells C: Comparison of mechanisms underlying carbohydrate intolerance in subclinical diabetic women during pregnancy and during postpartum oral contraceptive steroid treatment. J Clin Endocrinol 29:807, 1969

Bellina JH, Dougherty CM, Mickal A: Pyeloureteral dilation and pregnancy. Am J Obstet Gynecol 108:356, 1970

Bieniarz J, Branda LA, Maqueda E, Morozovsky J, Caldeyro-Barcia R: Aortacaval compression by the uterus in late pregnancy: III. Unreliability of the sphygmomanometric method in estimating uterine artery pressure. Am J Obstet Gynecol 102:1106, 1968

Bille-Brahe NE, Rørth M: Red cell 2, 3-diphosphoglycerate in pregnancy. Acta Obstet Gynecol Scand 58:19, 1979

Blechner JN, Stenger VG, Prystowsky H: Blood flow to the human uterus during maternal metabolic acidosis. Amer J Obstet Gynecol 121:789, 1975

Bleicher SJ, O'Sullivan JB, Freinkel N: Carbohydrate metabolism in pregnancy: V. The interrelations of glucose, insulin, and free fatty acids in late pregnancy and post-partum. New Engl J Med 271:866, 1964

Bonnar J: Hemostatic function and coagulopathy during pregnancy. In Wynn R (ed): Obstetrics and Gynecology Annual: 1978. New York, Appleton, p 195

Brown RD, Strott CA, Liddle GW: Plasma deoxycorticosterone in normal and abnormal human pregnancy. J Clin Endocrinol Metab 35:736, 1972

Browne JCM, Veall N: The maternal placental blood flow in normotensive and hypertensive women. J Obstet Gynaecol Br Emp 60:142, 1953

Burt CC: Forearm and hand blood flow in pregnancy. In Toxaemias of Pregnancy. Ciba Foundation Symposium. Philadelphia, Blakiston, 1950, p 151

Burt RL, Davidson IWF: Insulin half-life and utilization in normal pregnancy. Obstet Gynecol 43:161, 1974

Carsten ME: Regulation of myometrial composition, growth, and activity. In Assali NE (ed): Biology of Gestation: The Maternal Organism, Vol. I. New York, Academic 1968

Caton WL, Roby CC, Reid DE, Gibson JG: Plasma volume and extravascular fluid volume during pregnancy and the puerperium. Am J Obstet Gynecol 57:471, 1949

Chesley LC: Weight changes and water balance in normal and toxic pregnancy. Am J Obstet Gynecol 48:565, 1944

Chesley LC: Renal function during pregnancy. In Carey HM (ed): Modern Trends in Human Reproductive Physiology. London, Butterworth, 1963

Chesley LC, Sloan DM: The effect of posture on renal function in late pregnancy. Am J Obstet Gynecol 89:754, 1964

Chrétien FC: Ultrastructure and variations of human cervical mucus during pregnancy and the menopause. Acta Obstet Gynecol Scand 57:337, 1978

Combes B, Adams RH: Pathophysiology of the liver in pregnancy. In Assali NS (ed): Pathophysiology of Gestation, Vol I. New York, Academic, 1971

Combes B, Shibata H, Adams R, Mitchell BD, Trammell V: Alterations in sulfobromophthalein sodium-removal mechanisms from blood during normal pregnancy. J Clin Invest 42:1431, 1963

Coopland, A, Alkjaersig N, Fletcher AP: Reduction in plasma factor XIII (fibrin stabilization factor) concentration during pregnancy. J Lab Clin Med 73:144, 1969

Crisp WE, DeFrancesco S: The hand syndrome of pregnancy. Obstet Gynecol 23:433, 1964

Cutforth R, MacDonald CB: Heart sounds and murmurs in pregnancy. Am Heart J 71:741, 1966

Dahlström H, Ihrman K: A clinical and physiological study of pregnancy in a material from Northern Sweden. IV. Observations on the blood volume during and after pregnancy. Acta Soc Med Upsal 65:295, 1960

Danforth DN, Buckingham JC: Connective tissue mechanisms and their relation to pregnancy. Obstet Gynecol Survey 19:715, 1964

Davison JM, Hytten FE: Glomerular filtration during and after pregnancy. J Obstet Gynaecol Brit Commonw, 81:588, 1974

Davison JM, Hytten FE: The effect of pregnancy on the renal handling of glucose. Brit J Obstet Gynaecol 82:374, 1975

Dennis KJ, Bytheway WR: Changes in the body weight after delivery. J Obstet Gynaecol Br Commonw 72:94, 1965

Diczfalusy E, Troen P: Endocrine functions of the human placenta. Vitam Horm 19:229, 1961

Duenhoelter JH, Jimenez JM, Baumann G: Pregnancy performance of patients under fifteen years of age. Obstet Gynecol 46:49, 1975

Dunlop W: Investigations into influence of posture on renal plasma flow and glomerular filtration rate during late pregnancy. Br J Obstet Gynaecol 83:17, 1976

Edman CD, MacDonald PC, Gant NF: Placental clearance of maternal plasma androstenedione through estradiol formation. Proceedings of the Society for Gynecologic Investigation, p. 67, 1979 (abstract)

Efrati P, Presentey B, Margalith M, Rozenszajn L: Leukocytes of normal pregnant women. Obstet Gynecol 23:429, 1964

Fainstat T: Ureteral dilation in pregnancy: a review. Obstet Gynecol Survey 18:845, 1963

Fletcher AP, Alkjaersig N: Thromboembolism and contraceptive medications: incidence and mechanism. In Salhanick HA, Kipnis DM, Vande Wiele RL (eds): Metabolic Effects of Gonadal Hormones and Contraceptive Steroids. New York, Plenum, 1969

Friesen H, Hwang P, Guyda H, Tolis G, Tyson J, Myers R: A radioimmunoassy for human prolactin. In Prolactin and Carcinogenesis, Proceedings of the Fourth Tenovus Workshop Cardiff, March 1972. Cardiff, Wales, Alpha Omega Alpha, August 1972

Fulop M, Brazeau P: Increased ureteral back pressure enhances renal tubular sodium reabsorption. J Clin Invest 49:2315, 1970

Garcia-Bunuel R, Berek JS, Woodruff JD: Luteomas of pregnancy. Obstet Gynecol 45:407, 1975

Gee JBL, Packer BS, Millen JE, Robin ED: Pulmonary mechanics during pregnancy. J Clin Invest 46:945, 1967

Geelhoed GW, Vander AJ: Plasma renin activities during pregnancy and parturition. J Clin Endocrinol 28:412, 1968

Hahn PF, Carothers EL, Darby WJ, Martin M, Sheppard CW, Cannon RO, Beam AS, Densen PM, Peterson JC, McClellan GS: Iron metabolism in human pregnancy as studied with the radioactive istope Fe^{59}. Am J Obstet Gynecol 61:477, 1951

Hamolsky MW, Stein M, Freedberg AS: The thyroid hormone-plasma protein complex in man: II. A new in vitro method for study of "uptake" of labelled hormonal components by human erythrocytes. J Clin Endocrinol 17:33, 1957

Harbert GM, Cornell GW, Littlefield JB, Kayan JB, Thornton WN: Maternal hemodynamics associated with uterine contraction in gravid monkeys. Am J Obstet Gynecol 104:24, 1969

Hellman LM, Rosenthal AH, Kistner RW, Gordon R: Some factors influencing the proliferation of the reserve cells in the human cervix. Am J Obstet Gynecol 67:899, 1954

Hendricks CH, Barnes AC: Effect of supine position on urinary output in pregnancy. Am J Obstet Gynecol 69:1225, 1955

Hensleigh PA, Woodruff JD: Differential maternal-fetal response to androgenizing luteoma or hyperreactio luteinalis. Obstet Gynecol 33:262, 1978

Hershman JM, Starnes WR: Extraction and characterization of a thyrotropic material from the human placenta. J Clin Invest 48:923, 1969

Hillyard CJ, Stevenson JC, MacIntyre I: Relative deficiency of plasma-calcitonin in normal women. Lancet 2:961, 1978

Hodgkinson CP: Physiology of the ovarian veins in pregnancy. Obstet Gynecol 1:26, 1953

Horger EO III, Smythe AR II: Pregnancy in women over forty. Obstet Gynecol 49:257, 1977

Howard BK, Goodson JH, Mengert WF: Supine hypotensive syndrome in late pregnancy. Obstet Gynecol 1:371, 1953

Hutchinson DL, Westoner JL, Well DW: The destruction of the maternal and fetal pituitary glands in subhuman primates. Am J Obstet Gynecol 83:857, 1962

Hytten FE, Leitch I: The Physiology of Human Pregnancy, 2nd ed. Philadelphia, Davis, 1971

Hytten FE, Thomson AM: Maternal physiological adjustments. In Assali NS (ed): Biology of Gestation: The Maternal Organism, Vol I. New York, Academic 1968

Ihrman K: A clinical and physiological study of pregnancy in a material from northern Sweden. VII. The heart volume during and after pregnancy. Acta Soc Med Upsal 65:326, 1960

Ingerslev M, Teilum G: Biopsy studies on the liver in pregnancy: II. Liver biopsy on normal pregnant women. Acta Obstet Gynecol Scand 25:352, 1946

Jepson JH, Friesen HG: The mechanism of action of human placental lactogen on erythropoiesis. Br J Haematol 15:465, 1968

Kaplan NM: Successful pregnancy following hypophysectomy during the twelfth week of gestation. J Clin Endocrinol 21:1139, 1961

Kasper CK, Hoag MS, Aggelar PM, Stone S:

Blood clotting factors in pregnancy: Factor VIII concentrations in normal and AHF-deficient women. Obstet Gynecol 24:242, 1964

Katz R, Karliner JS, Resnik R: Effects of a natural volume overload state (pregnancy) on left ventricular performance in normal human subjects. Circulation 58:434, 1978

Kauppila A, Koskinen, Puolakka J, Tuimala R, Kuikka J: Decreased intervillous and unchanged myometrial blood flow in supine recumbency. Obstet Gynecol 55:203, 1980

Kerr MG: The mechanical effects of the gravid uterus in late pregnancy. J Obstet Gynaecol Br Commonw 72:513, 1965

Kim YJ, Felig P: Maternal and amniotic fluid substrate levels during caloric deprivation in human pregnancy. Metabolism 21:507, 1972

Klafen, Palugyay: Arch Gynaekol 131:347, 1927

Krause DE, Stembridge VA: Luteomas of pregnancy. Am J Obstet Gynecol 95:192, 1966

Künzel W, Kastendieck E, Böhme U, Feige A: Uterine hemodynamics and fetal response to vena caval occlusion in sheep. J Perinat Med 3:260, 1975

Laidlaw JC, Ruse JL, Gornall AG: The influence of estrogen and progesterone on aldosterone excretion. J Clin Endocrinol 22:161, 1962

Landau RL, Lugibihl K: The catabolic and natriuretic effects of progesterone in man. Recent Prog Horm Res 17:249, 1961

Lees MM, Scott DB, Slawson KB, Kerr MG: Haemodynamic changes during caesarean section. J Obstet Gynaecol Br Commonw 75:546, 1968

Liggins GC: Ripening of the cervix. In Oliver TK Jr, Kirschbaum TH (eds): Seminars in Perinatology, Vol. II, No. 3, 1978, p 261

Lund CJ, Fullerton RE, Tristan TA: Cinefluorographic studies of the bladder and urethra in women: II. Stress incontinence. Am J Obstet Gynecol 78:706, 1959

McLennan CE: Antecubital and femoral venous pressure in normal and toxemic pregnancy. Am J Obstet Gynecol 45:568, 1943

McLennan CE, Lowenstein JM, Sayler CB, Richards EM: Blood volume changes immediately after delivery. Stanford Med Bull 17:152, 1959

McLennan MT, McLennan CE: Failure of vaginal wall cytologic smears to predict abortion. Am J Obstet Gynecol 103:228, 1969

Manasc B, Jepson J: Erythropoietin in plasma and urine during human pregnancy. Can Med Assoc J 100:687, 1969

Margulis RR, Luzardre JH, Hodgkinson CP: Fibrinoylsis in labor and delivery. Obstet Gynecol 3:487, 1954

Massani ZM, Sanguinetti R, Gallegos R, Raimondi D: Angiotensin blood levels in normal and toxemic pregnancies. Am J Obstet Gynecol 99:313, 1967

Meisels A: Hormonal cytology in pregnancy. Clin Obstet Gynecol 11:1121, 1968

Mendenhall HW: Serum protein concentrations in pregnancy: I. Concentrations in maternal serum. Am J Obstet Gynecol 106:388, 1970

Metcalfe J, Romney SL, Ramsey LH, Reid DE, Burwell CS: Estimation of uterine blood flow in normal human pregnancy at term. J Clin Invest 34:1632, 1955

Migeon CJ, Bertrand J, Wall PE: Physiological disposition of 4-C[14] cortisol during late pregnancy. J Clin Invest 36:1350, 1957

Milne JS, Howie AD, Pack AI: Dyspnoea during normal pregnancy. Brit J Obstet Gynaecol 85:260, 1978

Möbius Wvon: Atmung und Schwangerschaft. Munch Med Wochenschr 103:1389, 1961

Mueller MN, Kappas A: Estrogen pharmacology: I. The influence of estradiol and estriol on hepatic disposal of sulfobromophthalein (BSP) in man. J Clin Invest 43:1905, 1964

Mulaisho C, Utiger, RD: Serum thyroxine-binding globulin: Determination by competitive ligand-binding assay in thyroid disease and pregnancy. Acta Endocrinol 85:314, 1977

Newton M: Postpartum hemorrhage. Am J Obstet Gynecol 94:711, 1966

Nolten WE, Lindheimer MD, Oparil S, Ehrlich EN: Desoxycorticosterone in pregnancy I. Sequential studies of the secretory patterns of desoxycorticosterone, aldersterone and cortisol. Am J Obstet Gynecol 132:414, 1978

Osathanondh R, Tulchinsky D, Chopra IJ: Total and free thyroxine and triiodothyronine in normal and complicated pregnancy. J Clin Endocrinol Metab 42:98, 1976

Page EW, Glendening MB, Dignam W, Harper HA: The causes of histidinuria in normal pregnancy. Am J Obstet Gynecol 68:110, 1954

Pitkin RM, Gebhardt MP: Serum calcium concentrations in human pregnancy. Am J Obstet Gynecol 127:775, 1977

Pitkin RM, Witte DL: Platelet and leukocyte counts in pregnancy. JAMA. In press, 1980

Potter JM, Nestel PJ: The hyperlipidemia of pregnancy in normal and complicated pregnancies. Am J Obstet Gynecol 133:165, 1979

Potter MG: Observations of the gallbladder and bile during pregnancy at term. JAMA 106:1070, 1936

Pritchard JA: Plasma cholinesterase activity in normal pregnancy and in eclamptogenic toxemias. Am J Obstet Gynecol 70:1083, 1955

Pritchard JA: Changes in the blood volume during pregnancy and delivery. Anesthesiology 26:393, 1965

Pritchard JA: Personal observations.

Pritchard JA, Adams RH: Erythrocyte production and destruction during pregnancy. Am J Obstet Gynecol 79:750, 1960

Pritchard JA, Hunt CF: A comparison of the hematologic responses following the routine prenatal administration of intramuscular and oral iron. Surg Gynecol Obstet 106:516, 1958

Pritchard JA, Mason RA: Iron stores of normal adults and their replenishment with oral iron therapy. JAMA 190:897, 1964

Pritchard JA, Scott DE: Iron demands during pregnancy. In Iron Deficiency-Pathogenesis: Clinical Aspects and Therapy. London, Academic, 1970, p 173

Pritchard JA, Barnes AC, Bright RH: The effect of the supine position on renal function in the near-term pregnant woman. J Clin Invest 34:777, 1955

Ratnoff OD, Colopy JE, Pritchard JA: The blood-clotting mechanism during normal parturition. J Lab Clin Med 44:408: 1954

Reitz RE, Thomas AD, Woods JR, Weinstein RL: Calcium, magnesium, phosphorus, and parathyroid hormone interrelationships in pregnancy and newborn infants. Obstet Gynecol 50:701, 1977

Rekonen A, Luotola H, Pitkänen M, Kuikka J, Pyörälä M: Measurement of intervillous and myometrial blood flow by an intravenous ^{133}Xe method. Brit J Obstet Gynaecol 83:723, 1976

Riggs LA, Lein A, Yen SSC: Pattern of increase in circulating prolactin levels during human gestation. Am J Obstet Gynecol 129:454, 1977

Rubi RA, Sala NL: Ureteral function in pregnant women: III. Effect of different positions and of fetal delivery upon ureteral tonus. Am J Obstet Gynecol 101:230, 1968

Russ EM, Raymunt J: Influence of estrogens on total serum copper and caeruloplasmin. Proc Soc Exp Biol Med 92:465, 1956

Russell DH, Durie BGM: Polyamines as Biochemical Markers of Normal and Malignant Growth. In Progress in Cancer Research and Therapy, Vol. 8. New York, Raven Press, 1978

Russell DH, Giles HR, Christian CD, Campbell JL: Polyamines in amniotic fluid, plasma, and urine during normal pregnancy. Am J Obstet Gynecol 132:649, 1978

Russell KP, Rose H, Starr P: Further observations on thyroxine interactions in the newborn at delivery and in the immediate neonatal period. Am J Obstet Gynecol 90:682, 1964

Salvatore CA: Cervical mucus crystallization in pregnancy. Obstet Gynecol 32:226, 1968

Sandiford I, Wheeler T: Basal metabolism before, during, and after pregnancy. J Biol Chem 62:329, 1924

Schulman A, Herlinger H: Urinary tract dilatation in pregnancy. Brit J Radiol 48:638, 1975

Schwabe C, Steinetz B, Weiss G, Segaloff A, McDonald JK, Byrne EO, Hochman G, Carriere B, Goldsmith L: Relaxin in Recent Prog Horm Res., Roy O Greep, (ed.), New York, Academic, p. 123, 1978

Scott DE, Pritchard JA: Iron deficiency in healthy young college women. JAMA 199:897, 1967

Sims EAH: The kidney in pregnancy. In Strauss MB, Welt LG (eds): Diseases of the Kidney. Boston, Little, Brown, 1963

Sjöstedt S: Acid-base balance of arterial blood during pregnancy, at delivery, and in the puerperium. Am J Obstet Gynecol 84:775, 1962

Song CS, Kappas A: The influence of estrogens, progestins and pregnancy on the liver. Vitam Horm 26:147, 1968

Spellacy WN, Buhi WC: Pituitary growth hormone and placental lactogen levels measured in normal term pregnancy and at the early and late postpartum periods. Am J Obstet Gynecol 105:888, 1969

Spellacy WN, Goetz FC: Plasma insulin in normal late pregnancy. New Engl J Med 268:988, 1963

Spellacy WN, Goetz FC, Greenberg BZ, Schoeller KL: Tolbutamide response in normal pregnancy. J Clin Endocrinol 25:1251, 1965

Spetz S: Peripheral circulation during normal pregnancy. Acta Obstet Gynecol Scand 43:309, 1964

Sternberg WH: Non-functioning ovarian neoplasms. In Grady HG, Smith DE (eds): International Academy of Pathology Monograph, No. 3, The Ovary. Baltimore, Williams & Wilkins, 1963

Stevenson JC, Hillyard CJ, MacIntyre I, Cooper H, Whitehead MI: A physiological role for calcitonin: Protection of the maternal skeleton. Lancet 2:769, 1979

Sturgeon P: Studies of iron requirements in infants: III. Influence of supplemental iron during normal pregnancy on mother and infant. A. The mother. Br J Haematol 5:31, 1959

Talbert LM, Langdell RD: Normal values of certain factors in the blood clotting mechanism in pregnancy. Am J Obstet Gynecol 90:44, 1964

Taylor GO, Modie JA, Agbedana EO: Serum free fatty acids, insulin and blood glucose in pregnancy. Brit J Obstet Gynaecol 85:592, 1978

Tyson JE, Austin K, Farinholt J, Fiedler J: Endocrine-metabolic response to acute starvation in human gastation. Am J Obstet Gynecol 125:1073, 1976

Ueland K: Maternal cardiovascular dynamics. VII. Intrapartum blood volume changes. Am J Obstet Gynecol 126:671, 1976

Ueland K. Hansen JM: Maternal cardiovascular dynamics: II. Posture and uterine contractions. Am J Obstet Gynecol 103:1, 1969

Ueland K, Metcalfe J: Circulatory changes in pregnancy. Clin Obstet Gynecol 18:41, 1975.

Ulmsten U, Sundström G: Esophageal manometry in pregnant and nonpregnant women. Am J Obstet Gynecol 132:260, 1978

Van Wagenen G. Jenkins RH: An experimental examination of factors causing ureteral dilatation of pregnancy. J Urol 42:1010, 1939

Verkauf BS, Reiter EO, Hernandez L, Burns SA: Virilization of mother and fetus associated with luteoma of pregnancy: A case report with endocrinologic studies. Am J Obstet Gynecol 129:274, 1977

Watanabe M, Meeker CI, Gray MJ, Sims EAH, Solomon S: Secretion rate of aldosterone in normal pregnancy. J Clin Invest 42:1619, 1963

Whalley PJ, MacDonald PC, Pritchard JA: Unpublished observations

Whalley PJ, Roberts AD, Pritchard JA: The effects of posture on renal function during pregnancy in a patient with diabetes insipidus. J Lab Clin Med 58:867, 1961

Wharton LR: Normal pregnancy with living children in women past the age of fifty. Am J Obstet Gynecol 90:672, 1964

Widdowson EM: Growth and composition of the fetus and newborn. In Assali NS (ed): Biology of Gestation: The Fetus and Neonate, Vol II. New York, Academic, 1968

Widdowson EM, Spray CM: Chemical development in utero. Arch Dis Child 26:205, 1951

Wilcox CF, Hunt AB, Owen CA: The measurement of blood lost during cesarean section. Am J Obstet Gynecol 77:772, 1959

Winkel, CA, Milewich L, Gant NF, MacDonald PC: The conversion of circulating progesterone to desoxycorticosterone (DOC). Proceedings of the Society of Gynecologic Investigation, 1979, p 140

Winters AJ, Colston C, MacDonald PC, Porter JC: Fetal plasma prolactin levels. J Clin Endocr Metab 41:626, 1975

Wintrobe MM: Clinical Hematology. Philadelphia, Lea & Febiger, 1961

Woodfield DG, Cole SK, Allan AGE, Cash JD: Serum fibrin degradation products throughout normal pregnancy. Br Med J 4:665, 1968

Wright HP, Osborn SB, Edmonds DG: Changes in rate of flow of venous blood in the leg during pregnancy, measured with radioactive sodium. Surg Gynecol Obstet 90:481, 1950

Yoshima T, Strott CA, Marshall JR, Lipsett MD: Corpus luteum function early in pregnancy. J Clin Endocrinol Metab 29:225, 1969

10

Diagnosis of Pregnancy

Every physician who assumes the responsibility for the medical care of any woman under the age of 50, irrespective of the physician's type of practice or special interest, must always raise the question, "Is she pregnant?" Failure to do so often leads to incorrect diagnoses, inappropriate therapy, and, at times, to medicolegal embroilment. Ordinarily, the diagnosis of pregnancy should offer little difficulty. Most often the woman is aware of the likelihood of pregnancy when she consults a physician, although she may not volunteer this information unless asked specifically. However, at times, the diagnosis of pregnancy is not easy, but rarely is it impossible if appropriate clinical and laboratory aids are employed.

Mistakes in diagnosis are made most frequently in the first several weeks of pregnancy while the uterus is still a pelvic organ. Although it is possible to mistake the pregnant uterus, even at term, for a tumor of some nature, usually such errors are the result of hasty or careless examination.

The diagnosis of pregnancy is based upon certain symptoms and signs found on careful physical examination and upon results of laboratory tests. The signs and symptoms of pregnancy are classified into three groups: positive signs, probable signs, and presumptive evidence.

POSITIVE SIGNS OF PREGNANCY

The three positive signs of pregnancy are (1) identification of the fetal heart action separately and distinctly from that of the mother's, (2) perception of active fetal movements by the examiner, and (3) recognition of the fetus radiologically or the embryo and fetus sonographically.

1. Identification of Fetal Heart Action. Hearing or observing the pulsations of the fetal heart assures the diagnosis of pregnancy. Contractions of the fetal heart can be identified by auscultation employing a special fetoscope (Fig. 17-2.A, p. 412), by use of the Doppler principle with ultrasound and by use of sonography (Chap. 14, p. 345). The heart beat of the fetus can be detected by auscultation with a stethoscope by 17 weeks gestation on the average and by 19 weeks in nearly all pregnancies (Jimenez et al., 1979). Normally, the fetal heart rate ranges from 120 to 160 beats a minute and is heard as a double sound resembling the tick of a watch under a pillow. It is not sufficient for establishing the diagnosis of pregnancy merely to "hear" the fetal heart; it must be proved to be distinctly different from the maternal pulse. During much of pregnancy the fetus moves freely in the amnionic fluid and consequently the site on the maternal abdomen where the fetal heart sounds can be heard best will vary with the position of the fetus.

Several instruments are available that make use of the *Doppler principle* to detect the action of the fetal heart. Employing these instruments, ultrasound is directed toward the moving blood. The sound reflected by the moving blood undergoes a shift in frequency, the echo of which is detected by a receiving crystal immediately adjacent to the transmitting crystal. Because of the difference in heart rates, pulsatile flow in the fetus is differentiated easily from that of the mother unless there is severe fetal bradycardia or maternal tachycardia. Fetal cardiac action can be detected with appropriate equipment that employs the Doppler principle almost always by the tenth to twelfth week of gestation.

Echocardiography can be used to detect fetal heart action as early as 48 days after the beginning of the last menses (Robinson, 1972).

Real time sonography can be employed to detect fetal heart action and fetal movement after the second month of pregnancy.

Upon auscultation of the abdomen in the later months of pregnancy, the examiner often may hear sounds other than those produced by fetal heart action, the most important of which are (1) the funic (umbilical cord) souffle, (2) the uterine souffle, (3) sounds resulting from movement of the fetus, (4) the maternal pulse, and (5) the gurgling of gas in the intestines of the mother.

The funic, or umbilical cord, souffle is caused by the rush of blood through the umbilical arteries. It is a sharp, whistling sound that is synchronous with the fetal pulse and can be heard in perhaps 15 percent of pregnancies. It is inconstant, sometimes being recognizable distinctly at one examination but not found in the same woman on other occasions.

The uterine souffle is heard as a soft, blowing sound, which is synchronous with the maternal pulse, and usually is heard most distinctly during auscultation of the lower portion of the uterus. This sound is produced by the passage of blood through the dilated uterine vessels and is characteristic not only of pregnancy but of any condition in which the blood flow to the uterus is increased greatly. Accordingly, a uterine souffle may be heard in nonpregnant women with large uterine myomas or large tumors of the ovaries.

Frequently the maternal pulse can be heard distinctly by auscultation of the abdomen, and in some women the pulsation of the aorta is unusually loud. Occasionally during examination, the pulse of the mother may become so rapid as to simulate the fetal heart sounds. In addition to the sounds described, it is not unusual to hear certain other sounds that are produced by the passage of gases or liquids through the pregnant woman's intestines.

2. Perception of Active Fetal Movements.

The second positive sign of pregnancy is the detection, by the physician, of movements by the fetus. After about 20 weeks gestation, active fetal movements can be felt at intervals by placing the examining hand on the mother's abdomen. These movements vary in intensity from a faint flutter early in pregnancy to brisk motions at a later period; the latter are sometimes visible as well as palpable. Occassionally, somewhat similar sensations may be produced by contractions of the intestines or the muscles of the abdominal wall of the pregnant woman, although these should not deceive an experienced examiner.

3. Recognition of the Fetus Radiologically.

Whenever the fetal skeleton can be distinguished radiologically, the diagnosis of pregnancy is certain. This third method of positive diagnosis is usually not valid until after 16 weeks of gestation. By x-ray examination, Bartholomew and co-workers (1921) were able to make a positive diagnosis of pregnancy by 20 weeks gestation in one-third of their women who were pregnant, in one-half by 24 weeks, and in almost all after this stage of gestation. Just how early the fetal skeleton is visible in the roentgenogram depends, in part, upon the thickness of the abdominal wall of the mother and the radiologic

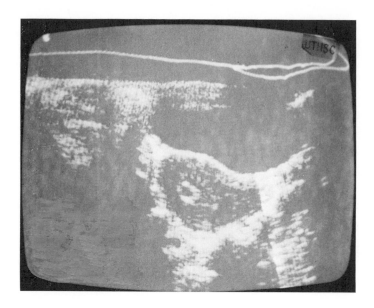

FIG. 10-1. Longitudinal sonogram in which a gestation sac at five to six weeks menstrual age is demonstrated. (Courtesy of Dr. R. Santos)

technic employed. Foci of ossification in the fetus have been demonstrated as early as 14 weeks although ordinarily the gestation must have reached 16 weeks or more before the fetal skeleton can be visualized. Roentgenography may be of value in differentiating the pregnant uterus from other abdominal tumors, especially when the fetus is more mature but dead.

4. Sonographic Examination. A normal intrauterine pregnancy may be demonstrable by pulse-echo sonography after only 5 weeks of amenorrhea (Fig. 10-1). After six weeks of amenorrhea, the small white gestational ring is so characteristic that failure to identify such raises doubts about pregnancy. Thus, there may be sonographic confirmation of pregnancy by the time that some of the common tests for human chorionic gonadotropin (hCG) in urine become positive. By careful scanning, distinct echoes from the embryo can be demonstrated within the gestational ring by eight weeks after commencement of the last menstrual period. Moreover, from the length of the embryo, the gesta-

tional age can be estimated quite accurately (Fig. 10-2).

In addition to the early identification of normal pregnancy, the findings of sonography may also allow the identification of those gestations in which there is a blighted ovum, i.e., the embryo is dead and abortion will occur ultimately. The characteristic features of a blighted ovum are (1) loss of definition of the gestational sac, (2) an unusually small gestational sac, and (3) the absence of echoes emanating from the fetus after eight weeks gestation (Fig. 24-3, p. 596).

By 11 weeks of amenorrhea, normally the pregnancy ring is no longer distinctly identifiable in the uterine cavity by sonography. By this time, however, fetal heart action usually can be detected with equipment that utilizes the Doppler effect or by real time sonography. By the 14th week, the fetal head and thorax can be identified and soon thereafter the placental site can be visualized by ultrasound technics.

During the latter half of pregnancy, ultrasonography can be employed to identify successfully the number of fetuses, the present-

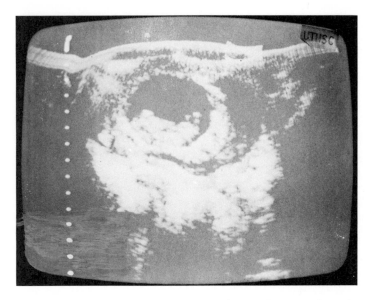

FIG. 10-2. Transverse sonographic view of amnionic sac that contains a fetus of 10 to 11 weeks gestation age of menstrual dates. (Courtesy of Dr. R. Santos)

ing part(s), various fetal anomalies, hydramnios, and to assess the rate of fetal growth by measuring serially the biparietal diameter of the fetal head, and, when indicated, the circumference of the fetal abdomen.

The findings of sonography often provide as much, and usually much more, information as do those of radiography without the potential, albeit undefined, risks of irradiation. To date no adverse effects on the human embryo and fetus have been identified from exposure to energies comparable to those employed for clinical sonographic examinations.

PROBABLE EVIDENCE OF PREGNANCY

These signs include (1) enlargement of the abdomen; (2) changes in the shape, size, and consistency of the uterus; (3) changes in the cervix; (4) Braxton Hicks' contractions; (5) ballottement; (6) outlining the fetus; and (7) results of endocrine tests.

1. Enlargement of the Abdomen. By 12 weeks of gestation, usually the uterus can be felt through the abdominal wall just above the symphysis as a tumor that thereafter increases gradually in size up to the end of pregnancy. In general, any enlargement of the abdomen during the childbearing period is strongly suggestive of pregnancy.

The abdominal enlargement usually is less pronounced in nulliparous than in multiparous women whose abdominal musculature has lost some of its tone; indeed in some multiparous women the abdominal wall is so flaccid that the uterus sags forward and downward, producing a pendulous abdomen. This difference in abdominal tone between first and subsequent pregnancies is so obvious that it is not rare for women in the latter part of a second pregnancy to suspect a twin pregnancy because of the increased size of their abdomen, as compared with that in the corresponding month of their previous pregnancy. The abdomen of the pregnant woman also undergoes significant changes in shape depending on her body position. The uterus is, of course, much less prominent when the woman is in the supine position.

2. Changes in Size, Shape, and Consistency of the Uterus. During the first few weeks of pregnancy, the increase in size of the uterus is limited principally to the anteroposterior diameter, but at a little later period, the body of the uterus becomes almost globular, attaining an average diameter of 8 cm by 12 weeks. On bimanual examination, the pregnant uterine body feels doughy or elastic and sometimes becomes exceedingly soft.

At about 6–8 weeks after the onset of the last period, Hegar's sign becomes manifest. With one hand on the abdomen and two fingers of the other hand in the vagina, the still firm cervix is felt, with the elastic body of the uterus above the compressible soft isthmus, which lies between the two. Occasionally the softening at the isthmus is so marked that the cervix and the body of the uterus seem to be separate. The inexperienced examiner may mistake the cervix for a small uterus, and the softened body of the fundus for a tumor of the ovaries or oviducts. Hegar's sign is not, however, positively diagnostic of pregnancy, since occasionally it may be present when the walls of the nonpregnant uterus are excessively soft.

3. Changes in the Cervix. At 6 to 8 weeks gestation, the cervix often becomes considerably softened. In primigravidas, the consistency of the cervix surrounding the external os is more similar to that of the lips of the mouth than to that of the nasal cartilage, as at other times. Other conditions, however, may bring about softening of the cervix. Estrogen-progestin contraceptives, for example, commonly cause some softening and congestion of the uterine cervix.

As pregnancy advances, the cervical canal may become sufficiently patulous as to admit the tip of the examining finger. In certain inflammatory conditions, as well as in carcinoma, the cervix may remain firm during pregnancy, yielding only with the onset of labor, if at all.

4. Braxton Hicks' Contraction. The uterus during pregnancy undergoes palpable but ordinarily painless contractions at irregular intervals from early stages of gestation. These may be enhanced by massaging the uterus. These Braxton Hicks' contractions, however, are not positive signs of pregnancy, since similar contractions sometimes are observed in uteri of women with hematometra and occasionally in uteri containing soft myomas, especially those of the pedunculated submucous variety. The presence of Braxton Hicks' contractions, however, may be of aid in excluding the existence of an ectopic abdominal pregnancy.

5. Ballottement. Near midpregnancy, the volume of the fetus is small compared to that of the amnionic fluid, and consequently sudden pressure exerted on the uterus may cause the fetus to sink in the amnionic fluid, then rebound to its original position and the tap is felt by the examining finger.

6. Outlining the Fetus. In the second half of pregnancy, the outlines of the fetal body may be palpated through the maternal abdominal wall, and the outlining of the fetus becomes easier the nearer that term is approached. Occasionally, subserous myomas may simulate the fetal head or small parts, or both, thus causing serious diagnostic errors. A positive diagnosis of pregnancy cannot be made, therefore, on this sign alone.

7. Endocrine Tests. The presence of hCG in maternal plasma and its excretion in urine provides the basis for the endocrine tests for pregnancy. hCG may be identified in body fluids by any one of a variety of immunoassay or bioassay technics. *Hormonal tests that are commonly performed in the physician's office or clinic or in clinical laboratories, do not identify absolutely the presence or absence of pregnancy.* This fact led Hobson (1969) to emphasize that the degree of accuracy attained by some laboratories with commonly used pregnancy tests is not greater than might be achieved by tossing a coin.

One potential problem in most assay procedures arises from the immunologic and biologic similarities between hCG formed by the trophoblast and luteinizing hormone (LH) secreted by the pituitary. In most test systems employing immunoassay procedures, LH cross-reacts with antibody to hCG; moreover, LH may induce a response similar to that of hCG in most methods of bioassay (see Chap. 7, p. 148). If the test employed is so sensitive that it detects very small amounts of hCG, the results may give rise to a positive test for pregnancy, especially in problem cases, because of the cross-reactivity of circulating or excreted LH. At the time of menopause, for example, amenorrhea not infrequently causes considerable fear of a possible pregnancy. At the same time, the levels of pituitary gonadotropins in plasma and urine usually are elevated and may be the cause of a falsely positive pregnancy test. If, however, the sensitivity of the pregnancy test is reduced in order to exclude a falsely positive result from LH, some pregnancies will not be identified because the levels of hCG are too low to be detected. The falsely negative test is most likely to be encountered during the first few days of pregnancy or after the fourth month, although with abnormal pregnancies, such as a tubal pregnancy, hCG may be present only in small amounts and therefore not identified by the less sensitive methods of testing.

The production of hCG begins very early in the course of pregnancy and indeed may even precede the time of nidation. Certainly with a sensitive test, e.g., the radioimmunoassay employing antibodies against the β-subunit of hCG (which is specific for hCG and does not cross-react significantly with LH), the pregnancy hormone can be demonstrated at least one week prior to the time of the anticipated menses in a fertile cycle.

The concentration of hCG in serum rises rapidly as pointed out in Chapter 7 (p. 148), and equivalent amounts are present in urine. A good rule of thumb is that the concentration of hCG contained in 1 liter of maternal plasma is equivalent to that contained in 24 hours of urine. Thus, if the urine excreted per 24 hours were 1 liter, the concentration of hCG in serum and in urine would be simi-

lar. Employing most of the newer immunologic tests for pregnancy using latex fixation, 75 to 100 milli-International Units (mIU) will be detected, while some of the hemagglutination inhibition tests will detect 50 mIU. Since these tests ordinarily make use of one drop of urine, this is equivalent to the concentration 0.5 to 1 International Unit (IU) per ml. If the rate of urine excretion during the time of collection were 1 liter per 24 hours, the detectable concentration would be equivalent to the concentration of 0.5 to 1 IU of hCG per ml of serum. Rarely do concentrations of LH reach this level even in postmenopausal women. Ordinarily, concentrations of LH at the time of the midcycle LH surge reach levels in the order of 40 to 60 mIU per ml of plasma. We have observed that nonspecific substances in urine, or even in tap water, are more likely to give rise to false positive pregnancy tests employing the latex fixation immunoassay procedures than is increased LH excretion either at midcycle or in the postmenopausal woman.

More specific tests for hCG, i.e., those utilizing the antibody to the β-subunit of hCG, are currently under investigation for potential marketing. Theoretically this test would provide greater specificity, since the β-subunit of hCG differs antigenetically from the β-subunit of LH. The antibodies developed to the β-subunit do not cross-react with those of the β-subunit of LH or with the total LH moiety. Thus, greater accuracy, but as yet undefined sensitivity, would be possible.

IMMUNOASSAY. Kerber and associates (1970) compared several of the commerically available immunologic tests for identifying chorionic gonadotropin. They found some methods of testing, at least those which use the technic of hemagglutination inhibition (Pregnosticon tube test or UCG test) to be quite sensitive and therefore very unlikely to yield a falsely negative result. The assay takes about 2 hours to complete. As a general all-purpose rapid pregnancy screening test, Kerber and associates found that one of the latex inhibition slide tests, the Pregnosticon slide test, which takes only a few minutes to perform, offered a number of advantages and a few disadvantages. Today there are four over-the-counter pregnancy tests that can be purchased for approximately $10 each for use at home. Each of the tests employs the principle of hemagglutination inhibition using sheep erythrocytes, antibodies to hCG, and the subject's urine. The experience to date has been that women who employed the test at home experienced a relatively low ($\simeq$ 5 percent) false positive rate, but a high false negative ($\simeq$ 20 percent) result. Physician opinion is divided concerning the wisdom of making pregnancy testing available to nonprofessionals. Some argue that such tests will give results that will prompt women to see physicians earlier. We are of the view that the reverse may be more likely in those complicated situations in which early physician consultation is urgently needed.

The kits commercially available to laboratories that employ failure of agglutination of latex particles to detect hCG in urine contain two reagents. One is a suspension of latex particles coated with hCG and the other contains a solution of hCG antibody. To test for hCG, one drop of urine is mixed with one drop of the antibody-containing solution on a black glass slide. If no hCG is present in the urine, antibody will remain available to agglutinate the hCG-coated latex particles which are added subsequently. Agglutination of the latex particles can be observed easily when a bright light source is employed against the dark background of the glass slide. If hCG were present in the urine, it would bind to the antibody and thus prevent agglutination of the hCG-coated latex particles. Therefore, the pregnancy test is positive if no agglutination occurs; the pregnancy test is negative when agglutination occurs.

Duenhoelter and associates (1979) evaluated five commercially available pregnancy tests: UCG (Wampole Laboratories), Pregnosticon (Organon Diagnostics), Pregnosis (Roche Diagnostics), Gravindex (Ortho Diagnostics), and Gestate (Fisher Scientific). The results obtained were compared to those obtained employing radioimmunoassay utilizing an antibody against the β-subunit of hCG. They found that the sensitivity of some of the tests was greater than that stated by the manufacturer but for others it was less (Table 10-1).

Duenhoelter and associates also conducted a systematic evaluation of the role of proteinuria in the production of falsely positive tests. They found that 28 percent of the results were falsely positive when they employed the more sensitive tests on urine specimens that contained 30 mg/dl or more of protein. They recommended that protein should be measured in every urine to be tested for the presence of hCG. Employing the 5 commercially available tests, they found false negative tests to be 2 to 3 percent with Gravindex and UCG when hCG was known to be present in concentrations of 1 IU/ml.

TABLE 10-1.
SENSITIVITY OF HCG ASSAYS (IU/ML)

| TEST KIT | SENSITIVITY DEMONSTRATED | | SENSITIVITY STATED BY MANUFACTURER |
	If Urine Protein Less Than 30 mg/dl	If Urine Protein 30 mg/dl or Greater	
Pregnosticon	7.7–8.8	4.4–5.8	1–2
UCG	2.2–2.8	0.5–1.7	2
Pregnosis	2.9–4.3	1.5–3.5	1.5–2.5
Gravindex	0.9–2.3	0.4–1.1	3.5
Gestate	6.0–8.8	3.0–7.0	2–4

From Duenhoelter and co-workers: *Dallas Med J* 64:232, 1979.

TABLE 10-2.
BIOLOGIC TESTS FOR PREGNANCY

NAME	TEST ANIMAL	END POINT	TIME OF TEST
Aschheim-Zondek	Mice or rats	Corpus luteum formation	5 days
Friedman	Rabbits	Corpus luteum formation	48 hr
Ovarian hyperemia			
(Beck and co-workers)	Rats	Hyperemia	12–18 hr
Frog test			
(Wiltberger, Miller)	Female	Extrusion of eggs	24 hr
Toad test			
(Galli Mainini, Shapiro)	Male	Extrusion of sperm	2–5 hr

RADIORECEPTOR ASSAY. Saxena and Landesman (1978) have reviewed the development and utilization of a radioreceptor assay for hCG. This assay makes use of the high affinity receptors on plasma membrane preparations of responsive tissues, e.g., bovine corpora lutea. The radioreceptor assay does not distinquish between LH and hCG. It requires the utilization of radio-iodine labeled HCG and approximately two hours to conduct. The test does offer the advantage of good accuracy and applicability to serum testing (Boyko, Russell, 1979).

BIOASSAY. Few of the many bioassay technics that have been employed in the past to detect hCG are still in use. Of these the rat ovarian hyperemia test was probably the most satisfactory for general pregnancy testing. Several of the previously employed bioassay methods are of some historical interest and are listed in Table 10-2.

Progesterone-induced and synthetic progestin-induced withdrawal uterine bleeding has been used in an attempt to differentiate pregnancy from other causes of amenorrhea. In the absence of pregnancy, withdrawal bleeding usually occurs 3 to 5 days after the last dose of the progestin in estrogen-producing anovulatory women. This response, of course, requires an estrogen-primed endometrium. Withdrawal of the progestin results in uterine bleeding if there is little or no endogenous progesterone production. If there is sufficient production of endogenous progesterone in the absence of pregnancy or if the endometrium is not estrogen-primed,

no bleeding occurs, resulting in a falsely positive test. In general, this method offers little that cannot be accomplished by evaluating carefully the woman's history and by ascertaining, at the time of pelvic examination, whether there is any cervical mucus and, if so, whether the spread and dried mucus crystallizes to form a fern or a cellular pattern (see Chap. 4, p. 87). If copious thin mucus is present and if a fern pattern develops on drying, early pregnancy is very unlikely and the patient almost certainly will sustain uterine bleeding after treatment and withdrawal from progestin. If little cervical mucus is present and a highly cellular pattern forms, she may or may not be pregnant. If not pregnant, she may or may not develop uterine bleeding after receiving progestin, depending upon her own supply of endogenous progesterone. Moreover, currently there is the fear that progestins are potential teratogens (see Chap. 40, p. 1020). While the evidence to support such a conclusion is not yet definitive, nonetheless considering the lack of utility of this procedure, progestin-induced withdrawal menses as a test of pregnancy cannot be recommended.

In summary, none of the chemical tests of pregnancy is sufficiently accurate to provide positive proof of pregnancy. Unfortunately the same or even greater error rate in tests conducted by women at home may give rise to false security or unnecessary alarm if she cannot evaluate the likely validity of the results of such tests in light of other signs or symptoms.

PRESUMPTIVE EVIDENCE
OF PREGNANCY

The presumptive evidence of pregnancy is comprised largely of subjective symptoms and signs that are appreciated by the woman. These signs include (1) cessation of menses, (2) changes in the breasts, (3) discoloration of the vaginal mucosa, and (4) increased skin pigmentation and the appearance of abdominal striae. The symptoms include (1) nausea with or with vomiting. (2) disturbances in urination, (3) fatigue, and (4) the perception of fetal movement.

1. Cessation of the Menses. In a healthy woman who previously has had spontaneous, cyclic, and predictable menstruation, the abrupt cessation of menstruation is strongly suggestive of pregnancy. Not until 10 days or more after the time of expected onset of the menstrual period, however, is the absence of menses a reliable indication of pregnancy. When the second period is missed, the probability is very much stronger.

Although cessation of menstruation is an early and very important indication of pregnancy, gestation may begin without prior menstruation; and uterine bleeding that is suggestive of menstruation to the woman is occasionally noted after conception. In certain Oriental countries where girls marry at a very early age, and in sexually promiscuous groups, pregnancy sometimes occurs before the menarche. Indeed we have managed the pregnancies of a girl who had four children without ever having a menstrual period. She delivered her fourth child at age 16, and conceived her first child at age 13 before menarche. Nursing mothers, who usually do not menstruate during lactation, sometimes conceive at that time and, more rarely, women who believe they have passed the menopause become pregnant. Conversely, during the first half of pregnancy, one or two episodes of bloody discharge, reminiscent of menstruation, are not uncommon, but almost without exception such bleeding is brief and scant. In a series of 225 consecutive gravidas who

did not abort, Speert and Guttmacher (1954) observed that macroscopic vaginal bleeding that occurred between the time of conception and the 196th day of pregnancy was reported by 22 percent of these women. In the absence of any cervical lesion, the bleeding began on or before the 40th day in 8 percent. Speert and Guttmacher interpreted such bleeding to be physiologic, the consequence of implantation. Bleeding during pregnancy was three times more frequent among multiparas than among primigravidas. Of 83 multiparas, 25 percent observed bleeding. Instances in which women are said to have "menstruated" every month throughout pregnancy are of questionable authenticity, and true uterine bleeding during pregnancy is undoubtedly the result of some abnormality of the reproductive organs. Bleeding per vagina at any time during pregnancy must be regarded as abnormal.

Absence of menstruation may result from a number of conditions other than pregnancy. Probably one of the most common causes of delay in the onset of the menstrual period is anovulation, which in turn may be the consequence of a number of factors including emotional disorders, particularly the fear of pregnancy. Environmental change as well as a variety of chronic disease processes may also suppress menstruation by inducing anestrogenic or estrogenic anovulation.

2. Changes in the Breasts. Generally, the breast changes that accompany pregnancy (see Chap. 9) are quite characteristic in primiparas but are less obvious in multiparas, whose breasts may contain a small amount of milk or colostrum for months or even years after their last delivery. Occasionally, changes in the breasts similar to those produced by pregnancy are found in women with prolactin-secreting pituitary tumors and in women taking certain tranquilizers which induce hyperprolactinemia. Instances have also been reported of such breast changes occurring in women with spurious or imaginary pregnancy (pseudocyesis, see p. 270) or after repeated stimulation of the breasts.

3. Discoloration of the Vaginal Mucosa.
During pregnancy, the vaginal mucosa frequently appears dark bluish or purplish-red and congested (Chadwick's sign). This appearance of the vagina is taken as presumptive evidence of pregnancy but is not conclusive, since such vaginal changes may be observed in any condition that causes intense congestion of the pelvic organs.

4. Increased Skin Pigmentation and the Appearance of Abdominal Striae.
These cutaneous manifestations are common to, but not absolutely diagnostic of, pregnancy. These signs may be absent during gestation and, conversely, may be associated with the use of estrogen-progestin contraceptives.

Symptoms

1. Nausea with or Without Vomiting.
Pregnancy is commonly characterized by disturbances of the digestive system, manifested particularly by nausea and vomiting. The so-called morning sickness of pregnancy usually commences during the early part of the day but passes off in a few hours, although occasionally it persists longer and may occur at other times. This disturbing symptom usually appears about 6 weeks after the commencement of the last menstrual period and disappears spontaneously 6 to 12 weeks later.

2. Disturbances in Urination.
During the first trimester of pregnancy, the enlarging uterus, by exerting pressure on the urinary bladder, may cause frequent micturition. Urinary frequency diminishes gradually during pregnancy as the uterus rises up into the abdomen. This symptom reappears, however, at or near the end of pregnancy when the fetal head descends into the maternal pelvis.

3. Fatigue.
Easy fatigability is such a frequent characteristic of early pregnancy that it affords a noteworthy diagnostic clue.

4. The Sensation of Fetal Movement.
Sometime between 16 and 20 weeks after the onset of the last menstrual period, the pregnant woman usually becomes conscious of slight fluttering movements in the abdomen and these movements gradually increase in intensity. These are caused by fetal activity, and the time that these are appreciated first by the mother is designated as "quickening," or the perception of life. This sign provides only corroborative evidence of pregnancy and in itself is of little diagnostic value.

Differential Diagnosis of Pregnancy

Often the uterus of pregnancy is mistaken for other tumors occupying the pelvis or abdomen; less frequently the opposite error is made. The uterine changes of the early weeks of pregnancy may be simulated by enlargement of the uterus caused by myomas, hematometra, adenomyosis, or by apparent enlargement that is actually due to a contiguous extrauterine mass or masses. As a rule, the enlarged uterus in these circumstances is firmer than it is in pregnancy and is less elastic and boggy. Except in hematometra, moreover, such conditions usually are not attended by cessation of the menses. However, if uncertainty remains, reexamination in a few weeks will usually allow for the correct diagnosis to be established.

Spurious Pregnancy

Imaginary pregnancy, or *pseudocyesis,* usually occurs in women nearing the menopause or in women who desire intensely to be pregnant. Such women may present all the subjective symptoms of pregnancy in association with a considerable increase in the size of their abdomen, caused either by deposition of fat, by gas in the intestinal tract, or by abdominal fluid. In such women, the menses do not as a rule disappear, but may become unpredictable in time of onset and in amount and duration of bleeding. Changes in the breasts, including enlargement, the appearance of galactorrhea, and increased arealor pigmentation, sometimes occur. In a majority of these women there is morning sickness, probably of psychogenic origin.

The ingestion of a variety of phenothiazines can lead to amenorrhea, breast enlargement, hyperprolactenemia and galactorrhea, and even false positive pregnancy tests. Obviously, the emotional problem being treated may be compounded by these changes.

The supposed fetal movements that are perceived by women with pseudocyesis can be ascribed to contractions of the woman's intestines or the muscles of her abdominal wall, but occasionally these are so marked as to deceive even physicians. Careful examination of such women usually leads to a correct diagnosis without great difficulty since the small uterus can be palpated on bimanual examination. The greatest difficulty encountered in the care of such women may be that of convincing her of the correct diagnosis. Psychotic women may persist for years in the delusion that they are pregnant.

Distinction Between First and Subsequent Pregnancies

Occasionally, it is of practical importance to ascertain whether a woman is having her first baby or has previously borne children. Ordinarily, but not always, there are indelible traces of a former pregnancy.

In a nullipara, the abdomen is usually tense and firm, and the uterus is felt through it with difficulty. The characteristic old abdominal striae and the distinctive changes in the breasts are absent. The labia majora are usually in close apposition and the frenulum is intact. The vagina is usually narrow and characterized by well developed rugae. The cervix is softened but usually does not admit the tip of the examiner's finger until the very end of pregnancy.

In multiparas, usually the abdominal wall is lax and, at times, pendulous, and through it the uterus is palpated readily. In addition to the pink abdominal striae associated with the present pregnancy, the silvery cicatrices of past pregnancies may also be present. Usually the breasts are not so firm as in women during their first pregnancy and frequently the skin over the breast tissue contains striae similar to those on the abdomen. The vulva of women who previously have delivered vaginally usually gapes open to some extent, the frenulum has disppeared, and the hymen is transformed into the myrtiform caruncles. In multiparas who had previously delivered vaginally, the external os, even in the early months of pregnancy, may admit the tip of the examiner's finger, which can be carried up to the internal os. Moreover the sites of healed lacerations of the cervix usually can be identified.

Identification of Fetal Life or Death

In the early months of pregnancy, the diagnosis of fetal death may present difficulty. Unless special ultrasonic technics are employed, the diagnosis of fetal death can be made with certainty only after it can be shown by repeated examinations that the uterus has remained stationary in size or has actually decreased in size over a number of weeks. Since the placenta may continue to produce hCG for several weeks after death of the embryo or fetus, a positive endocrine test for pregnancy is not necessarily an indication that the fetus is alive.

In the latter half of pregnancy, the cessation of fetal movements usually alerts the woman to the possibility of fetal death, but if fetal cardiac action can still be identified distinct from that of the mother, the fetus certainly is alive. However, if by careful auscultation the fetal heart tones are not heard, the fetus is probably dead. There is a possibility of error, of course, especially in pregnancies in which the fetal heart is remote from the examiner, for example, if the woman is obese or if hydramnios exists.

Ultrasonic instruments employing the Doppler shift principle, as described on page 262, are of considerable value in the evaluation of pregnancies in which the fetal heart cannot be heard by auscultation with a stethoscope. The use of Doppler ultrasound is especially valuable when fetal death was suspected but fetal heart action can be identified. If fetal heart action is not demonstrated after careful examination, very likely the fetus is dead. There are reports by some investigators of no errors in diagnosis in this circumstance. Other careful workers, however, have on occasion failed to identify fetal heart action yet the fetus was proven to be alive. Brown (1971), for example, reported four such instances of 106 evaluated; two of the mothers were obese and two had hydramnios. When restudied subsequently, however, fetal heart action was identified in each instance. Therefore, from the twelfth week on, an instrument that employs the Doppler principles is likely to be of aid in identifying correctly fetal cardiac action.

If the fetus has succumbed, usually it can be shown by careful examination that the uterus does not correspond in size to the estimated duration of pregnancy or actually that the uterus has become smaller than previously observed. With the death of the fetus, maternal weight gain usually ceases, and not infrequently there is even a slight decrease in her weight. At the same time, retrogressive changes usually have occurred in the breasts. Ordinarily, the diagnosis of fetal death cannot be made from the findings of a single examination, but fetal death certainly must be considered when the signs just mentioned are identified and fetal cardiac action cannot be detected.

Occasionally a positive diagnosis of fetal death can be established by palpating the col-

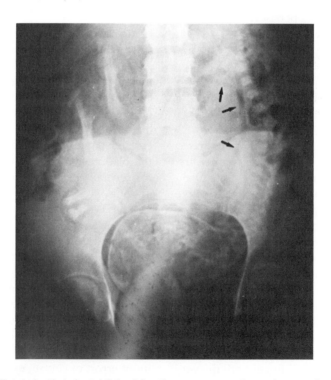

FIG. 10-3. Fetal death is established by the presence of gas in a major vessel. The close proximity to the fetal spine implies that the vessel is the aorta.

lapsed fetal skull through the partially dilated cervix; in that event the loose bones of the fetal head feel as though they were contained in a flabby bag.

There are three principal radiologic signs of fetal death:

1. Significant overlap of the skull bones (Spalding's sign), caused by liquefaction of the brain, a process that requires several days to develop. A similar sign may develop occasionally with a living fetus, e.g., when the fetal head is compressed in the maternal pelvis.
2. Exaggerated curvature of the fetal spine. Since the development of this sign depends on maceration of the spinous ligaments, its development also requires several days; moreover, mild degrees of curvature of the spine in living fetuses may be misleading.
3. Demonstration of gas in the fetus is an uncommon but reliable sign of fetal death (Fig. 10-3).

In instances in which the fetus has been dead for several days to weeks, the amnionic fluid is red to brown and usually turbid rather than nearly colorless and clear. The finding of such amnionic fluid is not absolutely diagnostic of fetal death, however, since prior hemorrhage into the amnionic sac, as sometimes occurs during amniocentesis, may lead to similar discoloration of the amnionic fluid even though the fetus is alive.

Kerenyi and Sarkozi (1974) demonstrated that creatine phosphokinase activity in amnionic fluid increases remarkably by the fifth day after the death of the fetus. Creatine phosphokinase activity was 30 milliunits per ml or less in amnionic fluid from normal pregnancies compared to 1,000 milliunits or more by the fourth to fifth day after fetal death. The epithelium and subcutaneous tissue of the fetus are rich sources of this enzyme.

REFERENCES

Bartholomew RA, Sale BE, Calloway JT: Diagnosis of pregnancy by the roentgen ray. JAMA 76:912, 1921

Boyko WL, Russell HT: Evaluation and clinical application of the quantitative radio receptor assay for serum hCG. Obstet Gynecol 54:737, 1979

Brown RE: Doppler ultrasound in obstetrics. JAMA 218:1395, 1971

Chadwick JR: Value of the bluish coloration of the vaginal entrance as a sign of pregnancy. Trans Am Gynecol Soc 11:399, 1886

Duenhoelter JH, Santos-Ramos R, Porter JC: Reliability of latex agglutination pregnancy tests. Dallas Med J 64:232, 1979

Hobson BM: Pregnancy diagnosis. Lancet 2:56, 1969

Jimenez JM, Tyson JE, Santos-Ramos R. Duenhoelter JH: Comparison of obstetric and pediatric evaluation of gestational age. Ped. Res. 13:498, 1979

Kerber IJ, Inclan AP, Fowler EA, Davis K, Fish SA: Immunologic tests for pregnancy: a comparison. Obstet Gynecol 36:37, 1970

Kerenyi T, Sarkozi L: Diagnosis of fetal death in utero by elevated amnionic fluid CPK levels. Obstet Gynecol 44:215,1974

Robinson HP: Detection of fetal heart movement in first trimester of pregnancy using pulsed ultrasound. Br Med J 4:66, 1972

Santos R: Personal communication, 1979

Saxena, BB, Landesman, R: Diagnosis and management of pregnancy by the radioreceptor assay of human chorionic gonadotropin. Am J Obstet Gynecol 131:97, 1978

Speert H, Guttmacher AF: Frequency and significance of bleeding in early pregnancy. JAMA 155:172, 1974

11

The Normal Pelvis

The mechanisms of labor are essentially processes of accommodation of the fetus to the bony passage through which it must pass. Accordingly, the size and the shape of the pelvis are of extreme importance in obstetrics. In both women and men, the pelvis forms the bony ring through which the body weight is transmitted to the lower extremities, but in women it assumes a special form that adapts it to childbearing (Fig. 11-1).

The adult pelvis is composed of four bones: the sacrum, the coccyx, and the two innominate bones. Each innominate bone is formed by the fusion of the ilium, the ischium, and the pubis. The innominate bones are joined firmly to the sacrum at the sacroiliac synchondroses, and to one another at the symphysis pubis. Consideration of the pelvis will be limited to those peculiarities of importance in childbearing.

PELVIC ANATOMY FROM THE OBSTETRIC POINT OF VIEW

The linea terminalis demarcates the *false pelvis* from the *true pelvis* (Fig. 11-2). The false pelvis lies above the linea terminalis and the true pelvis below this anatomic boundary.

The false pelvis is bounded posteriorly by the lumbar vertebrae and laterally by the iliac fossae; in front the boundary is formed by the lower portion of the anterior abdominal wall. The false pelvis varies considerably in size among women according to the flare of the iliac bones, but is of no particular obstetric significance.

The true pelvis lies beneath the linea terminalis and is the portion important in childbearing. The true pelvis is bounded above by the promontory and alae of the sacrum, the linea terminalis, and the upper margins of the pubic bones; and below by the pelvic outlet. The cavity of the true pelvis can be compared with an obliquely truncated, bent cylinder with its greatest height posteriorly, since its anterior wall at the symphysis pubis measures about 5 cm and its posterior wall about 10 cm (Figs. 11-3, 11-4). With the woman upright, the upper portion of the pelvic canal is directed downward and backward, and its lower course curves and becomes directed downward and forward.

The walls of the true pelvis are partly bony and partly ligamentous. The posterior boundary is furnished by the anterior surface of the sacrum, and the lateral limits are formed by the inner surface of the ischial bones and the sacrosciatic notches and sacrosciatic liga-

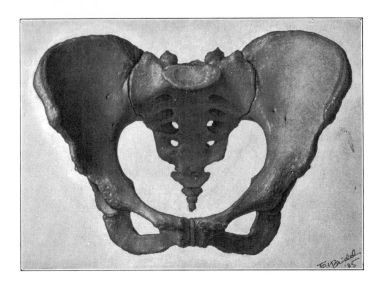

FIG. 11-1. Normal female pelvis.

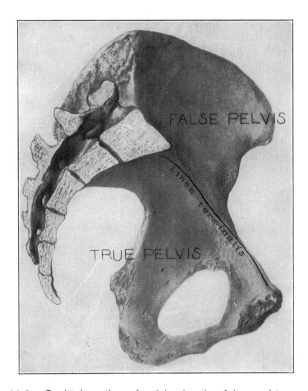

FIG. 11-2. Sagittal section of pelvis showing false and true pelvis.

ments. In front, the true pelvis is bounded by the pubic bones, the ascending rami of the ischial bones, and the obturator foramina which they partially enclose.

The side walls of the true pelvis of the normal adult woman converge somewhat; therefore, if the planes of the ischial bones of the pelvis of a normal adult woman were extended downward, they would meet near the knee. Extending from the middle of the posterior margin of each ischium are the ischial spines, which are of great obstetric im-

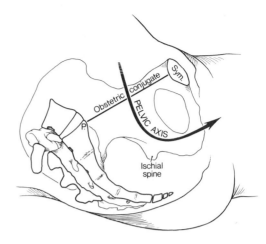

FIG. 11-3. The cavity of the true pelvis is comparable to an obliquely truncated, bent cylinder with its greatest height posteriorly. Note the curvature of the pelvic axis.

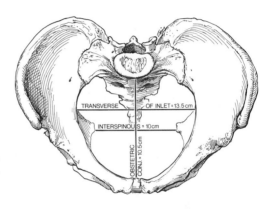

FIG. 11-4. Adult female pelvis demonstrating anteroposterior and transverse diameters of the pelvic inlet and transverse (interspinous) diameter of the midpelvis; the obstetric conjugate normally is greater than 10 cm.

portance, inasmuch as a line drawn between them typically represents the shortest diameter of the pelvic cavity. Moreover, since the ischial spines can be felt readily by vaginal or rectal examination, they serve as valuable landmarks in determining the level to which the presenting part of the fetus has descended into the pelvis.

The sacrum forms the posterior wall of the pelvic cavity. Its upper anterior margin, corresponding to the body of the first sacral vertebra and designated as the promontory, can be felt on vaginal examination and therefore provides a landmark for internal pelvimetry. Normally, the sacrum possesses a marked vertical and a less pronounced horizontal concavity, which, in abnormal pelves, may undergo important variations. A straight line drawn from the promontory to the tip of the sacrum usually measures 10 cm, whereas the distance along the concavity averages 12 cm.

In women the appearance of the pubic arch is characteristic. The descending rami of the pubic bones unite at an angle of 90 to 100 degrees to form a rounded arch under which the fetal head may readily pass (Fig. 11-1).

Planes and Diameters of the Pelvis. Because of the peculiar shape of the pelvis, it is difficult to describe the exact location of an object therein. For convenience, the pelvis has long been described as having four imaginary planes: (1) the plane of the pelvic inlet (superior strait), (2) the plane of the pelvic outlet (inferior strait), (3) the plane of greatest pelvic dimensions, and (4) the plane of the midpelvis (least pelvic dimensions).

PELVIC INLET. The pelvic inlet (superior strait) is bounded posteriorly by the promontory and alae of the sacrum, laterally by the linea terminalis, and anteriorly by the horizontal rami of the pubic bones and symphysis pubis (Figs. 11-1 and 11-4). The configuration of the inlet of the pelvis of women typically is more nearly round than ovoid. Caldwell and Moloy (1934) identified roentgenographically a nearly round or "gynecoid" pelvic inlet in 50 percent of the pelves of white women.

Four diameters of the pelvic inlet are usually described: the anteroposterior, the transverse, and two obliques. The obstetrically important anteroposterior diameter is the shortest distance between the promontory of the sacrum and the symphysis pubis and is designated the *obstetric conjugate* (Figs. 11-3, 11-4). Normally, the obstetric conjugate measures 10 cm or more, but it may be considerably shortened in abnormal pelves.

The transverse diameter is constructed at right angles to the obstetric conjugate and represents the greatest distance between the linea terminalis on either side. It usually intersects the obstetric conjugate at a point about 4 cm in front of the promontory (Fig. 11-4).

Each of the oblique diameters extends from one of the sacroiliac synchondroses to the iliopectineal eminence on the opposite side of the pelvis. They average just under 13 cm and are designated right and left, respectively, according to whether they originate at the right or left sacroiliac synchondrosis.

The anteroposterior diameter of the pelvic inlet that has been identified as the *true conjugate*, does not represent the shortest distance between the promontory of the sacrum and symphysis pubis (Fig. 11-5). The shortest distance is the *obstetric conjugate*, which is the shortest anteroposterior diameter through which the head must pass in descending through the pelvic inlet (Fig. 11-3–11-5).

The obstetric conjugate cannot be measured directly with the examining fingers, therefore, various instruments have been designed in an effort to obtain such a measurement, but none gives satisfactory results. For clinical purposes, therefore, it is sufficient to estimate the length of the obstetric conjugate indirectly by measuring the distance from the

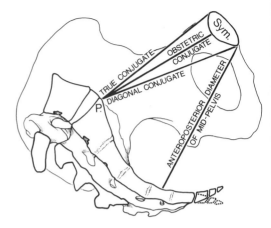

FIG. 11-5. Three anteroposterior diameters of the pelvic inlet are illustrated: the true conjugate, the obstetrically important obstetric conjugate, and the clinically measurable diagonal conjugate. The anteroposterior diameter of the midpelvis is also shown (P = sacral promontory; Sym = symphysis pubis).

lower margin of the symphysis to the promontory of the sacrum, that is, the *diagonal conjugate,* and subtracting 1.5 to 2 cm from the result, according to the height and inclination of the symphysis pubis (Fig. 11-5).

PELVIC OUTLET. The outlet of pelvis consists of two approximately triangular areas not in the same plane but having a common base which is a line drawn between the two ischial tuberosities. The apex of the posterior triangle is at the tip of the sacrum; the lateral boundaries are the sacrosciatic ligaments and the ischial tuberosities. The anterior triangle is formed by the area under the pubic arch. Three diameters of the pelvic outlet are usually described: the anteroposterior, the transverse, and the posterior sagittal. The anteroposterior diameter extends from the lower margin of the symphysis pubis to the tip of the sacrum (11.5 cm). The transverse diameter is the distance between the inner edges of the ischial tuberosities (10.0 cm). The posterior sagittal diameter extends from the tip of the sacrum to a right-angled intersection with a line between the ischial tuberosities (7.5 cm).

MIDPELVIS. The midpelvis at the level of the ischial spines (midplane, or plane of least pelvic dimensions) is of particular importance following engagement of the fetal head in obstructed labor. The interspinous diameter of 10.0 cm, or somewhat more, is usually the smallest diameter of the pelvis (Fig. 11-4). The shortest anteroposterior diameter, at the level of the ischial spines, normally measures at least 11.5 cm (Fig. 11-5). The posterior component (posterior sagittal diameter) between the sacrum and the intersection with the interspinous diameter, is usually at least 4.5 cm.

The *plane of greatest pelvic dimensions* has no obstetric significance. As the name implies, this plane represents the roomiest portion of the pelvic cavity. It extends from the middle of the posterior surface of the symphysis pubis to the junction of the second and third sacral vertebrae and passes laterally through the ischial bones over the middle of the acetabulum. Its anteroposterior and transverse diameters average about 12.5 cm. Since its oblique diameters terminate in the obturator foramina and the sacrosciatic notches, their length is indeterminate.

Pelvic Inclination. The normal position of the pelvis, in the erect woman, can be reproduced by holding a skeletal specimen with the incisures of the acetabula pointing directly downward. The same result is achieved when the anterior superior spines of the ilium and the pubic tubercles are placed in the same vertical plane.

Pelvic Joints. Anteriorly, the pelvic bones are joined together by the symphysis pubis, which consists of fibrocartilage, and by the superior and inferior pubic ligaments, the latter frequently designated the arcuate ligament of the pubis (Fig. 11-6). The symphysis has a certain degree of mobility, which increases during pregnancy, particularly in multiparas. This fact was demonstrated by Budin (1897), who somehow showed that if a finger were inserted into the vagina of a pregnant woman and she were to walk, the ends of the pubic bones could be felt moving up and down with each step. The

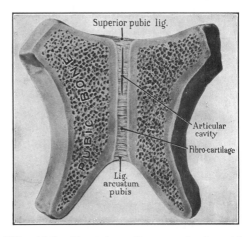

FIG. 11-6. Frontal section symphysis pubis. Lig. arcuatum pubis = arcuate pubic ligament. (From Spalteholz. *Hand-Atlas of Human Anatomy,* Vol. 1, Philadelphia, Lippincott)

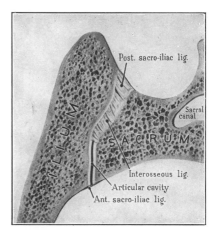

FIG. 11-7. Sacroiliac synchondrosis. (From Spalteholz. *Hand Atlas of Human Anatomy,* Vol. 1, Philadelphia, Lippincott)

articulations between the sacrum and innominate bones *(sacroiliac joints)* also have a certain degree of mobility (Fig. 11-7).

Relaxation of the pelvic joints during pregnancy is probably the result of hormonal changes. Abramson and co-workers (1934) observed that relaxation of the symphysis pubis commenced in women in the first half of pregnancy and increased during the last three months. These investigators observed that regression of relaxation began immediately after parturition and was completed within three to five months. Based on further observations, it is apparent that the symphysis pubis increases in width during pregnancy (more in multiparas than in primigravidas) and returns to normal soon after delivery. By careful roentgenographic studies, Borell (1957) demonstrated rather marked mobility of the pelvis of women at term that was caused by an upward gliding movement of the sacroiliac joint. The displacement, which is greatest in the dorsal lithotomy position, may cause an increase in the diameter of the outlet of 1.5 to 2 cm.

Because of the elasticity of the pelvic joints in pregnancy, formerly it was thought that positioning the woman in extreme hyperextension increased the obstetric conjugate. To obtain this objective, the woman was placed on her back with her buttocks extending slightly over the edge of the delivery table and with her legs hanging down by their own weight, the so-called Walcher's position. From results of roentgenologic studies, Young (1940) and Brill and Danielius (1941) showed clearly that this concept was erroneous and that no appreciable increase in pelvic size results from Walcher's position. The position is both useless and very uncomfortable for the mother.

The conversion of the pelvis of the fetus to the adult form, including sexual differences, is considered at the end of this chapter.

PELVIC SIZE AND ITS ESTIMATION

Diagonal Conjugate. In many abnormal pelves, the shortest anteroposterior diameter of the pelvic inlet (the obstetric conjugate) is considerably shortened. It is

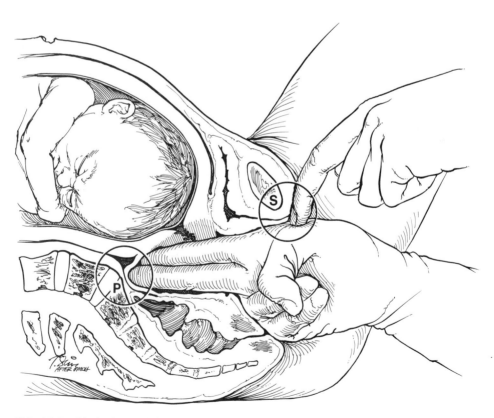

FIG. 11-8. Vaginal examination to determine the diagonal conjugate (P = sacral promontory; S = symphysis pubis).

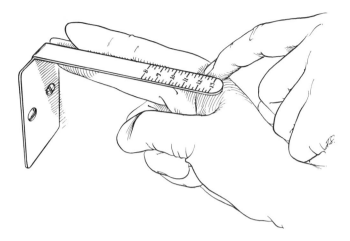

FIG. 11-9. Metal scale fastened to wall for measuring the diagonal conjugate diameter as ascertained manually.

therefore important to determine its length, but this measurement can be obtained only by roentgenologic technics. However, the distance from the sacral promontory to the lower margin of the symphysis pubis (the diagonal conjugate) can be measured clinically (Figs. 11-8, 11-9). *The diagonal conjugate measurement is most important, and every practitioner of obstetrics should be thoroughly familiar with the technic of its measurement and interpretation.*

For this purpose, the woman should be placed upon an examining table with her knees drawn up and her feet supported by suitable stirrups. If such an examination cannot be arranged conveniently, she should be brought to the edge of the bed where a firm pillow should be placed beneath her buttocks. The examiner introduces two fingers into the vagina; before measuring the diagonal conjugate, the mobility of the coccyx is evaluated and the anterior surface of the sacrum is palpated. The mobility of the coccyx is tested by palpating it with the fingers in the vagina and attempting to move it to and fro. The anterior surface of the sacrum is then palpated methodically from below upward and its vertical and lateral curvatures are noted. In normal pelves, only the last three sacral vertebrae can be felt without indenting the perineum, whereas in markedly contracted varieties the entire anterior surface of the sacrum usually

is readily accessible. Frequently the mobility of the coccyx and the anatomic features of the lower sacrum may be defined more easily by rectal examination.

Except in extreme degrees of contraction, in order to reach the promontory of the sacrum, the elbow must be depressed and the perineum forcibly indented by the knuckles of the examiner's third and fourth fingers. The index and the second fingers, held firmly together, are carried up over the anterior surface of the sacrum, where, by sharply depressing the wrist, the promontory is felt by the tip of the second finger as a projecting bony margin at the base of the sacrum. With the finger closely applied to the most prominent portion of the upper sacrum, the vaginal hand is elevated until it contacts the pubic arch, and the immediately adjacent point on the index finger is marked, as shown in Fig. 11-8. The hand is withdrawn and the distance between the mark and the tip of the second finger is measured. Because measurement using a pelvimeter often introduces an error of 0.5 to 1 cm, it is better to employ a rigid measuring scale attached to the wall, as shown in Fig. 11-9. The diagonal conjugate is thus determined and the obstetric conjugate is computed by deducting 1.5 to 2.0 cm, depending upon the height and inclination of the symphysis pubis, as illustrated in Figure

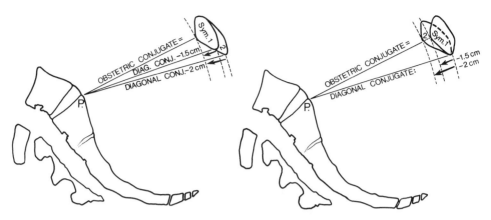

FIG. 11-10. Variations in length of diagonal conjugate dependent on height and inclination of the symphysis pubis.

11-10. If the diagonal conjugate is greater than 11.5 cm, it is justifiable to assume that the pelvic inlet is of adequate size for childbirth.

Objection to measurement of the diagonal conjugate is sometimes raised on the basis that it is painful to the patient. It probably causes mild momentary discomfort, but if properly performed and deferred until the latter half of pregnancy, when the distensibility of the vagina and perineum is greater,

women object to it no more than to venipuncture.

Transverse contraction of the inlet can be measured only by x-ray pelvimetry. Transverse contractions may exist even in the presence of an adequate anteroposterior diameter.

Engagement. Engagement is the descent of the biparietal plane of the fetal head to a level below that of the pelvic inlet (Figs.

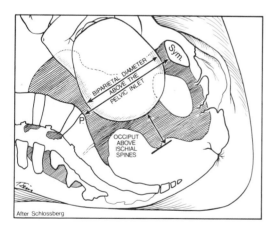

FIG. 11-11. When the lowermost portion of the fetal head is above the ischial spines, the biparietal diameter of the head is not likely to have passed through the pelvic inlet and therefore is not engaged (P = sacral promontory; Sym = symphysis pubis).

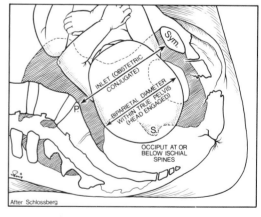

FIG. 11-12. When the lowermost portion of the fetal head is at or below the ischial spines, it is usually engaged. Exceptions occur when there is considerable molding or caput formation, or both (P = sacral promontory; Sym = symphysis pubis; S = ischial spine).

11-11, 11-12). In other words, when the biparietal or largest diameter of the normally flexed head has passed through the inlet, engagement has taken place, and the head is engaged. Although engagement is usually regarded as a phenomenon of labor (and will be discussed later in that connection), in nulliparas it commonly occurs during the last few weeks of pregnancy. When it does so, it is confirmatory evidence that the pelvic inlet is adequate for that particular fetal head. With engagement, the fetal head serves as an internal pelvimeter to demonstrate that the pelvic inlet is ample for that particular fetus.

Whether the head is engaged may be ascertained either by rectal or vaginal examination or by abdominal palpation. After gaining experience with vaginal examination, it becomes relatively easy to locate the station of the lowermost part of the fetal head in relation to the level of the ischial spines. If the lowest part of the occiput is at or below the level of the spines, the head is usually, but not always, engaged, since the distance from the biparietal plane of the pelvic inlet to the level of the ischial spines approximates 5 cm in most pelves, whereas the distance from the biparietal plane of the unmolded fetal head to the vertex is only about 3 to 4 cm. In these circumstances, the vertex cannot possibly reach the level of the spines unless the biparietal diameter has passed the inlet or unless there has been considerable elongation of the fetal head because of molding and formation of caput succedaneum (see Chap. 16, p. 403).

Engagement may be ascertained less satisfactorily by abdominal examination. If in a mature infant the biparietal plane has descended through the inlet, that plane so completely fills the inlet that the examining fingers cannot reach the lowermost part of the head. Hence, when pushed downward over the lower abdomen, the examining fingers will slide over that portion of the head proximal to the biparietal plane (nape of the neck) and diverge. Conversely, if the head is not engaged, the examining fingers can easily palpate the lower part of the head and will hence converge, as shown in Figure 11-13.

Fixation of the fetal head is descent of the head through the pelvic inlet to a depth that prevents its free movement in any direction when pushed by both hands placed over the lower abdomen; it is not necessarily synonymous with engagement. Although a head that is freely movable on abdominal examination cannot be engaged, fixation of the head is sometimes seen when the biparietal plane is a centimeter or more above the pelvic inlet, especially if the head is molded appreciably.

Although engagement is conclusive evidence of an adequate pelvic inlet for the fetus concerned, its absence is by no means always indicative of pelvic contraction. For instance, in Bader's study (1936), labor was entirely normal in 87 percent of the 499 primigravidas with unengaged fetal heads at the onset of labor. Nevertheless, the incidence of contraction of the inlet is higher in this group than in the obstetric population at large.

Outlet Measurements. The other important dimension of the pelvis that is accessible for clinical measurement is the diameter between the ischial tuberosities, variously called the *bisischial diameter,* the *intertuberous diameter,* and the *transverse diameter of the outlet.* With the woman in a lithotomy position, the measurement is made from the inner and low-

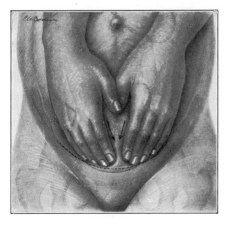

FIG. 11-13. If the fingers converge when palpating the lateral aspects of the fetal head, it is not engaged.

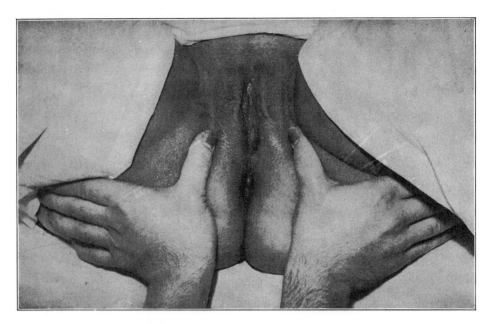

FIG. 11-14. Palpation of pubic arch.

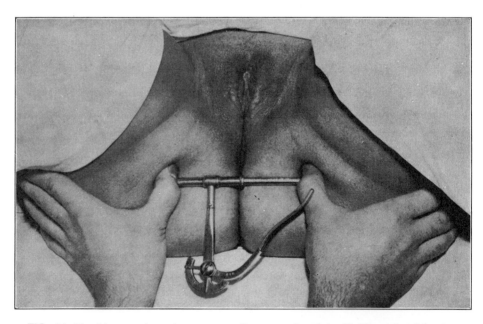

FIG. 11-15. Mensuration of transverse diameter of outlet with Thoms' pelvimeter.

ermost aspect of the ischial tuberosities, as shown in Figures 11-14 and 11-15. A measurement over 8 cm is considered to be normal. For measuring that diameter the pelvimeter devised by Thoms can be employed. The shape of the subpubic arch can be appreciated best if the pubic rami are palpated from the subpubic region to the ischial tuberosities.

Clinical Estimation of Midpelvic Size. Clinical estimation of midpelvic capacity by any direct form of measurement is not possible. If the ischial spines are quite prominent, or if the side walls of the pelvis are felt to converge, or if the concavity of the sacrum is very shallow, suspicion of contraction in this region is aroused, but only by roentgenologic studies can the midpelvis be precisely measured.

X-RAY PELVIMETRY

Status of X-ray Pelvimetry. Considerable difference of opinion about the value of x-ray pelvimetry remains. Some obstetricians consider it superfluous and even misleading. Others regard x-ray pelvimetry as the solution to all problems in the management of pelvic contraction. The logical view is something between these two extremes. The prognosis for successful labor in any given case cannot be established on the basis of x-ray pelvimetry alone, since the pelvic capacity is but one of several factors that determine the outcome. As enumerated by Mengert (1948), there are at least five factors concerned: (1) size and shape of the bony pelvis, (2) size of the fetal head, (3) force of the uterine contractions, (4) moldability of the head, and (5) presentation and position. Only the first of these factors is amenable to reasonably precise roentgenologic measurement, and it is the object of x-ray pelvimetry simply to eliminate this one factor from the category of the unknown. X-ray pelvimetry must hence be regarded merely as an adjunct in the management of the pregnancy in which the mother is suspected of having a contracted pelvis.

X-ray pelvimetry has the following advantages over manual estimation of pelvic size:

1. It provides precision of mensuration to a degree otherwise unobtainable. The clinical importance of such precision becomes evident when the shortcomings of the diagonal conjugate measurement are considered. When the diagonal conjugate exceeds 11.5 cm, the anteroposterior dimension of the inlet (the obstetric conjugate) is very rarely contracted. When the diagonal conjugate is under 11.5, however, it is not always a reliable index of the obstetric conjugate, since the difference between these two diameters, usually about 1.5 cm, may range from less than 1 to more than 2 cm. For example, two primigravidas may have diagonal conjugates of 10.5 cm, but one of the obstetric conjugate may be 10.2 cm and easy vaginal delivery follows, whereas in the other it may be 8.2 cm, in which case cesarean section is obligatory.

2. It provides exact mensuration of two important diameters not otherwise obtainable, namely, the transverse diameter of the inlet, and the interischial spinous diameter.

3. In the course of labor, if roentgenograms are obtained with the mother standing, precise information about the descent or lack of descent of the biparietal plane of the head is provided. This information is sometimes difficult to obtain by palpating the presenting part, because elongation of the head as a result of molding and caput succedaneum may make such digital findings misleading.

Indications for X-ray Pelvimetry. Because of the expenses involved, as well as radiologic hazards (p. 288), radiographic pelvic measurement is not feasible for all pregnant women, nor is it necessary in the great majority of cases. There are, however, certain clinical circumstances that point to the probability of pelvic contraction or potential dystocia and may, at times, make x-ray pelvimetry a part of good obstetric practice. These include the following circumstances:

1. Previous injury or disease likely to affect the bony pelvis
2. Ability of examiner to touch sacral promontory easily on vaginal examination (diagonal conjugate less than 11.5 cm)
3. Unusually prominent ischial spines with converging pelvic side walls or flattened sacrum

4. Markedly narrowed intertuberous diameter with narrow subpubic angle
5. Failure to progress in labor
6. Breech, face, and other abnormal presentations

Before obtaining x-ray pelvimetry, it is essential to ask a singularly important question: "Is the information to be obtained likely to affect the subsequent management of labor and delivery?" If cesarean section almost certainly is going to be performed irrespective of the roentgenographic revelations, the use of x-ray pelvimetry is difficult to justify. At a time in the not too distant past, hospital accreditation agencies demonstrated great concern over cesarean section rates and insisted that consultation be obtained before carrying out cesarean section. Such a formal

recommendation, by the way, was almost unique to this surgical procedure. In these circumstances, the presence of an x-ray report perhaps generated the appearance of the obstetrician doing all that was possible before performing a cesarean section to protect the fetus from further deterioration in utero or from some form of birth trauma. There should be no further need for this particular form of "defensive medicine."

PELVIC SHAPES

Pelvic roentgenography has also afforded an understanding of the general architecture or configuration of the pelvis, apart from its size. The findings of the classic studies of Caldwell

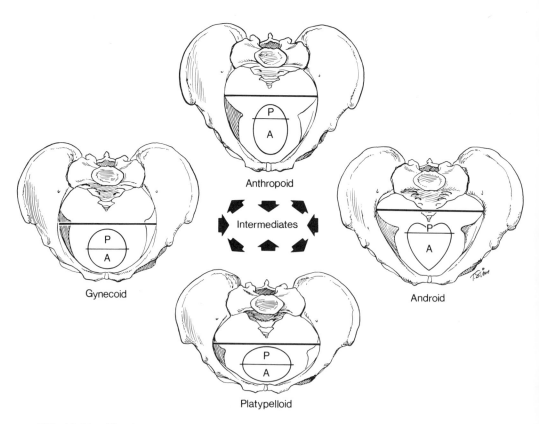

FIG. 11-16. The four parent pelvic types. A line passing through the widest transverse diameter divides the inlet into posterior (P) and anterior (A) segments.

and Moloy (1933) produced a now widely used classification of the pelvis according to shape.

Familiarity with such a classification contributes to the understanding of the mechanism of labor and to the intelligent management of labor in pregnancies with pelvic contraction. In that connection, study of pelvic shape has pointed up the importance of the pelvic shape actually available to the fetal head, as opposed to the total space indicated by absolute dimensions. For example, a spherical object can pass through a circular opening of smaller area than that occupied by the smallest rectangle that it could traverse, because the whole area is utilized by the object.

Caldwell-Moloy Classification. The type of posterior and anterior segments of the pelvic inlet are important determinants in this method of classification (Fig. 11-16). A line drawn through the greatest transverse diameter of the inlet divides the inlet into anterior and posterior segments. Many pelves are not pure but mixed types, as, for example, a gynecoid pelvic with android "tendency," meaning that the hindpelvis is gynecoid and the forepelvis is android.

GYNECOID PELVIS. This pelvis displays the anatomic characteristics ordinarily associated with that of women. The posterior sagittal diameter at the inlet is only slightly shorter than the anterior sagittal. The sides of the posterior segment are well rounded, and the forepelvis is also well rounded and wide. Since the transverse diameter of the inlet is either slightly greater than or about the same as the anteroposterior diameter, the inlet as a whole is either slightly oval or round. The side walls of the pelvis are straight; the spines are not prominent; the pubic arch is wide, with a transverse diameter at the ischial spines of 10 cm or more. The sacrum is inclined neither anteriorly nor posteriorly. The sacrosciatic notch is well rounded and never narrow. Caldwell and co-workers (1939) ascertained the frequency of

the four parent types by study of Todd's collection of pelves. They found the gynecoid pelvis was the most common type, occurring in almost one-half.

ANDROID TYPE. The posterior sagittal diameter at the inlet is much shorter than the anterior sagittal, limiting the use of the posterior space by the fetal head. The sides of the posterior segment are not rounded but tend to form, with the corresponding sides of the anterior segment, a wedge at their point of junction. The forepelvis is narrow and triangular. The side walls are usually convergent; the ischial spines are prominent; and the subpubic arch is narrowed. The bones are characteristically heavy. The sacrosciatic notch is narrow and high-arched. The sacrum is set forward in the pelvis and is usually straight, with little or no curvature, and the posterior sagittal diameter is decreased from inlet to outlet by the forward inclination. Not infrequently there is considerable forward inclination of the tip.

The extreme android pelvis presages a very poor prognosis for delivery through the vagina. The frequency of difficult forceps operations and stillbirths increases substantially when there is a small android pelvis. The android type makes up one-third of pure-type pelvis encountered in white women and one-sixth in nonwhite women in the Todd collection.

ANTHROPOID TYPE. This pelvis is characterized by an anteroposterior diameter of the inlet greater than the transverse, forming more or less an oval anteroposteriorly, with the anterior segment somewhat narrow and pointed. The sacrosciatic notch is large. The side walls are often somewhat convergent, and the sacrum usually has six segments and is straight, making the anthropoid pelvis deeper than the other types.

The ischial spines are likely to be prominent. The subpubic arch is frequently somewhat narrow but well shaped. The anthropoid pelvis is said to be more common in nonwhite women, whereas the android form is more frequent in white women. Anthropoid types make up one-fourth of pure-type pelves in white women, in comparison with nearly one-half in nonwhite women.

PLATYPELLOID TYPE. This pelvis is a flattened gynecoid pelvis, with a short antero-posterior and a wide transverse diameter. The latter is set well in front of the sacrum, as in the typical gynecoid form. The angle of the forepelvis is very wide, and the anterior puboiliac and posterior iliac portions of the iliopectineal lines are well curved. The sacrum is usually well curved and rotated backward. Thus, the sacrum is short and the pelvis shallow, creating a wide sacrosciatic notch. The platypelloid pelvis is the rarest of the pure varieties, occurring in less than 3 percent of women.

INTERMEDIATE TYPES. Intermediate or mixed types of pelves are much more frequent than the pure types. The character of the posterior segment determines the type, and that of the anterior segment the tendency.

HAZARDS OF DIAGNOSTIC RADIATION

An increasing awareness of the potential hazards of radiation has focused attention on the true value of diagnostic x-rays in obstetrics as compared with the potential damage to the mother, her fetus, and generations yet unborn. The recognized dangers to the fetus from diagnostic radiation are mutations and increased risk of malignancy after birth. Many, but not all, geneticists and radiobiologists believe, on the basis of animal experimentation, that the only entirely safe dose of irradiation is zero (Brent, Gorson, 1972; Gaulden, 1974). The possibility of malignancy was raised by the report of Stewart and associates in 1956, who identified an increase in leukemia in children of women x-rayed during pregnancy. Since then, there have been several more reports that are sup-

TABLE 11-1.
RISK OF LEUKEMIA AFTER RADIATION EXPOSURE IN UTERO FOR PELVIMETRY

	APPROXIMATE RISK PER FIRST 10 YRS	RELATIVE RISK
U.S. white children (Control)	1:2800	1
In utero during x-ray pelvimetry	1:2000	1.5
Siblings of leukemic children	1:720	4
Identical twin of leukemic child	1:3	1000

portive of the thesis that diagnostic radiation absorbed by the fetus increases the risk of subsequent development of leukemia and other malignant conditions. A comparison made by Brent (1974) of the apparent risk of leukemia developing in various groups with specific epidemiologic and pathologic characteristics is presented in Table 11-1. Oppenheim and associates (1975) point out that increased morbidity and mortality has not been identified uniformly among children exposed prenatally to diagnostic x-rays. If the mother underwent roentgenographic examination because of medical indication there was increased morbidity and mortality in the offspring compared to that found in offsprings of women in whom the irradiation was routine, for example, with pelvimetry. *The risk from x-ray pelvimetry seems justifiable whenever information critical to the welfare of the fetus or mother is likely to be obtained.*

Previously many groups, e.g., the National Council on Radiation Protection and Measurements and the International Commission on Radiation Protection adopted the 10-day or 14-day rule in the recommendation of guidelines to be followed in the utilization of irradiation of the uterus in women of childbearing age (Parker, Taylor, 1971). Namely, the following was recommended:

When radiologic procedures are planned on pregnant or potentially pregnant women, special consideration must be given to the relatively high radiosensitivity of the fetus in utero, particularly during the early phases of gestation. It is recommended that radiologic examinations of the abdomen and pelvis which do not contribute to the diagnosis or treatment of such women in relation to their current illness (e.g., low-back examinations for employment) be restricted to the first 14 days of the menstrual cycle in the case of potentially pregnant individuals and avoided entirely during known pregnancy. Examinations of other parts of the body may be done at any time provided such examinations are conducted under conditions carefully designed to limit the radiation exposure to an amount necessary for an adequate examination. Filtration, collimation of the radiation beam to the anatomic region of interest, and careful selection of technical exposure factors can significantly contribute to good radiologic practice and the reduction of radiation exposure to all tissue.

Examinations of the abdomen and pelvis that are deemed useful to patient care may be done at any time without regard for the phase of the menstrual cycle or fetal presence. In each case, the final decision to proceed or not to proceed must reside with the attending physician, in consultation with the radiologist, when such services are utilized; that is, the attending physician must retain full and complete discretion to decide each case according to his judgment.

More recently the 10-day or 14-day rule has been questioned on the grounds that there is no period, including the 10- to 14-day interval following the onset of menses during which radiologic examination of the pelvis of a woman of childbearing potential can be conducted without risk. This obtains since the risk is approximately the same from sometime *before conception* to term. However, the predominant biologic effects vary with the stage of pregnancy during which pregnancy occurs (Brown et al., 1974).

Based on these considerations, the American College of Obstetricians and Gynecologists in cooperation with the American College of Radiology, in 1977, issued a statement of policy in which the "Guidelines For Diagnostic X-ray Examination of Fertile Women" was enunciated. It was agreed that, "Attempts to schedule abdominal x-ray examinations in relation to a woman's menstrual cycle are of little value. The developing ovum

is at risk prior to ovulation as well as subsequently. Thus it is erroneous to assume that any time is 'safer' for radiation exposures than another."

The recommended guidelines were as follows:

1. The use of x-ray examinations should be considered on an individual basis. Concern over harmful effects should not prevent the proper use of radiation exposure when significant diagnostic information can be obtained. Preexamination consultation with a radiologist may be useful in obtaining optimal information from the x-ray exposure.
2. There is no measurable advantage to scheduling diagnostic x-ray examinations at any particular time during a normal menstrual cycle.
3. The degree of risk involved in an x-ray examination if the person is pregnant, or should become pregnant, should be explained to the patient and documented in her record.

Sexual Differences in the Adult Pelvis. The pelvis presents marked sexual differences. Generally, the pelvis of men is heavier, higher, and more conical than that of women. In men the muscular attachments are much more strongly marked, and the iliac bones flare less than in women. The pubic arch in men is more angular and presents an aperture of 70 to 75 degrees, as compared with 90 to 100 degrees in women. In men, the pelvic inlet is smaller and more nearly triangular, and the pelvic cavity is deeper and more conical; the sacrosciatic notch is narrower and the distance between the lower border of the sacrum and the ischial spine smaller than in the pelvis of women.

Pelvis of the Newborn Child. The mechanism by which the pelvis of the fetus is converted into the adult form is of interest since it affords important information about the mode of production of certain varieties of deformed pelves.

The pelvis of the child at birth is partly bony and partly cartilaginous (Fig. 11-17). The innominate bone does not exist as such, but is represented by the ilium, ischium, and pubis, which are united by a large Y-shaped cartilage, the three bones meeting in the acetabulum. The iliac crests and the acetabula, as well as the greater part of the ischiopubic rami, are entirely cartilaginous.

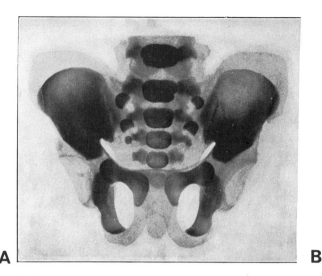
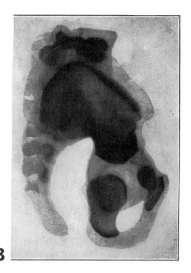

A   **B**

FIG. 11-17. Fetal pelvis near term. Frontal **(A)** and lateral **(B)** views showing extent of ossification.

The cartilaginous portions of the pelvis gradually give place to bone, but complete union in the acetabulum does not occur until about puberty, and occasionally even later. The innominate bones may not, in fact, become completely ossified until between 20 and 25 years of age.

TRANSFORMATION OF FETAL INTO ADULT PELVIS.   The evolution of the pelvic form is generally believed to involve two sets of factors: developmental and inherent tendencies, and mechanical influences. The process is not entirely the result of mechanical forces as manifested by the existence of sexual and racial differences in the adult pelvis. The mechanical influences that come into play after birth are identical in both sexes, but the sexual differences are, nevertheless, established during the pubertal process.

The part played by developmental and hereditary influences was demonstrated clearly by Litzmann (1861), who showed that the sacrum of women is markedly wider than that of men. At birth, in both sexes, the body of the first sacral vertebra is twice as broad as the alae (100 to 50), but in the adult the ratio becomes 100 to 76 in women, and 100 to 56 in men, indicating a much more rapid growth of the alae in women. Early investigators held that all the changes in the developing pelvis are similarly caused and that the influence of mechanical factors is merely accessory. The growth and development of that portion of the ilium forming the upper boundary of the great sacrosciatic notch profoundly affect the shape and size of the pelvic inlet.

Three mechanical forces are important in bringing about the final shape of the pelvis: body weight, the upward and inward pressure that is exerted by the heads of the femurs, and the cohesive force exerted by the symphysis pubis. So long as the child constantly remains in the recumbent position, these forces are not operative, but as soon as she sits up or walks, the body weight is transmitted through the vertebral column to the sacrum. Inasmuch as the center of gravity is anterior to the sacral promontory, the transmitted force is resolved into two components. One force is directed downward, and the other forward. Together the two tend to force the promontory of the sacrum downward and forward toward the symphysis pubis, a process that can be accomplished only by the sacrum rotating about its transverse axis. Its tip tends to become displaced both upward and backward. The strong sacrosciatic ligaments, however, resist this displacement and therefore permit only slight extension, with the result that the partly cartilaginous sacrum becomes bent upon itself just in front of its axis, that is, about the middle of its third vertebra, so that its anterior surface becomes markedly concave from above downward, instead of flat, as previously. At the same time, the body weight forces the bodies of the sacral vertebrae forward so that they project slightly beyond the alae, thereby diminishing the transverse concavity of the sacrum.

Since the anterior surface of the sacrum is wider than the posterior, the bone tends to sink into the pelvic cavity under the influence of the body weight and would prolapse completely into it were it not held in place by the strong posterior iliosacral ligaments that suspend it, as it were, from the posterior superior spines of the ilium. As the sacrum is pushed downward into the pelvic cavity, it exerts traction upon these ligaments, which in turn drag the posterior superior spines inward toward the midline and consequently tend to rotate the anterior portions of the innominate bones outward. Excessive outward rotation is prevented, however, partly by the cohesive force exerted at the symphysis but particularly by the upward and inward pressure exerted by the heads of the femurs. Practically, then, the iliac bone becomes converted into a two-armed level with the articular surface of the sacrum serving as a fulcrum; consequently, it bends at the point of least resistance, which is just anterior to the articulation, and thus gives the pelvis a greater transverse and a lesser anteroposterior diameter. At the same time, much of the transverse widening is more apparent than real and is caused by the relative shortening of the true conjugate by the downward and forward displacement of the promontory of the sacrum.

It is evident that the forces just mentioned must act in the same manner in the two sexes, so that whereas they may be important in the transformation of the fetal into the adult pelvis, they do not participate directly in the development of sexual differences in the adult pelvis.

The cohesive force exerted at the symphysis pubis cannot act alone, since it is manifested only when the force exerted by the body weight causes a tendency toward gaping of the pubic bones. The effect of the upward and inward force exerted by the femurs cannot act alone, since it comes into play only when it reacts against the body weight; nor has the action of the body weight alone ever been observed, though theoretically it might be noted in an individual presenting a split pelvis (congenital lack of union at the symphysis pubis) who has never walked. The action of the body weight, however, has been studied experimentally by Freund) (1885), who suspended a cadaver by the iliac crests after cutting through the symphysis and found that the innominate bones gaped widely.

The effect of the combined action of the body weight and the force exerted by the femurs has been studied by Litzmann (1861) in persons with congenital absence of the symphysis pubis. In such circumstances, there is a marked transverse widening of the posterior portion of the pelvis, while the force exerted by the femurs causes the anterior portions of the innominate bones to become almost parallel.

The action of the body weight and the cohesive force exerted at the symphysis without the upward and inward pressure exerted by the femurs can be studied in individuals whose lower extremities are absent and occasionally in persons with congenital dislocation of the hips. Holst (1869) described a case in which the lower extremities were congenitally absent and the pelvis was characterized by a marked increase in width and a marked decrease in its anteroposterior diameter. Because of the excessive pressure exerted upon the tubera ischii in the absence of the counteracting force exerted by the femurs, the innominate bones are inwardly rotated so as to turn their crests inward and the tubera ischii outward, thus producing a considerable transverse widening of the inferior strait. More or less similar changes may be observed in cases of congenital dislocation of the hip in individuals who have never walked. The effect of the various mechanical influences is exaggerated in the pelves softened by diseases such as rickets and osteomalacia. (See Chap. 31.)

REFERENCES

Abramson D, Roberts SM, Wilson PD: Relaxation of the pelvic joints in pregnancy. Surg Obstet Gynecol 58:595, 1934

American College of Obstetricians Gynecologists: Statement of Policy, "Guidelines for Diagnostic X-ray Examination of Fertile Women." Chicago, May, 1977

Bader A: The significance of the unengaged head in primiparous labor. Abstracted in Ber ges Gynak u Geburtsh 31:395, 1936

Borell U, Fernstrom I: Movements at the sacroiliac joints and their importance to changes in pelvic dimensions during parturition. Acta Obstet Gynecol Scand 36:42, 1957

Brent RL: Comment and Table on Editorial Page 14. J Reprod Med 12:6, 1974

Brent RL, Gorson RO: Radiation exposure in pregnancy. Curr Probl Radiol 2:1, 1972

Brill HM, Danielius G: Roentgen pelvimetric analysis of Walcher's position. Am J Obstet Gynecol 42:821, 1941

Brown R, Shaver J, Lamel D: A concept and proposal concerning the radiation exposure of women. Radiological Health Sciences Education Project. San Francisco, University of California, San Francisco Medical Center, 1974, unpublished contract report

Budin RC: X-radiography of a Naegele pelvis. Obstetrique Par 2:499, 1897

Caldwell WE, Moloy HC: Anatomical variations

in the female pelvis and their effect in labor with a suggested classification. Am J Obstet Gynecol 26:479, 1933

Caldwell WE, Moloy HC, D'Esopo DA: A roentgenologic study of the mechanism of engagement of the fetal head. Am J Obstet Gynecol 28:824, 1934

Caldwell WE, Moloy HC, Swenson PC: The use of the roentgen ray in obstetrics: I. Roentgen pelvimetry and cephalometry; technic of pelvioroentgenography. Am J Roentgenol 41: 305, 1939

Freund WA: On the so-called kyphotic pelvis. Gynaekol Klin Strassb I., 1, 1885

Gauldin ME: Possible effects of diagnostic X-rays on the human embryo and fetus. J Arkansas Med Soc 70:424, 1974

Holst: Description of the pelvis and the delivery of a 40-year-old female amelus. Holst's Beitrage, Hef. 2 pp 145–148, 1869

Litzmann CCT: Die Formen des Beckens. Berlin, G Reimer, 1861

Mengert WF: Estimation of pelvic capacity. JAMA 138:169, 1948

Oppenheim BE, Griem ML, Meier P: The effects of diagnostic X-ray exposure on the human fetus: An examination of the evidence. Radiology 114:529, 1975

Parker HM, Taylor LS: Basic radiation protection criteria. National Council on Radiation Protection and Measurements Report No. 39, 1971

Stewart A, Webb J, Giles D, Hewitt D: Malignant disease in childhood and diagnostic irradiation in utero. Lancet 2:447, 1956

Walsh JW: Diagnostic x-ray procedures in obstetrics. Obstet Gynecol 13:74, 1959

Young J: Relaxation of pelvic joints in pregnancy: Pelvic arthropathy of pregnancy. Br J Obstet Gynaecol 47:493, 1940

12

Presentation, Position, Attitude, and Lie of the Fetus

Fetal Posture. In the later months of pregnancy the fetus assumes a characteristic posture sometimes described as the *attitude* or *habitus* (Fig. 12-1). As a rule, the fetus forms an ovoid mass that corresponds roughly to the shape of the uterine cavity. The fetus becomes folded or bent upon himself in such a manner that the back becomes markedly convex; the head is sharply flexed so that the chin is almost in contact with the chest; the thighs are flexed over the abdomen; the legs are bent at the knees; and the arches of the feet rest upon the anterior surfaces of the legs. Usually the arms are crossed over the thorax or become parallel to the sides, and the umbilical cord lies in the space between them and the lower extremities. This characteristic posture results partly from the mode of growth of the fetus and partly from a process of accommodation to the uterine cavity.

Lie of the Fetus. The lie is the relation of the long axis of the fetus to that of the mother and is either *longitudinal* or *transverse.* Occasionally, the fetal and the maternal axes

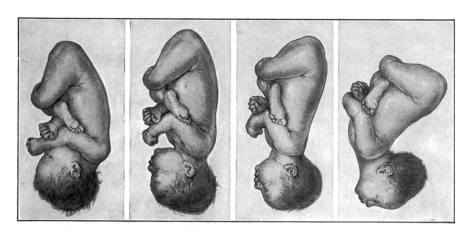

FIG. 12-1. Differences in attitude of fetus in vertex, sinciput, brow, and face presentations.

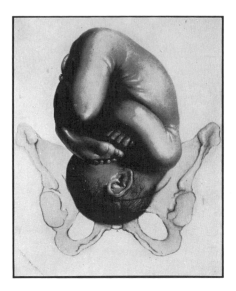

FIG. 12-2. Left occiput transverse (LOT), the most common position.

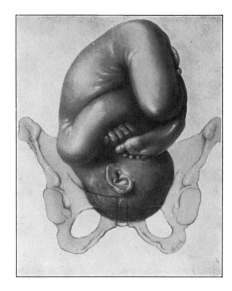

FIG. 12-3. Right occiput transverse (ROT), the second most common position.

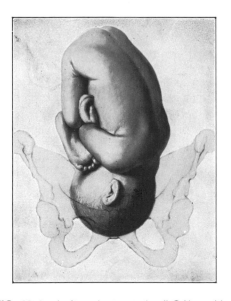

FIG. 12-4. Left occiput anterior (LOA) position.

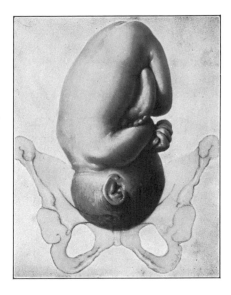

FIG. 12-5. Right occiput anterior (ROA) position.

may cross at a 45-degree angle, forming an *oblique* lie, which is unstable and always becomes longitudinal or transverse during the course of labor. Longitudinal lies are present in over 99 percent of labors at term.

Presentation and Presenting Part. The presenting part is that portion of the body of the fetus which is either foremost within the birth canal or in closest proximity to it and that which is felt through the cervix on vaginal examination. The presenting part determines the presentation. Accordingly, in longitudinal lies, the presenting part is either the fetal head or the breech, creating cephalic and breech presentations, respectively. When

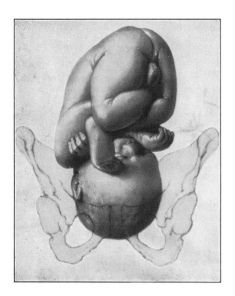

FIG. 12-6. Right occiput posterior (ROP) position.

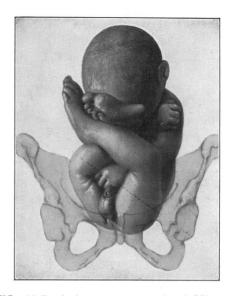

FIG. 12-7. Left sacrum posterior (LSP) position.

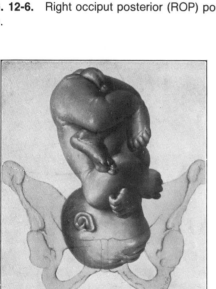

FIG. 12-8. Left mentoanterior (LMA) position.

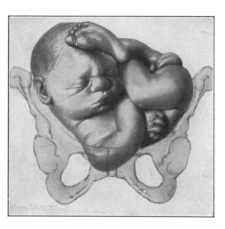

FIG. 12-9. Right acromiodorsoposterior (RADP) position. The shoulder of the fetus is to the mother's right, and the back is posterior.

the fetus lies with the long axis transversely, the shoulder is the presenting part, and a shoulder presentation obtains.

Cephalic presentations are classified according to the relation of the head to the body of the fetus (Fig. 12-1). Ordinarily, the head is flexed sharply so that the chin is in contact with the thorax. In this circumstance, the occipital fontanel is the presenting part,

although such a presentation is usually referred to as a *vertex* or *occiput presentation.* (The vertex actually lies in front of the occipital fontanel, and the occiput behind the fontanel, as illustrated in Figure 8-7). Much less commonly, the neck may be sharply extended so that the occiput and back come in contact and the face is foremost in the birth canal *(face presentation).* The fetal head may assume a position between these extremes, partially flexed in some cases with the anterior (large) fontanel, or bregma, presenting *(sinciput presentation),* or partially extended in other cases with the brow presenting *(brow presentation).* Perhaps the latter two should not be classified as distinct presentations, since these are usually transient. As labor progresses, sinciput and brow presentations are almost always converted into vertex or face presentations by flexion or extension, respectively.

When the fetus presents by the breech, the thighs may be flexed and the legs extended over the anterior surfaces of the body *(frank breech presentation);* or the thighs may be flexed on the abdomen and the legs upon the thighs *(complete breech presentation);* one or both feet, or one or both knees, are lowermost *(incomplete,* or *footling breech presentation).*

Position.   Position refers to the relation of an arbitrarily chosen portion of the fetus to the right or left side of the maternal birth canal. Accordingly, with each presentation there may be two positions, right or left. The occiput, chin, and sacrum are the determining points in vertex, face (mentum), and breech presentations, respectively (Figs. 12-2–12-9).

Variety.   For still more accurate orientation, the relation of a given portion of the presenting part to the anterior, transverse, or posterior portion of the mother's pelvis is considered. Since there are two positions, it follows that there must be six varieties for each presentation (Figs. 12-10–12-13).

Nomenclature.   Since the presenting part in any presentation may be in either the left or right position, there are left and right occipital, left and right mental, and left and right sacral presentations, which in abbreviated form may be written LO and RO, LM and RM, LS and RS, respectively. Since the presenting part in each of the two positions may be directed anteriorly (A), transversely (T), or posteriorly (P), there are six varieties of each of these three presentations.

In shoulder presentations, the acromion (or the scapula) is the portion of the fetus arbitrarily chosen to orient it with the maternal pelvis. One example of the terminology sometimes employed for this purpose is illustrated in Figure 12-9. The acromion or back of the fetus may be directed either posteriorly, anteriorly, superiorly, or inferiorly (see Chap. 30, p. 813). However, since it is impossible to differentiate exactly the several varieties of shoulder presentation by clinical examination and since such differentiation serves no practical purpose, it is customary to refer to all transverse lies of the fetus simply as shoulder presentations.

Frequency of the Various Presentations and Positions.   At or near term, the incidence of the various presentations is approximately as follows: vertex, 96 percent; breech, 3.5 percent; face, 0.3 percent; shoulder, 0.4 percent. About two-thirds of all vertex presentations are in the left position, and one-third in the right. The occiput is usually directed transversely.

Although the incidence of breech presentation is only a little over 3 percent at term, it is much greater earlier in pregnancy. White (1956) found the incidence of breech presentation to be 7.2 percent by x-ray examination at the end of the 34th week. A similar frequency has been identified sonographically (see Table 30-1). In about one-third of nulliparas and two thirds of multiparas, the breech converted to vertex spontaneously before delivery.

Reasons for the Predominance of Cephalic Presentations.   Of the several reasons that have been advanced to explain why the fetus at term usually presents by the vertex, the most logical seems to be related to the role of the piriform shape of the uterus. Although the fetal head at term is slightly larger than the breech, the entire podalic pole of the fetus, that is, the breech and its flexed extremities, is bulkier than the cephalic pole and more movable. The cephalic pole is comprised of the fetal head only, since the upper extremities are removed some distance and small and less protruding. Until about the 32nd week, the amnionic cavity is large compared to the fetal mass, and there is no crowding of the fetus by the uterine walls. At approximately that time, however, the ratio of amnionic volume to fetal mass alters by rela-

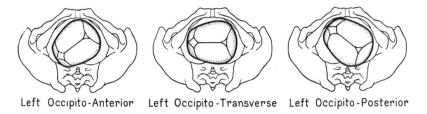

Left Occipito-Anterior   Left Occipito-Transverse   Left Occipito-Posterior

FIG. 12-10.   Left positions in occiput presentations, with fetal head viewed from below.

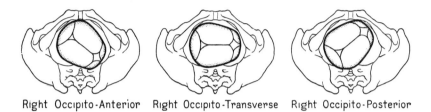

Right Occipito-Anterior   Right Occipito-Transverse   Right Occipito-Posterior

FIG. 12-11.   Right positions in occiput presentations.

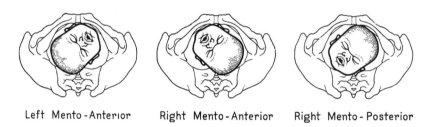

Left Mento-Anterior   Right Mento-Anterior   Right Mento-Posterior

FIG. 12-12.   Left and right positions in face presentations.

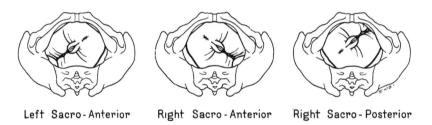

Left Sacro-Anterior   Right Sacro-Anterior   Right Sacro-Posterior

FIG. 12-13.   Left and right positions in breech presentations.

tive diminution of amnionic fluid. As a result, the uterine walls are apposed more closely to the fetal parts, and then the piriform shape of the uterus exerts its effect. The fetus, if presenting by the breech, changes its polarity in order to make use of the roomier fundus for its bulkier and more movable podalic pole. The high incidence of breech presentation in hydrocephalic fetuses is in accord with this theory, since in this circumstance the ce-

phalic pole of the fetus is definitely larger than the podalic pole.

The cause of breech presentation may be some circumstance that prevents normal version from taking place, for example, a septum that protrudes into the upper uterine segment. A peculiarity of fetal attitude, particularly extension of the vertebral column in frank breeches, may also prevent the fetus from turning.

DIAGNOSIS OF PRESENTATION AND POSITION OF THE FETUS

There are several diagnostic methods that can be used: abdominal palpation, vaginal and rectal touch, combined examination, auscultation, and, in certain doubtful cases, roentgenography or ultrasonography.

Obstetric Palpation.   In order to obtain satisfactory results, the examination should be conducted systematically employing the four maneuvers suggested by Leopold and Sporlin (1894). The mother should be on a firm bed or examining table, with her abdomen bared. During the first three maneuvers, the examiner stands at the side of the bed more convenient to him and faces the patient, but he reverses his position and faces her feet for the last maneuver (Figs. 12-14, 12-15).

FIRST MANEUVER.   After outlining the contour of the uterus and ascertaining how nearly the fundus approaches the xiphoid cartilage, the examiner gently palpates the fundus with the tips of the fingers of both hands in order to define which fetal pole is present in the fundus. The fetal breech gives the sensation of a large, nodular body, whereas the head feels hard and round and is freely movable and ballottable.

SECOND MANEUVER.   Having determined which pole of the fetus lies in the fundus, the palms of the examiner's hands are placed on either side of the abdomen and gentle but deep pressure is exerted. On one side, a hard resistant structure is felt, the back, and on the other, numerous nodulations, the small parts. In pregnant women with thin abdominal walls, the fetal extremities can be differentiated readily, but in obese women only irregular nodulations can be felt. In the presence of obesity or considerable amnionic fluid, the back is felt more easily by making deep pressure with one hand while palpating with the other. By next noting whether the back is directed anteriorly, transverely, or posteriorly, a more accurate picture of the orientation of the fetus is obtained.

THIRD   MANEUVER.   Employing the thumb and fingers of one hand, the examiner grasps the lower portion of the maternal abdomen, just above the symphysis pubis. If the presenting part is not engaged, a movable body will be felt, usually the fetal head. The differentiation between head and breech is made as in the first maneuver. If the presenting part is not engaged, the examination is almost complete; with the location of the fetal head, breech, back, and extremities known, all that remains to be defined is the attitude of the head. If by careful palpation it can be shown that the cephalic prominence is on the same side as the small parts, the head must be flexed, and therefore the vertex is the presenting part. When the cephalic prominence of the fetus is on the same side as the back, the head must be extended. However, if the presenting part is deeply engaged, the findings from this maneuver are simply indicative that the lower pole of the fetus is fixed in the pelvis; the details are then defined by the last maneuver.

FOURTH   MANEUVER.   The examiner faces the mother's feet and, with the tips of the first three fingers of each hand, makes deep pressure in the direction of the axis of the pelvic inlet. If the head presents, one hand is arrested sooner than the other by a rounded body, the cephalic prominence, while the other hand descends more deeply into the pelvis. In vertex presentations, the prominence is on the same side as the small parts, and in face presentations, on the same side as the back. The ease with which the prominence is felt is indicative of the extent to which descent has occurred. In many instances, when the fetal head has descended into the pelvis, the anterior shoulder of the fetus may be differentiated readily by the third maneuver. In breech presentations, the information obtained from this maneuver is less precise.

Abdominal palpation can be performed throughout the latter months of pregnancy and during the intervals between the contractions of labor. The findings provide information about the presentation and position of the fetus and the extent to which the present-

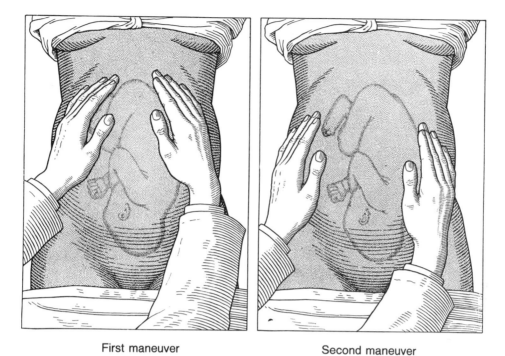

First maneuver

Second maneuver

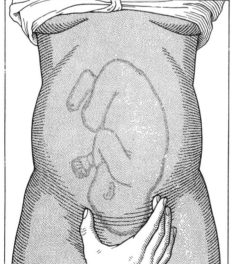

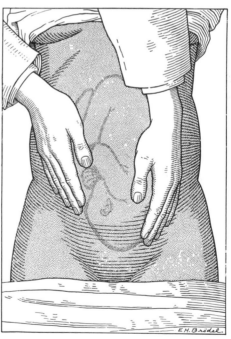

Third maneuver

Fourth maneuver

FIG. 12-14. Palpation in left occiput anterior position (maneuver of Leopold).

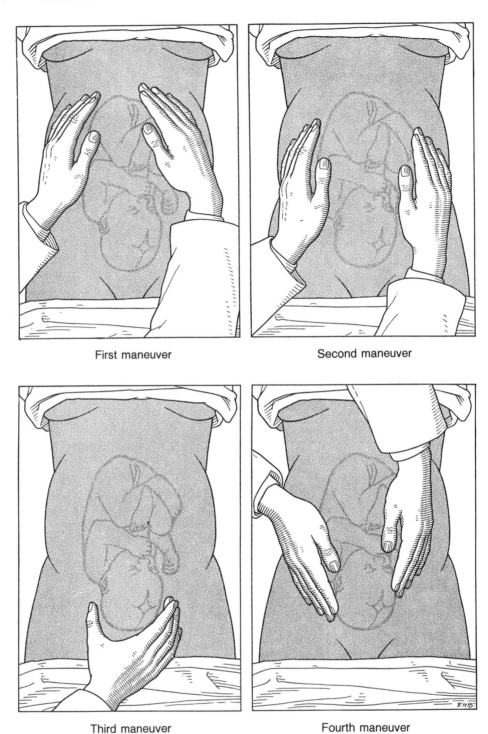

First maneuver

Second maneuver

Third maneuver

Fourth maneuver

FIG. 12-15. Palpation in right occiput posterior position.

ing part has descended into the pelvis. For example, so long as the cephalic prominence is readily palpable, the vertex has not descended to the level of the ischial spines. The degree of cephalopelvic disproportion, moreover, can be gauged by evaluating the extent to which the anterior portion of the fetal head overrides the mother's symphysis pubis. With experience, it is possible to estimate the size of the fetus and even to map out the presentation of the second fetus in a twin gestation.

During labor, palpation also may provide valuable information about the lower uterine segment. When there is obstruction to the passage of the fetus, a pathologic retraction ring sometimes may be felt as a transverse or oblique ridge extending across the lower portion of the uterus (see Chap. 29, p. 795). Moreover, even in normal cases, the contracting body of the uterus and the passive lower uterine segment may be distinguished by palpation. During a contraction, the upper portion of the uterus is firm or hard, whereas the lower segment feels elastic or almost fluctuant.

Vaginal Examination. Before labor, the diagnosis of fetal presentation and position by vaginal examination may be somewhat inconclusive, because the presenting part must be palpated through the lower uterine segment. During labor, however, after dilatation of the cervix, important information may be obtained. In vertex presentations, the position and variety are recognized by differentiation of the various sutures and fontanels; in face presentations, by the differentiation of the portions of the face; and in breech presentations, by the palpation of the sacrum and ischial tuberosities.

In attempting to determine presentation and position by vaginal examination, it is advisable to pursue a definite routine, comprising three maneuvers (Figs. 12-16, 12-17):

1. After the woman is prepared appropriately, as described in Chapter 17, two fingers of either gloved hand of the examiner are introduced into the vagina and carried up to the presenting part. The differentia-

tion of vertex, face, and breech then is accomplished readily.

2. If the vertex is presenting, the examiner's fingers are carried up behind the symphysis pubis and then are swept backward over the fetal head toward the maternal sacrum. During the performance of this movement, the examiner's fingers necessarily cross the sagittal suture. When it is felt, its course is outlined, with small and large fontanels at the opposite ends.

3. The positions of the two fontanels then are ascertained. The examiner's fingers are passed to the anterior extremity of the sagittal suture, and the fontanel encountered there is examined carefully and identified; then by a circular motion, the fingers are passed around the side of the head until the other fontanel is felt and differentiated.

Thus the various sutures and fontanels are located readily, and the possibility of error is lessened considerably. In face and breech presentations, errors are minimized, since the various parts are distinguished more readily.

Auscultation. Auscultation, by itself, does not provide very reliable information concerning the presentation and position of the fetus, but the findings of auscultation sometimes reinforce the results obtained by palpation. Ordinarily, the fetal heart sounds are transmitted through the convex portion of the fetus that lies in intimate contact with the uterine wall. Therefore, fetal heart sounds are heard best through the fetal back in vertex and breech and through the fetal thorax in face presentations. The region of the abdomen in which the fetal heart tones are heard most clearly varies according to the presentation and the extent to which the presenting part has descended. In cephalic presentations, the point of maximal intensity of fetal heart sounds usually is midway between the maternal umbilicus and the anterior superior spine of her ilium, whereas in breech presentations it is usually about level with the umbilicus. In occipitoanterior positions, the heart sounds usually are heard best

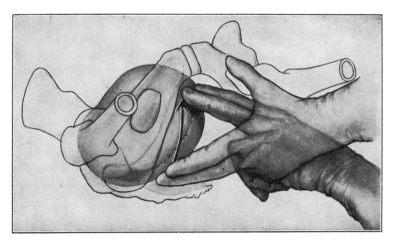

FIG. 12-16. Locating the sagittal suture on vaginal examination.

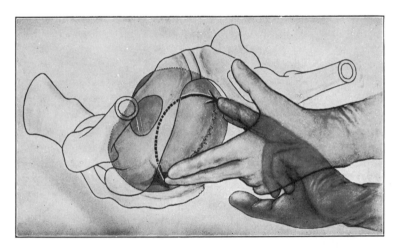

FIG. 12-17. Differentiating the fontanels on vaginal examination.

a short distance from the midline, in the transverse varieties they are heard more laterally, and in the posterior varieties well back in the mother's flank.

X-ray and Sonar. Improvements in roentgenographic technic have provided another diagnostic aid of particular value in doubtful cases. In obese women or in women whose abdominal walls are rigid, an x-ray examination may provide information to solve many diagnostic problems and lead to early recognition of a breech or shoulder presentation that might otherwise have escaped detection until late in labor. Employing ultrasonography, the fetal head and body can be located without the potential hazards of ionizing radiation (see Chap. 14, p. 344).

REFERENCES

Leopold and Sporlin: Conduct of normal births through external examination alone. Arch Gynaekol 45:337,1894

White AJ: Spontaneous cephalic version in the later weeks of pregnancy and its significance in the management of breech presentation. Br J Obstet Gynaecol 63:706,1956

13

Prenatal Care

The objective of prenatal care is to assure that every wanted pregnancy culminates in the delivery of a healthy baby without impairing the health of the mother.

Significance. Before the rise of present-day obstetrics, the pregnant woman usually had but a single antepartum interview with a physician. At that interview, often not much more was accomplished than an attempt to anticipate the date of delivery. When next seen by the physician, the woman might be in the throes of an eclamptic convulsion, or suffering severe chills and high fever from pyelonephritis, or struggling to expel a very large but dead fetus. Appropriate antepartum care has proven to be of great value in the prevention of such catastrophes.

It hardly needs saying that prenatal care should do no harm. Nonetheless, prenatal care, at times, has been a two-edged sword. Instead of improving pregnancy outcome, on occasion, the exact opposite was accomplished in a variety of ways, including inappropriate dietary advice to achieve rigid weight restriction, the unnecessary prescription of potentially dangerous drugs such as powerful diuretics, and by not encouraging

the immediate reporting of an abnormal event, but rather have the expectant mother wait to do so at the next scheduled office or clinic visit.

A priori pregnancy should be considered a normal physiologic state. Unfortunately, the complexity of the functional and anatomic changes that accompany gestation tends in the minds of some to stigmatize normal pregnancy as a disease process. For example, a hemoglobin concentration of 11.0 g per dl is abnormally low for the woman who is not pregnant but not if she is late in the second trimester of pregnancy, a plasma thyroxine level of 16 μg per dl is normal during pregnancy but is very strongly suggestive of hyperthyroidism in the absence of pregnancy unless the woman is receiving exogenous estrogen. At times, pregnancy imposes other changes that when modest in degree are normal, but when more intense are decidedly abnormal. An example, edema of the feet and ankles after ambulation, is the normal consequence of regional physical forces imposed by the large pregnant uterus and by gravity. Generalized edema obvious in the face, hands, and abdomen, however, is definitely abnormal. **Therefore, it is essential for the physician who assumes responsibil-**

ity for prenatal care to be very familiar with the changes in normalities as well as abnormalities imposed by pregnancy.

Good prenatal care is vital for the accomplishment of the objective stated at the outset, namely, the delivery of a healthy baby from a healthy mother. An attempt has been made in this chapter to delineate many of the ingredients essential to good prenatal care. Bad prenatal care may be worse than none. All to often, inadequate prenatal care provides the expectant mother with an unwarranted sense of security that allows her to ignore signs and symptoms for which, if left to her own instincts, she would have urgently sought advice.

GENERAL HEALTH CARE. Systematic health care beginning long before pregnancy undoubtedly proves quite beneficial to the physical and emotional health of the mother-to-be and, in turn, her child-to-be. Therefore, prenatal care ideally should be a continuation of a regimen of physician-supervised health care already established for the woman. As the consequence of such a program, acquired diseases and developmental abnormalities, for the most part, will have been recognized before pregnancy and appropriate steps can be taken to eradicate them or, at least, to minimize their deleterious effects. In any event, the mother should be seen as early in pregnancy as possible and at appropriate intervals thereafter.

TERMINOLOGY

Definitions

A *nulligravida* is a woman who is not now and never has been pregnant.

A *gravida* is a woman who is or has been pregnant irrespective of the pregnancy outcome. With the establishment of the first pregnancy, she becomes a primigravida and with successive pregnancies a multigravida.

A *nullipara* is a woman who has never completed a pregnancy to the stage of viability.

She may or may not have aborted previously.

A *primipara* is a woman who has been delivered once of a fetus or fetuses who reached the stage of viability. Therefore, the completion of any pregnancy beyond the stage of abortion (see Chap. 24, p. 587) bestows parity upon the mother.

A *multipara* is a woman who has completed two or more pregnancies to the stage of viability. It is the number of pregnancies reaching viability and not the number of fetuses delivered that determines *parity.* Parity is not greater if a single fetus, twins, or quintuplets were delivered, nor fewer if the fetus or fetuses were stillborn.

In certain clinics, it is customary to summarize the past obstetric history of a woman by a series of digits connected by dashes as follows: 6-1-2-6. The first digit refers to the number of term infants, the second to the number of premature infants, the third to the number of abortions, and the fourth to the number of children currently alive. For the example given of 6-1-2-6, the woman has had six term deliveries, one premature delivery, two abortions, and has six children alive at present. This series of digits obviously gives a more complete obstetric history than the mere designation *gravida 9, para 7.*

A *parturient* is a woman in labor.

A *puerpera* is a woman who has just given birth.

Normal Duration of Pregnancy. The average duration of pregnancy calculated from the first day of the last normal menstrual period averages very close to 280 days, or 40 weeks. Kortenoever (1950), in an analysis of 7504 pregnancies, found the average duration to be 282 days. Moreover, the mean value of 281 days was calculated from data of the Obstetrical Statistical Cooperative for 77,300 women who underwent spontaneous labor and whose infants weighed at least 2500 g. Nakano (1972) identified for 5596 pregnancies in Osaka, Japan, the mean duration to be 279 days from the first day of the last menstrual period with two standard deviations of ±17 days. All pregnancies that terminated before 28 weeks gestation were excluded by Nakano, as were breeches and multiple births.

It is customary to estimate the expected date of delivery by adding 7 days to the date of the first day of the last normal menstrual period and counting back 3 months (Naegele's rule). For example, if the woman's last menstrual period began on September 10, the expected date of delivery would be June 17. It is apparent that pregnancy "begins" on the average 2 weeks before ovulation if the duration of pregnancy is so calculated from the first day of the last menstrual period. Clinicians use *gestational age,* or *menstrual age,* calculated from the first day of the last menstrual period to identify temporal events in pregnancy; embryologists and other biologists more often employ *ovulatory age,* or *fertilization age,* which is typically 2 weeks shorter.

It has become customary to divide pregnancy into three equal parts, or *trimesters,* of slightly more than 13 weeks, or 3 calendar months, each. There are certain major obstetric problems that cluster in each of these time periods. For example, most spontaneous abortions occur during the first trimester, whereas practically all cases of pregnancy-induced hypertension become clinically evident during the third trimester. The clinical use of trimesters to describe the duration of a specific pregnancy should be abandoned, however. It is inappropriate in case of uterine hemorrhage, for example, to categorize the problem temporally as "third trimester bleeding." Appropriate management for the mother and her fetus will vary remarkably, depending upon whether the bleeding occurs early or late in the third trimester.

Precise knowledge of the age of the fetus is imperative for ideal obstetric management. Therefore, expert attention must be given to this important measurement. The clinically appropriate unit of measure is Weeks of Gestation Completed.

GENERAL PROCEDURES

Every word and every act by all who come in contact with the pregnant woman should impress upon her both the importance and the availability of prenatal care for her fetus and herself. All too often, especially in public clinics, the strong impression has been propagated that such care is not really available without great expenditure of physical and emotional effort, and, at times, of money beyond the woman's ability to pay. It is tragic when women and their fetuses are denied adequate prenatal care simply because of lack of funds. Over and above the humanitarian aspects, the cost for good prenatal care is modest compared to the expense of caring subsequently for serious, but preventable, complications in the mother and her fetus. It is also unfortunate that, among those who in one way or another come in contact with the pregnant woman who seeks prenatal care, there may be some who display an intolerance for the poor, for the unwed, and for the mother's particular ethnic group. In such circumstances, the best of medical care often goes to waste.

Initial Care.   Prenatal care should be initiated as soon as there is reasonable likelihood of pregnancy. This may be as early as a few days after a missed menstrual period, especially for the woman who desires an abortion, but it should be no later than the second missed period for anyone.

In order to initiate antepartum care early, the system that has been developed at Parkland Memorial Hospital has, in general, proved effective. The woman is seen any day of the week without an appointment. At this initial visit nurses with expertness in obstetric care identify the following: (1) the probability of pregnancy (including urine testing for hCG when indicated), (2) the woman's desire for the pregnancy to continue, (3) any current health problems, (4) any previous major illnesses, including those in previous pregnancies, (5) the outcomes of previous pregnancies, and (6) all medications being used.

The woman is instructed to bring with her at the next visit all drugs that she has been taking.

Initial physical evaluation by the nurse includes determination of blood pressure, height, and weight.

The following laboratory examinations are initiated at the first visit: *Blood:* Hemoglobin, hematocrit, red cell indexes, serologic test for syphilis, identification of blood types and abnormal antibodies, and rubella antibody titer if not performed previously. *Urine:* Glucose, protein, and quantitative culture of clean catch midstream urine to identify significant bacteriuria (at least 100,000 organisms per ml).

Physicians are continually available in the clinic and are consulted by the nurse whenever a problem is suspected that might require immediate attention. Any woman who is considering abortion is seen by a physician at this time. Moreover, every woman is asked specifically if she wishes to see a physician at this screening visit. Finally, she is given explicit instructions as to how to obtain information by phone and where to get help promptly in case of emergency.

It is difficult to convince the pregnant woman of the importance of prenatal care if, when she seeks it, the physician delays for many weeks her initial care! Even in the absence of identified pregnancy problems, all women are given appointments within 10 days, for completion by a physician of a comprehensive general health evaluation. Previous health records and all laboratory data are reviewed at that time.

INITIAL COMPREHENSIVE EVALUATION

Goals. The major goals of this examination are (1) to define the health status of the mother and fetus, (2) to determine the gestational age of the fetus, and (3) to initiate a plan for continuing obstetric care. Once the health status of the mother and fetus has been defined, the initial plan for subsequent care may range from relatively infrequent routine visits to either prompt therapeutic abortion or prolonged hospitalization because of serious maternal or fetal disease.

History. For the most part, the same essentials go into appropriate history taking from the pregnant woman as elsewhere in medicine. The history should be obtained unhurriedly in a reasonably private setting. This is the best time for the physician and for those who assist in providing care for the expectant mother and her fetus to establish the good rapport so necessary to a successful outcome of the pregnancy. Although it is undesirable for the woman to wait for protracted periods of time before interview, it is far worse for her to be hurriedly and indifferently interrogated without having her answers appropriately evaluated. **It is mandatory that all data important to the care of the mother and fetus be clearly recorded so that all members of the health care team that use the record can correctly interpret them.**

The *menstrual history* is extremely important. The woman who spontaneously menstruates regularly every 28 days or so is very likely to ovulate at midcycle. Thus, the gestational age (menstrual age) becomes simply the number of weeks since the onset of the last menstrual period. If her menstrual cycles were significantly longer than 28 to 30 days, ovulation more likely occurred well beyond 14 days or, if the intervals are much longer and irregular, anovulation may have characterized some of the episodes of vaginal bleeding. In the latter instance, the menstrual data are unreliable for calculating the duration of the gestation.

It is important to ascertain whether or not *steroidal contraceptives* were used before the pregnancy and, if so, when. It is now common for women who sustain regularly recurring withdrawal bleeding while using oral contraceptives cyclically to stop their use and to conceive with no further menstrual-like bleeding. Ovulation, however, may not have resumed two weeks after the onset of the last withdrawal bleeding but, instead, at an appreciably later date. The difficult problem of predicting the time of ovulation in this circumstance is similar to that in which pregnancy occurs following delivery or abortion prior to the reestablishment of normal menstrual periods.

The possibility of the presence of an *intrauterine device* should be ascertained, since certain pregnancy complications are increased by its presence in utero (see Chap. 40, p. 1026). Its fate must also be clearly recorded.

Physical Examination. The cervix is visualized employing a speculum lightly lubricated on the outside of each blade. Next, in order to identify cytologic abnormalities, a gentle swabbing from the lower half of the cervical canal and then a scraping from the squamocolumnar junction are obtained and spread on separate slides and fixed immediately in ether-alcohol or by a special aerosol fixative. The outer half of the cervical canal is again swabbed carefully for gonococci and the applicator stick is rolled over Trans-Grow medium or another suitable transport medium while the container is held vertically to prevent loss of the carbon dioxide-enriched air in the culture bottle. The specimens are labeled immediately and accurately and then processed appropriately.

Bluish-red passive hyperemia of the cervix characteristic of, but not diagnostic of, pregnancy is searched for. If the cervix is dilated, this may, at times, be identified by visualizing membranes through the speculum. The character of vaginal secretions is noted. A moderate amount of white mucoid discharge is normal. The presence of foamy yellow liquid in the vagina is strongly suggestive of *Trichomonas* while the presence of a curdlike discharge is consistent with *Candida* infection (p. 325). Material may be swabbed from the vagina for microscopic examination or for culture.

The speculum is removed and the internal pelvic examination is completed by palpation with special attention given to the consistency, length, and dilatation of the cervix; to the fetal presenting part, especially if late in pregnancy; to the bony architecture of the pelvis; and to any anomalies of the vagina and perineum, including cystocele, rectocele, and relaxed or torn perineum. The vulva and contiguous structures are carefully inspected. (The pelvic examination is described in more detail in Chapter 17, p. 406). All cervical, vaginal, and vulvar lesions should be evaluated further by appropriate use of colposcopy, biopsy, culture, or darkfield examination. Rectal examination should be done to identify hemorrhoids or other lesions.

Between 18 and 30 weeks of gestation, there is an excellent correlation between the height of the uterine fundus above the symphysis pubis and the age of the fetus which is, simply, the height in cm equals the gestational age in weeks. Therefore, it is important for the examiner to document carefully the height of fundus, as described below (p. 306).

The general physical examination includes evaluation of the teeth. Repair of carious teeth should be undertaken promptly. Varicose veins should be looked for and when identified, frequent postural drainage should be urged and elastic support stockings provided.

Further Instructions. After the history and physical examination have been completed, the expectant mother is instructed about diet, relaxation and sleep, bowel habits, exercise, bathing, clothing, recreation, general care, smoking, and drug and alcohol ingestion. Usually it is possible to assure her that she may anticipate an uneventful pregnancy followed by an uncomplicated delivery. **At the same time, she is tactfully instructed about the following danger signals, which must be reported immediately, day or night:**

1. Any vaginal bleeding
2. Swelling of the face or fingers
3. Severe or continuous headache
4. Dimness or blurring of vision

5. Abdominal pain
6. Persistent vomiting
7. Chills or fever
8. Dysuria
9. Escape of fluid from the vagina

Also, she is instructed precisely as to what steps she must take if a scheduled prenatal examination is missed.

Prognosis. All information obtained should be employed to identify accurately the gestational age of the fetus and to anticipate the kinds and the magnitude of morbidity, both maternal and fetal, that may develop subsequently. Often, when morbidity is anticipated, its intensity can be minimized by appropriate care.

SUBSEQUENT PRENATAL CARE

Return Visits. Traditionally, the timing of subsequent prenatal examinations have been scheduled at intervals of 4 weeks throughout the first 7 months, then every 2 weeks until the last month, and weekly thereafter. Rather often, however, important information can be gained from a more flexible appointment schedule. For example, at mid-pregnancy, certain clinically discernible events chacteristically occur that, when precisely identified, enhance greatly the reliability of the estimate of the gestational age of the fetus.

AUDIBLE FETAL HEART SOUNDS. In essentially all pregnancies the fetal heart may be first heard between 16 and 19 weeks of gestation when carefully listened for with a fetal stethoscope (see Chap. 10, p. 261).

FUNDAL HEIGHT. Measurement of the height of the uterine fundus above the symphysis can provide useful information. Jimenez and co-workers (1979) demonstrated that between the 18th and 30th weeks of gestation the fundal height in cm equals the gestational age in weeks. The top of the fun-

dus was identified by percussion, as well as palpation. They measured with a tape calibrated in centimeters and applied over the abdominal curvature the distance between the symphysis pubis and the top of the fundus. Distortion from urine in the bladder was eliminated by having the woman void before examination.

GESTATIONAL AGE. When the date of onset of the last normal menstrual period and fundal height are in temporal agreement, the duration of gestation can be firmly established. When gestational age cannot be clearly identified, sonography may prove to be of considerable value (see Chap. 14, p. 345).

Later in pregnancy precise knowledge of gestational age is likely to be of considerable importance since a number of pregnancy complications may develop, the optimal treatment for which will depend on fetal age. For example, with the development of maternal hypertension at 38 weeks, very often delivery is the treatment most beneficial to both mother and fetus. However, if the duration of gestation is only 30 weeks when hypertension develops, attempts at medical management with delayed delivery may be more beneficial for the quite premature fetus.

At each return visit steps are taken to identify the well-being of the expectant mother, as well as that of her fetus. Certain information, obtained by interrogation and by examination, is especially important in this regard:

Maternal
1. Blood pressure, actual and extent of change
2. Weight, actual and amount of change
3. Symptoms, including headache, altered vision, abdominal pain, nausea and vomiting, bleeding, fluid from vagina, dysuria
4. Height of uterine fundus above symphysis
5. Position, consistency, effacement, and dilatation of the cervix (late in pregnancy)

Fetal
1. Fetal heart rate(s)
2. Size of fetus(es), actual and rate of change

3. Amount of amnionic fluid
4. Presenting part and station (late in pregnancy)
5. Fetal activity

A carefully performed vaginal examination near term often provides valuable information:

1. Confirmation of the presenting part
2. Station (depth in the pelvis) of the presenting part (see Chap. 17, p. 407).
3. Clinical mensuration of the pelvis and an appreciation of its general configuration (see Chap. 11, p. 280).
4. The consistency, effacement, and dilatation of the cervix. Digital exploration must be conducted with care lest an undiagnosed low-lying placenta be separated, causing severe hemorrhage

SUBSEQUENT LABORATORY TESTS. If the initial results were quite normal, most of the procedures need not be repeated. Hematocrit determination and perhaps the serologic test for syphilis, should be repeated at 32 to 34 weeks gestation. A cervical culture for gonorrhea may be repeated at the time of the pelvic examination near term, especially if gonorrhea is relatively common in the population being cared for.

Routine urine examination at every clinic visit is rarely warranted. Practically all women who develop preeclampsia develop a significant rise in blood pressure, and many have a sudden gain in weight before proteinuria develops. Therefore, proteinuria need only be looked for selectively in those women who develop an increase in blood pressure or marked increase in weight. Fasting and postprandial plasma glucose levels are much more informative than are tests for glucosuria in the case of the woman with a strong family history of diabetes, or previous large infants, or, who during the current pregnancy, has an unusually large fetus. Even so, glucosuria cannot be ignored.

All pertinent information obtained at each visit must be recorded legibly in such a way that anyone who uses the pregnancy record

at any time can appreciate the significance of the information available.

NUTRITION DURING PREGNANCY

Throughout most of this century, the diets of pregnant women have been the subject of endless discussions that often resulted in considerable confusion. Various enthusiasts have urged pregnant women to adhere to a wide variety of diets, ranging from those that emphasize rigid caloric restriction to those that provide unusually large amounts of protein as well as calories. Faulty reasoning led some obstetricians to advise rigid caloric restriction, a recommendation that stemmed primarily from the observation that a prominent feature of preeclampsia and eclampsia was excessive weight gain. That the weight gain in preeclampsia and eclampsia actually results from edema rather than excessive caloric intake was not generally appreciated.

Meaningful studies of nutrition in human pregnancy are exceedingly difficult to design. Ethically, dietary deficiency must not be reproduced experimentally in pregnant women. In those instances in which severe nutritional deficiencies have been induced as a consequence of social, economic, or political disaster, coincidental events often have created many variables, the effects of which are not amenable to quantitation. Some past experiences suggest, however, that a state of near starvation must be induced to establish clear differences in pregnancy outcome, as for example, the starvation imposed on pregnant women during the occupation of the Netherlands late in World War II.

During the winter of 1944–45 nutritional deprivation of known intensity prevailed in a well-circumscribed area of the Netherlands. As pointed out by Stein and associates (1972), the type and the degree of nutritional deprivation during the famine was identified with a precision unequaled in any large population before or since. At the lowest point, rations reached 450 kcal per day, with generalized undernutrition rather than selective malnutrition. Shortly after the end of the war, Smith (1947) analyzed the outcomes of pregnancies that were in progress during this six-month period of famine. *The median birth weights of infants were decreased about 8 ounces. The weights rose again after food became available in a way that indicated that birth weight can be influenced significantly by starvation during the latter half of pregnancy.* The perinatal mortality rate, however, was not increased, nor was the incidence of malformations significantly increased.

Evidence of impaired brain development has been obtained in some animal fetuses whose mothers during pregnancy had been subjected to dietary deprivation. These animal studies, in turn, stimulated interest in the subsequent intellectual development of the now young adults in the Netherlands whose mothers had been starved during pregnancy. A comprehensive study by Stein and co-workers (1972) was made feasible by the fact that practically all males at age 19 undergo compulsory examination for military service. From their extensive analyses, Stein and associates concluded that the severe dietary deprivation during pregnancy caused no detectable effects on the mental performance of the surviving male offspring.

Caution must be exercised in extrapolating from one species to another. For example, severe protein deprivation of a few days duration in the pregnant rat, in which gestation is only 21 days and in which total fetal weight represents 25 percent of maternal weight, may lead to serious reproductive casualties. In human pregnancy, which lasts 266 days and in which fetal weight is only 5 percent that of the mother, failure to ingest protein for the same number of days could hardly be expected to produce an insult of the same intensity.

Weight Gain During Pregnancy. During a normal pregnancy with a single fetus, a weight gain of 20 pounds (9 kg) can be anticipated just on the basis of obvious pregnancy-induced physiologic changes. These include an increase of 11 pounds for intrauterine contents that include the fetus (7½ pounds), placenta and membranes (1½

pounds), and amnionic fluid (2 pounds), in addition to a maternal contribution of 8 pounds, resulting from increases in the weights of the uterus (2½ pounds), blood (3½ pounds), and breasts (2 pounds). Moderate expansion of interstitial fluid in the pelvis and lower extremities is a normal event attributable to the increased venous pressure created by the large pregnant uterus. In the ambulatory woman, it most likely amounts to at least 2 to 3 pounds. There is, therefore, a physiologic basis for a maternal weight gain of at least 20 pounds (9 kg).

For the woman whose weight is normal before pregnancy, a gain of 20 pounds appears to be associated with the most favorable outcome of pregnancy (Naeye, 1979). In most pregnant women, this result may be achieved by eating, according to appetite, a diet adequate in calories, protein, essential fatty acids, minerals, and vitamins. Seldom, if ever, should maternal weight gain be restricted deliberately below this level. **Indeed, failure of the pregnant woman to gain weight is an ominous sign.**

Eastman and Jackson (1968) carefully evaluated the relation between maternal weight gain and birth weight in term pregnancies and found that, in general, birth weight paralleled maternal weight gain. The full significance of this relationship is best appreciated when the fate of low-birth-weight infants is considered. The neonatal mortality rate for chronologically mature white newborns weighing 2500 g or less was 45.1 per 1000 live births, in contrast to 6.1 per 1000 lives births for those whose weight exceeded 2500 g.

Undoubtedly, failure of the mother to gain weight was caused in some instances by associated maternal disease rather than just imposed caloric restriction. Nonetheless, in spite of the experiences in the Netherlands, observations such as those of Eastman and Jackson, coupled with those from several well-controlled animal studies demonstrating deleterious effects on the offspring when severe maternal caloric restriction was imposed, point out that rigid caloric restriction during pregnancy can be dangerous to the fetus.

Eastman and Jackson found that the incidence of low birth weight was greatest in pregnant women whose weight was low before pregnancy and whose weight gain was low during gestation. Therefore, they recommend that women whose weight before pregnancy is less than 120 pounds be urged to eat according to appetite, at least during the first half of pregnancy. At about the 20th week, weight gain should be reviewed. If it is less than 10 pounds, someone who possesses nutritional expertise should evaluate the diet and make appropriate corrections so that weight gain approaches a pound a week.

A Task Force on Nutrition of the American College of Obstetricians and Gynecologists (1978) has emphasized that the nutritional status of the expectant mother is more likely to be compromised in any of the following circumstances:

1. She is under 16 years of age.
2. She is economically deprived.
3. She has had 3 or more pregnancies within 2 years.
4. Her past reproductive performance has been poor.
5. She consumes a therapeutic diet in the course of management of some preexisting disease.
6. She is a food faddist.
7. She smokes, drinks, or uses hard drugs.
8. She is appreciably underweight at the outset.
9. The hematocrit drops much below 33 or the hemoglobin concentration falls much below 11 g/dl.
10. Weight gain for any month during the second and third trimesters is less than 2 pounds.

Recommended Dietary Allowances.
Periodically, the Food and Nutrition Board of the National Research Council recommends dietary allowances for women, including those who are pregnant or lactating. Their recent recommendations are summarized in Table 13-1. For certain nutrients, the Board made higher recommendations for the nonpregnant teenager compared to older women of reproductive age. Where this oc-

curs, the recommended value for 15 to 18 years of age is given for each nutrient.

Calories. A daily caloric increase throughout pregnancy of 300 kcal has been recommended by the Food and Nutrition Board. Calories are necessary for energy production. Whenever caloric intake is inadequate, protein may be metabolized as a source of energy, rather than being spared for its vital role in growth and development. The importance of adequate caloric intake is emphasized by a relatively recent nutrition intervention study in Guatemala which identified infant birth weights to be larger when the marginal diets of the mothers were supplemented (Delgado et al., 1977). In two of four villages a high protein calorie supplement was made available; in the other two villages a drink that provided calories without protein was offered. Birth weights were influenced by the number of calories ingested rather than by the protein content of the supplements. For those pregnancies in which less than 10,000 supplemental kcal were ingested, birth weight averaged 2986 g and 18.3 percent of the infants weighed less than 2500 g. For those pregnancies in which more than 20,000 kcal were consumed in the form of supplements, the mean birth weight was 3120 g and only 9.4 percent, or one-half as many, infants weighed less than 2500 g at birth. These studies serve to emphasize the importance of caloric intake on birth weight.

Protein. To the basic protein needs of the nonpregnant woman for repair of her tissues are added the demands for growth and repair of the fetus, placenta, uterus and breasts, and increased maternal blood volume. During the last six months of pregnancy about 1 kg of protein, or 5 to 6 g per day, is deposited (Hytten, Leitch, 1971).

It is desirable that the majority of the protein be supplied from animal sources such as meat, milk, eggs, cheese, poultry, and fish, since they furnish amino acids in optimal combinations. Milk and milk products have long been considered nearly ideal sources of nutrients, especially protein and calcium, for pregnant or lactating women. Nonetheless,

TABLE 13-1.
RECOMMENDED DAILY DIETARY ALLOWANCES FOR WOMEN
163 CM (64") TALL AND WEIGHING 55 KG (121 LBS.)

NUTRIENT	NONPREGNANT	INCREASE	
		Pregnant	Lactating
Kilocalories	2100	300	500
Protein (g)	44*	30	20
Vitamin A (RE)†	800	200	400
Vitamin D (μg)‡	7.5	5	5
Vitamin E (mg T.E.)§	10	2	3
Ascorbic Acid (mg)	60	20	40
Folacin (mg)‖	0.4	0.4	0.1
Niacin (mg)#	14	2	5
Riboflavin (mg)	1.3	0.3	0.5
Thiamin (mg)	1.1	0.4	0.5
Vitamin B_6 (mg)	2.0	0.6	0.5
Vitamin B_{12} (μg)	3.0	1.0	1.0
Calcium (mg)	800	400	400
Phosphorus (mg)	800	400	400
Iodine (μg)	150	25	50
Iron (mg)	18	Supplement**	0
Magnesium (mg)	300	150	150
Zinc (mg)	15	5	10

* 46 g if under 19 years of age
† 1 μg retinol = 1 retinol equivalent (R.E.)
‡ As cholecalciferol; 100 International Units = 2.5 μg of cholecalciferol
§ T.E. = tocopherol equivalent
‖ Refers to dietary sources ascertained by Lactobacillus casei assay; pteroylglutamic acid may be effective in smaller doses
Includes dietary sources of the vitamin plus 1 mg equivalent for each 60 mg of dietary tryptophan
** Increased requirement cannot be met by ordinary diets; therefore supplementation recommended (see text)
From Recommended Dietary Allowances, 9th ed., National Academy of Sciences, Washington, D.C., 1979

milk (lactose) intolerance in the form of gastrointestinal disturbances that include bloating, flatulence, and cramps is a problem in some adults. For example, abnormal lactose tolerance was found in 81 percent of black adults compared to 12 percent of whites in the studies of Bayless and co-workers (1975). As little as 240 ml of milk caused the unpleasant symptoms.

A "high" protein diet has been urged by some enthusiasts who contend that most problems of pregnancy are amenable to manipulation of maternal diet. The desirability of consuming inordinately large amounts of protein must be questioned from the standpoint of safety, as well as economics. Analyses

of several studies by Stein and associates (1978) have failed to demonstrate an improvement in birth weight due specifically to a protein-rich supplement. In fact, they are concerned that the reverse might sometimes be the consequence. The Food and Nutrition Board has recommended for young nonpregnant women a protein intake of about 0.9 g per kg per day, and an additional 30 g of protein per day is recommended during pregnancy.

Minerals.   The intakes recommended by the Food and Nutrition Board for a variety of minerals are presented in Table 13-1 and discussed below. There is good evidence that only one mineral, iron, need be given to pregnant women as a supplement. Practically all diets that supply sufficient calories for appropriate weight gain will contain enough of the other minerals to prevent a mineral deficiency if iodized salt is used.

IRON. There are increased iron requirements during pregnancy, the reasons for which are discussed in Chapter 9 (p. 234). Of the approximately 300 mg of iron transferred to the fetus and placenta and the 500 mg incorporated into the expanding maternal hemoglobin mass, nearly all is utilized during the latter half of pregnancy. During that time, the average iron requirements imposed by the pregnancy itself are about 6 mg a day and, in addition, there is the need for nearly 1 mg to compensate for maternal excretion, or a total of about 7 mg of iron per day (Pritchard, Scott, 1970). Very few women have sufficient iron stores to supply this amount of iron. Moreover, the diet seldom contains enough iron to meet this demand. The recommendation by the Food and Nutrition Board (Table 13-1) of 18 mg of dietary iron per day for nonpregnant women represents the ceiling imposed by caloric requirements. To ingest any more iron from dietary sources would simultaneously provide an undesirable excess of calories. The Board has acknowledged that because of small iron stores the pregnant woman often will be unable to meet the iron requirements imposed by pregnancy and therefore has recommended supplementation.

Supplementation with medicinal iron is commonly practiced in the United States and elsewhere, although the merits of this practice continue to be questioned by a minority of investigators, as cited below. Scott and co-workers (1970) established that 30 mg of iron supplied in the form of a simple iron salt such as ferrous gluconate, sulfate, or fumarate, and taken regularly once each day throughout the latter half of pregnancy provided sufficient iron to meet the requirements of pregnancy and to protect any preexisting iron stores. Iron, 30 mg daily, as a simple salt, should also provide for the iron require-

ments of lactation. The pregnant woman who is large, who has twin fetuses, who is late in pregnancy, who takes iron irregularly, or whose hemoglobin level is somewhat depressed, may benefit from 60 to 100 mg of iron per day. The woman who is overtly anemic from iron deficiency responds well to 200 mg of iron per day in divided doses (see Chap. 28, p. 715).

Since iron requirements are slight during the first four months of pregnancy, it is not necessary to provide supplemental iron during this time. Withholding iron during early pregnancy avoids the risk of aggravating nausea and vomiting, which are common at that time. Ingestion of iron at bedtime will also minimize the possibility of an adverse gastrointestinal reaction. Keeping the container in proximity to toothpaste enhances the ability of the expectant mother to remember to ingest the supplement regularly. Iron-containing medications must be kept out of the reach of small children lest they ingest a large number of the usually quite attractive tablets or capsules.

DEFICIENCY VS. OVERSUFFICIENCY OF IRON.   Paintin and co-workers (1966), Taylor and Lind (1976), and others have contended that iron supplements stimulate hematologic changes in pregnant women even when they are iron sufficient. Moreover, Taylor and Lind question whether iron preparations can be given safely to all pregnant women because of the increase in mean red cell volume that is likely to follow. The results of a number of studies that refute both of these contentions were cited at the Ross Conference on Obstetrical Decisions and Neonatal Outcomes (Pritchard, 1979). In brief, there is good evidence that a higher hemoglobin concentration depends on whether or not iron is available, irrespective of whether or not it is derived from stores or from supplements, or from both. The similarity of the magnitude of the increases observed in several studies performed over the past quarter century is apparent in Table 13-2. Importantly, the average increase equals the hemoglobin content of 500 ml of normal donor

TABLE 13-2.
STUDIES OF THE EFFECTS
OF IRON SUPPLEMENTATION DURING PREGNANCY
ON HEMOGLOBIN CONCENTRATION, 1958–77

	HEMOGLOBIN (G/DL)		
	Unsupplemented	Supplemented	Difference
Chanarin et al. (1977)	11.2	12.8	+1.6
Taylor and Lind (1976)	11.0	12.3	+1.3
Paintin et al. (1966)	10.7	12.0	+1.3
DeLeeuw et al. (1966)	10.9	12.4	+1.5
Chisholm (1966)	11.2	12.4	+1.2
Pritchard and Hunt (1958)	11.3	12.5	+1.2
Average	11.05	12.40	+1.35

From Pritchard: Ross Laboratories Conference on Obstetrical Decisions and Neonatal Outcomes, Columbus, Ohio, 1979

blood. Especially in the nearly 20 percent of women who are now delivered by cesarean section, the presence or absence of such an increase may determine whether or not they are transfused.

The moderate increases in maternal mean red cell volume that concerned Taylor and Lind (1976) have a physiologic basis; recently synthesized red cells are larger than are older red cells.

CALCIUM. The expectant mother retains about 30 g of calcium during pregnancy, most of which is deposited in the fetus late in pregnancy (Pitkin, 1975). This amount of calcium represents only about 2.5 percent of the total maternal calcium, most of which is in bone, and which can be readily mobilized for fetal growth. Moreover, Heaney and Skillman (1971) demonstrated increased absorption of calcium by the intestine and progressive retention throughout pregnancy. In a few places in the world *osteomalacia* is still recognized in women who are reproducing but only under the very unusual circumstances of almost total avoidance of sunlight coupled with low vitamin D intake and low calcium intake for very long periods. Bound calcium levels, but probably not ionized calcium, fall slightly in maternal plasma as the concentration of albumin decreases.

One quart of cow's milk provides approximately 1 g of calcium. Although calcium sup-

plementation during pregnancy has been widely practiced in the United States, it is unlikely to be of any benefit even when the traditional quart of milk per day is not consumed.

PHOSPHORUS. The ubiquitous distribution of phosphorus assures an adequate intake during pregnancy. Plasma levels of inorganic phosphorus do not differ appreciably from nonpregnant levels.

ZINC. Deficiency of zinc may lead to poor appetite, suboptimal growth, and impaired wound healing. Profound zinc deficiency may cause dwarfism and hypogonadism. The rationale for increasing the recommended zinc intake during pregnancy is not altogether clear. There is not strong evidence at this time that dietary supplementation with zinc in the United States is of any benefit to the expectant mother or fetus. Plasma zinc levels are usually depressed in human zinc deficiency but hypozincemia does not necessarily indicate body depletion of zinc. Levels may become depressed with infection, hyperestrogenemia, and hypoalbuminemia. The decrease is quite variable in pregnancy (Hambidge, Mauer, 1978).

IODINE. The use of iodized salt by all pregnant women is recommended to offset the increased need for fetal requirements and probable increased loss through the maternal kidneys. Severe maternal iodine deficiency in expectant mothers predisposes their offspring to endemic cretinism, characterized by multiple severe neurological defects. In parts of New Guinea where this condition was endemic, the intramuscular injection of iodized oil into women very early in pregnancy or before, successfully prevented cretinism in the offspring (Pharoah et al., 1971). The ingestion of iodide in large (pharmacologic) amounts during pregnancy may depress thyroid function and induce a sizable goiter in the fetus. The consumption of large amounts of seaweed by food faddists may do the same.

MAGNESIUM. A deficiency of this element as the consequence of pregnancy has not been recognized. Undoubtedly, during prolonged illness with no magnesium intake, the plasma level might become critically low, as it would in the absence of pregnancy.

POTASSIUM. The concentration of potassium in maternal plasma normally is the same as in nonpregnant plasma or decreases slightly. Potassium deficiency develops in the same circumstances as when not pregnant. Prolonged nausea and vomiting may lead to hypokalemia and metabolic alkalosis. A previously rather common cause—the use of diuretics—has nearly disappeared.

SODIUM. A deficiency of sodium during pregnancy is most unlikely unless diuretics are prescribed or dietary sodium intake is reduced markedly. In general, salting food to taste will provide an abundance of sodium. The concentration of sodium in plasma normally decreases a few milliequivalents during pregnancy.

FLUORIDE. The value of supplemental fluoride during pregnancy has been questioned. Horowitz and Heifitz (1967) investigated the prevalence of caries in temporary and permanent teeth of children with the same postnatal exposure to optimally fluoridated water but different patterns of prenatal exposure. They concluded that there was no

meaningful additional benefits from the ingestion of fluoride in water by the expectant mother if the offspring ingested fluoridated water from birth. Glenn (1979), however, has reported a remarkably lower incidence of caries in children whose mothers ingested 2.2 mg of sodium fluoride daily during pregnancy when compared to those whose mothers used only fluoridated water. She strongly recommended that for structurally-superior and caries-free teeth, 2.2 mg of sodium fluoride be ingested daily while fasting, starting during the third month of pregnancy. Foods or supplements that contain calcium should be avoided for at least one hour after taking the sodium fluoride, since calcium fluoride is not absorbed.

Further investigations are needed to confirm the benefits claimed by Glenn and, at the same time, to detect deleterious effects, if any, from the fluoride.

Vitamins. Most evidence concerning the importance of various vitamins for successful reproduction has been obtained from animal experiments. Typically, severe deficiency has been produced in the animal either by withholding the vitamin completely beginning long before the time of pregnancy, or by giving a very potent vitamin antagonist. The administration of some vitamins in great excess to pregnant animals has been shown to exert deleterious effects on the fetus and newborn.

The practice of supplying vitamin supplements prenatally is a deeply ingrained habit of many obstetricians, even though scientific evidence to show that the usual vitamin supplements are of benefit to either the mother or her fetus is quite meager. The Committee on Maternal Nutrition of the National Research Council pointed out that in the majority of cases routine pharmaceutical supplementation of vitamin and mineral preparations to pregnant women is of doubtful value, except for iron and possibly folic acid. Such vitamin and mineral preparations should not be regarded as substitutes for food.

The increased requirements for vitamins

during pregnancy (Table 13-1) can in practically all circumstances be supplied by any natural diet that provides adequate numbers of calories and amounts of protein, including protein from animal sources. The possible exception is folic acid during times of unusually large requirements, such as pregnancy complicated by hemolytic anemia or pregnancy with multiple fetuses.

FOLIC ACID. Whereas the advantages to be gained from supplemental iron during pregnancy are quite straightforward, namely, protection against maternal iron deficiency and anemia, the benefits to be derived from folic acid supplementation are not nearly so distinct. Hibbard and associates (1969), Fraser and Watt (1964), Streif and Little (1967), and Stone and associates (1967) in the United States implicated maternal folate deficiency in a variety of reproductive casualties, including placental abruption, pregnancy-induced hypertension (toxemia of pregnancy), and fetal anomalies. Their findings, however, have not been confirmed (Alperin et al., 1969; Emery, 1977; Giles, 1966; Hall, 1977; Varadi, 1966; Whalley and associates, 1969; Pritchard, et al., 1969). To date, no one has been able to reduce significantly the frequency of these complications simply by administering folic acid during pregnancy.

Evidence is abundant, however, that maternal folate requirements are increased during pregnancy. In the United States, this increase frequently leads to lowered plasma folate levels, less often to hypersegmentation of neutrophils, infrequently to megaloblastic erythropoiesis, but only rarely to megaloblastic anemia. The amount of folic acid supplement that will prevent these changes varies considerably, depending primarily on the diet consumed by the pregnant woman. Since 1 mg of folic acid orally per day produces a vigorous hematologic response in pregnant women with severe megaloblastic anemia, this amount would almost certainly provide very effective prophylaxis (Pritchard and co-workers, 1969). Chanarin and assocites (1968) found that as little as 0.1 mg of folic

acid per day raised the blood folate level to the normal nonpregnant range. Food and Drug Administration regulations require that vitamin preparations that provide 1 mg of folic acid per day be dispensed only on prescription. Interestingly, those that contain 0.8 mg of folic acid or less do not now require a prescription. If folic acid is prescribed with iron, a desirable combination is a tablet that provides 30 to 60 mg of iron plus 0.3 to 1 mg of folic acid once daily.

VITAMIN B_{12}. The level of vitamin B_{12} in maternal plasma decreases variably in otherwise normal pregnancies (Sauberlich, 1978). The decrease, which is thought to result mostly from a reduction in plasma binders rather than depletion, is prevented only in part by supplementation. However, maternal vitamin B_{12} deficiency can develop in special circumstances. Vitamin B_{12} occurs naturally only in foods of animal origin. It is now established that *strict vegetarians* may give birth to infants whose vitamin B_{12} stores are low. Although vitamin B_{12} levels in cord plasma consistently are higher than in maternal plasma, both increase in parallel fashion. Moreover, since breast milk of a vegetarian mother will most likely contain little vitamin B_{12}, the deficiency may become profound in the breast fed infant (Higginbottom et al., 1978). Thus, the apparently increasing population of pregnant vegetarians should be identified by obtaining a careful dietary history and vitamin B_{12} should be provided as least during pregnancy and while breast feeding.

Excessive ingestion of vitamin C can also lead to a functional deficiency of vitamin B_{12}, as described below under Vitamin C.

VITAMIN B_6. A variety of biochemical changes induced by vitamin B_6 deficiency, including excessive excretion of xanthurenic acid after the ingestion of a tryptophan load, have been summarized by Sauberlich (1978). Several of the changes also accompany otherwise apparently normal pregnancy and have been identified in women who use estrogen-containing oral contraceptives.

Some investigators have related impaired glucose tolerance during pregnancy to altered metabolic pathways induced by low vitamin B_6 levels and, in turn, a lowering of the biological activity of endogenous insulin. However, neither the observations of Perkins (1977), nor those of Gillmer and Mazibuko (1979) provide support for this premise. Gillmer and Mazibuko investigated 13 pregnant women who had abnormal glucose tolerance tests and who excreted elevated amounts of xanthurenic acid after a tryptophan load. Treatment with pyridoxine, 100 mg daily for two to three weeks, restored the urinary excretion of xanthurenic acid to normal levels for nonpregnant individuals but improvement in the glucose tolerance test was observed in only 2 of the 13 pregnant women. There was no change in 5 and deterioration in 6.

As the consequence of some of these observations an appreciable increase in the recommended daily dietary allowance for pyridoxine intake during pregnancy has been urged by some. However, to modify some of the biochemical changes that imply a deficiency of vitamin B_6 during pregnancy requires appreciably more of the vitamin than is now recommended and would likely necessitate specific supplementation. For example, Cleary and associates (1975) emphasized that to raise pyridoxal phosphate levels in maternal plasma to those characteristic of normal nonpregnant women required a daily supplement of pyridoxine of more than 2.5 mg. In fact, in some pregnant women daily supplementation with 10 mg did not accomplish this objective. The benefits that might accrue from larger supplements do not appear at this time to warrant so vigorous an undertaking.

The latest recommendation by the Food and Nutrition Board of the National Research Council calls for 2.0 mg of pyridoxine daily for nonpregnant women and 2.6 mg per day when pregnant or lactating.

VITAMIN C. The recommended dietary allowance for vitamin C during pregnancy is 80 mg per day, or about one-third more than when nonpregnant (see Table 13-1). A reasonable diet should readily provide this amount. The maternal plasma level declines during pregnancy while the cord level is high compared to that of the mother, a phenomenon that is observed with most water-soluble vitamins.

The ingestion of 1 or more g of vitamin C for the prophylaxis of the common cold has become commonplace, even though there is no good evidence that vitamin C when so used is of any benefit and there is evidence that it may prove harmful during pregnancy. Scurvy has been identified in normally fed infants whose mothers had ingested large doses of vitamin C during pregnancy (Cochrane, 1965). Large dose of vitamin C can also interfere with vitamin B_{12} absorption and metabolism. This problem may not be overcome by supplementation with vitamin B_{12} (Herbert, Jacob, 1974).

Pragmatic Nutritional Surveillance. While the science of nutrition continues in its perpetual struggle to identify the ideal amount of protein and other nutrients for the pregnant woman and her fetus, those directly responsible for their care may best discharge their duties as follows:

1. In general, advise the expectant mother to eat what she wants in amounts she desires and salted to taste.
2. Make sure that there is ample food to eat, especially in the case of the socioeconomically deprived woman.
3. Make sure by serially weighing every expectant mother that she is gaining weight with a goal of at least 20 pounds.
4. At each prenatal visit, explore the food intake by dietary recall to uncover the ingestion of any bizarre diet. In this way the occasional nutritionally absurd diet will be discovered for example, the ingestion of a peck of grapes per day or a pound of Argo Gloss Starch.
5. Give tablets of simple iron salts that provide 30 to 60 mg of iron daily.

GENERAL HYGIENE

Exercise. Dangerous activities that carry a risk of bodily injury should be prohibited, but, in general, it is not necessary for the pregnant woman to limit exercise provided she does not become excessively fatigued. The current enthusiasm for jogging has also attracted a number of pregnant women to the endeavor. In fact, several women, even in late in pregnancy, have run in marathons of considerable distance without apparent harm to themselves or their fetuses. Presumably, all the expectant mothers were in excellent general health and were well conditioned for the event.

Regarding pregnancy as a malady, it is obviously undesirable for all pregnant women to abandon pleasurable activity. With some pregnancy complications, however, the mother and her fetus may benefit significantly from a very sendentary existence, for example, women with pregnancy-induced hypertension (see Chap. 27, p. 681). Women pregnant with two or more fetuses should be encouraged to lead a very sedentary life (see Chap. 26, p. 657).

Employment. It is estimated that more than one-third of all women of childbearing age in the United States are now in the labor force and even larger proportions of socioeconomically less fortunate women are working. Although most studies have not found that work in itself is deleterious to the outcome of pregnancy, certain safeguards are recommended. Any occupation that subjects the pregnant woman to severe physical strain should be avoided. Ideally, no work or play should be continued to the extent that undue fatigue develops. Adequate period of rest should be provided during the working day. Women with previous complications of pregnancy that are likely to be repetitive (for example, low-birth-weight infants) should minimize physical work.

Travel. The restriction of travel to short trips had been a rule for obstetric patients until World War II, when many women found it necessary to follow their husbands regardless of distance or mode of travel. The data compiled during that era are consistent with the conclusion that travel by the woman without complications has no harmful effect on pregnancy. Travel in properly pressurized aircraft offers no unusual risk. At least every two hours, the pregnant woman should walk about. Perhaps the greatest risk with travel is the development of pregnancy complication remote from facilities adequate for treating the complication.

Bathing. There is no objection to bathing at any time during pregnancy or the puerperium. During the last trimester of pregnancy, the heavy uterus usually upsets the balance of the pregnant woman and increases the likelihood of her slipping and falling in the bathtub. For that reason, tub baths at the end of pregnancy may be inadvisable. However, it is not true that wash water readily enters the vagina and thereby carries infection to the uterus.

Clothing. The clothing worn during pregnancy should be practical, attractive, and nonconstricting. Intricate, expensive supporting girdles and brassieres are rarely used today; constricting garters should be avoided during pregnancy because of the interference with venous return and the aggravation of varicosities.

The increasing mass of the breasts may make them pendulous and painful. In such instances well-fitting supporting brassieres are indicated.

Backache and pressure associated with lordotic posture and a pendulous abdomen may be relieved by a properly fitted maternity girdle. There is no real reason for insisting that the pregnant woman wear only low-heeled shoes, unless she develops backache from the increased lordosis that results from shoes with high heels or she is unable to maintain good balance.

Bowel Habits. During pregnancy, bowel habits tend to become more irregular presumably because of generalized relaxation of smooth muscle and compression of the lower bowel by the enlarging uterus early in pregnancy or by the presenting part of the fetus late in pregnancy. In addition to the discomfort caused by the passage of hard fecal material, bleeding and painful fissures in the edematous and hyperemic rectal mucosa may develop. There is also greater frequency of *hemorrhoids* and, much less commonly, of prolapse of the rectal mucosa.

Women whose bowel habits are reasonably normal in the nonpregnant state may prevent constipation during pregnancy by close attention to bowel habits, sufficient quantities of fluid, and reasonable amounts of daily exercise, supplemented when necessary by a mild laxative, such as prune juice, milk of magnesia, bulk-producing substances, or stool-softening agents. The use of nonabsorbable oil preparations has been discouraged because of their possible interference with the absorption of lipid-soluble vitamins. The use of harsh laxatives and enemas is not recommended.

Coitus. When abortion or premature labor threatens, coitus should be avoided. Otherwise, there is general agreement that in healthy pregnant women sexual intercourse usually does no harm before the last four to six weeks of pregnancy. It has long been the custom of many obstetricians to recommend abstinence from intercourse during the last four to six weeks of pregnancy, a recommendation undoubtedly not followed in many instances. Pugh and Fernandez (1953), in one of a few detailed studies to ascertain the effect of coitus on pregnancy, could not find that intercourse caused premature labor, rupture of the membranes, bleeding, or infection. They concluded that it is not necessary to abstain from coitus during the final weeks of gestation.

Goodlin and associates (1972) were more concerned about possible injurious effect from intercourse late in pregnancy. They identified graphically transient fetal bradycardia with increased uterine tension during maternal orgasms induced by vulval and vaginal manipulation at 39 weeks gestation. The painful uterine contractions ceased within 15 minutes after the last orgasm. Whether such changes commonly accompany orgasm and whether they are harmful to the fetus are not definitely known. Goodlin and associates have reported the incidence of orgasm after 32 weeks to have been significantly higher for women who subsequently delivered prematurely. Grudzinkas and co-workers (1979) found no association between gestational age at delivery and the frequency of coitus during the last 4 weeks of pregnancy. However, women who were sexually active in the last 4 weeks showed a a higher incidence of fetal distress.

On occasion, the couple's sexual drive in the face of the admonishment against intercourse late in pregnancy has led to unusual sexual practices with disastrous consequences. Aronson and Nelson (1967), for instance, describe fatal cases of air embolism late in pregnancy as a result of air blown into the vagina during cunnilingus.

Douches. If douching in pregnancy is desirable because of excessive vaginal secretions, the following precautions should be observed:

1. Hand bulb syringes must absolutely be forbidden, since several deaths in pregnancy from air embolism have followed their use (Forbes, 1944).
2. The douche bag should be placed not more than 2 feet above the level of the hips to prevent high fluid pressure.
3. The nozzle should not be inserted more than 3 inches through the vulva.

Care of Breasts and Abdomen. Special care of the breasts during pregnancy is often advised to increase the ability to nurse, to toughen the nipples and thereby reduce the incidence of cracking, and to effect enlargement and eversion of the nipples. From the available data it is concluded that ointments, massage, and traction on the nipples do not always improve these functions, but such practices are usually harmless. Massages and ointments do not alter significantly the incidence of striae on the breasts or abdomen. In general, the extent of striation is proportional to the size of the uterus and the weight gain of the woman.

Smoking. Mothers who smoke during pregnancy frequently bear smaller infants than do nonsmokers. There also is evidence that smoking mothers have a significantly greater number of unsuccessful pregnancies because of an increase in perinatal deaths. Goldstein (1977) estimated that about 4600 infants die in the United States every year because their mothers smoke. Many of the data to support these statements were presented in the publication, Smoking and Health, Report to the Surgeon General of the Public Health Service (1979).

To explain these adverse effects from smoking various investigators have implicated the following: (1) carbon monoxide and its functional inactivation of fetal and maternal hemoglobin, (2) vasoconstrictor action of nicotine causing reduced perfusion of the placenta, (3) reduced appetite and, in turn, reduced caloric intake by women who smoke, (4) a peculiarity of certain women which persists even when they do not smoke.

Astrup and associates (1972) implicated carbon monoxide in the genesis of low birthweight on the basis of their studies on both women and rabbits. D'Souza and co-workers (1978) identified the hemoglobin level in cord blood to average 17.8 g/dl if the mother smoked during pregnancy compared to 16.3 g/dl if she did not smoke; a plausible explanation to account for these differences in hemoglobin concentrations is bone marrow stimulation from chronic fetal hypoxia. Lehtovirta and Forss (1978) reported intervillous blood flow to be acutely reduced during smoking and for 15 minutes afterwards. Rush (1974) and Davies and co-workers (1976) have contended that the lower birthweight of infants whose mothers smoke is primarily the consequence of lower pregnancy weight gain by smoking mothers. Yerushalmy (1972), however, implicated the smoker and not the smoke in the genesis of low birth weight. He reported lower birth weights for infants

whose mothers had not yet smoked when the infants were born but who began to smoke subsequently. Most other investigators have not confirmed Yerushalmy's findings. Interestingly, the incidence of preeclampsia has been reported to be somewhat lower in women who smoke (Duffus, MacGillivray, 1968; Underwood and co-workers, 1967).

Hardy and Mellits (1973) could not identify any harmful long-term effects in children of smoking mothers even though they weighed on the average 250 g less and were shorter at birth. Butler and Goldstein (1973), however, based on a sample of several thousand children 7 to 11 years of age, found slight retardation for reading, mathematics, and general ability in children whose mothers smoked during pregnancy.

In the past, a limitation of smoking to no more than 10 cigarettes per day during pregnancy was recommended. In view of the obvious dangers to people who smoke, cigarettes should be avoided completely by women, irrespective of any deleterious effects on pregnancy.

Alcohol. Excessive ingestion of alcohol by the expectant mother can produce abnormal changes in the fetus. A few cases of the syndrome of acute withdrawal of alcohol (delerium tremens) have been described in newborn infants of mothers who consumed excessive amounts of alcohol (Nichols, 1967). The affected newborn is depressed at birth but soon becomes extremely hyperactive with sweating, tremors, and episodes of generalized twitching of the face and extremities. At the same time, the mother also suffers delirium tremens.

Chronic alcoholism may lead to fetal maldevelopment, commonly referred to as the *fetal alcohol syndrome.* Jones and associates (1974, 1975), described a common pattern of craniofacial, limb, and cardiovascular defects associated with prenatal and postnatal growth retardation in the offspring of alcoholic mothers. All the children subsequently demonstrated impaired fine and gross motor function. The perinatal mortality rate was 17 percent. At seven years of age 44 percent of the survivors had an IQ below 80, compared to 9 percent in a control group.

Women with chronic and severe drinking problems should be discouraged from becoming pregnant until these problems are brought under control. Serious consideration should be given to early pregnancy termination in alcoholic women.

Hopefully, the adverse affects of alcohol on the pregnancy do not persist after the woman stops drinking. However, a child with most of the stigmas of the fetal alcohol syndrome has been born to parents who drank heavily in the past but denied any consumption of alcohol while members of Alcoholics Anonymous for 1½ years (Scheiner et al., 1979).

"Hard" Drugs. Chronic use by the expectant mother of "hard" drugs, including opium derivatives, barbiturates, and amphetamines, in large doses, is harmful to the fetus. Intrauterine distress, low birth weight, and serious compromise as the consequence of drug withdrawal soon after birth have been well documented. Often the mother who uses hard drugs does not seek prenatal care and even if she does she is unlikely to volunteer that she uses such substances. Detection of scars from venipunctures may be the first clue. As emphasized elsewhere (see Chap. 38, p. 981), the management of pregnancy and delivery and successful care of the newborn infant may be extremely difficult. Abortion should be considered for the addicted early pregnant woman who wants to try to "kick the habit."

Care of the Teeth. In general, pregnancy does not contraindicate required dental treatment. The concept that dental caries are aggravated by pregnancy is unfounded.

Immunization. There has been some concern over the safety of various immunization technics during pregnancy. The recommendations of the American College of Obstetricians and Gynecologists (1973) with appropriate updating for specific immunizations during pregnancy are summarized below:

Tetanus-diphtheria	Give if no primary series, or no booster in 10 years
Poliomyelitis	Not recommended routinely for adults but mandatory in epidemic
Mumps	Contraindicated
Rubella	Contraindicated
Typhoid	Recommended if traveling in endemic region
Smallpox	No need; smallpox has been eradicated
Yellow fever	Immunize before travel in high risk area; risk of yellow fever to mother and fetus greater than risk from immunization
Cholera	Only to meet travel requirements
Rabies	Same as nonpregnant
Hepatitis-A	After exposure or before travel in developing countries
Influenza	Evaluate pregnant women for immunization according to criteria applied to other persons

Medications. With rare exception, any drug that exerts a systemic effect in the mother will cross the placenta to reach the embryo and fetus. The effects on the embryo and fetus cannot be predicted accurately either from the effects or lack of effects in the mother or from the effects or lack of effects on the embryo or fetus in animal species. Moreover, widespread use of a medication during pregnancy without recognized adverse effects on the fetus does not guarantee the safety of the medication. An especially pertinent example of delayed recognition of adverse effects by a drug that was widely used in obstetrics for a number of years is the induction of vaginal cancer in young women whose mothers ingested diethylstilbestrol during that pregnancy (Herbst, Scully, and Robboy, 1975).

Only after many years of use was it established that diphenylhydantoin (Dilantin) and phenobarbital given to women to control epilepsy may both induce fetal malformation

(Meadow, 1968) and impair synthesis by the fetus and newborn infant of the vitamin K-dependent coagulation factors II, VII, IX, and X (Mountain et al., 1970). An association between cleft lip and use of diazepam during the first trimester was suggested, at least, by the findings of Safra and Oakley (1975).

Even the use of aspirin by the mother has been demonstrated to cause a variety of adverse effects not previously suspected. Maternal ingestion of aspirin induces a degree of platelet dysfunction and diminishes factor XII activity (Bleyer, Breckenridge, 1970; Corby, Schulman, 1971). Shapiro and associates (1976) could find no evidence that the use of aspirin during pregnancy caused perinatal death or reduced birthweight. Moreover, aspirin does not appear to be teratogenic (Slone et al., 1976). However, Australian workers reported that persistent maternal ingestion of analgesic compounds containing salicylates in combination with caffeine or phenacetin or both is associated with an increased incidence of anemia, hemorrhage, prolonged gestation, perinatal mortality, and low birth weight (Collins, Turner 1975; Turner, Collins, 1974).

Because of aspirin's potentially adverse effects on the hemostatic mechanism of the fetus and its displacement of bilirubin from protein-binding sites, the use of aspirin should be discouraged, especially late in pregnancy. Acetamenophen has been suggested as a safer alternative; however, we have observed severe maternal hepatic and renal failure and fetal death from acetamenophen toxicity.

The administration of prostaglandin synthetase inhibitors, such as indomethacin, will sometimes arrest premature labor but may also cause premature closure of the ductus arteriosus in the fetus.

All physicians should develop the habit early of ascertaining the likelihood of pregnancy before prescribing drugs for any woman, since a number of medications in common use can be injurious to the embryo and the fetus. Package inserts provided by the pharmaceutical company and approved by the Food and Drug Administration should be consulted before drugs are prescribed for pregnant women. **If a drug is administered during pregnancy, the advantages to be gained must clearly outweigh any risks inherent in its use.**

COMMON COMPLAINTS

Nausea and Vomiting. Nausea and vomiting are common complaints during the first half of pregnancy. Typically, nausea and vomiting commence between the first and second missed menstrual period and continue until about the time of the fourth missed period. Nausea and vomiting are usually worse in the morning but may continue throughout the day.

The genesis of pregnancy-induced nausea and vomiting is not clear. Possibly the hormonal changes of pregnancy are responsible. Chorionic gonadotropin, for instance, has been implicated on the basis that its levels are rather high at the same time that nausea and vomiting are most common. Moreover, in women with hydatidiform mole, in which levels of chorionic gonadotropin typically are very much higher than in normal pregnancy, nausea and vomiting are often prominent clinical features.

Emotional factors undoubtedly can contribute to the severity of the nausea and vomiting of pregnancy, which at times may become so intense or so protracted as to cause serious metabolic derangements in the mother and fetus. Very infrequently, vomiting may be so very severe that dehydration, electrolyte and acid-base disturbances, and starvation become serious problems.

Seldom is the treatment of nausea and vomiting of pregnancy so successful that the affected expectant mother is afforded complete relief. However, the unpleasantness and discomfort usually can be minimized. Eating small feedings at more frequent intervals but stopping short of satiation is of value. Since the smell of certain foods often precipitates or aggravates the symptoms, such foods should be avoided as much as possible.

In more recent years at Parkland Memorial Hospital a combination of the antihistaminic doxylamine succinate and pyridoxine in a specially coated tablet (Bendectin) has been prescribed for pregnancy-induced nausea and vomiting. Usually two tablets taken when retiring, and if necessary, another taken upon arising, seem to have provided a measure of relief. Shapiro and associates (1977) found no evidence that such medication taken during the first four months of pregnancy predisposed to congenital malformations, increased perinatal mortality rate, lower birth weight, or lower intelligence quotient score at four years of age.

Meclizine (Bonine) and meclizine with pyridoxine (Bonadoxin), which have been used widely in an effort to control nausea and vomiting, also seem to provide some benefit. The suggestion has been made that meclizine might be teratogenic, but the evidence in support of this view is not convincing (Yerushalmy, Milkovich, 1965).

A great variety of other agents have been recommended for treatment. Fairweather (1975), for example, in his comprehensive review of nausea and vomiting in pregnancy, tabulated such bizarre and diverse treatments as hibernotherapy, intravenously administered honey, husband's blood, and the husband's sex hormone (testosterone).

Fortunately, effective psychologic support can be offered in the form of reassurance to the pregnant woman that these symptoms nearly always will disappear by the fourth month, and, moreover, that pregnancies in which nausea and vomiting occur are more likely to have a favorable outcome than are those without nausea and vomiting (Yerushalmy, Milkovich, 1965).

The syndrome of nausea and vomiting of great intensity and commonly requiring hospitalization for successful management is referred to as *hyperemesis gravidarum.* Prompt correction of fluid and electrolyte imbalances usually relieves the symptoms. Today therapeutic abortion is rarely required.

Backache. Backache occurs to some extent in most pregnant women. Minor degrees follow excessive strain or fatigue and excessive bending, lifting, or walking. Mild backache usually requires little more than elimination of the strain and occasionally a lightweight maternity girdle.

Severe backaches should not be dismissed as caused simply by pregnancy until a thorough orthopedic examination has been conducted. Muscular spasm and tenderness, which are often classified clinically as acute strain or fibrositis, respond well to analgesics, heat, and rest.

In some women, motion of the symphysis pubis and lumbrosacral joints, and general relaxation of pelvic ligaments may be demonstrated. In severe cases, the pregnant woman may be unable to walk or even remain comfortable without support furnished by a heavy girdle and prolonged periods of rest. Occasionally anatomic defects are found, either congenital or traumatic, which may precipitate the complaints. Pain caused by herniation of an intervertebral disc occurs during pregnancy with about the same frequency as at other times.

Varicosities. Varicosities, generally resulting from congenital predisposition, are exaggerated by prolonged standing, pregnancy, and advancing age. Usually varicosities become more prominent as pregnancy advances, as weight increases, and as the length of time spent upright is prolonged.

The symptoms produced by varicosities vary from cosmetic blemishes on the lower extremities and mild discomfort at the end of the day to severe pain that requires prolonged rest with the feet elevated.

The treatment of varicosities of the lower extremities is generally limited to periodic rest with elevation of the legs, or elastic stockings, or both. Surgical correction of the condition during pregnancy generally is not advised, although the symptoms rarely may be so severe that injection, ligation, or even stripping of the veins is necessary in order to allow the pregnant woman to remain ambulatory. In general, these operations should be postponed until after delivery. Varicosities of the vulva may be aided by application of a foam rubber pad suspended across the vulva by a belt of the type used with a perineal pad. Rarely, large varicosities may rupture, resulting in profuse hemorrhage.

Hemorrhoids. Varicosities of hemorrhoidal veins occasionally first appear during pregnancy. More often, pregnancy causes an exacerbation or recurrence of previous symptoms. The development or aggravation of hemorrhoids during pregnancy is related undoubtedly to increased pressure in the hemorrhoidal veins caused by obstruction of venous return by the large pregnant uterus, and to the tendency toward constipation during pregnancy. Usually pain and swelling are relieved by topically applied anesthetics, warm soaks, and agents that soften the stool. Thrombosis of a hemorrhoidal vein can cause considerable pain, but the clot can usually be evacuated by incising the wall of the involved vein with a scalpel under topical anesthesia.

Bleeding from hemorrhoidal veins occasionally may result in loss of sufficient blood to cause iron deficiency anemia. The loss of only 15 ml of blood results in the loss of 6 to 7 mg of iron, an amount equal to the daily requirements for iron during the latter half of pregnancy. If bleeding is persistent, hemorrhoidectomy may be required. In general, however, hemorrhoidectomy is not desirable during pregnancy, since most often hemorrhoids become asymptomatic soon after delivery.

Heartburn. Heartburn, one of the most common complaints of pregnant women, usually is caused by reflux of gastric or duodenal contents into the lower esophagus. The increased frequency of regurgitation during pregnancy most likely results from the upward displacement and compression of the stomach by the uterus combined with decreased gastrointestinal motility. In some pregnant women, the cardia actually herniates through the diaphragm.

Antacid preparations may provide considerable relief. Aluminum hydroxide, magnesium trisilicate, or magnesium hydroxide, alone or in combination (for example, Amphojel, Gelusil, Maalox, and milk of magnesia), should be used in preference to sodium bicarbonate. The pregnant woman who tends to retain sodium can become edematous as the result of the ingestion of excessive amounts of sodium bicarbonate. Antacids that contain magnesium and aluminum hydroxides impair absorption of iron somewhat but otherwise appear to be quite innocuous (Gant et al., unpublished).

Pica. Occasionally during pregnancy bizarre cravings for strange foods develop and at times for materials hardly considered edible, such as laundry starch, clay, and even dirt. For example, at Parkland Memorial Hospital, interrogation of recently delivered mothers in a single day disclosed that the following items were craved and consumed by them during the current pregnancy: Argo Gloss Starch, flour, baking powder, baking soda, clay, baked dirt, powdered bricks, and frost scraped from the refrigerator.

The ingestion of starch (amylophagia) or clay (geophagia) or related items, is practiced more often by socioeconomically less privileged pregnant women. It is quite unlikely, however, that the craving for these materials is simply the result of hunger but is rather, in part at least, a social custom. In this country pica involving lump laundry starch or clay appears to have long been prevalent among black women in the South; with their migration, the custom spread throughout most of the United States. Since young women are constantly introduced to the practice by older women, the custom is not dying out. McGanity and co-workers (1969), for instance, reported that one-half of the teen-age pregnant women cared for in their clinic admitted to pica.

The desire for dry lump starch, clay, chopped ice, or even refrigerator frost has been considered by some to be triggered by severe iron deficiency. Although women with severe iron deficiency sometimes crave these items, and although the craving is at times ameliorated after correction of the iron deficiency, not all women with pica are necessarily iron-deficient.

Minnich and associates (1968) found that the ingestion of clay, especially Turkish clay and to a lesser extent clays from Georgia and Mississippi, impaired absorption of iron. In Dallas, however, we were unable to demonstrate that either of two Texas clays studied or Argo Gloss Starch reduced absorption of iron significantly (Talkington et al., 1970).

The consumption of starch in sufficient quantities to provide a significant portion of the calories ingested or to cause ptyalism is not healthful nor is the ingestion of clay to the extent that the intestine is sufficiently filled to cause obstruction of labor or fecal impaction. Nonetheless, it is quite unlikely that either laundry starch or clay free of parasites is distinctly harmful to the pregnancy if consumed in moderation and if the diet is nutritionally adequate.

Ptyalism. Women during pregnancy are occasionally distressed by profuse salivation. The cause of the ptyalism sometimes appears to be stimulation of the salivary glands by the ingestion of starch. This cause should be looked for and eradicated if found.

Fatigue and Somnolence. Early in pregnancy, most women complain of fatigue and desire excessive periods of sleep. The condition usually remits spontaneously by the fourth month of pregnancy and has no special significance.

Headache. Headache early in pregnancy is a frequent complaint. A few cases may result from sinusitis or ocular strain caused by refractive errors. In the vast majority, however, no cause can be demonstrated. Treatment is largely symptomatic. By the middle of pregnancy, most of these headaches decrease in severity or disappear. The pathological significance of headaches later in pregnancy is considered in Chapter 27 (p. 680).

Leukorrhea. Pregnant women commonly develop increased vaginal discharge, which in many instances has no pathologic cause. Increased formation of mucus by cervical glands in response to hyperestrogenemia is undoubtedly a contributing factor. If the secretion is troublesome, the woman may be advised to douche with water mildly acidified with vinegar. The precautions for douching listed on page 319 should be stressed.

Occasionally, troublesome leukorrhea is the result of an infection caused by *Trichomonas vaginalis* or *Candida albicans.*

TRICHOMONAS VAGINALIS. This organism can be identified in as many as 20 percent of women during prenatal examination; however, the infection is symptomatic in a much smaller percentage of pregnant women. Trichomonal vaginitis is characterized by foamy leukorrhea with pruritus and irritation. Trichomonads are readily demonstrated in fresh vaginal secretions as flagellated, pearshaped, motile organisms that are somewhat larger than leukocytes.

Metronidazole (Flagyl) has proved effective in eradicating *Trichomonas vaginalis.* The drug may be administered both orally and vaginally. When ingested by the mother, metronidazole crosses the placenta and enters the fetal circulation; the possibility of teratogenicity persists if metronidazole is ingested during the first trimester.

CANDIDA ALBICANS. Candida (Monilia) can be cultured from the vagina in about 25 percent of women approaching term. Asymptomatic vaginal candidiasis requires no treatment. However, it may sometimes cause an extremely profuse irritating discharge. Gentian violet applied as a 1 percent aqueous solution has been a dependable local therapeutic agent, although it may stain the skin and clothing and produce local edema. Miconazole nitrate, 2 percent, in a vaginal cream, has been claimed to be highly effective for the treatment of candidiasis during pregnancy (McNellis et al., 1977). Candidiasis is likely to recur, thereby requiring repeated treatment during pregnancy, but usually it subsides at the end of gestation.

REFERENCES

Alperin JB, Haggard ME, McGanity WJ: Folic acid, pregnancy, and abruptio placentae. Am J Clin Nutr 22:1359, 1969

American College of Obstetricians and Gynecologists Technical Bulletin, No. 20, March, 1973: Immunization During Pregnancy.

Aronson ME, Nelson PK: Fatal air embolism in pregnancy resulting from an unusual sex act. Obstet Gynecol 30:127, 1967

Astrup P, Olsen HM, Trolle D, Kjeldsen K: Effect of moderate carbon-monoxide-exposure on fetal development. Lancet 2:1220, 1972

Bayless TM, Rothfeld B, Massa C, et al.: Lactose and milk intolerance: clinical implications. New Engl J Med 292:1156, 1975

Bleyer WA, Breckenridge RT: Studies on the detection of adverse drug reactions in the newborn. JAMA 213:2049, 1970

Butler NR, Goldstein H: Smoking in pregnancy and subsequent child development. Br Med J 3:573, 1973

Center for Disease Control: Influenza vaccine: Preliminary statement. Ann Intern Med 89:373, 1978

Chanarin I, Rothman D, Ward A, Perry J: Folate status and requirements in pregnancy. Br Med J 2:390, 1968

Cleary RE, Lumeng L, Li Y-K: Maternal and fetal plasma levels of pyridoxal phosphate at term: Adequacy of vitamin B_6 supplementation during pregnancy. Am J Obstet Gynecol 121:25, 1975

Cochrane WA: Overnutrition in prenatal and neonatal life: A problem? Can Med Assoc J 93:893, 1965

Collins E, Turner G: Maternal effects of regular salicylate ingestion in pregnancy. Lancet 2:335, 1975

Corby DG, Schulman I: The effect of antenatal drug administration on aggregation of platelets of newborn infants. J Pediatr 79:307, 1971

Davies DP, Gray OP, Ellwood PC, Abernethy M: Cigarette smoking in pregnancy: Associations with maternal weight gain and fetal growth. Lancet 1:385, 1976

De Leeuw NK, Lowenstein L, Hsieh YS: Iron deficiency and hydremia in normal pregnancy. Medicine 45:291, 1966

Delgado H, Lechtig A, Yarbrough C, Martorell R, Klein RE, Irwin M: Maternal nutrition— its effects on infant growth and development and birthspacing. In Moghissi KS, Evans TN (eds.): Nutritional Impacts On Women. Hagerstown, Md, Harper & Row, 1977, p 133

D'Souza SW, Black PM, Williams N, Jennison RF: Effect of smoking during pregnancy upon the haematological values of cord blood. Br J Obstet Gynaecol 85:495, 1978

Duffus G, MacGillivray I: The incidence of pre-eclamptic toxemia in smokers and non-smokers. Lancet 1:994, 1968

Eastman NJ, Jackson E: Weight relationships in pregnancy: I. The bearing of maternal weight gain and pre-pregnancy weight on birth weight in full term pregnancies. Obstet Gynecol Survey 23:1003, 1968

Emery AEH: Folates and fetal central-nervous-system malformations. Lancet 1:703, 1977

Fairweather DV: Nausea and vomiting in pregnancy. Am J Obstet Gynecol 102:135, 1968

Food & Nutrition Board Position Paper on the Relationship of Nutrition to Brain Development and Behavior. Washington, DC, National Academy of Sciences, 1973

Forbes G: Air embolism as complication of vaginal douching in pregnancy. Br Med J 2:529, 1944

Fraser JL, Watt HJ: Megaloblastic anemia in pregnancy and the puerperium. Am J Obstet Gynecol 89:532, 1964

Gant NF, Scott DE, Pritchard JA: Unpublished observations.

Giles C: An account of 335 cases of megaloblastic anaemia of pregnancy and the puerperium. J Clin Pathol 19:1, 1966

Gillmer MDG, Mazibuko D: Pyridoxine treatment of chemical diabetes in pregnancy. Am J Obstet Gynecol 133:499, 1979

Glenn FB: Immunity conveyed by sodium-fluoride supplement during pregnancy: Part II. J Dent Child Jan-Feb:17, 1979

Goldstein H: Smoking in pregnancy: some notes on the statistical controversy. Br J Prevent Soc Med 31:13, 1977

Goodlin RC, Keller DW, Raffin M: Orgasm during late pregnancy: Possible deleterious effects. Obstet Gynecol 38:916, 1971

Goodlin RC, Schmidt W, Creevy DC: Uterine tension and fetal heart rate during maternal orgasm. Obstet Gynecol 39:125, 1972

Grudzinkas JG, Watson C, Chard T: Does sexual intercourse cause fetal distress? Lancet 2:692, 1979

Hall MH: Folates and the fetus. Lancet 1:648, 1977

Hambidge KM, Mauer AM: Trace elements. In laboratory indices of nutritional status in pregnancy. Washington, DC, The National Research Council—National Academy of Sciences, 1978, p 157

Hardy JB, Mellits ED: Does maternal smoking during pregnancy have a long-term effect on the child? Lancet 2:1332, 1973

Heaney RP, Skillman TG: Calcium metabolism in normal human pregnancy. J Clin Endocrinol 33:661, 1971

Herbert V, Jacob E: Destruction of vitamin B_{12} by ascorbic acid. JAMA 230:241, 1974

Herbst AL, Scully RE, Robboy SJ: Effects of maternal DES ingestion on the female genital tract. Hosp Prac 10:51, 1975

Hibbard BM, Hibbard ED, Jeffcoate TNA: Folic acid and reproduction. Acta Obstet Gynecol Scand 44:375, 1969

Higginbottom MC, Sweetman L, Nyhan WL: A syndrome of methylmalonic aciduria, homocystinuria, megaloblastic anemia and neurologic abnormalities in a vitamin B_{12}-deficient breast-fed infant of a strict vegetarian. New Engl J Med 299:317, 1978

Horowitz HS, Heifetz SB: Effects of prenatal exposure to fluoridation on dental caries. Pub Health Rep 82:297, 1967

Hytten FE, Leitch I: The Physiology of Human Pregnancy, 2d ed. Oxford, Blackwell, 1971

Jiminez JM, Tyson JE, Santos-Ramos R, Duenhoelter JH: Comparison of obstetric and pediatric evaluation of gestational age. Ped Res 13:498, 1979

Jones KL, Smith DW: The fetal alcohol syndrome. Teratology 12:1, 1975

Jones KL, Smith DW, Streissguth AP, Myrianthopoulos NC: Incidence of the fetal alcohol syndrome in offspring of chronically alcoholic women. Pediatr Res 8:440, 1974

Jones KL, Smith DW, Ulleland CN, Streissguth P: Pattern of malformation in offspring of chronic alcoholic mothers. Lancet 1:7815, 1974

Kortenoever ME: Pathology of pregnancy: Pregnancy of long duration and postmature infant. Obstet Gynecol Surv 5:812, 1950

Lehtovirta P, Forss M: The acute effect of smoking on intervillous blood flow of the placenta. Br J Obstet Gynaecol 85:729, 1978

McGanity WJ, Little HM, Fogelman A, Jennings L, Calhoun E, Dawson EB: Pregnancy in the adolescent: I. Preliminary summary of health status. Am J Obstet Gynecol 103:773, 1969

McNellis D, McLeod M, Lawson J, Pasquale SA: Treatment of vulvovaginal candidiasis in pregnancy. Obstet Gynecol 50:674, 1977

Meadow SR: anticonvulsant drugs and congential abnormalities. Lancet 2:1296, 1968

Medical Letter, 15 (16), 1973

Minnich V, Okcuoglu A, Tarcon Y, Arcasoy A, Cin S, Yorukoglu O, Renda F, Demirag B: Pica in Turkey: II. Effect of clay upon iron absorption. Am J Clin Nutr 21:78, 1968

Mountain KR, Hirsh J, Gallus AS: Neonatal coagulation defect due to anticonvulsant drug treatment in pregnancy. Lancet 1:265, 1970

Nakano R: Post-term pregnancy. Acta Obstet Gynecol Scand 51:217, 1972

Naeye R: Weight gain and the outcome of pregnancy. Am J Obstet Gynecol 135:3, 1979

Nichols MM: Acute alcohol withdrawal syndrome in a newborn. Am J Dis Child 113:714, 1967

Paintin DB, Thomson AM, Hytten FE: Iron and the haemoglobin level in pregnancy. J Obstet Gynaecol Brit Commonw 73:181, 1966

Perkins RP: Failure of pyridoxine to improve glucose tolerance in gestational diabetes mellitus. Obstet Gynecol 50:370, 1977

Pharoah POD, Buttfield IH, Hetzel BS: Neurological damage to the fetus resulting from severe iodine deficiency during pregnancy. Lancet 1:308, 1971

Pitkin RM: Calcium metabolism in pregnancy: A review. Am J Obstet Gynecol 121:724, 1975

Pritchard JA: Antenatal Care and Nutrition in Pregnancy. 78th Ross Conference on Pediatric Research, Obstetric Decisions and Neonatal Outcome, San Diego, CA, 1979

Pritchard JA, Hunt CF: A comparison of the hematologic responses following the routine prenatal administration of intramuscular and oral iron. Surg Gynecol Obstet 106:516, 1958

Pritchard JA, Scott DE: Iron demands during pregnancy. In Hallberg L, Harwerth H-G, Vannotti A (eds): Iron Deficiency: Pathogenesis, Clinical Aspects, Therapy. New York, Academic, 1970

Pritchard JA, Whalley PJ: High risk pregnancy and reproductive outcome. In Gluck, L (ed) Modern Perinatal Medicine. Chicago, Year Book, 1974

Pritchard JA, Scott DE, Whalley PJ: Folic acid requirements in pregnancy induced megaloblastic anemia. JAMA 208:1163, 1969

Pugh WE, Fernandez FL: Coitus in late pregnancy. Obstet Gynecol 2:636, 1953

Recommended Dietary Allowances, 9th ed. Food and Nutrition Board. Washington, DC, National Research Council-National Academy of Sciences, 1979

Rush D: Lower weight gain among smokers explains most of the effect of smoking on birthweight. Pediatr Res 8:450, 1974

Safra MF, Oakley G Jr: Association between cleft lip with or without cleft palate and prenatal exposure to diazepam. Lancet 2:478, 1975

Sauberlich HE: Vitamin indices. In Laboratory Indices of Nutritional Status in Pregnancy. Washington, DC, National Research Council Committee on Nutrition of the Mother and Preschool Child, National Academy of Sciences, 1978, p. 109

Scheiner AP, Donovan CM, Bartoshesky LE: Fetal alcohol syndrome in child whose parents had stopped drinking. Lancet 2:478, 1979

Scott DE, Pritchard JA, Saltin A-S, Humphryes SM: Iron deficiency during pregnancy. In Hallberg L, Harwerth H-G, Vannotti A (eds): Iron Deficiency: Pathogenesis, Clinical Aspects, Therapy. New York, Academic, 1970

Shapiro S, Monson RR, Kaufman DW, Siskind V, Heinonen OP, Slone D: Perinatal mortality and birth-weight in relation to aspirin taken during pregnancy. Lancet 1:1375, 1976

Shapiro S, Heinonen OP, Siskind V, Kaufman DW, Monson RR, Slone D: Antenatal exposure to doxylamine succinate and dicyclomine hydrochloride (Bendectin) in relation to congenital malformations, perinatal mortality rate, birth weight, and intelligence quotient score. Am J Obstet Gynecol 128:480, 1977

Slone D, Heinonen OP, Kaufman DW, Siskind V, Monson RR, Shapiro S: Aspirin and congenital malformations. Lancet 1:1373, 1976

Smith CA: Effects of maternal undernutrition upon the newborn infant in Holland (1944–1945). Am J Obstet Gynecol 30:229, 1947

Stein Z, Susser M, Rush D: Prenatal nutrition and birth weight: Experiments and quasi-experiments in the past decade. J Reprod Med 21:287, 1978

Stein Z, Susser M, Saenger G, Marolla F: Nutrition and mental performance. Science 178:708, 1972

Stone ML, Luhby AL, Feldman R, Gordon M, Cooperman JM: Folic acid metabolism in pregnancy. Am J Obstet Gynecol 99:638, 1967

Streif RR, Little AB: Folic acid deficiency in pregnancy. New Engl J Med 276:776, 1967

Talkington KM, Gant NF, Scott DE, Pritchard JA: Effect of ingestion of starch and some clays on iron absorption. Am J Obstet Gynecol 108:262, 1970

Task Force Report. Am College Obstet Gynecol Assessment of Maternal Nutrition. Chicago, 1978

Taylor DJ, Lind T: Haemotological changes during normal pregnancy: Iron induced macrocytosis. Br J Obstet Gynaecol 83:760, 1976

Turner G, Collins E: Fetal effects of regular salicylates ingestion in pregnancy. Lancet 2:338, 1975

Underwood PB, Hester LL, Lafitte T Jr, Gregg KV: The relationship of smoking empirically related to pregnancy outcome. Obstet Gynecol 29:1, 1967

Varadi S, Abbott D, Elwis A: Correlation of peripheral white cell and bone marrow changes with folate levels in pregnancy and their clinical significance. J Clin Pathol 19:33, 1966

Whalley PJ, Scott DE, Pritchard JA: Maternal folate deficiency and pregnancy wastage: I. Placental abruption. Am J Obstet Gynecol 105:670, 1969

Yerushalmy J: Infants with low birth weight born before their mothers started to smoke cigarettes. Am J Obstet Gynecol 112:277, 1972

Yerushalmy J, Milkovich L: Evaluation of the teratogenic effect of meclizine in man. Am J Obstet Gynecol 93:553, 1965

14

Technics to Evaluate Fetal Health

Until relatively recently, the intrauterine sanctuary of the embryo and fetus was held to be inviolate. The mother was the patient to be cared for, whereas the fetus was but another, albeit transient, maternal organ. The philosophy prevailed that "good maternal care" would automatically provide what was best for the products of conception. Ideally, labor would not occur until the fetus weighed more than 2500 g (once the widely accepted definition of fetal maturity), except in instances of gross developmental abnormality when, it was hoped, the embryo or nonviable fetus might be expelled spontaneously. If, however, spontaneous abortion did not ensue, society decreed the only alternative to be that the parents, or at times some governmental agency, must try to care for the subsequently liveborn but malformed offspring.

During the past two decades, remarkably intimate knowledge of the human fetus and his or her immediate environment has accumulated (see Chap. 8). As did maternal health earlier in this century, fetal health, or fetal medicine, has come to be appreciated not merely as an exciting arena for research but as a clinical discipline with great potential for influencing favorably the quality of human offspring. Indeed, the fetus is no longer dealt with as a maternal appendage ultimately to be shed at the whim of biologic forces beyond control. Instead, the fetus has rightfully achieved the status of the second patient, a patient who usually faces much greater risks of serious morbidity and mortality than does the mother.

A variety of technics that may be of value for appraising the health of the embryo and fetus are considered especially, but certainly not totally, in this chapter. The technics include (1) amniocentesis, amnioscopy, and fetoscopy; (2) ultrasonography; (3) radiography, including amniography and fetography; (4) measurements of certain hormones and enzymes in maternal plasma, urine, or both; (5) antepartum fetal heart "stress" and "nonstress" tests; and (6) intrapartum surveillance of fetal heart action, uterine contractions, and physicochemical properties of fetal blood.

The use of newer biochemical and electronic procedures should be regarded, *as their value is proved,* as worthy additions to existing clinical procedures already available to help identify the fetus at risk. It is emphasized at the outset that these procedures may impose some risk of morbidity and mortality to the fetus and the mother, or impose significant expense, or both. Therefore, their use should provide benefits that clearly outweigh both the potential risks and the costs. Certainly the physician who orders them must be prepared to acknowledge the results and to use them objectively.

There is no doubt but what pregnancy outcomes have improved during the time that most, if not all, of the technics described in this chapter have been available to try to identify the presence or absence of fetal well-being. In 1969, for the first time, the perinatal death rate dropped to below 30 per 1000. It has continued to fall and in 1977 was 19.6 per 1000. Although it is tempting to do so, it is inappropriate to ascribe the dramatic decrease solely to the availability of more and better technics to evaluate fetal health. A multiplicity of important factors have undoubtedly contributed to this accomplishment:

1. Less unplanned and unwanted pregnancies as the consequence of federally funded family planning programs and the legalization of elective abortion
2. Pregnant women taking greater advantage of antepartum care
3. The elimination by selective abortion of some pregnancies in which the fetus or neonate was at increased risk of dying
4. More liberal use of hospitalization in an attempt to prolong gestation safely
5. Greater attention paid to the fetus, including the use of a variety of technics to try to monitor fetal well-being or lack of same
6. Increased use of cesarean section to try to minimize fetal trauma and asphyxia
7. Availability of excellent neonatal care
8. As emphasized by Schiffrin (1979), Factor X, or *tender loving care*

AMNIOCENTESIS

The ability to enter the amnionic sac without appreciable risk to the mother or fetus has remarkably influenced obstetric care in a variety of ways that are illustrated in Figure 14-1. The aspiration of a sample of amnionic fluid provides for a variety of diagnostic tests that are indicative of fetal well-being.

Aspirated amnionic fluid typically is separated by appropriate centrifugation into cell-rich and cell-free fractions. The supernatant is used for a variety of biochemical procedures and, at times, microbiologic studies while the cellular fraction may be used without prior cell culture to identify the sex of the fetus and for certain enzyme studies. Much more often, however, the cells are placed in culture and when of sufficient number in a few weeks, the replicated cells are studied cytogenetically and biochemically.

Technics. Beginning early in the 2nd trimester, after the exocoelomic space between amnion and chorion has been obliterated, the chorion laeve has fused with the uterine decidua, and the uterus is enlarged sufficiently to be easily palpated above the symphysis, amnionic fluid may be aspirated transabdominally. After locally anesthetizing the abdominal wall, a 20- or 22-gauge needle 3 to 6 inches long, depending upon the thickness of the abdominal wall, the size of the uterus, and the site of puncture, is carefully inserted into the amnionic sac. When cells from amnionic fluid are desired for culture, up to 30 ml of amnionic fluid is withdrawn at 15 to 18 weeks gestation.

Risks. The three major risks from amniocentesis are readily deduced: (1) trauma to the fetus, to the placenta, or less often, to the umbilical cord or to maternal structures; (2) infection; and (3) abortion or premature labor. Surgical asepsis is mandatory to avoid infection not only in the mother and fetus but also in the aspirated amnionic fluid, especially when it is to be used for cell culture or microbiologic studies.

As well as causing hemorrhage into the placenta and into the amnionic sac (Fig. 14-2), perforation of the placenta may lead to

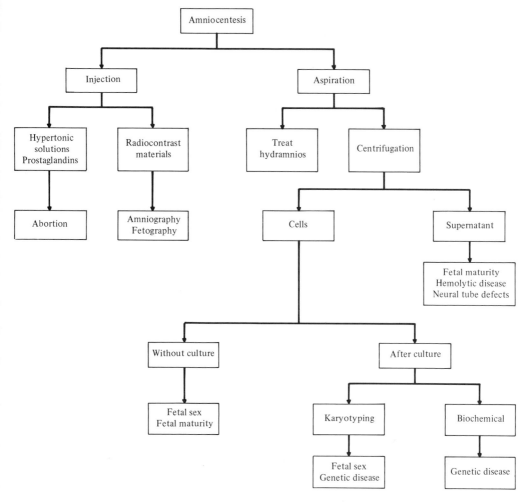

FIG. 14-1. The various clinical applications of amniocentesis.

significant transfer of fetal blood to the mother, which may incite or enhance maternal isoimmunization and, in turn, hemolytic disease in the fetus. Therefore, sonographic localization of the placenta before amniocentesis has been widely recommended. While sonographic localization of the placenta before amniocentesis reduces the likelihood of perforating the placenta during insertion of the needle, unfortunately, it does not always preclude appreciable fetal to maternal bleeding (Blajchman et al., 1974; Harrison et al., 1975). Consequently, anti-Rho globulin is commonly administered to nonsensitized Rh

negative women at the time of amniocentesis (see Chap. 38, p. 963).

Freda (1973) pointed out that late in pregnancy there is little risk of perforating the placenta if the transabdominal puncture is performed suprapubically, as shown in Figure 14-3. The experiences of Leach and co-workers (1978) further attest to the suprapubic site being the most favorable one for amniocentesis performed late in pregnancy. Whether such a low puncture site enhances the risk of a leak of amnionic fluid is not clear. It has been our experience that, if the fetus can be easily palpated immediately be-

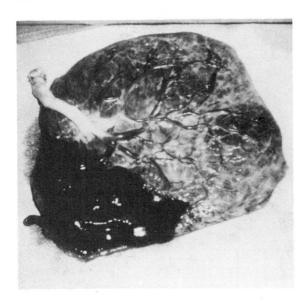

FIG. 14-2. Hemorrhage from perforation of a fetal vessel in the placenta at the time of amniocentesis.

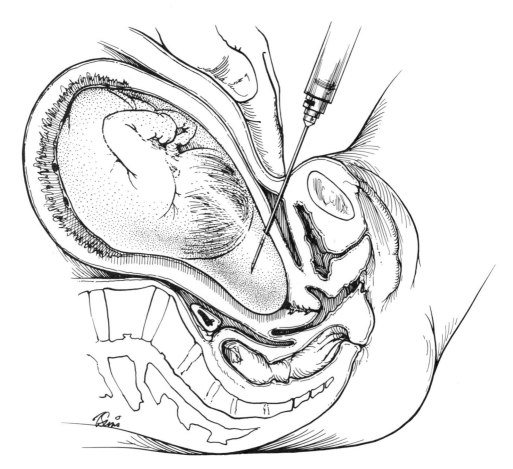

FIG. 14-3. Amniocentesis late in pregnancy, performed suprapubically.

neath the proposed site of transabdominal puncture, the placenta is implanted elsewhere. If, however, fetal parts cannot be easily palpated immediately beneath the proposed site of puncture, sonographic localization of the placenta is indicated.

Trauma to the umbilical cord is more likely if the cord is around the neck of the fetus and entry into the amnionic space is attempted adjacent to the fetal head and shoulder. Injury to the fetus is more common when the volume of amnionic fluid is small compared to the size of the fetus, or when the amnionic fluid is thick and does not flow freely through the needle. These later conditions are more likely to be encountered late in pregnancy and especially in the postterm pregnancy. Repeated taps after failure to obtain amnionic fluid increase the risk of trauma to the fetus.

After amniocentesis, the fetus who is sufficiently mature to have reasonable potential for survival if delivered should be closely evaluated for evidence of deterioration by observing the fetal heart rate, especially if the tap was thought possibly to be traumatic. Immediately after delivery all infants should be carefully examined for any evidence of needle puncture. Rapidly fatal pneumothorax following delivery has been observed; death could have been prevented by detection of the needle wound in the thorax and prompt treatment.

Several attempts have been made to identify the overall risk of amniocentesis performed near midpregnancy for the purpose of detecting hereditary disease or congenital defects in the fetus. In one study (National Institute of Child Health and Human Development, 1976) no significant differences were found in fetal loss rate, birth weights, birth defects, neonatal complications, or growth and development at 1 year of age. The overall fetal loss was 3.5 percent for the amniocentesis group and 3.2 percent for the control group. The overall accuracy of prenatal diagnosis was 99.4 percent. Similar results were obtained in a Canadian study (Simpson et al., 1976). In a British study, however,

(Working Party on Amniocentesis, 1978) a higher fetal loss rate of 2.6 percent was identified in the amniocentesis group, compared to an unusually low value of 1.1 percent in the control group. Of concern, there was an apparent increase in certain abnormalities in the newborn infants, especially respiratory problems at birth and orthopedic postural deformities. The abnormalities are suggestive that amniocentesis, at times, resulted in loss of amnionic fluid volume sufficient to restrict pulmonary excursion and to create abnormal fetal postures. In all studies, complications were greater when a large needle (18-gauge or larger) was used and when more than two taps were made to obtain fluid.

BLOODY TAP. Erythrocytes contaminating amnionic fluid may complicate appreciably the technics for study and the interpretation of the results. Erythrocytes may inhibit the replication in culture of fetal cells from amnionic fluid. Moreover, blood may change the apparent level of various constituents of amnionic fluid under study. Gibbons and coworkers (1974) have studied the effects of adding up to 4 percent maternal blood to fresh amnionic fluid which was then promptly centrifuged. The addition to amnionic fluid of blood concentrations of 1 percent or more produced a lowering of the lecithin to sphingomyelin (L/S) ratio and a slight decrease in creatinine concentration. Thus, the changes were in a direction that would lead to the prediction of a less mature fetus for reasons considered below. Buhi and Spellacy (1975) identified maternal serum to have a L/S ratio of 1.3 to 1.5, and they found that its addition to amnionic fluid influenced the ratio accordingly; meconium also lowered the L/S ratio somewhat. In general, if the "hematocrit" of the spun amnionic fluid exceeds 3 percent, the sample should be considered unsatisfactory for measurement of L/S ratio. Minute amounts of fetal, but not maternal, blood can lead to falsely high levels of α-fetoprotein in amnionic fluid. Therefore, if the amnionic fluid appears bloody, it should not be used for such analysis if the red cells are of fetal origin.

Amnionic Fluid Surfactant.

Amniocentesis was initially employed primarily to estimate the concentration of bilirubin or bilirubin-like pigment in amnionic fluid and thereby to identify hemolytic disease in the fetus. Currently, it is probably used most often to determine the relative concentration of surfactant-active phospholipids to try to identify the fetus that is at risk of developing respiratory distress if delivered at that time.

So-called type II pneumocytes of fetal lung alveoli produce surface-active phospholipids that are essential for the maintenance of effective respiration immediately after birth (see Chap. 8, p. 188). Without appropriate surfactant activity, the lung literally collapses with each expiration because of the high surface tension at air–fluid interfaces, and the syndrome of idiopathic respiratory distress develops (see Chap. 38, p. 957).

The specific lecithin dipalmitoyl phosphatidylcholine plus phosphatidylinnositol and especially phosphatidylglycerol are critically important in the formation and stabilization of the surface-active layer which prevents alveolar collapse and the development of respiratory distress. These compounds are contained in lamellar bodies which are released from the type II cell into the alveolar space from which appreciable amounts are transported to the surrounding amnionic fluid. An important consequence of the containment of most of the surfactant in the lamellar bodies is that after too vigorous centrifugation the precipitate is likely to contain most of the lecithin, while most of the sphingomyelin remains in the supernatant to give a falsely low lecithin to sphingomyelin ratio.

LECITHIN-SPHINGOMYELIN (L/S) RATIO.

Measurement of the L/S ratio demands a well-monitored laboratory, since slight variations in technic can appreciably affect the accuracy of the results. Especially critical steps are centrifugation at appropriate speed, acetone precipi-

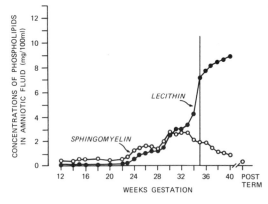

FIG. 14-4. Changes in mean concentrations of lecithin and sphingomyelin in amnionic fluid during gestation in normal pregnancy. (From Gluck and Kulovich. *Am J Obstet Gynecol* 115:541, 1973)

tation, and densitometric measurement of the charred lecithin and sphingomyelin. If the analysis is not performed promptly, the specimen should be refrigerated.

Before 34 weeks gestation, lecithin and sphingomyelin are present in amnionic fluid in approximately equal amounts. At about 34 weeks, the concentration of lecithin relative to sphingomyelin begins to rise (Fig. 14-4).

It has been shown by Gluck and co-workers (1971), and confirmed by others, that for pregnancies of unknown duration, but otherwise uncomplicated, the risk of respiratory distress in the newborn is very slight whenever the concentration of lecithin in amnionic fluid is at least twice that of sphingomyelin whereas there is increased risk of respiratory distress when the L/S ratio is below 2. Harvey et al. (1975) have combined the data from 25 reports in which L/S ratios were measured by similar technics on amnionic fluid collected within 72 hours of delivery. The results are shown in Table 14-1. With an L/S ratio greater than 2.0, the risk of respiratory distress was found to be slight unless the mother had diabetes (see Chap. 28, p. 748). If the L/S ratio was 1.5 to 2.0, respiratory distress was identified in 40 percent, and if below 1.5, in 73 percent. Even though 73

TABLE 14-1.
RELATIONSHIP OF
LECITHIN-SPHINGOMYELIN RATIO
TO DEVELOPMENT OF
RESPIRATORY DISTRESS

L/S RATIO	INFANTS (NO.)	RESPIRATORY DISTRESS (PERCENT)	
		All Cases	Deaths
> 2.5	543	0.9	0
> 2.0	1596	2.2	0.1
1.5–2.0	223	40	4
< 1.5	162	73	14

Adapted from Harvey, Parkinson, and Campbell: *Lancet* 1:42, 1975

percent of infants did develop respiratory distress when the L/S ratio was below 1.5, it proved fatal in but 14 percent (Table 14-1).

The recent experiences at Parkland Memorial Hospital have been that respiratory distress did not develop in some instances in which the L/S ratio was as low as 0.6. Moreover, infants for whom the L/S ratio in amnionic fluid was as low as 0.3 have survived after suffering respiratory distress (Herbert et al., 1979). When the L/S ratio was greater than 0.50 deaths from respiratory distress were actually quite low (Table 14-2). Obviously, there are times when the risk to the fetus from a hostile intrauterine environment will be greater than the risk of death from

respiratory distress even though the L/S ratio is less than 2.

Unfortunately, with some pregnancy complications, for example, class A and B maternal diabetes, erythroblastosis fetalis, or most any event which causes the infant to be metabolically seriously compromised at birth, an L/S ratio of 2 or more does not necessarily preclude the development of respiratory distress. Surfactant action insufficient to prevent respiratory distress, even though the L/S ratio is 2 or more, is thought to be due usually to lack of *phosphatidylglycerol* and the enhancement of surface-active properties that phosphatidylglycerol provides. The indentification of phosphatidylglycerol in amnionic fluid provides assurance that respiratory distress will not develop (Hallmann et al., 1977). Moreover, phosphatidylglycerol has not been detected in blood, meconium, or vaginal secretions; consequently, these contaminants do not confuse the interpretation. Importantly, the absence of phosphatidylglycerol is not necessarily a strong indicator that respiratory distress is likely to develop after delivery; its absence serves to indicate only that the infant *may* develop respiratory distress.

The possibility has been raised that the location of the needle in the amnionic sac may influence the L/S ratio. Worthington and Smith (1978) contend that fluid collected remote from the location of the fetal mouth and nares may have an L/S ratio appreciably

TABLE 14-2.
RELATIONSHIP BETWEEN L/S RATIO, IDIOPATHIC RESPIRATORY
DISTRESS, VENTILATOR THERAPY, AND NEONATAL MORTALITY AT
PARKLAND MEMORIAL HOSPITAL

L/S RATIO	INFANTS (NO.)	RESPIRATORY DISTRESS	VENTILATOR RX	DIED
≤ 0.50	13	13	13	10
0.51–1.00	17	6	4	2
1.01–1.50	14	1	1	0
1.51–1.99	22	0	0	0

From Herbert, Tyson, and Jimenez: *Ped Res* 13:497, 1979

lower than that collected in close proximity to the mouth and nares. This observation has not been confirmed.

FOAM STABILITY (SHAKE) TEST. To reduce the time and effort inherent in precise measurement of the L/S ratio, the foam stability test, or so-called shake test, was introduced by Clements and associates (1972). The test depends upon the ability of surfactant in amnionic fluid when mixed appropriately with ethanol to generate stable foam at the air–liquid interface. The technic takes no more than one-half hour to complete.

Into one chemically clean 13 × 100 mm glass tube with a Teflon-lined plastic screw cap are added 1.0 ml of recently collected amnionic fluid and 1 ml of 95 percent ethanol (prepared by diluting 19.0 parts absolute alcohol with 1 part of distilled water) and into another tube 0.5 ml of amnionic fluid, 0.5 ml of 0.9 percent saline, and 1 ml of the 95 percent ethanol. Each tube is vigorously shaken for 15 sec and placed upright in a rack for 15 min. The persistence of an intact ring of bubbles at the air–liquid interface after 15 min is a positive test.

If the ring of foam persists for 15 min in both tubes, the risk of respiratory distress is very low. For example, Schleuter and coworkers (1979), identified but one instance of respiratory distress developing out of 205 pregnancies in which the test was positive for amnionic fluid diluted with an equal volume of saline. There are, however, two problems with the test: (1) Slight contamination of amnionic fluid, reagents, or glassware, or errors in measurement may alter the test results markedly. (2) A falsely negative test is rather common, i.e., failure of the ring of foam to persist intact for 15 min in the tube containing diluted amnionic fluid seldom is associated with respiratory distress. At least that is the experience at our institution.

FLUORESCENT POLARIZATION (MICROVISCOMETRY). Another approach to the identification of surfactant activity in am-

nionic fluid has been evaluated by Blumenfeld et al., (1978), Elrad et al., (1978), and Golde and coworkers (1979). The microviscosity of lipid aggregates in the amnionic fluid may be assayed by mixing the fluid with a specific fluorescent dye which incorporates into the hydrocarbon region of the lipids in surfactant. The intensity of the fluorescence induced by polarized light is then measured. The technic is rapid and appears simple to perform but the instrument is expensive.

Amnionic Fluid Bilirubin. Hemolysis yields bilirubin, most of which remains unconjugated by the fetus. How unconjugated bilirubin reaches the amnionic fluid from the fetus is uncertain, since there is essentially none in the fetal urine and the fetal skin appears to be impermeable to free bilirubin during the latter half of pregnancy. The respiratory tract and the amnion over the placenta and umbilical cord are possible but unproven pathways. The concentration of bilirubin in amnionic fluid normally falls progressively during the latter half of pregnancy, usually to become essentially zero as the fetus reaches maturity. Typically, the bilirubin level and the rate of decrease during the last several weeks of pregnancy are so slight and problems inherent in analysis are sufficiently great to preclude its use as a sensitive test of fetal maturity. In case of fetal hemolytic disease, however, the concentration of bilirubin for any given fetal age usually reflects the intensity of the hemolysis (see Chap. 38, p. 966).

It is not always appreciated that bilirubin in the amnionic fluid need not be of fetal origin. An elevated maternal plasma concentration of free bilirubin, as for example with sickle cell anemia, is reflected in an elevation in the amnionic fluid.

Amnionic fluid supernatant is best analyzed for bilirubin using a continuously recording spectrophotometer. There is a characteristic absorption peak at 450 nm, the correct height of which, when measured as an increase in optical density above baseline, is proportional to the bilirubin concentration (Fig. 38-4), p. 964). In current symbolism, the value is usually expressed as Δ OD 450. Measurement of bilirubin by ordinary chemical methods is not satisfactory because of the low concentration in amnionic fluid.

Other Amnionic Fluid Indicators of Fetal Maturity.   Evaluation of many other constituents or properties of amnionic fluid has been suggested to try to identify fetal maturity. Those that have been cited often are the concentration of creatinine, the osmolality, and the presence of appropriate amounts of cells that are lipid-stainable. While these constituents or properties change as the fetus matures, the rate and the degree of change often are so slight or so variable that their measurements do not provide an acceptable level of precision for identification of fetal maturity. Moreover, results that imply functional maturity for one organ system should not be interpreted to imply functional maturity of another. For example, remarkable variation was demonstrated for quintuplets born at Parkland Memorial Hospital 222 days after the onset of the last menstrual period. Within the limits of measurement the creatinine concentration and the osmolality were identical in amnionic fluid from each sac, 2 mg per dl and 265 mOsmol per liter, respectively. These values imply fetal maturity as pointed out below. At the same time the L/S ratio in amnionic fluid from each sac ranged from less than 2 to greater than 5. Respiratory distress was associated with the low but not the high L/S ratios.

AMNIONIC FLUID CREATININE.   During the latter half of pregnancy, the concentration of creatinine in amnionic fluid slowly rises until near term, when the increase is more rapid. The rise most likely is the consequence of increased excretion of creatinine by the maturing fetal kidneys. A level of 2.0 mg per dl in amnionic fluid not treated to remove nonspecific chromogens most often indicates fetal maturity. There are two problems inherent in the test: (1) pulmonary function may prove to be mature even though the creatinine concentration is less than 2 mg

per dl; (2) an increase in maternal plasma creatinine will cause an increase in the amnionic fluid creatinine although the fetus is not mature. Therefore, although measurement of creatinine in amnionic fluid has been urged, at least by some, to identify fetal maturity, others have regarded it as unreliable. If creatinine concentration is to be used, it is essential to ascertain that the mother's plasma creatinine level is not elevated. According to Teoh and co-workers (1973), measurement of uric acid offers no advantage over creatinine, while urea is even less reliable as an indicator of fetal maturity. Pitkin (1974) rightfully emphasized that none of these laboratory tests is a substitute for rational clinical judgment.

AMNIONIC FLUID OSMOLALITY.   Early in pregnancy, the osmolality of amnionic fluid and fetal serum are the same. From 20 weeks onward, however, the osmolality of amnionic fluid decreases at the rate of approximately 1 mOsmol per liter per week, presumably as the consequence of dilution by nonprotein nitrogen-rich, but hypotonic, fetal urine. The rate of decrease, in osmolality, however, is too gradual and too variable to allow a precise prediction of fetal maturity.

LIPID-STAINING OF CELLS IN AMNIONIC FLUID.   Staining of amnionic fluid aspirate with Nile blue sulfate discloses two categories of cells or cell particles. Blue-stained bodies represent shed fetal epithelial cells, while the orange-stained bodies originate from sebaceous glands. In the later stages of gestation, an increase in orange bodies appears to reflect maturity of the sebaceous glands. Bishop and Corson (1968) claimed that orange bodies in excess of 10 percent indicate the gestational age of the fetus to be a least 35 weeks, and, when in excess of 30 percent, fetal age most likely is more than 36 weeks. Nonetheless, two major problems arise from the use of the Nile blue sulfate technic to identify fetal maturity: (1) The orange-colored bodies tend to clump, which makes quantification difficult.

(2) Lower percentages of orange-colored bodies do not necessarily indicate prematurity.

Amniocentesis to Identify Inherited Disorders. Amniocentesis allows access to fetal somatic cells and fluid that can be used to identify the cytogenetic constitution of the fetus or to assess a variety of abnormal biochemical processes. To identify a genetic disorder in the fetus, chromosomal analysis is more commonly employed:

1. Pregnancies in women 35 years of age or older.
2. A previous pregnancy that resulted in the birth of a chromosomally abnormal offspring.
3. Chromosomal abnormality in either parent, including
    (a) balanced translocation carrier state
    (b) aneuploidy
    (c) mosaicism
4. Down syndrome or other chromosomal abnormality in a close family member.
5. Pregnancy after three or more spontaneous abortions.
6. A previous infant with multiple major malformations but no cytogenetic study was performed.
7. Fetal sex determination in pregnancies at risk of a serious X-linked hereditary disorder.
8. Biochemical studies in pregnancies at risk of a serious autosomal or X-linked recessive disorder.
9. A previous child or a parent with a neural tube defect or on routine screening maternal serum α-fetoprotein level is abnormally high.

The amnionic fluid is aspirated at 15 to 18 weeks gestation when there is likely to be sufficient fetal cells present to allow successful cell culture. There is the possibility that the fluid collected at this time is urine from the maternal bladder rather than amnionic fluid. Elias and co-workers (1979) have pointed out that the two fluids usually can be quickly differentiated by the presence

TABLE 14-3.
FREQUENCY OF SELECTED CHROMOSOME ABNORMALITIES IN THE NEWBORN

Trisomy 21	1 in 800–1000 births
Trisomy 18	1 in 8000 births
Trisomy 13	1 in 20,000 births
XXY	1 in 1000 male births
XYY	1 in 1000 male births
XXX	1 in 950 female births
XO	1 in 10,000 female births

From *Antenatal Diagnosis.* NIH Publication Number 79–1973, April, 1979

of crystallization when the amnionic fluid is dried on a glass slide and examined microscopically under low power.

The frequencies of the more common significant cytogenetic abnormalities in newborn infants in the United States are listed in Table 14-3. From these data, it is estimated that each year in the United States 15,000 infants are born with a chromosomal abnormality (Antenatal Diagnosis, 1979). Moreover, there are probably 175,000 spontaneous abortions of chromosomally abnormal fetuses annually.

The most common abnormality in the infant who is liveborn is trisomy 21, or Down syndrome (Table 14-3), even though it is estimated that two thirds of conceptuses with trisomy 21 do not survive the pregnancy. Whereas the risk of a liveborn offspring with Down syndrome is one in 885 at maternal age 30, it increases to 1 in 365 at age 35, to 1 in 109 at age 40, and 1 in 32 at age 45 (Table 39-3, p. 996). The frequencies of most other trisomies and sex chromosome aneuploidies also increase with maternal age.

Cytogenetic studies are being widely recommended for all women who are 35 or older, although any age limit is arbitrarily selected rather than being decided on the basis of a sudden biologic difference between women immediately above or below a certain age. The magnitude of the problem created by attempting to provide genetic counseling and cytogenetic screening of fetuses of all women who are 35 or older becomes readily apparent when it is appreciated that in 1979 there were 142,000 births by women 35 or older, compared to but 25,000 births by women who were 40 or older. Moreover, it is predicted that within a decade the number of births by women 35 or older will exceed 200,000 annually (Antenatal Diagnosis, 1979).

When a parent is the carrier of a balanced chromosomal translocation, there is a 4 to 20 percent risk that the fetus will be abnormal (see Chap. 39, p. 996).

With X-linked recessive diseases for which no specific prenatal diagnostic test is readily available to differentiate affected from unaffected male fetuses, at least the sex of the fetus can be identified accurately, and when female and the father is not affected, the risk of an affected offspring is eliminated.

FETAL SEX. At 15 to 18 weeks gestation, the sex of the fetus can be determined by (1) demonstrating the nuclear sex chromatin mass (Barr body), (2) Y chromosome staining, and (3) cell culture and karyotyping. With very careful studies to identify the presence or absence of nuclear sex chromatin in uncultivated, directly stained amnionic fluid cells, the overall accuracy is about 95 percent (Milunsky, 1973). Staining for the Y chromosome in uncultured cells from amnionic fluid, Valenti and co-workers (1972) reported an accuracy of about 97 percent. Thus, the test did not improve the accuracy significantly over the sex chromatin method, and when the prediction of sex is crucial, they recommend that confirmation be derived by karyotyping cultured amnionic fluid cells.

Identification of the sex of the fetus has been attempted by measuring testosterone and FSH in amnionic fluid. In one study, overlap of values for female and male fetuses was sufficient that in 7 percent neither determination was indicative of fetal sex (Belisle et al., 1977).

OTHER INHERITABLE DISORDERS. A great variety of inheritable disorders of metabolic function have been detected by appropriate study of amnionic fluid contents, especially using cells grown in culture. Listings of many such disorders are presented in Table 14-4.

Approximately 75 recessively inherited X-sex chromosome-linked or autosomal metabolic disorders are now detectable in somatic cell systems and therefore are approachable in the fetus through amniocentesis. The risk of an autosomal recessive disorder in the fetus may have become apparent from either the previous birth of an affected infant or from screening of the parents for the carrier state. If both parents are carriers, the risk of the fetus being homozygous and therefore seriously affected is 25 percent, whereas for X-linked disease, if the mother is a carrier, the risk of male offspring being affected is 50 percent but for female offspring it is zero, unless the father is affected. Unfortunately, the carrier state for several recessive conditions cannot be detected except by birth of an affected infant. One which can be detected, however, is Tay-Sachs disease in which screening programs have been established especially among Jewish couples for Tay-Sachs disease, since it is 100 times more frequent in Jews. The affected fetus of heterozygous parents can be detected through biochemical studies on cells cultured from amnionic fluid.

Parents who are heterozygous for the gene for production of hemoglobin S or for beta thalassemia can be readily identified. However, to date, the identification of the homozygous state in the fetus has necessitated obtaining fetal red cells (p. 347).

DETECTION OF ELEVATED α-FETO-PROTEIN. The value of measurement of α-fetoprotein in amnionic fluid between 16 and 20 weeks gestation to detect fetal abnormality, especially open neural tube defects, is now established.

The site of production of most, if not all, of the increased α-fetoprotein is the fetus. It is the major protein in serum of the embryo and early fetus. Initially, it is produced in the yolk sac but by the end of the first trimester it is nearly all of hepatic origin. In both

TABLE 14-4.

OTHER INHERITABLE DISORDERS IDENTIFIABLE BY APPROPRIATE
STUDY OF AMNIONIC FLUID CONTENTS

DISORDER	ENZYME ACTIVITY DEFICIENCY	PRENATAL DIAGNOSIS
Prenatal Diagnosis of Inborn Errors of Lipid Metabolism*		
Cholesterol ester	Acid lipase	Possible
Fabry's disease	α-galactosidase A	Achieved
Farber's disease	Ceramidase	Potentially possible
Gaucher's disease	β-glucosidase	Achieved
GM$_1$ Gangliosidoses		
Type I–generalized gangliosidoses	β-galactosidase (A, B, and C)	Achieved
Type II–juvenile GM$_1$ gangliosidosis	β-galactosidase (B and C only)	Achieved
GM$_2$ Gangliosidoses		
Type I–Tay-Sachs disease	Hexosaminidase A	Achieved
Type II–Sandhoff's disease	Hexosaminidase A and B	Achieved
Type III–juvenile GM$_2$ gangliosidosis	Partial deficiency	Possible
Krabbe's disease (globoid cell leukodystrophy)	Galactocerebroside β-galactosidase	Achieved
Lactosyl ceramidosis	Lactosyl ceramidase	Possible
Metachromatic leukodystrophy	Aryl sulfatase A	Achieved
Mucolipidosis type II (I cell disease)	Multiple lysosomal hydrolases	Achieved
Mucolipidosis type III (Pseudopolydystrophy)	Multiple lysosomal hydrolases	Possible
Mucolipidosis IV	Multiple lysosomal hydrolases	Achieved
Neimann-Pick disease	Aphingomyelinase	Achieved
Refsum's disease	Phytanic acid α-hydrolase	Possible
Wolman's disease	Acid lipase	Possible
Prenatal Diagnosis of Mucopolysaccharidoses		
Type I H–Hurler syndrome	α-L-iduronidase	Achieved
Type I S–Scheie syndrome	α-L-iduronidase	Possible
Type I H/S– Hurler/Scheie	α-L-iduronidase	Possible
Type II–Hunter syndrome†	Iduronic acid sulfatase	Achieved
Type IIIa–Sanfilippo A	Heparin sulfamidase	Achieved
Type IIIb–Sanfilippo B	α-N-acetyl-glucosaminidase	Possible
Type IV–Morquio	N-acetyl-galactosamine-6-sulfatase	Possible
Type VI–Mara-teaux-Lamy	Arylsulfatase B	Achieved
Type VII–β-glucuronidase deficiency	β-glucuronidase	Possible

(Continued)

TABLE 14-4. (Continued)

DISORDER	ENZYME ACTIVITY DEFICIENCY	PRENATAL DIAGNOSIS
Prenatal Diagnosis of Inborn Errors of Carbohydrate Metabolism‡		
Fucosidosis	α-fucosidase	Possible
Galactokinase deficiency	Galactokinase	Potentially possible
Galactosemia	Galactose-1-phosphate uridyl transferase	Achieved
Glucose-6-phosphate dehydrogenase deficiency	Glucose-6-P-dehydrogenase	Possible
Glycogen storage diseases		
Type II–Pompe's disease	α-1, 4-glucosidase (acid maltase)	Achieved
Type III–Debrancher deficiency	Amylo-1, 6-glucosidase	Possible
Type IV–Brancher deficiency	Amylo-1, 4 to 1, 6-transglucosidase	Possible
Glycogen storage disease with phosphorylase kinase deficiency	Phosphorylase kinase	Possible
Mannosidosis	α-mannosidase	Possible
Phosphohexose isomerase deficiency	Phosphohexose isomerase	Possible
Pyruvate decarbosylase deficiency	Pyruvate decarbosylase	Potentially possible
Pyruvate dehydrogenase deficiency	Pyruvate dehydrogenase	Potentially possible
Prenatal Diagnosis of Amino Acid and Related Metabolic Disorders§		
Argininosuccinic aciduria	Argininosuccinase	Achieved
Aspartylglucosaminuria	Aspartylglucosaminidase	Possible
Citrullinemia	Argininosuccinate synthetase	Achieved
Cystathioninuria	Cystathionase	Potentially possible
Cystinosis	↑ Intracellular cystine content	Achieved
Histidinemia	Histidase	Possible
Homocystinuria	Cystathionine synthetase	Achieved
Hypervalinemia	Valine transaminase	Potentially possible
Maple syrup urine disease		
Severe infantile form	Branched-chain ketoacid decarboxylase	Achieved
Intermittent form	Branched-chain ketoacid decarboxylase	Potentially possible
Methylmalonic acidemia I B$_{12}$ unresponsive	Methylmalonic-CoA mutase	Achieved
Methylmalonic acidemia II B$_{12}$ responsive	Partial defect in vitamin B$_{12}$ coenzyme	Achieved
Ornithinemia	Ornithine-α-ketoacid transaminase	Possible

(Continued)

TABLE 14-4. (Continued)

DISORDER	ENZYME ACTIVITY DEFICIENCY	PRENATAL DIAGNOSIS
Propionic acidemia (ketonic hypergly- cinemia)	Propionyl CoA carboxylase	Achieved

Other Metabolic Disorders in which Prenatal Diagnosis is Applicable‖

Acatalasemia	↓ Catalase	Potentially possible
Adenosine deaminase deficiency	↓ Adenosine deaminase	Achieved
α-thalassemia	Deletion of α-globin structural genes	Achieved
Adrenogenital syndrome (congenital adrenal hyperplasia)	21-hydroxylase defi- ciency (one of many types)	Possible
Chediak-Higashi disease	Not known	Potentially possible
Congenital erythropoietic porphyria	↓ Uroporphyrinogen III cosynthetase	Achieved
Congenital nephrotic syndrome	↑ α-Fetoprotein amniotic fluid	Achieved
Familial hypercholes- terolemia	Abnormal feedback sup- pression of 3-hydroxy- 3-methyl glutaryl coenzyme A reductase	Possible
Hypophosphatasia	↓ Alkaline phosphatase	Achieved
Lesch-Nyhan syndrome‖	↓ Hypoxanthine-guanine phosphoribosyl trans- ferase	Achieved
Lysosomal acid phosphatase deficiency	↓ Lysosomal acid phosphatase	Achieved
Menkes' disease‖	↑ Copper accumulation	Achieved
Myotonic dystrophy‖	Linkage analysis possible in some families	Possible
Orotic aciduria	↓ Orotidylic pyrophos- phorylase ↓ Orotidylic decarboxy- lase	Potentially possible
Sulfite oxidase	↓ Sulfite oxidase	Possible
Xeroderma pigmentosa	Defective DNA repair	Achieved

From Miles and Kaback: Prenatal diagnosis of hereditary disorders. *Ped Clin North Am* 25:593, 1978

* The inheritance of each of these disorders is autosomal recessive except Fabry's disease which is X-linked recessive.

† The inheritance is autosomal recessive for each disorder except for Type II—Hunter syndrome, which is X-linked recessive

‡ The inheritance is autosomal recessive except for glucose-6-phosphate dehydrogenase defi- ciency and glycogen storage disease with phosphorylase kinase deficiency, in which it is X-linked recessive.

§ The inheritance of each of these disorders is autosomal recessive.

‖ Inheritance is autosomal recessive except for Lesch-Nyhan syndrome and Menkes' disease in which it is X-linked recessive, and myotonic dystrophy in which it is autosomal dominant.

fetal serum and amnionic fluid the concentration of α-fetoprotein is highest around the 13th week of gestation (Fig. 14-5). The concentration of fetal serum is about 100 times that of amnionic fluid. Apparently the normal source of the protein in amnionic fluid is fetal urine (Seppälä, 1978). Some of that protein, in turn, crosses the fetal membranes to enter the maternal circulation (Haddow et al., 1979).

After 13 weeks the levels in both fetal serum and amnionic fluid decrease rapidly in essentially parallel fashion. Since the level in amnionic fluid decreases sharply, correct interpretation requires precise knowledge of gestational age. The concentration of α-fetoprotein levels in maternal serum are only one-hundredth to one-thousandth those of fetal serum. The low maternal levels normally rise slowly during the 2nd trimester to reach a plateau early in the 3rd trimester.

The level of α-fetoprotein in amnionic fluid, maternal serum, or both, may be elevated in a number of circumstances which include the following:

1. Open neural tube defects (anencephaly, open spina bifida)
2. Congenital nephrosis
3. Bladder neck obstruction
4. Esophageal and duodenal atresia
5. Exomphalos
6. Sacrococcygeal teratoma
7. Pilonidal sinus
8. Turner syndrome (45, XO)
9. Fetal death
10. Fetal blood in amnionic fluid
11. Feto-maternal hemorrhage

OPEN NEURAL TUBE DEFECTS. Experiences with screening for open neural tube defects are now considerable, especially in Great Britain. As one consequence, considerable enthusiasm has been generated for measuring near midpregnancy the level of α-fetoprotein in the serum of most or all pregnant women. When levels are sufficiently elevated to suspect the possibility of a neural tube defect, then amniocentesis is performed to look for definitely elevated levels in amnionic

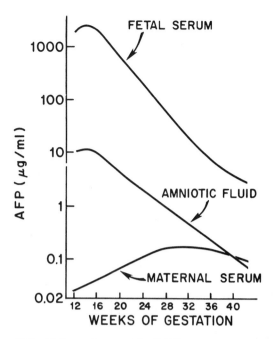

FIG. 14-5. α-fetoprotein (AFP) concentrations in fetal serum, amnionic fluid, and maternal serum throughout gestation. (From Seppälä. *Amniotic Fluid, 2nd ed.* (Ed) New York, Excerpta Medica, 1978)

fluid. Moreover, the fetus is usually carefully scanned sonographically for evidence of abnormality, especially anencephaly and spina bifida.

Ferguson-Smith and associates (1978) in Glasgow have reported their experiences from screening 11,585 pregnant women between 16 and 20 completed weeks of gestation for elevated serum levels of α-fetoprotein. A serum level sensitive enough to detect 93 percent of afflicted fetuses was found in 1.7 percent of women. Three-fourths of the false-positives were eliminated by repeat measurement of α-fetoprotein or by sonography. As the result, in only 73 of 11,585 pregnancies originally screened (0.63 percent) was amniocentesis performed and elevated levels of α-fetoprotein were found in 34 (47 percent). There were no terminations of pregnancies as the consequence of false-positive amnionic fluid α-fetoprotein results. The birth of 96 percent of infants with anencephaly, a fatal lesion (see Chap. 39, p. 997), was avoided, but only 56 percent of those with open spina bifida were detected. Wald and associates (1979) correctly identified a higher percentage of fetuses with open spina bifida but at the apparent expense of interrupting two normal pregnancies.

Ferguson-Smith and co-workers (1978), on the basis of their extensive experiences, emphasize the following:

1. So that they can make their own decisions, expectant mothers and their husbands should be appropriately counseled about the test, about amniocentesis, and about termination of pregnancy.
2. A high standard of sonography is required for identifying accurately gestational age, multiple fetuses, a dead fetus, a fetal abnormality, and for performing safe amniocentesis.
3. An efficient organization is mandatory for immediate recall of women for further diagnostic tests and counseling. Since in their study, amniocentesis was accomplished before 20 weeks gestation in only 60 percent of cases, it is important in such instances to be able to perform an abortion after 20 weeks gestation.

CONGENITAL NEPHROSIS. Children with congenital nephrosis, although severely handicapped, may live for as long as 2 or 3 years. The abnormality is inherited as an autosomally recessive trait. In case of a previous infant born with congenital nephrosis, or a strong family history, an affected fetus may be identified through measurements of α-fetoprotein in maternal serum and especially in amnionic fluid (Aula et al., 1978).

ROUTINE SCREENING FOR α-FETO-PROTEIN. It is the consensus of a group of experts that at this time the measurement of α-fetoprotein in maternal serum is not justified for all pregnancies (Antenatal Diagnosis, 1979). Further studies may more clearly establish the worth, or lack of same, of routinely measuring the protein in maternal sera. However, if an amniocentesis is being performed at 15 to 19 weeks for some other purpose, it is probably wise also to measure α-fetoprotein.

AMNIONIC FLUID ACETYLCHOLINESTERASE ACTIVITY. Raised levels of acetylcholinesterase have been found by Smith and co-workers (1979), and others, in amnionic fluid in most instances of open neural tube defects. These findings suggest that the measurement of this enzyme in amnionic fluid may complement the measurement of α-fetoprotein and hopefully help reduce the number of falsely positive and negative diagnoses of open neural tube defects.

SONOGRAPHY

The impact of the use of pulse-echo ultrasonography on the practice of obstetrics has been great. Given but one choice from the many biochemical and biophysical technics that have been developed in more recent years to try to improve pregnancy outcome, sonography would seem the best. Methods for evaluating the health of the fetus that apply pulse-echo ultrasound are now widely employed for the very good reasons summarized below and illustrated frequently throughout this text. Sonographic technics that are now available, when carefully performed and accurately interpreted, can supply vital information about the status of the fetus, with no known risks from the ultrasound.

Intermittent high-frequency sound waves are generated by applying an alternating current to a transducer made of a piezoelectric material. The transducer is "connected" to the abdominal wall by placing a coupling agent—usually mineral oil—on the skin to diminish the loss of ultrasound waves at the interface between the transducer and the skin. The transducer so applied emits a pulse of sound waves that passes through soft tissue until an interface between structures of different tissue densities is reached. When this occurs, some of the energy, proportional to the difference in densities at the interface, is reflected, or echoed, back to the transducer. This, in turn, stimulates the transducer while in the listening state to generate a small electrical voltage which is then amplified and displayed on a fluorescent screen.

The pulse-echo technic serves to identify the location of anatomic structures by measuring the transition time for ultrasound waves to reach the structure, be reflected at the interface, and return to the detector. This basic technic can be applied in a number of ways: (1) to measure the size of structures (A-scan) such as the fetal head; (2) to provide a visual cross-sectional picture that will allow identification of size, shape, and location of structures (B-scan); (3) to observe actual movement of structures (Real time). With Real time ultrasonography, a special transducer is employed which generates multiple pulse-echo systems that are activated in sequence and thereby detect movement, including breathing, cardiac actions, and vessel pulsations.

Clinical Application. Sonography has proved valuable for monitoring the products of conception in a variety of ways that include:

1. Very early identification of intrauterine pregnancy
2. Demonstration of the size and the rate of growth of the amnionic sac and the embryo, and, at times, resorption or expulsion of the embryo
3. Identification of multiple fetuses, including conjoined twins
4. Measurements of the biparietal diameter of the fetal head to help identify the duration of gestation for the normal fetus or, when measured sequentially, to help identify the growth-retarded fetus
5. Comparison of fetal head and chest or abdominal circumference to identify hydrocephaly, microcephaly, or anencephaly
6. Detection of fetal anomalies such as marked distension of the fetal bladder, ascites, polycystic kidneys, renal agenesis, ovarian cyst, intestinal obstruction, meningomyelocele, or limb defects
7. Demonstration of hydramnios or oligohydramnios by comparing the size of the fetus to the amnionic space surrounding the fetus
8. Location of the placenta
9. Demonstration of placental abnormalities such as hydatidiform mole, as well as the location of the placenta
10. Identification of uterine tumors or anomalous development
11. Detection of a foreign body (intrauterine device).

FETAL MOTION. It is established unequivocally that the fetus breathes throughout most of pregnancy (see Chap. 8, p. 198). The movements can be witnessed by use of Real time sonography. Using Real-time sonography fetal heart beat has been demonstrated as early as 7 weeks gestation, trunk movement as early as 8 weeks, and limb movement as early as 9 weeks (Shawker et al, 1980).

FETAL URINATION. Bladder filling and emptying, and in turn estimation of the rate of urine formation, have been identified by serial sonography (see Chap. 8, p. 187). The procedure has not been generally applied in clinical practice, however.

RADIOGRAPHY, AMNIOGRAPHY, FETOGRAPHY

A variety of diagnostic radiologic technics have long been applied in obstetrics. In recent years, however, there has been growing concern over the possibility of radiation-induced carcinogenic and teratogenic effects, and also of mutagenic effects on future generations. The magnitude of the risks has not yet been clearly identified.

It is of interest to note the change in the use of diagnostic x-ray that has taken place with the advent of sonography. Whitehouse and associates, for example, reported for their department in 1958 that more than half of the x-ray requests for obstetric conditions were for determination of fetal age or for placental localization. With the advent of sonography, both determinations are now performed sonographically with much greater precision and probably greater safety.

Simple Roentgenogram. A roentgenogram of the abdomen and pelvis after 16 weeks gestation most often will identify fetal skeletal parts. During the latter half of pregnancy, the number of fetuses can usually be quantified. Gross skeletal abnormalities such as anencephaly and marked hydrocephaly are usually easily identified during the 3rd trimester. During the second half of pregnancy characteristic x-ray changes usually develop in the fetus sometime after death (see Chap. 10, p. 273).

Neither the age of the fetus nor his size can be identified with precision by use of simple radiography. Studies that have shown the best correlation between fetal age and the time of appearance of *lower limb ossification centers* typically have evaluated the limb radiologically after birth (Chan et al., 1972). Identification of ossification centers radiologically while in utero is often more difficult, however, since (1) maternal osseous structures may overlie and obscure the limb centers; (2) soft-tissue shadows from mother, fetus, amnionic fluid, and placenta may prevent visualization of the ossification centers; or (3) the fetus may move and blur the image. (X-ray pelvimetry is considered in Chapter 11, p. 285).

Amniography. Radiopaque agents may be injected into the amnionic sac to identify certain characteristics of the amnionic fluid, fetus, and placenta. Amniography, using water-soluble, iodinated radiocontrast material such as Urografin or Hypaque to opacify the amnionic fluid, may be employed to demonstrate abnormal amounts of amnionic fluid, the abnormally located placenta, the soft-tissue silhouette of the fetus, and, after a few hours of swallowing, the fetal gastrointestinal tract. Caterini and associates (1976) have described their generally favorable experiences

with amniography, the technic used by them, and an estimate of the doses of radiation that resulted. They emphasized that meconium staining of the amnionic fluid may follow amniography, particularly if the fetus is approaching maturity, but this should not be interpreted to indicate fetal distress. Moreover, the contrast agent is excreted into the maternal urine for the next 2 to 3 days following amniography and may cause erroneously low estriol values, at least with some methods. The water-soluble contrast media used in amniography may also falsely raise the L/S ratio in amnionic fluid (Knox et al., 1977).

Hydatidiform moles very often produce a diagnostic honey-combed x-ray pattern when water-soluble, iodinated contrast material is injected into the uterine cavity. However, sonography provides a simpler and usually more accurate technic for identification of a hydatidiform mole (Fig. 23-10, p. 563).

Fetography. Fetography involves the use of a heavily iodinated, lipid-soluble agent such as Ethiodol. When injected into the amnionic sac, the iodinated lipid adheres to the vernix on the skin of the near-mature fetus and thereby may outline the fetus much more vividly than do water-soluble radiopaque agents. This provides a capability for diagnosing some external soft-tissue anomalies and other pathologic states such as the cutaneous edema of hydrops fetalis (Wiessenhann, 1972).

Sonography carefully performed usually provides most of the information that may be afforded by amniography or fetography without using diagnostic x-rays, invading the amnionic sac, or injecting possibly harmful chemical agents.

AMNIOSCOPY

Saling (1973) has reported extensively on the visualization of amnionic fluid through the membranes when the cervix is sufficiently dilated. Amnioscopy to identify meconium-staining of amnionic fluid may be of value in late pregnancy complicated by (1) maternal hypertension, (2) apparently prolonged pregnancy, (3) suspected fetal growth retardation, (4) previous unexplained stillbirth, and (5) lack of orderly cervical dilatation or descent of the presenting part during the first stage of labor. Problems associated with amnioscopy are (1) the cervix must be accessible for visualization, i.e., neither too far posterior nor too far anterior; (2) the cervix must be dilated enough to visualize the membranes and the fluid behind them; (3) the membranes may be ruptured inadvertently during the examination; and (4) the intravaginal and intracervical manipulations may lead to infection of the products of conception and the upper genital tract. Amnioscopy to try to visualize amnionic fluid for meconium staining has not become popular in the United States.

Use of an amnioscope to obtain fetal blood is described on page 358 and demonstrated in Figure 14-10.

FETOSCOPY

There is considerable interest in instrumentation that provides for direct visualization of the fetus and the placenta. Development of such a laparoamnioscope hopefully will allow detection of externally located fetal anomalies and will provide tissue from the fetus or fetal blood vessels in the placenta for identification of serious fetal disease without appreciable risk to the fetus or the mother.

A technic currently employed to try to observe the fetus for gross anomalies or to obtain fetal blood is described: The position of the fetus and placenta are localized employing sonography, a site of entry for the fetoscope is chosen, and the abdominal wall at that site is anesthetized with a local anesthetic. A small skin incision is made, a cannula with a sharp trocar is inserted into the amnionic sac, and the trocar is replaced by the fetoscope.

The view of the fetus at any instant is lim-

ited to 2 to 4 cm of fetal surface. Nonetheless, Rodeck and Campbell (1978), and others, have reported the correct identification of neural tube defects in fetuses examined directly by fetoscopy at 16 to 18 weeks gestation.

A minute biopsy of skin may be made through the fetoscope to provide living cells for culture and subsequent biochemical or chromosomal studies. The safest place to obtain fetal blood is from a fetal vessel in the placenta immediately beneath the amnion. A 26- or 27-gauge needle may be inserted and blood collected directly or the needle may simply perforate the vessel after which the amnionic fluid in the vicinity of the hemorrhage is collected as the blood spurts from the needle hole (Hobbins, 1979). Fetal blood, either collected directly (Mibashan, 1979), or contained in amnionic fluid, has been used to identify classic hemophilia (Firshein et al., 1979), and to identify von Willebrand's disease (Hoyer et al., 1979).

Fetal blood cells obtained through the fetoscope as just described, or by simple needle aspiration of the placenta, have been used to identify a serious sickle cell hemoglobinopathy or the homozygous state for beta-thalassemia. A census performed by Alter served to identify 500 attempts made throughout the world as of September, 1978, to try to diagnose these conditions in utero (450 for beta-thalassemia and 50 for sickle cell anemia). Only 8 diagnostic errors were known to have been made (cited in Antenatal Diagnosis, 1979).

Fetoscopy must still be regarded as a research procedure because of the limitations of the fetoscope and the increased risks to the fetus and the mother compared to other methods of prenatal screening and diagnosis (Hobbins, 1979).

FETAL CELLS FROM MATERNAL BLOOD. Fetal cells potentially usable for prenatal diagnosis have been sorted from maternal blood samples collected as early as 15 weeks of gestation (Herzenberg et al., 1979). The potential for screening of pregnancies for abnormalities is apparent.

HORMONE AND ENZYME ASSAYS

Pregnancy-induced changes in a variety of hormones and enzymes have been extensively investigated with the hope of discovering practical tests to ascertain fetal age and fetal well-being.

Placental Lactogen and Estriol.
Placental lactogen (hPL) in maternal plasma, and especially estriol in maternal plasma and urine have been claimed to provide important predictive information concerning fetal well-being or lack of same. The use and abuse of measurements of these hormones are considered in Chapter 7 (p. 149 and p. 159), along with their production, distribution, metabolic functions, and clearance.

Chorionic Gonadotropin.
This hormone, normally produced by trophoblast and of clinical value for identifying early pregnancy, is considered in Chapter 7, page 147 and Chapter 10, page 265. Its measurement to identify persistent trophoblastic neoplasia is discussed in Chapter 23, p. 567.

Other Hormonal Tests.
Raja and co-workers (1974) reported that estradiol-17β rose appreciably in peripheral plasma before the onset of premature labor, while progesterone levels showed no consistent trend. They suggest that the measurement of estradiol-17β might prove to be of value to identify pregnancies in which premature labor is likely to occur. Their observations await confirmation.

Measurements of *progesterone levels* in maternal plasma have uncovered no constant pattern of change in pregnancies complicated by hypertension, diabetes, Rh isoimmunization, fetal growth retardation, or impending fetal death (Lindberg et al., 1974).

Measurement of the increase in *urinary estriol* excretion following intravenous injection of dehydroisoandrosterone has been evaluated as a test of placental function but appears to have little clinical value.

The metabolic clearance rate of *dehydroisoandrosterone sulfate* for young women destined to develop pregnancy-induced hypertension is somewhat greater early in pregnancy and then significantly lower than in normal pregnant women (Gant et al., 1971). Measurement of the metabolic clearance of dehydroisoandrosterone sulfate has not been demonstrated to have practical clinical utility.

Enzymes in Maternal Serum.
The activities of a number of enzymes change appreciably in maternal serum during pregnancy. Measurements of heat stable and total alkaline phosphatase, oxytocinase, and diamine oxidase have been urged by some to monitor fetal well-being, or to identify fetal maturity, or to do both. Such measurements have, in general, provided little information of value clinically.

FETAL BODY MOVEMENT AND WELL-BEING

Normally, throughout the second half of pregnancy expectant mothers are cognizant of frequent movement by the fetus. Ehrström (1979) identified in normal pregnancies fetal movements to increase from a median value of 86 per 12 hours in the 24th week to a maximum of 132 in the 32nd week. Activity then decreased to a median 12-hour value of 107 movements during the 40th week. It should be emphasized that there was considerable individual variation among the normal pregnancies that were studied.

Reduced Fetal Movements.
The fetus who late in pregnancy is felt by the mother to move consistently most often is healthy. Conversely, a sudden decrease in fetal movements is an ominous sign of loss of fetal well-being. The absolute number of movements per day appears to be less important in prognosis than is the degree of change in the frequency of fetal movements. In the case of cessation of fetal movements, fetal heart

sounds have been observed commonly to disappear within the next 24 hours. Sadovsky and Polishak (1977) found loss of fetal movement to be more reliable than measurements of urinary estriol for predicting impending fetal death.

Increased Fetal Movements. In some circumstances of sudden, severe fetal hypoxia, such as produced by abruptio placentae or severe cord compression, vigorous fetal movements are felt transiently by the mother. The increased movement is soon followed by loss of movement unless fetal hypoxia is promptly relieved, usually by delivery.

ELECTRONIC FETAL STRESS AND NONSTRESS TESTS

Two technics have emerged in which subtle changes in the fetal heart rate are searched for to try to evaluate fetal well-being. One is commonly referred to as the contraction stress test, or oxytocin challenge test, and the other as the nonstress test, or fetal heart acceleration test.

Contraction Stress Test. Hammacher (1966) appears to be the first to suggest that the fetal heart rate response to uterine contractions be used antepartum as a test of fetal well-being. Subsequently, in this country, Ray and co-workers (1972), and several others (see Huddleston and Freeman, 1977), have recommended the use of the contraction stress test, or oxytocin challenge test, for this purpose.

INDICATIONS AND CONTRAINDICATIONS. The following conditions may contraindicate the use of oxytocin to perform a contraction stress test: (1) threatened preterm labor, (2) placenta previa, (3) hydramnios, (4) multiple fetuses, (5) rupture of the membranes, (6) previous preterm labor, (7) and previous classical cesarean section. Otherwise, the proponents of the contraction stress test recommend that it be implemented during the 3rd trimester whenever the fetus is suspected of being in jeopardy. If the test is negative, it is usually repeated weekly thereafter as long as it remains negative.

TECHNIC. The contraction stress test usually takes 1 to 2 hours when performed as follows: With the mother lying on her back, but with her head and shoulders raised somewhat ("semi-Fowler" position), the fetal heart rate is recorded from an externally placed detector. Most often an ultrasound transducer (Fig. 14-6) is used since both phonocardiography and fetal electrocardiography when attempted through maternal tissue usually prove unsatisfactory (p. 354). Uterine activity is identified with an external tocographic transducer. As the uterus contracts and moves forward, a sensor pin attached to a strain gauge is pushed in by the change in shape of the abdominal wall. The change in electric current so generated is amplified and recorded. Although intrauterine pressure is not recorded, the onset, the time of maximum intensity, and the cessation of the contraction are identified with reasonable precision. To try to detect any reduction in placental perfusion as the consequence of aortocaval compression by the pregnant uterus while the mother is recumbent and thereby avoid a false-positive test, the maternal blood pressure is recorded initially and at least every 10 min thereafter during the procedure. Baseline uterine activity and fetal heart rate are recorded for 15 to 30 min. If spontaneous uterine contractions that last 40 to 60 sec and recur approximately three times in 10 min are detected, the response of the fetal heart rate to the contractions is evaluated as described below. In the absence of demonstrable spontaneous uterine activity and of abnormalities of fetal heart rate, oxytocin is then administered intravenously. The initial rate of infusion of 0.5 mU/min through a constant-speed infusion pump is doubled every 15 to 20 min until uterine contractions lasting 40 to 60 sec with a frequency of three per 10 min are established.

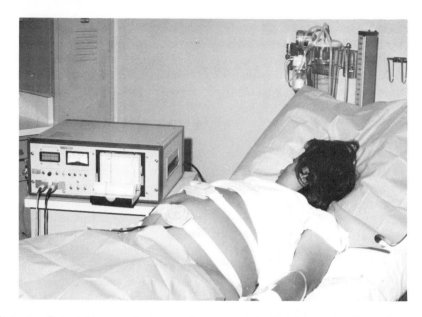

FIG. 14-6. External tococardiography. The upper detector strapped to the abdomen senses uterine contractions from the change in the curvature of the abdomen. The lower one detects fetal heart action using the Doppler principle and ultrasound. During the monitoring, the mother should not be restricted to the supine position.

INTERPRETATION. Freeman (1975) has categorized the results of the oxytocin challenge test as follows:

Positive: There is consistent and persistent late deceleration of the fetal heart rate, i.e., slowing of the heart rate develops sometime after the onset of the uterine contraction, the nadir for the heart rate is reached after the peak of uterine contraction, and recovery occurs after the contraction is completed (p. 356 and Fig. 14-7).

Negative: At least three contractions in 10 min, each lasting at least 40 sec, are observed without late deceleration of the fetal heart rate.

Suspicious: There is inconstant late deceleration that does not persist with subsequent contractions.

Hyperstimulation: If uterine contractions are more frequent than every 2 min, or last longer than 90 sec, or persistent uterine hypertonus is suspected, late deceleration does not necessarily indicate uteroplacental disease.

Unsatisfactory: The frequency of contractions is less than three per 10 min or the tracing is poor.

FALSE-NEGATIVE TESTS. It is now apparent that a negative contraction stress test *usually, but not always,* is compatible with uteroplacental function sufficient to maintain the fetus alive in utero for at least one more week. For example, Evertson and associates (1978) in one study identified the fetal death rate from all causes to be 7 out of 680, or 1 percent, within the next 7 days after a negative contraction stress test and Gal and coworkers (1979) in another reported three antepartum fetal deaths among 584 pregnancies within one week of a negative oxytocin challenge test.

FALSE-POSITIVE TESTS. The high false positive rate with the contraction stress test is even more troublesome. To avoid interrupting pregnancy prematurely when the test is positive, most advocates of the test recommend the application of other tests, especially measurements of amnionic fluid L/S ratio and urinary estriol, to try to identify more pre-

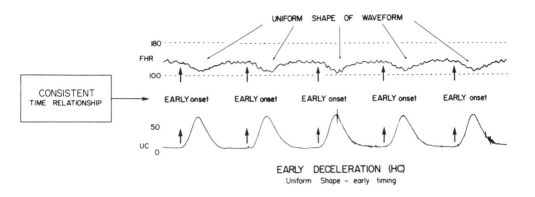

EARLY   DECELERATION   (HC)
Uniform   Shape - early   timing

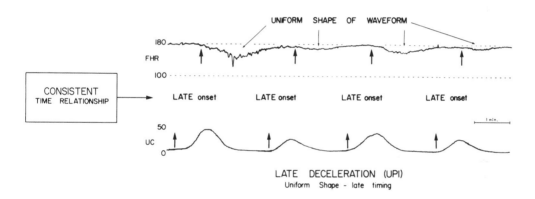

LATE   DECELERATION   (UPI)
Uniform   Shape - late   timing

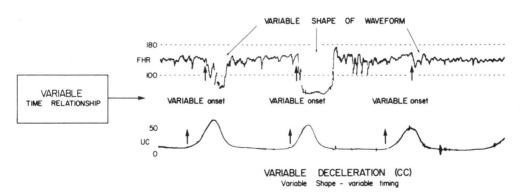

VARIABLE   DECELERATION   (CC)
Variable   Shape - variable   timing

FIG. 14-7.   Fetal heart rate decelerations in relation to the time of onset of uterine contractions. (From Hon. *An Atlas of Fetal Heart Rate Patterns.* New Haven, Harty Press, 1968)

cisely the status of the fetus. For example, when the contraction stress test is positive, Freeman (1975), considers active intervention if the L/S ratio is greater than 2.0, and even when the L/S ratio is less than 2.0 if urinary estriol is low or falling. Because of the likelihood in their experience that labor will be tolerated by the fetus, although the contraction stress test was recently positive, they recommend a trial of labor. As soon as the presenting part has descended into the pelvis and the cervix is dilated sufficiently to allow amniotomy a fetal scalp electrode is applied and an intrauterine pressure catheter is inserted, as described below.

Nonstress Test. Fetal movement typically is accompanied by transient acceleration of the fetal heart rate. This phenomenon, observed and reported by Hammacher and associates (1968), Kubli and co-workers (1969), and more recently by many others, serves as the basis for the "nonstress test" or fetal heart acceleration test.

TECHNIC. An ultrasonic transducer to detect the fetal heart beat is placed as described for the oxytocin test. Each time fetal movement is felt by the mother she presses a button to record the instant of movement on the same moving paper strip that the heart rate is recorded.

INTERPRETATION. The test is generally considered normal when three or more fetal movements are accompanied by acceleration of the fetal heart rate of at least 10 beats per minute. Lack of acceleration with fetal movement is considered abnormal. No fetal movement is considered unsatisfactory for testing but, if lacking for a prolonged period, may, in itself, be ominous (p. 348).

Several investigators have reported that acceleration of the fetal heart rate during and immediately after fetal movement is as good a prognosticator of fetal well-being as is a negative contraction stress test. Koller and Curet (1978), for example, found 99.5 percent of oxytocin challenge tests to be negative when performed soon after demonstrating ac-

celeration of the fetal heart rate with fetal movement. Lack of acceleration with fetal movement, however, was followed by a positive oxytocin challenge test in only 12 percent of their cases. Therefore, they considered lack of response to fetal movement to be unreliable and to require an oxytocin challenge test be performed and interpreted as described above. Observations reported to date imply that acceleration of the fetal heart with fetal movement, as with the oxytocin challenge test, most often, but not always, indicates that the fetus will survive in utero for at least one more week.

Other Antepartum Fetal Heart Rate Tests. Read and Miller (1977) have reported that sound of 105 to 120 decibels intensity delivered for 5 seconds through a microphone closely applied to the lower abdomen of the mother evoked acceleration of the fetal heart rate in instances where the oxytocin challenge test was negative. No response to the sound, however, was frequently associated with a suspicious or positive oxytocin challenge test. Harrigan and Marino (1978) have claimed that acceleration of the fetal heart rate in response to insertion of the needle during transabdominal amniocentesis is a favorable sign of fetal well-being whereas the reverse is usually true for decelerations that accompany amniocentesis. Possibly more "fetal fright tests" using other stimuli noxious at least to the fetus will be described.

INTRAPARTUM SURVEILLANCE OF THE FETUS

A major goal to be constantly strived for during labor is the preservation of fetal well-being by early detection and relief of fetal distress. To monitor means simply to watch or check on a person or thing. In the minds of many people, however, the word "monitor" in recent years has come to mean specifically surveillance of the fetal heart and uterine activity by some sort of an electronic detecting and recording device. It is sometimes lost sight of that clinical monitoring has produced meritorious results when conscientiously applied during labor and delivery by appropriately trained individuals (Haverkamp et al., 1976, 1979).

Electronic Monitoring of Fetal Heart Rate and Uterine Contractions. With each uterine contraction, there is a variable, temporary reduction in the flow of oxygenated maternal blood through the placental intracotyledonary spaces. Hon (1974) aptly pointed out that labor is a stress test for the fetus who may be handicapped by (1) intrinsic fetal disease, (2) placental disease, (3) cord compression, (4) maternal disease, (5) drugs administered for analgesia and anesthesia, or (6) maternal hypotension from the supine position, conduction anesthesia, or both. To detect fetal distress during labor, he and others urge that continuous beat-to-beat recording of the fetal heart rate be made comcomitant with the pressure changes generated by the uterine contractions. To this end, Hon and others perfected sophisticated electronic detection and recording equipment that is widely used for monitoring the fetal heart and uterine contractions (Fig. 14-6).

INTERNAL MONITORING OF FETAL HEART. The fetal heart rate may be identified beat by beat by attaching a unipolar electrode directly to the fetus and another electrode to the mother and, after appropriate filtration and amplification, recording each contraction of the fetal heart on a time-calibrated moving-strip recorder.

The spiral electrode in common use, developed by Hon and associates (1972), is shown in Figure 14-8. Electrical contact with the fetus is established by twisting the driving tube, which propels the spiral electrode through the skin. To be able to attach the electrode to the fetus the cervix needs to be dilated at least 1 cm, and, of course, the membranes above the cervix must be ruptured. It is important that the electrode be attached

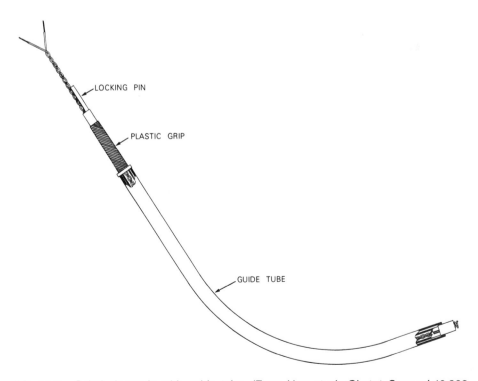

LOCKING PIN

PLASTIC GRIP

GUIDE TUBE

FIG. 14-8. Spiral electrode with guide tube. (From Hon et al. *Obstet Gynecol* 40:362, 1972)

to the fetus at a relatively benign site, avoiding such critical areas as the eyes. Thus, it is imperative that not only the presenting part be identified but that the site of attachment be precisely known.

The electrocardiographic signal picked up by the electrode inserted through the fetal skin is amplified sufficiently that typically the fetal R wave can be identified by a threshold detector which excludes all artifacts of lesser intensity. Good electrode placement that provides a high amplitude fetal electrocardiographic signal yields the best "signal-to-noise" ratio. In practice, each detected R wave (and any electronic noise of equal intensity) is recorded on a calibrated moving paper strip.

INTRAUTERINE PRESSURE MEASUREMENTS. Measurements of intrauterine pressure, i.e., the pressure in amnionic fluid, between and during contractions, are made by directly coupling the fluid to some sort of recording device. In clinical practice, a fluid-filled plastic catheter is positioned in utero so that the distal tip is located in amnionic fluid above the presenting fetal part (Fig. 14-9A and B). First, a plastic catheter guide that contains the distal portion of the catheter is inserted just through the cervical internal os and then the catheter is gently pushed beyond the guide into the uterine cavity. To minimize risk to the placenta from the catheter tip, Patel (1979), has recommended that when the site of placental implantation is known, the tip of the catheter inserter be positioned so that the catheter is likely to be inserted away from the placental site. The opposite end of the catheter, filled with saline, is connected to a strain-gauge pressure sensor adjusted to the same level as the catheter tip in the uterus. The amplified electrical signal produced in the strain-gauge by variations in pressure within the fluid system is recorded on a calibrated moving paper strip, usually simultaneously with the recording of the fetal heart rate. Free communication between amnionic fluid and fluid in the catheter is essential for meaningful pressure measurements. If the catheter tip becomes obstructed, it usually can be re-

lieved by injecting a small volume of sterile saline from a syringe through the catheter. To avoid damage to the transducer, it must be isolated from the system during this maneuver.

External (Indirect) Electronic Monitoring. The necessity for rupture of the membranes and invasion of the uterus may be avoided by use of external detectors to detect fetal heart action and to identify uterine activity (Fig. 14-6). External monitoring does not provide the precision of measurement of fetal heart rate or of uterine pressure afforded by internal monitoring.

The fetal heart rate may be detected in a number of ways through the maternal abdominal wall overlying the uterus. The easiest technic to use during the antepartum and early intrapartum periods utilizes the *ultrasound Doppler principle*. Ultrasonic waves undergo a shift in frequency as they are reflected from moving fetal heart valves and from fetal blood cells ejected in pulsitile fashion by cardiac systole. The unit for detecting fetal heart action consists of a transducer that emits ultrasound, typically with a frequency of 2 mHz, and a sensor to detect a shift in frequency of the reflected sound. The detector is placed on the abdomen at a site where fetal heart action is best detected. A coupling gel must be applied to the maternal skin, since air conducts ultrasound poorly. The device is held in position by an abdominal belt (Fig. 14-6).

Phonocardiography using a sensitive microphone may be tried to detect the sound generated by fetal heart action. Unfortunately, in clinical practice, extraneous sounds often create technical difficulties that limit the utility of this technic. The fetal *electrocardiogram* may, at times, be detected through electrodes attached to the maternal abdomen. The signal strength typically is quite weak and therefore is difficult to separate from extraneous electrical interference, including the maternal electrocardiogram.

REMOTE DISPLAY FROM ELECTRONIC MONITORS. Observation of the fetal heart rate and uterine contraction patterns of labor-

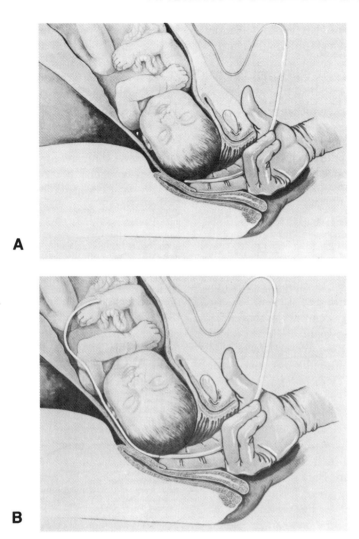

FIG. 14-9.A. A sagittal view demonstrating placement of the catheter guide and catheter just within the cervix. **B.** A sagittal view showing the catheter inserted beyond the guide and within the amnionic sac. (From Chan, Paul, Toews. *Obstet Gynecol* 41:7, 1973)

ing women by means of centrally located electronic display units is becoming popular. Although this enables a single individual to observe these recorded functions at a distance from the laboring women, other aspects of intrapartum surveillance that are equally important may be neglected as a consequence.

Terminology To Describe Fetal Heart Rate. Since the fetal heart rate is rarely fixed, but instead, shows frequent periodic variations, standardized terminology has been proposed to try to describe more pre-cisely both baseline activity and periodic variations from the baseline (ACOG Technical Bulletin No. 32, 1975):

Baseline fetal heart rate refers to the modal rate that prevails apart from any periodic accelerations or decelerations associated with uterine contractions. A baseline rate between 120 and 160 beats per min is considered *normal*, a rate of 100 to 120 *mild bradycardia*, and a rate of less than 100 *marked bradycardia*. Tachycardia is considered *mild* if the baseline rate is 161 to 180 beats per min and *marked* if 180 or more.

Periodic fetal heart rate refers to deviations from baseline that are related to uterine contractions. *Acceleration* refers to an increase in fetal heart rate above baseline and *deceleration* to a decrease below the baseline rate. Three major patterns of deceleration are described: (1) *Uniform patterns of deceleration* reflect the shape of the simultaneously recorded uterine contractions. With the uniform pattern of *early deceleration,* the onset, nadir, and recovery of the fetal heart rate to baseline coincide with the onset, peak, and end of the uterine contraction. Early decelerations, sometimes referred to as Type I or early dips, are usually attributed to compression of the fetal head, although the stimulus to early deceleration may be more ominous. With the other uniform pattern, that of *late deceleration,* the onset of slowing occurs as the contraction intensity peaks, the nadir in heart rate is reached well after the peak, and recovery is not achieved until after the uterine contraction has terminated (Fig. 14-7). Late decelerations, also called Type II or late dips, are likely to be the consequence of uteroplacental insufficiency. (2) *Variable patterns of deceleration,* or *nonuniform decelerations,* are characterized by a decrease in heart rate beginning at no fixed time in relation to the uterine contractions and by wave forms that differ in shape from those of the uterine contractions and from each other, and may be nonrepetitive (Fig. 14-7). Variable decelerations may be the consequence of cord compression. (3) *Combined (mixed) patterns of deceleration,* as the term implies, exhibit the characteristics of two or more of the patterns described above.

The *pattern of early deceleration,* characterized by slowing of the heart rate at the onset of the contraction (Fig. 14-7), is likely to be the consequence of a transient increase in intracranial pressure from head compression, which stimulates the vagus nerve, thereby slowing the heart. Early decelerations may, however, have a more ominous origin. Mendez-Bauer and co-workers (1978), for example, have demonstrated early deceleration to be, at times, the consequence of compression of the umbilical cord.

Prompt sterile vaginal examination to identify the status of the cervix and the presenting part, and to rule out prolapsed cord, is indicated. Treatment includes acertaining that the mother is reclining comfortably on her side and checking the monitor, especially if external, to make sure that it is functioning properly. Early decelerations from head compression may be eliminated by the administration of atropine to the mother. Early decelerations that are severe and prolonged or persistent, and certainly if accompanied by gross meconium staining of the amnionic fluid, must not be ignored.

The *pattern of late deceleration* (Fig. 14-7) is likely to be the consequence of hypoxia and associated metabolic derangement from uteroplacental insufficiency. After termination of the uterine contractions, the heart rate may return to or transiently above normal baseline in the less severely affected fetus, or remain low in the severely affected fetus. The fetus stressed to an intermediate degree may demonstrate tachycardia between contractions. Delivery can be safely delayed only if the uteroplacental insufficiency is promptly corrected, as for example, the relief of uterine overactivity by immediately stopping oxytocin stimulation or by correcting maternal hypotension. Otherwise, prompt delivery is usually indicated.

The *pattern of variable deceleration (nonuniform deceleration)* is likely to be the consequence of compression of the umbilical cord. Vaginal examination should be done promptly to search for cord prolapse and to determine the degree of cervical dilatation and the station and position of the presenting part. The position of the mother should then be changed so that she is lying on her side or turned to the opposite side. If decelerations persist, either immediate measurement of fetal scalp blood pH (p. 359) or prompt delivery is indicated.

It is becoming apparent that these various deceleration patterns just described do not always reflect the causes ascribed to them. While the classification presented has served as a guide to the interpretation of various patterns of fetal heart response during labor, its rigid application, unfortunately, has led, at times, to erroneous diagnosis and treatment (Editorial, 1978).

Beat-to-Beat Variation in Fetal Heart Rate. Late in pregnancy there is normally a beat-to-beat variation in the fetal heart rate, i.e., the time interval between the same locus, for example, the R wave, in consecutive electrical systoles is not fixed. The variation, caused by the continuous interaction of accelerator and decelerator cardiovascular reflexes (Hon, 1974), when present, can be demonstrated by internal electronic monitoring. Unfortunately, recordings made with externally applied detecting devices are unreliable for identifying the presence or absence of beat-to-beat variation. Absence of beat-to-beat variability in some circumstances late in pregnancy may be indicative of fetal compromise. In fact, Boehm (1977) has maintained that fetal heart rate variability has become the most important aspect of the overall clinical evaluation of the fetus in utero. It should be emphasized that the otherwise normal premature fetus or the fetus who is "asleep" may not demonstrate beat-to-beat variability. Moreover, medications in doses commonly used during labor and in preparation for delivery, may ablate beat-to-beat variability. These include meperidine, morphine, alphaprodine, barbiturates, general and conduction anesthesia, diazepam, phenothiazines, atropine, scopolamine, and perhaps magnesium sulfate in large doses (Babaknia and Niebyl, 1978; Boehm, 1977; Cohen and Schifrin, 1977).

Sinusoidal Fetal Heart Rate Pattern. A sinusoidal fetal heart rate pattern is characterized by uniform oscillations of 3 to 5 cycles per min. Gal and associates (1978), as well as some others, consider it to be an alarming sign of fetal distress and attribute it to lack of control of the heart rate by the central nervous system. While a sinusoidal pattern of fetal heart rate has been described especially in fetuses who are severely anemic, Mueller-Heuback and co-workers (1978) have observed such a pattern to develop after

successful intrauterine transfusion and a favorable fetal outcome. Moreover, Gray and associates (1978) describe the development of a sinusoidal fetal heart rate pattern in nearly one-half of pregnancies in which the mothers received alphoprodine (Nisentil) for relief of labor discomfort. In their experience, fetal outcome did not appear to be adversely affected by the presence of a sinusoidal heart rate pattern.

Persistent Fetal Tachycardia or Bradycardia. Tachycardia without deceleration may be the consequence of febrile illness or, more ominous for the fetus, a response to hypoxia, or rarely to fetal thyrotoxicosis. Mild bradycardia without deceleration or acceleration is not necessarily caused by fetal distress. Young and associates (1979) found no evidence of acidosis during labor and delivery in 11 fetuses who demonstrated persistent bradycardia in the range of 100 to 120 beats per min. The neonatal outcomes were good. Interestingly, an occiput posterior or transverse position was identified in each instance. They ascribed the moderate bradycardia to a vagal response induced by persistent head compression.

More severe bradycardia may be the consequence of congenital heart lesions or severe hypoxia. An association has recently been identified between heart block in the fetus and newborn infant and maternal collagen vascular diseases, especially lupus erythematosus (Chap. 28, page 769). Viral infections of the fetus may also cause congenital heart block (Lewis and coworkers, 1980). We have also observed fetal bradycardia to accompany marked maternal hypothermia; the heart rate rose from 90 to 136 when the mother became euthermic. Fetal bradycardia has also been associated with sudden lowering of the blood pressure from excessive administration of hydralazine to a severely hypertensive woman not in labor.

An important cause of presumed fetal bradycardia is fetal death, with the maternal heart rate being recorded by the monitor, and therefore likely to be considered to be the fetal heart rate (Odendaal, 1976). An illustration of this phenomenon is seen in Figure 21-8. (p. 503). Maternal tachycardia, as occurs with sepsis or with concealed hemorrhage from abruptio placentae, may spuriously provide a recording of what appears to be a normal fetal heart rate even though the fetus is dead. *Especially before performing any heroic treatment on the basis of electronic monitoring data, it is always wise to listen carefully to the fetal heart with an appropriate stethoscope while simultaneously checking the maternal pulse rate.*

Fetal Cardiac Arrhythmias.   Intermittently recurring cardiac arrhythmias of ectopic origin may cause concern. The experience of Sugarman and associates (1978), as well as the earlier reports of others, however, indicate that the arrhythmias are likely to be innocuous and that the generally favorable neonatal outcome is not improved by pregnancy intervention or attempts at pharmacologic treatment in utero. Shenker (1979) has provided an extensive review.

Normal Fetal Heart Rate Pattern.   The absence of an ominous fetal heart rate pattern is generally, but not absolutely, predictive of a good fetal outcome. Hayashi and Fox (1975) and others since have documented cardiac arrest and death of the fetus without detecting a preceding ominous fetal heart rate pattern.

Fetal Blood Sampling.   Measurements of the pH of appropriately collected capillary blood may help to identify the fetus in serious distress. A suitably illuminated endoscope is inserted through the sufficiently dilated cervix and ruptured membranes so as to press firmly against fetal skin, usually the scalp (Fig. 14-10). The skin is wiped clean with a cotton swab, sprayed with ethyl chloride to induce hyperemia, and coated with a silicone gel to cause the blood to accumulate as discrete globules. One or two incisions are made through the skin to a calibrated depth with a special blade on an appropriately long handle. When a drop of blood forms on the surface, it is

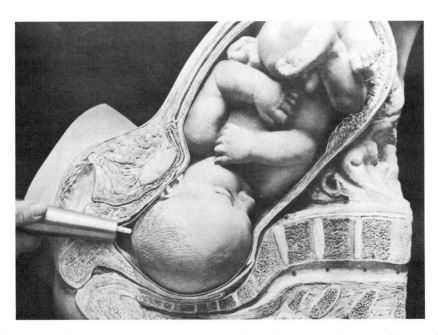

FIG. 14-10.   The technique of fetal scalp sampling utilizing an endoscope. Note end of endoscope displaced from fetal vertex approximately 2 cm to show disposable blade against the fetal scalp before incision. (From Hamilton and McKeown. In Wynn RM (ed): *Obstetrics and Gynecology Annual: 1973.* New York, Appleton, 1974)

immediately collected into a heparinized glass capillary tube and the pH of the blood is promptly measured. The pH of fetal capillary blood usually is lower than arterial blood and approaches that of venous blood.

Saling (1964) initially proposed a pH of 7.20 as the critical value for identification of serious fetal distress, while Mann (1978) and some others have recommended immediate delivery whenever scalp blood pH is 7.25 or less. Zalar and Quilligan (1979) employ the following protocol to try to identify fetal distress through use of fetal scalp sampling: If pH is greater than 7.25, labor is observed. If pH is between 7.20 and 7.25, the pH measurement is repeated within 30 min. If pH is less than 7.20, another scalp blood sample is immediately collected and the mother is taken to an operating room and prepared for surgery. Cesarean section is promptly performed if the low pH is confirmed. Otherwise, labor is allowed to continue and scalp blood samples are repeated periodically.

One expert committee considers a pH of 7.25 or greater to be normal, 7.20 through 7.24 borderline, and less than 7.20 abnormal (ACOG Bulletin No. 42, 1976). An accompanying dictum from the committee is: "Never Act On A Single Determination." In following this dictum, the obstetrician must be careful not to allow repetition of laboratory tests to lead to dangerous clinical procrastination.

Too close adherence to a critical pH value may in actual practice be disadvantageous, since it will tend to allay suspicion of early hypoxic acidosis. A fall in pH is a relatively late effect of hypoxia and, when samples of fetal blood are obtained intermittently, detection of hypoxia of rapid onset may be unduly delayed. It must also be kept in mind that the pH of fetal capillary blood need not accurately reflect the degree of hypoxia in the fetus, since the pH will be influenced appreciably by that of the mother. The severely hypoxic fetus becomes overtly acidotic, which is reflected by a low blood pH except when the mother is alkalotic, for example, from hyperventilation. Conversely, the fetus may have a low blood pH without being remark-

ably hypoxic if the mother is acidotic. Rooth and associates (1973) have emphasized the impact of maternal pH on fetal scalp blood pH. They have suggested that clinically important fetal acidosis be identified by demonstrating the value for the fetus to be at least 0.20 pH units less than that of the mother.

Measurements of blood PO_2 and PCO_2 require more blood but probably do not provide enough additional information to justify their determination. In fact, hypoxic danger to the fetus is better assessed by pH determinations, which reflect metabolic reactions to hypoxia, rather than by isolated measurements of blood gases, which may vary rapidly and remarkably with transient circulatory changes.

Continuous transcutaneous monitoring of fetal oxygen has been described: Through a cervix dilated at least 3 cm, an electrode about 2 cm in diameter was attached by a tissue glue to a shaved region of the fetal scalp. The electrode was integrally heated to 44 C to effect vasodilatation. Using this technic, Huch and co-workers (1978) report a number of observations of clinical interest: Fetal transcutaneous PO_2 rose when the mother was given oxygen. It fell, however, during maternal hypoventilation subsequent to hyperventilation, and it fell during uterine contractions when the mother was kept supine. Moreover, it was low when severe decelerations of the fetal heart rate were evident and low when the basal fetal heart rate was less than 100 or greater than 180 beats per min. Unexpectedly, loss of baseline variability of fetal heart rate was not always accompanied by a low transcutaneous PO_2.

Continuous monitoring of scalp tissue pH has also been described (Lauersen et al., 1979; Weber et al., 1978; Wood et al., 1978). Generally, the pH readings were similar to those obtained on fetal scalp blood. Wood and associates pointed out that practical use of their equipment may be limited by skill required to use it. It is emphasized that both procedures remain experimental.

Complications from Internal Electronic and Physicochemical Monitoring. There are potential dangers inherent in monitoring the fetal heart rate by direct application of an electrode to the fetus, in measuring uterine pressure by inserting an indwelling catheter into the uterine cavity, or in incising the fetal scalp to measure blood pH. A strong orientation toward universal use of internal monitoring technics is likely to predispose to *early amniotomy* and its potential dangers, including cord prolapse, infection, and possibly more stress to the fetus when not cushioned by amnionic fluid during labor (Schwarcz et al., 1973). In this regard the studies performed on late pregnant monkeys by Gabbe and associates (1976) and similar studies in sheep serve to reemphasize the protective cushion against cord compression provided by amnionic fluid. Acute reduction in amnionic fluid volume was accompanied by periodic fetal heart rate decelerations variable in pattern. Restoration of the amnionic fluid volume eliminated the abnormal pattern.

Another potential morbidity is *trauma*. Injury to the fetal scalp induced by the electrode is rarely a major problem, although application at some other site, for example, the eye in case of a face presentation, can prove serious. A fetal vessel in the placenta may be ruptured inadvertently by the placement of the catheter. Trudinger and Pryse-Davies (1978) observed four such accidents, two of which led to death of the fetus or newborn infant from exsanguination. Moreover, they identified one instance of severe cord compression from entanglement with the intrauterine catheter. Others have had similar experiences. Penetration of the placenta causing hemorrhage and perforations of the uterus during insertion of the catheter for pressure recording do occur and have led to serious morbidity, as well as to spurious recordings that led to inappropriate management of labor and delivery.

Both the fetus and the mother may be at increased risk of *infection* as the consequence of internal electronic monitoring. Scalp wounds from the electrode may become infected by organisms of the vaginal flora (Okada et al., 1977). Infection of the newborn infant with Herpes hominis type 2 virus has been identified following use of scalp electrodes; systemic viral disease, as well as chronic scalp infection, resulted (Adams et al., 1975). Infants born after internal electronic monitoring appear more likely to have been colonized by maternal group B streptococcus (Davis et al., 1979).

An increase in maternal infections following the use of internal electronic monitoring has not been a uniform finding. Perhaps a decrease in the frequency and therefore the number of vaginal examinations for the woman who is being so monitored offsets the undoubtedly increased risk imposed by rupture of the membranes and the placement and persistence of the catheter and wires in utero. Gassner and Ledger (1976) found an increased frequency of infection in women so monitored who subsequently underwent cesarean section. Perloe and Curet (1979) similarly identified febrile morbidity to be more common in women whose labors were so monitored and then underwent cesarean section, especially when the membranes had been ruptured for 12 hours or more.

The fluid-filled intrauterine pressure transducer may harbor potentially pathogenic organisms which on occasion enter the catheter fluid and, in turn, the uterine cavity. The organisms are likely to be those associated with standing water, especially species of *Pseudomonas, Flavobacterium, Achromobacter,* and *Alcaligines faecalis* (Baker et al., 1979).

While external monitoring technics avoid the necessity of ruptured membranes and invasion of the uterus, as well as direct trauma to the fetus, their use, unless meticulously guarded against, commonly results in the mother's lying in the supine position most of the time so as to protect the placement of the external detectors. The supine position, by causing aortocaval compression, is likely to be deleterious to the fetus if the fetus is already in jeopardy for other reasons, fetal or maternal.

Three major complications resulting from fetal scalp blood sampling are infection, blade breakage, and bleeding. Blade breakage must be excluded by inspecting the blade after each puncture. If vaginal bleeding is encountered at any time following scalp blood sampling, fetal bleeding must be ruled out. Marked deficiencies of vitamin-K-dependent coagulation factors have been implicated in the genesis of such hemorrhage in some infants (Hull, 1972), and hemophilia has been subsequently diagnosed in a few others. The negative pressure from use of a vacuum extractor to effect delivery after scalp blood sampling may incite troublesome hemorrhage (Roberts and Stone, 1978).

ASSESSMENT OF RESULTS FROM ELECTRONIC MONITORING

In the United States, Hon, Quilligan, Paul, and Freeman are prominent among the names of obstetricians who have long championed continuous electronic recording of the fetal heart during labor. They have observed somewhat lower perinatal mortality rates at Los Angeles County Hospital for labors in which the fetal heart rate was continuously recorded even though the group so monitored was selected because of pregnancy complications recognized to predispose to a poorer outcome for the fetus (Paul et al., 1977). Beard (1974) of Great Britain has considered electronic monitoring limited only to so-called high-risk pregnancies to be unsound, and has urged that electronic monitoring be used for all labors. In his experience, in terms of the number of fetuses who became acidotic during labor, there was little difference between the identified high-risk pregnancies and those considered normal. He emphasized that only by so monitoring all labors will intrapartum asphyxial damage be eliminated.

At the same time that considerable enthusiasm has been generated for in-hospital, intrapartum intensive care with continuous electronic fetal monitoring, there has been an enthusiastic renewal of interest, at least in some areas of the United States, in delivery at home supervised by the family physician and midwife. Whitt and associates (1974), for example, have been quoted as stating that four-fifths of 450 deliveries attended by them during a 3-year period were in the home and that their experience confirmed this not to

be a reckless or dangerous choice. Most obstetricians and neonatologists, for many good medical reasons, certainly do not subscribe to their conclusions.

While several groups have stated, or at least implied, a significant reduction in fetal mortality rates with continuous electronic monitoring, one study, now repeated, has demonstrated as good an outcome for high-risk pregnancies using systematic clinical monitoring. Trained nursing personnel monitored clinically the mother and fetus in a standardized fashion throughout labor until the actual delivery of the infant (Haverkamp et al., 1976, 1979). The fetal heart was checked routinely every 15 minutes during the first stage, and every 5 minutes during the second stage, and more often if an abnormality was suspected. Uterine contractions were evaluated frequently by palpation and the mother was observed continuously. In the group so monitored clinically, the Apgar scores were as high as in the group routinely subjected to continuous electronic monitoring, while the cesarean section was appreciably lower.

It cannot be overemphasized that the technics for continuous recording of fetal heart rates and uterine pressures do not by themselves provide continuous surveillance of the fetus. Appropriately trained personnel must be immediately available to activate the electronic technics, to inspect and analyze almost continuously the data that are being recorded, and to act promptly on the findings.

For many obstetric services, but not all, the increasing use of electronic fetal monitoring has been accompanied by an appreciable increase in cesarean section rate (Antenatal Diagnosis, 1979). Whether the two phenomena are directly related is not clear in many instances. However, in the case of the two studies by Haverkamp and co-workers cited above, cesarean section with electronic monitoring of labor, when compared to clinical monitoring carried out as described, was either two times or three times as high, depending upon whether or not scalp sampling to measure fetal blood pH was performed in conjunction with electronic monitoring.

Recently, a Task Force concerned with the

various facets of the difficult problem of predicting intrapartum fetal distress has provided certain conclusions about monitoring the fetus electronically during labor (Antenatal Diagnosis, 1979). These are provided below:

Conclusions of Task Force On Predictors of Fetal Distress

1. Intrapartum events are currently estimated to account for 20 percent of stillbirths, 20 to 40 percent of cerebral palsy, and approximately 10 percent of severe mental retardation, less than estimates based upon earlier retrospective studies. Nevertheless, adverse intrapartum events continue to be an important source of potentially preventable death and damage. Neonatal morbidity and mortality secondary to intrapartum asphyxia is well known, but the precise magnitude of these problems is not certain. The possibility of subclinical neurologic dysfunction has been suggested in animal studies, but current outcome parameters are inadequate to assess subclinical effects of intrapartum hypoxia in humans.

2. Intrapartum hypoxic events may occur in any pregnancy, but are more common in women defined as high-risk during either the antepartum or intrapartum periods. Unfortunately, current risk assessment profiles do not predict all instances of intrapartum morbidity and mortality.

3. Intermittent methods of fetal surveillance during labor (auscultation of the fetal heart every 15 min in the first stage and every 5 min during the second stage, in both instances for a period of 30 sec immediately after a uterine contraction) provides an acceptable basis for intrapartum monitoring in the low-risk patients. This intensive supervision requires an adequate number of well-trained personnel at the patient's bedside.

4. A normal fetal heart rate pattern on continuous electronic fetal monitoring indicates a greater than 95 percent probability of fetal well-being. Laboratory and clinical studies have demonstrated that fetal hypoxia reliably produces changes in fetal heart patterns; however, these abnormal patterns may occur in the absence of fetal distress.

5. Fetal distress in labor cannot be assessed by considering a single parameter such as intermittent or continuous fetal heart rate. Because fetal heart rate patterns suggestive of hypoxia may occur in the absence of fetal distress, intermittent and continuous fetal heart rate assessment are screening, rather than diagnostic, techniques. Failure to appreciate this limitation may lead to inappropriate clinical decisions.

6. Intervention in labor to alleviate fetal hypoxia requires careful consideration of all available information. Fetal heart rate data indicating fetal distress require support from other clinical and laboratory information, including fetal scalp blood pH determination, when indicated, before a firm basis for intervention can be established.

7. The weight of present evidence from prospective and retrospective analyses show no apparent effect of electronic fetal monitoring upon perinatal mortality and morbidity in low-risk patients.

   As maternal and fetal risk increases, there is a trend suggesting a beneficial effect of electronic fetal monitoring upon intrapartum and neonatal morbidity and mortality. Specific obstetric risk factors especially amenable to intervention via electronic fetal monitoring have not been completely enumerated.

8. Maternal and fetal complications of electronic fetal monitoring have been reported. The most frequently reported fetal complication of internal monitoring is scalp abscess at the site of electrode application. Internal fetal monitoring by itself does not appear to be an important factor in the incidence of maternal postpartum infection. Other complications less frequently reported relate predominantly to errors in application of the fetal scalp electrode or intrauterine pressure catheter. The known risks of the external mode of fetal monitoring at present are minimal. There are no conclusive data on the long-term effects of continuous ultrasound application.

9. The effect of electronic fetal monitoring upon the incidence of cesarean section may vary with the manner in which the data are interpreted. Four randomized clinical trials in teaching hospital settings have demonstrated increased rates of primary cesarean section in monitored women. The increase in cesarean sections for fetal distress was statistically significant in two of the four trials. Several large retrospective studies in teaching hospitals have found this increase in cesarean section rate for fetal distress to be independent of the use of electronic fetal monitoring. The

effect of electronic fetal monitoring upon the cesarean delivery rate in any particular hospital may depend upon the clinical use and norms of practice in that hospital. There is evidence that the simultaneous use of fetal scalp blood sampling provides additional information and may reduce the incidence of monitoring-associated cesarean section. The ideal use of electronic fetal monitoring in influencing more appropriate cesarean delivery has yet to be determined.

10. A number of additional promising fetal assessment techniques are currently under investigation. These include the use of computers and microprocessors in combination with heart rate monitors, telemetry systems, continuous monitoring of fetal scalp pH, transcutaneous monitoring of fetal oxygen tension, evaluation of fetal movements, and electroencephalography. None of these has been sufficiently evaluated to merit introduction into obstetrical practice.

11. Techniques introduced into obstetric practice in the last decade may conflict with the concept of family centered childbirth. Although limited research in this area has been done, currently available data suggest that electronic fetal monitoring need not diminish the human experience of childbirth when properly employed and explained by knowledgeable and supportive medical personnel. This early research also suggests that pregnant women who have an opportunity to discuss the potential uses and limitations of electronic fetal monitoring are less likely to have negative reaction to its use.

12. Many of the ethical issues presented by electronic fetal monitoring are related to uncertainties about its risks and benefits, and to the unique psychological situation of a woman in labor. Both increase the difficulties of achieving truly informed decision making. Other such issues arise from the current concern over increased medical malpractice litigation, the increasing use of technology in childbirth, and questions of social justice and allocation of scarce resources. Future research to define proper use of electronic fetal monitoring may disclose additional issues.

13. Under present methods of application, electronic fetal monitoring increases the cost of obstetrical services, though not by a large amount. These costs must be considered against the economic savings and benefits generated by electronic fetal monitoring. The development of more reliable estimates of these benefits must await definitive studies of the impact of electronic monitoring on perinatal morbidity and mortality.

14. Courts of law should recognize that intrapartum hypoxia is only one of many factors involved in the development of handicaps and perinatal death, and that current research and clinical data do not allow a comprehensive definition of antepartum and intrapartum risk, nor of means to reduce risk of adverse outcome.

CLINICAL MONITORING

The status of the fetus can be satisfactorily monitored clinically by appropriately trained individuals as described above under "Assessment of Results From Electronic Monitoring" and especially in Chapter 17. In summary, the fetal heart rate is determined carefully at close intervals during and immediately after a uterine contraction until the infant is actually delivered; the frequency and intensity of uterine contractions are carefully estimated; and the rate of cervical dilatation and descent of the presenting part are determined periodically (Haverkamp et al., 1976, 1979).

Normally, the fetal heart rate between contractions will average about 140 and will range from no less than 120 to no more than 160 beats per min. Typically, the fetal heart rate drops somewhat during a uterine contraction but recovers promptly as the contraction ends. The fetal heart rate may be determined using a specialized stethoscope or an instrument that utilizes the Doppler principle and ultrasound to detect fetal heart action, as shown in Figure 17-2. A and B, p. 412.

For some time, we have been using this model of Doppler instrument to identify fetal heart sounds continuously. The holder for the transducer is affixed with a washable rubber belt to the maternal abdomen in the vicinity of the fetal heart. By simply depressing a button and rotating the handle on the transducer holder, the transducer can be aimed to provide for optimum pickup of fetal heart actions. The mother need not be kept on her back in order to detect the fetal heart and the fetal heart most often can be identified continuously right up to the time the infant is born.

Intrapartum Surveillance of the Fetus at Parkland Memorial Hospital

In two-thirds of labors, the fetus is monitored clinically as described above and in Chapter 17. Continuous electronic monitoring is reserved for the following circumstances:

1. Variations in the fetal heart rate detected by auscultation *and for which immediate delivery is not considered necessary*
2. Meconium in amnionic fluid
3. Induction or augmentation of labor
4. Increased likelihood of uteroplacental insufficiency or compromised fetus:
   a. Hypertension
   b. Bleeding
   c. Preterm and postterm pregnancies
   d. Small fetus, possibly growth-retarded
   e. Abnormal presentations
   f. Previous unexplained stillbirth
   g. Sickle cell hemoglobinopathies
   h. Hemolytic disease of the fetus
   i. Diabetes

While the application of continuous electronic monitoring cannot by itself be credited for any remarkable reduction in intrapartum or neonatal mortality at Parkland Memorial Hospital, it has provided an elegant means for demonstrating to physicians in training, medical students, nurses, obstetric associates, physician's assistants, and others the normal and abnormal forces of labor and the cardiac responses of the fetus.

REFERENCES

ACOG Technical Bulletin No. 32. Fetal Heart Rate Monitoring. Guidelines for Monitoring, Terminology and Instrumentation. Chicago, American College of Obstetricians and Gynecologists, 1975

ACOG Technical Bulletin No. 42. Fetal Blood Sampling. Chicago, American College of Obstetricians and Gynecologists, 1976

Adams G, Purohit D, Bada H, Andrews B: Neonatal infection by Herpes hominis type 2, a complication of intrapartum fetal monitoring. Clin Res 23:69A, 1975

Antenatal Diagnosis. Report of a Consensus Development Conference Sponsored by the National Institute of Child Health and Human Development, NIH Publication Number 79–1973. Washington, D.C., U.S. Gov Print Off, 1979

Aula P, Rapola J, Karjalainen O, Lindgren J, Hartikainen AL, Seppälä M: Prenatal diagnosis of congenital nephrosis in 23 high-risk families. Am J Dis Child 132:984, 1978

Babaknia A, Niebyl JR: The effect of magnesium sulfate on fetal heart rate baseline variability. Obstet Gynecol 51(Suppl):2, 1978

Baker DA, Mead PB, Gallant JM, Hayward RG, Hamel AJ: Water-borne contamination of intrauterine pressure transducers. Am J Obstet Gynecol 133:923, 1979

Beard RW: The detection of fetal asphyxia in labor. Pediatrics 53:157, 1974

Belisle S, Fencl MD, Tulchinsky D: Amniotic fluid testosterone and follicle-stimulating hormone in the determination of fetal sex. Am J Obstet Gynecol 128:514, 1977

Bishop EH, Corson S: Estimation of fetal maturity by cytologic examination of the amniotic fluid. Am J Obstet Gynecol 102:654, 1968

Blajchman MA, Mandsley RF, Uchida I, Zipursky A: Diagnostic amniocentesis and fetal-maternal bleeding. Lancet 1:993, 1974

Blumenfeld TA, Stark RI, James LS, George JD, Dyrenfurth I, Freda VJ, Shinitzsky M: Determination of fetal lung maturity by fluorescence polarization of the amniotic fluid. Am J Obstet Gynecol 102:782, 1978

Boehm FH: FHR variability: key to fetal well-being. Contemp Ob/Gyn 9:57, 1977

Buhi WC, Spellacy WN: Effects of blood or meconium on the determination of the amniotic fluid lecithin/sphingomyelin ratio. Am J Obstet Gynecol 121:321, 1975

Caterini H, Sama J, Iffy L, Harrigan J, Pelosi M, Tiku J: A reevaluation of amniography. Obstet Gynecol 47:373, 1976

Chan WF, Ang AH, Soo YS: The value of lower limb ossification centres in the radiological estimation of fetal maturity. Aust NZ J Obstet Gynaecol 12:55, 1972

Clements JA, Platzker ACG, Tierney DF, Hobel CJ, Creasy RK, Margolis AJ, Thibeault DW,

Tooley WH, Oh W: Assessment of the risk of respiratory distress syndrome by a rapid test for surfactant in amniotic fluid. N Engl J Med 286:1077, 1972

Cohen WR, Schifrin BS: Diagnosis and treatment of fetal distress. In Bolognese RJ, Schwarz RH (eds): Perinatal Medicine. Baltimore, Williams & Wilkins, 1977, p 131

Davis JP, Moggio MF, Klein D, Tiosejo LL, Welt SI, Wilfert CM: Vertical transmission of group B Streptococcus: Relation to intra-uterine fetal monitoring. JAMA 242:42, 1979

Editorial: Reappraisal of fetal heart rate patterns. J Perinat Med 6:65, 1978

Ehrström C: Fetal movement monitoring in normal and high-risk pregnancy. Acta Obstet Gynecol 80 (Suppl), 1979

Elias S, Martin AO, Patel VA, Gerbie A, Simpson JL: Analysis for amniotic fluid crystallization in second-trimester amniocentesis. Am J Obstet Gynecol 133:401, 1979

Elrad H, Beydoun SN, Gagen JH, Cabalum MT, Aubry RH, Smith C: Fetal pulmonary maturity as determined by fluorescent polarization of amniotic fluid. Am J Obstet Gynecol 132:681, 1978

Evertson LR, Gauthier RJ, Collea JV: Fetal demise following negative contraction stress tests. Obstet Gynecol 51:671, 1978

Ferguson-Smith MA, May HM, Vince JD, Robinson HR, Rawlinson HA, Tait HA, Gibson AAM, Ratcliffe JG: Avoidance of anencephalic and spina bifida births by maternal serum-alphafetoprotein screening. Lancet 1:1330, 1978

Firshein SI, Hoyer LW, Lazarchick JL, Forget BG, Hobbins JC, Clyne LP, Pitlick FA, Muir WA, Merkatz IR, Mahoney MJ: Prenatal diagnosis of classic hemophilia. N Engl J Med 300:937, 1979

Freda V: Hemolytic disease. Clin Obstet Gynecol 16:72, 1973

Freeman RK: The use of the oxytocin challenge test for antepartum clinical evaluation of utero-placental respiratory function. Am J Obstet Gynecol 121:481, 1975

Gabbe SG, Ettinger BB, Freeman RK, Martin CB: Umbilical cord compression associated with amniotomy: Laboratory observations. Am J Obstet Gynecol 126:353, 1976

Gal D, Neuhoff S, Lilling MI, Tancer ML: False negative oxytocin challenge test: Report of three cases. Am J Obstet Gynecol 133:111, 1979

Gant NF, Hutchinson HT, Siiteri PK, MacDonald PC: Study of the metabolic clearance rate of dehydroisoandrosterone sulfate in pregnancy. Am J Obstet Gynecol 111:555, 1971

Gassner CB, Ledger WJ: The relationship of hospital-acquired maternal infection to invasive intrapartum monitoring techniques. Am J Obstet Gynecol 126:33, 1976

Gibbons JM Jr, Huntley TE, Corral AG: Effect of maternal blood contamination on amniotic fluid analysis. Obstet Gynecol 44:657, 1974

Gluck L, Kulovich MV, Borer RC Jr, Brenner PH, Anderson GG. Spellacy WN: Diagnosis of the respiratory distress syndrome by amniocentesis. Am J Obstet Gynecol 109:440, 1971

Golde SH, Vogt JF, Gabbe SG, Cabal LA: Evaluation of the FELMA microviscometer in predicting fetal lung maturity. Obstet Gynecol 54: 639, 1979

Gray JH, Cudmore DW, Luther ER, Martin TR, Gardner AJ: Sinusoidal fetal heart rate pattern associated with alphaprodine administration. Obstet Gynecol 52:678, 1978

Haddow JE, Macri JN, Munson M: The amnion regulates movement of fetally derived alpha-fetoprotein into maternal blood. J Lab Clin Med 94:344, 1979

Hallmann M, Feldman BH, Kirkpatrick E, Gluck L: Absence of phosphatidylglycerol in respiratory distress syndrome in the newborn. Pediatr Res 11:714, 1977

Hammacher K: Früherkennung intrauteriner gefahrenzustände durch electrophonokardiographie und fokographie. In Elert R, Hüter KA (eds): Prophylaxe Frühkindlicher Hirnshäden. Stuttgart, Georg Theime Verlag, 1966, p 120

Hammacher K, Hüter KA, Bokelmann J, Werners PH: Foetal heart frequency and perinatal condition of the foetus and newborn. Gynaecologia 166:349, 1968

Harrigan JT, Marino JF: Fetal heart rate reaction to amniocentesis as an indicator of fetal well-being. Am J Obstet Gynecol 132:49, 1978

Harrison R, Campbell S, Craft I: Risks of fetomaternal hemorrhage resulting from amniocentesis with and without ultrasound placental localization. Obstet Gynecol 46:389, 1975

Harvey D, Parkinson CE, Campbell S: Risk of respiratory-distress syndrome. Lancet 1:42, 1975

Haverkamp AD, Thompson HE, McFee JE, Cetrulo C: The evaluation of continuous fetal heart rate monitoring in high risk pregnancy. Am J Obstet Gynecol 125:310, 1976

Haverkamp AD, Orleans M, Langendoerfer S, McFee JG, Murphy J, Thompson HE: A controlled trial of the differential effects of intrapartum fetal monitoring. Am J Obstet Gynecol 134:399, 1979

Hayashi RH, Fox ME: Unforeseen sudden intrapartum fetal death in a monitored labor. Am J Obstet Gynecol 122:786, 1975

Herbert WNP, Tyson JE, Jimenez JM: Absence of hyaline membrane disease at low lecithin to sphingomyelin ratios. Pediatr Res 13:497, 1979

Herzenberg LA, Bianchi DW, Schröder J, Cann HM, Iverson GM: Fetal cells in the blood of pregnant women: Detection and enrichment by fluorescence-activated cell sorting. Proc Natl Acad Sci 76:1453, 1979

Hobbins JC: Diagnosing with fetoscope. Contemp Ob/Gyn 13:143, 1979

Hon EH: Fetal heart rate monitoring. In Modern Perinatal Medicine, L Gluck ed, Year Book Publishers, Chicago, 1974

Hon EH, Paul RH, Hon RW: Electronic evaluation of fetal heart rate. XI. Description of spiral electrode. Obstet Gynecol 40:362, 1972

Hoyer LW, Linsten J, Blombäck M, Hagenfeldt L, Cordesius E, Strömberg P, Gustavii B: Prenatal evaluation of fetus at risk for severe von Willebrand's disease. Lancet 2:191, 1979

Huch A, Huch R, Schneider H, Lucey JF: Monitoring fetal arterial oxygen continuously during labor. Contemp Ob/Gyn 12:73, 1978

Huddleston JF, Freeman RK: The use of the oxytocin challenge test for the management of pregnancies at risk for uteroplacental insufficiency. In Bolognese RJ, Schwarz RH (eds): Perinatal Medicine. Baltimore, Williams & Wilkins, 1977, p 68

Hull MGR: Perinatal coagulopathies complicating fetal blood sampling. Br Med J 3:319, 1972

Knox E, Todd K, Cassady G: The effect of amniography on amniotic fluid L/S ratio. Obstet Gynecol 49:154, 1977

Koller WS Jr, Curet LB: Fetal activity determinations and oxytocin challenge tests for the assessment of fetal well-being. Obstet Gynecol 52:176, 1978

Kubli FW, Kaeser O, Hinselmann M: Diagnostic management of chronic placental insufficiency. In Pecile A, Finzi C (eds): The Foeto-Placental Unit. Amsterdam, Excerpta Medica Foundation, 1969, p 323

Lauersen NH, Miller FC, Paul RH: Continuous intrapartum monitoring of fetal scalp pH. Am J Obstet Gynecol 133:44, 1979

Leach G, Chang A, Morrison J: A controlled trial of puncture sites for amniocentesis. Br J Obstet Gynaecol 85:328, 1978

Lewis PE, Cefalo RC, Zaritsky AL: Fetal heart block due to cytomegalo-virus. Am J Obstet Gynecol. In press

Lindberg BS, Nilsson BA, Johansson EDB: Plasma progesterone levels in normal and abnormal pregnancies. Acta Obstet Gynecol Scand 53:329, 1974

Mann L: Intrapartum fetal monitoring: scalp blood pH is a useful tool. Contemp Ob/Gyn 11:25, 1978

Mendez-Bauer C, Ruiz Canseco A, Andujar Ruiz M, Menendez A, Arroya J, Gardi RD, Sastry V, Zamarriego Crespo J: Early decelerations of the fetal heart rate from occlusion of the umbilical cord. J Perinat Med 6:69, 1978

Mibashan RS, Thumpston JK, Singer JD, Rodeck CH, Edwards RJ, White JM, Campbell S: Plasma assay of fetal factors VIII C and IX for prenatal diagnosis of haemophelia. Lancet 1:1309, 1979

Milunsky A: The Prenatal Diagnosis of Hereditary Disorders. Springfield, Ill. Thomas, 1973

Mueller-Heubach E, Caritas SN, Edelstone DI: Sinusoidal fetal heartrate pattern following intrauterine fetal transfusion. Obstet Gynecol 52:435, 1978

National Institute of Child Health and Human Development, National Registry for Amniocentesis Study Group: Midtrimester amniocentesis for prenatal diagnosis: Safety and accuracy. JAMA 236:1471, 1976

Odendaal HJ: False interpretation of fetal heart rate monitoring in cases of intra-uterine death. South Afr Med J 50:1963, 1976

Okada DM, Chow AW, Bruce VT: Neonatal scalp abscess and fetal monitoring: factors associated with infection. Am J Obstet Gynecol 129:185, 1977

Patel N: Personal communication, 1979

Paul RH, Huey JR Jr, Yaeger CF: Clinical fetal monitoring. Postgrad Med 61:160, 1977

Perloe M, Curet CB: The effect of internal fetal monitoring on cesarean section morbidity. Obstet Gynecol 53:354, 1979

Pitkin RM: Amniotic fluid in estimating fetal maturity. Contemp Ob/Gyn 4:13, 1974

Ray M, Freeman R, Pine S, Hesselgesser R: Clinical experience with the oxytocin challenge test. Am J Obstet Gynecol 114:1, 1972

Raja RLT, Anderson AMB, Turnbull AC: Endocrine changes in premature labor. Br Med J 4:67, 1974

Read JA, Miller FC: Fetal heart rate acceleration in response to acoustic stimulation as a measure of fetal well-being. Am J Obstet Gynecol 129:512, 1977

Roberts IF, Stone M: Fetal hemorrhage: Complications of vacuum extractor after fetal blood sampling. Am J Obstet Gynecol 132:109, 1978

Rodeck CH, Campbell S: Early prenatal diagnosis of neural-tube defects by ultrasound-guided fetoscopy. Lancet 1:1128, 1978

Rooth G, McBride R, Ivy BJ: Fetal and maternal pH measurements. Acta Obstet Gynecol Scand 52:47, 1973

Sadovsky E, Polishuk WZ: Fetal movements in utero: Nature, assessment, prognostic value, timing of delivery. Obstet Gynecol 50:49, 1977

Saling E: Die Blutgasverhaltnisse und der saure Basen-Haushalt der Feten bei ungerstörtem geburtsablauf. Z Gerburtsh Gynaekol 161:262, 1964

Saling EZ, Dudenhausen JW: The present situation of clinical monitoring of the fetus during labor. J Perinat Med 1:75, 1973

Schifrin BS: The non-stress test. Presented at the Seventy-eighth Ross Conference on Pediatric Research (Obstetrical Decisions and Neonatal Outcome), San Diego, Ca., May 30, 1979

Schlueter MA, Phibbs RH, Creasy RK, Clements JA, Tooley WH: Antenatal prediction of graduated risk of hyaline membrane disease by amniotic fluid foam test for surfactant. Am J Obstet Gynecol 134:761, 1979

Schwarcz R, Althabe O, Belitzky R, Lanchares JL, Alvarez R, Berdaguer P, Capurro H, Belizan JM, Sabatino JH, Abusleme C, Caldeyro-Barcia R: Fetal heart rate patterns in labors with intact and with ruptured membranes. J Perinat Med 1:153, 1973

Seppälä M: Alpha-fetoprotein in the amniotic fluid in relation to neural tube defects and other congenital/genetic disorders of the fetus. In Fairweather DVI, Eskes TKAB, (eds): Amniotic Fluid: Research and Clinical Application, 2nd ed. New York, Excerpta Medica, 1978

Shawker TH, Schuette WH, Whitehouse W, Rifka SM: Early fetal movement: A real-time ultrasound study. Obstet Gynecol 55:194, 1980

Shenker L: Fetal cardiac arrhythmias. Obstet Gynecol Survey 34:561, 1979

Simpson H, Dallaire L, Miller J, Simonovitch L, Hamerton J: Prenatal diagnosis of genetic disease in Canada: Report of a collaborative study. Can Med Assoc J 115:739, 1976

Smith AD, Wald NJ, Cuckle HS, Stirrat GM, Bobrow M, Lagercrantz H: Amniotic-fluid acetylcholinesterase as a possible diagnostic test for neural-tube defects in early pregnancy. Lancet 1:685, 1979

Sugarman RG, Rawlinson KF, Schifrin BS: Fetal arrhythmias. Obstet Gynecol 52:301, 1978

Teoh ES, Lau YK, Ambrose A, Ratnam SS: Amniotic fluid creatinine, uric acid and urea as indices of gestational age. Acta Obstet Gynecol Scand 52:323, 1973

Trudinger BJ, Pryse-Davies J: Fetal hazards of the intrauterine pressure catheter: Five case reports. Br J Obstet Gynaecol 85:567, 1978

Valenti C, Lin CC, Baum A, Masobrio M: Prenatal sex determination. Am J Obstet Gynecol 112:890, 1972

Wald NJ, Cuckle HS, Boreham J, Brett R, Stirrat GM, Bennett MJ, Turnbull AC, Solymar M, Jones N, Bobrow M, Evans CJ: Antenatal screening in Oxford for fetal neural tube defects: Br J Obstet Gynaecol 86:91, 1979

Weber T, Hahn-Pedersen S, Bock JE: Continuous fetal tissue pH recordings during labour. A preliminary report. Br J Obstet Gynaecol 85:770, 1978

Whitehouse WM, Simmons CS, Evans TN: Reduction of radiation hazard in obstetric roentgenography. Am J Roentgenol 80:690, 1958

Whitt M: quoted in Ob Gyn News, February 1, 1974

Wiessenhaan PF: Feography. Am J Obstet Gynecol 113:819, 1972

Wood C, Anderson I, Reddy S, Shekleton P: Continuous measurement of tissue pH in the human fetal scalp. Br J Obstet Gynaecol 85:668, 1978

Working Party on Amniocentesis: An assessment of the hazards of amniocentesis: Report to the M.R.C. Br J Obstet Gynaecol 85 (Suppl):2, 1978

Worthington D, Smith BT: The site of amniocentesis and the lecithin-sphingomyelin ratio. Obstet Gynecol 52:552, 1978

Young BK, Katz M, Klein SA, Silverman F: Fetal blood and tissue pH with moderate bradycardia. Am J Obstet Gynecol 135:45, 1979

Zalar RW, Quilligan EJ: The influence of scalp sampling on the cesarean section rate for fetal distress. Am J Obstet Gynecol 135:239, 1979

15

Physiology of Labor

CAUSE OF LABOR

The cause of labor remains unknown. Several attractive theories concerned with the mechanism for the onset of parturition in the human, therefore, are to varying degrees still viable.

Oxytocin Stimulation Theory. Parenterally administered oxytocin, especially to women near term, usually stimulates the uterus to contract and, in turn, to expel the products of conception. For this reason, it was tempting to implicate endogenous oxytocin in the onset of spontaneous labor. To date, however, no convincing evidence has been presented to support a role for maternal or fetal oxytocin in the onset of spontaneous parturition. Increased plasma levels of oxytocin in the maternal circulation are ordinarily found only during the second stage of labor. Based on this finding, Chard (1973) deduced that the role of oxytocin was to facilitate contraction of the uterus after delivery, a process that would serve to reduce postpartum uterine bleeding.

Progesterone Withdrawal Theory. For many years, theories have been proposed that involve progesterone withdrawal as an important event in the initiation of human labor. This theory evolved primarily from observations made years ago on pregnant rabbits. In rabbits, withdrawal of progesterone is, indeed, followed promptly by evacuation of the contents of the pregnant uterus. Conversely, the administration of progesterone will inhibit evacuation long beyond the normal time for delivery. The results of most studies on women, however, have not provided evidence that progesterone levels, at least in maternal blood, necessarily fall before labor. *Nonetheless, in all likelihood, for reasons presented below, progesterone does play an important role, albeit indirect, in the control of the length of gestation and, in turn, the onset of labor.*

Fetal Cortisol Theory. More recently, an attractive new hypothesis has emerged that has gained considerable support. From the results of the elegant studies of Liggins (1973), we have learned the importance of the function of the brain (hypothalamus), pituitary, and adrenal cortex of the fetus in the preparation for, or in the initiation of, the biochemical events of parturition. Using the pregnant sheep as a model, Liggins found that hypophysectomy, or adrenalectomy, or transection of the hypophysial portal vessels of the fetus resulted in prolonged gestation.

Conversely, Liggins observed that the infusion into the fetus of either cortisol or ACTH caused premature parturition in the ewe. On the other hand, hypophysectomy or adrenalectomy of the pregnant ewe did not cause prolonged gestation, nor did treatment of the ewe with ACTH or cortisol cause premature parturition.

In human pregnancy, there appears to be a naturally occurring anomaly analogous to Liggins' sheep model. In 1933, the British obstetrician Malpas documented the occurrence of prolonged gestation in human pregnancy with an anencephalic fetus. Even then, Malpas suggested that the defect in the initiation of parturition in pregnancies with an anencephalic fetus resided in faulty fetal brain-pituitary-adrenal function. The adrenal gland of the anencephalic fetus is very small compared to that of a normal fetus. Indeed, the adrenal of the anencephalic fetus at term may weigh only 5 to 10 percent of that of a normal fetus. The smallness of the gland is due largely to failure of development of the fetal zone, the structure that accounts for most of the mass of the fetal adrenal. It has been confirmed and reconfirmed that some human pregnancies with an anencephalic fetus, at least those without hydramnios, may be characterized by prolonged gestation and a degree of refractoriness to the induction of labor.

These observations, together with those made in the sheep, have prompted numerous investigators to suggest a key role for fetal cortisol in the initiation of parturition. To date, however, there has been no well-documented instance of the initiation of premature parturition in human pregnancy by the injection of either cortisol or ACTH into the fetus and earlier reports of the induction of labor by injecting corticosteroids into the amnionic sac have not been confirmed (Katz et al., 1979). Furthermore, several naturally occurring instances of failure of cortisol production in the human fetus do not result in prolonged gestation, for example, defects in steroid 21-hydroxylation, 17 α-hydroxylation, 11 β-hydroxylation, and 3 β-hydroxysteroid dehydrogenase in the adrenal cortices of the developing fetus, which preclude augmented cortisol production by the fetus.

Conversely, of the more than a dozen cases of placental sulfatase deficiency that have been reported and the others that are known to exist, many have been associated with prolonged gestation or refractoriness to oxytocin induction of labor. Presumably, placental sulfatase deficiency does not result in deficient production of cortisol by the fetal adrenal. Furthermore, the level of ACTH in fetal blood does not increase before parturition but rather appears to decrease somewhat during the course of human gestation. Indeed, the concentration of ACTH in cord blood of infants delivered near term is similar irrespective of whether the fetus was delivered vaginally following normal spontaneous labor, or delivered by elective repeat cesarean section prior to the onset of labor, or by vaginal delivery following oxytocin induction of labor (Winters et al., 1974). In addition, human pregnancy appears to differ from that of the animal model in that a discordance seems to exist between lung maturation and the onset of parturition in the human. In the sheep, cortisol administered to the lamb induces premature lung maturation as well as premature parturition (Liggins, 1973). However, in those instances of prolonged gestation in the human, best exemplified by anencephaly, but also perhaps represented by placental sulfatase deficiency and by adrenal hypoplasia, there is no consistent retardation in lung maturation. Thus, there is no evident common thread for a central role for cortisol in the maturation of the human fetal lung and the initiation of human parturition. Nonetheless, the analogy between the anencephalic fetus and the hypophysectomized or adrenalectomized lamb model in Liggins' classic studies is suggestive of the possibility of a common phylogenetic corollary.

Fetal Membrane Glycerophospholipid Arachidonic Acid-Prostaglandin Theory. The formation of prostaglandins by the fetal membranes and uterine decidua vera appears to be an exciting possibility as the finale in the biochemical events that herald parturition. It has been amply demonstrated that prostaglandin $F_{2\alpha}$ or prostaglandin E_2 will evoke myometrial contractions at any stage of gestation whether administered by intravenous, intra-amnionic, or extraovular routes (Karim, 1972). These observations, together with the demonstration that the multienzyme complex, prostaglandin synthetase, exists in human fetal membranes and decidua vera are strongly suggestive, at least, that prostaglandins occupy a key role in the initiation of myometrial contractions. Further substantiating this possibility is the observation that levels of prostaglandins are increased in the amnionic fluid of laboring women, and indeed prostaglandins, or their metabolic products, are increased in the peripheral blood of women just before and during labor.

ARACHIDONIC ACID. Since the eventual formation of prostaglandins in decidua vera may be the initiator of myometrial contractions in the parturient woman, a careful examination of the biochemical mechanisms involved in prostaglandin formation is of immediate interest. It is clearly established that prostaglandins of the -2- series can be formed biosynthetically only from the nonesterified, polyunsaturated, essential fatty acid, arachidonic acid. No other fatty acid can serve as the precursor of prostaglandin $F_{2\alpha}$ or prostaglandin E_2.

With this stipulation in mind, an in-depth study of the role of arachidonic acid in the initiation of parturition has been undertaken (MacDonald et al., 1974, 1978). It should be emphasized that it is arachidonic acid in its free form that serves as the obligatory precursor of prostaglandin $F_{2\alpha}$. Specifically, esterified arachidonic acid, such as that which exists in glycerophospholipids, cannot be utilized for prostaglandin synthesis. Thus, it is believed that the release of free arachidonic acid is the rate-limiting step in the biosynthesis of prostaglandins in most tissues. For this reason it was of interest to compare the concentration of free arachidonic acid in the amnionic fluid of women not in labor to the concentration of free arachidonic acid in the amnionic fluid of women in active labor.

There was a sixfold increase in the concentration of arachidonic acid in the amnionic fluid of laboring women. This observation is suggestive that the release of arachidonic acid from an esterified storage form may be a key event in controlling prostaglandin synthesis and, in turn, labor in the human (MacDonald et al., 1974).

FETAL MEMBRANE GLYCEROPHOS-PHOLIPID. Arachidonic acid is commonly incorporated into the *sn*-2 position of glycerophospholipids. Therefore, a possible preparatory even for human parturition may be the specific incorporation of arachidonic acid into a particular glycerophospholipid that serves as the storage depot for prostaglandin precursor.

A possible anatomic site for the storage of esterified arachidonic acid is the fetal membranes (amnion and chorion laeve). Obstetricians have long recognized that damage to the fetal membranes through premature rupture, infection, or even exposure to hypertonic solutions commonly results in premature parturition in women. Furthermore, the fetal membranes occupy a large surface area contiguous to the metabolically active uterine decidua vera, a known site of prostaglandin synthetase activity. Finally, by analysis of fetal membranes from women near term, Schwarz and co-workers (1975) found an extremely high arachidonic acid content in the fetal membranes, namely, 18 percent of the total fatty acids was arachidonic acid, whereas that in the maternal parietal peritoneum was 0.4 percent. Thus, it appears that there is specific and preferential storage in the human fetal membranes of the obligatory prostaglandin precursor, namely, arachidonic acid.

More recently, Okita and co-workers (1979) found that a particular glycerophospholipid, namely, phosphatidylethanolamine, of the amnion and chorion laeve, is especially enriched in arachidonic acid. Indeed, 50 percent of the fatty acid content of phosphatidylethanolamine in amnion and chorion laeve is arachidonic acid, and 60 percent of the fetal membrane arachidonic acid is found in phosphatidylethanolamines, even though

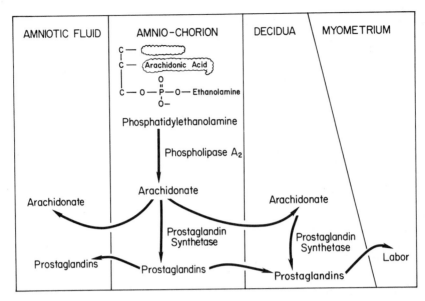

FIG. 15-1. Model of the metabolic relationships envisioned to exist between the fetal membranes (amnio-chorion), decidua vera, and myometrium in the initiation of human parturition. (Courtesy of Drs. J. Okita, B. Schwarz, and J. Johnston)

phosphatidylethanolamines constitute only 30 percent of the glycerophospholipids of fetal membrane tissue.

FETAL MEMBRANE PHOSPHOLIPASE A₂. Since arachidonic acid is stored principally in the *sn-2* position of glycerophospholipids (especially in the *sn-2* position of phosphatidylethanolamines), and since unesterified arachidonic acid is the obligate prostaglandin precursor, it is essential to ascertain the mechanisms by which the arachidonic acid becomes available for utilization in prostaglandin synthesis. The enzyme *phospholipase A₂* catalyzes the hydrolysis of the *sn-2* esters of the glycerophospholipids giving rise to a free fatty acid (e.g., arachidonic acid) and *sn-1*-lysoglycerophospholipid. Therefore, phospholipase A₂ is envisioned as occupying a crucial role in the liberation of arachidonic acid from its esterified form. Okazaki and colleagues (1978) have demonstrated that human fetal membranes possess a phospholipase A₂ that has specificity for phosphatidylethanolamines and greatest specificity for arachidonoyl esters of phosphatidylethanolamines. No such substrate specificity was demon-

strated for the phospholipase A₂ activity of decidua vera. The sequence of events by which arachidonic acid is released from its storage form, viz, phosphatidylethanolamine in the amnio-chorion, and converted to prostaglandins is illustrated in Figure 15-1.

DECIDUA VERA. A similar mechanism, but having its origin in the uterine decidua, was suggested by Gustavii (1972) and by Liggins (1973). Phospholipase A₂ action in other tissues has been shown to be the rate-limiting step in prostagladin formation. Commonly, phospholipase A₂ activity is a lysosomal enzyme. Therefore, the release (or the expression) of phospholipase A₂ activity from fetal membrane lysosomes (or decidual lysosomes as proposed by Gustavii and by Liggins) is an attractive possibility as one of the final steps in the provision of nonesterified arachidonic acid from its storage form for utilization by decidua vera in the synthesis of prostaglandin F₂α or prostaglandin E₂ or both.

LYSOSOMAL STABILIZATION–LABILIZATION. A key question in this entire hypothesis, therefore, may be the mechanism of stabilization of the fetal membrane lyso-somes before term, and labilization at term. Such a mechanism is essential to provide for the expression of lysosomal phospholipase A_2 activity which catalyzes the hydrolysis of glycerophospholipids (phosphatidylethanola-mines) to provide arachidonic acid from its esterified form. It is tempting to speculate that certain steroids, of either fetal or mater-nal origin, may participate in the metabolic expression of enzyme activity of lysosomes in the fetal membranes. Schwarz and co-workers (1976) found that progesterone is avidly bound to a subcellular fraction of fetal membranes that appeared in differential ul-tracentrifugation samples in the same fraction as certain marker enzymes for lysosomes (β-glucuronidase, acid phosphatase, aryl-sulfa-tase). This finding is suggestive that proges-terone becomes intimately associated with fe-tal membrane lysosomes.

ANALOGY TO MENSTRUATION. Fur-ther support of this hypothesis is provided by the observations that during the course of the luteal phase of the menstrual cycle there is an increase in both the size and num-ber of lysosomes of the endometrium (Fe-renczy, Richart, 1974), and these lysosomes are disrupted following progesterone with-drawal at the end of the ovarian cycle. Events analogous to those postulated for parturition occur thereafter, i.e., the formation of prosta-glandins as evidenced by their occurrence in both the menstrual fluid and the bloodstream of menstruating women. Gustavii (1972), for example, has referred to labor as "delayed menstruation." All these observations are suggestive that the withdrawal of, or interfer-ence with the production of, or changes in the metabolism of, progesterone at the level of fetal membranes or the decidua may be important in the unmasking or accelerated expression of lysosomal phospholipase A_2 ac-tivity and, in turn, the liberation of arachi-donic acid, and finally the formation of pros-taglandins in fetal membranes or uterine decidua. Further support for this hypothesis comes from the observations of Okita and co-workers (1979). They found a striking re-

duction in the arachidonic acid content of phosphatidylethanolamines in fetal mem-branes during the course of human labor. Moreover, Schwarz and co-workers (1979) demonstrated that the rate of release of lyso-somal enzymes by amnions obtained from la-boring women was much greater than that of amnions obtained before labor began.

PROPOSED ROLE FOR ESTROGENS. The following theory has been proposed to amalgamate the hypotheses relative to the participation of the fetus (through activities in the fetal brain, i.e., hypothalamus, pitui-tary, and adrenal cortex) with those of the presumed final event, prostaglandin forma-tion: The fetal adrenal cortical secretions re-sult ultimately in preparatory biochemical events, or fetal adrenal secretory products ul-timately effect a change in the stabilization–labilization of membrane lysosomes, or both events are operative. Considering the proper-ties of estrogens for initiating phospholipid metabolism and in modulating systems con-cerned with progesterone action, it is tempt-ing to speculate that the human fetal adrenal participates in parturition as follows: Placen-tal estrogen precursors (see Chap. 7, p. 152) are elaborated by the fetal adrenal and the resultant estrogens produced—perhaps es-triol, which is so abundant in pregnancy—are important in the storage of arachidonic acid in the fetal membranes. Ultimately, the estrogens may serve a critical role in bringing about the expression of phospholipase A_2 ac-tivity in fetal membranes (or decidua), an activity that may have been held latent through pregnancy by progesterone stabiliza-tion of the lysosomal membrane.

PROSTAGLANDIN AS LABOR INITIA-TOR. While the key role of prostaglandin production as the initiator of parturition in the human has not been established, it is in-teresting to note that the administration of aspirin to the human gravida has resulted in prolonged gestation (Collins, Turner, 1975). This observation is consistent with prosta-glandin formation being the initiator of myometrial contractions. This obtains since aspirin is known to inhibit the conversion of arachidonic acid to prostaglandin. Furthermore, indomethacin, a compound which also inhibits prostaglandin synthetase activity, has been shown to prolong gestation in the subhuman primate (Novy et al., 1974). Moreover, the intra-amnionic instillation of nonesterified arachidonic acid into the amnionic sac during the second trimester of apparently normal pregnancies, or late in pregnancies with a dead fetus, causes the uterus to contract and expel its contents (MacDonald et al., 1974). The introduction of unesterified arachidonic acid into the amnionic sac would make available to the decidua, by diffusion, the obligatory prostaglandin precursor and thus would sidestep the necessity of cleavage of arachidonic acid from phospholipid by phospholipase A_2.

These diverse observations led to a consideration of the amnionic fluid (fetal membranes) decidua vera complex as a metabolically active communications unit that may, in fact, transmit and respond to signals that lead to the onset of labor in normal human pregnancy. Whereas most previous investigations of the determinants of labor initiation were concerned primarily with the placenta and uterus, there is a certain teleologic preference for considering the fetus and fetal membranes as the central source of such a signal. It would seem to be preferable to generate uterine contractions in myometrium contiguous to the fetal membranes rather than at the placental implantation site. Moreover, direct communication is established between the fetus and fetal membranes by steroids and/or other substances which originate in the fetus and are excreted into the amnionic fluid in fetal urine, in lung secretions, or through the skin.

While it may seem remarkable that exact biochemical events that herald human parturition are not yet defined precisely, nonetheless, in the past decade great strides have been made in interpreting definitive biochemical events that appear to be of signal importance in this previously inexplicable event.

PHYSIOLOGY OF UTERINE CONTRACTIONS

Evidence, which is considered below, has accrued that is suggestive, at least, that the final event in initiating a myometrial contraction is the release of calcium from its repository form in the sarcoplasmic reticulum. The consequence of this event is to elevate the concentration of intracellular free calcium, which may then become associated with the myofibril of the uterine muscle. This interaction will give rise to uterine contractions, whereas the ATP-energy-dependent translocation of calcium back to a stored form in the sarcoplasmic reticulum is associated with uterine relaxation.

Contractile Elements of Uterus. Ultimately, the stimulus for uterine contractions must act on the contractile elements of the uterus, specifically the myometrium. It is likely that such a mechanism involves a requirement for an increased intracellular concentration of *free calcium* to effect the contraction of the smooth muscle of the uterus just as free calcium is required to induce contraction in striated muscle. The accumulated evidence is suggestive that calcium exists in one or more bound forms in smooth muscle. One of these calcium storage or sequestering sites is the sarcoplasmic reticulum.

SARCOPLASMIC RETICULUM. The sarcoplasmic reticulum surrounds the myofibril and constitutes a storage system from which calcium can be released to the myofibril, effecting a muscle contraction following which the calcium is returned to the *sarcoplasmic reticulum*. Carsten (1968) isolated a calcium-binding membrane system from the myometrium and she pointed to its resemblance to sarcoplasmic reticulum from other muscle systems. Indeed, a well-developed sarcoplasmic reticulum in human uterine muscle at term has been demonstrated by electron microscopy.

Considering both the importance of liberated calcium in initiating uterine muscle contractions and the demonstration of a calcium-binding site in human uterine muscle, namely, the sarcoplasmic reticulum, it appears to be of signal importance to examine the release of calcium from the sarcoplasmic reticulum for transport to the myofibril for the initiation of uterine contractions. In this regard, Carsten also demonstrated, through elegant studies, that prostagladin E_2 and $F_{2\alpha}$ inhibit the ATP-dependent binding of calcium to the sarcoplasmic reticulum. On the other hand, prostaglandin $F_{1\beta}$, which has no physiologic effect on the myometrium, does not inhibit the ATP-dependent calcium-binding to the sarcoplasmic reticulum. It is likely, therefore, that the action of prostaglandin E_2 and prostaglandin $F_{2\alpha}$ in the initiation of uterine contractions is related to their capability of inhibiting calcium-binding to the sarcoplasmic reticulum. Such an action would give rise to an increased concentration of intracellular free calcium which may interact with the regulatory proteins of the myofibril eventuating in uterine contractions. Conversely, the binding, storage, or sequestration of calcium by the sarcoplasmic reticulum will decrease the concentration of intracellular calcium, resulting in uterine muscle relaxation.

Carsten also demonstrated that oxytocin will inhibit the ATP-dependent storage of calcium to the sarcoplasmic reticulum. Interestingly, there is a marked difference in the capability of oxytocin to effect this inhibition in preparations of uterine muscle obtained from nonpregnant women. On the other hand, only a modest difference in the capability of prostaglandin $F_{2\alpha}$ or prostaglandin E_2 to inhibit storage of calcium between uterine preparations of pregnant and nonpregnant women was observed. These findings may provide an explanation for the susceptibility of the myometrium to the effects of certain prostaglandins at all stages of gestation, whereas it is known that there is a relative refractoriness of the human uterus to oxytocin-induced contractions until late in gestation. Whether or not oxytocin and the prostaglandins effect calcium release by precisely the same mechanism is not yet established.

THREE STAGES OF LABOR

Labor is customarily, and for good clinical reasons, divided into three distinct stages.

The first stage of labor commences when uterine contractions (myometrial forces) reach sufficient *frequency, intensity,* and *duration* to bring about readily demonstrable effacement and dilatation of the cervix. The first stage ends when the cervix is fully dilated, i.e., when the cervix is sufficiently dilated to allow the fetal head to pass through. The first stage of labor, therefore, is primarily the stage of *cervical effacement* and *dilatation.*

The second stage of labor begins when dilatation of the cervix is complete and ends with delivery of the infant. The second stage of labor is the stage of *expulsion of the fetus.*

The third stage of labor begins with delivery of the infant and ends with the delivery of the placenta. The third stage of labor is the stage of *separation and expulsion of the placenta.*

In addition to these classic three stages of labor, some obstetricians categorize a period of *prelabor* and a *latent phase of labor* that precede the first stage, and a *fourth stage of labor* that follows delivery of the placenta. Hendricks (1970), for example, identified *prelabor* as the period of increased uterine activity that occurs for a few weeks before clinical labor. During this period, the increased uterine activity is believed to stimulate softening of the cervix, some cervical effacement, slight-to-modest cervical dilatation, and expansion of the lower uterine segment. Friedman (1955) described a *latent phase of labor* of several hours before active labor (see Chap. 29, p. 787). During the latent phase, uterine contractions typically are infrequent, produce some discomfort, and may be irregular, but apparently generate sufficient force to cause slow dilatation and some effacement of the cervix.

A fourth stage of labor has been identified by some obstetricians as that period of an hour or so after delivery of the placenta during which myometrial contraction and retraction, along with vessel thrombosis, effectively controls bleeding from the placental implantation site. Prelabor, the latent phase of labor, and the fourth stage of labor lack the precision of definition and ease of identification that characterize the three classic stages of labor, but are of undoubted importance in human parturition.

CLINICAL COURSE OF LABOR

"Lightening." A few weeks before the onset of labor, the abdomen of the pregnant woman commonly undergoes a change in shape. The fundal height decreases somewhat, and this event at times is described by the mother as "the baby dropped." This phenomenon is the consequence of the development of a well-formed lower uterine segment, the descent of the fetal head to or even through the pelvic inlet, and to some degree a reduction in the volume of amnionic fluid.

False Labor. For a variable period of time before the establishment of true or effective labor, women may experience so-called false labor. The uterine contractions of false labor are characterized by irregularity and brevity, and the discomfort produced most often is confined to the lower abdomen and groin. In contrast, the discomfort produced by uterine contractions characteristic of true labor begins first in the fundal region and then radiates over the uterus and through to the lower back.

Uterine irritability that causes discomfort but that does not represent true labor (in that cervical dilatation does not occur) may develop at any time during pregnancy. False labor is most common late in pregnancy and in parous women. It often stops spontaneously but may convert rapidly to the effective contractions of true labor. Therefore, the complaints of relatively infrequent and brief but uncomfortable uterine contractions cannot be dismissed summarily. All too frequently when this is done, delivery takes place without benefit of the assistance of professional personnel or facilities essential for optimal care of the mother and fetus-infant.

"Show." A rather dependable sign of the approach of labor (provided no rectal or vaginal examination has been performed in the preceding 48 hours) is "show" or "bloody show," which consists of the discharge from the vagina of a small amount of blood-tinged mucus, representing the extrusion of the plug of mucus that has filled the cervical canal during pregnancy. "Show" is a late sign, for labor usually ensues during the next several hours to a few days. Normally, only a few drops of blood escape with the mucous plug; more substantial bleeding is suggestive of an abnormal condition.

CHARACTERISTICS OF UTERINE CONTRACTIONS IN LABOR

Alone among physiologic muscular contractions, those of labor are painful. Therefore, the common designation in many languages for such a contraction is "pain." The cause of the pain is not known definitely, but the following hypotheses have been suggested: (1) hypoxia of the contracted myometrium (as in angina pectoris); (2) compression of nerve ganglia in the cervix and lower uterus by the tightly interlocking muscle bundles; (3) stretching of the cervix during dilatation; and (4) stretching of the overlying peritoneum. Compression of nerve ganglia in the cervix and lower uterine segment by the contracting myometrium is an especially attractive hypothesis, since paracervical infiltration with a local anesthetic typically produces appreciable relief of pain during subsequent uterine contractions (see Chap. 18, p. 446).

Uterine contractions are involuntary and, for the most part, independent of extrauterine control. Neural blockage from caudal or epidural anesthesia, if initiated quite early in labor, sometimes reduces the frequency and intensity of uterine contractions but not after labor is well established. Moreover, paraplegic women have normal though painless contractions, as do women after bilateral lumbar sympathectomy. Thus far attempts to initiate labor in women by electrical stimulation have been only partially successful (Theobald, 1968).

Ivy, Hartman, and Koff (1931) believed that the uterus has pacemakers that initiate uterine contractions and control their rhythmicity. As pointed out by Carsten (1968), however, in a comprehensive review of myometrial composition, growth, and activity, the cells participating in the pacemaker activities, unlike those of the heart, do not differ anatomically from the surrounding myocytes. Pacemaker activity is not confined to a specific site (Wolfs, van Leeuwen, 1979). It requires only a group of highly excitable myometrial cells and it may start in a variety of sites. The contractile rhythm of one pacemaker may reinforce or block that of another. Since electric current does not flow easily from one myometrial cell to another, activation of individual myometrial cell membranes almost certainly serves to propagate the impulse throughout the myometrium. In women, the pacemaker sites most often appear to be near the uterotubal junctions.

Mechanical stretching of the cervix enhances uterine activity in several species, including man. This phenomenon has been referred to as the *Ferguson reflex*. The exact mechanism by which mechanical dilatation of the cervix causes increased myometrial contractility is not clear. Release of oxytocin was suggested as the cause by Ferguson (1941) but this has not been proved. Spinal or epidural anesthesia effectively blocks the stimulatory effect of stretching the cervix, according to Sala and associates (1970).

The interval between contractions diminishes gradually from about 10 minutes at the onset of the first stage of labor to as little as 1 minute in the second stage. Periods of relaxation between contractions are essential to the welfare of the fetus, since unremitting contractions may interfere with uteroplacental blood flow sufficiently to produce fetal hypoxia. The duration of each contraction ranges from 30 to 90 seconds, averaging about 1 minute. There is appreciable variability in the intensity of uterine contractions during apparently normal labor, as emphasized

by Schulman and Romney (1970). They recorded the amnionic fluid pressures generated by uterine contractions in women during spontaneous labor; the pressures averaged 40 mm Hg but varied from 20 to 60 mm Hg.

Differentiation of Myometrial Activity. With labor, the uterus differentiates into two distinct parts. The actively contracting upper segment becomes thicker as labor advances. The lower portion, comprising the lower segment of the uterus and the cervix, is relatively passive compared to the upper segment, and it develops into a much thinner-walled muscular passage for the fetus. The lower uterine segment is the greatly expanded and thinned-out isthmus of the nonpregnant uterus. Its formation is not solely a phenomenon of labor. The lower segment develops gradually as pregnancy progresses and then thins remarkably during labor (Fig. 15-2A,B). On abdominal palpation, even before rupture of the membranes, the two segments can be differentiated during a contraction. The upper uterine segment is quite firm or hard, whereas the lower uterine segment feels much less firm. The former represents the actively contracting part of the uterus; the latter is the distended, normally much more passive portion.

If the entire sac of uterine musculature, including the lower uterine segment and cervix, were to contract simultaneously and with equal intensity, the net explosive force would be decreased markedly. Therein lies the importance of the division of the uterus into an actively contracting upper segment and a more passive lower segment which differ not only anatomically but also physiologically. The upper segment contracts, retracts, and expels the fetus. In response to the force of contractions of the upper segment, the lower uterine segment and cervix dilate and thereby form a greatly expanded, thinned-out muscular and fibromuscular tube through which the fetus can pass.

The myometrium of the upper uterine segment after contracting does not relax to its original length. Rather, it becomes relatively fixed at a shorter length, the tension, how-

378

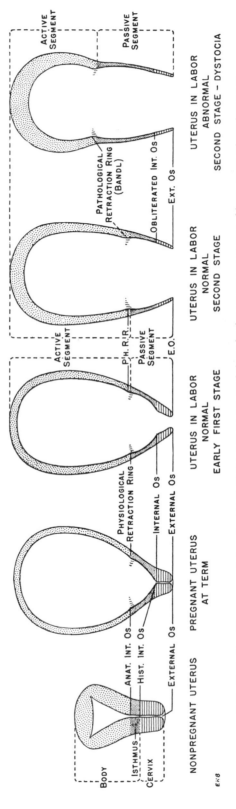

FIG. 15-2. A. Sequence of development of the segments and rings in the pregnant uterus. Note comparison between the nonpregnant uterus, uterus at term, and uterus in labor. The passive lower segment of the uterine body is derived from the isthmus; the physiologic retraction ring develops at the junction of the upper and lower uterine segments. The pathologic retraction ring develops from the physiologic ring. (Anat. Int. Os = anatomic internal os; Hist. Int. Os = histologic internal os; Ph. R. R. = physiologic retraction ring; E.O. = external os.)

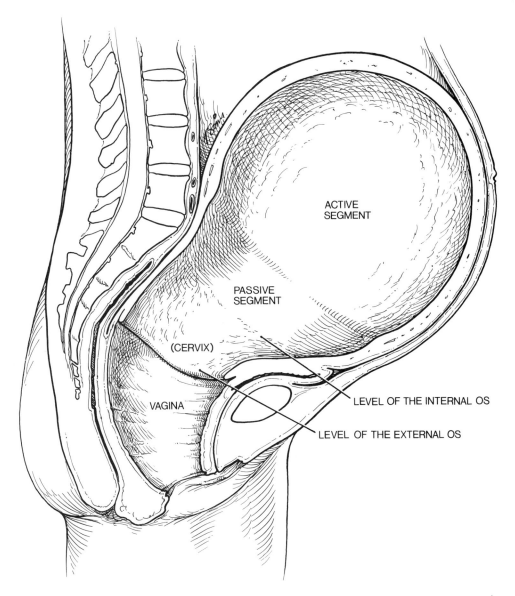

FIG. 15-2. B. The uterus at the time of vaginal delivery. The active upper segment of the uterus retracts about the fetus as the fetus descends through the birth canal. The passive lower segment has considerably less myometrial tone.

ever, remaining the same as before the contraction. The purpose of the ability of the upper portion of the uterus, or active segment, to contract down on its diminishing contents with myometrial tension remaining constant is to take up slack, i.e., to hold the advantage gained, and to maintain the uterine musculature in firm contact with the intrauterine contents. As the consequence of retraction, each successive contraction starts where its predecessor left off, so that the upper part of the uterine cavity becomes slightly smaller with each successive contraction. Because of the successive shortening of its muscular fibers with each contraction, the upper uterine segment (Active Segment, Fig. 15-2A) becomes progressively thickened throughout the first and second stages of labor and tremendously thickened immediately after the birth of the baby. The phenomenon of retraction of the upper uterine segment is contingent upon a decrease in the volume of its contents. For its contents to be diminished, particularly early in labor when the entire uterus is virtually a closed sac with only a minute opening at the cervix, requires that the musculature of the lower segment stretch, permitting increasingly more of the intrauterine contents to occupy the lower segment. Indeed, the upper segment retracts only to the extent that the lower segment distends and the cervix dilates.

The relaxation of the lower uterine segment is by no means complete relaxation, but rather the opposite of retraction. The fibers of the lower segment become stretched with each contraction of the upper segment, after which they do not return to their previous length but remain relatively fixed at the longer length, the tension, however, remaining essentially the same as before. The musculature still manifests tone, still resists stretch, and still contracts somewhat on stimulation.

The successive lengthening of the muscular fibers in the lower uterine segment as labor progresses is accompanied in thinning, normally to only a few mm in its thinnest part. As a result of the thinning of the lower

uterine segment and the concomitant thickening of the upper, the boundary between them is marked by a ridge on the inner uterine surface, the *physiologic retraction ring.* When the thinning of the lower uterine segment is extreme, as in obstructed labor, the ring is very prominent, forming, in extreme cases, a *pathologic retraction ring* (Bandl's ring), an abnormal condition demonstrated in Figure 15-2.A. and discussed further in Chapter 29, p. 795.

Quantitative measurements of the difference in behavior of the upper and lower parts of the uterus during normal labor have disclosed normally a gradient of diminishing physiologic activity from the fundus to the cervix. Several ingenious devices have been used, including the tokodynamometer, intrauterine receptors, and intramyometrial catheters.

The tokodynamometer employs three strain guages set in heavy brass ring mountings, which may be placed anywhere on the abdomen. When the uterus contracts, the increased convexity of the local arc of uterus underlying the ring pushes upward on the gauge and applies a strain to its elements proportional to the local force of the uterine contraction. A record is obtained electro-

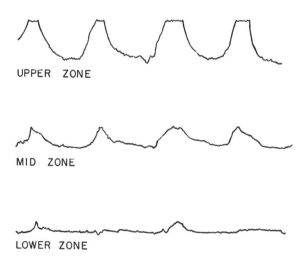

UPPER ZONE

MID ZONE

LOWER ZONE

FIG. 15-3. Uterine contractions in various parts of the uterus recorded by Reynolds' toko-dynamometer. The lower zone probably corresponds to the lower uterine segment. The patient was a primigravida in active labor, with cervix 5 cm dilated, and contractions about 3 minutes apart. The original tracings have been inked over for clearer reproduction. (From Reynolds, Hellman, and Bruns. *Obstet Gynecol Surv* 3:629, 1948)

metrically, an example of which is shown in Figure 15-3. It is evident from these tracings that the intensity of each contraction is greater in the fundal zone than in the midzone, and greater in the midzone than lower down. Equally noteworthy is the differential in the duration of the contractions; those in the midzone are much briefer than those above, whereas the contractions in the lower zone are extremely brief and sometimes absent. This subsidence of contraction in the midzone while the upper zone is still contracting indicates that the upper part of the corpus, throughout a substantial portion of each contraction, exerts pressure caudally on the more relaxed parts of the uterus. Occasionally, when labor is not progressing, this gradient is absent, and both the intensity and the duration of the contractions may be the same in all three zones.

These findings of Reynolds (1949) were confirmed through use of an entirely different apparatus by Karlson (1949). His technic measured the internal pressure in the uterus at any point by means of so-called receptors (metal capsules about 12 mm long with a diameter of 4.5 mm), in the middle of which is a small aperture. On the inner side of this aperture is a membrane that is sensitive to pressure. Pressure exerted against the window is carried and registered electrometrically; an example of one of Karlson's tracings is shown in Figure 15-4. Here again there is a gradient of diminishing activity from the fundus to the lower uterine segment. Karlson's other tracings, like those of Reynolds, indicate that in the absence of this gradient, that is, when the intensity of contraction of the lower segment equals or exceeds

that of the fundus, cervical dilatation may cease. Similar results were obtained by Caldeyro-Barcia, Alvarez, and Reynolds (1950), who inserted either small intramyometrial ballons or open-ended catheters at various levels and recorded the pressures during contractions.

Change in Uterine Shape. Each contraction produces an elongation of the uterine ovoid with a concomitant decrease in horizontal diameters. This change in shape has two important effects on the process of labor:

1. The decrease in horizontal diameter produces a straightening of the fetal vertebral column, pressing its upper pole firmly against the fundus of the uterus, while the lower pole is thrust farther downward into the pelvis. The lengthening of the fetal ovoid thus produced has been estimated as between 5 and 10 cm. The pressure so exerted is known as fetal axis pressure.
2. With the lengthening of the uterus, the longitudinal fibers are drawn taut; and since the lower segment and cervix are the only parts of the uterus that give, they are pulled upward over the lower pole of the fetus. This effect on the musculature of the lower segment and on the cervix is an important factor in cervical dilatation. The round ligaments also contain smooth muscle, which can contract and pull the

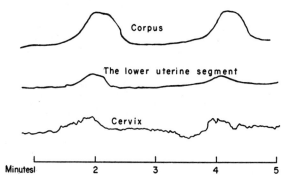

FIG. 15-4. Uterine contractions in various parts of the uterus recorded by Karlson by means of intrauterine receptors. The patient was in early labor, but from the time this tracing was made progress was rapid. To permit clearer reproduction, the background of the original record has been eliminated and the tracings inked over corpus–upper uterine segment. (Modified from Karlson. *Acta Obstet Gynecol Scand* 28:209, 1949)

uterus forward. They are not essential for successful labor and delivery, however.

OTHER FORCES CONCERNED IN LABOR

Intra-abdominal Pressure.   After the cervix is dilated fully, the chief force that expels the fetus is increased intra-abdominal pressure created by contraction of the abdominal muscles simultaneous with forced respiratory efforts with the glottis closed. In obstetric jargon, this is usually referred to as "pushing." The force produced is similar to that involved in defecation but usually much more intense. The important role played by intra-abdominal pressure in fetal expulsion is most plainly attested to by the labors of paraplegic women. Such women suffer no pain, although the uterus may contract vigorously. Cervical dilatation, solely the result of uterine contractions, proceeds normally, but expulsion of the infant is rarely possible except when the woman is instructed to bear down and can do so at the time that the obstetrician identifies uterine contractions. Although increased intra-abdominal pressure is required for the spontaneous completion of labor, it is futile until the cervix is fully dilated. In other words, it is necessary auxiliary to uterine contractions in the second stage of labor, but "pushing" accomplishes little in the first stage but fatigue of the mother.

Intra-abdominal pressure may also be important in the third stage of labor, especially if the parturient is unattended. After the placenta has separated, its spontaneous expulsion is aided by the mother's bearing down, i.e., by an increase in intra-abdominal pressure.

Resistance.   Labor is work, and mechanically work is the generation of motion against resistance. The forces involved in labor are those of the uterus and the abdomen that expel the infant and that must overcome the resistance offered by the cervix to dilatation and the friction created by the birth canal during passage of the presenting part. In addition, forces of resistance may be exerted by the muscles of the pelvic floor. The work involved in labor, according to Gemzell and others (1957), is only a fraction of the maximal funtional capacity of the normal woman.

Changes Induced in the Cervix.   The effective force of the first stage of labor is the uterine contraction which, in turn, exerts hydrostatic pressure through the membranes against the cervix and lower uterine segment. In the absence of intact membranes, the presenting part is forced directly against the cervix and lower uterine segment. As the result of the action of these forces, two fundamental changes, effacement and dilatation, take place in the cervix.

THE MECHANISM OF CERVICAL EFFACEMENT.   Effacement of the cervix ("obliteration" or "taking up") is the shortening of the cervical canal from a structure approximately 2 cm in length to one in which the canal is replaced by a mere circular orifice with almost paper-thin edges. The process takes place from above downward; it occurs as the muscular fibers in the vicinity of the internal os are pulled upward, or "taken up," into the lower uterine segment, while the condition of the external os remains temporarily unchanged. As illustrated in Figures 15-5 through 15-8, the edges of the internal os are drawn upward several cm to become functionally part of the lower uterine segment. Effacement may be compared to a funneling process in which the whole length of a narrow cylinder is converted into a very obtuse flaring funnel with only a small circular orifice for an outlet. As the result of increased myometrial activity during "prelabor" or the "latent phast of labor," appreciable effacement of the cervix sometimes is attained before true labor begins. Such effacement usually facilitates expulsion of the mucus plug from the cervical canal as the canal shortens.

THE MECHANISM OF CERVICAL DILATATION.   In order for the head of the average fetus at term to be able to pass through

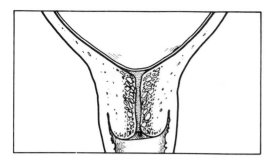
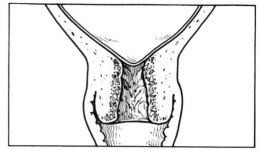

FIG. 15-5. Cervix near the end of pregnancy but before labor. *Left,* primigravida; *right,* multipara.

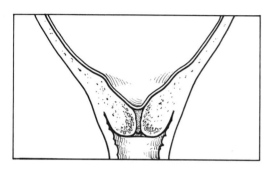
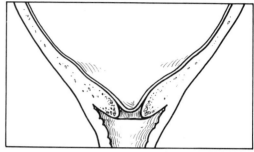

FIG. 15-6. Beginning effacement of cervix. Note dilatation of internal os and funnel-shaped cervical canal. *Left,* primigravida; *right,* multipara.

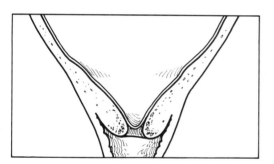
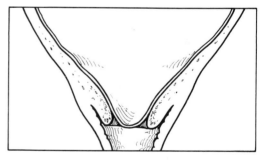

FIG. 15-7. Further effacement of cervix. *Left,* primigravida; *right,* multipara.

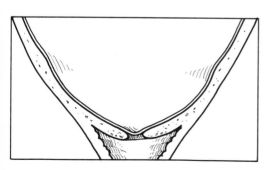
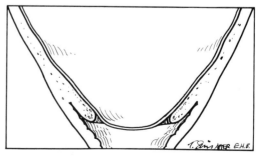

FIG. 15-8. Cervical canal obliterated, i.e., the cervix is completely effaced. *Left,* primigravida; *right,* multipara.

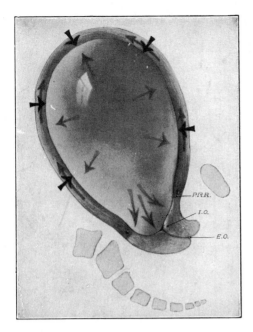

FIG. 15-9. Hydrostatic action of membranes in effecting cervical effacement and dilatation. In absence of intact membranes, the presenting part applied to the cervix and forming the lower uterine segment (P.R.R.) acts similarly. In this and the next two illustrations note changing relations of external os (E.O.), internal os (I.O.), and physiologic retraction ring (P.R.R.).

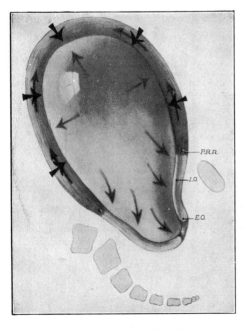

FIG. 15-10. Hydrostatic action of membranes at completion of effacement.

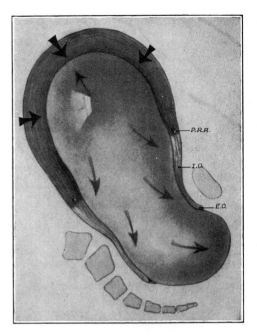

FIG. 15-11. Hydrostatic action of membranes at full cervical dilatation.

the cervix, the canal must dilate to a diameter of about 10 cm. When dilatation has reached a diameter sufficient for the head to pass through, the cervix is said to be "completely dilated" or "fully dilated."

Compared to the body of the uterus, the lower uterine segment and cervix are regions of lesser resistance. Therefore, during a contraction, these structures are subjected to distension, in the course of which a centrifugal pull is exerted on the cervix (Figs. 15-9 to 15-11). As the uterine contractions exert pressure on the membranes, the hydrostatic action of the amnionic sac, in turn, dilates the cervical canal in the manner of a wedge. In the absence of intact membranes, the pressure of the presenting part against the cervix and lower uterine segment is similarly effective. Early rupture of the membranes ("dry birth") does not retard cervical dilatation so long as the presenting part of the fetus exerts pressure against the cervix and lower uterine segment.

The decidua of the lower uterine segment is thin and poorly developed. The slightest movement of the underlying muscle, therefore, might allow the fetal membranes to slip

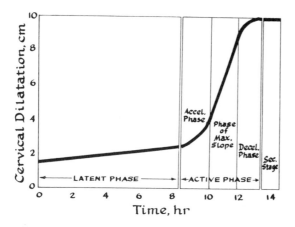

FIG. 15-12. Composite of the average dilatation curve for nulliparous labor based on analysis of the data derived from the patterns traced by a large, nearly consecutive series of gravidas. The first stage is divided into a relatively flat latent phase and a rapidly progressive active phase. The active phase has three identifiable component parts—an acceleration phase, a linear phase of maximum slope, and a deceleration phase. (From Friedman. *Labor: Clinical Evaluation and Management,* 2nd ed. New York, Appleton, 1978)

back and forth over the decidua. This loosening of the membranes in the lower segment is a normal feature of early labor and a prerequisite to successful cervical dilatation. Membranes that slide readily over the lower segment and partly through the cervix are much more efficacious dilators than are those which are more firmly attached. The little that is known of the physicochemical changes that accompany cervical dilatation is considered on page 386 and in Chapter 9.

There may be no fetal descent during cervical effacement, but as a rule, the station of the presenting part descends somewhat as the cervix dilates. During the second stage, descent typically occurs rather slowly but steadily in nulliparas. In multiparas, however, particularly those of high parity, descent may be very rapid.

Pattern of Cervical Dilatation. Friedman (1978) in his elegant treatise on labor, stated correctly that, "The clinical features of uterine contractions—namely, frequency, intensity, and duration—cannot be relied upon as measures of progression in labor nor as indices of normality. . . . Except for cervical dilatation and fetal descent, none of the clinical features of the parturient patient appears to be useful in assessing labor progres-

sion." The pattern of cervical dilatation that takes place during the course of normal labor takes on the shape of a sigmoid curve (Fig. 15-12). As depicted in Figure 15-12, two phases of cervical dilatation can be defined: the latent phase and the active phase. The active phase has been subdivided further as the acceleration phase, phase of maximum slope, and the deceleration phase (Friedman, 1978). The duration of the latent phase is more variable and subject to sensitive changes by extraneous factors and by sedation (prolongation of latent phase) and myometrial stimulation (shortening of latent phase). The duration of the latent phase has little bearing on the subsequent course of labor, whereas the characteristics of the accelerated phase usually are predictive of the outcome of a particular labor. Friedman (1978) considers the maximum slope as a "good measure of the overall efficiency of the machine," whereas the deceleration phase is more reflective of fetopelvic relationships. The completion of cervical dilatation during the active phase of labor is accomplished by cervical retraction about the presenting part of the fetus. After complete cervical dilatation, the second stage of labor commences and thereafter only progressive descent is available to assess the progress of labor.

Pattern of Descent. In many nulliparas, engagement of the fetal head is achieved prior to the onset of labor and further descent does not occur until late in labor. In others in whom engagement initially is not so extensive, further descent occurs during the first stage of labor. The descent pattern of normal labor traces a typical hyperbolic curve when the station of the fetal head is plotted as a function of the duration of labor. Active descent usually takes place after cervical dilatation has progressed for some time. In nulliparas, increased rates of descent are observed ordinarily during the phase of maximum slope of cervical dilatation. At this time the speed of descent increases to a maximum (Friedman, 1978), and this maximal rate of descent is maintained until the presenting fetal part reaches the perineal floor.

NORMAL LABOR

Based upon the findings of a scholarly analysis of the labor patterns of a large number of women, Friedman (1978) also sought to select criteria that would delimit normal labor and thus be able to identify significant abnormalities of labor. The limits, admittedly arbitrary, appear to be logical and clinically useful.

The group of women studied were nulliparas and multiparas, with no fetopelvic disporportion, no fetal malposition or malpresentation, no multiple pregnancy, and not treated with heavy sedation or conduction anesthesia, oxytocin, or operative intervention; all had normal pelves and were at term with vertex presentations and delivered average size infants. From these studies, Friedman developed the concept of three functional divisions of labor—preparatory, dilatational, and pelvic—to describe their physiologic objectives (Fig. 15-13). He found that the preparatory division of labor may be sensitive to sedation and anesthesia. While little cervical dilatation occurs during this phase, considerable changes take place in the ground substance, i.e., collagen and other connective tissue components, of the cervix (Danforth

et al., 1960). The dilatational division of labor, during which time dilatation is occurring at its most rapid rate, is principally unaffected by sedation or anesthesia employed for analgesia. The pelvic division of labor commences with the deceleration phase of cervical dilatation. The classic mechanisms of labor involving the cardinal movements of the fetus take place principally during the pelvic division of labor. In actual practice, however, the time of onset of the pelvic division of labor is seldom clearly identifiable separate from the dilatational division of labor. Moreover, the rate of cervical dilatation does not always decelerate as full dilatation is approached; in fact, it may accelerate.

RUPTURE OF MEMBRANES. Spontaneous rupture of the membranes most often occurs sometime during the course of active labor. Typically, rupture of the membranes is manifested by a sudden gush of a variable quantity of normally clear or slightly turbid, nearly colorless fluid. Infrequently, the membranes remain intact until the time of delivery of the infant. If by chance the membranes remain intact until completion of delivery, the fetus is born surrounded by them, and the portion covering his head is sometimes referred to as the *caul*.

Changes in the Vagina and Pelvic Floor. The birth canal is supported and is closed functionally by a number of layers of tissues that together form the pelvic floor. From within outward, these tissues are (1) peritoneum, (2) subperitoneal connective tissue, (3) internal pelvic fascia, (4) levator ani and coccygeus muscles, (5) external pelvic fascia, (6) superficial muscles and fascia, (7) subcutaneous tissue, and (8) skin.

ANATOMY OF PELVIC FLOOR. Of these structures, the most important are the levator ani and the fascia covering its upper and lower surfaces, which for practical purposes may be considered the pelvic floor (Fig. 2-6, p. 20). This muscle (or group of muscles) closes the lower end of the pelvic cavity as a diaphragm and thereby presents a concave upper and a convex lower surface, as illustrated in Figures 15-14 and 15-15.

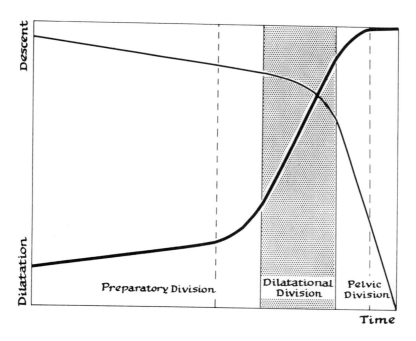

FIG. 15-13. Labor course divided functionally on the basis of expected evolution of the dilatation and descent curves into *(1)* a preparatory division, including latent and acceleration phases, *(2)* a dilatational division, occupying the phase of maximum slope of dilatation, and *(3)* a pelvic division, encompassing both deceleration phase and second stage while concurrent with the phase of maximum slope of descent. Recognizing these distinctive functional divisions proves useful in clinical practice. (From Friedman. *Labor: Clinical Evaluation and Management,* 2nd ed. New York, Appleton, 1978)

On either side, the levator ani consists of a pubic and iliac portion. The former is a band 2 to 2.5 cm in width arising from the horizontal ramus of the pubis 3 to 4 cm below its upper margin and 1 to 1.5 cm from the symphysis pubis. Its fibers pass backward to encircle the rectum and possibly give off a few fibers that pass behind the vagina. The greater or iliac portion of the muscle arises on either side of the pelvis from the white line (the tendinous arch of the pelvic fascia) and from the ischial spine at a distance of about 5 cm below the margin of the pelvic inlet. The greater part of the muscle passes backward and unites with that from the other side of the rectum; the posterior portions meet in a tendinous raphe in front of the coccyx, with the most posterior fibers attached to the bone itself. The posterior and lateral portions of the pelvic floor, which are not filled out by the levator ani, are occupied by the piriformis and coccygeus muscles on either side (Fig. 2-6, p. 20).

The levator ani varies from 3 to 5 mm in thickness, though it margins encircling the rectum and vagina are somewhat thicker. During pregnancy

the levator ani usually undergoes hypertrophy. On vaginal examination, the internal margin of the muscle can be felt as a thick band extending backward from the pubis, encircling the vagina about 2 cm above the hymen. On contraction, the levator ani draws both the rectum and vagina forward and upward in the direction of the symphysis pubis and thereby acts to close the vagina, for the more superficial muscles of the perineum are too delicate to serve more than an accessory function.

The internal pelvic fascia, which forms the upper covering of the levator ani, is attached to the margin of the pelvic inlet, where it is joined by the fascia of the iliac fossa, and by the transverse fascia of the obturator internus and is attached firmly to the periosteum covering the lateral wall of the pelvis. The white line is indicative of its point of deflection from the periosteum. From there the internal pelvic fascia spreads out over the upper surface of the levator ani and coccygeus muscles.

The inferior fascial covering of the pelvic diaphragm is divided into two parts by a line drawn between the ischial tuberosities. The posterior por-

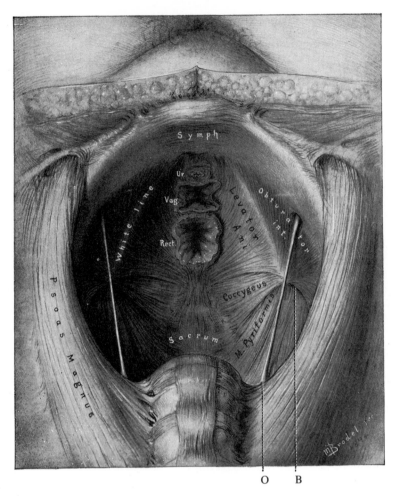

O   B

FIG. 15-14. The pelvic floor seen from above. Uterus, tubes, ovaries, peritoneum, support-ing ligaments, and internal fascial coverings have been removed. O = obturator nerve; B = border of great sciatic foramen; symph = symphysis; Ur = urethra; Vag = vagina; Rect = rectum. (From Kelly. *Operative Gynecology.* New York, Appleton, 1906)

tion consists of a single layer, which, taking its origin from the sacrosciatic ligament and the is-chial tuberosity, passes up over the inner surface of the ischial bones and the obturator internus to the white line, in the formation of which it takes part. From this tendinous structure, it is re-flected at an acute angle over the inferior surface of the levator ani; the space included between the latter and the lateral pelvic wall forms the *ischiorectal fossa.* The structure filling out the trian-gular space between the pubic arch and a line joining the ischial tuberosities is known as the *urogenital diaphragm,* which, exclusive of skin and subcutaneous fat, consists principally of three lay-ers of fascia: (1) the deep perineal fascia, which

covers the anterior portion of the inferior surface of the levator ani muscle and is continuous with the fascia just described; (2) the middle perineal fascia, which is separated from the former by a narrow space in which are situated the pubic ves-sels and nerves; (3) the superficial perineal fascia, which, together with the layer just described, forms a compartment in which lie the superficial perineal muscles, with the exception of the sphinc-ter ani, the rami of the clitoris, the vestibular bulbs, and the vulvovaginal glands (see Fig. 2-6, p. 20).

The superficial perineal muscles consist of the bulbocavernosus, the ischiocavernosus, and the su-perficial transverse perineal muscles. These mus-

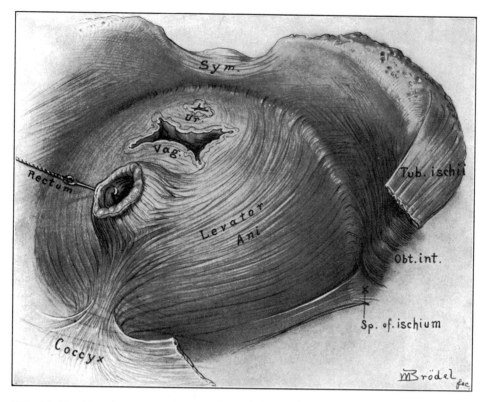

FIG. 15-15. The deep muscles of the pelvic floor seen from below. Sym = symphysis; Ur = urethra; Vag = vagina; Sp. of Ischium = ischial spine; Obt. int. = obturator internus muscle; Tub. ischii = ischial tuberosity.

cles are delicately formed and are of no major obstetric importance except that the superficial transverse perineal muscles are always torn in perineal lacerations.

In the first stage of labor, the membranes and presenting part of the fetus play a role in dilating the upper portion of the vagina. After the membranes have ruptured, however, the changes in the pelvic floor are caused entirely by pressure exerted by the presenting part of the fetus. The most marked change consists of the stretching of the fibers of the levator ani muscles and the thinning of the central portion of the perineum, which becomes transformed from a wedge-shaped mass of tissue 5 cm in thickness to, in the absence of episiotomy, a thin almost transparent membranous structure less than 1 cm in thickness. When the perineum is distended maximally, the anus becomes dilated mark-

edly and presents an opening, varying from 2 to 3 cm in diameter, through which the anterior wall of the rectum bulges.

The extraordinary increase in the number and size of the blood vessels supplying the vagina and pelvic floor increases greatly the magnitude of blood loss when the tissues are torn.

THIRD STAGE OF LABOR

The third stage of labor, which begins immediately after delivery of the fetus, involves the separation and expulsion of the placenta.

The Phase of Placental Separation. As the baby is born, the uterus spontaneously contracts down on its diminishing contents. Normally, by the time the infant is com-

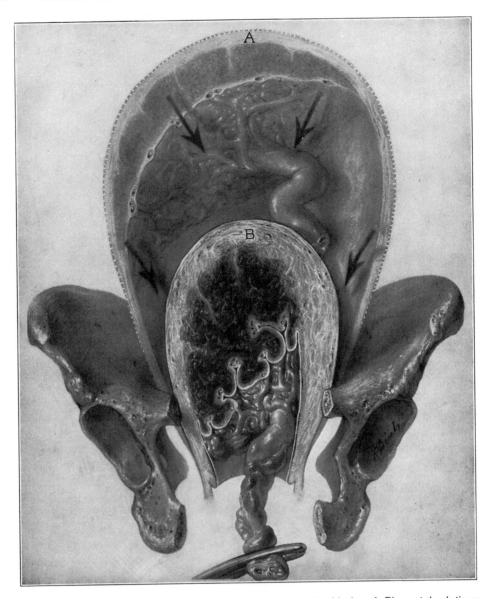

FIG. 15-16.   Diminution in size of placental site after birth of baby. *A.* Placental relations before birth of infant. *B.* Placental relations after birth of infant.

pletely delivered, the uterine cavity is nearly obliterated and the organ consists of an almost solid mass of muscle, the walls of which are several cm thick above the lower segment, and the fundus of which lies just below the level of the umbilicus. This sudden diminution in uterine size inevitably is accompanied by a decrease in the area of the placental implantation site (Fig. 15-16). In order to accommodate itself to this reduced area, the placenta increases in thickness, but because of its limited elasticity it is forced to buckle. The resulting tension causes the weakest layer of the decidua, the spongy layer or decidua spongiosa, to give way, and cleavage takes place at that site. Therefore, separation of the placenta results primarily from a disproportion created between the unchanged size of the placenta and the reduced size of the underlying implantation site. During cesarean section, this phenomenon may be observed directly when the placenta is implanted posteriorly.

Cleavage is facilitated greatly by the loose structure of the spongy decidua, which may be likened to the row of perforations between postage stamps. As separation proceeds, a hematoma forms between the separating placenta and the remaining decidua. Formation of the hematoma is usually the result, rather than the cause, of the separation, since in some cases bleeding is negligible. The hematoma may, however, accelerate the process of cleavage. Since the separation of the placenta is through the spongy layer of the decidua (see Chap. 6, p. 123), part of the decidua is cast off with the placenta, while the rest remains attached to the myometrium (Fig. 15-17). The amount of decidual tissue retained at the placental site varies.

Most investigators have found that placental separation occurs within a very few minutes after delivery. Brandt (1933) and others, based on results obtained in combined clinical and roentgenologic studies, supported the idea that since the periphery of the placenta is probably the most adherent portion, separation usually begins elsewhere. Occasionally, some degree of separation begins even before the third stage of labor commences, probably accounting for certain cases of fetal distress just before expulsion of the infant.

SEPARATION OF AMNIO-CHORION. The great decrease in the surface area of the cavity of the uterus simultaneously causes the fetal membranes (amniochorion) and the parietal decidua to be thrown into innumerable folds that increase the thickness of the layer from less than a millimeter to 3 to 4 mm. The lining of the uterus, as illustrated in Figure 15-18, early in the third stage, is indicative that much of the parietal layer of decidua vera is included between the folds of the festooned amnion and chorion laeve.

The membranes usually remain in situ until the separation of the placenta is nearly completed. They are then peeled off the uterine wall, partly by the further contraction of the myometrium and partly by traction exerted by the separated placenta, which lies in the flabby lower uterine segment or in the upper portion of the vagina. The body of the uterus at that time normally forms an almost solid mass of muscle, the anterior and posterior walls of which, each measuring 4 to 5 cm in thickness, lie in close apposition such that the uterine cavity is almost obliterated.

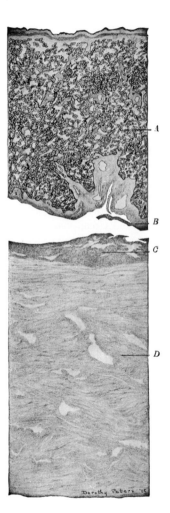

FIG. 15-17. Separation of placenta with cleavage of the decidua. *A.* Placenta. *B.* Decidua cast off with placenta. *C.* Decidua retained in utero. *D.* Myometrium.

The Phase of Placental Extrusion.
After the placenta has separated from its implantation site, the pressure exerted upon it by the uterine walls causes it to slide down-

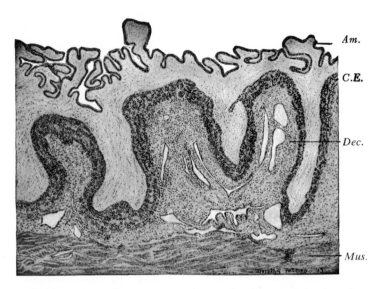

FIG. 15-18. Folding of membranes as uterine cavity decreases in size. Am. = amnion; C.E. = epithelium of chorion laeve; Mus. = myometrium; Dec. = decidua vera.

ward into the flaccid lower uterine segment or the upper part of the vagina. In some cases, the placenta may be expelled from those locations by an increase in abdominal pressure, but women in the recumbent position frequently cannot expel the placenta spontaneously. Therefore, an artificial means of completing the third stage generally is required. The usual method employed is to alternately compress and elevate the fundus, while exerting *gentle* traction on the umbilical cord (see Chap. 17, p. 423).

MECHANISMS OF PLACENTAL EXTRUSION. When the central, or usual, type of placental separation occurs, the retroplacental hematoma is believed to push the placenta toward the uterine cavity, first the central portion and then the rest. The placenta, thus inverted and weighted with the hematoma, then descends. Since the surrounding membranes are still attached to the decidua, the placenta can descend only by dragging after it the membranes, which peel off its periphery. Consequently, the sac formed by the membranes is inverted, with the glistening fetal surface of the placenta presenting at the vulva. The retroplacental hematoma either follows the placenta or is found within the inverted sac. In this process, known as *Schultze's mechanism* of placental expulsion, blood from the placental site pours into the

inverted sac, not escaping externally until after extrusion of the placenta.

The other method of placental extrusion is known as the *Duncan mechanism,* in which separation of the placenta occurs first at the periphery, with the result that blood collects between the membranes and the uterine wall and escapes from the vagina. In this circumstance, the placenta descends to the vagina sideways, and the maternal surface appears first at the vulva.

REFERENCES

Brandt ML: Mechanism and management of the third stage of labor. Am J Obstet Gynecol 25:662, 1933

Caldeyro-Barcia R, Alvarez H, Reynolds SRM: A better understanding of uterine contractility through simultaneous recording with an internal and a seven channel external method. Surg Gynecol Obstet 91:641, 1950

Carsten ME: Regulation of myometrial composition, growth, and activity. In Assali NS (ed): Biology of Gestation, Vol I, The Maternal Organism. New York, Academic, 1968

Chard T: The role of the posterior pituitaries of mother and foetus in spontaneous parturition. In Comline KS, Cross, KW, Dawes GS (eds): Foetal and Neonatal Physiology. Cambridge, Cambridge University Press, 1973

Collins E, Turner G: Maternal effects of regular salicylate ingestion in pregnancy. Lancet 2:335, 1975

Danforth DN, Buckingham JC, Roddick JW: Connective tissue changes incident to cervical effacement. Am J Obstet Gynecol 80:939, 1960

Ferenczy A, Richart, RM: Female Reproductive System: Dynamics of Scan and Transmission Electron Microscopy. New York, Wiley, 1974

Ferguson JKW: A study of the motility of the intact uterus at term. Surg Gynecol Obstet 73:359, 1941

Friedman EA: Graphic appraisal of labor: a study of 500 primigravidas. Bull Sloan Hosp Women 1:42, 1955

Friedman EA: Labor: Clinical Evaluation and Management, 2nd ed. New York, Appleton, 1978

Gemzell CA, Robbe H, Stern B, Strom G: Observation on circulatory changes and muscular work in normal labour. Acta Obstet Gynecol Scand 36:75, 1957

Gustavii B: Labour: a delayed menstruation? Lancet 2:1149, 1972

Hendricks CH, Brenner WE, Kraus G: The normal cervical dilatation pattern in late pregnancy and labor. Am J Obstet Gynecol 106:1065, 1970

Ivy AC, Hartman CG, Koff A: The contractions of the monkey uterus at term. Am J Obstet Gynecol 22:388, 1931

Karim SMM: The Prostaglandins. New York, Wiley-Interscience, 1972

Karlson S: On the motility of the uterus during labour and the influence of the motility pattern on the duration of the labour. Acta Obstet Gynecol Scand 28:209, 1949

Katz Z, Lancet M, Levani E: The efficacy of intra-amniotic steroids for induction of labor. Obstet Gynecol 54:31, 1979

Liggins GC: Fetal influences on myometrial contractility. Clin Obstet Gynecol 16:148, 1973

MacDonald PC, Porter JC, Schwarz BE, Johnston JM: Initiation of parturition in the human female. Semin Perinatol 2:273, 1978

MacDonald PC, Schultz FM, Duenhoelter JH, Gant NF, Jimenez JM, Pritchard JA, Porter JC, Johnston JM: Initiation of human parturition: I. Mechanisms of action of arachidonic acid. Obstet Gynecol 44:629, 1974

Malpas P: Postmaturity and malformation of the fetus. J Obstet Gynaecol Br Emp 40:1046, 1933

Novy MJ, Cook MJ, Manaugh L: Indomethacin block of normal onset of parturition in primates. Am J Obstet Gynecol 118:412, 1974

Okazaki T, Okita JR, MacDonald PC, Johnston JM: Initiation of human parturition: X. Substrate specificity of phospholipase A_2 in human fetal membranes. Am J Obstet Gynecol 130:432, 1978

Okita JR, Okazaki T, MacDonald PC, Johnston JM: Alterations in phospholipid content of human fetal membranes during parturition. San Diego, Soc Gynecol Invest, Abstract 188: 114, 1979

Reynolds SRM: Physiology of the Uterus with Clinical Correlations, 2d ed. New York, Hoeber, 1949

Sala NL, Schwarcz RL, Althabe O, Fisch L, Fuente O: Effect of epidural anesthesia upon uterine contractility induced by artificial cervical dilatation in human pregnancy. Am J Obstet Gynecol 106:26, 1970

Schulman H, Romney SL: Variability of uterine contractions in normal human parturition. Obstet Gynecol 36:215, 1970

Schwarz BE, Johnston JM, Athey R, Milewich L, MacDonald PC: Progesterone binding protein in human chorion and amnion. Gynecol Invest 7:46, 1976

Schwarz BE, MacDonald PC, Johnston JM: Initiation of human parturition: XI. Lysosomal enzyme release *in vitro* obtained from amnions of laboring and nonlaboring women. Submitted Am J Obstet Gynecol, in press

Schwarz BE, Schultz FM, MacDonald PC, Johnston JM: III. Fetal membrane content of prostaglandin E_2 and $F_{2\alpha}$ precursor. Obstet Gynecol 46:564, 1975

Theobald GW: Nervous control of uterine activity. Clin Obstet Gynecol 11:15, 1968

Winters AJ, Oliver C, Colston C, MacDonald PC, Porter JC: Plasma ACTH levels in the human fetus and neonate as related to age and parturition. J Clin Endocrinol Metab 39:269, 1974

Wolfs GMJA, van Leeuwen M: Electromyographic observations on the human uterus during labour. Act Obstet Gynecol Scand suppl 90, 1979

16

Mechanism of Normal Labor in Occiput Presentation

Occiput (vertex) presentations occur in about 95 percent of all labors.

DIAGNOSIS OF OCCIPUT PRESENTATION

The presentation of the fetus is most commonly ascertained during pregnancy by abdominal palpation and confirmed sometime before or at the onset of labor by vaginal examination. In the majority of cases, the vertex enters the pelvis with the sagittal suture in the transverse pelvic diameter.

Occiput Transverse Positions. For diagnosis by abdominal examination, the four maneuvers of Leopold are employed (see Chap. 12). With the fetus in the left occiput transverse position (LOT), the following findings are obtained by abdominal examination:

First maneuver: Fundus occupied by the breech.
Second maneuver: Resistant plane of the back felt directly to the right, readily palpated through the mother's flank.

Third maneuver: Negative if the head is engaged (biparietal diameter through pelvic inlet); otherwise, the movable head is detected at or above the pelvic inlet.
Fourth maneuver: Negative if head is engaged; otherwise cephalic prominence on the right.

In the right occiput transverse position (ROT) palpation yields similar information, except that the fetal back is in the right flank and the small parts and cephalic prominence are on the left.

On vaginal examination, the sagittal suture occupies the transverse diameter of the pelvis more or less midway between the sacrum and the symphysis. In left occiput transverse positions, the smaller posterior fontanel is to the left in the maternal pelvis and the larger anterior fontanel is directed to the opposite side. In right occiput transverse positions, the reverse holds true. The fetal heart in right and left positions is usually heard in the right and left flank, respectively, at or slightly below the level of the mother's umbilicus.

Occiput Anterior Positions. In occiput anterior positions, the head either enters the pelvis with the occiput rotated 45 degrees anteriorly from the transverse position or subsequently does so. This degree of anterior rotation produces only slight differences on abdominal examination. The mechanism of labor usually is very similar to that in transverse positions of the occiput.

Occiput Posterior Positions. The incidence of occiput posterior positions is approximately 10 percent and the right occiput posterior position (ROP) is much more common than the left (LOP). Evidence from radiographic studies indicates that posterior positions more often are associated with a narrow forepelvis.

On vaginal or rectal examination in the occiput right posterior position, the sagittal suture occupies the right oblique diameter; the small fontanel is felt opposite the right sacroiliac synchondrosis; and the large fontanel is directed toward the left iliopectineal eminence. In the left position, the reverse obtains. In many cases, particularly in the early part of labor, because of imperfect flexion of the head, the large fontanel lies at a lower level than in anterior positions and is more readily felt.

CARDINAL MOVEMENTS OF LABOR IN OCCIPUT PRESENTATION

Because of the irregular shape of the pelvic canal and the relatively large dimensions of the mature fetal head, it is evident that not all diameters of the head can necessarily pass through all diameters of the pelvis. It follows that a process of adaptation or accommodation of suitable portions of the head to the various segments of the pelvis is required for completion of childbirth. These positional changes of the presenting part constitute the mechanism of labor. *The cardinal movements of labor are (1) engagement, (2) descent, (3) flexion, (4) internal rotation, (5) extension, (6) external rotation, and (7) expulsion.* They are shown in Figure 16-1.

For purposes of instruction, the various movements are often described as though they occurred separately and independently. In reality, the mechanism of labor consists of a combination of movements that are going on at the same time. For example, as part of the process of engagement, there is both flexion and descent of the head. It is manifestly impossible for the movements to be completed unless the presenting part descends simultaneously. Concomitantly, the uterine contractions effect important modifications in the attitude, or habitus, of the fetus, especially after the head has descended into the pelvis. These changes consist principally in a straightening of the fetus, with loss of its dorsal convexity and closer application of the extremities and small parts to the body. As a result, the fetal ovoid is transformed into a cylinder with normally the smallest possible cross section passing through the birth canal.

Engagement. As discussed on page 282 of Chapter 11, the mechanism by which the biparietal diameter, the greatest transverse diameter of the head in occiput presentations, passes through the pelvic inlet is designated *engagement.* This phenomenon may take place during the last few weeks of pregnancy or may not do so until after the commencement of labor. In many multiparous and some nulliparous women, at the onset of labor the fetal head is freely movable above the pelvic inlet into the iliac fossae. In this circumstance, the head is sometimes referred to as "floating." A normal-sized head usually does not engage with its sagittal suture directed anteroposteriorly. Instead it enters the pelvic inlet either in the transverse diameter, as usually occurs, or in one of the oblique diameters.

ASYNCLITISM.   Although the fetal head tends to accommodate to the transverse axis of the pelvic inlet, the sagittal suture, while remaining parallel to that axis, may not lie exactly midway between the symphysis and sacral promontory. The sagittal suture is frequently deflected either posteriorly toward the promontory or anteriorly toward the symphysis, as shown in Figure 16-2. Such lateral

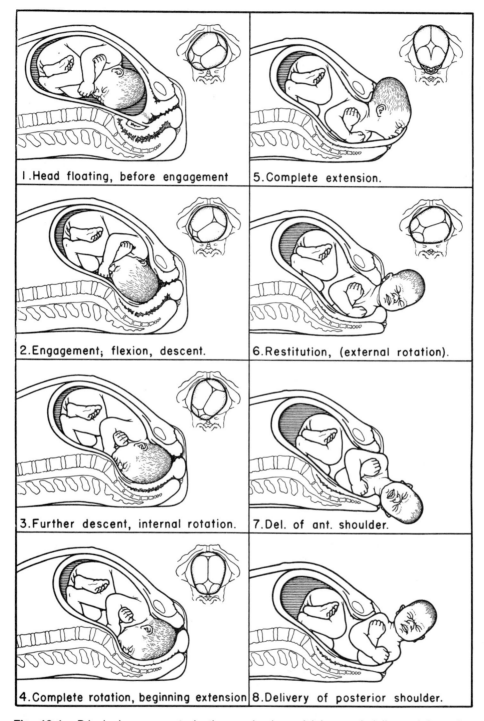

1. Head floating, before engagement

5. Complete extension.

2. Engagement; flexion, descent.

6. Restitution, (external rotation).

3. Further descent, internal rotation.

7. Del. of ant. shoulder.

4. Complete rotation, beginning extension

8. Delivery of posterior shoulder.

Fig. 16-1. Principal movements in the mechanism of labor and delivery, left occiput anterior position.

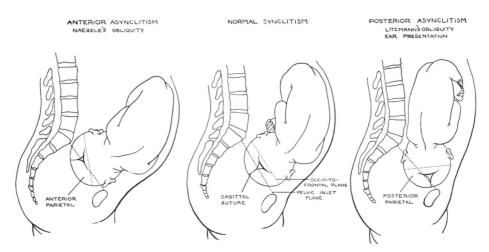

FIG. 16-2. Synclitism and asynclitism.

deflection of the head to a more anterior or posterior position in the pelvis is called *asynclitism*. If the sagittal suture approaches the sacral promontory, more of the anterior parietal bone presents itself to the examining fingers and the condition is called *anterior asynclitism*. If, however, the sagittal suture lies close to the symphysis, more of the posterior parietal bone will present and the condition is called *posterior asynclitism*. Moderate degrees of asynclitism are the rule in normal labor. Successive changes from posterior to anterior asynclitism facilitate descent by allowing the fetal head to take advantage of the roomiest areas of the pelvic cavity.

Descent. The first requisite for the birth of the infant is descent. With the nulliparous woman, engagement may occur before the onset of labor, and further descent may not necessarily follow until the onset of the second stage of labor. In multiparous women, descent usually begins with engagement. Descent is brought about by one or more of four forces: (1) pressure of the amnionic fluid; (2) direct pressure of the fundus upon the breech; (3) contraction of the abdominal muscles; and (4) extension and straightening of the fetal body.

Flexion. As soon as the descending head meets resistance, whether from the cervix, the walls of the pelvis, or the pelvic floor,

flexion of the head normally results. In this movement, the chin is brought into more intimate contact with the fetal thorax, and the appreciably shorter suboccipitobregmatic diameter is substituted for the longer occipitofrontal diameter (Figs. 16-3, 16-4).

Internal Rotation. This movement is a turning of the head in such a manner that the occiput gradually moves from its original position anteriorly toward the symphysis pubis or, less commonly, posteriorly toward the

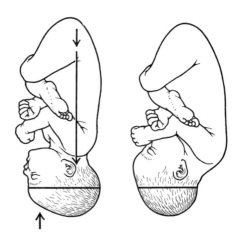

FIG. 16-3. Lever action producing flexion of head; conversion from occipitofrontal to suboccipitobregmatic diameter typically reduces the anteroposterior diameter from nearly 12 cm to 9.5 cm.

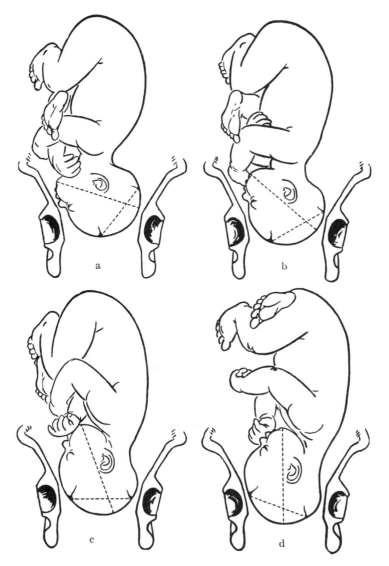

FIG. 16-4. Four degrees of head flexion. One dotted line indicates the occipitomental diameter and the other line connecting the center of the anterior fontanel with the posterior fontanel: **a.** Flexion poor. **b.** Flexion moderate. **c.** Flexion advanced. **d.** Flexion complete. Note with flexion complete the chin is on the chest and the suboccipitobregmatic diameter, the shortest anteroposterior diameter of the fetal head, is passing through the pelvic inlet. (From Rydberg. *The Mechanism of Labour.* Springfield, Ill., Thomas, 1954)

hollow of the sacrum (Figs. 16-5, 16-6). Internal rotation is essential for the completion of labor, except when the fetus is abnormally small. Internal rotation, which is always associated with descent of the presenting part, is usually not accomplished until the head has reached the level of the spines and therefore is engaged.

Calkins (1939) studied more than 5000 patients in labor to ascertain when internal rotation occurs. He concluded that in approximately two-thirds of all women internal rotation is complete by the time the head reaches the pelvic floor; in about one-fourth, internal rotation is completed very shortly after the head reaches the pelvic floor; and in about 5 percent, rotation to the anterior does not take place. When rotation fails to occur until

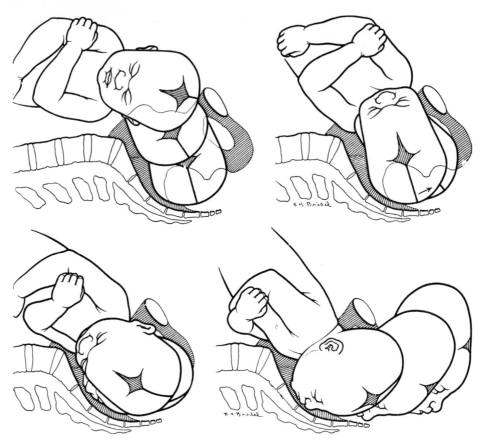

FIG. 16-5. Mechanism of labor for left occiput transverse position lateral view. Posterior parietal presentation (posterior asynclitism) at the brim followed by lateral flexion, resulting in anterior parietal presentation (anterior asynclitism) after engagement, further descent, rotation, and extension. (From Steele and Javert. *Surg Gynecol Obstet* 75:477, 1942)

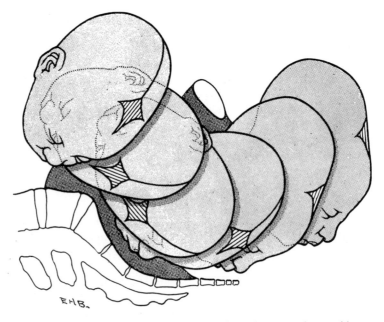

FIG. 16-6. Mechanism of labor for left occiput anterior position.

the head reaches the pelvic floor, it takes place during the next one or two contractions in multiparas, and in nulliparas during the next three to five. Rotation before the head reaches the pelvic floor is definitely more frequent in multiparas than in nulliparas, according to Calkins.

Extension. When, after internal rotation, the sharply flexed head reaches the vulva, it undergoes another movement that is essential to its birth, namely, extension, which brings the base of the occiput into direct contact with the inferior margin of the symphysis pubis. Since the vulvar outlet is directed upward and forward, extension must occur before the head can pass through it. If the sharply flexed head, on reaching the pelvic floor, did not extend but was driven farther downward, it would impinge upon the posterior portion of the perineum and, if the vis a tergo were sufficiently strong, would eventually be forced through the tissues of the perineum. When the head presses upon the pelvic gutter, however, two forces come into play. The first, exerted by the

uterus, acts more posteriorly, and the second, supplied by the resistant pelvic floor, acts more anteriorly. The resultant force is in the direction of the vulvar opening, thereby causing extension.

With increasing distension of the perineum and vaginal opening, an increasingly large portion of the occiput gradually appears. The head is born by further extension as the occiput, bregma, forehead, nose, mouth, and finally the chin pass successively over the anterior margin of the perineum. Immediately after its birth, the head drops downward so that the chin lies over the maternal anal region.

External Rotation. The delivered head next undergoes restitution. If the occiput was originally directed toward the left, it rotates toward the left ischial tuberosity, and in the opposite direction if originally directed toward the right. The return of the head to the oblique position (restitution) is followed by completion of external rotation to the transverse position, a movement that corre-

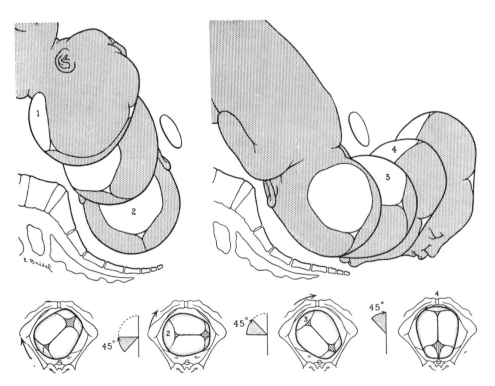

FIG. 16-7. Mechanism of labor for right occiput posterior position, anterior rotation.

sponds to rotation of the fetal body, serving to bring its bisacromial diameter into relation with the anteroposterior diameter of the pelvic outlet. Thus one shoulder is anterior behind the symphysis and the other is posterior. This movement is brought about apparently by the same pelvic factors that effect internal rotation of the head.

Expulsion. Almost immediately after external rotation, the anterior shoulder appears under the symphysis pubis, and the perineum soon becomes distended by the posterior shoulder. After delivery of the shoulders, the rest of the body of the child is quickly extruded.

Labor in Persistent Occiput Posterior Position. In the great majority of labors in the occiput posterior positions, the mechanism of labor is identical with that observed in the transverse and anterior varieties, except that the occiput has to rotate to the symphysis pubis through 135 degrees instead of 90 degrees and 45 degrees, respectively (Fig. 16-7).

With effective contractions, adequate flexion of the head, and a fetus of average size, the great majority of posteriorly positioned occiputs rotate promptly as soon as they reach the pelvic floor and labor is not appreciably lengthened. In perhaps 5 to 10 percent of cases, however, these favorable circumstances do not obtain. For example, with poor contractions or faulty flexion of the head or both, rotation may be incomplete or may not take place at all especially if the fetus is large. If rotation is incomplete, *transverse arrest* results. If rotation toward the symphysis does not take place, the occiput usually rotates to the direct occiput posterior position, a condition known as *persistent occiput posterior.* Both transverse arrest and persistent occiput posterior represent deviations from the normal mechanisms of labor, and are considered further in Chapter 30, page 818.

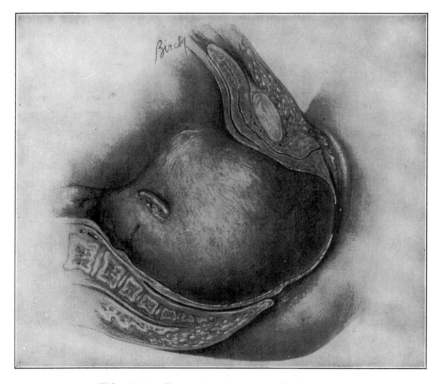

FIG. 16-8. Formation of caput succedaneum.

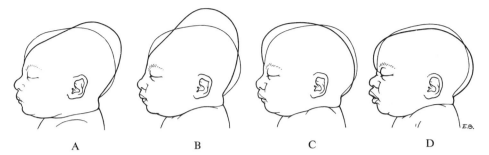

FIG. 16-9. Molding of head in cephalic presentations. **A.** Occiput anterior. **B.** Occiput posterior. **C.** Brow. **D.** Face.

CHANGES IN THE SHAPE OF THE FETAL HEAD

Caput Succedaneum. In vertex presentations, the fetal head undergoes important characteristic changes in shape as the result of the pressures to which it is subjected during labor. In prolonged labors before complete dilatation of the cervix, the portion of the fetal scalp immediately over the cervical os becomes edematous, forming a swelling known as the *caput succedaneum* (Fig. 16-8). It usually attains a thickness of only a few millimeters, but in prolonged labors it may be sufficiently extensive to prevent the differentiation of the various sutures and fontanels. More commonly, the caput is formed when the head is in the lower portion of the birth canal and frequently only after the resistance of a rigid vaginal outlet is encountered. Since it occurs over the most dependent portion of the head, in left occiput transverse position it is found over the upper and posterior extremity of the right parietal bone, and in right positions over the corresponding area of the left parietal bone. Hence, it follows that often after labor the original position may be ascertained by noting the location of the caput succedaneum.

Molding. Of considerable importance is the degree of molding that the head undergoes. Because the various bones of the skull are not firmly united, movement may occur at the sutures. Ordinarily the margins of the occipital bone, and more rarely those of the frontal bone, are pushed under those of the parietal bones. In many cases, one parietal bone may overlap the other, the anterior parietal usually overlapping the posterior. These changes are of greatest importance in contracted pelves, when the degree to which the head is capable of molding may make the difference between successful vaginal delivery and a major obstetric operation (Fig. 16-9). Molding may account for a diminution in biparietal and suboccipitobregmatic diameters of 0.5 to 1.0 cm, or even more in neglected cases.

REFERENCES

Calkins LA: The etiology of occiput presentations. Am J Obstet Gynecol 37:618, 1939

17

Conduct of Normal Labor and Delivery

PSYCHOLOGIC CONSIDERATIONS

The pregnant woman very often approaches labor with two major fears: "Will my baby be all right?" "Will labor and delivery be painful?" Her concerns should also be uppermost in the mind of everyone who participates in caring for the mother and her fetus. Everything possible should be done to make the answer to the first question "Yes, your baby will be all right." And to the second, "No, as long as the method for pain relief does not harm the fetus."

Is labor easy because a woman is calm, or is she calm because her labor is easy? Is a woman pained and frightened because her labor is difficult, or is her labor difficult and painful because she is frightened? After scrutinizing many cases, the late British obstetrician Read concluded: "Fear is in some way the chief pain-producing agent in otherwise normal labor." Quite likely, fear may exert a deleterious effect on the quality of uterine contractions and on cervical dilatation.

It is not an easy task to dispel the age-old fear of pain during labor and delivery, but from the first prenatal visit a conscious effort should be made on the part of all persons involved in the care of the mother and

her unborn child to make the point that labor and delivery are normal physiologic processes. Everyone who is involved in caring for the mother and her fetus must demonstrate professional competence but also instill the feeling that he or she is the mother's friend, sincerely desirous of sparing her all possible pain within the limit of safety for her and her child. Physicians, nurses, and students should note especially that the morale of a woman in labor may sometimes be destroyed by careless remarks or actions. Casual comments outside the labor room are often overheard by her and misinterpreted. Laughter is frequently interpreted as directed toward her.

Physiologic Childbirth. To eliminate the harmful influence of fear in labor, a school of thought has developed emphasizing the advantages of "natural childbirth" or "physiologic childbirth." Natural or physiologic childbirth entails antepartum education designed to eliminate fear; exercises to promote relaxation, muscle control, and breathing; and adroit management throughout labor with a nurse or physician skilled in reassurance of the mother constantly in attendance.

Most proponents of physiologic childbirth have never claimed that labor can be made devoid of pain or that delivery should be conducted without anesthetic aids. With natural childbirth, most patients experience some pain, and analgesics and anesthetics are not withheld when they are indicated. Physiologic, or psychoprophylactic, childbirth is also considered in Chapter 18 (p. 453).

ADMITTANCE PROCEDURES

The woman should be urged to report early in labor rather than to procrastinate until delivery is imminent for fear that she might be experiencing false labor.

Identification of Labor. Although the differential diagnosis between false and true labor is difficult at times, it can usually be made on the basis of the following features:

Contractions of True Labor
  Occur at regular intervals
  Intervals gradually shorten
  Intensity gradually increases
  Discomfort in back and abdomen
  Cervix dilates
  Not stopped by sedation

Contractions of False Labor
  Occur at irregular intervals
  Intervals remain long
  Intensity remains same
  Discomfort chiefly in lower abdomen
  Cervix does not dilate
  Usually relieved by sedation

The general condition of the mother and her fetus must be quickly but accurately ascertained by means of history and physical examination. Inquiry is made as to the frequency and intensity of the uterine contractions and when they first became uncomfortable. The degree of discomfort that the mother displays is noted. The heart rate, presentation, and size of the fetus are evaluated abdominally. *The fetal heart rate should be checked especially at the end of a contraction and immediately thereafter to identify pathologic bradycardia.* Inquiries

are made particularly about the status of the membranes including the question of whether fluid has leaked from the vagina and if so, how much, and when the leakage first commenced.

Admittance Vaginal Examination. Most often, *unless there has been bleeding in excess of bloody show,* a vaginal examination under aseptic conditions is performed as described below. Careful attention to the following items is essential in order to obtain the greatest amount of information and to minimize bacterial contamination from multiple examinations:

1. *Amnionic fluid.* If there is question of rupture of the membranes, the vulva and vaginal introitus are cleansed, a sterile speculum is carefully inserted, and fluid is looked for in the posterior vaginal fornix. Any fluid is observed for vernix or meconium and, if the source of the fluid remains in doubt, it is collected on a swab for further study as described below (p. 407).
2. *Cervix.* Softness, degree of effacement, extent of dilatation, and location of the cervix with respect to the presenting part are ascertained as described below. The presence of membranes with or without amnionic fluid below the presenting part often can be felt by careful palpation.
3. *Presenting part.* The nature of the presenting part should be positively determined and, ideally, its position, as described in Chapter 12 (p. 294).
4. *Station.* The degree of descent of the presenting part into the birth canal is identified as described below and, if the fetal head is high in the pelvis (above the level of the ischial spines), the effect of firm fundal pressure on descent of the fetal head is tested.
5. *Pelvic architecture.* The diagonal conjugate, ischial spines, pelvic sidewalls, and sacrum are reevaluated for adequacy (See Chap. 11, p. 290).
6. *Vagina and perineum.* The distensibility of the vagina and the firmness of the perineum are assessed.

CERVICAL EFFACEMENT. The degree of effacement of the cervix is usually expressed in terms of the length of the cervical canal compared to that of an uneffaced cervix (see Chap. 15, p. 382). When the length of the cervix is reduced by one-half, it is 50 percent effaced; when the cervix becomes as thin as the adjacent lower uterine segment, it is completely, or 100 percent, effaced.

CERVICAL DILATATION. The amount of cervical dilatation is ascertained by estimating the average diameter of the cervical opening. The examining finger is swept from the margin of the cervix on one side to the opposite side, and the diameter traversed is expressed in cm. The cervix is said to be fully dilated when the diameter of the opening measures 10 cm, for the presenting part usually can pass through a cervix so widely dilated (see Chap. 15, p. 385).

POSITION OF CERVIX. The relationship of the cervical os to the fetal head is categorized as posterior, midposition, or anterior. The posterior position is suggestive of premature labor.

STATION. When conducting a vaginal examination, it is valuable to identify the level of the presenting fetal part in the birth canal. The ischial spines are about halfway between the pelvic inlet and the pelvic outlet. When the lowermost portion of the presenting fetal part is at the level of the ischial spines, it is designated as being at zero station. The long axis of the birth canal above the ischial spines is arbitrarily divided into thirds. If the presenting part is at the level of the pelvic inlet, it is at −3 station; if it has descended one-third the distance from the pelvic inlet to the ischial spines, it is at −2 station; if it has reached a level two-thirds the distance from the inlet to the spines, it is at −1 station. The long axis of the birth canal between the level of the ischial spines and the outlet of the pelvis is similarly divided into thirds. If the level of the presenting part in the birth canal is one-third or two-thirds of the distance between the ischial spines and

the pelvic outlet, it is at +1 station or +2 station, respectively. When the presenting fetal part reaches the perineum, its station is +3. If the vertex is at 0 station or below, most often engagement of the head has occurred, that is, the biparietal plane of the head has passed through the pelvic inlet. *If the head is unusually molded, or if there is an extensive formation of caput, or both, engagement might not have taken place even though the vertex is at 0 station.* Progressive cervical dilatation with no change in the station of the presenting part suggests fetopelvic disproportion.

An alternative method for designating the station of the fetal head has been used by some obstetricians (Friedman, 1978). Five levels, rather than 3 levels, are identified above and below the ischial spines. Each of the 5 levels differs from the adjacent level by approximately 1 cm. It is important that the two systems not be confused in the course of management of labor.

Detection of Ruptured Membranes. The pregnant woman should be well coached antepartum to observe for leakage of fluid from the vagina and to report such an occurrence promptly. The significance of rupture of the membranes is great for three reasons: First, if the presenting part is not fixed in the pelvis, the possibility of prolapse of the cord and cord compression is greatly increased. Second, labor is likely to occur quite soon if the pregnancy is at or near term. Third, if the fetus remains in utero upward of 24 hours or more after the rupture of the membranes, there is real likelihood of intrauterine infection that may be especially harmful to the fetus even though antibiotics are administered to the mother.

A firm diagnosis of rupture of the membranes is not always easy to make unless amnonic fluid is seen or felt escaping from the cervical os by the examiner. Although several diagnostic tests for the detection of ruptured membranes have been recommended, none is completely reliable. Perhaps the most widely employed procedures involve testing the acidity or alkalinity of the vaginal fluid. The basis for these tests is that normally the pH of the vaginal secretion ranges between

4.5 and 5.5, whereas that of the amnionic fluid is usually 7.0 to 7.5.

NITRAZINE TEST.   The use of the indicator nitrazine for the diagnosis of ruptured membranes was first suggested by Baptisti (1938) and is a simple and fairly reliable method. Test papers are impregnated with the dye, and the color of the reaction is interpreted by comparison with a standard color chart. The pH of the vaginal secretion is estimated by inserting a sterile cotton-tipped applicator deeply into the vagina and then touching it to a strip of the nitrazine paper and comparing the color of the paper with the chart. Color changes are interpreted as follows:

Probably intact membranes
   Yellow   pH 5.0
   Olive-yellow   pH 5.5
   Olive-green   pH 6.0

Ruptured membranes
   Blue-green   pH 6.5
   Blue-gray   pH 7.0
   Deep blue   pH 7.5

Baptisti (1938)pointed out that a false reading is likely to be encountered in women with intact membranes who have an unusually large amount of bloody show, since blood, like amnionic fluid, is not acidic. A more extended study of the nitrazine test by a slightly different technic was made by Abe (1940), who found the nitrazine test to be correct in 98.9 percent of women with known rupture of membranes and in 96.2 percent of women with intact membranes. In clinical practice, however, these tests will not yield such accurate results as those just described, because they are used in questionable cases in which the amount of fluid is small and therefore more susceptible to a change in pH by admixed blood and vaginal secretions.

Other Evaluation.   The maternal blood pressure, temperature, pulse, and respiratory rate are checked for any abnormality, and these are recorded. The Pregnancy Record is promptly reviewed to identify complica-

tions. Any problem identified previously during the antepartum period, as well as any that were anticipated, should be prominently displayed in the Pregnancy Record, along with the plan of management.

Preparation of Vulva and Perineum.   The woman is placed on a bedpan with her legs widely separated. While washing the region, the attendant holds a sponge to the woman's introitus to prevent wash water from running into the vagina. Scrubbing is directed from above downward and away from the introitus. Attention should be paid to careful cleansing of the vulvar folds during this procedure. As the scrub sponge passes over the anal region, it is discarded immediately. In many hospitals the hair at least on the lower half of the vulva and perineum is removed either by shaving or by clipping.

Vaginal   vs.   Rectal   Examinations.   Ideally, after the vulvar and perineal regions have been prepared properly, and the examiner has donned sterile gloves, the thumb and forefinger of one hand separate the labia widely to expose the vaginal opening and prevent the examining fingers from coming in contact with the inner surfaces of the labia. The index and second fingers of the other hand are then introduced into the vagina (Fig. 17-1 A, B, C). During vaginal examination, a precise routine of evaluation should be followed as described above. It is important not to withdraw the fingers from the vagina until the examination is entirely completed.

Rectal examinations were once considered to be much safer than vaginal because they were less likely to carry bacteria from the introitus into the cervix and above. A vaginal examination, *properly performed with appropriate preparation and care,* is probably not much more likely than a rectal to carry pathogenic bacteria through the dilating cervix into the uterus. In spite of past reports that vaginal examinations during labor do not contribute to morbidity, clinical experience in certain circumstances is strongly suggestive of the opposite. The likelihood of an injurious effect

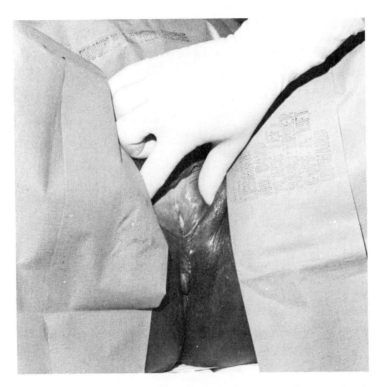

FIG. 17-1. A. Vaginal examination. The labia are separated with a sterile gloved hand.

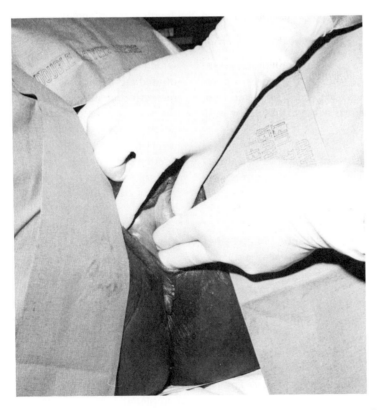

FIG. 17-1. B. Vaginal examination. The first and second fingers of the other sterile gloved hand are carefully inserted through the introitus.

409

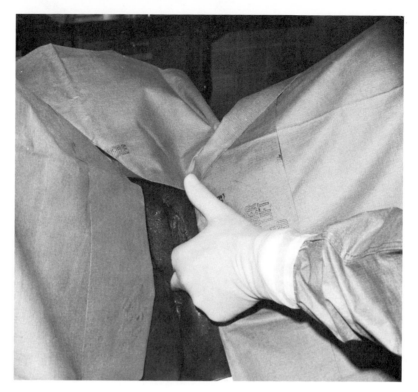

FIG. 17-1. C. During vaginal examination, the fourth and fifth fingers should not contact the anus.

from repeated vaginal examinations seems most apparent in the case of early rupture of the membranes followed by repeated vaginal examinations casually performed by multiple examiners.

Enema. Early in labor, a cleansing enema is generally given to minimize subsequent contamination by feces which otherwise may be a problem, especially during delivery. A ready-to-use enema solution of sodium phosphates in a disposable container (Fleet enema) has proved satisfactory at Parkland Memorial Hospital. Enemas are not used to stimulate labor. The infamous "3-H" enema ("High, Hot, and Hell of a Lot") has no place in obstetrics.

Laboratory. When admitted in labor, most often the hematocrit, or hemoglobin concentration, should be rechecked. The hematocrit can be measured easily and quickly. Blood may be collected in a plain tube from

which a heparinized capillary tube is filled immediately. Employing a small microhematocrit centrifuge in the labor-delivery unit, the value can be obtained in 3 minutes. The labeled tube of blood is allowed to clot and is kept on hand for blood cross match, if needed, or otherwise used for routine serology. A voided urine specimen, as free as possible of debris, is examined for protein and glucose.

SUBSEQUENT MANAGEMENT OF FIRST STAGE

As soon as possible after admittance, the remainder of the general physical examination is completed. The physician can reach a conclusion about the normalcy of the pregnancy only when all the examinations have been completed. The physician must then draw upon the information obtained from these results, as well as all information previously compiled during the antepartum period. A rational plan for monitoring labor can then be established based on the needs of the fetus and the mother. If no abnormality is identified or suspected, the mother should be assured that all is well. Although the average duration of the first stage of labor in nulliparous women is about 8 hours, and in parous women about 5 hours, there is marked individual variation. Most often, therefore, any precise statement as to the duration of her labor is unwise. Obstetricians and others who venture to make precise statements will find that their predictions are likely to be faulty and the mother and family are made more anxious needlessly.

Monitoring Labor. The word *monitor* currently is equated in the minds of some only with continuous electronic recording of the fetal heart rate and intrauterine pressures. The desirability, not alone the necessity, for such monitoring for all labors has certainly not been established, as pointed out elsewhere (see Chap. 14, p. 353).

It is mandatory, however, that for a good pregnancy outcome, a well-defined program be established that provides careful surveillance of the well-being of both the mother and the fetus. All observations must be appropriately recorded. The frequency, intensity, and duration of uterine contractions, and the response of the fetal heart rate to the contractions are of considerable concern. These features can be promptly evaluated in logical sequence:

FETAL HEART RATE. The heart rate of the fetus may be identified with a suitable stethoscope or any of a variety of Doppler ultrasonic devices (Fig. 17-2A, B). Changes in the fetal heart rate that are most likely to be ominous almost always are detectable immediately after a uterine contraction. Therefore, it is imperative that the fetal heart be monitored by auscultation immediately after a contraction. To avoid confusing maternal and fetal heart actions, the maternal pulse should be counted as the fetal heart rate is counted. Otherwise maternal tachycardia may be misinterpreted to be a normal fetal heart rate.

Fetal distress, i.e., loss of fetal well-being, is suspected if the fetal heart rate immediately after a contraction is repeatedly below 120 per minute. Fetal distress very likely exists if the rate is heard to be less than 100 per minute, even though there is recovery to a rate in the 120 to 160 range before the next contraction. When decelerations of this magnitude are found after a contraction, the fetus may be in jeopardy and further labor, if allowed, is often best monitored electronically as described in Chapter 14 (p. 356).

During the first stage of labor, in the absence of any abnormalities, the fetal heart rate should be checked immediately after a contraction every 15 minutes.

The findings of the study by Benson and associates (1968) have been quoted widely as evidence that auscultation of the fetal heart during labor is unreliable for detecting fetal distress save in an extreme degree. Their study by design ignored the determination of the fetal heart rate for at least the first 30 seconds after a contraction, a critical period for identifying ominous decelerations (see Chap. 14, p. 362). Moreover, the protocol for evaluating the fetal heart every 15 minutes during the first stage of labor and every 5 minutes during the second stage frequently was not followed.

UTERINE CONTRACTIONS. The examiner with the palm of the hand lightly on the uterus determines the time of onset of the contraction. The intensity of the contraction is gauged from the degree of firmness the uterus achieves. At the acme of effective contractions, the finger or thumb cannot readily indent the uterus. Next, the time that the contraction disappears is noted. This sequence is repeated with the following contraction in order to evaluate the frequency, duration, and intensity of uterine contractions. It is inappropriate simply to describe ongoing uterine contractions, or labor as "good." "Good" uterine contractions can be identified only retrospectively, i.e., if the contractions produced orderly effacement and

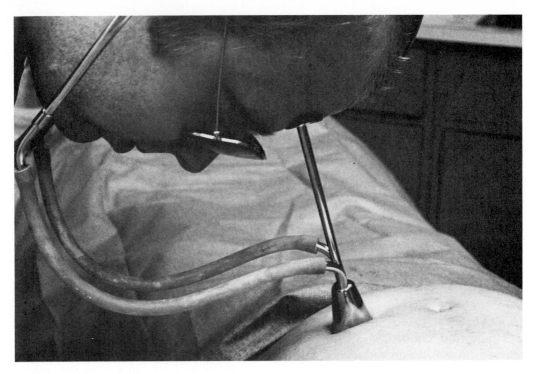

FIG. 17-2. A. Monitoring the fetal heart rate with a DeLee-Hillis fetoscope. The bell of the stethoscope is firmly applied to the uterine wall to improve the transmission of sound.

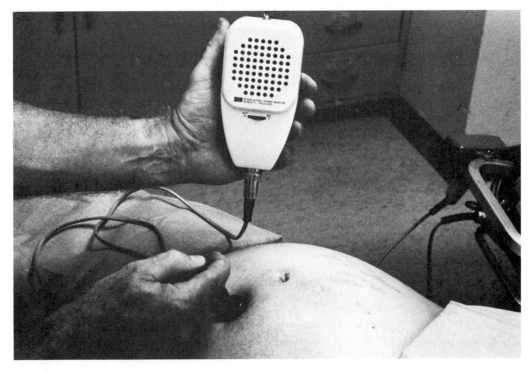

FIG. 17-2. B. Monitoring the fetal heart rate by use of ultrasound and the Doppler effect. The transducer may be held in an appropriate place on the abdomen by a comfortable rubber strap yet allow the mother to be free to move about.

dilatation of the cervix with descent of the presenting part followed by uncomplicated delivery of an uncompromised infant.

ATTENDANCE IN LABOR. Ideally, the person who performs these measurements is able to remain with the mother throughout labor to provide psychologic support as well as discern promptly any fetal or maternal abnormalities. Haverkamp and co-workers (1976, 1979) have demonstrated that an equally satisfactory outcome for the fetus can be achieved without continuous electronic monitoring of the fetal heart rate, continuous intrauterine pressure recording, and fetal scalp blood pH measurement *if the mother and fetus are closely attended by appropriately trained labor room personnel.* Given a choice, many women would probably prefer the reassurance of the nearly continuous presence of the obstetrician or of a compassionate welltrained obstetric associate to that of a metal cabinet and its wires and tubes that invade her and her fetus.

Maternal Position During Labor. The normal mother and fetus need not be confined to bed early in labor prior to use of analgesia. A comfortable chair may be beneficial psychologically and perhaps physiologically. In bed, the mother should be allowed to assume the position she finds most comfortable, which will be lateral recumbent most of the time. She must not be restricted to lying supine.

Flynn and co-workers (1978), in a small randomized prospective study of women thought to be in spontaneous labor, found that the duration of labor was shorter, there was less need for pharmacologically augmenting labor, less need for analgesia, and Apgar scores of infants were higher for women who labored while ambulatory rather than recumbent. All ambulatory women whose membranes had not ruptured early underwent amniotomy so that the fetal heart and uterine pressures could be monitored by radiotelemetry. Conventional bedside internal monitoring was used in the recumbent women. Of great interest would be the findings of a larger study designed to confirm or refute the suggested benefits from ambulation without either amniotomy with invasion of the uterus or the restraints on movement imposed on the recumbent women by "conventional" internal monitoring.

Subsequent Vaginal Examinations. During the first stage of labor, the need for subsequent vaginal examinations to identify the status of the cervix and the station and position of the presenting part will vary considerably. When the membranes rupture, the examination should be repeated immediately if the fetal head was not definitely engaged at the previous vaginal examination. In either situation, the fetal heart rate should be checked immediately to identify cord compression during a contraction.

Analgesia. Most often, analgesia is initiated on the basis of the woman's discomfort, a uterine contraction pattern of established labor, and cervical dilatation of at least 2 cm. The kinds of analgesia, the amounts, and the frequency of administration should be based on the need to allay pain on the one hand and the likelihood of delivering a depressed infant on the other (see Chap. 18, p. 437).

The timing, the method of administration, and the size of initial and subsequent doses of analgesic agents are based to a considerable degree on the anticipated interval of time until delivery. A repeat vaginal examination is often appropriate, therefore, before administering more analgesia. With the onset of symptoms characteristic of the second stage of labor, i.e., an urge to bear down or "push," the status of the cervix and the presenting part should be reevaluated. A common tendency, especially at large, busy public institutions, has been too little "laying on of hands" to gauge the quality of labor and too much "putting in of hands" to identify cervical dilatation.

Maternal Vital Signs. The mother's temperature, blood pressure, and pulse are evaluated every 1 to 2 hours. If membranes have been ruptured for many hours before the onset of labor or if there is a borderline elevation, the temperature should be checked hourly during labor. Moreover, with prolonged rupture of the membranes, the pregnancy should be considered high risk. The blood pressure is taken between contractions, since the blood pressure normally rises during a contraction (Kjeldsen, 1979).

Amniotomy. If the membranes are thought to be intact, there is great temptation even during normal labor to perform an amniotomy. The presumed benefits are more rapid labor and perhaps earlier detection of instances of meconium staining of amnionic fluid. Amniotomy may shorten the length of labor slightly but there is no evidence that shorter labor is necessarily beneficial to the fetus or to the mother. Indeed, the reverse may be true (Caldeyro-Barcia et al., 1974). If amniotomy is performed, aseptic technic must be employed and the fetal head must not be dislodged from the pelvis to hasten the escape of amnionic fluid; to do so invites prolapse of the umbilical cord.

Oral Intake. In essentially all circumstances, food and oral fluids should be withheld during active labor and delivery. Gastric emptying time typically is remarkably prolonged once labor is established and analgesics are administered. As the consequence, ingested substances, including most medications, remain in the stomach and are not absorbed.

Intravenous Fluids. Although it has become customary in many hospitals to establish an intravenous infusion system routinely early in labor, there is seldom any real need for such in the normally pregnant woman at least until analgesia is administered. An intravenous infusion system is advantageous during the immediate puerperium in order to administer oxytocin prophylactically and at times therapeutically when uterine hypotonicity persists. Moreover, with longer labors the administration of glucose, some salt, and water to the otherwise fasting woman at the rate of 60 to 120 ml per hour is efficacious.

Urinary Bladder Function. Bladder distension must be avoided, since it can lead both to obstructed labor and to subsequent hypotonia and infection. In the course of each abdominal examination, the suprapubic region should be palpated in order to detect a filling bladder. If the bladder is readily palpated above the symphysis, the woman should be encouraged to void. At times she can ambulate with assistance to a toilet and successfully void, even though she could not void on a bedpan. If the bladder is distended and she cannot void, catheterization is indicated. During labor, it may be less traumatic to catherize again rather than to leave an indwelling catheter in place.

MANAGEMENT OF SECOND STAGE

Identification. With full dilatation of the cervix, which signifies the onset of the second stage of labor, the woman typically begins to bear down and with descent of the presenting part she develops the urge to defecate. Uterine contractions and the accompanying expulsive forces may last 1½ minutes and recur at times after a myometrial resting phase of no more than a minute.

Duration. The median duration of the second stage (complete dilatation of the cervix) is 50 minutes in nulliparas and 20 minutes in multiparas, but it can be highly variable. In a woman of higher parity with a stretched vagina and perineum, two or three expulsive efforts after the cervix is fully dilated may suffice to complete the delivery of the infant. Conversely, in a woman with a contracted pelvis or with impaired expulsive efforts from conduction anesthesia, the second stage may become abnormally long.

Fetal Heart Rate. It is essential to good care that the status of the fetal heart be identified at 5-minute intervals during this critical period. Slowing of the fetal heart rate induced by compression of the fetal head is common during a contraction and the accompanying maternal expulsive efforts. If re-

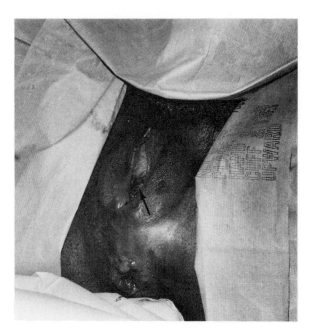

FIG. 17-3. Scalp (arrow) appearing at vulva during a contraction.

covery of the fetal heart rate is prompt after the contraction and expulsive efforts cease, if similar events did not complicate the first stage of labor, and if delivery can be accomplished soon, labor is allowed to continue. Not all instances of slowing of the fetal heart during the second stage of labor are the consequence of head compression, however. The vigorous force generated within the uterus by its contraction and by the woman's expulsive efforts may reduce placental perfusion appreciably. Descent of the fetus through the birth canal towards the perineum and the consequent reduction in uterine volume may trigger some degree of premature separation of the placenta with further compromise of fetal well-being. Descent of the fetus is even more likely to tighten a loop or loops of umbilical cord sufficiently to obstruct umbilical blood flow. Maternal tachycardia, which is common during the second stage, must not be mistaken for a normal fetal heart rate.

Maternal Expulsive Efforts. In most cases, bearing-down efforts are reflex and spontaneous in the second stage of labor, but occasionally the woman does not employ her

expulsive forces to good advantage and coaching is desirable. Her legs should be half-flexed so that she can push with them against the mattress. Instructions should be to take a deep breath as soon as the next uterine contraction begins and, with her breath held, to exert downward pressure exactly as though she were straining at stool. Usually these bearing-down efforts are rewarded by increasing bulging of the perineum, that is, by further descent of the fetal head. The mother should be informed of such progress, for encouragement at this stage is very important. During this period of active bearing-down, the fetal heart sounds should be auscultated immediately after the contraction.

As the head descends through the pelvis, small particles of feces are frequently expelled; as they appear at the anus, they should be sponged off with large pledgets soaked in diluted soap solution. As the head descends still farther, the perineum begins to bulge and the overlying skin becomes tense and glistening. Now the scalp of the fetus may be visible through the slitlike vulvar opening (Fig. 17-3). At this time, or before in instances where little perineal resistance to ex-

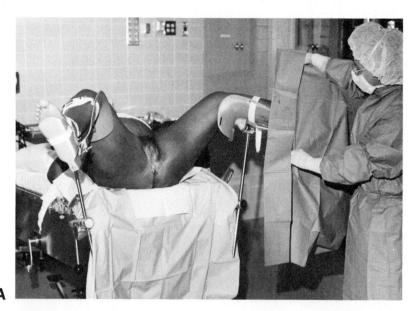

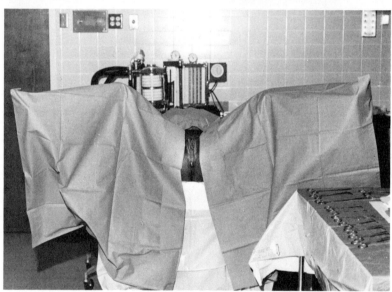

FIG. 17-4. A. The vulva, perineum, and adjacent regions have been thoroughly scrubbed. Sterile disposable drapes are being applied. **B.** The field is sterile-draped in preparation for delivery.

pulsion is anticipated, the woman and her fetus are formally prepared for delivery.

Preparation for Delivery. No one should be permitted in the delivery room without a scrub suit, a mask covering both nose and mouth, and a cap that completely covers the hair. Preparation for actual delivery entails thorough vulvar and perineal scrubbing and covering with sterile drapes in such a way that only the immediate area about the vulva is exposed (Fig. 17-4 A,B).

In placing the legs in leg-holders, care should be taken not to separate the legs too widely and not to place one leg higher than the other. The popliteal region should rest comfortably in the proximal portion and the heel in the distal portion of the leg-holder.

Too often the leg is forced to conform to the existing setting. Cramps in the leg may develop in the second stage of labor in part because of pressure by the baby's head on nerves in the pelvis. Such cramps may be relieved by changing the position of the leg or by brief massage, but leg cramps should never be ignored.

Scrubbing and Gloving. Since sterile rubber gloves are punctured easily or tear occasionally, the necessity for meticulously cleansing the hands before putting on gloves is apparent. Even with these precautions, the possibility of disseminating bacteria within the genital tract is not eliminated entirely, since the organisms may be carried up from the vaginal outlet by the gloved finger. In all cases, the hands should be cleansed as carefully as for a major surgical operation:

1. The fingernails are cut and cleaned before starting to scrub.
2. Using a antiseptic soap, both hands and forearms to 5 cm above the elbows are washed for 1 minute. The mixture is then rinsed off with running lukewarm water.
3. A sterile orangewood or plastic stick is next employed to clean thoroughly beneath the fingernails.
4. Utilizing a sterile hand brush and the antiseptic solution, each hand is then vigorously scrubbed for 2 minutes; each forearm to 5 cm above the elbow is then scrubbed for 1 minute. The hands, followed by the forearms, are now rinsed with warm water.

This technic involves a total of 6 minutes after the initial 1-minute wash. When the birth of the baby becomes imminent or in any emergency the time is shortened accordingly.

After the hands are scrubbed, a sterile gown is donned in such a manner that the hands do not touch its outer surface. Likewise, the gloves are put on in such a manner that the ungloved hands never touch the outer surface of the gloves.

SPONTANEOUS DELIVERY

Delivery of the Head. With each contraction, the perineum bulges increasingly and the vulvovaginal opening becomes more and more dilated by the fetal head (Fig. 17-5), gradually forming an ovoid and finally an almost circular opening. With the cessa-

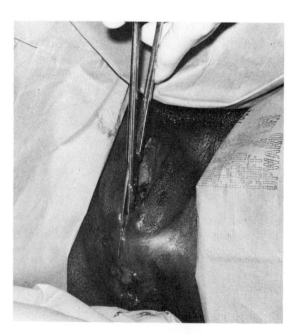

FIG. 17-5. Vulva partially distended by fetal head. Midline episiotomy being made.

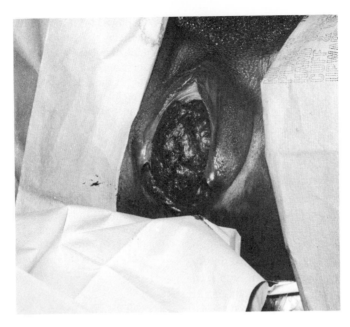

FIG. 17-6. Birth of head. The occiput is being kept close to the symphysis by moderate pressure to the fetal chin at the tip of the maternal coccyx.

tion of each contraction, the opening becomes smaller as the head recedes. As the head becomes increasingly visible, the vaginal outlet and vulva are stretched further until they ultimately encircle the largest diameter of the baby's head (Fig. 17-6). This encirclement of the largest diameter of the fetal head by the vulvar ring is known as *crowning.*

Unless an episiotomy has been made already, as described on page 430, the perineum by now is extremely thin, and almost at the point of rupture with each contraction. At the same time the anus becomes greatly stretched and protuberant, and the anterior wall of the rectum may be easily seen through it. Failure to perform an episiotomy by this time only invites perineal lacerations and some degree of permanent relaxation of the pelvic floor with its possible sequelae of cystocele, rectocele, and uterine prolapse.

RITGEN MANEUVER. By the time the head distends the perineum during a contraction to a diameter of 5 cm or so, it is desirable to drape a towel over one hand to protect it from the anus and then exert forward pressure on the chin of the fetus through the perineum just in front of the coccyx while the other hand exerts pressure superiorly against the occiput (Fig. 17-7). Although this maneuver is simpler than that originally described by Ritgen (1855), it is customarily designated the Ritgen maneuver or the modified Ritgen maneuver. It allows the physician to control the delivery of the head. It also favors extension, so that the head is delivered with its smallest diameters passing through the introitus and over the perineum (Fig. 17-8). The head is delivered slowly with the base of the occiput rotating around the lower margin of the symphysis pubis as a fulcrum, while the bregma (anterior fontanel), brow, and face pass successively over the perineum (Fig. 17-9).

To minimize the likelihood of aspiration of amnionic fluid debris and blood that might occur once the thorax is delivered and the infant could inspire, the face is quickly wiped and the nares and mouth are aspirated with a bulb syringe as demonstrated in Fig. 20-1, (p. 475). Next the finger should be passed to the neck of the fetus to ascertain whether it is encircled by one or more coils of the

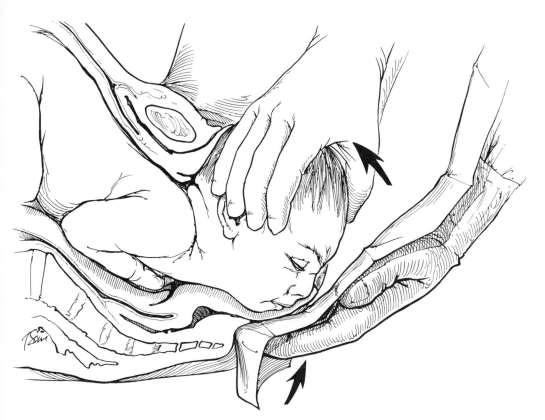

FIG. 17-7. Near completion of the delivery of the fetal head by the modified Ritgen maneuver. Moderate upward pressure is applied to the fetal chin by the posterior hand while the suboccipital area of the fetal head is held against the symphysis.

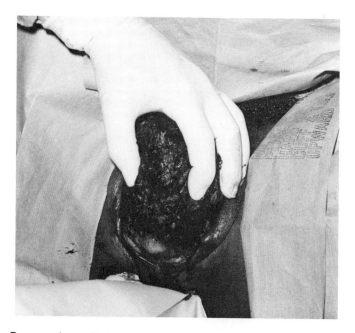

FIG. 17-8. Pressure is applied through the towel covering the hand to the underside of the chin of the infant as soon as the occiput is beyond the symphysis. This extends the head. At the same time, the fingers of the other hand simultaneously elevate the scalp to help extend the head.

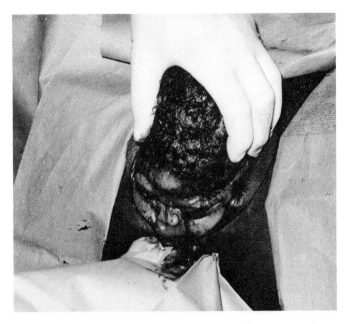

FIG. 17-9.   Birth of head; the mouth is appearing over perineum.

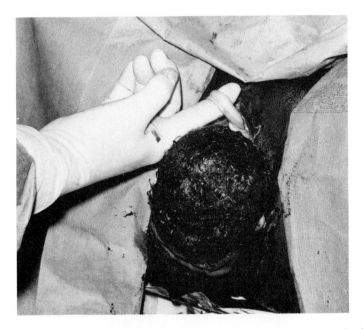

FIG. 17-10.   Cord identified around the neck. It readily slipped over the head.

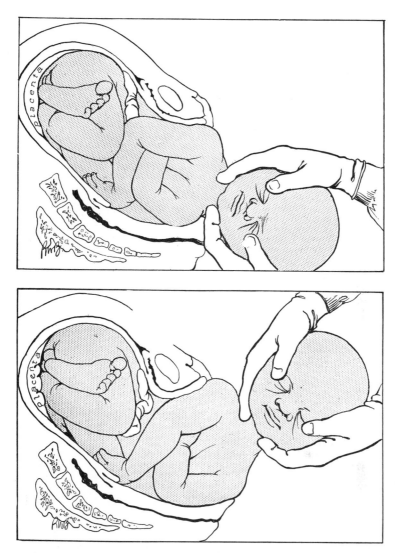

FIG. 17-11. Gentle downward traction to bring about descent of anterior shoulder (top). Delivery of anterior shoulder completed; gentle upward traction to deliver the posterior shoulder (bottom).

umbilical cord (Fig. 17-10). Coils occur in about 25 percent of cases and ordinarily do no harm, but occasionally they may be so tight that constriction of the umbilical vessels and consequent hypoxia result. If a coil is felt, it should be drawn down between the fingers and, if loose enough, slipped over the infant's head. If it is applied too tightly to the neck to be slipped over the head, it should be cut between two clamps and the infant delivered promptly.

Delivery of Shoulders. After its birth, the head falls posteriorly, bringing the face almost into contact with the anus. As described in Chapter 16, the occiput promptly turns toward one of the maternal thighs so that the head assumes a transverse position. The successive movements of restitution and external rotation are indicative that the bisacromial diameter (transverse diameter of thorax) has rotated into the anteroposterior diameter of the pelvis.

In most cases, the shoulders appear at the vulva just after external rotation and are born spontaneously. Occasionally, a delay occurs and immediate extraction may appear advisable. In that event, the sides of the head are grasped with the two hands and *gentle* downward traction applied until the anterior shoulder appears under the pubic arch. Then, by an upward movement, the posterior shoulder is delivered and the anterior shoulder usually drops down from beneath the symphysis. An equally effective method entails completion of delivery of the anterior shoulder before that of the posterior (Fig. 17-11).

The rest of the body almost always follows the shoulders without difficulty, but in case of prolonged delay its birth may be hastened by *moderate* traction on the head and pressure on the uterine fundus. Hooking the fingers in the axillae should be avoided, however, since it may injure the nerves of the upper extremity, producing a transient or possibly even a permanent paralysis. Traction, furthermore, should be exerted only in the direction of the long axis of the child, for if applied obliquely it causes bending of the neck and excessive stretching of the brachial plexus.

Immediately after extrusion of the infant, there is usually a gush of amnionic fluid, often tinged with blood, but not grossly bloody.

Clamping the Cord. The umbilical cord is cut between two clamps such as pean clamps placed 4 or 5 cm from the abdomen, and subsequently, about 2 cm from the abdomen, a formal cord clamp is applied. A plastic clamp that is safe, efficient, easy to sterilize, and fairly inexpensive is shown in Figure 17-12.

TIMING OF CORD CLAMPING.   If after delivery the infant is placed at the level of the vaginal introitus or below and the fetoplacental circulation is not immediately occluded by clamping the cord, as much as 100 ml of blood may be shifted from the placenta to the infant.

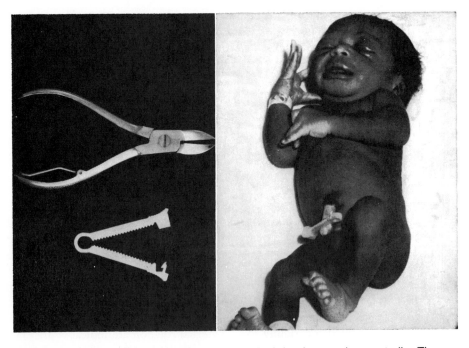

FIG. 17-12. Plastic cord clamp. These clamps lock in place and cannot slip. They are removed on the second or third day simply by cutting the plastic at the loop, or they can be allowed to drop off with the cord.

Yao and Lind (1969, 1974), measured the residual volume of placental blood in response to positioning the infant at precisely measured distances above or below the introitus for varying periods of time before clamping the cord. They observed that placing the infant within 10 cm above or below the introitus for 3 minutes resulted in the shift of about 80 ml of blood from the placenta to the infant. Lowering to 40 cm below the introitus for only 30 seconds effected the same degree of transfer. If the infant was held 50 to 60 cm above the introitus, however, transfer of blood to the infant was negligible even after 3 minutes.

One benefit to be derived from placental transfusion is that the hemoglobin in 80 ml of placental blood that shifts to the fetus eventually provides about 50 mg of iron to the infant's stores and no doubt reduces the frequency of iron-deficiency anemia later in infancy. In the presence of accelerated destruction of erythrocytes, as occurs with maternal alloimmunization, the bilirubin formed from the added erythrocytes contributes further to the danger of hyperbilirubinemia (see Chap. 38, p. 972). Although theoretically the risk of circulatory overloading from gross hypervolemia is formidable, especially in premature infants, the addition of placental blood to the infant's circulation does not ordinarily cause difficulty.

Our policy is to clamp the cord after first thoroughly clearing the infant's airway, all of which usually takes upwards of 30 seconds. The infant is not elevated above the introitus at vaginal delivery nor above the maternal abdominal wall at cesarean section.

MANAGEMENT OF THE THIRD STAGE

Immediately after delivery of the infant, the height of the uterine fundus and its consistency are ascertained. As long as the uterus remains firm and there is no unusual bleeding, watchful waiting until the placenta is separated is the usual practice. No massage is practiced; the hand is simply rested on the fundus frequently, to make certain that the organ does not become atonic and filled with blood behind a separated placenta.

Since attempts to express the placenta prior to its separation are futile and possibly dangerous, it is most important that the following signs of placental separation be recognized:

1. The uterus becomes globular and, as a rule, firmer. This sign is the earliest to appear.
2. There is often a sudden gush of blood.
3. The uterus rises in the abdomen because the placenta, having separated, passes down into the lower uterine segment and vagina, where its bulk pushes the uterus upward.
4. The umbilical cord protrudes farther out of the vagina, indicating that the placenta has descended.

These signs sometimes appear within about a minute after delivery of the infant and usually within 5 minutes. When the placenta has separated, the physician first ascertains that the uterus is firmly contracted. The mother, if she is not anesthetized, may be asked to bear down, and the intra-abdominal pressure so produced may be adequate to expel the placenta. If these efforts fail, or if spontaneous expulsion is not practicable because of anesthesia, the physician, again having made certain that the uterus is contracted firmly, exerts pressure with the hand on the fundus and to propel the detached placenta into the vagina (Figs. 17-13, 17-14).

Delivery of the Placenta. Placental expression should never be forced before placental separation lest the uterus be turned inside out. Inversion of the uterus is one of the grave accidents associated with delivery (see Chap. 34, p. 888). As pressure is applied to the fundus, the umbilical cord is kept slightly taut (Fig. 17-13). *Traction on the cord, however, must not be used to pull the placenta out of the uterus.* As the placenta passes through the introitus, fundal pressure is stopped. The placenta is then gently lifted away from the introitus (Fig. 17-14). Care is taken to pre-

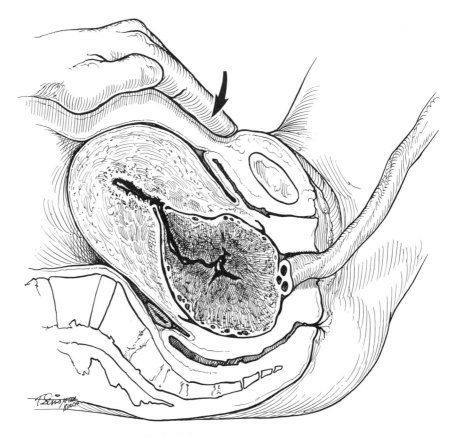

FIG. 17-13. Expression of placenta.

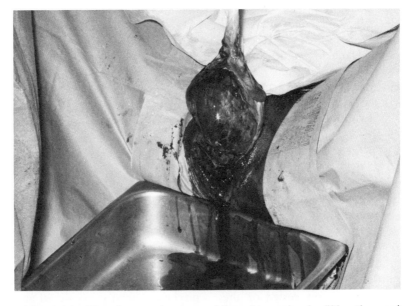

FIG. 17-14. The placenta is removed from the vagina by lifting the cord.

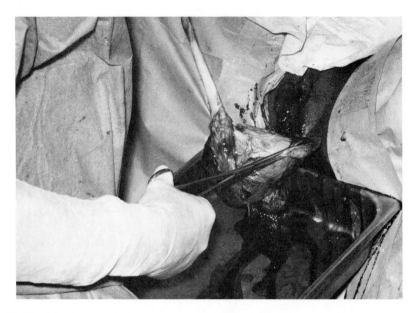

FIG. 17-15. Membranes that were somewhat adherent to the uterine lining are separated by gentle traction with a ring forceps.

vent the membranes from being torn off and left behind. If the membranes start to tear, they are grasped with a clamp and removed by gentle traction (Fig. 17-15). The placenta should be examined carefully to ascertain whether it has been delivered in its entirety from the uterine cavity.

If at any time there is brisk bleeding and the placenta cannot be delivered by these technics, manual removal of the placenta is indicated, with all of the safeguards described in Chapter 34 (p. 880).

Occasionally, the placenta will not separate promptly. A question to which there is still no definite answer concerns the length of time that should elapse in the absence of bleeding before the placenta is manually removed. If the placenta has not separated within 3 to 5 minutes after the birth of the baby, the genital tract is satisfactorily anesthetized, and there has been no contamination of the operative field, manual removal of the placenta should be carried out. The principle advantage of this approach is the reduction of blood loss during the third stage, whereas the main disadvantage is the possibility of introducing infection into the uterine cavity.

ROUTINE MANUAL REMOVAL OF THE PLACENTA. Management of the retained placenta has varied considerably. Manual removal of the placenta is rightfully practiced much sooner and more often than in the past. In fact, some obstetricians practice routine manual removal of any placenta that has not separated spontaneously by the time they have completed delivery of the infant and care of the cord. The majority, however, do not resort so promptly to manual removal of the placenta, although the procedure must be performed whenever bleeding is excessive.

Routine manual removal of the placenta has proved to be a safe procedure only in the following circumstances: (1) if few vaginal examinations were performed during labor and if they were accompanied by a minimum of bacterial contamination; (2) if the vulva, perineum, and adjacent regions were carefully prepared and draped prior to delivery; (3) if delivery was accomplished without contaminating the genital tract; and (4) if regional or general anesthesia is satisfactory. In other circumstances, since the risks of immediate manual removal of the placenta outweigh the advantages, the procedure should be restricted to instances in which hemorrhage threatens.

The placenta, membranes, and umbilical cord should be examined for completeness and for anomalies, as described in Chapter 23, (p. 551).

The hour immediately following delivery of the placenta is a critical period and has been designated by some obstetricians as the "fourth stage of labor." Even though oxytocics are administered, as described below, postpartum hemorrhage as the result of uterine relaxation is most likely to occur at this time. As emphasized in Chapter 19 (p. 467), it is mandatory that the uterus be evaluated very frequently throughout this period by a competent attendant, who keeps a hand on the fundus and massages it at the slightest sign of relaxation. At the same time, the vaginal and perineal region is also inspected frequently to identify promptly any excessive bleeding.

OXYTOCIC AGENTS

After the uterus has been emptied and the placenta has been delivered, the primary mechanism by which hemostasis is achieved at the placental site is vasoconstriction produced by a well-contracted myometrium (see Chap. 21, p. 489). Oxytocin (Pitocin, Syntocinon), ergonovine maleate (Ergotrate), and methylergonovine maleate (Methergine) are employed in various ways in the conduct of the third stage of labor, principally to stimulate myometrial contractions and thereby reduce the blood loss.

Oxytocin. The synthetic form of the octapeptide oxytocin is commercially available in the United States as Syntocinon and Pitocin; 1 mg of oxytocin is equal to about 500 USP units. Each ml of injectable oxytocin contains 10 USP units of oxytocin, which is not effective by mouth. The half-life of intravenously infused oxytocin is very short, perhaps 3 minutes.

Before delivery, the spontaneously laboring uterus is very likely to be exquisitely sensitive to oxytocin. Even with an intravenous dose of a few milliunits per minute, the pregnant uterus may contract so violently as to kill the fetus, rupture itself, or both (see Chap. 29, p. 791). After delivery of the fetus, these dangers no longer exist. Nonetheless, at this time there are other potentially grave dangers from inappropriate use of oxytocin.

CARDIOVASCULAR. Deleterious effects may on occasion follow the intravenous injec-

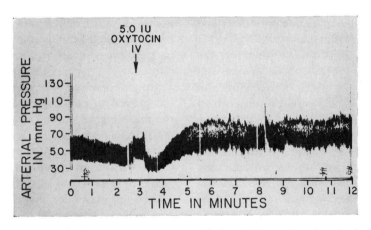

FIG. 17-16. Adverse effect of the intravenous bolus of five units of oxytocin in a case of postpartum hemorrhage 18 minutes postdelivery. The hypotension worsened to a level of 44/26 mm Hg until saline was infused rapidly. (From Hendricks and Brenner. *Am J Obstet Gynecol* 108:751, 1970)

tion of a bolus of oxytocin. Hendricks and Brenner (1970), for example, demonstrated with the rapid intravenous injection of 5 units (0.5 ml) of oxytocin that the uterus contracted tetanically for several minutes but maternal blood pressure decreased simultaneously. In one dramatic instance of hypotension from uterine bleeding following delivery of twins, they noted that the injection of 5 units of oxytocin intravenously was followed promptly by a further decrease in blood pressure from 70/42 mm Hg to 44/26 mm Hg (Fig. 17-16). After rapid administration of 500 ml of saline, the blood pressure rose and the mother again became responsive.

Secher and co-workers (1978) consistently found in healthy women after an intravenous bolus of 10 units of oxytocin a transient but marked fall in arterial blood pressure that was followed rapidly by an abrupt increase in cardiac output. They too conclude that these hemodynamic changes could be dangerous to women whose circulation was already compromised by hypovolemia or who had cardiac disease which limits cardiac output or is complicated by right to left shunts. Oxytocin should not, therefore, be given intravenously as a large bolus, but rather as a much more dilute solution by continuous intravenous infusion as described on page 429, or be injected intramuscularly in a dose of 10 units.

ANTIDIURESIS. Another important adverse effect of oxytocin is antidiuresis, caused primarily by reabsorption of free water. Abdul-Karim and Assali (1961) demonstrated clearly that in both pregnant and nonpregnant women oxytocin possesses antidiuretic activity. In women who are undergoing diuresis in response to the administration of water, the continuous intravenous infusion of 20 milliunits of oxytocin per minute usually produces a demonstrable decrease in urine flow. When the rate of infusion is raised to 40 to 50 milliunits per minute, urinary flow is strikingly reduced. With doses of this magnitude, it is possible to produce water intoxication if the oxytocin is administered

in a large volume of electrolyte-free aqueous dextrose solution (Liggins, 1962; Whalley, Pritchard, 1963; Eggers, Fliegner JR, 1979).

The hyponatremic, hypoosmotic state is not limited to just the mother. Schwartz and Jones (1978), for example, described convulsions in both the mother and her newborn infant following the administration of 6.5 liters of 5 percent dextrose solution and 36 units of oxytocin predelivery. The concentration of sodium in cord plasma was 114 mEq/l.

In general, if oxytocin is to be administered at a relatively high rate of infusion for a considerable period of time, increasing the concentration of the hormone is preferable to increasing the rate of flow of the more dilute solution. The antidiuretic effect of intravenously administered oxytocin disappears within a few minutes after the infusion is stopped. Oxytocin injected intramuscularly in doses of 5 to 10 units (0.5 to 1 ml) every 15 to 30 minutes also causes antidiuresis, but the possibility of water intoxication is not nearly so great, since large volumes of electrolyte-free aqueous solution are not required as a vehicle (Whalley, Pritchard, 1963).

OTHER EFFECTS. Oxytocin causes milk ejection by inducing contractions of the myoepithelial cells of the mammary gland (Chap. 19, p. 464). This phenomenon is not seen in nonpregnant women, but from very early in pregnancy the gland becomes progressively more sensitive to the hormone. During the second half of pregnancy, a demonstrable effect can be elicited with as little as 1 milliunit of oxytocin (Sala, 1964). The milk-ejecting effect induced by oxytocin is about 40 to 50 times greater than that of vasopressin. The intravenous injection of 10 milliunits of oxytocin per kg is followed by an appreciable increase in the concentration of free fatty acids in the plasma and sizable decreases in the levels of blood glucose in very recently pregnant and nonpregnant women (Burt et al., 1963). The significance of these effects, however, is not clear. Oxytocin is without effect when taken orally because of its rapid destruction in the gastrointestinal tract. Slight oxytocic and milk-ejection effects can sometimes be induced by applying oxytocin to the nasal mucosa in the form of a pledget or a spray; a very small amount, however, may be absorbed when continuously applied to the buccal mucosa.

Posterior pituitary extract (Pituitrin) is a mixture of both the oxytocic and vasopressor-antidiuretic principles from the pituitary glands of domestic animals. It is mentioned here only to condemn its use. Along with oxytocic action, there is the potent vasopressor effect of vasopressin. If given in large doses parenterally, especially if administered intravenously, it can produce profound shock. Pituitrin shock probably results in large part from constriction of coronary arteries by the rapid injection of large amounts of vasopressin. Oxytocin should have long since completely replaced Pituitrin in all hospitals.

Ergonovine and Methylergonovine.
Ergonovine is an alkaloid obtained either from ergot, a fungus that grows upon rye and some other grains, or synthesized in part from lysergic acid. Methylergonovine is a very similar alkaloid, also made from lysergic acid.

The alkaloids are dispensed as the maleate (Ergotrate and Methergine, respectively) either in solution for parenteral use or in tablets for oral use.

EFFECTS. There is no convincing evidence of any appreciable difference in the actions of ergonovine and methylergonovine; therefore, these will be considered together. Whether given intravenously, intramuscularly, or orally, ergonovine and methylergonovine are powerful stimulants of myometrial contraction, exerting an effect that may persist for hours. The sensitivity of the pregnant uterus to ergonovine and methylergonovine is very great. In pregnant women, an intravenous dose of as little as 0.1 mg, or an oral dose of only 0.25 mg, results in a tetanic contraction that occurs almost immediately after intravenous injection of the drug and within a few minutes after intramuscular or oral administration. Moreover, the response is sustained with little tendency toward relaxation. The tetanic effect of ergonovine and methylergonovine is effective for the prevention and control of postpartum hemorrhage but is very dangerous for the fetus and the mother prior to delivery.

The parenteral administration of these alkaloids, especially by the intravenous route, sometimes initiates transient but severe hypertension. Such a reaction is most likely to occur when conduction anesthesia is used for delivery and in women who are prone to develop hypertension. Browning (1974) has vividly described four instances of serious side effects postdelivery attributable to 0.5 mg of ergonovine administered intramuscularly. Two women promptly became severely hypertensive, the third became hypertensive and convulsed, and the fourth woman suffered a cardiac arrest. Because of the frequency of hypertension among our obstetric population, these alkaloids are seldom used at Parkland Memorial Hospital. Nausea is another troublesome feature.

HISTORY.   The history of *ergot* is fascinating. For centuries it has been recognized that ergot could cause severe pain, convulsions, extensive gangrene of the extremities, and death. Repeated epidemics of ergotism plagued Europe until ergot was proved to be their cause and they were then brought under control. A local outbreak, nevertheless, occurred in France a little more than a decade ago.

Centuries ago ergot was recognized as capable of producing uterine contractions, and early in the nineteenth century Pulvis Parturiens was introduced into medicine. A letter by John Stearns published in the *Medical Repository of New York* in 1808 is presented in part (quoted from Goodman and Gilman, 1965): "It expedites lingering parturition and saves to the accoucheur a considerable portion of time, without producing any bad effects on the patient. . . . Previous to its exhibition it is of the utmost consequence to ascertain the presentation . . . as the violent and almost incessant action which it induces in the uterus precludes the possibility of turning. . . . If the dose is large it will produce nausea and vomiting. In most cases you will be surprised with the suddenness of its operation; it is, therefore, necessary to be completely ready before you give the medicine. . . . Since I have adopted the use of this powder I have seldom found a case that detained me more than three hours."

After a flurry of widespread administration it became apparent that powdered ergot was capable of producing violent uterine contractions with fetal and maternal death. Moir (1932), has pointed out that such has been the history of most uterine stimulants. There was initial surprise and pleasure on discovering the uterine-stimulating effect; the cautious employment of the drug clinically to initiate or stimulate labor followed. Favorable reports were soon followed by uncritical and dangerous use with extensive fetal and maternal injuries and deaths. Finally the way to safe use of the drug evolved or, if there was none, it was discarded.

Ergot as a powder or as the fluid extract was recognized until recently in official compendiums of drugs. Attempts to standardize the oxytocic activity of ergot were based on assays that compared its ability to produce gangrene of a rooster's comb with that of a standard preparation. This bioassay measured the activity of the wrong constituents, since the alkaloids that produced the gangrene possessed little or no oxytocic activity, and vice versa. The alkaloid with potent oxytocic properties, ergonovine, was isolated in 1935.

Oxytocics During and After Delivery.

Oxytocin, ergonovine, and methylergonovine are all employed widely in the conduct of the normal third stage of labor, but the timing of their administration differs in various institutions. Oxytocin and especially ergonovine given before delivery of the placenta will decrease blood loss somewhat according to the measurements of Sorbe (1978), who employed single intravenous injections of 10 units of oxytocin or 0.2 mg of ergonovine. With oxytocin he observed no fall in blood pressure and no subjective side effects. He did observe and emphasize the known side effects of ergonovine, i.e., the possibility of a steep rise in blood pressure, generalized uterine spasm, and the likelihood of partial placental separation with bleeding and entrapment unless active intervention was employed quickly. Of considerable concern, the use of oxytocin, and especially ergonovine or methylergonovine, before delivery of the placenta may entrap an undiagnosed and therefore undelivered second twin. This may prove injurious, if not fatal, to the entrapped fetus. In most cases following uncomplicated vaginal delivery, the third stage of labor can be conducted with reasonably small blood loss without using oxytocin or these alkaloids of ergot.

If an intravenous infusion is in place, standard practice at Parkland Memorial Hospital has been to add 20 units (2 ml) of oxytocin per liter, which is administered after delivery of the placenta at a rate of 10 ml per minute for a few minutes until the uterus remains firmly contracted and the bleeding is controlled. Then the infusion rate is reduced to 1 to 2 ml per minute until the mother is ready for transfer from the recovery suite to the postpartum unit, when it is usually discontinued.

Lacerations of the Birth Canal.

Lacerations of the vagina and perineum are classified as first, second, or third degree. Such lacerations most often are preventable with an appropriate episiotomy and avoidance of midforceps delivery.

First-degree lacerations involve the fourchet, the perineal skin, and vaginal mucous membrane but not the underlying fascia and muscle.

Second-degree lacerations (Fig. 17-17) involve, in addition to skin and mucous membrane, the fascia and muscles of the perineal body but not the rectal sphincter. These tears usually extend upward on one or both sides of the vagina, forming an irregular triangular injury.

Third-degree lacerations extend through the skin, mucous membrane, and perineal body, and involve the anal sphincter. Not infrequently, these third-degree lacerations may also extend a distance up the anterior wall of the rectum.

A so-called fourth-degree laceration is distinguished by some. This designation is applied to third-degree tears that extend through the rectal mucosa to expose the lumen of the rectum. The term *fourth-degree laceration* will not be used in the ensuing discussion. Instead, when third-degree lacerations with rectal wall extension are mentioned, they will be so designated. Tears in the region of the urethra are also likely to occur unless an adequate episiotomy is performed, and they may bleed profusely.

Since the repair of perineal tears is virtually the same as that of episiotomy incisions, albeit often more difficult because of irregular

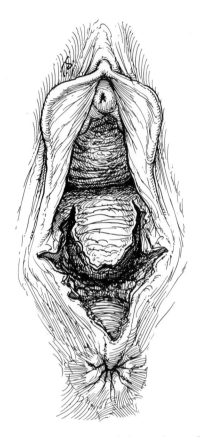

FIG. 17-17. Deep second-degree laceration of perineum and vagina.

lines of tissue cleavage, the technic of repairing them will be discussed in the following section.

EPISIOTOMY AND REPAIR

Episiotomy, in a strict sense, is incision of the pudenda. Perineotomy is incision of the perineum. In common parlance, however, episiotomy is often used synonymously with perineotomy, a practice that will be followed here. The incision may be made in the midline (median episiotomy), or it may be begun in the midline but directed laterally and downward away from the rectum (mediolateral episiotomy).

Purposes of Episiotomy. Except for cutting the umbilical cord, episiotomy is the most common operation in obstetrics. The reasons for its popularity among obstetricians are clear. It substitutes a straight, neat surgical incision for the ragged laceration that otherwise frequently results. It is easier to repair and heals better than a tear. It spares the fetal head the necessity of serving as a battering ram against perineal obstruction. If prolonged, the pounding of the fetal head against the perineum may cause intracranial injury. Episiotomy shortens the second stage of labor. Finally, with mediolateral episiotomy, the likelihood of lacerations into the rectum is reduced.

More recently, the advantages provided by episiotomy have been questioned by some individuals (Coogan and Edmunds, 1977), as have most aspects of obstetric care. It can be said with certainty that, since the era of in-hospital deliveries with episiotomy, there has been an appreciable decrease in the number of women subsequently hospitalized for treatment of symptomatic cystocele, rectocele, uterine prolapse, and stress incontinence!

The important questions for the obstetrician concerning episiotomy are:

1. How long before delivery should it be performed?
2. Should a median or mediolateral incision be made?
3. Should the incision be sutured before or after expulsion of the placenta?
4. What are the best suture materials and technic to employ?

Timing of the Episiotomy. If episiotomy is performed unnecessarily early, bleeding from the gaping wound may be considerable during the interim between the incision and the birth of the baby. If episiotomy is performed too late, the muscles of the perineal floor already will have undergone excessive stretching, and one of the objectives of the operation is defeated. It is common practice to perform episiotomy when the head is visible during a contraction to a diameter of 3 to 4 cm (Fig. 17-5).

In this connection, the question arises whether episiotomy should be performed before or after the application of forceps. Application and articulation of forceps with widely separated shanks, as with Simpson forceps, may cause tearing of the introitus (see Chap. 41, p. 1050). The application of those with narrow overlapping shanks, such as Tucker McLane forceps, before episiotomy is not likely to be so traumatic. Although it is slightly more awkward to perform episiotomy with the forceps in place, blood loss from the episiotomy wound is somewhat less with this technic, since immediate traction on the forceps can be exerted, and the resultant tamponade of the perineal floor by the fetal head is effected earlier than could otherwise be achieved.

MEDIAN (MIDLINE) VS. MEDIOLATERAL EPISIOTOMY. The advantages and disadvantages of the two types of episiotomy may be enumerated as follows:

Median Episiotomy
1. Easy to repair
2. Faulty healing rare
3. Less painful in puerperium
4. Dyspareunia rarely follows
5. Anatomic end results almost always excellent
6. Blood loss smaller
7. Extension through the anal sphincter and into rectum is rather common

Mediolateral Episiotomy
1. More difficult to repair
2. Faulty healing more common
3. Pain in one-third of cases for a few days
4. Dyspareunia occasionally follows
5. Anatomic end results more or less faulty in some 10 percent of cases (depending on operator)
6. Blood loss greater
7. Extension through sphincter is uncommon

With proper selection of cases, it is possible to secure the advantages of median episiotomy and at the same time reduce to a minimum its one disadvantage, the greater risk of third-degree extension. The size of the perineal body is related to the likelihood of third-degree laceration, since the accident is naturally more likely to occur if the perineal body is short. The possibility of extension of a median episiotomy into the rectal sphincter is also much greater when the fetus is large, when the occiput is posterior, in midforceps deliveries, and in breech deliveries. It is good practice, in general, to use mediolateral episiotomy in the circumstances mentioned but to employ the median incision otherwise. Even with this selection of cases, however, the total number of third-degree lacerations sustained with this policy is probably greater than with routine mediolateral episiotomy. In any case, pointed scissors should not be used lest the posterior (internal) blade inadvertently penetrate the rectum.

Benyon (1974) described her experiences with a policy of mandatory midline episiotomy. Of 1166 nulliparas who underwent a midline episiotomy, there was extension through the sphincter with involvement of *the rectum in 8.0 percent.* The technic of repair was similar to that described below. She emphasized that the episiotomies and repairs were performed primarily by house officers in training. Following repair, there was no special emphasis on bowel action. Suppositories, rectal tubes, and enemas were not allowed and rectal examinations were avoided. All were followed after primary repair and in only one woman was a rectovaginal fistula subsequently identified. Therefore, a third-degree laceration as the consequence of a median episiotomy need not be a major catastrophe. Despite its one drawback, the median episiotomy is a satisfactory procedure for most deliveries.

TIMING OF THE REPAIR OF EPISIOTOMY. The most common practice is to defer repair of the episiotomy until after the placenta has been delivered. That policy permits the obstetrician to give undivided attention to the signs of placental separation and to deliver the organ just as soon as it has separated. Early delivery of the placenta is believed to decrease the loss of blood, since it prevents the development of extensive retroplacental bleeding. A further advantage of this practice is that the episiotomy repair is not interrupted or disrupted by the obvious

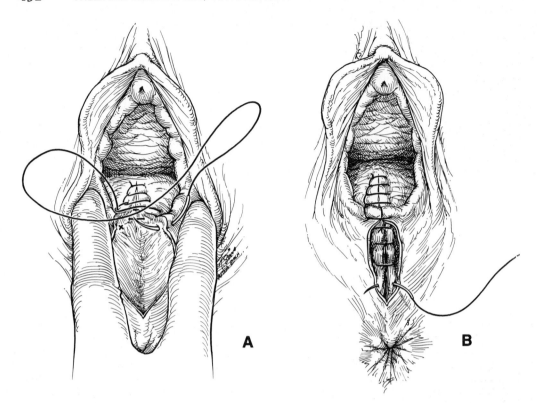

FIG. 17-18. Repair of median episiotomy. **A.** Chromic catgut 00, or preferably 000, is used as a continuous suture to close the vaginal mucosa and submucosa. **B.** After closing the vaginal incision and reapproximating the cut margins of the hymeneal ring, the suture is tied and cut. Next three or four interrupted sutures of 00 or 000 catgut are placed in the fascia and muscle of the incised perineum. *(continued)*

necessity of delivering the placenta, especially if manual removal must be performed.

TECHNIC. There are many ways to close the episiotomy incision, but *hemostasis and anatomic restoration without excessive suturing are essential* for success with any method. A technic that is commonly employed in episiotomy repair is shown in Figure 17-18A–E. The suture material ordinarily used is 00 or preferably 000 chromic catgut.

THIRD-DEGREE LACERATION. The technic of repairing a third-degree laceration with extension into the wall of the rectum is shown in Figure 17-19. Here again various technics have been recommended, but all emphasize careful approximation of the torn edges of the rectal wall with stitches about 0.5 cm apart, then covering this layer with a layer

of fascia, and finally, careful isolation and suture of the anal sphincter with two or three interrupted stitches. The remainder of the repair is the same as for episiotomy. If the rectal mucosa was involved, stool softeners should be prescribed for a week. Enemas, of course, should be avoided. The value of prophylactic antibiotics has not been established.

PAIN AFTER EPISIOTOMY. For the relief of episiotomy pain, a heat lamp has been a standard remedy, but during the summer months especially it may produce more discomfort than relief. An ice collar applied early tends to reduce swelling and allay discomfort. Aerosol sprays containing a local anesthetic are helpful at times. Analgesics such as codeine give considerable relief. *Since pain may be a signal of a large vulvar, paravaginal,*

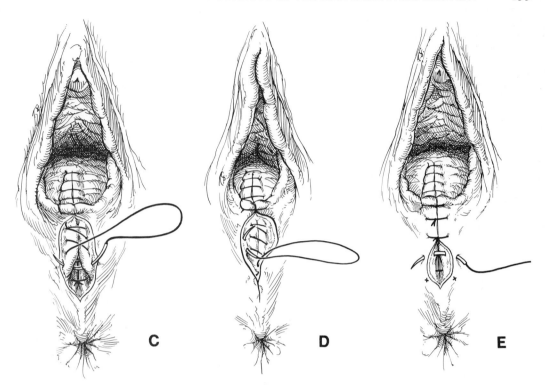

C   D   E

FIG. 17-18 (cont.). Repair of median episiotomy, continued. **C.** A continuous suture is now carried downward to unite the superficial fascia. **D.** Completion of repair. The continuous suture is carried upward as a subcuticular stitch. An alternative method of closure of skin and subcutaneous fascia is illustrated in E. **E.** Completion of repair of median episiotomy. A few interrupted sutures of 000 chromic catgut are placed through the skin and subcutaneous fascia and loosely tied. This closure avoids burying two layers of catgut in the more superficial layers of the perinium.

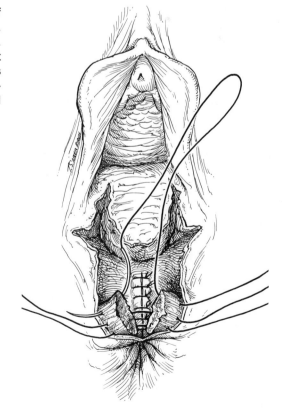

FIG. 17-19. (Right). Repair of complete perineal tear. The rectal mucosa has been repaired with interrupted, fine chromic catgut sutures. The torn ends of the sphincter ani are next approximated with two or three interrupted chromic catgut sutures. The wound is then repaired, as in a second-degree laceration or an episiotomy.

or ischiorectal hematoma or abscess, it is essential to examine these sites carefully if pain is severe or persistent. Management of these complications is discussed in Chapter 36.

REFERENCES

Abdul-Karim R, Assali NS: Renal function in human pregnancy: V. Effects of oxytocin on renal hemodynamics and water and electrolyte excretion. J Lab Clin Med 57:522, 1961

Abe T: The detection of the rupture of fetal membranes with the nitrazine indicator. Am J Obstet Gynecol 39:400, 1940

Baptisti A: Chemical test for the determination of ruptured membranes. Am J Obstet Gynecol 35:688, 1938

Benson RC, Shubeck F, Deutschberger J, Weiss W, Berendes H: Fetal heart rate as a predictor of fetal distress. A report from the Collaborative Project. Obstet Gynecol 32:259, 1968

Benyon CL: Midline episiotomy as a midline procedure. J Obstet Gynaecol Br Commonw 81:126, 1974

Browning DJ: Serious side effects of ergometrine and its use in routine obstetric practice. Med J Austral 1:957, 1974

Burt RL, Leake NH, Dannenburg WN: Effect of synthetic oxytocin on plasma nonesterified fatty acids, triglycerides, and blood glucose. Obstet Gynecol 21:708, 1963

Caldeyro-Barcia R, Schwarcz R, Belizan JM, et al.: Adverse perinatal effects of early amniotomy during labor. In Gluck L (ed): Modern Perinatal Medicine. Chicago, Year Book, 1974

Coogan R, Edmunds EP: The unkindest cut? Contemp Ob/Gyn 9:55, 1977

Eggers TR, Fliegner JR: Water intoxication and syntocinon intoxication. Aust NZ J Obstet Gynaecol 19:59, 1979

Flynn AM, Kelly J, Hollins G, Lynch PF: Ambulation in labour. Br Med J 2:591, 1978

Friedman EA: Labor, Clinical Evaluation and Management, 2nd ed. New York, Appleton, 1978

Goodman LS, Gilman A: The Pharmacological Basis of Therapeutics. New York, Macmillan, 1965

Haverkamp AD, Thompson HE, McFee JG, Cetrulo C: The evaluation of continuous fetal heart rate monitoring in high risk pregnancy. Am J Obstet Gynecol, 125:310, 1976

Haverkamp AD, Orleans M, Langendoerfer S, et al.: A controlled trial of the differential effects of intrapartum fetal monitoring. Am J Obstet Gynecol, 134:399, 1979

Hendricks CH, Brenner WE: Cardiovascular effects of oxytocic drugs used postpartum. Am J Obstet Gynecol 108:751, 1970

Kjeldsen J: Hemodynamic investigations during labour and delivery. Acta Obstet Gynecol Scand suppl 89, 1979

Liggins GC: Treatment of missed abortion by high dosage syntocinon intravenous infusion. J Obstet Gynaecol Br Commonw 69:277, 1962

Moir JC: Clinical comparison of ergotoxine and ergotamine. Br Med J 1:1022, 1932

Ritgen G: (Concerning his method for protection of the perineum. Monatschrift für Geburtskunde 6:21, 1855). See English translation, Wynn RM: Am J Obstet Gynecol 93:421, 1965

Sala NL: The milk-ejecting effect induced by oxytocin and vasopressin during human pregnancy. Am J Obstet Gynecol 89:626, 1964

Schwartz RH, Jones RWA: Transplacental hyponatremia due to oxytocin. Br Med J 1:152, 1978

Secher NJ, Arnsbo P, Wallin L: Haemodynamic effects of oxytocin (Syntocinon) and methyl ergometrine (Methergin) on the systemic and pulmonary circulations of pregnant anaesthetized women. Acta Obstet Gynecol Scand 57:97, 1978

Sorbe B: Active pharmacologic management of the third stage of labor. A comparison of oxytocin and ergometrine. Obstet Gynecol 52:694, 1978

Whalley PJ, Pritchard JA: Oxytocin and water intoxication. JAMA 186:601, 1963

Yao AC, Lind J: Effect of gravity on placental transfusion. Lancet 2:505, 1969

Yao AC, Lind J: Placental transfusion. Am J Dis Child 127:128, 1974

18

Analgesia and Anesthesia

Labor is a painful process that for the nulliparous woman may be the most painful event that she has ever experienced. Fortunately, it often proves to be the most rewarding. The relief of pain in labor presents special problems, which may be best appreciated by reviewing the several important differences between obstetric and surgical anesthesia and analgesia:

1. In surgical procedures, there is but one patient to consider, whereas in parturition there are two, the mother and the fetus-infant. The respiratory center of the infant is highly vulnerable to sedative and anesthetic drugs and, since these agents, if given systemically, regularly traverse the placenta, they may jeopardize respiration after birth. This consideration is more than a mere theoretical possibility, as some degree of respiratory depression can be observed in infants whose mothers have received sedation during labor. The sensitivity of the fetus to the effects of almost all forms of maternal anesthesia poses one of the most difficult problems in obstetrics.
2. In major surgery, anesthesia is essential to the safe, satisfactory, and humane execution of the technical procedures.

Whereas anesthesia is mandatory in many abnormal deliveries, it is not absolutely necessary in spontaneous vaginal delivery, because the baby can be born satisfactorily without any medication, albeit the mother may suffer severe pain. Hence, in the strictest sense, an anesthetic death in obstetrics is usually an unnecessary death.

3. Surgical anesthesia is administered for the duration of the operation, which lasts in most cases for not more than an hour or two. Efficient pain relief in labor must cover not only the delivery ("obstetric anesthesia") but also a preceding period of from 1 to 12 hours or even longer ("obstetric analgesia").
4. In both obstetric analgesia and anesthesia, it is important that the agents used exert little deleterious effect on uterine contractions and maternal voluntary expulsive efforts. If they do, the progress of labor may stop, or if uterine contractility is depressed immediately after delivery, postpartum hemorrhage is likely to occur.
5. In the majority of surgical operations, there is ample time to prepare the patient for anesthesia, especially by withholding food and fluids for 12 hours. Since most labors begin without warning, obstetric anesthesia is often administered within a

few hours after a full meal. Moreover, gastric emptying is likely to be delayed appreciably during labor, especially after analgesics for pain relief (Nimmo et al., 1975). Vomiting with aspiration of gastric contents is, hence, a frequent threat and a major cause of morbidity and mortality in obstetric anesthesia.

Because of these inherent difficulties, no completely safe and satisfactory method of pain relief in obstetrics has yet been developed. It is therefore sometimes falsely alleged that the hazards of pain relief in labor offset its advantages. On the contrary, vast experience has shown that obstetric analgesia and anesthesia, when judiciously employed by skilled personnel, are in general beneficial rather than detrimental to both baby and mother. Pain relief forestalls the importunities of the parturient and her family for premature operative interference. Formerly, premature and injudicious operative delivery, thus provoked, constituted a common cause of trauma to both mother and infant. Such injuries were occasionally fatal to the mother and frequently so to the baby. The relief of pain itself, however, although desirable, does not justify the use of anesthetic procedures that are potentially lethal if administered by untrained individuals or with inadequate equipment.

Personnel and Facilities. The Joint Commission on Accreditation of Hospitals has urged that skilled personnel and appropriate equipment be immediately available to provide obstetric anesthesia: "Obstetric anesthesia must be considered as emergency anesthesia demanding a competence of personnel and equipment similar to or greater than that required for elective procedures." The societal benefits to be derived from modifying existing priorities for utilization of trained anesthesia personnel have been succinctly stated by Jacoby (1974): "Young women with babies are far more important to society than old people with irreversible disease. If we cannot do justice to both, then we should concentrate on the obstetrical patients."

According to the survey conducted by the American College of Obstetricians and Gynecologists, as recently as 1970 only 8 percent of hospital obstetric services had 24-hour anesthesia coverage by anesthesiologists. There has been some improvement since then. It is to be hoped that the increase in number of physicians now being graduated will help meet this need in the near future.

GENERAL PRINCIPLES

As stressed in another connection (see Chap. 17, p. 405), the proper psychologic management of the mother throughout the antepartum period and labor is a valuable basic tranquilizer. A woman who is free from fear and who has complete confidence in the obstetric staff that cares for her usually enjoys a relatively comfortable first stage of labor and requires only a modest amount of medication.

Three essentials of obstetric pain relief are preservation of fetal homeostasis, simplicity, and safety. Fetal homeostasis must not be impaired by the analgesic or anesthetic method. Most important is the transfer of oxygen, which is dependent on the concentration of inhaled oxygen, uterine blood flow, the oxygen gradient across the placenta, and umbilical blood flow. Impaired fetal oxygenation most often is the consequence of either compression of the umbilical cord or prolonged or repeated falls in placental perfusion. Prominent causes of the latter are hypertonic uterine contractions, severe pregnancy-induced hypertension, hemorrhage, premature separation of the placenta, and hypotension from spinal or epidural anesthesia.

The woman who receives any form of analgesia requires close supervision. If unattended and under heavy sedation, she may throw herself out of bed or against a wall, or she may vomit and aspirate the gastric contents. Numerous injuries and a few deaths as a result of such negligence are on record. Similarly, safe spinal and epidural anesthesia demands assiduous attention to the blood pressure and anesthetic levels.

It is practically impossible for an obstetrician to achieve expertise in the use of all the currently available technics for obstetric analgesia and anesthesia. He should, however, master an effective method of systemic analgesia such as provided by meperidine (Demerol) plus promethazine (Phenergan), and become expert in local, pudendal, paracervical, and low spinal ("saddle block") anesthesia. He should also have immediately available general anesthesia appropriate for laparotomy such as that produced by the combination of thiopental (Pentothal), nitrous oxide, and succinylcholine. Continuous lumbar or caudal epidural analgesia and anesthesia are niceties that, when skillfully administered in appropriately selected circumstances, provide elegant and safe relief from the discomfort of parturition. General anesthesia that will effectively and rapidly relax the uterus, such as provided by halothane (Fluothane), may be needed when intrauterine manipulation of the fetus is required to effect delivery or, even more rarely, when the acutely inverted uterus must be replaced.

ANALGESIA AND SEDATION DURING LABOR

Once labor is established, i.e., once the cervix is dilating and uterine contractions cause discomfort, medication for pain relief with a narcotic analgesic drug, such as meperidine, plus one of the tranquilizer drugs, such as promethazine, is usually indicated. With a successful program of analgesia and sedation, the mother should rest quietly between contractions, and although discomfort is felt at the acme of an effective uterine contraction, the pain is not unbearable. Finally, she does not recall labor as a horrifying experience. Appropriate drug selection and administration should accomplish these objectives for the great majority of women in labor without risk to them or their infants.

Meperidine and Promethazine. Meperidine, 50 to 100 mg, with promethazine, 25 mg, can be administered intramuscularly at intervals of 3 to 4 hours. In general, a

smaller dose given more frequently is preferable to a larger one administered less often. Then, if delivery occurs during the next hour or so after injection, the infant is less likely to be depressed by the medication. The size of the mother should also be taken into account in determining the size of the dose.

For predictable effects, it is essential that these and all other medications for intramuscular injection actually be injected into muscle and not subcutaneously. Dundee and co-workers (1974), for example, have reported an illustrative study in which diazepam (Valium) was ordered to be injected intramuscularly. Nurses often used relatively fine (23-gauge), short (3-cm) needles and subsequent drug levels were often low. Undoubtedly, the drug was commonly injected subcutaneously rather than intramuscularly.

A more rapid effect is achieved by giving the agents intravenously, but, in general, not more than 50 mg of meperidine or more than 25 mg of promethazine should be given at one time by this route. Whereas analgesia is maximal about 45 minutes after intramuscular administration, it develops much more rapidly, about 5 minutes, when given intravenously. The times for the depressant effect to develop in the fetus are not far behind. Some physicians advocate the intravenous administration be made during a uterine contraction when, theoretically, blood flow to the uterus and, therefore, the amount of drug delivered to the placenta are reduced.

EFFECT OF MEPERIDINE ON LABOR. Fear has been expressed by some that administration of meperidine to provide obstetric analgesia might at times prolong or even arrest labor. Certainly, with the doses usually used for analgesia, there is no convincing evidence that this occurs. Riffel and co-workers (1973), for example, have quantitatively evaluated the effects of meperidine alone and meperidine plus promethazine on labor, and they observed not a decrease but a slight increase in uterine activity following their injection, confirming and extending the earlier observations by DeVoe and co-workers (1969).

Other Drugs for Relief of Labor Pain.
Other narcotic analgesics, e.g., alphaprodine (Nisentil), are used to provide pain relief during labor, but meperidine is the most popular. A great variety of sedative and tranquilizer agents are administered with a narcotic analgesic or, at times, alone. It is important to recognize that all narcotics and tranquilizers cross the placenta to reach the fetus, where their effects may be deleterious; yet at times the effects are so subtle as to delay their recognition.

Morphine during labor has been nearly abandoned after a period of popularity in which it was used with scopolamine to produce so-called twilight sleep. The combination produced excellent analgesia and amnesia, but the mother sometimes became quite excited, delirious, and hallucinated. Moreover, at birth the infant was more likely to demonstrate apnea, which at times persisted dangerously long.

Narcotic Antagonists.   The administration of meperidine or other narcotics to a woman in labor may impair respiratory function in the newborn infant. Naloxone hydrochloride (Narcan) is a narcotic antagonist capable of reversing respiratory depression induced by opioid narcotics by displacing the narcotic from specific receptors in the central nervous system. Unfortunately, it concomitantly inhibits the analgesia and the euphoria produced by the narcotic. In fact, withdrawal symptoms may be precipitated in recipients who are physically dependent on narcotics. The suggested dose for the newborn infant is 10 μg per kg injected into the umbilical vein. When so injected, naloxone usually acts within two minutes and its beneficial effects persist for at least 30 minutes. Since the depressant action of meperidine may persist beyond this time, the injection of naloxone may have to be repeated after 30 to 45 minutes (Wiener et al., 1977).

In the absence of narcotics, naloxone exhibits little, if any, adverse activity and thereby differs from levallorphan (Lorphan) and nalorphine (Nalline). The last two compounds may, if fact, enhance respiratory depression not caused by narcotic drugs. Therefore, naloxone is the drug of choice for treating narcotic depression in the newborn. Although narcotic antagonists may help relieve respiratory depression from opioid drugs in the newborn infant, it is best to avoid, as much as possible, the administration of narcotics to the mother at times when they might cause respiratory depression in the newborn.

GENERAL ANESTHESIA

The placenta is not a barrier to general anesthetics. Without exception, all anesthetic agents that depress the central nervous system of the mother cross the placenta and depress the central nervous system of the fetus. Another constant hazard with any general anesthetic is aspiration of gastric contents. Fasting before the time of anesthesia is not always an effective safeguard, since fasting gastric juice that is free of particulate matter but strongly acidic can produce fatal aspiration pneumonitis. At the same time, endotracheal intubation is valuable to ensure a satisfactory airway and to minimize the risk of aspiration. With inhalation anesthesia, the concentration of the agent increases in the lung of the pregnant women somewhat more rapidly because the functional residual capacity and residual volume of the lung are reduced (see Chap. 9, p. 240). For the same reason, the residual oxygen in the lung after expiring is appreciably less, a factor of importance when there is delay in intubation and oxygenation after muscle paralysis.

Trained personnel and specialized equipment are mandatory for the safe use of general anesthesia. Airway obstruction and hypoxia must be avoided. General anesthesia should not be induced until all steps preparatory to actual delivery have been completed, so as to minimize transfer of the anesthetic agent to the fetus and, in turn, lessen the likelihood of depression of the newborn.

A unique use for acute obstruction of the airway of the laboring woman is cited by Vogel (1970) in his treatise *American Indian Medicine.* The treatment of protracted labor in Indian women allegedly included binding a cloth tightly over the mouth and nose to bring on partial suffocation. From the struggles that ensued, ''she was in a few seconds delivered." It is hoped that modern women and their infants are never so "aided," inadvertently or otherwise.

Gas Anesthetics. Two anesthetic gases, nitrous oxide and cyclopropane, are used currently in obstetrics.

NITROUS OXIDE. Nitrous oxide is the one gas that is used to provide relief of pain during labor as well as at delivery. This agent produces analgesia and altered consciousness but by itself does not provide true anesthesia. Nitrous oxide does not prolong labor or interfere with uterine contractions. When appropriately administered, satisfactory analgesia often is obtained with a concentration of 50 percent nitrous oxide and 50 percent oxygen, but its satisfactory use requires that personnel be in close attendance. During the second stage of labor, when the woman indicates that a uterine contraction is beginning, a well-fitting mask is placed on her face and she is encouraged to take three deep breaths of the mixture and then to bear down. The concentration of nitrous oxide mixed with oxygen for analgesia should not exceed 70 percent, since concentrations higher than 70 percent may result in maternal as well as fetal hypoxia.

CYCLOPROPANE. At one time cyclopropane was popular in obstetric practice. There are several disadvantages inherent in the use of cyclopropane for abdominal or vaginal delivery. *The gas is highly explosive and must always be given in a closed system.* It is not likely to relax the myometrium sufficiently to allow intrauterine manipulation of the fetus. Unless the time of anesthesia is kept very short, resuscitation of the infant is required.

Volatile Anesthetics. Of the volatile anesthetics, ether, halothane (Fluothane), methoxyflurane (Penthrane), and enflurane (Ethrane) merit consideration. These agents cross the placenta readily and are capable of producing narcosis in the fetus.

ETHER. Since in the hands of inexperienced anesthetists the margin of safety was

usually greater with diethyl ether than with any other general anesthetic, it enjoyed considerable popularity in former years but not now. Ether is unpleasant to the mother; it depresses the fetus-infant; it causes the uterus to relax, thereby enhancing hemorrhage immediately after delivery; and it is explosive. Therefore, it is little used.

HALOTHANE. This potent, nonexplosive agent is of limited use for obstetric anesthesia. Halothane produces remarkable uterine relaxation and should be restricted to those very uncommon situations in which uterine relaxation is a requisite rather than a hazard. Therefore, it is the anesthetic agent of choice for the now very uncommon procedures of internal podalic version, breech decomposition, and replacement of the acutely inverted uterus. As soon as the maneuver has been completed, the administration of halothane should be stopped and immediate efforts made to promote myometrial contraction and retraction to minimize hemorrhage from the placental implantation site. Because of its cardiodepressant and hypotensive effects, halothane may intensify the adverse effects of maternal hypovolemia.

Blood loss associated with abortion has also been found to be increased appreciably when halothane is used for anesthesia (Cullen et al., 1970).

METHOXYFLURANE. This agent is pleasant to take and may be self-administered in low concentration to provide analgesia during the first and second stages of labor, and during delivery. Overdose may be a major complication when methoxyflurane is self-administered for analgesia. Unless the woman is kept under very close surveillance, she may, at times, cover the inhaler and her head with a pillow or sheet and thereby increase appreciably the concentration inhaled. Methoxyflurane may depress myometrial contractility and thereby increase blood loss from the placental implantation site. In the small series studied by Enrile and associates (1973), uterine inertia or atony from methoxyflurane was frequently troublesome.

There is also convincing evidence of dose-related methoxyflurane nephrotoxicity.

Shnider (1979) summarizes the use of methoxyflurane as follows:

It seems advisable to limit the use of methoxyflurane to a relatively small total dose, such as 15 ml, for labor and delivery. Even so, patients with pre-existing renal impairment (such as those with toxemia), and those taking enzyme inducing agents or nephrotoxic drugs, may still be at risk. If dosage limits are observed and patients are carefully selected, the use of methoxyflurane in low concentrations for relatively short periods, seem to be free from hazard.

ENFLURANE. The dose of enflurane which provides analgesia is likely to cause unconsciousness. Also, like halothane, it may cause myometrial depression and increased hemorrhage. It should not be given to anyone suspected of impaired renal function.

TRICHLOROETHYLENE. This compound is no longer available in this country. When a closed circuit system with soda lime was used to provide anesthesia, trichlorethylene formed toxic products. Moreover, deaths were recorded from trichloroethylene self-administered for analgesia during labor.

Intravenous Anesthesia. Intravenous thiopental in obstetrics offers the advantages of ease and extreme rapidity of induction, ample oxygenation, ready controllability, minimal postpartum bleeding, and promptness of recovery without vomiting. The first and last of these advantages make it very popular with patients. Thiopental and similar compounds are poor analgesic agents, and the administration of enough of the drug alone to maintain anesthesia in the mother may cause appreciable depression of the newborn infant. Therefore, the intravenous barbiturates are seldom employed as sole anesthetic agents but are now used in small doses to induce sleep along with nitrous oxide for analgesia and a muscle relaxant. A commonly used technic is the following:

Atropine is given through a well-functioning intravenous system. The mother remains awake breathing oxygen until the operative field is suit-ably scrubbed and draped and the obstetrician is ready to begin vaginal delivery or cesarean section. During this interval, if she is in labor and quite uncomfortable, 50 to 70 percent nitrous oxide plus oxygen may be administered. A small dose of D-tubocurarine is injected intravenously to block muscle fasciculations, followed by thiopental in a dose sufficient to produce unconsciousness. To prevent regurgitation, pressure on the cricoid cartilage is carefully applied by an associate. A paralyzing dose of succinylcholine is now injected. Under direct vision, a cuffed endotracheal tube is placed between the vocal cords into the trachea, the cuff is promptly inflated, and 50 percent to never more than 70 percent nitrous oxide plus oxygen is administered. Delivery—abdominal or vaginal—is now begun. As the uterus is entered for cesarean section, or the head is about to be delivered vaginally, oxygen only is inhaled until the umbilical cord is clamped. After the cord has been clamped, a variety of agents can be used to provide effective analgesia and lack of awareness in the mother. Inhalation of the original concentrations of nitrous oxide plus oxygen, enhanced by a potent analgesic such as morphine or meperidine, very often proves quite effective. Fentanyl (Sublimaze), a narcotic analgesic with a short duration of action, is currently popular for this purpose. Throughout the procedure, succinylcholine is infused as needed.

ASPIRATION DURING GENERAL ANESTHESIA

Pneumonitis from inhalation of gastric contents has been the most common cause of anesthetic death in obstetrics. For example, a survey in Great Britain reported by Crawford (1972) identified inhalation of gastric contents to be associated with at least one-half of all obstetric deaths. The aspirated material from the stomach may contain undigested food and thereby cause airway obstruction which, unless promptly relieved, may prove rapidly fatal. After fasting, gastric juice is likely to be free of particulate matter but extremely acidic and thereby capable of inducing a lethal chemical pneumonitis. The aspiration of strongly acidic gastric juice is probably more common and more dangerous than is the aspiration of gastric contents that contain particulate matter but are somewhat buffered by the food.

Prophylaxis.   Important to effective prophylaxis are (1) fasting, (2) neutralization of gastric acidity before anesthesia, (3) skillful endotracheal intubation, and (4) at the completion of the procedure, extubation with the patient awake and lying on her side with head lowered.

FASTING.   Withholding food for 12 hours should rid the stomach of undigested food but not necessarily of acidic liquid. If general anesthesia is necessary soon after eating, the stomach contents may be emptied by provoking emesis. Many consider such prophylactic treatment to be cruel, yet it may protect the life of the mother and the fetus. Unfortunately, use of apomorphine as an emetic may cause respiratory depression while use of a nasogastric tube with suction to empty the stomach of particulate matter is unpleasant, time-consuming, and not totally effective.

ANTACIDS.   Ingestion of antacids shortly before induction of anesthesia can reduce appreciably the acidity of the gastric juice. It is essential that the antacid disperse promptly throughout all of the gastric contents to neutralize the hydrogen ion effectively, but it is equally important that the antacid, if aspirated, not incite comparably serious pulmonary pathologic problems. A number of antacids are now being used. Magnesium hydroxide suspension (milk of magnesia) is an effective neutralizer (Wheatley et al., 1979). Its laxative effect usually is not marked and therefore not a contraindication to its use. At Parkland Memorial Hospital, 30 ml of magnesium hydroxide suspension is given up to one-half hour before the anticipated time of induction of anesthesia. In theory, 1 ml of milk of magnesia will neutralize nearly 3 mEq of acid, or about 25 ml of gastric juice of pH 1.

INTUBATION.   Various positions have been tried to minimize aspiration before and during intubation and inflation of the cuff, but the disadvantages from positions other than supine outweigh any advantage. Cricoid pressure from the time of induction of anesthesia until intubation is worthwhile but requires a skilled associate. Intubation may be attempted with the mother awake, but to intubate without local anesthesia is barbaric; yet the use of local anesthesia may obtund the laryngeal reflex sufficiently to allow aspiration.

EXTUBATION.   At the completion of the procedure, the endotracheal tube may be safely removed only if the patient is conscious and has been placed in the lateral recumbent position with her head lowered.

Pathology.   Aspiration pneumonia associated with obstetric anesthesia was clearly described by Mendelson in 1946. Teabeaut (1952) demonstrated experimentally that if the pH of aspirated fluid was below 2.5, severe chemical pneumonitis developed. It is of interest that in one study the pH of gastric juice of nearly one-half of women tested intrapartum was below 2.5 (Taylor, Pryse-Davies, 1966).

The right main bronchus usually offers the simplest pathway for aspirated material to reach the lung parenchyma and therefore the right lower lobe is most often involved. In severe cases, there is bilateral widespread involvement.

The woman who aspirates may develop evidence of respiratory distress immediately or as long as several hours after aspiration, depending in part upon the material aspirated, the severity of the process, and the acuity of the attendants. Aspiration of a large amount of solid material causes obvious signs of overt respiratory obstruction. Smaller particles without acidic liquid may lead to patchy atelectasis and later to bronchopneumonia. When highly acidic liquid is inspired, tachypnea, bronchospasm, rhonchi, rales, atelectasis, cyanosis, tachycardia, and hypotension are likely to develop. At the sites of injury, protein-rich fluid containing numerous erythrocytes exudes from capillaries into the lung interstitium and alveoli to cause decreased pulmonary compliance, shunting of blood, and severe hypoxemia. Roentgenographic changes may appear relatively late and be quite variable. Therefore chest x-ray alone should not be used to exclude aspiration of a significant amount of strongly acidic gastric contents.

Cameron and associates (1973) report the overall mortality rate with documented aspiration in a heterogeneous population to be 62 percent and with involvement of more than one lobe, 90 percent!

Treatment. In recent years, the methods recommended for treatment of aspiration have changed appreciably, indicating that previous therapy was not very successful. Suspicion of aspiration of gastric contents demands very close monitoring of the patient for evidence of any pulmonary damage.

SUCTION AND BRONCHOSCOPY. As much as possible of the inhaled fluid should be immediately wiped out of the mouth and removed from the pharynx and trachea by suction. Saline lavage, rather than being beneficial, probably further disseminates the acid throughout the lung. If large particulate matter is inspired, prompt bronchoscopy is indicated to relieve airway obstruction. Otherwise, bronchoscopy not only is unnecessary but may contribute to morbidity and mortality.

CORTICOSTEROIDS. There has been considerable enthusiasm for administering corticosteroids in very large pharmacologic doses in an attempt to maintain cell integrity in the presence of strong acid. There is no clinical evidence that such therapy is unequivocally beneficial (Bynum, Pierce, 1976), nor do experimental studies support the thesis that appreciable benefits accrue from the use of corticosteroids. Nonetheless, the clinical impression of some has been that the immediate intravenous administration of 500 mg of methylprednisolone sodium succinate (Solu-Medrol), with repeated doses of 250 mg every 8 hours for 24 hours, is beneficial.

OXYGEN AND VENTILATION. Oxygen delivered through an endotracheal tube in increased concentration by intermittent positive pressure is often required to raise and maintain the arterial PO_2 at 60 mm Hg. Frequent suction is necessary to remove secretions including edema fluid. Mechanical ventilation that produces positive end-expiratory pressure may prove beneficial by preventing on expiration the complete collapse of the now surfactant-poor lung and by retarding the outpouring of protein-rich fluid from pulmonary capillaries into the interstitium and alveoli.

ANTIBIOTICS. Although the likelihood of bacterial contamination and infection from aspiration is appreciable, the use of antibiotics prophylactically remains controversial (Bynum, Pierce, 1976). Bartlett et al. (1974) identified anaerobic bacteria in 50 of 54 cases of pneumonia that was caused by aspiration. They concluded that anaerobes play a key role in most cases of infection after aspiration and suggested the use of clindomycin or chloramphenicol for those anaerobes that are not sensitive to penicillin.

Anesthetic Gas Exposure and Pregnancy Outcome. Sufficient data have accumulated to create concern over the welfare of the embryo and fetus of pregnant women who work in operating rooms where they are exposed chronically to anesthetic gases. In some reports, but not all, the abortion rate is about twice that for unexposed personnel and the malformation rate about 1½ times greater (Knill-Jones et al., 1975). More recently in England and Wales, a comparison has been made between pregnancy outcomes of women doctors exposed to anesthetic gases during pregnancy and those working but not so exposed. Conception that occurred while the woman was actively engaged in anesthesiology resulted in somewhat smaller babies (3347 g vs. 3388 g), an increased frequency of cardiovascular malformation (1.4 percent vs. 0.4 percent), and of stillbirth (1.7 percent vs. 0.8 percent). Spontaneous abortions were the same (13.8 percent) in both groups (Pharoah et al., 1977). Ericson and Källén (1979) found no differences in pregnancies of operating room workers in Sweden.

SENSORY INNERVATION OF GENITAL TRACT

Innervation of Uterus. Pain in the first stage of labor stems largely from the uterus, the sensory innervation of which is derived primarily from the sympathetic nervous system. Visceral sensory fibers from the uterus, cervix, and upper vagina traverse from the uterus, travel through *Frankenhäuser's ganglion* to the pelvic plexus, and thence to the middle and superior hypogastric plexuses. From there, the fibers travel in the lumbar and lower thoracic sympathetic chains to enter the spinal cord through the white rami communicantes associated with the tenth, eleventh, and twelfth thoracic and first lumbar nerves. Early in the first stage of labor, the pain of uterine contractions is transmitted through predominantly the eleventh and twelfth thoracic nerves.

The motor pathways leave the spinal cord at the level of the seventh and eighth thoracic vertebrae. Theoretically, any method of sensory block that does not also block the motor pathways to the uterus can be used for obstetric analgesia.

Innervation of Lower Genital Tract. Although painful contractions of the uterus continue during the second stage of labor, much of the pain of vaginal delivery arises in the lower genital tract. Painful stimuli from the lower genital tract are transmitted in large part through the *pudendal nerve,* the peripheral branches of which provide sensory innervation to the perineum, anus, and the more medial and inferior parts of the vulva and clitoris. The pudendal nerve passes across the posterior surface of the sacrospinous ligament just as the ligament attaches to the ischial spine (Figs. 18-1,2). The sensory fibers of the pudendal nerve are derived from the ventral branches of the second, third, and fourth sacral nerves.

REGIONAL ANALGESIA AND ANESTHESIA

Anesthetic Agents. A variety of compounds are currently used in obstetrics to produce local or regional analgesia and anesthesia. While their appropriate use almost

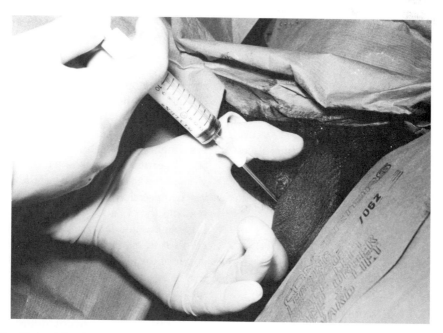

FIG. 18-1. Injecting local anesthetic in immediate vicinity of pudendal nerve beneath the left ischial spine.

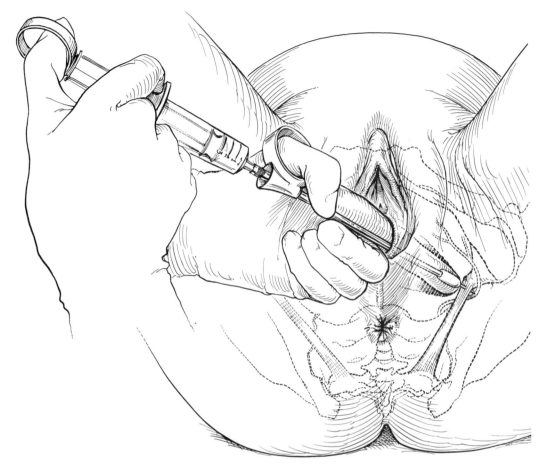

FIG. 18-2. Local infiltration of the pudendal nerve. Transvaginal technic showing needle passing through the sacrospinous ligament. A needle guard is usually used.

always proves to be safe for both the mother and the fetus-infant, the potential exists for toxic reactions that may prove life-threatening. Perhaps the least common toxic reaction, but often terrifying, is the induction of convulsions from high circulating levels of the compound. Since convulsions may follow any route of administration, management of this complication is considered now.

CENTRAL NERVOUS SYSTEM TOXICITY. Symptoms include lightheadedness, dizziness, slurred-speech, metallic taste, numbness of tongue and mouth, muscle fasciculation, loss of consciousness, and generalized convulsions. Quickly and simultaneously the convulsions should be controlled, an airway established, and oxygen delivered. Succi-

nylcholine abolishes the peripheral manifestations of the convulsions and allows endotracheal intubation. Thiopental or diazepam acts centrally to inhibit convulsions. Maternal hypotension and impaired uteroplacental perfusion is combatted by turning the woman toward the left side to relieve aortocaval compression, the rapid intravenous administration of balanced salt solution, and the intravenous administration of ephedrine. Fetal distress, manifested by either late decelerations of the heart rate or persistent bradycardia, may develop as the consequence of maternal hypoxia and lactic acidosis induced by the convulsions and of drug-induced fetal cardiac depression, hypotension, and impaired uteroplacental perfusion. With arrest of the convulsions, the administration of oxygen and the application of the other supportive measures outlined above, the fetus is likely to recover more quickly in utero than if immediately delivered by cesarean section. Moreover, maternal well-being is usually better served by waiting until the intensity of the hypoxia and metabolic acidosis have diminished. If after several minutes the status of the fetus has not improved in response to the above measures, delivery is usually indicated. Personnel and facilities for instituting cardiopulmonary resuscitation should be immediately available for both the mother and the infant.

The various groups of local anesthetic agents, their structure-activity relationship, disposition, and toxicity have been considered in detail by Fishburne (1975), Salts and associates (1976), and Covino (1978).

Local Infiltration. This technic is of negligible value for analgesia during labor but has been employed for delivery. From the standpoint of safety, local infiltration anesthesia is preeminent. Its advantages have been summarized by Greenhill (1943) as follows:

> There is practically no anesthetic mortality. Fetal mortality or hypoxia from direct effect of the anesthetic agent is absent. Simplicity of administration is obvious. Uterine contractions are not impaired. There is no need to hurry through an operation. The toxic effects are minimal.

Unfortunately, pain relief with vaginal delivery and especially with laparotomy is usually far from complete.

Transvaginal Pudendal Block. A tubular director that allows 1.0 to 1.5 cm of a 22-gauge needle that is 15-cm long to protrude from its tip is used to guide the needle into position over the pudendal nerve (Fig. 18-1). The end of the director is placed against the vaginal mucosa just beneath the tip of the ischial spine. The needle is inserted through the mucosa and a submucosal wheal is made with 1 ml of 1 percent lidocaine solution or an equivalent dose of another local anesthetic with similar high tissue penetration

and rapid action. Aspiration is attempted before this and all subsequent injections to guard against intravascular infusion. The needle is then advanced until it touches the sacrospinous ligament, which is infiltrated with 3 ml of 1 percent lidocaine solution. The needle is advanced further, and as it pierces the loose areolar tissue behind the ligament, the resistance of the plunger decreases (Fig. 18-2). Another 3 ml of the anesthetic solution is injected in the region. Next, the needle is withdrawn into the guide, the tip of the guide is moved to just above the ischial spine, and the needle is inserted through the mucosa. After again aspirating to avoid intravascular injection, the rest of the 10 ml of solution is deposited.

Within 3 to 4 minutes from the time of injection, the successful pudendal block will allow pinching of the lower vagina and posterior vulva bilaterally without pain. It is often of benefit before pudendal block to infiltrate directly the fourchette, perineum, and adjacent vagina at the site where the episiotomy is to be made with 5 to 10 ml of 1 percent lidocaine solution. Then, if delivery occurs before pudendal block becomes effective, an episiotomy can be made without pain.

Pudendal block usually works well for spontaneous delivery but is not likely to provide adequate anesthesia for forceps delivery. Moreover, anesthesia limited to pudendal block is inadequate after delivery for complete visualization of the cervix and upper vagina or manual exploration of the uterine cavity. Under these circumstances, the addition of an intravenously administered narcotic analgesic such as 50 mg of meperidine, may provide appreciable, although not total, relief from the pain of examination. *With such an approach, caution must be exercised not to give narcotics and sedatives in doses or combinations that might so obtund the woman that she would suffer airway obstruction or aspiration.* Instead, general anesthesia should be administered by trained individuals.

COMPLICATIONS. The intravascular injection of the local anesthetic may cause serious systemic toxicity characterized by stimulation of the cerebral cortex leading to convulsions and depression of the medulla to cause respiratory depression. A troublesome hematoma, the consequence of perforation of a blood vessel, is most likely to occur when there is defective coagulation such as that induced by heparin or by severe placental abruption. Rarely, a severe infection may originate at the injection site. The infection tends to spread to the region posterior to the hip joint, into the gluteal musculature, or into the retroposal space (Svancarek and associates, 1977). Deaths and severe permanent impairment in some survivors have been recorded (Wenger, Gitchell, 1973).

Paracervical Block. This technic serves to relieve pain of uterine contractions, but inasmuch as the pudendal nerves are not blocked, additional anesthesia is required for delivery. Since the anesthetic is relatively short-acting, the paracervical block may have to be repeated during labor.

TECHNIC.   Asepsis is essential. A tubular director that allows no more than 0.5 cm of the tip of a 20-gauge, 15-cm (6-inch) needle to protrude beyond the guard's tip is placed in the lateral vaginal fornix and the needle is passed through the director and vaginal mucosa. After aspirating to make sure that the needle has not entered the maternal circulation, including that of a low-lying placenta, and making certain to avoid the presenting part of the fetus, the local anesthetic solution is injected into one of the lateral fornices in the immediate vicinity of Frankenhäuser's ganglion to block visceral afferent pain fibers. The fetal heart rate is then monitored for 5 minutes and, if there is no fetal bradycardia, the injection is repeated on the opposite side. It seems to make little difference whether the injections are made at the "3 o'clock" and "9 o'clock" position, or somewhat more posterior nearer the uterosacral ligaments. The duration of action typically is 1 to 2 hours. The more commonly used anesthetic solutions are 1 percent lidocaine or mepivacaine (Carbocaine), or a 0.25 percent bupivacaine (Marcaine), with 5 to no more than 10 ml injected on each side. Jägerhorn (1975) recommended an injection depth of

no more than 3 mm and the use of two injection sites on each side to reduce the possibility of a larger bolus being injected into a parametrial vein or the fetal scalp.

COMPLICATIONS.   While good to excellent pain relief is usually achieved from paracervical block during the first stage of labor, *fetal bradycardia* is a complication. Most reports indicate a 10 to 25 percent incidence of this complication. While several investigators stress that fetal bradycardia is not a sign of fetal asphyxia, since the bradycardia is usually transient and the newborns are in most instances vigorous at birth, there are reports in which fetal scalp blood pH and Apgar scores were found at times to be lower than in the control group. The effect on the fetus may be the consequence of transplacental transfer of the anesthetic agent or its metabolites and, in turn, a depressant effect on the heart. Greiss and co-workers (1976) and Fishburne and co-workers (1979), however, based on studies in pregnant ewes, believe that the fetal bradycardia results from decreased placental perfusion as the consequence of drug-induced uterine vasoconstriction and myometrial hypertonus. Teramo (1971) has concluded that 200 mg of mepivacaine can be injected for paracervical block with relatively great safety provided the fetus is in no way compromised before the application of the block. At Parkland Memorial Hospital, paracervical block is restricted to labors in which fetal compromise is neither suspected nor anticipated. Serious adverse effects from paracervical block have thus far been avoided.

Paracervical anesthesia to accomplish dilatation and curettage for abortion is described elsewhere (see Chap. 24, p. 604).

Spinal Anesthesia.   Introduction of a local anesthetic into the subarachnoid space to effect spinal anesthesia continues to be popular for both uncomplicated cesarean section and vaginal delivery of normal women of low parity. It must be always kept in mind that because of the smaller subarachnoid space during pregnancy, the same amount of anesthetic agent in the same volume of solution produces a much higher spinal blockade in parturients than in nonpregnant women. The smaller subarachnoid space is the consequence most likely of engorgement of the internal vertebral venous plexus which, in turn, is the consequence of compression by the uterus of the inferior vena cava and adjacent large veins below the level of the diaphragm.

VAGINAL DELIVERY. A popular form of anesthesia for delivery is low spinal block with a level of anesthesia to the tenth thoracic dermatome (T10), which normally corresponds at the midline to the level of the umbilicus. Blockade to T10 provides excellent relief from the pain of uterine contractions. The term *saddle block* has been applied to this level of anesthesia, but incorrectly since the area of skin anesthetized is appreciably greater than that which would be in contact with a saddle.

Nearly all local anesthetic agents have been used for spinal anesthesia, but for many years one that has proved quite satisfactory for vaginal delivery is tetracaine (Pontocaine) in a dose of 4 mg already dissolved in 2 ml of 6 percent solution of dextrose in water. The anesthetic should not be administered for vaginal delivery until the cervix is fully dilated and all other criteria for safe forceps delivery have been fulfilled. Spinal anesthesia is not recommended before this time because of the frequency of disruption of orderly labor by the anesthetic and, as the consequence, a complicated delivery traumatic to the infant and the mother. With 4 mg of tetracaine, satisfactory anesthesia in the lower vagina and perineum persists for about an hour.

CESAREAN SECTION. For cesarean section, a higher level of spinal sensory blockade is essential to at least the level of the eighth thoracic dermatome (T8), which in the midline is just below the xiphoid process of the sternum. Therefore, a somewhat larger dose of anesthetic agent *relative to that used for vaginal delivery* is necessary. This increases the frequency and the intensity of the complications just cited. Depending upon the mother's size, 8 to 10 mg, but most often 8 mg,

of tetracaine is administered. Undue delay between intrathecal injection of anesthetic agent and delivery of the infant should be avoided if a safe dose of the anesthetic drug is to be used yet have spinal anesthesia of sufficient intensity and duration to allow completion of abdominal delivery without serious discomfort. Therefore, catheterization of the bladder and the shaving of the operative field should be done before the anesthetic is administered.

TECHNIC. While receiving an isotonic salt solution through an 18-gauge needle or plastic catheter to minimize hypotension from sympathetic blockade, the woman is placed in either the sitting, or less often the lateral, decubitus positon. The lower back is then scrubbed and draped in sterile fashion. With a stock solution of 1 percent lidocaine and a standard 26-gauge needle on a 2-ml syringe, a skin wheal is raised in the midline over the interspace between the third and fourth lumbar vertebrae. Then, a 22-gauge needle and the same syringe may be used to infiltrate the interspace to the depth of the ligamentum flavum. Next, a diminution of the lumbar spinal curvature is effected by an assistant holding the woman in complete flexion. A midline intrathecal puncture is made with a 22- to 26-gauge, 3½-inch spinal needle with the bevel directed downward. While continuing to observe strict asepsis the anesthetic solution, in the absence of a uterine contraction, in injected in a steady stream with constant pressure over about 5 seconds. The spinal needle is removed and the woman is immediately placed in the supine position for cesarean section. The desirable level of anesthesia is obtained by manipulating the head of the table above or below the horizontal plane.

For vaginal delivery, since a lower level of block is desired, the woman is allowed to sit up for about 45 seconds and then placed supine.

COMPLICATIONS WITH SPINAL ANESTHESIA. A number of complications may ensue:

HYPOTENSION.   Maternal   hypotension

may occur very soon after the injection of the anesthetic agent. The hypotension is the consequence of vasodilatation from sympathetic blockade compounded by obstructed venous return because of compression by the uterus of the vena cava and adjacent large veins. Importantly, in the supine position, even in the absence of maternal hypotension, placental blood flow is reduced significantly (Kaupilla et al., 1980). Marx and co-workers (1969) have provided confirmatory evidence that the infant at birth is better biochemically as well as clinically when hypotension from spinal anesthesia for cesarean section is prevented rather than treated. Important to prophylaxis and to treatment of spinal hypotension are (1) uterine elevation and displacement to the left of the abdomen, (2) acute hydration with a balanced salt solution, and (3) at the first sign of a decrease in blood pressure, the intravenous injection of 10 to 15 mg of ephedrine.

TOTAL SPINAL BLOCKADE. Complete spinal blockade with respiratory paralysis may complicate spinal anesthesia. Most often total spinal blockade is the consequence of administration of a dose of anesthetic agent far in excess of that tolerated by pregnant women. Hypotension and apnea promptly develop and must be immediately treated to prevent cardiac arrest. The undelivered woman should be turned toward her left side. Effective ventilation is urged, through an endotracheal tube, when possible, to protect against aspiration. When the woman is hypotensive, ephedrine is urged. Elevation of the legs will increase venous return and help combat hypotension. Preparations should be made for cardiac resuscitation in the event of cardiac arrest.

ANXIETY AND DISCOMFORT. It is imperative that everyone in the operating room remember at all times that the woman under regional anesthesia is awake. In every case, great care must be exercised over what is said and how the many activities associated with care of the mother and fetus are performed lest the mother interpret remarks or actions as an indication that she or her fetus is in jeopardy, or that there is inappropriate concern for her welfare. The woman is usually aware of the surgical manipulation, identifying each surgical maneuver as a feeling of pressure. She is, of course, painfully quite aware of any manipulation above the level of the spinal sensory blockade.

At times, the degree of pain relief from the spinal anesthetic is inadequate, making the operation a most unpleasant experience. In this circumstance, a significant measure of relief can be provided before delivery of the infant by administering 50 to 70 percent nitrous oxide with oxygen. Immediately after clamping the cord, a variety of technics can be employed to provide effective analgesia. Morphine, meperidine, or fentanyl given intravenously at this time often provides excellent analgesia and euphoria as the operation is being completed.

SPINAL (POSTPUNCTURE) HEADACHES. Leakage of cerebrospinal fluid from the site of puncture of the meninges is the major factor in the genesis of spinal headache. Presumably, when the woman sits or stands, the diminished volume of cerebrospinal fluid allows traction on pain-sensitive central nervous system structures. The likelihood of this unpleasant complication can be reduced by using a small-gauge spinal needle and avoiding multiple punctures of the meninges. Placing the woman absolutely flat on her back for many hours has been recommended to prevent postspinal headache, but there is no good evidence that this procedure is very effective. Hyperhydration has been claimed to be of value, without compelling evidence to support its use. Creation of a "blood patch" has been reported to be efficacious; in this, a few milliliters of the woman's blood without anticoagulant is injected epidurally at the site of the spinal tap. Saline similarly injected in larger volumes has also been claimed to provide relief. Abdominal support with a girdle or abdominal binder does seem to afford relief and is worth trying (Beck, 1973). At Parkland Memorial Hospital, treatment of spinal headache consists of (1) a full explanation to the woman of the cause of the headache, (2) bed rest, (3) the use of analgesics such as codeine orally or meperidine intramuscularly, and (4) the application of an abdominal binder. Typically, the headache is remarkably improved by the third day and absent by the fifth.

BLADDER DYSFUNCTION. With spinal anesthesia, bladder sensation is likely to be obtunded and bladder emptying impaired during the first few hours after delivery. As a consequence, bladder distension is a frequent complication of the puerperium, especially if appreciable volumes of intravenous fluid have been or are being administered. The combination of (1) infusion of a liter or more of aqueous fluid, (2) neural blockade from epidural or spinal anesthesia, (3) antidiuretic effect of oxytocin infused for a time after delivery and then stopped, (4) discomfort from a sizable episiotomy, (5) failure to observe the woman very closely for bladder distension, and (6) failure to relieve bladder distension promptly by catheterization is very likely to lead to quite troublesome bladder dysfunction and urinary tract infection.

OXYTOCICS AND HYPERTENSION. Paradoxically, hypertension from ergonovine (Ergotrate) or methylergonovine (Methergine) injected following delivery is most common in women who have received a spinal or epidural block.

ARACHNOIDITIS AND MENINGITIS. No longer are the ampules of local anesthetic stored in alcohol, formalin, or other highly toxic media. Needles and catheters are now rarely subjected to cleaning by chemical treatment so that they can be reused. Instead, one-time disposable equipment is used. These current practices, coupled with strict aseptic technic, have made meningitis and arachnoiditis rarities.

CONTINUOUS SPINAL ANESTHESIA. Use of continuous spinal anesthesia, in which an indwelling catheter is inserted into the subarachnoid space, allows the anesthetic to be administered in fractional doses. This technic minimizes the likelihood of many of the serious adverse effects that may promptly follow a larger dose of anesthetic by single injection, especially total spinal block. Also, for longer procedures, the anesthetic drug can be replenished as needed. A hole through the meninges large enough initially for a needle containing the indwelling catheter and the perpetuation of the hole by the continued presence of the catheter are very likely to predispose to troublesome postspinal headache.

CONTRAINDICATIONS TO THE USE OF SPINAL ANESTHESIA. The common serious complication from spinal anesthesia is hypotension. The supine position late in pregnancy commonly predisposes to a reduction in return of blood from veins below the level of the large pregnant uterus and, in turn, a reduction in cardiac output (see Chap. 9, p. 238). Moreover, sympathetic blockade from spinal anesthesia is usually extensive and leads to further pooling of blood in dilated blood vessels below the level of the blockade, especially in the lower extremities. Therefore, obstetric complications that in themselves predispose to maternal hypovolemia and hypotension are contraindications to the use of spinal anesthesia. *Severe falls in blood pressure can be predicted when spinal anesthesia is used in the presence of hemorrhage or overt pregnancy-induced hypertension.*

The cardiovascular effects of spinal anesthesia in the presence of acute blood loss but in the absence of the hemodynamic effects of pregnancy have been investigated by Kennedy and co-workers (1968). In 15 nonpregnant volunteers, spinal anesthesia to a T5 sensory level was induced twice, the second time after a phlebotomy of 10 ml per kg. In the case of subarachnoid block without hemorrhage, the mean arterial blood pressure fell 10 percent, while cardiac output rose slightly. In the case of hemorrhage without subarachnoid block, the mean blood pressure fell to the same degree and again the cardiac output rose slightly. However, when there was subarachnoid block after a modest hemorrhage, the mean arterial pressure fell 29 percent and cardiac output fell 15 percent. Undoubtedly, the presence of a large pregnant uterus serves only to magnify appreciably these deleterious changes from spinal anesthesia after hemorrhage.

Disorders of coagulation and defective hemostasis preclude the use of spinal anesthesia. Spinal anesthesia is contraindicated when the skin or underlying tissues at the site of needle entry is infected and neurologic disorders are usually considered to be a contraindication, if for no other reason than exacerbation of the neurologic disease might be attributed to the spinal anesthetic.

EPIDURAL (PERIDURAL) BLOCK

Relief from the pain of uterine contractions and delivery, vaginal or abdominal, can be accomplished by injecting a suitable local anesthetic agent into the epidural or peridural space. The epidural space, in effect, is a potential space that contains areolar tissue, fat, lymphatics, and the internal venous plexus, which becomes engorged during pregnancy so that it reduces appreciably the volume of the epidural space. It is limited peripherally by the ligamentum flavum and centrally by the dura matter, and it extends from the base of the skull to almost the end of the sacrum. The portal of entry into the epidural space for obstetric analgesia and anesthesia is through either a lumbar intravertebral space or through the sacral hiatus and sacral canal. The injection may be solitary or, much more often, repetitive through an indwelling plastic catheter.

Continuous Lumbar Epidural Block.
Complete anesthesia for the pain of labor and vaginal delivery necessitates a block from T10 to S5. For abdominal delivery, a block is essential from at least T8 to S1. The spread of epidural anesthesia will depend upon the location of the catheter tip, the dose and volume of anesthetic agent used, and whether the woman is placed in the head-down, hori-

zontal, or head-up position. It is important that the meninges not be perforated. Otherwise, the injected anesthetic enters the subarachnoid space, and in the dose used to achieve epidural anesthesia it may rapidly produce total spinal blockade.

TECHNIC.   The patient is placed on her left side with shoulders parallel and legs partially flexed. No attempt is made to keep the spinal column convex, since that position reduces the peridural space and stretches the dura, rendering it more susceptible to puncture. If the interspaces of the patient are small, the sitting position may be more advantageous.

The back is cleaned and draped as for a spinal puncture. The skin, the interspinous ligament, and the ligamentum flavum are successively infiltrated with the same anesthetic solution that is used for the continuous block. An 18-gauge thin-walled Tuohy needle is introduced into any of the lumbar interspaces. The needle is blunted, but has a sharp stylet in place to facilitate piercing the skin, subcutaneous tissue, and interspinous ligament. The site chosen is frequently the lumbar area, since the largest peridural spaces are found there. The needle should be placed directly into the center of the interspace without anterior or posterior deviation. The needle should engage the ligamentum flavum, which is the most important landmark for a peridural injection. Unless the needle pierces the middle of the ligamentum flavum, the center of the peridural space will not be entered, and a catheter cannot be passed with ease.

The "air-rebound" method for ascertaining the depth of insertion of the needle for peridural anesthesia is regarded by some anesthesiologists as the most reliable sign. The needle is inserted and guided by palpation into an interspace until the blunt bevel impinges on the ligamentum flavum. The location is then verified by injection of a small amount of air. If the needle is situated properly on the ligament, there is rebound of the plunger of the syringe, and the depth of the needle at the ligament is reasonably certain; its advancement approximately another millimeter results in entry into the extradural space. Air may then be injected with ease and no cerebrospinal fluid can be aspirated.

When air is injected into the peridural space, however, the plunger of the syringe actually falls into place. As the needle is advanced through the ligamentum flavum, frequent minute "air tests" are made with a small syringe to ascertain when the negative pressure in the peridural space is encountered. Entrance into the peridural space is often evidenced by the release of resistance as the blunt Tuohy needle passes through the dense ligamentum flavum.

When the Tuohy needle has been properly placed and no spinal fluid is aspirated, a plastic catheter is introduced through the needle into the peridural space. The catheter is directed either cephalad or caudad, depending upon the somatic segments involved in transmitting the painful impulses. Its passage sometimes elicits a distinct hyperesthetic response in the leg, hip, or back, if the soft tip of the catheter touches a nerve in the peridural space. Indications of proper placement of the catheter in the peridural space include the following:

1. The ease with which air can be injected after the ligamentum has been penetrated.
2. Hyperesthesia upon passage of the catheter into the peridural space in the absence of spinal fluid.
3. Easy passage of the catheter either up or down the peridural space in the absence of spinal fluid.
4. Absence of somatic anesthesia following a test dose of anesthetic agent to rule out spinal anesthesia. Shnider and associates (1979) recommended two test doses.
5. Prompt somatic anesthesia after a larger dose of anesthetic.

Continuous Caudal Analgesia and Anesthesia. At the lower end of the sacrum, on its posterior surface, there is a foramen resulting from the nonclosure of the laminae of the last sacral vertebra. It is screened by a thin layer of fibrous tissue. This foramen, called the sacral hiatus, leads to the caudal canal or caudal space, which is actually the lowest extent of the epidural, or peridural, space. Through the caudal space, a rich network of sacral nerves passes downward after having emerged from the dural sac a few inches higher. The dural sac separates the caudal canal from the spinal cord and its surrounding fluid.

A suitable anesthetic solution that fills the caudal canal may abolish the sensation of pain carried via the sacral nerves and anesthetize the pelvis, producing anesthesia suitable for vaginal delivery. Higher levels with continu-

ous caudal technic provide both analgesia in the first and second stages and anesthesia for delivery.

TECHNIC. When the patient is in active labor with the cervix at least 3 to 4 cm dilated, she is placed on her side in the Sims position. The sacral and coccygeal areas are prepared with an antiseptic solution. Considerable experience is necessary for accurate palpation of the sacral hiatus. A small skin wheal is made over the area with an anesthetic solution. Using a slightly longer needle, the solution is carried down and injected into the fascia over the sacral hiatus. A thin-walled 18-gauge needle with a short bevel is directed toward the sacral hiatus and through the sacrococcygeal membrane. The procedure must not be attempted if the sacral hiatus is not clearly identified. Otherwise, the needle may bypass the sacrum and penetrate the head of the fetus with disastrous consequences. The needle is then depressed and inserted into the canal superiorly for a distance of approximately 3 cm. The stylet is removed and a polyethylene or polyvinyl catheter is then passed through the needle and into the caudal canal for a distance of 5 cm. Once the catheter has passed the tip of the needle, care should be taken not to withdraw the catheter through the needle lest the catheter be severed. After placement of the catheter, the needle is withdrawn. The catheter is then attached to a closed system for administration of almost any of the local anesthetics. The catheter is taped in place. The patient is then permitted free movement. A test dose of one of the anesthetic solutions is injected slowly and after 5 minutes the patient is tested for spinal anesthesia. If she can move both legs freely and there is no sensory impairment, the caudal analgesia dose is then administered. The dose is repeated as necessary.

COMPLICATIONS. Both lumbar and caudal epidural analgesia for labor and anesthesia for delivery may provide most pleasant relief from the pain of labor. There are certain problems inherent in their use, however:

1. *Inadvertent Spinal Anesthesia.* Puncture of the dura along with inadvertent spinal anesthesia is always a potential complication, so personnel and facilities must be immediately available to manage the complications of high spinal anesthesia. Postspinal

headache is a less serious but troublesome complication of inadvertent entry into the subarachnoid space.

2. *Ineffective Anesthesia.* The extent to which pain relief can be obtained with lumbar epidural analgesia varies. In the best of circumstances, according to Crawford (1979), about 85 percent of parturient women are free of pain, 12 percent experience partial relief, and 3 percent have no relief whatsoever. Nonetheless, establishment of effective pain relief with maximum safety takes time. Consequently, in case of rapid labor, the potential for pain relief during labor and for delivery is not realized. Therefore, epidural anesthesia for women of higher parity in active labor is likely to prove not worth the bother, risk, and expense.

If the epidural anesthesia is allowed to dissipate before another injection of anesthetic drug, subsequent anesthesia may be delayed, incomplete, or both.

At times, perineal anesthesia for delivery is difficult to obtain, especially with the lumbar epidural technic. When this condition is encountered, Akamatsu and Bonica (1974) recommend use of a second catheter to achieve low caudal block. Insertion of a second catheter, of course, increases many of the risks being described. For this problem, others have suggested addition of low spinal ("saddle block") anesthesia, pudendal block, or systemic analgesia or anesthesia.

3. *Hypotension.* Epidural anesthesia by blocking the sympathetic tracts may cause hypotension. In the nonhypertensive and normally hypervolemic pregnant woman, hypotension induced by epidural anesthesia usually can be prevented by rapid infusion of balanced salt solution or treated successfully as described for spinal anesthesia. It is important that with each injection of anesthetic the blood pressure be measured every 2 minutes for the next 20 minutes. Ueland and co-workers (1972) have confirmed by a number of physiologic measurements that hypotension with epidural anesthesia in *normal*

pregnant women usually is modest and easily corrected.

4. *Central Nervous Stimulation.* Convulsions are an uncommon but serious complication, the immediate management of which has been described above. Tahir and co-workers (1975) have emphasized that late in pregnancy epidural veins are thin-walled and engorged which predisposes to perforation by the catheter and intravenous injection of the anesthetic agent. Treatment is described above.

5. *Effect on Labor.* Epidural block induced prior to well-established labor may be followed by desultory labor. The precise role played by epidural anesthesia in this phenomenon is not clear, since this sequence of events is seen in the absence of epidural analgesia. Lowensohn and co-workers (1974) report significant depression of uterine activity for about 30 minutes following the epidural injection of lidocaine. Akamatsu and Bonica (1974) suggest that epinephrine injected with the anesthetic agent may impair labor. During the second stage of labor, epidural anesthesia that provides effective pain relief is likely to reduce appreciably maternal explusive efforts. As a consequence, epidural anesthesia may lead to delay, or less frequently to failure of the descent of the presenting part and spontaneous rotation to the most favorable position for delivery, i.e., the occiput anterior position. Therefore, with epidural anesthesia there is likely to be an increased incidence of deliveries by use of midforceps and forceps rotations.

CONTRAINDICATIONS. As with spinal anesthesia, these include actual or anticipated *maternal hemorrhage, overt hypertension, infection* at or near the sites for puncture, and suspicion of *neurologic disease.*

Disagreements persist over the use of epidural anesthesia in the presence of *hypertension.* Some obstetric anesthesiologists urge regional analgesia and anesthesia for women with overt hypertension. Marx (1974), for example, has contended that by use of regional anesthesia maternal circulatory and cerebrospinal fluid pressure responses to painful uterine contractions are reduced and the hazard of hypertensive crisis is minimized. For slowly progressing labor, she recommends a double catheter extradural block, but for labor with rapid progress, possibly a spinal block. The intrigue for the use of regional anesthesia in hypertensive states complicating pregnancy undoubtedly stems from the fact that the mother is hypertensive and the blood pressure is very often lowered by the regional anesthetic. This attitude prevails even though the mechanism by which the blood pressure is lowered is probably no more physiologic than phlebotomy and causes a fall in *blood flow* through vital organs. For this reason, in over 150 consecutive cases of antepartum or intrapartum *eclampsia* at Parkland Memorial Hospital, regional anesthesia has been deliberately avoided. Instead, local or pudendal block plus nitrous oxide analgesia were used for easy vaginal deliveries and general anesthesia with thiopental, succinylcholine, and nitrous oxide was used for the occasional difficult vaginal delivery and for cesarean sections. All mothers survived (Chap. 27, p. 691).

Psychoprophylaxis for Pain Relief.
In 1944 Grantley Dick Read provided a text in which he emphasized that the intensity of pain with labor is related to a large degree to emotional tensions. He urged that women be well informed about the physiology of parturition and the various hospital procedures to which they would be subjected during labor and delivery. He also urged training in breathing and muscle relaxation be instituted well in advance of labor.

Subsequently, Lamaze (1970) described his psychoprophylactic method of childbirth which emphasizes that childbirth is a natural physiologic process and that pain can be minimized by appropriate training in breathing and appropriate psychologic support.

Read and Lamaze, through their pioneer writings and the "satisfied customers" who have used their methods, have had considerable impact on the use of potent analgesic, sedative, and amnesic drugs during labor and

general anesthesia for delivery. Undoubtedly, by minimizing fear, the discomfort from contractions is minimized. The presence of an involved, supportive father, of a conscientious labor attendant, and a considerate obstetrician who instills confidence contributes greatly to accomplishing this goal (see Chap. 17, p. 405).

Although psychoprophylaxis will not be completely successful in many women, it should be available for those who desire it and are willing to make the effort. At the same time, women who attempt psychoprophylaxis but find the discomforts of labor to be too great should not be denied relief provided by appropriate analgesics. It is not unusual for Lamaze prepared women in the United States to receive some narcotic analgesia during labor and nerve block anesthesia for delivery, usually local, pudendal, or epidural (Hughey et al., 1978).

Abdominal Decompression. In 1959, Heyns introduced a large plastic shield that produced negative pressure when applied to the abdomen of the parturient. He claimed that the device reduced the pain and duration of labor and increased the oxygenation of the fetus, thus producing infants with high IQs. These claims have not been substantiated. Castellanos and colleagues (1968) were unable to show that the decompression apparatus relieved the pains of labor. Liddicoat (1968), in a controlled study, was unable to find a difference in IQs between children born to mothers who used the apparatus and those who did not.

Acupuncture. Although the contemporary American woman is likely to be subjected to a multitude of needle punctures during labor and delivery, so far there are few reports concerned with formal application of acupuncture. Bonica (1974) commented that in one small group of obstetric patients relief of pain was good in about one-third, partial in a third, and poor in a third. Nineteen of the 21 laboring women studied by Wallis and co-workers (1974) regarded acupuncture as unsuccessful in providing analgesia for labor and delivery.

Conclusions. It is evident that no single method is entirely satisfactory for the alleviation of pain during labor and delivery. At the same time, there has been an increasing demand by the laity for relief of suffering associated with childbirth. Such relief of pain is desirable, provided it carries no danger to mother or infant. Safety must remain the prime consideration.

Anesthesia is playing a more prominent role in maternal mortality. Aspiration of vomitus with general anesthesia and unusually high levels with spinal anesthesia are the prime offenders. These deaths are doubly tragic insofar as they are largely preventable in the hands of experienced personnel.

REFERENCES

ACOG National Study of Maternity Care Survey of Obstetric Practice and Associated Services in Hospitals in the United States. A report of the Committee on Maternal Health. Chicago, The American College of Obstetricians and Gynecologists, 1970

Akamatsu TJ, Bonica JJ: Spinal and extradural analgesia-anesthesia for parturition. Clin Obstet Gynecol 17:183, 1974

Bartlett JG, Gorbach SL, Finegold SM: The bacteriology of aspiration pneumonia. Am J Med 56:202, 1974

Beck WW Jr: Prevention of the postpartum spinal headache. Am J Obstet Gynecol 115:354, 1973

Bonica JJ: Acupuncture anesthesia in the People's Republic of China: implications for American medicine. JAMA 229:1317, 1974

Bynum LJ, Pierce AK: Pulmonary aspiration of gastric contents. Am Rev Respir Dis 114:1129, 1976

Cameron JL, Mitchell WH, Ziudema GD: Aspiration pneumonia: clinical outcome following documented aspiration. Arch Surg 106:49, 1973

Castellanos R, Aguero O, deSoto E: Abdominal decompression: a method of obstetric analgesia. Am J Obstet Gynecol 100:924, 1968

Covino BG: Pharmacology of local anesthetic agents. Surgical Rounds, July, 1978, p.44

Crawford JS: Maternal mortality associated with anesthesia. Lancet 2:918, 1972

Crawford JS: Continuous lumbar epidural analgesia for labour and delivery. Br Med J 1:72, 1979

Cullen B, Margolis AH, Eger EI II: The effects of anesthesia and pulmonary ventilation on blood loss during elective therapeutic abortion. Anesthesiology 32:108, 1970

DeVoe SJ, DeVoe K Jr, Rigsby WC, McDaniels BA: Effects of meperidine on uterine contractility. Am J Obstet Gynecol 105:1004, 1969

Dundee JW, Gamble JAS, Assof RAE: Plasma-diazepam levels following intramuscular injection by nurses and doctors. Lancet 2:1461, 1974

Enrile LL Jr, Roux JF, Wilson R, Lebherz TB: Methoxyflurane (Penthrane) inhalation in labor. Obstet Gynecol 41:860, 1973

Ericson A, Källén B: Survey of infants born in 1973 or 1975 to Swedish women working in operating rooms during their pregnancies. Anesth Analg 58:302, 1979

Fishburne JI: Local anesthetics in obstetrics. Contemporary Ob/Gyn 6:101, 1975

Fishburne JI Jr, Greiss FC Jr, Hopkinson R, Rhyne AL: Response of the gravid uterine vasculature to arterial levels of local anesthetic agents. Am J Obstet Gynecol 133:753, 1979

Greenhill JP: Use of local infiltration anesthesia in obstetrics and gynecology. Surg Clin North Am 23:143, 1943

Greiss FC Jr, Still JG, Anderson SG: Effects of local anesthetic agents on the uterine vasculatures and myometrium. Am J Obstet Gynecol 124:889, 1976

Heyns OS: Abdominal decompression in the first stage of labor. Br J Obstet Gynaecol 66:220, 1959

Hughey MJ, McElin TW, Young T: Maternal and fetal outcome of Lamaze prepared patients. Obstet Gynecol 51:643, 1978

Jacoby J: Anesthesia for normal vaginal delivery. Anesth Rev 1:11, 1974

Jägerhorn M: Paracervical block in obstetrics: an improved injection method. Acta Obstet Gynecol Scand 54:9, 1975

Kaupilla A, Koskinen M, Puolakka J, Tuimala R, Kuikka J: Decreased intervillous and unchanged myometrial blood flow in supine recumbency. Obstet Gynecol 55:203, 1980

Kennedy WF Jr, Bonica JJ, Akamatsu TJ, et al.: Cardiovascular and respiratory effects of subarachnoid block in the presence of acute blood loss. Anesthesiology 29:29, 1968

Knill-Jones RP, Newman BJ, Spence AA: Anaesthetic practice and pregnancy. Lancet 2:807, 1975

Lamaze F: Painless Childbirth: Psychoprophylactic Method. Chicago, Henry Regnery, 1970

Liddicoat R: The effects of maternal antenatal decompression treatment on infant mental development. S Afr Med J 42:203, 1968

Lowensohn RI, Paul RH, Fales S, Yet S-Y, Hon EH: Intrapartum epidural anesthesia: an evaluation of effects on uterine activity. Obstet Gynecol 44:388, 1974

Marx GF: Obstetric anesthesia in the presence of medical complications. Clin Obstet Gynecol 17:165, 1974

Marx GF, Cosmi EV, Wollman SB: Biochemical status and clinical condition of mother and infant at cesarean section. Anesth Analg (Cleveland) 48:986, 1969

Medical Letter, Naloxone hydrochloride (Narcan): a new narcotic antagonist. 14 (1): 2, (Jan) 1972

Mendelson CL: The aspiration of stomach contents into the lungs during obstetric anesthesia. Am J Obstet Gynecol 52:191, 1946

Nimmo WS, Wilson J, Prescott LF: Narcotic analgesics and delayed gastric emptying during labor. Lancet 1:890, 1975

Pharoah POD, Alberman E, Doyle P: Outcome of pregnancy among women in anaesthetic practice. Lancet 1:34, 1977

Read GD: Childbirth Without Fear. New York, Harper, 1944, p 192

Riffel HD, Nochimson DJ, Paul RH, Hon EHG: Effects of meperidine and promethazine during labor. Obstet Genecol 42:738, 1973

Salts L, Ott M, Walson PD: Local anesthetic agents—pharmacologic basis for use in obstetrics: A review. Anesth Analg 55:829, 1976

Schultz JH, Luthe W: Autogenic Training. New York, Grune & Stratton, 1959

Shnider SM, Levinson G: Anesthesia for Obstetrics. Baltimore, Williams and Wilkins, 1979.

Svancarek W, Chirino O, Schaefer G Jr, Blythe JG: Retropsoas and subgluteal abscesses following paracervical and pudendal anesthesia JAMA 237:892, 1977

Tahir AH, Adriani J, Naraghi M: Acute systemic toxicity from bupivicaine during epidural anesthesia in obstetric patients. South Med J 68:1377, 1975

Taylor G, Pryse-Davies J: The prophylactic use of antacids in the prevention of the acid pulmonary aspiration syndrome. Lancet 1:288, 1966

Teabeaut JR II: Aspiration of gastric contents: an experimental study. Am J Pathol 28:51, 1952

Teramo K: Effects of obstetrical paracervical blockade on the fetus. Acta Obstet Gynecol Scand (suppl) 16:6, 1971

Ueland K, Akamatsu TJ, Eng M, Bonica JJ, Hansen JM: Maternal cardiovascular dynamics: I. Cesarean section under epidural anesthesia without epinephrine. Am J Obstet Gynecol 114:775, 1972

Vogel VJ: American Indian Medicine. Norman, OK, University of Oklahoma Press, 1970

Wallis L, Shnider SM, Palahniuk RJ, Spivey HT: An evaluation of acupuncture analgesia in obstetrics. Anesthesiology 41:596, 1974

Wenger DR, Gitchell RG: Severe infections following pudendal block anesthesia: need for orthopaedic awareness. J Bone Joint Surg (Am) 55:202, 1973

Wheatley RG, Kallus FT, Reynolds RC, Giesecke AH: Milk of magnesia is an effective pre-induction antacid in obstetrical anesthesia. Anesthesiology 50:514, 1979

Wiener PC, Hogg MIJ, Rosen M: Effects of naloxone on pethidine-induced neonatal depression. Br Med J 2:228, 1977

19

The Puerperium

Definition. Although the puerperium is literally defined as the period of confinement during and just after birth, it came to include the subsequent weeks during which the reproductive tract returns to a normal nonpregnant state. The plan for follow-up care that has been generally practiced by most obstetricians, at least until recently, has resulted commonly in the first 6 weeks being considered the puerperium. During this time, the reproductive tract returns anatomically to a normal nonpregnant state, which includes those permanent structural changes in the cervix, vagina, and perineum that were acquired as the consequence of labor and delivery. Moreover, by 6 weeks after delivery, or not long thereafter, in most nonnursing mothers pituitary-ovarian synchrony will have been reestablished appropriate for ovulation.

INVOLUTION OF THE GENITAL AND URINARY TRACTS

Involution of the Body of the Uterus. Immediately after expulsion of the placenta, the fundus of the contracted body of the uterus is about midway between the umbilicus and symphysis, or slightly higher. The body of the uterus now consists of mostly myometrium covered by serosa and lined by basal decidua. The anterior and posterior walls, in close apposition, each measure 4 to 5 cm in thickness. Because its vessels are compressed by the contracted myometrium, the puerperal uterus on section appears ischemic, compared to the reddish-purple hyperemic pregnant organ. During the next 2 days, the uterus remains approximately the same size, and then atrophies, so that within 2 weeks it has descended into the cavity of the true pelvis and can no longer be felt above the symphysis. It normally regains its previous nonpregnant size, or very close to it, within 5 to 6 weeks. The rapidity of the process is remarkable. The freshly delivered uterus weighs about 1000 to 1200 g. As the consequence of *involution,* one week later it weighs about 500 g, decreasing at the end of the second week to about 300 g, and soon thereafter to 100 g or even less. The total number of muscle cells does not decrease appreciably; instead, the individual cells decrease markedly in size. The mechanism by which the individual muscle cell divests itself of excess cytoplasm, including contractile protein, remains to be elucidated. The involution of the connective tissue framework occurs equally rapidly (Woessner, 1968).

Since the separation of the placenta and membranes involves primarily the spongy layer of the decidua, the basal portion of the decidua remains in the uterus. The decidua that remains presents striking variations in thickness, an irregular jagged appearance, and infiltration with blood, especially at the placental site.

REGENERATION OF ENDOMETRIUM. Within 2 or 3 days after delivery, the decidua remaining in the uterus becomes differentiated into two layers. The superficial layer becomes necrotic, whereas the basal layer adjacent to the myometrium does not. The former is cast off in the lochia, and the latter, which contains the fundi of the endometrial glands, is the source of new endometrium. The endometrium arises from proliferation of the endometrial glandular remnants and the stroma of the interglandular connective tissue.

The process of endometrial regeneration is rapid, except at the placental site. Elsewhere, the free surface becomes covered by epithelium within a week or 10 days, and the entire endometrium is restored during the third week. Sharman (1953), in an extensive study of postpartum uteri, identified fully restored endometrium in all biopsy specimens obtained from the 16th day onward. The endometrium was normal except for occasional hyalinized decidual remnants and leukocytes. The so-called endometritis identified histologically in the reparative days of the puerperium is but part of the normal process of repair.

INVOLUTION OF THE PLACENTAL SITE. According to Williams (1931), complete extrusion of the placental site takes up to 6 weeks. This process is of great clinical importance, for when it is defective late puerperal hemorrhage may ensue. Immediately after delivery, the placental site is about the size of the palm of the hand but it rapidly decreases in size. By the end of the second week, it is 3 to 4 cm in diameter. Very soon after the termination of labor, the placental site normally consists of many thrombosed

vessels (Fig. 19-1) that undergo typical organization of the thrombus.

If involution of the placental site comprised only these events, each pregnancy would leave a fibrous scar in the endometrium and subjacent myometrium, thus eventually limiting the number of future pregnancies. In his classic investigations, Williams (1931) explained involution of the placental site as follows:

> Involution is not effected by absorption in situ, but rather by a process of exfoliation which is in great part brought about by the undermining of the placental implantation site by the growth of endometrial tissue. This is effected partly by extension and down growth of endometrium from the margins of the placental site and partly by the development of endometrial tissue from the glands and stroma left in the depths of the decidua basalis after the separation of the placenta . . . such a process of exfoliation should be regarded as very conservative, and as a wise provision on the part of nature; otherwise great difficulty might be experienced in getting rid of the obliterated arteries and organized thrombi which, if they remained in situ, would soon convert a considerable part of the uterine mucosa and subadjacent myometrium into a mass of scar tissue with the result that after a few pregnancies it would unlikely be possible for it to go through its usual cycle of changes, and the reproductive career would come to an end.

Anderson and Davis (1968), on the basis of their studies of involution of the placental site, concluded that exfoliation of the placental site is brought about as the consequence of a necrotic slough of infarcted superficial tissues followed by a reparative process not unlike that which takes place on any denuded epithelium-covered structure.

CHANGES IN THE UTERINE VESSELS. A successful pregnancy requires a great increase in uterine blood flow. To provide for this, arteries and veins that transport blood to and from the uterus and those that convey blood within the uterus, especially to the pla-

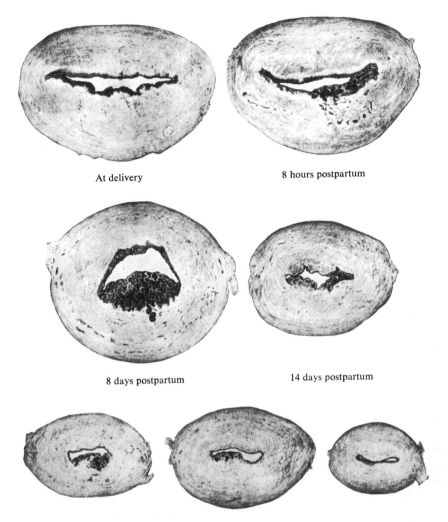

At delivery   8 hours postpartum

8 days postpartum   14 days postpartum

FIG. 19-1. Cross sections of the uterus made at the level of the involuting placental site at varying times after delivery. (From Williams. *Am J Obstet Gynecol* 22:664, 1931)

cental site, change remarkably. Transport vessels to and from the uterus dilate remarkably (see Chap. 9, p. 221). Within the uterus both dilatation of preexisting vessels and growth of new vessels provide for the increase in blood flow. After delivery the caliber of the extrauterine vessels decrease to equal, or at least approach, that of the prepregnant state.

Within the puerperal uterus, for the most part, the blood vessels are obliterated by hyaline changes and vessels that are smaller develop in their place. The resorption of the hyaline is accomplished by processes similar to those observed in the ovaries subsequent to ovulation and corpus luteum formation. Minor vestiges, however, may persist for years, affording under the microscope a means of differentiating between the uteri of parous and nulliparous women.

Changes in the Cervix and Lower Uterine Segment. Immediately after the completion of the third stage of labor, the cervix and lower uterine segment are thin, collapsed, flabby structures. The outer margin of the cervix that corresponds to the external os usually is lacerated, especially laterally. The cervical opening contracts slowly. For a few days immediately after labor, it readily admits two fingers, but by the end of the first week it has become so narrow as to render difficult the introduction of one finger. As the cervical opening narrows, the cervix thickens and a canal is reformed. At the completion of involution, however, the external os does not resume its pregravid appearance completely. It remains somewhat wider, and, typically, bilateral depressions at the site of lacerations remain as permanent changes that characterize the parous cervix (Fig. 2-11, p. 23).

After delivery, the markedly thinned out myometrium of the lower uterine segment contracts and retracts but not as forcefully as the body of the uterus. Over the course of a few weeks the lower segment is converted from a clearly evident structure large enough to contain most of the head of the term fetus to a barely discernable uterine isthmus located between the body of the uterus above and the internal os of the cervix below (Fig. 2-8, p. 22).

Vagina and Vaginal Outlet. The vagina and vaginal outlet in the first part of the puerperium form a capacious smooth-walled passage that gradually diminishes in size but rarely returns to the nulliparous dimensions. The rugae begin to reappear about the third week. The hymen is represented by several small tags of tissue, which during cicatrization are converted into the myrtiform caruncles characteristic of parous women.

Changes in the Peritoneum and Abdominal Wall. As the myometrium contracts and retracts after delivery and for a few days after, the peritoneum covering much of the uterus is thrown into folds and wrinkles. The broad and round ligaments are much more lax than in the nonpregnant condition, and they require considerable time to recover from the stretching and loosening to which they have been subjected during pregnancy.

As a result of the rupture of the elastic fibers of the skin and the prolonged distension caused by the enlarged pregnant uterus, the abdominal walls remain soft and flabby for a while. The return to normal of these structures requires several weeks. Recovery is aided by exercise. Except for silvery striae, the abdominal wall usually resumes its pre-pregnancy appearance, but when the muscles are atonic, it may remain lax. There may be a marked separation, or diastasis, of the rectus muscles. In that condition, the abdominal wall in the vicinity of the midline is formed simply by peritoneum, attenuated fascia, subcutaneous fat, and skin.

Changes in the Urinary Tract. Cystoscopic examination soon after delivery shows not only edema and hyperemia of the bladder wall, but, frequently, submucous extravasation of blood. In addition, the puerperal bladder has an increased capacity and a relative insensitivity to intravesical fluid pressure. Therefore, overdistension, incomplete emptying, and excessive residual urine must be watched for closely. The paralyzing effect of anesthesia, especially conduction anesthesia, and the temporarily disturbed neural function of the bladder are undoubtedly contributory factors. Residual urine and bacteriuria in a traumatized bladder, coupled with the dilated renal pelves and ureters create optimal conditions for the development of urinary tract infection (see Chap. 28, p. 701). After delivery, the dilated ureters and renal pelves return to normal within about 8 weeks (see Chap. 9, p. 245). The stretching and dilatation during pregnancy do not cause permanent changes in the renal pelves and ureters unless infection has supervened.

CHANGES IN THE MAMMARY GLANDS

Anatomy of the Breasts. The anlage of the mammary glands are contained in the ectodermal ridges that form on the ventral

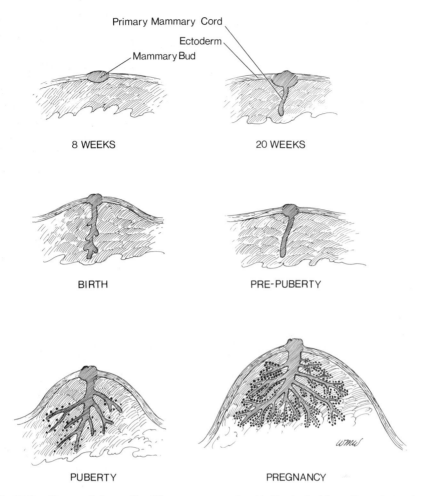

Primary Mammary Cord
Ectoderm
Mammary Bud

8 WEEKS   20 WEEKS

BIRTH   PRE-PUBERTY

PUBERTY   PREGNANCY

FIG. 19-2.   Sequential growth of the mammary gland is illustrated from 8 weeks embryonic age through puberty and during pregnancy. (Courtesy of Dr. John C. Porter)

surface of the embryo and extend from fore-limb to hindlimb bilaterally. The multiple pairs of buds normally all disappear from the embryo except for one pair in the pectoral region which eventually develops into the two mammary glands (Fig. 19-2). At times, however, the buds elsewhere may not completely disappear, but, instead, may participate to a lesser degree in the pattern of growth that characterizes the two normal mammary glands. This condition of *polymastia* has been reviewed by Garcia and co-workers (1978). At mid-pregnancy, each of the two mammary buds in the fetus destined to form the breasts begin to grow and divide with

the formation of 15 to 25 secondary buds which provide the basis for the duct system in the mature breast. Each secondary bud elongates into a cord, bifurcates, and differentiates into two concentric layers of cuboidal cells and a central lumen. The inner layer of cells eventually gives rise to the secretory epithelium which synthesizes the milk, while the outer layer becomes myoepithelium, which provides the mechanism for milk ejection (Fig. 19-3.A).

Thelarche, the onset of rapid increase in breast size from estrogen stimulation, begins about the time of puberty when estrogen production rises. The previously infantile mammary glands respond to estrogen with growth and development of the mammary ducts and the deposition of fat. With the onset of ovulation, progesterone is produced which stimulates development of the alveoli of the mammary gland and sets the stage for future lactation.

Anatomically, each mature mammary gland is made up of 15 to 25 lobes which arose from the secondary mammary buds described above. The lobes are arranged more or less radially and are separated from one another by a varying amount of fat. Each lobe consists of several lobules, which in turn are made up of large numbers of alveoli (Fig. 19-3A). Every lobule is provided with a small duct that joins others to form a single larger duct for each lobe. These lactiferous ducts make their way to the nipple and open separately upon its surface, where they may be distinguished as minute but distinct orifices. The alveolar secretory epithelium synthesizes the various constituents of the milk (Fig. 19-3B).

Lactation. By the second postpartum day, a modest amount of colostrum can be expressed from the nipples.

COLOSTRUM. Compared with the mature milk that is ultimately secreted by the breasts, colostrum contains more protein, much of which is globulin, and more minerals, but less sugar and fat. Colostrum, nevertheless, contains rather large fat globules in so-called colostrum corpuscles, which are thought by some to be epithelial cells that have undergone fatty degeneration and by others to be mononuclear phagocytes containing considerable fat. The secretion of colostrum persists for about a week, with gradual conversion to mature milk. Antibodies are readily demonstrable in colostrum. Its content of IgA may offer protection to the newborn infant against enteric infection as described below. Other host resistance factors, as well as immunoglobulins, have been described in human colostrum and milk. These include components of complement, macrophages, lymphocytes, lactoferrin, lacto-

peroxidase, and lysozyme (Goldman and Smith, 1973).

MILK. The major components of milk are proteins, lactose, water, and fat. The major *proteins* in milk—casein, α-lactalbumin, and β-lactoglobulin—are synthesized in the rough endoplasmic reticulum of the alveolar secretory cell. The essential amino acids are derived from the blood; nonessential amino acids are derived in part from the blood or synthesized in the mammary gland. The proteins of milk are unique proteins not found elsewhere.

The synthesis of lactose from glucose in the alveolar secretory cells is catalyzed by lactose synthetase. Some lactose spills into the maternal circulation and may be excreted by the kidney and detected in the urine. Milk is isotonic with plasma; lactose, rather than protein, provides much of the osmotic pressure.

Fatty acids are synthesized in the alveoli from glucose. Fat droplets are secreted by an apocrine-like process.

All vitamins except vitamin B_{12} are present in variable amounts in milk. Milk contains very little ascorbic acid and vitamin D, and is a poor source of iron. The mammary gland, like the thyroid gland, concentrates iodine which appears in the milk.

The approximate concentrations of the more important components of human colostrum, human mature milk and cow's milk are presented in Table 19-1.

ENDOCRINOLOGY OF LACTATION. The precise humoral and neural mechanisms involved in lactation are obviously complex. Progesterone, estrogen, and placental lactogen, as well as prolactin, cortisol, and insulin appear to act in concert to stimulate the growth and development of the milk-secreting apparatus of the mammary gland (Porter, 1974). With the delivery of the placenta, there is an abrupt and profound decrease in the levels of progesterone and estrogen, which somehow serves to initiate lactation. It is very likely that lactation is not initiated until the end of pregnancy because the high

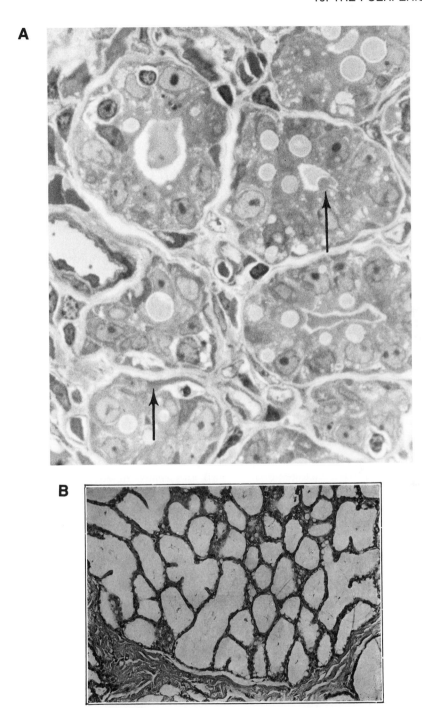

FIG. 19-3.A. Histology of maternal breast at 32 weeks gestation in preparation for lactation. Secretions are evident in the lumen of each alveolus. Myoepithelial cells are evident around alveoli (lower left arrow). Secretions are being delivered by exocytosis into the lumen of one alveolus (upper right arrow) **B.** Section of breast during lactation. The alveoli are distended and the cells are filled with fat. (From Bell. *Textbook of Pathology.* Philadelphia, Lea & Febiger)

TABLE 19-1.

APPROXIMATE CONCENTRATIONS (PER DL) OF COMPONENTS OF
HUMAN COLOSTRUM, HUMAN MATURE MILK, AND COW'S MILK

	HUMAN COLOSTRUM	HUMAN MATURE MILK	COWS' MILK
Water (g)	—	88	88
Lactose (g)	5.3	6.8	5.0
Casein: lactalbumin ratio	—	1:2	3:1
Fat (g)	2.9	3.8	3.7
Linoleic acid	—	8.3% of fat	1.6% of fat
Sodium (mg)	92	15	58
Potassium (mg)	55	55	138
Chloride (mg)	117	43	103
Calcium (mg)	31	33	125
Magnesium (mg)	4	4	12
Phosphorus (mg)	14	15	100
Iron (mg)	0.09*	0.15*	0.10*
Vitamin A (μg)	89	53	34
Vitamin D (μg)	—	0.03*	0.06*
Thiamine (μg)	15	16	42
Riboflavine (μg)	30	43	157
Nicotinic acid (μg)	75	172	85
Ascorbic acid (μg)	4.4†	4.3†	1.6*

From Edwards (ed.): *Research in Reproduction*, Vol. 6. November, 1974
* Poor source
† Just adequate

levels of estrogen and progesterone during pregnancy interfere with the lactogenic actions of prolactin and adrenal steroids.

In otherwise normal circumstances, the intensity and the duration of lactation are subsequently controlled in large part by the repetitive stimulus of nursing. Prolactin is essential for lactation; women with extensive pituitary necrosis, as in Sheehan's disease, do not lactate (see Chap. 34, p. 879). Although plasma prolactin falls after delivery to appreciably lower levels than during pregnancy, each act of suckling triggers a rise in prolactin levels (Tyson et al., 1972). Presumably a stimulus from the breast curtails the release of prolactin-inhibiting factor from the hypothalamus which, in turn, induces transiently an increased secretion of prolactin by the pituitary.

The neurohypophysis secretes oxytocin, which stimulates the expression of milk from a lactating breast by causing contraction of myoepithelial cells in the alveoli and the small milk ducts. In fact, this mechanism has been utilized to assay oxytocin activity in biologic fluids. The ejection, or "letting down," of milk is a reflex initiated especially by suckling, which stimulates the neurohypophysis to liberate oxytocin. It may be provoked just by the cry of the infant or inhibited by fright or stress. Successful lactation in some cases of diabetes insipidus suggests, however, that an intact posterior pituitary is not absolutely necessary for lactation in women (Sende et al., 1975).

IMMUNOLOGIC CONSEQUENCES OF BREAST FEEDING. An intriguing story appears to be emerging concerning the role of the mother's milk in the immunocompetence of the newborn. The status of these issues were summarized by Beer and Billingham (1976). Antibodies are present in human colostrum and milk but none are absorbed from the infant's gut. Indeed, no Rho antibodies have been detected in the sera of infants fed milk containing a high titer of Rho antibodies. This circumstance however, does not mitigate necessarily against the importance of at least some of the antibodies in breast milk. The predominant immunoglobin in milk is secretory IgA, a macromolecule that is believed to be important in antimicrobial processes in the mucous membranes across which it is secreted. In this context it is envisioned that secretory IgA contained in mother's milk may act locally within the infant's gastrointestinal tract. Human breast milk contains secretory IgA antibodies against *Escherichia coli,* and it is known that breast-fed babies are less prone to enteric infections than are bottle-fed babies. It has been suggested that IgA exerts its antimicrobial action by preventing attachment of bacteria to cells on mucosal surfaces, preventing their penetration into tissues.

In addition to the role of antibodies in human milk, much attention is being directed to an elucidation of the role of maternal lymphocytes in breast milk in fetal immunologic processes. It has been reported that human milk contains both T and B lymphocytes. Lymphocytes in colostrum undergo blastoid transformation in vitro following exposure to specific antigens. In studies of experimental animals, Beer and Billingham have obtained evidence that there is transmission of viable lymphocytes from mother to infant through the breast milk.

Nursing. An ideal food for the newborn child is the milk of the mother. In most instances, even though the supply of milk at first appears insufficient, it becomes adequate if suckling is continued. Nursing also accelerates involution of the uterus, since repeated stimulation of the nipples through release of oxytocin from the neurohypophysis leads to increased contractions of the myometrium.

Most drugs given to the mother are secreted in the milk. Many factors influence their excretion, including the concentration of drugs in plasma, the degree of protein binding of the drug, plasma and milk pH, degree of ionization, lipid solubility, and molecular weight. In general, water-soluble drugs are excreted in higher concentration into colostrum, whereas lipid-soluble drugs are excreted in greater concentration into breast milk. Further consideration of factors involved in the secretion into milk of drugs administered to the mother and the possible effects on the infant have been provided by Anderson (1979).

CLINICAL ASPECTS OF THE PUERPERIUM

Temperature. Breast engorgement on the third or fourth day of the puerperium was once thought to cause a rise in temperature. This so-called milk fever was regarded as physiologic. Although no such entity is clearly recognized today, on occasion perhaps, extreme vascular and lymphatic engorgement may cause a sharp rise in fever but it does not last more than 24 hours at the most. *Any rise of temperature in the puerperium implies an infection, most likely somewhere in the genitourinary tract.*

Afterpains. In primiparas, the puerperal uterus tends to remain tonically contracted unless blood clots, fragments of placenta, or other foreign bodies are retained in its cavity, causing hypertonic contractions in an effort to expel them. In multiparas especially, the uterus often contracts vigorously at intervals, the contractions giving rise to painful sensations that are known as "afterpains" and that occasionally are sufficiently severe to require an analgesic. In some patients, they may last for days. Afterpains are particularly noticeable when the infant is put to the breast, presumably because of the release of oxytocin. Ordinarily, however, they decrease in intensity and become quite mild by the third day after delivery.

Lochia. Early in the puerperium, there is normally a variable amount of uterine discharge, the lochia. Microscopically, the lochia consists of erythrocytes, leukocytes, shreds of decidua, epithelial cells, and bacteria. Microorganisms can always be demonstrated in lochia pooled in the vagina and are present in most cases even when the discharge has been obtained from the uterine cavity.

For the first few days after delivery, the

content of blood in the lochia is sufficient to color it red, or *lochia rubra*. After 3 or 4 days, the lochia becomes progressively paler, or *lochia serosa*. After the 10th day, because of a marked admixture with leukocytes and a reduced fluid content, it assumes a white or yellowish-white color, or *lochia alba*. Foul-smelling lochia suggests, but does not prove, infection.

Adams and Flowers (1960) measured the lochia of 120 women during the first 5½ days after delivery. During this period, the lochial weight in nursing and nonnursing women averaged 251 and 277 g, respectively. Similar patients also received 0.2 mg of methylergo-novine maleate (Methergine) orally every 4 hours for the first 3 days after delivery. There was no appreciable difference in the amount of lochia between the women who received methylergonovine maleate and those who did not. The morbidity rates during the puerperium were the same, and the height of the fundus was identical in both the treated and untreated groups. The only real observed difference related to the mother's discomfort. Those who received the drug suffered much more from uterine cramping. These investigators concluded that the routine use of such medication was unwarranted. Newton and Bradford (1961) similarly concluded that after the immediate period following delivery the routine administration of intramuscular oxytocin to normal women was of no value in decreasing blood loss or hastening involution of the uterus.

In many instances, a reddish color in the lochia is maintained for a longer period. When it persists for more than 2 weeks, however, it indicates either the retention of small portions of the placenta or imperfect involution of the placental site, or both.

Urine. Diuresis regularly occurs between the 2nd and 5th days, even when intravenous fluids were not vigorously infused during labor and delivery. Normal pregnancy is associated with an appreciable increase in extracellular water. The puerperal diuresis represents a reversal of this process as the fluid-retaining stimuli of pregnancy-in-duced hyperestrogenism and elevated venous pressure in the lower half of the body are removed, and as any residual hypervolemia is dissipated. In preeclampsia, both retention of fluid antepartum and diuresis postpartum may be greatly increased (see Chap. 27, p. 676).

Occasionally, substantial amounts of sugar may be found in the urine during the first weeks of the puerperium. The sugar is lactose, which, fortunately, is nonreducing in test systems using glucose oxidase.

After a long labor, acetone may be identified in the urine as the consequence of starvation.

Blood. Rather marked leukocytosis occurs during and after labor, the leukocyte count sometimes reaching levels as high as 30,000 per mm³ (see Chap. 9, p. 236). The increase is made up predominantly of granulocytes. There is a relative lymphopenia and an absolute eosinopenia.

Normally, during the first few days after delivery, the hemoglobin, hematocrit, and erythrocyte count vary moderately. In general, however, if they fall much below the level present just before or during early labor, the patient has lost a considerable amount of blood (see Chap. 21, p. 487). By one week after delivery, the blood volume has returned to near the usual nonpregnant level.

The pregnancy-induced changes in blood coagulation factors persist for variable periods of time after delivery. The elevation of plasma fibrinogen is maintained at least through the first week of the puerperium. As a consequence, the elevated sedimentation rate normally found during much of pregnancy normally remains high during the early part of the puerperium.

Loss of Weight. In addition to the loss of about 11 pounds as the consequence of evacuation of the contents of the uterus, there is generally further loss of body weight during the puerperium of about 5 pounds. This weight loss is accounted for by fluid lost chiefly through urination, as described above.

Chesley and co-workers (1959) have demonstrated a decrease in the sodium space of about 2 liters, or nearly 5 pounds, during the first week after delivery.

CARE OF THE MOTHER DURING THE PUERPERIUM

Attention Immediately after Labor. After delivery of the placenta, the uterus should be firm, with its upper margin below the umbilicus. As long as it remains in this condition, there is no danger of postpartum hemorrhage *from uterine atony.* To guard against such an occurrence, the uterus should be gently palpated through the abdominal wall starting immediately after the conclusion of the second stage of labor and the maneuver repeated at frequent intervals during and after the completion of the third stage of labor, i.e., delivery of the placenta. If the size and consistency of the uterus remain unaltered, it should be left alone. If any relaxation is detected, however, the uterus should be massaged through the abdominal walls until it remains contracted, and usually an oxytocic agent should be administered. Blood may accumulate within the uterus without external evidence of bleeding. This condition may be detected early by identifying uterine enlargement through frequent palpation of the fundus during the first few hours postpartum. *Even in normal cases, a trained attendant should remain with the mother for at least 1 hour after completion of the third stage of labor.*

Care of the Vulva. Shortly after completion of the third stage of labor and perineal repair, the drapings and soiled linen beneath the mother are removed, provided there is no excessive bleeding or other reason to keep her in the lithotomy position and on the delivery table. The external genitalia and buttocks are flushed with soap and water in such a way that all of the liquid drains from the vulva and perineum down over the anus, rather than in the reverse direction. A sterile vulvar pad is then applied over the genitalia and replaced by a clean pad as necessary. After each bowel movement and before any local treatment or examination, the external genitalia should be similarly cleansed.

Subsequent Discomfort. The discomfort from cesarean section, its causes and its management are considered in Chapter 43, (p. 1098). During the first few days after vaginal delivery, the mother may be uncomfortable for a variety of reasons which include afterpains, episiotomy and lacerations, breast engorgement, and, at times postspinal headache. It is prudent to provide codeine, 60 mg, or aspirin, 0.6 g, at intervals as frequent as every 3 hours during the first few days after delivery. Uterine contractions are commonly accentuated during nursing, giving rise at times to troublesome afterpains.

The repaired espisiotomy or lacerations may be uncomfortable, as discussed in Chapter 17, page 432. Early application of an ice bag to the perineum may minimize the swelling and discomfort. The majority of women also appear to obtain a measure of relief from the periodic application of a local anesthetic spray to the site of episiotomy or laceration. Severe discomfort may mean that a sizable hematoma has formed in the genital tract. Therefore, careful examination is warranted, especially whenever ordinary orally-ingested analgesics do not provide appreciable relief. The episiotomy incision is usually firmly healed and nearly asymptomatic by the third week after delivery.

DEPRESSION. It is also fairly common for a mother to exhibit some degree of depression a few days after delivery. The transient depression, or "postpartum blues," most likely is the consequence of a number of factors. Prominent in its genesis are (1) the emotional let-down that follows the excitement and fears which most women experience during pregnancy and delivery, (2) the discomforts of the early puerperium that have been described above, (3) fatigue from loss of sleep during labor and postpartum in most hospital settings, (4) anxiety over her capabilities for caring for her infant after leaving the hospital, and (5) fears that she has become less attractive to her husband. In the great majority of cases effective treatment need be nothing more than anticipation, recognition, and reassurance.

Early Ambulation. Immediately after World War II, important changes began to take place in the management of the puerperium in the direction of early ambulation. Women are now out of bed well within the first 24 hours after vaginal delivery. The many advantages of early ambulation are confirmed by numerous well-controlled studies. Women state that they feel better and stronger after early ambulation. Bladder complications and constipation are less frequent. Early ambulation has also reduced materially the frequency of thrombosis and pulmonary embolism during the puerperium. For the first ambulation, at least, an attendant should be present to help prevent injury if the woman were to become syncopal.

Abdominal Wall Relaxation. An abdominal binder is unnecessary, although it was formerly believed to aid involution and help restore the mother's figure. It is now the consensus that it has no effect on involution. If the abdomen is unusually flabby or pendulous, an ordinary girdle is often more satisfactory than an abdominal binder. Exercises to help restore tone to the abdominal wall may be started at any time after vaginal delivery and as soon as the soreness diminishes after cesarean section.

Diet. It was formerly customary to restrict the diet of the puerperal woman who has been delivered vaginally, but at present an attractive general diet is recommended. If at the end of two hours after vaginal delivery there are no complications that are likely to necessitate another anesthetic, she should be given something to drink if thirsty and, if hungry, something to eat. The diet of the lactating mother, compared with that consumed during pregnancy, should be increased somewhat, especially in calories and protein, as recommended by the Food and Nutrition Board of the National Research Council (see Table 13-1, page 312). If the mother does not breast-feed the infant, her dietary requirements are the same as for a normal nonpregnant woman. There is absolutely no rationale for restricting fluids for women who do not desire to nurse.

It is standard practice at Parkland Memorial Hospital to continue iron supplementation for one month after delivery. The hematocrit is also checked at the time of the postpartum check routinely performed during the third week of the puerperium.

Bladder Function. The rate of accumulation of urine in the bladder after delivery may be quite variable. Currently, intravenous fluids are nearly always infused during labor and subsequently. Oxytocin, in doses that are antidiuretic, most often is infused intravenously after the third stage of labor and then stopped an hour or so later. As the consequence of the volume of fluid infused and the sudden withdrawal of the antidiuretic effect of oxytocin, rapid filling of the bladder is common. Moreover, both bladder sensation and the capability of the bladder to empty spontaneously may be appreciably diminished by anesthesia, especially conduction anesthesia, and by painful lesions in the genital tract, such as extensive episiotomy, lacerations, or hematomas. It is not surprising, therefore, that urinary retention with overdistension of the bladder is a nagging complication of the early puerperium. Once overdistension occurs, bladder function becomes further impaired and ascending infection of the urinary tract is a common consequence.

Prevention of overdistension demands close observation of the bladder after delivery to make sure that it does not overfill and that with each voiding it empties adequately. The bladder may be palpated as a cystic mass suprapubically, or the enlarged bladder may be evident abdominally only indirectly, the full bladder having elevated the uterine fundus to well above the umbilicus.

If the woman has not voided within four hours after delivery, it is likely that she cannot do so. Ambulation to a commode usually should be tried before resorting to catheterization. The woman who has trouble voiding initially is likely to have further trouble. At times, an indwelling catheter is necessary, as described in Chapter 36, page 917. Especially in those instances in which conduction anesthesia cannot be held responsible for urinary retention, the likelihood of hematomas of the genital tract must be kept in mind whenever the woman cannot void following delivery. Whenever the bladder has become overdistended, an indwelling catheter for a day, until the factors causing the retention have, for the most part, abated is likely to be beneficial.

Bowels. At times, the lack of a bowel movement is no more than the expected consequence of an efficient cleansing enema administered a few hours before delivery and little being eaten subsequently. With both early ambulation and early feeding of a general diet, constipation has become much less of a problem in the puerperium.

Care of the Breasts and Nipples. The nipples require little attention in the puerperium other than cleanliness and attention to fissures. Since dried milk is likely to accumulate and irritate the nipples, cleansing of the areolae with water and mild soap is helpful before and after nursing. Occasionally, with irritated nipples, it is necessary to resort to a nipple shield for 24 hours or longer. A nursing brassiere which provides support without constriction is desirable. Suppression of lactation in the woman who does not nurse her infant is considered in Chapter 36, page 918.

Immunizations. The Rho negative woman who is not isoimmunized and whose baby is Rho positive is given 300 μg of Rho immune globulin shortly after delivery (see Chap. 38, p. 963). Women who are not already immune to rubella (see Chap. 13, p. 321) and who are going to use a contraceptive agent are excellent candidates for vacci-

nation before discharge. At Parkland Memorial Hospital the mother also receives a tetanus booster injection at this time, unless it is contraindicated.

Time of Discharge. Puerperal women are usually up and about shortly after the birth of their children and see no reason after vaginal delivery for hospitalization normally beyond 3 days. Moreover, the increase in the prevalance of antiobiotic-resistant organisms militates against keeping well babies and well mothers in institutions. Finally, the cost of prolonged hospitalization has for many families become prohibitive.

Return of Menstruation and Ovulation. If the woman does not nurse her child, the menstrual flow will probably return within 6 to 8 weeks after labor. At times, however, it is difficult clinically to assign a specific date to the first menstrual period after delivery. A minority of women bleed small to moderate amounts intermittently, starting soon after delivery. Menses may not appear so long as the infant is nursed but great variations are observed, for in lactating women, the first period may occur as early as the second, or as late as the 18th month after delivery.

Sharman (1951) noted that at 3 months after childbirth, menstrual function had returned in 91 percent of the nonlactating primiparas, whereas only one-third of the lactating primiparas had menstruated. In lactating multiparas, however, there is a greater tendency for menstruation to reestablish itself within 3 months. The bleeding may occur in an ovulatory or an anovulatory cycle. Sharman (1966), by means of histologic dating of the endometrium, identified ovulation as early as 42 days after delivery, and Perez and associates (1972) did so as early as 36 days. Moreover, a corpus luteum has been observed 6 weeks after delivery at the time of sterilization (Chester, 1979). The necessity for avoiding delay in instituting contraceptive technics by the sexually active woman is obvious.

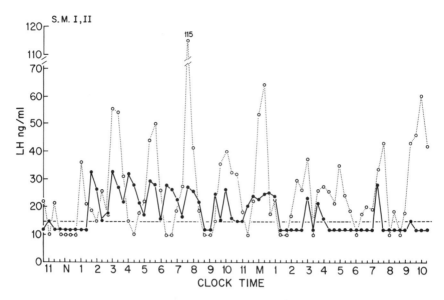

FIG. 19-4.A. Comparison of the 24 hour secretory patterns of LH in the lactating woman. The closed circles denote plasma LH levels during the period of amenorrhea. The open circles correspond to the plasma LH concentrations after menses had resumed. *(Continued)*

It has long been appreciated that ovulation is much less frequent in women who nurse their infants compared to those who do not. Nonetheless, pregnancy can occur while lactating. Hefnawi and Badraoui (1977) have provided the following quantitative information for women who nurse: Of 340 lactating Egyptian women who used no contraception after delivery, 26.4 percent had conceived again within the next 12 months. Of those who became pregnant, one-fourth had never menstruated since delivery. Onset of menses increased from 7.6 percent the first month after delivery to 60.5 percent by 12 months. Among those who menstruated, ovulation, identified by examinations of cervical mucus and endometrial biopsies, rose from 2.9 percent at one month to 58.8 percent at 12 months.

It is generally thought that amenorrhea during the period of lactation is the consequence of lack of appropriate ovarian stimulation by pituitary gonadotropins. In keeping with this concept, and as illustrated in Figure 19-4A and B, the levels of luteinizing hormone (LH) and follicle stimulating hormone (FSH) in one carefully studied lactating wo-

man were appreciably lower during the time of amenorrhea than they were after the resumption of menstruation (Madden et al., 1978).

While Keettel and Bradbury (1961), in a much earlier study, noted very low pituitary gonadotropic activity, as anticipated, in the urine of some lactating women with amenorrhea, they also detected by bioassay normal or even elevated amounts of gonadotropins in the urine of others. They concluded that in the latter circumstance the absent or very limited estrogenic effect on the vaginal epithelium, as well as the amenorrhea and anovulation, resulted from the failure of the ovaries to respond to the gonadotropins. The observations of Bonnar and co-workers (1975) have provided an explanation. In some women who were breast-feeding in their study, plasma estrogens did not increase despite a rise in FSH. The lack of response was attributed to an inhibitory effect of the increased prolactin levels on follicular development.

Follow-up Care. By the time of discharge from the hospital after a vaginal delivery and a normal in-hospital puerperium, the

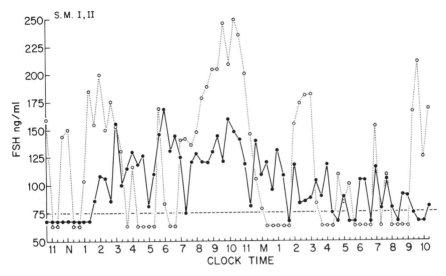

FIG. 19-4.B (Cont.).   Comparison of the 24 hour secretory patterns of FSH in the lactating woman. The closed circles denote plasma FSH levels during the period of amenorrhea. The open circles correspond to the plasma FSH concentrations after menses had resumed. (From Madden et al. *Am J Obstet Gynecol*, 132:436, 1978.)

mother can resume most activities, including bathing, driving, and household functions. Although it has been customary to recommend that she not resume employment or return to school for several weeks, there is no evidence that to do so earlier causes any physical harm. Ideally, it would appear that much of the care and attention received by the very young infant should be provided by the mother, amply augmented by the father; for her to do so precludes early return by the mother to full-time work or school.

Recommendations as to the time of resumption of sexual intercourse have varied considerably. It is most unlikely that there are increased risks from intercourse as early as two weeks after delivery except perhaps for dyspareunia which can be minimized by careful repair of the episiotomy (Richardson et al., 1976). As stated at the outset, delay of examination of the mother until 6 weeks postpartum became routine in the practice of obstetrics. From the standpoint of optimal clinical care, however, the reasons for selecting that time are not altogether clear. Since 1969, at Parkland Memorial Hospital, puerperal women typically have been given ap-

pointments for follow-up examination during the third week following delivery. The third week has proven quite satisfactory both to identify any abnormalities of the later puerperium and to initiate contraceptive practices. Estrogen plus progestin oral contraceptives started at this time have proved effective without increased morbidity. Moreover, the frequencies of uterine perforation, expulsions, and pregnancies when intrauterine devices were inserted during the third week postpartum were no greater than when the devices were inserted 3 months or more postpartum (Pritchard and Pritchard, unpublished). Family planning technics and follow-up care are discussed further in Chapter 40 (p. 1009).

REFERENCES

Adams H, Flowers CE: Oral oxytocic drugs in the puerperium. Obstet Gynecol 15:280, 1960

Anderson PO: Drugs and breast feeding. In Vorherr H (ed): Seminars in Perinatology, Vol 3. 1979, p 271

Anderson WR, Davis J: Placental site involution. Am J Obstet Gynecol 102: 23, 1968

Beer AE, Billingham RE: The Immunobiology of Mammalian Reproduction. Englewood Cliffs, N.J., Prentice-Hall, 1976, p 198

Bonnar J, Franklin M, Nott PN, McNeilly AS: Effect of breast-feeding on pituitary-ovarian function after childbirth. Br Med J 4:82, 1975

Chesley LC, Valenti C, Uichanco L: Alterations in body fluid compartments and exchangeable sodium in early puerperium. Am J Obstet Gynecol 77:1054, 1959

Chester D: Personal communication, 1979

Garcia JJ, Verkauf BS, Hochberg CJ, Ingram JM: Aberrant breast tissue of the vulva. Obstet Gynecol 52:225, 1978

Goldman AS, Smith CW: Host resistance factors in human milk. J Pediatr 82:1082, 1973

Hefnawi F. Badraoui MHH: The benefits of lactation amenorrhea as a contraceptive. Fertil Steril 28:320, 1977

Hervada A, Feit E, Sagraves R: Drugs in breast milk. Perinatal Care 2:19, 1978

Keettel WC, Bradbury JT: Endocrine studies of lactation amenorrhea. Am J Obstet Gynecol 82:995, 1961

Madden JD, Boyar R, MacDonald PC, Porter JC: Analysis of secretory patterns of prolactin and gonadotropins during twenty-four hours in a lactating woman before and after resumption of menses. Am J Obstet Gynecol 132:436, 1978

Newton M, Bradford WM: Postpartal blood loss. Obstet Gynecol 17:229, 1961

Perez A, Vela P, Masnic GS, Potter RG: First ovulation after childbirth: The effect of breastfeeding. Am J Obstet Gynecol 114:1041, 1972

Porter JC: Hormonal regulation of breast development and activity. J Invest Dermatol 63:85, 1974

Pritchard JA, Pritchard SA: Unpublished observations.

Richardson AC, Lyon JB, Graham EE, Williams NL: Decreasing postpartum sexual abstinence time. Am J Obstet Gynecol 126:416, 1976

Sende P, Pantelakis N, Suzuki K, Bashore R: Plasma oxytocin level in pregnancy with diabetes insipidus. Clin Res 23:242A, 1975

Sharman A: Menstruation after childbirth. J Obstet Gynaecol Br Emp 58:440, 1951

Sharman A: Postpartum regeneration of the human endometrium. J Anat 87:1, 1953

Sharman A: Ovulation in the post-partum period. Excerpta Medica International Congress Series, No. 133, 1966, p 158

Tyson JE, Friesen HG, Anderson MS: Human lactational and ovarian response to endogenous prolactin release. Science 177:897, 1972

Williams JW: Regeneration of the uterine mucosa after delivery with especial reference to the placental site. Am J Obstet Gynecol 22:664, 1931

Woessner JF: Postpartum involution of the uterus connective tissue framework. Ob/Gyn Digest July 1968, p 14

20

The Newborn Infant

The First Breath of Air. As the infant is born and the fetoplacental circulation ceases to function, the infant is subjected to rapid and profound physiologic changes (see Chap. 8, p. 180). The baby's survival demands a prompt and orderly interchange of oxygen and carbon dioxide between his new environment and the pulmonary circulation. For efficient interchange, the fluid-filled alveoli of the lungs must fill with air, the air must be exchanged by appropriate respiratory motion, and a vigorous microcirculation must be established in close proximity to the alveoli.

INTRAUTERINE RESPIRATION. Until recently, it was widely held that only at times of hypoxic stress did the fetus breathe in utero. This view was so strongly championed by some eminent fetal physiologists that observations to the contrary most often were promptly rejected as being the consequence of abnormal stimulation, most likely hypoxia, during the course of the experiment. In recent years, however, conclusive evidence of episodic respiratory movements in utero has been obtained during normal human pregnancy, as well as in the rabbit, sheep, and monkey (Boddy, Mantell, 1972; Dawes, 1974; Duenhoelter, Pritchard, 1973, 1976;

Martin et al., 1974; Yuan et al., 1974). Pressure changes during inspiration recorded in monkey fetuses by Martin and co-workers appear sufficiently intense to induce movement of amnionic fluid into and out of the fetal lungs, as demonstrated in both monkey and human fetuses by Duenhoelter and Pritchard (1976). It is of clinical interest that general anesthesia and surgery to terminate the pregnancy do not appear to stimulate the inspiration of amnionic fluid, but rather, the opposite.

Initiation of Air Breathing. Very soon after birth, the breathing pattern shifts from one of shallow episodic inspirations that characterize fetal breathing to that of regular deeper inhalations. It is now apparent that aeration of the newborn lung is not the inflation of a collapsed structure, but instead, the rapid replacement of bronchial and alveolar fluid by air.

In the lamb, and presumably in the human infant, residual alveolar fluid after delivery is cleared through the pulmonary circulation and to a lesser degree through pulmonary lymphatics (Chernick, 1978). Delay in the removal of the fluid from the alveoli probably contributes to the syndrome of *transient tachypnea of the newborn* (Avery et al., 1966).

As the fluid is replaced by air, there is considerable reduction in pulmonary vascular compression and, in turn, lowered resistance to blood flow. With the fall in pulmonary arterial blood pressure, the ductus arteriosus normally closes. Closure of the foramen ovale is more variable.

High negative intrathoracic pressures are required to bring about the initial entry of air into fluid-filled alveoli. Normally, from the first breath after birth progressively more residual air accumulates in the lung, and with each successive breath lower pulmonary opening pressure is required. In the mature normal infant, by about the fifth breath of air, the pressure-volume changes achieved with each respiration are very similar to those of the normal adult.

ALVEOLAR SURFACE TENSION AND LUNG SURFACTANT. The successful filling of the lungs with air and the rapid establishment of a physiologic pattern of pressure-volume changes on inspiration and expiration require the presence of surface-active material that will lower surface tension in the alveoli and thereby prevent the collapse of the lung with each expiration. Lecithin and phosphatidyl glycerol synthesized by the alveolar type 2 cells are important components of the pulmonary surfactant system (see Chap. 8, p. 188). Lack of sufficient surfactant leads to the prompt development of the respiratory distress syndrome (see Chap. 38, p. 957).

The Stimuli to Breathe Air. Normally, the newborn infant begins to breathe and cry almost immediately after birth, indicating the establishment of active respiration. All the factors involved in the first breath of air have been difficult to elucidate, undoubtedly because many individually subtle stimuli contribute simultaneously. Some noteworthy explanations follow:

PHYSICAL STIMULATION. The handling of the infant during delivery and contact with various relatively rough surfaces are believed to provoke respiration through stimuli reaching the respiratory center reflexly from the skin.

COMPRESSION OF FETAL THORAX INCIDENT TO DELIVERY. The compression of the thorax during the second stage of labor forces some fluid from the respiratory tract. For example, Saunders (1978) found that considerable pressure is often produced by compression of the chest during vaginal delivery and estimated that lung fluid is expelled equivalent to one-fourth to one-third of ultimate functional residual capacity. While babies born by cesarean section usually cry satisfactorily and sometimes just as quickly as babies born vaginally, they are likely to have more fluid and less gas in their lungs throughout the first six hours after birth (Milner et al., 1978). The compression of the thorax incident to vaginal delivery and the expansion that follows delivery may, nevertheless, be an auxiliary factor in the initiation of respiration.

DEPRIVATION OF OXYGEN AND ACCUMULATION OF CARBON DIOXIDE. It was the opinion of Barcroft and associates (1939), based on animal experimentation, that lack of oxygen caused respiration after birth. Observations on both animals and human beings, however, have shown that profound lack of oxygen produces apnea. If minor degrees of hypoxia produce the first respiration after birth, certain observations become difficult to explain. For example, there is no relation between the concentration of oxygen in the blood at birth and the onset of respiration except possibly that infants with normal levels of oxygen breathe more readily than those with extremely low levels who are often apneic. Blood samples obtained from catheters implanted into fetal vessels of experimental animals for prolonged periods of time without interruption of the pregnancy have revealed that PO_2 is low by adult standards. A further decrease in PO_2 diminishes or abolishes fetal respiratory motion, whereas elevation of PCO_2 increases the frequency and magnitude of fetal breathing movements

(Dawes, 1974). The fetus-infant most likely responds to hypoxia and to hypercapnea the same way in utero and after birth.

Immediate Care.   As the head of the infant is delivered, either vaginally or by cesarean section, the face is immediately wiped and the mouth and nares suctioned (Fig. 20-1). A soft rubber ear syringe or its equivalent inserted with care is quite suitable for the purpose. Before clamping and severing the cord, while the infant is still being held head down, it may be beneficial to aspirate the mouth and pharynx again. Once the cord has been divided, as described in Chapter 17 (p. 422), the infant is immediately placed supine with the head lowered and turned to the side in a heated unit with appropriate thermal regulation and equipped for immediate intensive care (Fig. 20-2).

Evaluation of the Infant.   Before and during delivery, careful consideration must be given to the following determinants of well-being for the infant: (1) health status of the mother; (2) fetal (gestational) age; (3) duration of labor; (4) duration of rupture of the membranes; (5) kinds, amounts, times,

and routes of administration of analgesics; (6) kind and duration of anesthesia; and (7) degree of difficulty encountered in effecting delivery. The obstetrician is responsible for having this information available and effectively disseminating it. The obstetrician inspects the infant for any visible abnormalities during delivery and until the cord is severed and the infant handed over to a trained associate for further care.

The person immediately in charge of caring for the infant should observe respirations closely and identify the heart rate. The heart rate can be determined by auscultation over the chest or by palpating the base of the umbilical cord. A readily discernible heart beat of a hundred or more is acceptable. Persistent bradycardia requires prompt resuscitation. The mouth, nares, and pharynx are carefully suctioned.

Most normal infants take a breath within a few seconds of birth and cry within half a minute. If respirations are infrequent, suction of the mouth and pharynx, followed by light slapping of the soles of the feet and rubbing of the back, usually together serve to stimulate breathing. Prolongation of these intervals beyond 1 and 2 minutes, respectively,

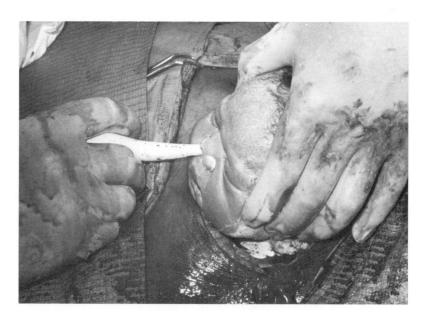

FIG. 20-1.   Aspirating the nose and mouth immediately after delivery of the head.

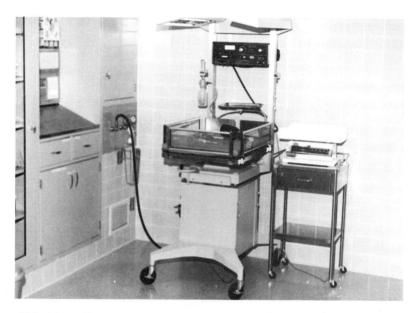

FIG. 20-2. Thermostatically controlled infant care unit in delivery room.

indicates an abnormality. Continued lack of breathing indicates either marked central depression or mechanical obstruction and demands active resuscitation. "Tubbing," "jackknifing," and dilatation of sphincters are condemned as wasteful of valuable time and may cause serious injury.

LACK OF EFFECTIVE RESPIRATIONS. Important causes of failure to establish effective respirations include the following: (1) fetal hypoxemia from any cause; (2) drugs administered to the mother; (3) gross immaturity of the fetus; (4) upper airway obstruction; (5) pneumothorax; (6) other lung abnormalities, either intrinsic (e.g., hypoplasia) or extrinsic (e.g., diaphragmatic hernia); (7) aspiration of amnionic fluid grossly contaminated with meconium, and (8) central nervous system injury.

APGAR SCORE. A useful aid in the evaluation of the infant is the Apgar Scoring System applied at 1 minute and again at 5 minutes after birth (Table 20-1). In general, the higher the score, up to a maximum of 10, the better is the condition of the infant. The one-minute Apgar score determines the need for immediate resuscitation. Most infants are in excellent condition, as indicated by Apgar scores of 7 to 10, and require no aid other than perhaps simple nasopharyngeal suction. *Mildly to moderately depressed infants* score 4 to 7 at one minute, demonstrating depressed respirations, flaccidity, and pale to blue color. Heart rate and reflex irritability, however, are good. *Severely depressed infants* score 0 to 4 with heart rate slow to inaudible and reflex response depressed to absent. Resuscitation, including artificial ventilation, should be started immediately. A low Apgar score at 5 minutes after birth is indicative of increased risk of infant mortality and morbidity.

Resuscitation. Although resuscitative measures beyond the stimulation provided by suctioning the mouth and nares, patting the feet, and rubbing the back are needed by only a small percentage of infants, more active measures, skillfully performed, are lifesaving for that small group. Common errors in the resuscitation of newborn are listed.

1. Failure to check resuscitation equipment beforehand
   damaged resuscitation bag

TABLE 20-1.
APGAR SCORING SYSTEM

SIGN	0	1	2
Heart rate	Absent	Slow (below 100)	Over 100
Respiratory effort	Absent	Slow, irregular	Good, crying
Muscle tone	Flaccid	Some flexion of extremities	Active motion
Reflex irritability	No response	Grimace	Vigorous cry
Color	Blue, pale	Body pink, extremities blue	Completely pink

laryngoscope with dull or flickering light

unsterile insertion of umbilical catheter
2. Use of a cold resuscitation table
3. Unsuccessful intubation
   hyperextension of neck
   inadequate suctioning
   excessive force
4. Inadequate ventilation
   improper head position
   improper application of mask
   placement of tube into esophagus or right mainstem bronchus
   failure to secure tube
5. Failure to detect and determine cause of poor chest movement or persistent bradycardia
6. Failure to detect and treat hypovolemia
7. Failure to perform cardiac massage

Successful active resuscitation requires (1) skilled personnel who are immediately available; (2) a suitably heated, well lighted, appropriately large work area (Fig. 20-2); (3) equipment to deliver oxygen by intermittent positive pressure through a face mask and to carry out endotracheal intubation with endotracheal suction and positive-pressure oxygenation (Fig. 20-3); and (4) drugs, syringes, needles, and catheters for possible intravenous administration of naloxone (Narcan), sodium bicarbonate, and rarely intracardiac injection of epinephrine. The site of every delivery, vaginal or abdominal, must be so

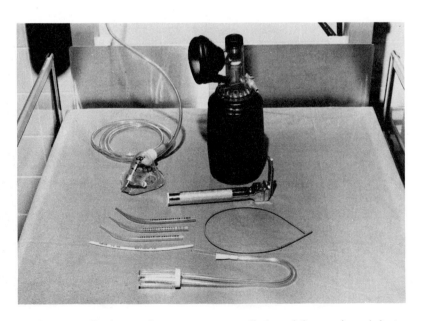

FIG. 20-3. Equipment for emergency ventilation of the newborn infant.

equipped for resuscitation, and the equipment should be thoroughly checked before each delivery.

VENTILATION BY MASK. Inadequate respirations that persist much beyond a minute lead to a falling heart rate and decreased muscle tone and call for a quick but careful physical examination, especially of the mouth, nose, pharynx, neck, and chest, and the administration of oxygen. If the mouth and pharynx are free of liquid and foreign material and no physical obstruction to breathing is identified, oxygen may be delivered through a well-fitting mask at a pressure of about 20 cm of water in 1- to 2-second bursts to deliver oxygen into the bronchi. If this maneuver does not *promptly* stimulate breathing and correct the evidence of hypoxia, endotracheal intubation is necessary under direct visualization with an appropriate laryngoscope.

ENDOTRACHEAL INTUBATION. The head of the supine infant is kept level. The laryngoscope is introduced into the right side of the mouth and then directed posteriorly toward the oropharynx (Fig. 20-4). The laryngoscope is next gently moved into the space between the base of the tongue and the epiglottis. Gentle elevation of the tip of the laryngoscope will pick up the epiglottis and expose the glottis and the vocal cords. The endotracheal tube is entered through the right side of the mouth and is inserted through the vocal cords until the shoulder of the tube reaches the glottis. Care must be exercised to make sure that the tube is in the trachea and not in the esophagus. The laryngoscope is then removed. Any foreign material encountered is immediately removed by suction. Meconium, blood, mucus, and particulate debris in amnionic fluid or in the birth canal may have been inhaled in utero or in the vagina. The resuscitator fills his mouth from an oxygen line and repeatedly puffs oxygen-rich air into the endotracheal tube at 1- to 2-second intervals with force adequate to lift gently the infant's chest wall. Pressures of 25 to 35 cm of water are desired to expand the alveoli yet not cause pneumothorax or pneumomediastinum. If the stomach expands, the tube is almost certainly in the esophagus rather than in the trachea.

As soon as adequate spontaneous respirations have been established, the tube is usually removed. Endotracheal tubes fitted with

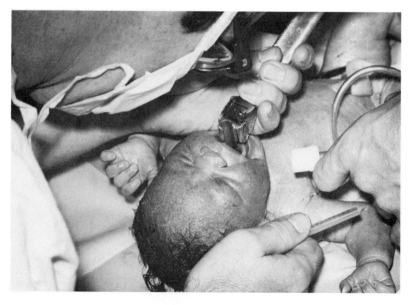

FIG. 20-4.   Use of laryngoscope to insert endotracheal tube under direct vision. Oxygen is being delivered from curved tube held by an assistant.

appropriate adapters may be connected to various mechanical systems for delivering oxygen or air-oxygen mixtures.

ACIDOSIS. Sodium bicarbonate, 1 mEq per kg is injected (after dilution with an equal volume of water) through the umbilical vein of the severely depressed, hypoxic newborn infant who does not respond promptly to establishment of an airway and positive-pressure oxygen administration. This dose may be repeated if favorable clinical response is not soon achieved. It is essential that the infant be ventilated effectively so that carbon dioxide from the bicarbonate can be dissipated. Otherwise, respiratory acidosis will develop, as well as a metabolic acidosis. Further administration of sodium bicarbonate is dependent upon results of measurements of blood gases and pH.

DEPRESSION FROM OPIOID DRUGS. Meperidine (Demerol) and similar drugs given to the mother an hour or less before delivery may cause respiratory depression in the newborn infant. If this appears to be the case, naloxone (Narcan) may be given in a dose of 10 μg per kg (see Chap. 18, p. 438).

HYPOVOLEMIA. Some severely depressed newborn infants are hypovolemic. Hypovolemia may occur without fetal hemorrhage having been detected, for example, with sepsis, fetal to maternal hemorrhage, trauma to the placenta, cord compression with obstruction of the umbilical vein and pooling of blood in the placenta, and twin-to-twin transfusion. At least partial restoration of intravascular volume and correction of anemia are essential for improvement in the volume-depleted infant.

CARDIAC MASSAGE. If fetal heart action was present just before delivery but cannot be demonstrated after birth, or the heart stops after birth, external cardiac massage may be initiated. Immediately, the airway must be cleared, the trachea intubated, and adequate pulmonary ventilation established. External cardiac massage is effected with pressure from two fingers applied to the anterior chest wall in the lower midline at a rate of about 120 per minute. Four compressions of the chest are alternated with each inflation of the lung. Several minutes delay in cardiac massage most likely will result in an unfortunate outcome, either death or permanent marked impairment of central nervous system function.

Epinephrine may be of value in resuscitating the arrested heart. Epinephrine, 0.1 ml per kg of a 1:10,000 dilution, is injected directly into the heart. A 22- or 24-gauge needle is inserted through the fourth intercostal space just to the left of the sternum; blood is aspirated to assure appropriate position of needle tip and the drug is injected as a bolus. Serious trauma from intracardiac injection is always a possibility but an intravenous injection may never reach the heart.

Estimation of Fetal (Gestational) Age. A rapid yet rather precise estimate of gestational age of the newborn infant may be made very soon after delivery by examining (1) sole creases, (2) breast nodules, (3) scalp hair, (4) ear lobe, and (5) in case of the male, testes, and scrotum, as outlined in Table 20-2. A more definitive estimate can be made in a few days with the help of neurologic examination (see Chap. 37, p. 928).

Care of the Eyes. Because of the possibility of infection of the eyes of the newborn during passage through the vagina of a mother with gonorrhea, Credé, in 1884, introduced the practice of instilling into each eye immediately after birth one drop of a 1 percent solution of silver nitrate, which was later washed out with saline. This procedure led to a marked decrease in the frequency but not the elimination of *gonorrheal ophthalmia* and resulting blindness. Some form of prophylaxis is mandatory within the first hour after birth. Several states by law, or health department regulations with the status of law, require effective prophylaxis be used for all deliveries, including cesarean section. At last count, 10 states still required that *silver nitrate* be the agent used.

Technic for Using Silver Nitrate. As a preliminary precaution, the region about each eye

TABLE 20-2.
RAPID ESTIMATION OF GESTATIONAL AGE OF THE NEWBORN

SITES	GESTATIONAL AGE		
	36 Weeks or Less	37 to 38 Weeks	39 Weeks or More
Sole creases	Anterior transverse crease only	Occasional creases anterior two-thirds	Sole covered with creases
Breast nodule diameter	2 mm	4 mm	7 mm
Scalp hair	Fine and fuzzy	Fine and fuzzy	Coarse and silky
Ear lobe	Pliable, no cartilage	Some cartilage	Stiffened by thick cartilage
Testes and scrotum	Testes in lower canal; scrotum small; few rugae	Intermediate	Testes pendulous Scrotum full; extensive rugae

should be irrigated with sterile water applied to the nasal side of the eye and allowed to run off the opposite side. The lower lid should then be drawn down and the 1 percent silver nitrate solution dropped into the lower cul-de-sac.

The silver nitrate produces a discernible chemical conjunctivitis in over half the cases, manifested by redness, edema, or discharge which develops in 24 hours and lasts two to three days.

Penicillin serves as an alternate to silver nitrate in prophylaxis of ophthalmia neonatorum, and for many years at the Johns Hopkins Hospital and the Kings County Hospital penicillin ointment in the strength of 100,000 units per g has been placed in the eyes of all newborn babies. Some institutions use a single dose of penicillin injected intramuscularly. Penicillin so administered to the neonate *may* reduce the frequency of sepsis from Group B streptococcus. Further studies are awaited.

Tetracycline ointment containing the antibiotic in a concentration of 1 percent, liberally instilled into each eye with the lids held apart, has afforded effective prophylaxis in more than 100,000 neonates cared for at Parkland

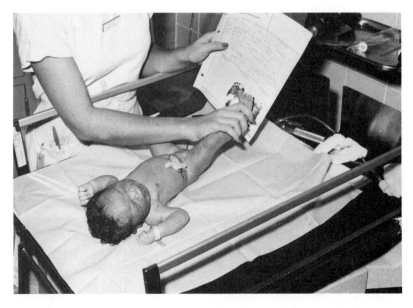

FIG. 20-5. Making a permanent record of the newborn infant's footprints.

Memorial Hospital. Tetracycline does not always prevent chlamydial conjunctivitis.

In summary, Credé prophylaxis with silver nitrate appears to be an anachronism which should be replaced with tetracycline ointment or another equally effective antibiotic regimen.

Permanent Infant Identification. Proper identification of each infant is of prime importance. A foolproof system must be operative at all hours. It should prevent separation of infant from his mother until identification is complete, and it should provide a record easily recognized by the mother, such as an identification band or row of beads that spell the infant's name. It is crucial, furthermore, that a permanent record, such as footprints, be kept on file at the hospital (Fig. 20-5).

The definitive ridges on the palms, fingers, and feet of human beings begin to form several months before birth and remain throughout life. Most hospitals today use footprints rather than fingerprints or palmprints in identifying infants, because the ridges in the feet are more pronounced, and it is easier to obtain prints from them in newborn infants.

Temperature. The temperature of the infant drops rapidly immediately after birth. If the naked newborn is left exposed in the usual air-conditioned delivery room, chilling so produced incites shivering and increases oxygen requirements. Consequently, the infant must be cared for in a warm crib in which temperature control is regulated closely. During the first few days of life, the infant's temperature is unstable, responding to slight stimuli with considerable fluctuations above or below the normal level.

Vitamin K. Routine use of Vitamin K is described in Chapter 38 (p. 976).

Umbilical Cord. Loss of water from Wharton's jelly leads to mummification of the cord shortly after birth. Within 24 hours, it loses its characteristic bluish white, moist appearance and soon becomes dry and black. Gradually the line of demarcation appears just beyond the skin of the abdomen, and in a few days the stump sloughs, leaving a small, granulating wound, which after healing forms the umbilicus. Separation usually takes place within the first two weeks after birth, most frequently around the 10th day, but occasionally only after several weeks.

Formerly the care of the cord was considered trivial. Disregard for asepsis in management of the cord, however, frequently resulted in serious infection transmitted through the umbilical vessels, and at times it caused death of the infant. Even today serious umbilical infections are sometimes encountered, usually, but not always, indicating gross lack of care. The offending organisms often are *Staphylococcus aureus, Escherichia coli,* or group B *Streptococcus.* Since the umbilical stump in such cases may present no outward sign of infection, the diagnosis cannot be made with certainty except by autopsy. Whenever infants die within three weeks after birth without an obvious cause, such an infection should be suspected. Examination of the intra-abdominal portion of the umbilical vessels at autopsy sometimes reveals purulent thrombi, in which pyogenic microorganisms can be demonstrated. Strict aseptic precautions should, therefore, be observed in the immediate care of the cord. The umbilical cord dries more quickly and separates more readily when exposed to the air, and therefore a dressing is not recommended.

Care of the Skin. Infants should be promptly patted dry to minimize heat loss caused by evaporation. In most hospitals, not all the vernix caseosa is removed, but the excess, as well as blood and meconium, is gently wiped off. The vernix caseosa is readily absorbed by the baby's skin and disappears entirely within 24 hours. It is unwise to wash a newborn infant until his temperature has stabilized. Handling of the baby should be minimized.

Stools and Urine. For the first two or three days after birth, the contents of the colon are composed of soft, brownish-green *meconium,* which is comprised of desquamated epithelial cells from the intestinal tract, mucus, and epidermal cells and lanugo (fetal hair) that have been swallowed with the amnionic fluid. The characteristic color results from fetal bile pigments. During intrauterine life and for a few hours after birth, the intestinal contents are sterile, but bacteria soon gain access to them. The passage of meconium and urine in the minutes immediately after birth or during the next few hours indicates patency of the gastrointestinal and urinary tracts. Of all newborn infants, 90 percent pass meconium within the first 24 hours; most of the rest do so within 36 hours. Voiding may not occur until the second day of life. Failure of the infant to eliminate meconium or urine after these times suggests a congenital defect such as imperforate anus or a urethral valve.

After the third or fourth day, as the consequence of ingesting milk, the meconium disappears and is replaced by light yellow homogeneous feces with a characteristic odor. For the first few days, the stools are unformed, but after a short time they assume their characteristic cylindric shape.

Icterus Neonatorum. About one-third of all babies, between the second and fifth day of life, develop so-called *physiologic jaundice of the newborn.* There is a hyperbilirubinemia at birth of 1.8 to 2.8 mg per dl of serum. It increases during the next few days but with wide individual variation. Between the third and fourth day, the bilirubin in mature infants commonly reaches somewhat more than 5 mg per dl of serum, the concentration at which jaundice usually becomes noticeable. Most of the bilirubin is free, or unconjugated. One cause, but not the sole cause, of the hyperbilirubinemia is immaturity of the hepatic cells, resulting in slight conjugation of bilirubin with glucuronic acid and reduced excretion of the conjugate in the bile (Chap. 38, p. 972). Reabsorption of free bilirubin as the consequence of the enzymatic splitting of bilirubin glucuronide by intestinal conjugase activity in the newborn intestine also appears to contribute significantly to the transient hyperbilirubinemia (Poland, Odell, 1971). In premature infants, jaundice is more common and usually more severe and prolonged than in term infants because of greater hepatic enzymatic immaturity. Infants that are small for gestational age, however, metabolize bilirubin in a manner similar to mature infants. Increased erythrocyte destruction from any cause contributes to hyperbilirubinemia (see Chap. 38, p. 972).

Initial Loss of Weight. Because the infant may receive little nutriment for the first three or four days of life and at the same time produces a considerable amount of urine, feces, and sweat, he progressively loses weight until the flow of maternal milk or other feeding has been established. Premature infants lose relatively more weight and regain their birth weight more slowly than do term infants. Infants that are small for gestational age, however, regain their initial weight more quickly, when fed, than do premature infants.

If the infant is nourished properly, the birth weight is usually regained by the end of the 10th day. Subsequently, the weight normally increases steadily at the rate of about 25 g a day for the first few months, to double the birth weight by the time the child is five months of age, and to triple it by the end of the first year.

Frequency of Feeding. Despite the small quantity of colostrum available, it is advisable, because of the stimulating effect of nursing on mother and baby, to commence regular nursing within the first 12 hours postpartum. Most mature infants thrive best when fed at intervals of about four hours. Premature or growth-retarded infants require feedings at shorter intervals; in most instances a three-hour interval is satisfactory.

Duration of Feeding. The proper length of each feeding depends on several factors, such as the quantity of breast milk, the readiness with which it can be obtained from the breast, and the avidity with which the infant nurses. It is generally advisable to allow the baby to remain at the breast for 10 minutes at first; 4 to 5 minutes are sufficient for some infants, however, and 15 to 20 minutes are required by others. It is satisfactory for the baby to nurse for 5 minutes at each breast for the first 4 days, or until the mother has a supply of milk. After the 4th day, the baby nurses up to 10 minutes on each breast. A baby receiving proper nourishment should increase steadily in weight.

Circumcision. There is no absolute medical indication for routine circumcision of the newborn, as emphasized in the report of the Ad Hoc Task Force on Circumcision to the American Academy of Pediatrics (1975). Nonetheless, this procedure has been very popular. For example, according to the Commission on Professional and Hospital activities, in 1974 the ratio of circumcisions of male infants (below two years of age) to the number of births of male infants was in excess of 0.8.

The following advantages are commonly claimed for circumcision of the newborn infant: (1) phimosis is prevented; (2) the incidence of balanitis is markedly reduced; (3) penile cancer is virtually eliminated; and (4) it has become traditional to circumcise male infants in the United States. Lack of circumcision of the male sex partner does not appear to increase the risk of carcinoma of the cervix, as previously thought (Terris et al., 1973).

Circumcision, if it is to be done at all, should not be performed at delivery but rather a day or two later, after the infant has been demonstrated to be healthy. Prematurity, neonatal illness, most congenital anomalies of the penis, and coagulation defects are contraindications to circumcision.

Within the past few years, a flurry of reports critical of routine circumcision have appeared. The adverse comments range from psychologic trauma to subsequent hypesthesia of the glans. The subjective nature of these allegations makes them difficult to prove. Objectively, operative complications can be minimized by attention to surgical technic. Proper use of the Gomco (Yellen) clamp (Fig. 20-6) (Woodside, 1980) provides an additional safeguard against accidents.

Circumcision with Gomco Clamp. The healthy infant who has fasted for 4 hours is fastened supine to a clean, padded, rigid, x-shaped form of appropriate size using clean, soft fabric around the arms, legs, and abdomen. The genitalia and surrounding region are scrubbed and the operating field draped, usually using a small sterile towel with a central opening. The prepuce is very carefully separated from the glans penis. To do so, the margins of the opening in the prepuce are grasped bilaterally with two small hemostats and a small curved hemostat is inserted between the inner surface of the foreskin and the glans with particular care to avoid entering the urethral meatus. The jaws of the curved clamp are opened circumferentially. The prepuce, after being separated from the glans, is incised superiorly; the length of the incision corresponds to the amount of foreskin to be removed (Fig. 20-6. A.). It is preferred by some to remove only one-half to two-thirds of the foreskin. The incised prepuce is next pushed back and any adherence to the glans that might persist is relieved.

The cone of a Gomco clamp of appropriate size is inserted between the foreskin and glans, and the margins of the foreskin are drawn through the beveled hole in the platform of the clamp. *This maneuver is especially critical, since it is possible to pull skin that normally covers the shaft of the penis through the beveled hole and inadvertently denude much or all of the penis.* The opposite end of the cone and the elevator arm of the clamp are now engaged and the nut is tightened firmly.

After 5 minutes to effect hemostasis, with the use of a scalpel the foreskin is excised immediately above the platform of the clamp (Fig. 20-6. B.). The clamp is disassembled, and the cone of the clamp is removed from over the glans (Fig. 20-6. C.). In the demonstration case provided in Figure 20-6, sufficient foreskin remains to cover part of the glans (Fig. 20-6. D.), yet can be easily pushed back to allow thorough cleansing (Fig. 20-6. E.). If there is no bleeding, and there should be none, the baby is returned to his crib with no dressing other than the diaper. Healing is normally prompt.

ANESTHESIA FOR CIRCUMCISION? Kirya and Werthmann (1978) raise the question, "Why not anesthesia for neonatal circumcision?" and, in turn, describe their experiences with regional nerve block from injected lidocaine. Perhaps a more pertinent question is, "Why routine neonatal circumcision in the first place?"

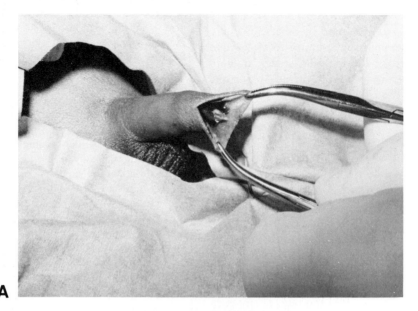

A

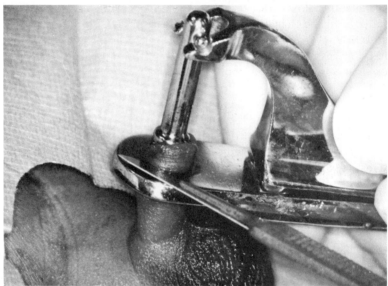

B

FIG. 20-6. A. The foreskin has been carefully separated from the glans and incised superiorly. The length of the incision corresponds to the amount of foreskin to be removed. The cone of the Gomco clamp is now inserted (see **C**). **B.** The foreskin is excised immediately above the base of the Gomco clamp. Five minutes before excision, the cone of the clamp was placed between foreskin and glans; the stem was then directed through the hole in the base; an appropriate amount of foreskin was carefully pulled over the cone through the hole in the base; the stem and fulcrum were engaged; and the nut on the opposite end of the clamp was firmly tightened. **C.** Approximately one-half of the foreskin has just been excised and the clamp removed except for the cone still in position between prepuce and glans. **D.** The cone has been removed. The foreskin that remains covers about one-half of the glans. **E.** The foreskin is easily retracted to expose all of the glans. *(Continued)*

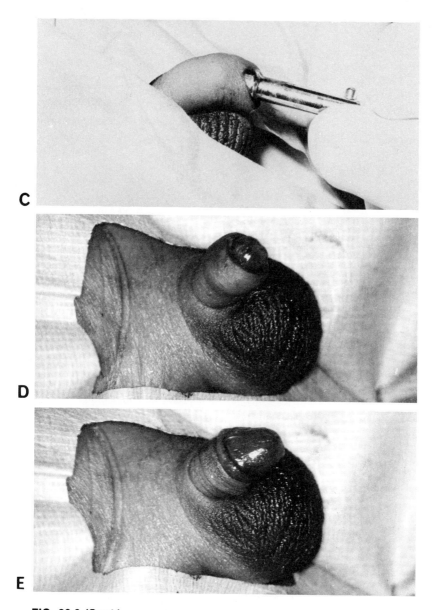

C

D

E

FIG. 20.6 (Cont.)

Rooming-in.   Rooming-in involves keeping the infant in a crib at the mother's bedside rather than in the nursery, which permits the mother to take care of the baby. This practice stems in part from a trend to make all phases of childbearing as "natural" as possible and to foster proper mother-child relationships at an early date. By the end of 24 hours, the mother is generally fully ambulatory and thereafter, with rooming-in, she can conduct for herself and for the infant practically all the routine care. An advantage of this program is the mother's increased ability, when she arrives at home, to assume full care of the baby.

Abnormalities of the Newborn Infant.   These are considered throughout the text and especially in Chapters 37, 38, and 39.

REFERENCES

Avery ME, Gatewood OB, Brumley G: Transient tachypnea of the newborn. Am J Dis Child 111:380, 1966

Barcroft J, Kramer K, Millikan GA: The oxygen in the carotid blood at birth. J Physiol 94:571, 1939

Boddy K, Mantell CD: Observations of fetal breathing movements transmitted through maternal abdominal wall. Lancet 2:1219, 1972

Chernick V: Fetal breathing movements and the onset of breathing at birth. Clin Perinatol 5:257, 1978

Credé CSF: Die Verhütung der Augenentzündung der Neugeborenen. Berlin, Hirschwald, 1884

Dawes GS: Breathing before birth in animals or man. New Engl J Med 290:557, 1974

Duenhoelter JH, Pritchard JA: Human fetal respiration. Obstet Gynecol 42:746, 1973

Duenhoelter JH, Pritchard JA: Fetal respiration: Quantitative measurements of amnionic fluid inspired near term by human and rhesus fetuses. Am J Obstet Gynecol 125:306, 1976

Kirya C, Werthmann MW Jr: Neonatal circumcision and penile dorsal route nerve block—a painless procedure. J Pediatr 92:998, 1978

Martin CB Jr, Murata Y, Petrie RH, Parer JT: Respiratory movements in fetal rhesus monkeys. Am J. Obstet Gynecol 119:939, 1974

Milner AD, Saunders RA, Hopkins IE: The effects of delivery by caesarean section on lung mechanics and lung volume in the human neonate. Arch Dis Child 53:545, 1978

Poland RL, Odell GB: Physiologic jaundice: the enterohepatic circulation of bilirubin. New Engl J Med 284:1, 1971

Report of the Ad Hoc Task Force on Circumcision. Pediatrics 56:610, 1975

Saunders RA: Pulmonary pressure/volume relationships during the last phase of delivery and the first postnatal breaths in human subjects. J Pediatr 93:667, 1978

Terris M, Wilson F, Nelson JH Jr: Relation of circumcision to cancer of the cervix. Am J Obstet Gynecol 117:1056, 1973

Woodside JR: Necrotizing fasciatis after neonatal circumcision. Am J Dis Child 134:301, 1980

Yuan L, Pericelli A, Gitlin D: The normal aspiration of amniotic fluid by the conceptus. Pediatr Res 8:453/179, 1974

21

Obstetric Hemorrhage

BLOOD LOSS AND REPLACEMENT THERAPY

Mortality from Hemorrhage. Obstetrics is "bloody business." Even though the maternal mortality rate has been reduced dramatically by hospitalization for delivery and the availability of blood for transfusion, death from hemorrhage remains prominent in most mortality reports. For example, 111 of 309 maternal deaths in Texas during 1969 to 1973 were attributed to hemorrhage (Gibbs, 1975). In Oklahoma, during the decade preceding 1975, 31 of 99 maternal deaths were the consequence of hemorrhage (Jimerson, Crosby, 1978).

Blood Loss at Parturition. Loss of 500 ml or more of blood after completion of the third stage of labor is a persistent definition of postpartum hemorrhage (Hughes, 1972). Nonetheless, nearly one-half of all women shed, as the consequence of parturition, that amount of blood or more, as emphasized by Newton (1966) and by Pritchard and coworkers (1962) (Fig. 21-1. A.).

The woman who develops a normal degree of pregnancy hypervolemia usually increases her blood volume by a factor of one-third to two-thirds, which for an individual of average size, amounts to 1000 to as much as 2000 ml (Pritchard, 1965). Most often she will tolerate, without any remarkable decrease in hematocrit, blood loss at delivery that approaches the volume of blood that was added during pregnancy (Fig. 21-1. B.). Data from a specific case that serve to dramatize the protective nature of pregnancy hypervolemia are in Table 21-1. In spite of a blood loss of 2200 ml, as the consequence of abdominal delivery plus radical hysterectomy and pelvic lymphadenectomy, hypervolemia was effectively combatted with only 500 ml of blood augmented by sufficient lactated Ringer's solution to maintain urine output. The hematocrit postpartum decreased only slightly, since total blood loss was not much greater than the sum of the 500 ml of blood replaced and the 1700 ml of pregnancy-induced normal hypervolemia.

The tolerance to hemorrhage at parturition that is normally induced by pregnancy undoubtedly allowed the human race to survive before the era of hospitalization and blood banks. Nonetheless, deaths from hemorrhage were common because of the number of obstetric complications that predisposed to severe hemorrhage and death in the absence of expert management, including blood replacement therapy.

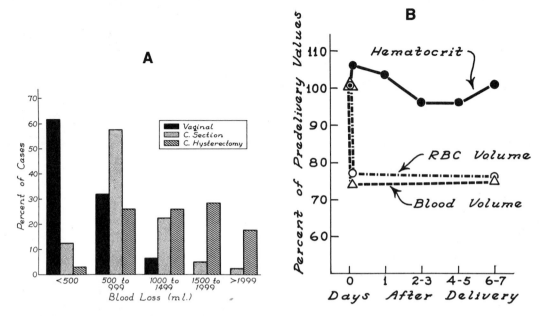

FIG. 21-1. A. *(above left)* Blood loss associated with vaginal delivery, repeat cesarean section, and repeat cesarean section plus total hysterectomy. **B.** *(above right)* In a group of women undergoing cesarean section, the hematocrit postpartum changed insignificantly from the predelivery value in spite of an average blood loss of 1000 ml. At the same time, the blood volume and total erythrocyte volume dropped nearly 25 percent. (From Pritchard et al. *Am J Obstet Gynecol* 84:1271, 1962)

TABLE 21-1.
PATIENT 37 WEEKS PREGNANT, CARCINOMA OF CERVIX,
RADICAL HYSTERECTOMY, AND PELVIC LYMPHADENECTOMY

| DAY | HEMATOCRIT | VOLUME | | LOSS | |
		Blood	RBC	RBC	Blood
−1	34.0	5444	1850		
Surgery	Transfused 500 ml blood				
+1	34.0	3835	1304	746*	2200
+2	30.5				
+4	30.5				
+6	29.0				
+8	31.0	4023	1247	813	2400
+84	42.0	3755	1577		

* Includes 200 ml of transfused RBC.

Listed below are the many clinical circumstances in which risk of obstetric hemorrhage is appreciably increased. It is apparent that serious obstetric hemorrhage may occur at any time throughout pregnancy and the puerperium.

OBSTETRIC HEMORRHAGE: IDENTIFICATION OF WOMEN AT INCREASED RISK

A. Abnormal Placental Implantation or Development
   1. Placenta previa

2. Placental abruption
3. Placenta accreta
4. Ectopic pregnancy
5. Late abortion
6. Hydatidiform mole
B. Trauma During Labor or Delivery
1. Vaginal delivery other than spontaneous or outlet forceps
2. Cesarean section or cesarean hysterectomy
3. Uterine rupture
(a) Previously scarred uterus
(b) High parity
(c) Obstructed labor
(d) Intrauterine manipulation to effect delivery (breech, version, destructive procedures on fetus)
C. Uterine Atony
1. Overdistended uterus
(a) Multiple fetuses
(b) Hydramnios
2. Exhausted myometrium
(a) Vigorous (tumultuous) labor
(b) Prolonged labor
(c) Oxytocin-stimulated labor
3. Anesthesia
(a) Ether and most halogenated agents
(b) Conduction anesthesia with hypotension and atony
4. Previous postpartum hemorrhage
D. Small Maternal Blood Volume
1. Small women
2. Pregnancy hypervolemia not yet maximum
3. Pregnancy hypervolemia obtunded
(a) Severe pregnancy-induced hypertension (especially eclampsia)
(b) Shrunken extracellular fluid volume (sodium restriction, diuretics, vomiting, diarrhea)
(c) Severe megaloblastic anemia
E. Coagulation Defects
1. Conditions predisposing to impaired coagulation
(a) Placental abruption
(b) Prolonged retention of dead fetus
(c) Amnionic fluid embolism
(d) Sepsis
(e) Gross intravascular hemolysis
(f) Massive hemorrhage treated with stored blood
(g) Eclampsia and severe preeclampsia
(h) Abnormalities of coagulation coincidental to pregnancy

The time of bleeding in pregnancy is widely used to classify obstetric hemorrhage, especially bleeding during the third trimester. The term *third trimester bleeding* serves only one useful purpose and that is to warn people *not* to proceed in routine fashion with pelvic examination on the bleeding woman for fear of inciting severe hemorrhage from placenta previa. The term otherwise is so imprecise for describing gestational (fetal) age and, in turn, intelligent management of the pregnancy that it ought to be abandoned.

Etiology of Obstetric Hemorrhage. Obstetric hemorrhage is the consequence of excessive bleeding from the placental implantation site, or trauma to the genital tract and adjacent structures, or both.

BLEEDING FROM PLACENTAL SITE. Near term, it is estimated that approximately 600 ml per minute of maternal blood flows through the intracotyledonary spaces of the placenta. With separation of the placenta, the many arteries and veins that carry blood to and from the intracotyledonary spaces are severed abruptly. Effective hemostasis demands that the patency of these vessels be quickly obliterated. Elsewhere in the body hemostasis in the absence of surgical ligation depends upon intrinsic vasospasm and formation of blood clot locally.

At the placental implantation site, much more important to hemostasis than intrinsic vasospasm and clotting, are contraction and retraction of the myometrium to compress the severed vessels and obliterate their lumens. Adherent pieces of placenta or large blood clots, as well as a hypotonic myometrium, are likely to prevent effective contraction and retraction of the myometrium and thereby impair hemostasis at the implantation site. Fatal postpartum hemorrhage can occur from a hypotonic uterus while the maternal blood coagulation mechanism is quite normal. Conversely, if the myometrium at and adjacent to the denuded implantation site contracts and retracts vigorously, fatal hemorrhage from the placental implantation site is unlikely even though the blood coagulation mechanism may be severely impaired.

BLEEDING FROM SITES OF TRAUMA. Lacerated or incised blood vessels in the reproductive tract other than in the body of the uterus lack the unique mechanism for obliterating vessel patency that is provided by a vigorously contracting and retracting myometrium. Consequently, oxytocic drugs and uterine massage are ineffective in controlling hemorrhage if the hemorrhage is not of uterine origin. Therefore, persistent hemorrhage from the genital tract following delivery of an intact placenta and with the uterus firmly contracted and retracted is indicative almost certainly of bleeding from lacerations of the genital tract.

Management of Hemorrhage. Whenever there is any suggestion of excessive blood loss from the genital tract, irrespective of apparent cause, it is essential that steps be taken immediately to identify the presence of uterine atony, retained placental fragments, and trauma to the genital tract. It is imperative that at least one, and in the presence of frank hemorrhage two, intravenous infusion systems of large caliber be established immediately to allow rapid administration of aqueous crystalloid solutions, of which lacatated Ringer's solution is especially appropriate, and blood, as one or both are needed. (Guidelines for their use are described below under "Fluid Replacement for Hemorrhage.") An operating room and surgical team, including an anesthesiologist, must be immediately available.

Magnitude of Hemorrhage. A number of techniques are employed to estimate the magnitude of the hemorrhage, most of which by themselves may yield grossly erroneous values, especially when hemorrhage is external but brisk or when hemorrhage is concealed, as with placental abruption or hemoperitoneum.

VISUAL ESTIMATE. Visual inspection is resorted to most often but is notoriously inaccurate. The estimates may be greatly excessive or, more likely, dangerously low. Furthermore, part or all of the hemorrhage may be concealed.

BLOOD PRESSURE AND PULSE. These vital signs may be quite misleading. Overt hypotension is, of course, a dangerous sign that cannot be ignored but the converse is not necessarily true. **A blood pressure reading in the normal range, or even hypertension, does not preclude dangerous hypovolemia.** Hypertension, either pregnancy-induced or chronic, is not unusual in pregnant women and therefore serious hemorrhage and the resultant hypovolemia may in this circumstance result in a fall in blood pressure only to normotensive levels. The normotensive reading may create a false sense of security with delay in identification of compromised perfusion of vital organs.

The pulse rate can be equally misleading since it may be elevated in circumstances where the degree of hemorrhage is negligible or normal or even low in the presence of severe hypovolemia (Jansen, 1978).

"TILT TEST." The woman who has bled appreciably but whose blood pressure and pulse rate are normal when recumbent may, when placed in the sitting position, become hypotensive, or develop tachycardia, or both. This so-called tilt test should be interpreted with caution: For the woman who is already hypotensive when recumbent, the tilt test is needless and potentially dangerous. The parturient who has not yet fully recovered from the sympathetic blockade of conduction anesthesia, especially spinal, may become hypotensive when placed in the sitting position without necessarily having suffered serious hemorrhage. Finally, the hypervolemic pregnant woman may lose a large amount of blood before demonstrating orthostatic hypotension.

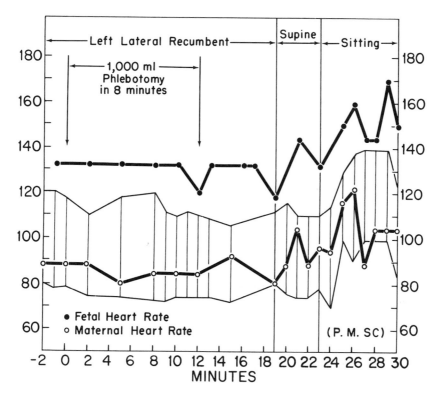

FIG. 21-2. Responses late in pregnancy to phlebotomy and changes in posture following phlebotomy. Partial exchange transfusion was being carried out in a woman with sickle cell-hemoglobin C disease; her pregnancy-induced hypervolemia amounted to 1400 ml. Systolic and diastolic blood pressures are plotted as light lines and each reading is interconnected. The open circles connected by a heavy line demonstrate the maternal pulse rate and the solid dots so connected are the fetal heart rates.

The immediate effects from appreciable hemmorrhage demonstrated in Figure 21-2 seem paradoxical. The woman with sickle cell-hemoglobin C disease near term underwent phlebotomy for exchange transfusion. Her measured blood volume was 6 liters and hematocrit 38. One liter of blood was removed over 8 minutes while she was very carefully observed lying on her side. Her blood pressure and pulse, as well as the fetal heart rate, were monitored continuously. During the 20 minutes following hemorrhage until infusion of packed erythrocytes was begun, she was observed first laterally recumbent, then supine, and finally sitting. Her blood pressure was unchanged until she sat up, when it rose moderately, as did the maternal and fetal heart rates. Thus the initial response to appreciable hemorrhage in the late pregnant woman may be a rise in blood pressure similar to that observed at times in normal non-pregnant individuals.

URINE FLOW. When carefully measured, the rate of urine formation *in the absence of potent diuretics* reflects the adequacy of renal perfusion and, in turn, the perfusion of other vital organs, since renal blood flow is especially sensitive to changes in effective blood volume. With potentially serious hemorrhage, an indwelling catheter is promptly inserted first to empty the bladder completely and then to collect quantitatively all urine formed.

Unfortunately, a potent diuretic such as furosemide is very likely to invalidate the relationship between urine flow and renal perfusion. This need not be a handicap to management of the woman who is hemorrhaging, however, since there are no proven benefits to be derived from the use of furosemide in this setting. Actually, the reverse is true;

there is the potential for harm. Furosemide very rapidly induces venodilatation and thereby further reduces venous return and cardiac output (Dikshit et al., 1973; Heinemann, 1978).

Measurements of Blood Volume. For identification of the magnitude of hemorrhage and the need for replacement therapy, measurements of blood volume have proved to be difficult to interpret for several reasons. For the individual pregnant woman, the ideal blood volume is not known. This is especially true during the intrapartum or early postpartum period, since the size of the intravascular compartment normally undergoes remarkable change then as the consequence of delivery (Pritchard, 1965). Moreover, in the presence of brisk hemorrhage, the blood volume changes so rapidly as to render any measurement invalid by the time it is completed.

Fluid Replacement for Hemorrhage. Treatment of serious hemorrhage demands prompt and adequate refilling of the intravascular compartment. Two general guidelines have proved to be invaluable for determining the amounts and the kinds of fluids that are needed to combat hypovolemia from obstetric hemorrhage irrespective of cause:

1. Lactated Ringer's solution and whole blood are given in such amounts and in such proportions that (1) urine flow is at least 30 ml per hour and ideally approaches 60 ml per hour, or 1 ml per minute, and (2) the hematocrit reading is maintained at 30 percent or slightly higher.
2. If initial vigorous therapy with the aqueous fluid and whole blood does not restore urine flow, the central venous pressure is then monitored as more fluids are given.

Two precautions require emphasis: (1) Urine flow after administration of a potent diuretic does not necessarily bear any relationship to the level of renal perfusion. Therefore, if the rate of urine flow is to be used successfully to identify adequate perfusion of the kidney and, in turn, other vital organs, diuretic agents such as furosemide should not be given. (2) Insertion of the catheter for monitoring central venous pressure may lead to troublesome bleeding at the site of venipuncture if significant coagulation defects exist. Hence, in circumstances where there may be coagulation defects, rather than insert the central venous pressure catheter into the subclavian vein, a vein in the antecubital fossa should be used since bleeding can be controlled by pressure and a dangerous expanding hematoma avoided. Further support for the recommendation above that the hematocrit be raised to and kept at 30 or slightly higher has been provided recently by Czer and Shoemaker (1978). In their series of 94 critically ill postoperative patients, oxygen availability and consumption increased significantly after transfusion whenever the pretransfusion hematocrit was much below 32. Importantly, mortality rates were lowest with hematocrit values between 27 and 33.

WHOLE BLOOD AND BLOOD FRACTIONS. Fresh compatible whole blood, rather than stored blood, would be more nearly ideal for treatment of hypovolemia from serious acute hemorrhage, since stored blood soon suffers from loss of functional platelets and decreased activities of factors V and VIII. After one day of storage, platelets and granulocytes are no longer viable. Moreover, as the length of storage time increases, the concentrations of potassium, ammonia, free acid, and hemoglobin rise in the plasma and that of 2, 3-diphosphoglycerate in the erythrocyte drops, causing increased oxygen affinity. In spite of these disadvantages, the policy of the Obstetrics Service and the Blood Bank at Parkland Memorial Hospital, dictated by the practicalities of blood banking, has long been to treat hypovolemia from hemorrhage with any readily available blood that is compatible by adequate cross-match. In the infrequent situation where immediate blood replacement is necessary, type-specific blood is used until appropriately crossmatched blood is available. So far, no serious problems from incompatibility have been created by this course of action. The so-called universal donor who has type 0 Rho-negative erythrocytes and low anti-A and anti-B titers is a rare individual, and therefore such blood is seldom available.

After the infusion of many units of stored whole blood, generalized bleeding may develop as the consequence of intense thrombocytopenia, or less likely, from low levels of factors V and VIII. To treat hemorrhage believed to be the direct consequence of severe thrombocytopenia, platelets should be administered from 8 to 10 units of blood that has been obtained very recently from donors of the same blood type as the recipient. If the platelets from an Rh-positive donor are given to an Rh-negative recipient who might conceive again, immune globulin containing Rho-antibody should be administered promptly in amounts sufficient to provide circulating free antibody. Factor V and VIII levels that are low after repeated transfusion with stored blood can be improved by administering fresh frozen plasma. The use of fibrinogen, as well as its nonuse since it is seldom required, is discussed under those obstetric diseases in which severe hypofibrinogenemia is sometimes found (p. 505).

Blood component therapy consisting of fresh platelet packs and previously frozen, freshly thawed erythrocytes and plasma will be used more often in the future but not to the exclusion of whole blood. Fresh frozen plasma provides higher levels of unstable coagulation factors than does stored whole blood. Very recently thawed and washed erythrocytes are essentially free of leukocyte antigens, as well as extracellular potassium, ammonia, and hemoglobin. Platelet packs hopefully supply functional platelets in appropriate numbers.

ACQUIRED COAGULATION DEFECTS

Gross derangement of the coagulation mechanism as the direct consequence of a variety of obstetric accidents, or less commonly as the result of a coincidental disease, may incite or enhance obstetric hemorrhage (p. 494). The subject has been reviewed by Bonnar and co-workers (1969), by Pritchard (1973), by Levin and Algazy (1975), and others. Pregnancy normally induces appreciable increases in the concentrations in plasma of coagulation factors I (fibrinogen), VII, VIII, IX, and X. Other plasma factors and platelets do not change so remarkably. Plasminogen levels are increased considerably, yet plasmin activity during the antepartum period is normally decreased compared to the nonpregnant state. Various stresses incite activation of plasminogen to plasmin including delivery and especially activation of the coagulation mechanism.

Investigations originally of a variety of accidents of pregnancy led to recognition of the entity of acquired intravascular coagulation, more recently referred to as consumptive coagulopathy, or disseminated intravascular coagulation (DIC). Reid, McKay, and co-workers in Boston, Page and associates in San Francisco (1951), Schneider (1951) in Detroit, and Ratnoff and colleagues (1955) in Cleveland during the 1950s provided many of the early critical observations.

PATHOLOGIC ACTIVATION OF COAGULATION MECHANISM. Undoubtedly, existing knowledge of the intricacies of the coagulation mechanisms is far from complete. There are very likely more mechanisms than primary activation of factor VII and the so-called extrinsic pathway, or of factor XII and the intrinsic pathway, by which some clotting factors may be activated and removed from the circulation.

Typically, coagulation incites the activation of plasminogen to plasmin which can lyse fibrinogen, fibrin monomer, and fibrin polymer to form a series of fibrinogen-fibrin degradation products, or split products. The degradation products, depending upon their size, may contribute to defective hemostasis by blocking the action of thrombin on fibrinogen (prolonged thrombin time), by impairing platelet function (impaired clot retraction), and by causing defective fibrin clot formation through their incorporation into fibrin polymer (impaired clot retraction and stability).

SIGNIFICANCE OF CONSUMPTIVE CO-AGULOPATHY.

Observations of consumptive coagulopathy were initially confined almost totally to obstetrics but more recently have been made in nearly all branches of medicine. Management commonly recommended in obstetrics and in other areas of medicine has often unduly emphasized (1) heroic attempts to replace the deficient clotting factors, especially fibrinogen; (2) injection of heparin in the hope of blocking further intravascular coagulation; (3) administration of ϵ-aminocaproic acid to try to block fibrinolysis; or (4) some combination of the first three. Not infrequently, the precise nature of the underlying disease has not been considered thoroughly, and it has even been ignored. The use of heparin, for example, has been urged by some in circumstances in which the likelihood of benefit would appear to be slight but the risk of potentiating hemorrhage great. More specifically, a disease such as placental abruption, in which the process of intravascular coagulation ceases at delivery, if not before, rarely, if ever, justifies the use of heparin. It is perplexing that recommendations for treatment of obstetric hemorrhage with heparin have commonly been made in general medical textbooks and journals, as well as in those works concerned primarily with obstetrics, by authors who cite no significant data, either personally accumulated or gleaned from the publications of others. This has been particularly true for placental abruption.

While the injection of coagulation factors, the blocking of fibrin formation with heparin, and use of drugs to inhibit fibrinolytic activity have been unduly stressed, the value of vigorous restoration and maintenance of the circulation to combat intravascular coagulation has not received appropriate attention. **With adequate perfusion of vital organs, activated coagulation factors and soluble fibrin and fibrin degradation products are much more promptly removed by the reticuloendothelial system. At the same time,** **synthesis of procoagulants is promoted, especially by the liver.**

The likelihood of hemorrhage in obstetric situations complicated by defective coagulation will depend not only on the extent of the coagulation defects, but of great importance, on whether or not the vasculature is intact or disrupted, and if it is disrupted, the magnitude of the disruption. With gross derangement of blood coagulation, there may be fatal hemorrhage when vascular integrity is disrupted, yet no hemorrhage as long as all blood vessels remain intact. Moreover, each category of disease must be considered separately, and for each case in any category the intensity of the intravascular coagulation and the dangers therefrom must be carefully measured before a decision is made to employ a therapy as potentially dangerous as heparin, fibrinogen, or ϵ-aminocaproic acid. A variety of factors must be considered that include "When will delivery be accomplished and by what route?" It cannot be overemphasized that the laboratory identification of possible stigmas of intravascular coagulation such as thrombocytopenia, fibrin degradation products in serum, or distorted erythrocytes in a blood smear suggesting microangiopathic hemolytic anemia, should *not* in themselves serve as indications for the prompt use of heparin, fibrinogen, or ϵ-aminocaproic acid. It also must be kept in mind that impaired synthesis may be the cause of pathologically low levels of some procoagulants rather than abnormal consumption.

Signs of Defective Hemostasis. Excessive bleeding at sites of modest trauma characterizes defective hemostasis. Persistent bleeding from venipuncture sites, nicks incurred from shaving the perineum or abdomen, trauma from insertion of a catheter, as well as spontaneous bleeding from the gums or nose, serve to alert the physician to probable defects in the coagulation mechanism.

If serious *hypofibrinogenemia* is present, as may be the case with severe placental abruption, especially, the clot formed from whole blood in a glass tube may be soft initially but not necessarily remarkably reduced in volume. Then, over the next one-half hour or so, it becomes quite small so that many of the erythrocytes are extruded and the volume of liquid clearly exceeds that of the clot. The addition of thrombin to hasten the conversion of circulating fibrinogen to fibrin has practical utility.

THROMBIN CLOT TEST. One drop of fresh bovine thrombin, 5,000 units per ml, is placed into each of a series of clean, small, plain glass tubes which are then stoppered and promptly frozen. As needed, a frozen thrombin tube is obtained and about 2 ml of venous blood (a column about 1 inch high) is promptly ejected from a syringe into the tube without foam. The time and date are marked on the tube, which is then taped upright and inspected at intervals of 5 to 10 minutes over the next half hour or so. The important feature is the size of the clot that evolves and persists and not the rate with which the clot forms.

Intense *thrombocytopenia* is likely if petechiae are present, or a large clot fails to retract over a period of an hour or so, or platelets are rare in a stained blood smear. Confirmation is provided by actual platelet count.

Prolonged *partial thromboplastin time* or *prothrombin time* may be the consequence, singly or in combination, of appreciable reductions in those coagulants essential for generating thrombin, of fibrinogen concentration below a critical level of about 100 mg per dl, or of appreciable amounts of circulating fibrinogen–fibrin degradation products. A long *thrombin time* may be the consequence of low fibrinogen, of appreciable amounts of fibrinogen-fibrin degradation products, or of both. Moreoever, in some cases of severe preeclampsia, and especially eclampsia, the thrombin time may be prolonged for reasons not readily apparent (Pritchard, Cunningham, and Mason, 1976). Heparin in the circulation will, of course, prolong all three tests.

PLACENTAL ABRUPTION

Nomenclature. The separation of the placenta from its site of implantation in the uterus before the delivery of the fetus has been called variously placental abruption, abruptio placentae, ablatio placentae, and premature separation of the normally implanted placenta.

The term *premature separation of the normally implanted placenta* is most descriptive, since it differentiates the placenta that separates prematurely but is implanted a distance from the cervical internal os from one that is implanted over the cervical internal os, i.e., placenta previa. It is cumbersome, however, and hence the shorter term *abruptio placentae,* or *placental abruption,* has been employed. The Latin *abruptio placentae,* which means a rending asunder of the placenta, denotes a sudden accident, a clinical characteristic of most cases of this complication. *Ablatio placentae* means a carrying away of the placenta, analogous to ablatio retinae; this term is not extensively used. The term frequently employed in Great Britain for this complication is *accidental hemorrhage.* The rationale for its use is that the condition is an "accident" in the sense of an event that takes place without expectation, in contrast to the "unavoidable" hemorrhage of placenta previa, in which bleeding is inevitable because of the anatomic relations between the placenta and dilating cervix. Since the term *accidental hemorrhage* may suggest an element of trauma, which is rarely a factor in these cases, it may be misleading and is rarely employed in the United States.

Some of the bleeding of placental abruption usually insinuates itself between the membranes and uterus, escapes through the cervix, and appears externally, causing an *external hemorrhage* (Fig. 21-3). Less often, the blood does not escape externally but is retained between the detached placenta and the uterus, leading to *concealed hemorrhage* (Figs. 21-3, 21-4). Placental abruption with concealed hemorrhage carries with it much greater maternal hazards because the extent of the hemorrhage is not appreciated, so blood replacement commonly has been "too little too late."

Frequency and Intensity. The incidence of placental abruption ranged from 1 in 78 deliveries to 1 in 206, and averaged 1 in 120, in the several reports reviewed by Knab (1978). In recent years in the Dallas community, the frequency of diagnosis of pla-

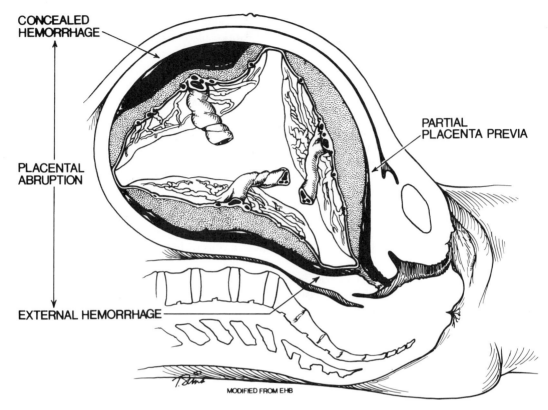

CONCEALED
HEMORRHAGE

PARTIAL
PLACENTA PREVIA

PLACENTAL
ABRUPTION

EXTERNAL HEMORRHAGE

MODIFIED FROM EHB

FIG. 21-3. Hemorrhage from premature placental separation: *Upper left,* extensive placental abruption but with the periphery of the placenta and the membranes still adherent, resulting in completely concealed hemorrhage. *Lower,* placental abruption with the placenta detached peripherally and with the membranes between the placenta and cervical canal stripped from underlying decidua, allowing external hemorrhage. *Right,* partial placenta previa with placental separation and external hemorrhage.

cental abruption has been 1 in 86 deliveries, or 0.5 percent. In this connection, it should be noted that of all cases of antepartum hemorrhage in the latter half of pregnancy, no more than half can be ascribed positively to either placental abruption or placenta previa, i.e., placental implantation in the immediate vicinity of the cervix. Of those remaining, a small number can be traced to lesions of the cervix, whereas bleeding in the rest is of uncertain origin. In all probability, much of this bleeding may result from minute marginal separations of the placenta, which are impossible to recognize with certainty either clinically or pathologically.

Using the criterion of placental abruption so extensive as to kill the fetus, the incidence

at Parkland Memorial Hospital has been 1 in 500 deliveries (Pritchard and Brekken, 1967). As the parity of women cared for has decreased in very recent years, the frequency of placental abruption has also decreased somewhat.

All degrees of premature separation of the placenta may occur, from an area only a few mm in diameter to the entire placenta. The placenta separating at its margin may disrupt the marginal sinus. Although *marginal sinus rupture* was formerly classified as a separate clinical entity, it simply represents placental separation limited to the margin.

Etiology.   The primary cause of placental abruption is unknown, but the following

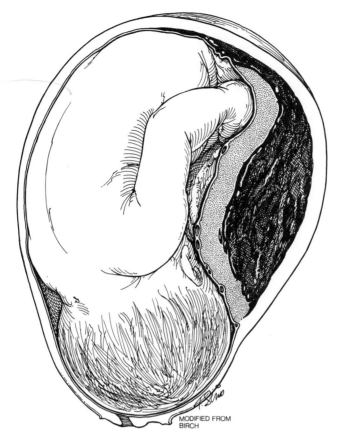

MODIFIED FROM
BIRCH

FIG. 21-4. Total placental abruption with concealed hemorrhage. The fetus is now dead.

conditions have been evoked as etiologic factors: trauma, shortness of the umbilical cord, sudden decompression of the uterus, uterine anomaly or tumor, compression or occlusion of the inferior vena cava, pregnancy-induced or chronic hypertension, pressure by the enlarged uterus on the inferior vena cava, and dietary deficiency.

In the Parkland study of 201 cases of placental abruption so severe as to kill the fetus, *maternal hypertension* was apparent in almost half of the cases once the depleted intravascular compartment was adequately refilled (Pritchard and co-workers, 1970). Nearly one-half of the hypertensive women had chronic vascular disease; in the remainder, the hypertension appeared to be pregnancy-induced. So high a frequency of maternal hypertension in pregnancies complicated by placental abruption has not been observed by

all (Paterson, 1979). It appears that there is not an increased incidence of hypertension in pregnancies with lesser degrees of placental abruption, whereas severe placental abruption is much more likely associated with maternal hypertension.

External trauma, an unusually short cord, or a uterine anomaly or tumor could be implicated only rarely in cases of severe placental abruption cared for at Parkland Memorial Hospital. Hydramnios with sudden uterine decompression and placental abruption was also uncommon (Pritchard and co-workers, 1970).

Lesser degrees of abruption may occur shortly before delivery of a singleton fetus when the amnionic fluid has drained from the uterus and the fetus has descended until the head is on the perineum. With twins, decompression following delivery of the first fetus may lead to premature separation of the placenta that endangers the second fetus (see Chap. 26, p. 661).

Experimental obstruction of the inferior vena cava and ovarian veins has been reported to produce placental abruption. There are, however, several recorded instances of ligation of ovarian veins and the inferior vena cava during the third trimester of pregnancy without subsequent placental abruption (Stone et al., 1968).

The Hibbards and some others have contended that folic acid deficiency has an etiologic role in placental abruption (see Chap. 13, p. 316). The hypothesis has been carefully examined by Menon and colleagues (1966), and by Kitay (1969), as well as by Whalley and associates (1969), Alperin and colleagues (1969), and others even more recently. These investigators found no evidence to support such a relationship.

Recurrence. Of considerable importance in the prognosis of the woman with a placental abruption, the risk of recurrence in a subsequent pregnancy is much higher than is the risk for the general population. Paterson (1979) noted a recurrence rate of 1 in 18 pregnancies; Pritchard and co-workers (1970) identified a recurrence rate of 1 in 10 pregnancies; and Hibbard and Jeffcoat (1976) observed the remarkably high rate of 1 in 6 pregnancies. Indeed, the likelihood of recurrence makes a subsequent pregnancy a high-risk pregnancy. Management of the subsequent pregnancy is made difficult by the fact that the placental separation may suddenly occur at any time, even remote from term. Beischer and associates (1970) found that normal levels of urinary estriol provided no assurance against imminent severe placental abruption. Moreover, Seski and Compton (1976) documented both accelerations of the fetal heart rate with fetal movement and no decelerations of the fetal heart rate in response to oxytocin-induced contractions 4 hours before the onset of placental abruption so severe that it killed the fetus.

Pathology. Placental abruption is initiated by hemorrhage into the decidua basalis.

The decidua then splits, leaving a thin layer adherent to the myometrium. Consequently, the process in its earliest stages consists of the development of a decidual hematoma that leads to separation, compression, and ultimate destruction of function of placenta adjacent to it. In its early stage, there may be no clinical symptoms. The condition is discovered only upon examination of the freshly delivered organ, which will present on its maternal surface a circumscribed depression measuring a few cm in diameter and containing dark, clotted blood.

In some instances, a decidual spiral artery ruptures to cause a retroplacental hematoma which, as it expands, disrupts more vessels to separate more placenta with more bleeding and, in turn, more separation. The area of separation becomes more extensive and reaches the margin of the placenta. Since the uterus is still distended by the products of conception, it is unable to contract and compress the torn vessels supplying the placental site. The escaping blood may dissect the membranes from the uterine wall and eventually appear externally (Fig. 21-3), or may be completely retained within the uterus (Fig. 21-4).

CONCEALED HEMORRHAGE. Retained, or concealed, hemorrhage is likely to occur when (1) there is an effusion of blood behind the placenta but its margins still remain adherent; (2) the placenta is completely separated, yet the membranes retain their attachment to the uterine wall; (3) the blood gains access to the amnionic cavity after breaking through the membranes; and (4) the fetal head is so closely applied to the lower uterine segment that the blood cannot make its way past it. In the majority of such cases, however, the membranes are gradually dissected off the uterine wall, and a variable amount of the blood eventually escapes from the cervix.

CHRONIC PLACENTAL ABRUPTION. Most often, hemorrhage from the placental implantation site persists either until delivery following which the blood vessels are successfully constricted by the contracting and retracting myometrium or until the woman dies. In a small minority of cases, however,

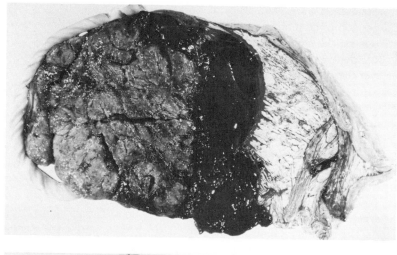

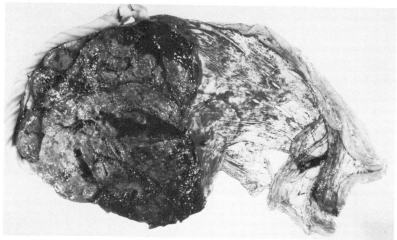

FIG. 21-5. A. Partial placental abruption with adherent blood clot. The fetus died from massive hemorrhage chiefly into the maternal circulation. **B.** The adherent blood clot has been removed. Note the laceration of the placenta. **C.** Smear of maternal blood after fetal death. The dark cells are fetal red cells whereas the empty cells are maternal in origin. Hemoglobin A has been eluted from the maternal cells by treatment with acid while hemoglobin F remains in the red cells of fetal origin.

C

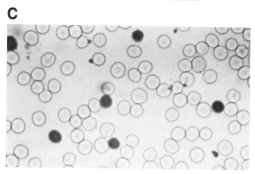

hemorrhage with retroplacental hematoma formation is somehow completely arrested without delivery having taken place. We have been able to document this phenomenon by labeling maternal red cells with a chromium isotope and showing that blood concealed within the uterus at delivery some days to weeks later contained no chromium (Cun-

ningham, Pritchard, unpublished observations).

Fetal to Maternal Hemorrhage. Massive bleeding from the fetus into the maternal circulation as the consequence of placental abruption has been rare in our experience. However, the placenta from such a case is shown in Figures 21-5. A. and 21-5. B. At 33 weeks gestation, the mother was forcefully thrown against the steering wheel during an auto accident even though she was wearing an over-the-shoulder seat belt. The fetal heart was not heard when listened for 20 minutes later. Spontaneous labor developed 22 hours after the accident. At that time, the maternal blood contained at least 75 ml of fetal erythrocytes, or 115 ml of fetal blood, calculated from the percentage of red cells rich in fetal homoglobin found in maternal blood (4.5 percent; Fig. 21-5. C.), the maternal blood volume (4500 ml), and hematocrit. The macerated fetus weighed 2140 g. The placenta contained a long rent that extended to the chorionic plate. The clot adherent to the placenta at the site of partial placental abruption contained nearly all maternal red cells. Moreover, these red cells had been shed before the onset of labor, since they contained none of the chromium used to measure the maternal blood volume at the onset of labor.

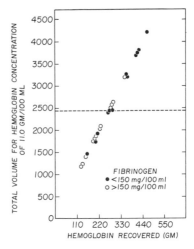

FIG. 21-6. Volumes of hemorrhage concealed within the uterus until delivery in women with extensive placental abruption. The dotted line identifies the median value; the open circles represent cases with severe hypofibrinogenemia. (From Pritchard JA, Brekken AL. *Am J Obstet Gynecol* 97:681, 1967)

Clinical Diagnosis. The findings in a typical case of severe abruptio placentae are (1) some vaginal bleeding, (2) increased uterine tone, (3) uterine tenderness, which may be localized or general, (4) absence of the fetal heart sounds, and (5) variable evidence of hypovolemia. Many deviations from this typical picture occur, however. For example, unless more than half of the placenta has been separated, the fetal heart tones are usually audible, although the rate may be abnormal. In concealed hemorrhage, of course, there is no external bleeding, but uterine rigidity and tenderness are likely to be pronounced. Pain is variable; it may be entirely absent or with severe abruption may be excruciating.

SHOCK. It has long been held that the shock sometimes seen in placental abruption is out of proportion to the amount of hemorrhage. An explanation proposed for this disparity has been that thromboplastin from decidua and placenta enters the maternal circulation at the site of placental separation and incites intravascular coagulation and, in turn, acute cor pulmonale. Admittedly, the sudden intravenous injection of large doses of thromboplastic material into experimental animals can cause profound shock, as shown by Schneider (1954). Despite Schneider's observations, the weight of evidence is that the intensity of shock is not out of proportion to the maternal blood loss. Pritchard and Brekken (1967), for example, studied the blood loss in 141 gravidas with placental abruption so severe as to kill the fetus and found blood loss often to be one-half of the pregnant blood volume (Fig. 21-6). Oliguria caused by inadequate renal perfusion but responsive to treatment of hypovolemia is frequently observed in these circumstances.

Although the severe case of placental abruption is usually, but not always, marked by such classic signs and symptoms that the diagnosis is at once obvious, the milder and more common forms are difficult to recognize clinically, and the diagnosis is often made by exclusion. Thus, in the face of persistent vaginal bleeding in the last trimester, it often becomes necessary to rule out placenta previa

and other causes of bleeding by clinical inspection and sonographic study. Unfortunately, there are neither tests nor diagnostic
methods to detect lesser degrees of separation of the placenta, and the cause of the
vaginal bleeding at times remains obscure
even after delivery.

Classic placental abruption with pain,
shock, uterine rigidity, and absent fetal heart
sounds may occur in the middle trimester of
pregnancy. These cases present the same
complications as do more advanced pregnancies, and may cause the death of the woman
unless she is appropriately treated.

**Consumptive Coagulopathy with Pla-
cental Abruption.** The most common
cause of consumptive coagulopathy in pregnancy is placental abruption. Overt hypofibrinogenemia (less than 150 mg per dl of
plasma), along with elevated levels of fibrinogen-fibrin degradation products, and variable
decreases in other coagulation factors, occurs
in about 30 percent of cases with abruption
severe enough to kill the fetus. Such coagulation defects are found very uncommonly in
those cases in which the fetus survives. *The
experience at Parkland Memorial Hospital is that
serious coagulopathy, when it develops, most often
is evident by the time the woman is hospitalized.*

The major mechanism in the genesis of
the coagulation defects of placental abruption
almost certainly is the induction of coagulation intravascularly and to a lesser degree
retroplacentally. Although an appreciable
amount of fibrin is commonly deposited
within the uterine cavity in cases of severe
placental abruption and hypofibrinogenemia,
the amounts are insufficient to account for
all of the fibrinogen missing from the circulation (Pritchard, Brekken, 1967). Moreover,
Bonnar and co-workers (1969) have shown
the levels of fibrin degradation products to
be higher in serum from peripheral blood
than in serum from blood contained in the
uterine cavity. The reverse would be anticipated in the absence of significant intravascular coagulation.

An important consequence of intravascular coagulation is the activation of plasminogen to plasmin which lyses microemboli of
fibrin, thereby maintaining patency of the microcirculation.

Renal Failure. Acute renal failure that
persists for any length of time is rare with
lesser degrees of placental abruption but is
seen in the severe forms when there is delayed or incomplete treatment of hypovolemia. Renal failure, usually renal cortical necrosis, was identified in six of 10 fatal cases
of placental abruption reported by Krupp and
associates (1970). The precise cause of the
renal damage that may be associated with placental abruption is not clear, but the major
etiologic factor very likely is severe intrarenal
vasospasm as the consequence of massive
hemorrhage. Even when placental abruption
is complicated by intravascular coagulation,
vigorous treatment of hemorrhage with
blood and balanced salt solution most often
prevents serious renal failure.

During the past 23 years at Parkland Memorial Hospital, more than 300 cases of placental abruption so severe as to kill the fetus
have received fluid replacement therapy consisting of whole blood and lactated Ringer's
solution, as outlined earlier for treatment of
obstetric hemorrhage (p. 492). In no instance has dialysis for renal failure been necessary.

Proteinuria is common, especially with
more severe forms of placental abruption.

**Uteroplacental Apoplexy (Couvelaire
Uterus).** In the more severe forms of placental abruption, widespread extravasations
of blood often take place into the uterine
musculature and beneath the uterine serosa
(Figs. 21-7. A, 21-7. B). Such effusions of
blood are also seen occasionally beneath the
tubal serosa, in the connective tissue of the
broad ligaments, in the substance of the ovaries, as well as free in the peritoneal cavity,
presumably from bleeding through the oviducts.

The phenomenon *uteroplacental apoplexy,*
first described by Couvelaire early in this century and now frequently called *Couvelaire
uterus,* was thought at one time to impair

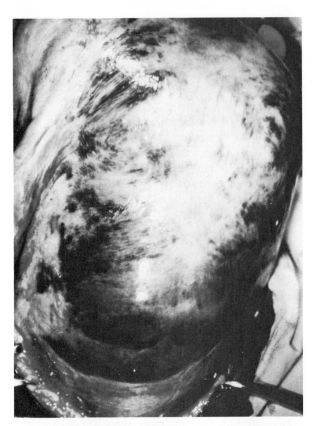

FIG. 21-7. A. "Couvelaire" uterus; a uterus with total placental abruption before being emptied by cesarean section. Blood had markedly infiltrated much of the myometrium to reach the serosa.

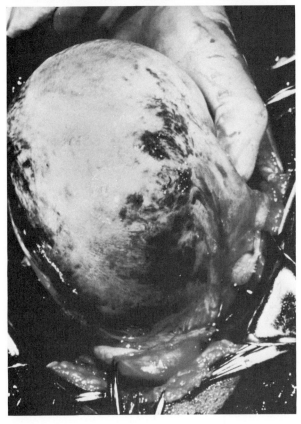

FIG. 21-7. B. Same uterus as in 21-7. A. after being emptied and closed. Note that it is well contracted even though there has been extensive hemorrhage into the myometrium.

uterine contractility after delivery with severe uterine hemorrhage as the consequence. These myometrial hematomas seldom interfere with uterine contractions sufficiently to produce postpartum hemorrhage. Shown in Figure 21-7. A. is a Couvelaire uterus just before cesarean section early in the third trimester. In Figure 21-7. B, the same uterus is seen well contracted after being emptied, appropriately sutured, and stimulated to contract with intravenuos oxytocin. The infiltration of blood characteristic of the Couvelaire uterus, therefore, is not an indication for hysterectomy. It is impossible to give an accurate estimate of the incidence of Couvelaire uterus because the condition can only be demonstrated conclusively at laparotomy.

Treatment.   The hemorrhage of placental abruption and the hypovolemia it causes demand immediate treatment. Prompt restoration of an effective circulation by the intravenous administration of appropriate fluids, especially whole blood, is the first consideration.

METHOD OF DELIVERY.   If the fetus is alive but distressed, rapid delivery is the next consideration. Rapid delivery of the fetus that is alive but in distress practically always means cesarean section. It is emphasized that an electrode applied directly to the fetus to record the fetal EKG may provide misleading information, as in the case of severe placental abruption illustrated in Figure 21-8. At first impression, at least, fetal bradycardia of 80 to 90 beats per minute with a degree of beat to beat variability is evident. The fetus, however, was dead. There were no audible fetal heart sounds and the maternal pulse rate was identical to that recorded through the fetal scalp electrode. Emergency cesarean section at this time might have proved disastrous to the mother, since she was profoundly hypo-

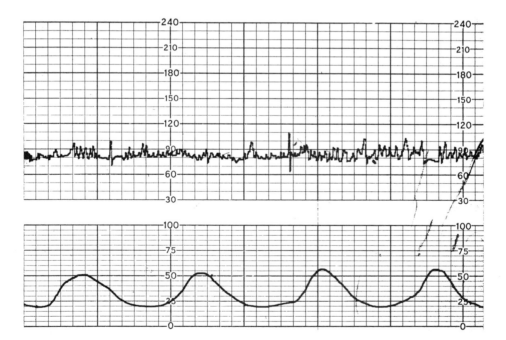

FIG. 21-8. A recording of uterine pressures and presumed fetal heart rate in a case of placental abruption so severe as to have killed the fetus. The scalp electrode conducted the maternal EKG signal. Note the increased uterine basal tone. Commonly, in cases of severe placental abruption both the basal tone and the maximum uterine pressure are greater than illustrated here.

volemic and had developed severe hypofibrinogenemia.

If the fetus is alive but cesarean section
is not immediately carried out, the fetus must
be monitored closely for evidence of distress
and be delivered whenever distress is detected. Therefore, appropriate facilities and
staff for cesarean section must be continuously available whenever placental abruption
is suspected.

If the separation is so severe that there
is no evidence of fetal life, vaginal delivery
is preferred unless hemorrhage is so brisk
that it cannot be successfully managed even
by vigorous blood replacement or there are
other obstetric complications that contraindicate vaginal delivery.

HEMORRHAGE AND HYPOVOLEMIA.
To combat hypovolemia successfully whole

blood must be available in large quantities.
As much as 10 liters of blood has been administered to a woman with severe placental
abruption at Parkland Memorial Hospital.

The basic rule for treating obstetric hemorrhage is applied. Blood and balanced salt
solution (lactated Ringer's solution) are infused in such proportions that the hematocrit
is maintained at 30 percent or slightly higher
and urine flow precisely measured is at least
30 ml per hour, and preferably about 60 ml
per hour, or 1 ml per minute. For the oliguric
patient, the dangers from mannitol or furosemide outweigh any advantages, actual or
theoretical, that might accrue from their use.
If vigorous fluid therapy does not promptly
relieve oliguria, the central venous pressure
should be monitored as more fluids are administered. Since central venous pressure
measurement might not detect early pulmo-

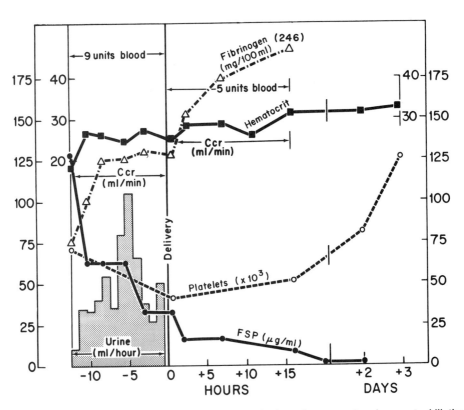

FIG. 21-9. Serial data from a case of placental abruption so extensive as to kill the
fetus and induce serious consumptive coagulopathy as well as severe anemia. Ccr =
creatinine clearance; FSP = fibrin degradation products. (From Cunningham and Pritchard,
unpublished observations)

nary congestion, the woman must also be observed for other signs, especially dyspnea, cough, and rales.

COAGULATION DEFECTS. Much concern has often been expressed over the rate of development of coagulation defects, as well as their intensity. The extensive experiences at Parkland Memorial Hospital have been that coagulation defects most often occur within the first few hours after the onset of pain or bleeding and usually do not worsen subsequently, except for the dilution effects from vigorous transfusion with stored whole blood and lactated Ringer's solution (Fig. 21-9). *If the clot observation test yields a very small or absent clot, the usual coagulation studies will be grossly abnormal and will provide very little useful information with the possible exception of a platelet count.* Even though *platelet counts* have been recommended to identify disseminated intravascular coagulation, very low *fibrinogen* levels may develop with placental abruption, yet the platelet count simultaneously may be well above 100,000 per mm^3. With extensive placental abruption, elevated levels of *fibrin degradation products* are so common as to be anticipated; therefore, their measurement provides little help in clinical management. The experience at Parkland Memorial Hospital has been that erythrocyte distortion or fragmentation characteristic of *fragmentation* or *microangiopathic hemolysis* is uncommon unless renal failure supervenes.

FIBRINOGEN THERAPY. Therapy with fibrinogen in cases of placental abruption with severe hypofibrinogenemia has been widely practiced for years. More recently, concern has been expressed that such use of fibrinogen simply adds "fuel to the fire" of disseminated intravascular coagulation with the dire consequences of fibrin deposition and obstruction of the microcirculation in vital organs, especially the kidney, adrenal, pituitary, and brain. There is no good evidence, however, that effective doses of 4 to 8 g of fibrinogen do so. For example, after 4 g of fibrinogen, adminstered intravenously in less than 10 minutes to a woman with se-

vere hypofibrinogenemia very soon before cesarean section, we observed no changes in central venous pressure, arterial blood pressure, pulse rate, or respiratory rate. Moreover, apprehension, a common occurrence with embolization to the lungs, did not develop. Typically, 4 g of fibrinogen will raise the fibrinogen concentration in plasma about 100 mg/dl.

The major problem from use of commercially available fibrinogen is the likelihood of hepatitis B, since each lot is prepared commercially from plasma from thousands of donors (Phillips, 1965). Cryoprecipitate from relatively few donors supplies fibrinogen with very much less risk of hepatitis. To supply 4 g of fibrinogen, 15 to more likely 20 bags of cryoprecipitate, each from an individual donor, are required. Ness and Perkins (1979), for example, found an average fibrinogen content of 0.27 g of fibrinogen per bag of cryoprecipitate but the content ranged from 0.06 to 0.42 g per bag.

ALTERNATIVE TO FIBRINOGEN. For the past several years at Parkland Memorial Hospital, fibrinogen has been used very infrequently. To avoid its use, trauma to the genital tract was kept to a minimum through simple vaginal delivery, most often spontaneous, of the dead fetus. No episiotomy was made if the fetus was small or the perineum was relaxed; otherwise, a midline episiotomy was made and carefully repaired. The emptied and intact uterus was immediately stimulated with oxytocin, 100 to 200 milliunits per minute intravenously, and the uterine fundus was continuously monitored and massaged when not firmly contracted. Effective *uterine massage* necessitated that the fundus of the uterus be clearly identified. If abnormally enlarged, the uterus was compressed to evacuate blood clots. Next a hand was placed over the anterior surface of the uterus with the fingers extending over the top of the fundus, and the uterus was now firmly rubbed to induce and maintain a contracted myometrium. An effective analgesic, such as meperidine, improved the mother's tolerance to this procedure.

Blood loss immediately postpartum probably has been somewhat greater than if fibrinogen had been given but the overall risks and costs very likely have been less.

With laparotomy for delivery, fibrinogen has been given only if there was gross evidence of disruption of the coagulation mechanism, including uncontrollable bleeding from all sites of trauma. With lesser amounts of bleeding, ligation of all bleeding points with, at times, drainage of the abdominal incision subfacially with Penrose drains has proved satisfactory. Most often, however, delivery of the woman with severe placental abruption and a dead fetus has been accomplished vaginally.

Following delivery, the coagulation defects repair spontaneously within 24 hours or so, except for platelets which, if very low, take two to four days to reach the normal range.

HEPARIN. The infusion of heparin to try to block disseminated intravascular coagulation associated with placental abruption is mentioned only to condemn its use. Heparin should not be used for the following reasons: (1) No one has reported more than a few anecdotal experiences in which heparin did not appear to make hemorrhage worse. (2) The stimulus to active intravascular coagulation ceases after delivery. In fact, the intense phase of intravascular coagulation occurs most often during and very soon after the placental separation. (3) Heparin is a potent anticoagulant that can be predicted to aggravate hemorrhage when there has been gross disruption of the vasculature. (4) Excellent results have been achieved with the plan of management described above. For example, more than 300 cases so severe as to kill the fetus have been managed without renal impairment that necessitated dialysis.

AMNIOTOMY. Rupture of membranes as early as possible has long been championed in the management of placental abruption. The rationale for amniotomy is that the escape of amnionic fluid might both decrease bleeding from the implantation site and reduce the entry into the maternal circulation of thromboplastin and perhaps activated coagulation factors from the retroplacental clot. There is no evidence, however, that either is accomplished by amniotomy. If the fetus is reasonably mature, rupture of the membranes may hasten delivery. If the fetus is immature, the intact sac may be more efficient in promoting cervical dilatation than will a small fetal part poorly applied to the cervix.

LABOR. With lesser degrees of placental separation, uterine contractions usually are of normal frequency, duration, and intensity, and uterine tone between contractions is low. With extensive placental abruption, the uterus is likely to be persistently hypertonic. Minimum intra-amnionic pressure may be 25 to 50 mm Hg with rhythmic increases up to 75 to 100 mm Hg. Because of persistent hypertonus, it is difficult at times to determine by palpation if the uterus is contracting and relaxing to any degree, although periodic complaints by the woman of increased pain often signals cyclic increases in uterine activity.

Sher (1977, 1978) has emphasized that in his experience uterine inertia refractory to usual therapy develops in about one out of 5 cases of placental abruption complicated by severe consumptive coagulopathy. He claimed that in this circumstance the administration of Trasylol resulted in rapid recovery of uterine activity. Trasylol is an inhibitor of proteases such as plasmin, and also possesses antithromboplastin and antikallikrein effects. In our extensive experiences with severe placental abruption, hypertonicity has characterized myometrial function in women with placental abruption complicated by gross disruption of the coagulation mechanism. Therefore, the need for Trasylol, which is not available for clinical use in the United States, is questioned. In fact, we have been looking for an agent to decrease safely myometrial activity somewhat in these circumstances. Magnesium sulfate has not proved to be effective for this purpose.

If severe placental abruption occurs before cervical effacement and dilatation, the subsequent pattern of change in the cervix typically is one of progressive effacement with little dilatation until effacement is complete. Dilatation is then usually rapid. Therefore, failure of the cervix to dilate while obviously effacing should not be considered as lack of progress.

OXYTOCIN. Uterine stimulation with oxytocin to effect vaginal delivery appears to provide benefits that override the risks. Care must be exercised not to provoke the uterus into self-destruction, especially in women of high parity or with fetopelvic disproportion. The use of oxytocin has been challenged on the basis that it might enhance the escape of thromboplastin into the maternal circulation and thereby initiate or enhance consumptive coagulopathy. There is no evidence to support this fear (Pritchard, Brekken, 1967).

Timing of Delivery after Abruption.
In some of the previous editions of this book, delivery within six hours was advocated. This recommendation arose from the general clinical impression that maternal morbidity and mortality were less when delivery was thus accomplished. Experiences at both the University of Virginia and Parkland Memorial Hospitals indicate that the outcome depends upon the diligence with which adequate fluid replacement therapy, especially blood, is pursued rather than the time to delivery (Brame et al., 1968; Pritchard, Brekken, 1967). At the University of Virginia Hospital, women with severe placental abruption, who were transfused for 18 hours or more before delivery, experienced complications that were neither more numerous nor greater in severity than did the group in which delivery was accomplished sooner. Serial observations on one of the most severe cases at Parkland Memorial Hospital in terms of the prolonged interval between onset of symptoms and delivery and the necessity of transfusing a large volume of blood are summarized in Figure 21-9 and a brief case summary follows:

The nulliparous woman was hospitalized 14 hours after the onset of abdominal pain and 12 hours

before delivery. Her hematocrit was 18.5 compared to 34 two weeks before. There was scant urine in the bladder even though she had not voided for several hours. Her blood pressure appeared normal. However, when vigorous fluid therapy was instituted the blood pressure rose to hypertensive levels and urine flow was reestablished. From the time of admittance until delivery 4500 ml of compatible whole blood and 3000 ml of lactated Ringer's solution were infused. During the interval until delivery, the measured creatinine clearance (Ccr) was 121 ml per minute; the hematocrit increased from 18.5 to range from 26 to 29; the plasma fibrinogen rose from 75 mg per dl to 128 mg per dl and fibrin degradation products (FSP) in serum dropped from 130 μg per ml to 30 μg per ml; the platelet count during transfusion dropped from 74,000 per mm^3 to 46,000. Oxytocin was infused during most of this time in dilute solution in an attempt to hasten delivery.

Until delivery, external bleeding was negligible. During spontaneous delivery of a stillborn infant over a midline episiotomy with local infiltration anesthesia plus nitrous oxide, blood and clots were collected from the uterus that contained 700 g of hemoglobin equivalent to 6400 ml of blood with a hemoglobin concentration of 11.0 g per dl. Fundal massage kept the uterus rather well contracted; otherwise, without massage, bleeding from the uterus was appreciable during the first 6 hours after delivery. Blood so lost during and after delivery was replaced and the hematocrit was raised to 32 by giving 2500 ml of stored whole blood. The creatinine clearance remained normal during this time.

The mother lactated early in the puerperium and was discharged on the third postpartum day. Normal menstrual function soon was reestablished. The creatinine clearance remote from pregnancy was 120 ml per minute, and blood volume was 3765 ml. The volume of blood concealed within the uterus at delivery was nearly twice her nonpregnant blood volume!

Consumptive Coagulopathy in the Infant.
Although we have never observed the phenomenon, changes in the coagulation mechanism of the newborn infant characteristic of those of intravascular coagulation have been described to accompany placental abruption (Edson et al., 1968; Nielsen, 1970). However, a variety of conditions predispose to the development of disseminated

intravascular coagulation in the newborn in the absence of placental abruption, including prematurity, hypoxia, and sepsis (Woods et al., 1979).

PLACENTA PREVIA

Definition. In placenta previa, the placenta, instead of being implanted in the body of the uterus well away from the cervical internal os, is located over or very near the internal os. Four degrees of the abnormality are recognized:

1. *Total Placenta Previa.* The cervical internal os is covered completely by placenta (Fig. 21-10).

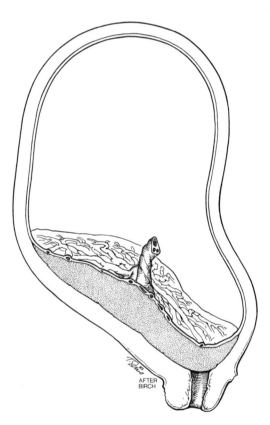

FIG. 21-10. Total placenta previa. Even with the modest cervical dilatation illustrated, copious hemorrhage would be anticipated.

2. *Partial Placenta Previa.* The internal os is partially covered by placenta (Fig. 21-11. A).
3. *Marginal Placenta Previa.* The edge of the placenta is at the margin of the internal os (Fig. 21-3).
4. *Low-lying Placenta.* The region of the internal os is encroached upon by the placenta, so that the placental edge may be palpated by the examining finger when introduced through the cervix.

The degree of placenta previa will depend in large measure on the cervical dilatation at the time of examination. For example, a low-lying placenta at 2-cm dilatation may become a partial placenta previa at 8-cm dilatation because the dilating cervix has uncovered placenta. Conversely, a placenta previa that appears to be total before cervical dilatation may become partial at 4-cm dilatation because the cervix dilates beyond the edge of the placenta (Fig. 21-11. A and B). Since exploration digitally of the region of the internal os in placenta previa is one of the most dangerous undertakings in obstetrics, it is unwise to attempt to ascertain these changing relations between the edge of the placenta and the internal os as the cervix dilates.

In both the total and partial varieties, a certain degree of separation of the placenta is an inevitable consequence of the formation of the lower uterine segment and the dilatation of the cervix. It is always associated with hemorrhage from blood vessels so disrupted and which cannot be effectively constricted by the myometrium until after the uterus has been emptied.

Frequency. Placenta previa is a serious but uncommon complication. In the Dallas community, in recent years, placenta previa was diagnosed once in every 260 deliveries, or 0.4 percent. Brenner and co-workers (1978) identified during the latter half of pregnancy an incidence of placenta previa of 0.6 percent, or 1 per 167 pregnancies; 20 percent were of the complete, or total, variety.

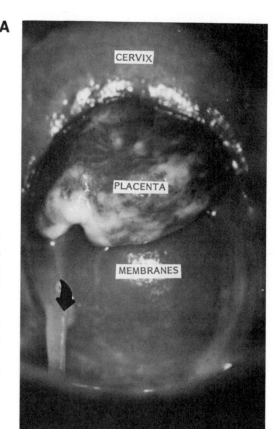

FIG. 21-11. A. Partial placenta previa seen through a cervix 3 to 4 cm dilated at 22 weeks gestation. The arrow points to mucus dropping from the cervix. Uterine cramping was evident but earlier intermittent bleeding had stopped one month before. The fetus weighed 410 g when delivered vaginally the next day. Blood loss was not massive. **B.** Gray scale longitudinal midline sonogram obtained the day after the photo in Figure 21-11. A. The upper arrow points to a partial placenta previa from an anteriorly implanted placenta. The lower arrow points to the amnionic sac bulging through the cervix. (Courtesy of Dr. R. Santos)

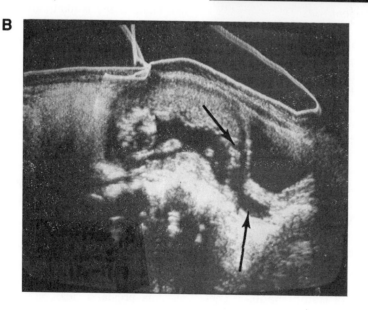

Contradictory statistics on the incidence of the various degrees of placenta previa reflect mostly the lack of precision in definition and identification for the reasons discussed above. A question difficult to answer is "Should painless bleeding from focal separation of a placenta implanted in the lower uterine segment but away from a partially dilated cervical os be classified as placenta previa or placental abruption?"

Etiology.   Multiparity and advancing age appear to favor placenta previa. One factor in the development of placenta previa is said to be defective vascularization of the decidua, the possible result of inflammatory or atrophic changes. Another is a large placenta, which spreads over a large area of the uterus as seen with fetal erythroblastosis and with multiple fetuses. In so doing, the lower portion of the placenta occasionally appoaches the region of the internal os, completely or partially overlapping it.

Rarely, placenta previa is associated with *placenta accreta* or one of its more advanced forms, *placenta increta* or *percreta* (see Chap. 34, p. 883). Such abnormally firm attachment of the placenta might be anticipated because of poorly developed decidua in the lower uterine segment.

Signs and Symptoms.   The most characteristic event in placenta previa is painless hemorrhage, which usually does not appear until near the end of the second trimester or after. Many abortions, however, probably result from abnormal locations of the developing placenta. Ultrasonic investigations of early pregnancies that eventually abort disclose an unexpectedly large number of low-lying embryos (Kobayashi et al., 1970). Not all that do not abort eventuate in placenta previa, however. As the placenta and uterus both grow, the placenta may eventually be located some distance from the cervix, as described on page 511.

Character of the Hemorrhage.   The hemorrhage from placenta previa occurs frequently without warning in a pregnant woman who appeared previously in perfect health. Occasionally, it makes its first appearance while she is asleep; on awakening, she is surprised to find herself in a pool of blood. Fortunately, the initial bleeding is rarely so profuse as to prove fatal. It usually, but certainly not always, ceases spontaneously, only to recur when least expected. In some cases, particularly with placentas implanted near but not over the cervical os, bleeding does not appear until the onset of labor, when it may vary from slight to profuse hemorrhage.

The cause of the hemorrhage is reemphasized. When the placenta is located over the internal os, the formation of the lower uterine segment and the dilatation of the internal os result inevitably in tearing of placental attachments, followed by hemorrhage from the uterine vessels. The bleeding is augmented by the inability of the myometrial fibers of the lower uterine segment to contract and retract and thereby compress the torn vessels, as occurs normally when the placenta separates from the otherwise empty uterus during the third stage of labor.

As the result of abnormal adherence, i.e., placenta accreta, or an excessively large area of attachment, the process of placental separation is sometimes impeded, and then excessive hemorrhage is likely after the birth of the infant. Hemorrhage from the placental implantation site in the lower uterine segment may continue after delivery of the placenta, since the lower uterine segment is more prone to contract poorly than is the body of the uterus and, as a consequence, there is less compression of the vessels that traverse the lower segment. Bleeding may result from lacerations in the friable cervix and lower uterine segment, especially with attempts at manual removal of a somewhat adherent placenta.

COAGULATION DEFECTS.   Whereas coagulation defects characteristic of consumptive coagulopathy are rather common with placental abruption, they are rare with placenta previa, at least until such time as large volumes of stored donor blood have been transfused. Then thrombocytopenia, and, less commonly, serious deficiencies of factors V and VIII can be anticipated, since stored donor blood usually is deficient in these components.

Diagnosis. In women with uterine bleeding during the latter half of pregnancy, placenta previa or abruptio placentae should always be suspected. The possibility of placenta previa should not be dismissed until appropriate evaluation, including sonography, has clearly proved its absence, in which case the diagnosis of placental abruption must be considered. The diagnosis of placenta previa rarely can be firmly established by clinical examination unless a finger is passed through the cervix and the placenta is palpated. **Such examination of the cervix is never permissible unless the woman is in an operating room with all preparations for immediate cesarean section, since even the gentlest examination of this sort can cause torrential hemorrhage. Furthermore, such an examination should not be made unless delivery is planned, for the trauma may cause bleeding of such a degree that immediate delivery becomes necessary even though the fetus is immature.**

After the fetus has reached a gestational age of 37 weeks or more, the neonatal mortality rate is not greatly improved by further intrauterine development. In such cases, the cause of vaginal bleeding may be ascertained by pelvic examination but only under those conditions emphasized above. If placenta previa is identified, delivery could be accomplished forthwith. In the presence of severe hemorrhage, the diagnosis must be made quickly by direct examination, so that the bleeding can be controlled by delivery.

Direct examination is withheld in women with premature fetuses for whom delay of delivery is advisable. In such instances, location of the placenta may be useful information, but it does not alter management remarkably, since those women who have bled must be carefully watched in any event. With proof that the placenta is normally located, the obstetrician may be more willing to discharge the mother from the hospital. However, whether at home or hospitalized, all women with bleeding are to be followed closely until delivery.

LOCALIZATION BY SONOGRAPHY. The simplest, most precise, and safest method of placental localization is provided by sonography, which locates the placenta with considerable accuracy (Figs. 21-11. B.–14). For example, Bowie and associates (1978) reported an accuracy of 93 percent for 164 pregnant women referred for examination because of placenta previa. There was one false-negative error in 13 cases of proven placenta previa and 10 false-positive errors in 151 women without placenta previa. Others have reported accuracies of 94 to 98 percent (Table 21-2). The false-positive results very likely were contributed to by bladder distension. Therefore, the ultrasonic scans in apparently positive cases should be repeated after nearly emptying the bladder.

Since the report of King (1973) the peripatetic nature of the placenta has come to be generally appreciated. Wexler and Gottesfeld (1977), for example, demonstrated sonographically that sometime during the second trimester 45 percent of pregnancies were characterized by a low-lying placenta. Young (1978) reached a similar conclusion after localizing the placenta utilizing arteriography. Therefore, placentas that lie in the vicinity of the internal cervical os during the second trimester or even early in the third trimester are likely to migrate subsequently toward the fundus. Rizos and associates (1979) recommend observation of the initially low-lying placenta with ultrasound at six- to eight-week intervals until the placenta moves away from the internal cervical os or the woman delivers. Since the great majority of cases of asymptomatic placenta previa found at midpregnancy are "cured" by placental migration, they do not recommend restriction of activity unless the placenta previa persists beyond 30 weeks or becomes clinically apparent.

LOCALIZATION BY ISOTOPES AND BY ROENTGENOGRAPHY. Several technics

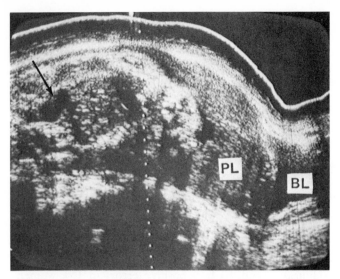

FIG. 21-12. Gray scale sonogram of total placenta previa at 30 weeks gestation. (BL = partly filled maternal bladder; PL = total placenta previa; arrow on left points to full fetal bladder). (Courtesy of Dr. R Santos)

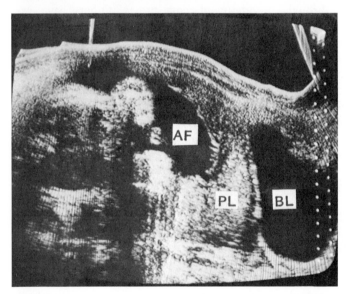

FIG. 21-13. Gray scale sonogram of total placenta previa at 33 weeks gestation. (BL = maternal bladder; PL = total placenta previa; AF = somewhat excessive amnionic fluid). (Courtesy of Dr. R Santos)

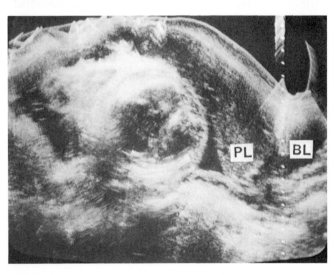

FIG. 21-14. Gray scale sonogram of partial placenta previa at 37 weeks gestation. (BL = partly filled maternal bladder; PL = partial placenta previa). (Courtesy of Dr. R Santos)

TABLE 21-2.
ACCURACY OF PLACENTAL LOCALIZATION
BY ULTRASOUND

AUTHORS	YEAR	RESULTS
Gottesfeld et al. (Denver)	1966	112 cases: accuracy rate 97% 18 cesarean sections with two wrong predictions
Donald, Abdulla (Glasgow)	1968	613 cases: accuracy rate 94% 107 cesarean sections
Campbell, Kohorn (London)	1968	72 cases: accuracy rate 94% 9 cesarean sections 38 patients, no confirmation obtained 29 exploration of the uterus
Kobayashi et al. (Brooklyn)	1970	100 cases: accuracy rate 95% 92 cesarean sections, 4 errors 8 hysterotomies, 1 error
Sunden (Sweden)	1970	107 cases: accuracy rate 95.6% 45 cesarean sections, 2 wrong predictions
Santos et al. (Dallas)	1978	100 cases: accuracy rate 98% at cesarean section
Bowie et al. (Chicago)	1978	164 cases: accuracy rate 93% missed 1 of 13 proven placenta previas

dependent upon radiation have been used to localize the placenta. They include (1) soft-tissue roentgenograms, (2) intravenous injection of radioactive isotopes to locate an area of maximum radioactivity, (3) contrast material injected into the amnionic sac, and (4) retrograde arteriography. Perhaps the most innocuous of these 4 procedures, soft-tissue roentgenography, is the least accurate, giving

a correct diagnosis in not more than 85 percent of cases. The method often fails when most needed, as in multiple pregnancy and obesity. Furthermore, diagnosis of posteriorly located placentas must be made by exclusion.

Isotopic procedures do not always differentiate between anteriorly and posteriorly located placentas or between merely a somewhat low-implanted placenta and actual placental previa. These methods have the added inconvenience of requiring a readily available isotope. Dunster and colleagues (1976) compared the use of ultrasound and of radionuclide imaging for localizing the placenta. While errors in diagnosis were made with both technics, they concluded that ultrasound was more likely to provide the correct diagnosis.

With amniography, the placenta, including fetal vessels, may be punctured during amniocentesis, causing fetal hemorrhage. Moreover, the hypertonic contrast medium may cause labor.

Angiography has the disadvantages of requiring an injection of a bolus of contrast material into the maternal femoral artery immediately followed by serial roentgenograms.

Management. Women with placenta previa may be assigned to the following groups: (1) those in whom the fetus is premature but there is no pressing need for delivery, (2) those in whom the fetus is within three weeks of term, (3) those in whom labor is in progress, and (4) those in whom hemorrhage is so severe as to necessitate evacuation of the uterus despite the immaturity of the fetus.

With placenta previa, the procedures available for delivery fall into two main categories: (1) vaginal methods, the rationale for which, it is hoped, is to be able to press the detached placenta against the implantation site during labor and thereby tamponade the bleeding vessels; and (2) cesarean section, the rationale for which is twofold. First, cesarean section, through immediate delivery, allows the uterus to contract and to stop the bleeding, and second, it forestalls the possibility of cervical lacerations, a complication of vaginal delivery in total and partial placenta previa.

CESAREAN SECTION. Cesarean section is the accepted method of delivery in practically all cases of placenta previa. In justifying cesarean section in the presence of a dead fetus, it is again necessary to understand that abdominal delivery is done primarily for the mother.

When the placenta lies far enough posteriorly that the lower uterine segment can be incised transversely without encountering placenta, and when the fetus is cephalic, the transverse incision is preferred. If, however, such an incision were to be made through the placenta, bleeding, both maternal and fetal, could be severe, and extension of the incision to involve one or both uterine arteries could occur with surprising ease. Therefore, with anterior placenta previa, a vertical uterine incision is often safer. When placenta previa is complicated by degrees of placenta accreta that render control of bleeding from the placental bed difficult by conservative means, total hysterectomy is usually the procedure of choice (see Chap. 34, p. 886).

VAGINAL METHODS. There are four "compression," or "tamponade," methods for vaginal delivery, although only simple rupture of the membranes is now in general use. Willett's forceps, insertion of a Voorhees' bag, and Braxton Hicks' version have all but disappeared from modern practice for a variety of reasons mentioned below.

1. Rupture of the membranes usually allows the head to drop down against the placenta and is often an efficacious procedure in multiparas with low-lying placentas and no bleeding until after onset of labor.
2. To put additional pressure on the placenta, a T-shaped clamp (Willett's forceps) was formerly attached to the fetal scalp and a weight of 1 or 2 pounds applied to the clamp over a pulley. This procedure caused little more compression than simple rupture of the membranes and frequently inflicted severe damage to the fetal scalp. It has fallen into disuse except in rare instances of fetal death associated with lesser degrees of hemorrhage from placenta previa.
3. Historically, a 10-cm Voorhees' bag filled with water and applied through the cervix was once employed to try to compress the placenta against the implantation site. This procedure has been abandoned because the manipulations necessary to insert the bag frequently traumatized the friable and vascular lower uterine segment, or caused further separation of the placenta, or both. Additional disadvantages were the frequent failure of the bag to cause full dilatation, the danger of infection, and the high perinatal mortality rate associated with its use.
4. The Braxton Hicks' version was not directed at immediate delivery. Rather, its objective was the utilization of the fetal buttocks and thigh for tamponade of the placenta. It differed from conventional version and extraction in several important respects: Braxton Hicks' version was done at a 4- to 8-cm dilatation. Two fingers and not the whole hand were inserted into the uterus to grasp the foot of the fetus, and after a foot had been delivered, no further effort at extraction was made, but simply enough traction exerted on the leg to control the bleeding. Only with complete dilatation was extraction effected. This procedure, too, has fallen into disrepute because of the difficulty of the operation, the high incidence of rupture of the friable lower uterine segment, the likelihood of further separation of the placenta during the intrauterine manipulation, and the almost inevitable death of the fetus.

Prognosis. A marked reduction in the rate of maternal mortality has been achieved, a trend that began in 1927 when Arthur Bill advocated adequate transfusion and cesarean section in the treatment of placenta previa. Since 1945, when Macafee and Johnson independently suggested expectant therapy for cases remote from term, a similar trend has been evident in perinatal loss. Half the cases are already near term when bleeding occurs, but prematurity still poses a formidable problem for the remainder, since not all women with placenta previa and a premature fetus can be treated expectantly. Delivery is forced by profuse hemorrhage in many and labor in some.

PROBABILITY OF A PATIENT WITH PLACENTA PREVIA
DELIVERING WITHIN THE NEXT 1, 2, OR 4 WEEKS

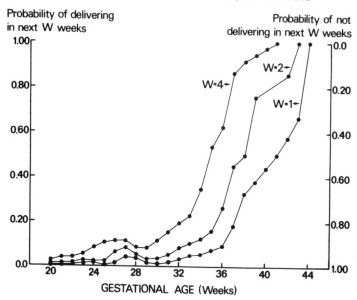

FIG. 21-15. Graphed is the probability that a woman with placenta previa will be delivered within 1 week (W = 1), 2 weeks (W = 2), and 4 weeks (W = 4) at each week of gestation during the latter half of pregnancy. (From Brenner, Edelman, Hendricks. *Am J Obstet Gynecol* 132:180, 1978)

Prematurity is a major cause of perinatal death even though expectant management of placenta previa is practiced. Moreover, for any fetal weight, perinatal mortality is likely to be greater with placenta previa than in the general population. Serious fetal malformations are also more common. The prognosis for achieving fetal maturity with expectant management of placenta previa has been calculated by Brenner and colleagues (1978) based on 178 cases studied by them. For a woman who has been diagnosed to have placenta previa, the probability of delivery within one week, two weeks, and four weeks, is plotted in Figure 21-15.

FETAL DEATH AND DELAYED DELIVERY

In general, during the past two decades, the management of a patient whose fetus has died and who fails to go into labor spontaneously has changed from watchful waiting to more active intervention. Although most women will eventually go into labor spontaneously, the psychologic stress imposed upon the mother carrying a dead fetus, the dangers of blood coagulation defects, and the advent of more effective methods of induction of labor have increased the desirability of early delivery. Because the generally available methods of early diagnosis of fetal death still lack certainty (see Chap. 10, p. 271), and since the majority of women will deliver within two weeks (Goldstein et al., 1963; Tricomi, Kohl, 1957) it is recommended that in the absence of other complications, attempts to evacuate the uterus generally be delayed for that period of time but not too much longer.

Coagulation Changes. Weiner and associates first pointed out in 1950 that some isoimmunized Rh-negative women who car-

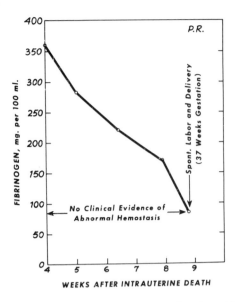

FIG. 21-16.   Slow development of maternal hypofibrinogenemia following fetal death and delayed delivery. (From Pritchard. *Obstet Gynecol*
14:574, 1959)

ried a dead fetus developed coagulation defects. An anterospective study indicated that
gross disruption of the maternal coagulation
mechanism rarely developed in less than one
month after fetal death (Pritchard, 1959,
Pritchard, Ratnoff, 1955). If the fetus was
retained for longer periods of time, however,
about 25 percent of the cases demonstrated
significant changes in the coagulation mechanism. Thus the "old wives' tale" that the dead
baby would poison the mother, although
scoffed at by physicians for a long time,
proved to be true. Maternal isoimmunization
with fetomaternal blood incompatibility is
not essential to the development of the coagulation changes as originally thought by
Weiner and associates (1950). Extrauterine
pregnancy with fetal death and delayed delivery may also be complicated by acquired hypofibrinogenemia (Dehner, 1972).

A few cases have been described with abrupt alterations in the plasma fibrinogen concentration, the values vacillating repeatedly
between normal and very low over the course
of a few days (Goldstein, Reid, 1963). Experience in Dallas and Cleveland, however, has

been that typically in all women the fibrinogen concentration falls from levels that are
normal for pregnancy to levels that are normal for the nonpregnant state, but in some
cases the decrease continues gradually to
reach potentially dangerous concentrations of
100 mg per dl or less (Pritchard, Ratnoff,
1955). The rate of decrease commonly found
is demonstrated in Figure 21-16. Simultaneously, fibrin degradation products are elevated in serum. The platelet count tends to
be reduced in these instances but, in our experience, severe thrombocytopenia seldom
develops, even though the fibrinogen level
is quite low (Fig. 21-17. A). Spontaneous
correction of the coagulation defects seldom
occurs until the dead products of conception
are evacuated (Jennison, Walker, 1956;
Pritchard, 1959).

PATHOGENESIS.   A series of reports
clearly establish that consumptive coagulopathy, presumably mediated by thromboplastin
from the dead products of conception, is operational in these cases (Lerner, et al., 1967;
Sherman, Middleton, 1958). As shown in
Figure 21-18, heparin, infused alone over a
few days, can correct the coagulation defects
but ε-aminocaproic acid does not. While
these observations serve to establish the
cause, they do not precisely identify the site
where fibrinogen is converted to fibrin. The
placenta from such a case commonly contains
much insoluble protein (Fig. 21-17. B.) that
can be made soluble by treatment with bovine fibrinolysin (Pritchard, 1973), but, most
likely, considerably more fibrinogen has been
converted to fibrin, presumably intravascularly, than can be recovered from the placenta.

USE OF HEPARIN.   Correction of coagulation defects has been accomplished using
heparin *under carefully controlled conditions in
women with an intact circulation.* Heparin appropriately adminstered can block further
pathologic consumption of fibrinogen and
other clotting factors and thereby allow the
coagulation mechanism to repair spontaneously. Once this has been accomplished and

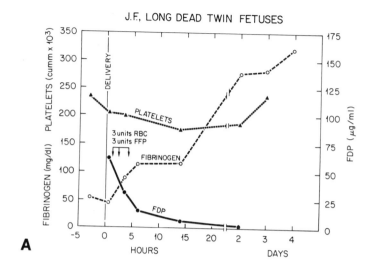

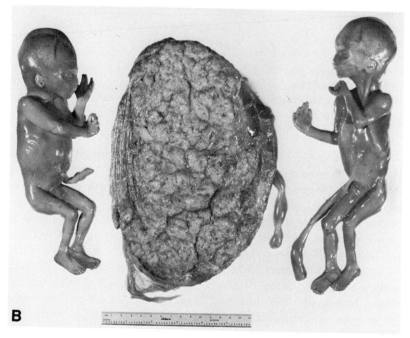

FIG. 21-17. **A.** Data from a case of fetal death and delayed delivery treated on an emergency basis at Parkland Memorial Hospital. The twin fetuses (Fig. 21-17. **B.**) had been dead for 8 weeks or more. Spontaneous delivery after spontaneous labor was followed by appreciable bleeding which was treated with intravenous oxytocin, uterine massage, and blood transfusion. (Blood fractions were used because of nonavailability of type-specific blood.) Initially there was marked hypofibrinogenemia and elevation of fibrin degradation products without thrombocytopenia. Recovery was uneventful; the hematocrit at discharge was 29. In retrospect, hypofibrinogenemia was apparent from the very small clot in blood drawn for serology after admittance to the hospital. (FDP = fibrin degradation products in maternal serum). **B.** Long-dead twin fetuses from case described in Figure 21-17. A. The placenta contains much fibrin.

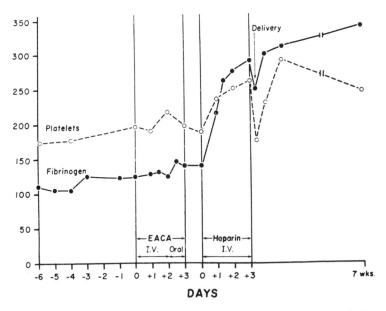

FIG. 21-18. Coagulation defects with prolonged retention of a dead fetus. Fibrinogen concentration and platelet count rose during intravenous infusion of heparin, 1500 μ per hour, but not during administration of ε-aminocaproic acid (EACA). (From Jimenez and Pritchard. *Obstet Gynecol* 32:449, 1968)

the heparin infusion is stopped, steps are promptly taken to evacuate the dead products of conception (Jimenez, Pritchard, 1968). It is emphasized that for heparin to be used safely to block the consumptive coagulopathy and thereby allow spontaneous repair of the coagulation mechanism, it is essential that the maternal circulatory system be intact. Otherwise, heparin most likely will incite or enhance hemorrhage. Moreover, once the dead products of conception have been evacuated, spontaneous repair will soon occur, so there is no good reason to give heparin at that time.

Treatment of Active Hemorrhage. If serious hemorrhage is encountered as the products of conception are being expelled or surgically removed and overt hypofibrinogenemia and associated coagulation defects are now identified, treatment with heparin almost certainly will enhance the bleeding. In this circumstance, effective primary treatment is blood and lactated Ringer's solution, according to the guidelines for treatment of

hemorrhage described under "Fluid Replacement Therapy." This approach has proved to be very successful just as it has for placental abruption.

Fibrinogen has been used to help control hemorrhage during and following evacuation of products of conception from women with hypofibrinogenemia (Pritchard, 1959; Pritchard, Ratnoff, 1955), but the disadvantage from its use is significant risk of hepatitis. If used, it should be given as cryoprecipitate (p. 505). Although ε-aminocaproic acid has been recommended to block fibrinolysis (Pfeffer, 1966), its use seems irrational and potentially dangerous.

Pregnancy Termination with Dead Fetus. Near term, intravenously administered oxytocin usually is effective, although it may have to be repeated (see Chap. 24, p. 607). Remote from term, however, it is less likely to prove effective unless given in high concentration on more than one occasion. It is not unusual for the infused oxytocin to initiate some palpable contractions which then abate even though the amount infused is increased. The oxytocin appears at times to influence the uterus subsequently to contract spontaneously, since, during the next 24 hours or so after oxytocin infusion, it is not unusual for spontaneous evacuation to take place. One or more laminaria tents placed in the cervical canal before the use of oxytocin may enhance expulsion of the dead products. The magnitude of risk of infection from use of laminaria in the presence of dead products of conception has not yet been identifed.

Water intoxication as the consequence of the antidiuretic effect of oxytocin administered with large volumes of aqueous dextrose has been documented repeatedly since first described in these circumstances by Liggins (1962). Administration of small volumes of lactated Ringer's solution, rather than large volumes of aqueous dextrose solution, avoids this problem.

Numerous observers have been favorably impressed by the fairly prompt abortifacient action provided by prostaglandin E$_2$ as a vaginal suppository (Bailey et al., 1975; Kent, Goldstein, 1976). Almost all women develop nausea, vomiting, and diarrhea after prostaglandin suppositories are inserted intravaginally; fever is also common (Phelan, Cephalo, 1978). Complications that have been reported also include uterine rupture (Schulman et al., 1979) and myocardial infarction (Patterson et al., 1979).

Orr and co-workers (1979) have emphasized that failure of prostaglandin E$_2$ suppositories to expel the dead products of conception must raise the question of extrauterine fetal death and cite four such experiences. Fetal death with delayed delivery should always provide the stimulus for asking the question, "Is the pregnancy extrauterine?"

The intrauterine injection of hypertonic saline is not recommended for evacuation of dead products of conception, since the volume of amnionic fluid is often reduced and the potentially highly toxic salt solution therefore is difficult to inject quantitatively into the sac. Coagulation defects may be enhanced by intraamnionic hypertonic saline (p. 609).

AMNIONIC FLUID EMBOLISM

Pathogenesis. Entry of amnionic fluid into the maternal circulation in some circumstances may prove fatal. Essential to the development of amnionic fluid embolism are (1) a rent through the amnion and chorion, (2) opened maternal veins, and (3) a pressure gradient sufficient to force the fluid into the venous circulation. Marginal separation of the placenta, or laceration of the uterus or cervix, serves to create an opening into the maternal circulation. Vigorous labor, including that induced with oxytocin, is more likely to provide the pressure. These events may also distress the fetus, leading to defecation of meconium in utero, thereby markedly potentiating the toxic nature of amnionic fluid if it should enter the maternal circulation.

In the typical case of amnionic fluid embolism, the woman is laboring vigorously, or having just done so, is in the process of being delivered when she develops varying degrees of respiratory distress and circulatory collapse. If the woman does not die immediately, serious hemorrhage with severe coagulation defects is soon evident from the genital tract and all other sites of trauma. The clinical features and the pathologic findings in 40 fatal cases have been reviewed by Peterson and Taylor (1970).

TOXICITY OF AMNIONIC FLUID. The lethality of intravenously infused amnionic fluid appears to vary remarkably depending upon the particulate matter contained. The suddenness and the intensity of cardiorespiratory problems that develop in many cases of amnionic fluid embolism and the histologic findings in the pulmonary vessels at autopsy strongly suggest, at least, that the likelihood of infused amnionic fluid proving to be lethal is greatest when it has been appreciably enriched with particulate debris. Moreover, it is not uncommon for amnionic fluid embolism to occur in circumstances that lead to fetal distress with the escape of meconium from the fetal colon into the amnionic sac.

Schneider (1955) showed that the lethal nature of human amnionic fluid infused in-

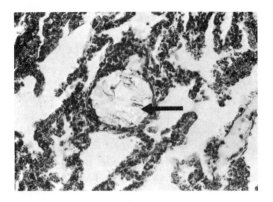

FIG. 21-19. Fetal squames (arrow) packed into small pulmonary artery in fatal cases of amnionic fluid embolism. (From Sparr and Pritchard. *Surg Gynecol Obstet* 107:560, 1958)

travenously into dogs was enhanced very greatly by the addition of meconium. Under these circumstances, it is envisioned that the particulate matter shed previously into the amnionic fluid or contained in the meconium, including shed fetal squamous cells (squames) (Fig. 21-19), fetal hairs (lanugo), vernix caseosa, and mucin, is pumped by a vigorous contraction from the disrupted amnionic sac into a maternal uterine vein. Severe pulmonary vascular obstruction from the particulate matter and possibly from fibrin deposition at this time causes *acute cor pulmonale* (Schneider, Henry, 1968). Abruptly, hypoxia and reduced cardiac output develop, and if not immediately fatal, hemorrhage from coagulation defects is soon evident, especially from traumatized blood vessels. Severe thrombocytopenia develops and the blood typically is incoagulable when treated with thrombin or, at most, there is formed a small, mushy clot which may lyse promptly. Plasma from such a case, mixed with normal plasma and recalcified or thrombin added, has been observed by us to clot but very promptly lyse, whereas the clotted normal plasma alone did not do so for days. Moreover, when fibrinogen was injected into the circulation, the thrombin-clottable protein promptly disappeared. These observations imply potent fibrinolytic activity, in some

cases at least, as well as consumptive coagulopathy.

COAGULATION INITIATED BY AMNIONIC FLUID. The clot-accelerating activity of amnionic fluid is greater at term than early in the third trimester, an observation that led Hastwell (1974) to suggest its measurement as an index of fetal maturity. Even at term, however, the activity normally is not great. The clot accelerator principle appears to behave more like Russell's viper venom than tissue thromboplastin, in that factor VII is not essential for the clot-accelerating action of amnionic fluid (Courtney, Allington, 1972; Phillips, Davidson, 1972). Of significance, amnionic fluid at times contains appreciable amounts of mucus which, in case of amnionic fluid embolism, might incite or aggravate intravascular coagulation. Extracts of human mucus have been shown in vitro and in vivo to induce coagulation, apparently by activation of factor X (Pineo et al., 1973).

EXPERIMENTAL AMNIONIC FLUID EMBOLISM.   Studies by Hanzlik and Karsner (1924) indicated that the injection of finely divided particulate matter, such as suspensions of charcoal particles or India ink, produced not only altered coagulability of the blood but also dramatic systemic phenomena, such as restlessness, tremors, marked dyspnea, convulsions, and often death. In the experiments of Halmagyi and co-workers (1962), after human amnionic fluid was injected into sheep, pulmonary hypertension, arterial hypoxia, and a marked fall in pulmonary compliance were noted. These changes, however, are similar to those found in pulmonary embolism of other cause, and they failed to occur when the amnionic fluid was filtered. Moreover, they were not completely prevented by heparin. Stolte and co-workers (1967) could not produce the syndrome in monkeys, nor could Spence and Mason (1974) do so in rabbits. Attwood (1964) caused the death of only 5 of 15 dogs by the intravenous injection of 50 ml of amnionic fluid and Pritchard and Capps (unpublished observations) noted an even lower mortality rate in dogs when sterile human amnionic fluid obtained at repeat cesarean section was used. However, a suspension of human meconium injected into dogs has been shown to be highly lethal, (Schneider, 1955).

AMNIONIC FLUID EMBOLISM WITH ABORTION. Fatal presumed amnionic fluid embolism associated with induced abortion has been reported by Grimes and Cates (1977). One pregnancy reported by them had reached 35 weeks gestation (hardly an abortion); death followed the injection of hypertonic saline. Another death followed the injection of 345 ml of 25 percent sodium chloride solution, allegedly into a uterus at 12 to 14 weeks gestation. Another death occurred at 16 to 17 weeks gestational age shortly after the uterus was opened at hysterotomy and the anterior placenta was separated. It is doubtful that normal amnionic fluid during the first half of pregnancy is very toxic, since it contains little or no particulate matter or mucin. Amnionic fluid contaminated with bacterial products, especially endotoxin, would almost certainly prove very toxic if it entered the maternal circulation. The same is very likely true for amnionic fluid enriched with cytolytic products from a long-dead fetus, as in one case described by Grimes and Cates.

Treatment. There almost certainly have been women with amnionic fluid embolism who survived, although the diagnosis is always open to question without identification of obvious amnionic fluid debris within blood vessels examined in sections of lung or at least the buffy coat of blood from the right side of the heart. Tuck (1972) has described the identification of squames presumed to be from amnionic fluid in sputum stained with Nile blue sulfate. Confirmatory experiences with this technique are needed.

Therapy for amnionic fluid embolism is notoriously unsuccessful. When treatment is successful, the diagnosis may be challenged. Vigorous treatment of the hypoxia is mandatory and usually necessitates mechanical ventilation. Blood replacement therapy is equally essential (Resnik and coworkers, 1976), but the patient with cor pulmonale tolerates any deficit or excess in blood volume very poorly. Use of fibrinogen, heparin, fibrinolytic agents, and antifibrinolytic agents has been described in various case reports but it is very

difficult to evaluate their efficacy (Chung, Merkatz, 1973; Gregory, Clayton, 1973; Kates, Schifrin, 1976; Pritchard, Dugan, 1956; Woodfield et al., 1971).

HEMORRHAGE WITH ABORTION

Etiology of Hemorrhage. Remarkable blood loss, both acute and chronic, may occur as the consequence of abortion. Hemorrhage during the first trimester is less likely to be severe unless the procedure was traumatic. When the pregnancy is more advanced, the mechanisms responsible for the hemorrhage most often are the same as those described for placental abruption and placenta previa. At times, appreciable changes in the coagulation mechanism complicate abortion.

Coagulation Defects. Serious disruption of the coagulation mechanism may develop as the consequence of (1) prolonged retention of a dead fetus, as described above; (2) sepsis, a notorious cause; and (3) the intrauterine instillation of hypertonic saline or urea solutions, which may incite consumptive coagulopathy and induce serious hemorrhage (Burkman et al., 1977; Stander et al., 1971).

HYPERTONIC SOLUTIONS. The kinds of changes in coagulation that have been identified with abortion induced with markedly hypertonic solutions imply, at least, that thromboplastin is released from placenta, fetus, decidua, or all three by the necrobiotic effect of the hypertonic solutions which then initiates coagulation within the maternal circulation. Intravascular hemolysis has also been identified with consumptive coagulopathy induced by hypertonic saline-induced abortion (Adachi et al., 1975). Prostaglandins to induce abortion so far have not been implicated in the production of coagulation defects except in association with prolonged retention of a dead fetus (Filshie, 1971).

SEPTIC ABORTION AND COAGULOPATHY. Gross disruption of the coagulation mechanism has been an uncommon but serious complication among women with septic abortion cared for at Parkland Memorial Hospital. The incidence has been highest in those with *Clostridium perfringens* sepsis and intense intravascular hemolysis (Pritchard, Whalley, 1971). In the presence of gross intravascular hemolysis, plasma fibrinogen concentrations ranged from normal to low, as did the platelet counts, while fibrin degradation products in serum were variably elevated. It has long been recognized that intense intravascular hemolysis is capable of inciting disseminated intravascular coagulation which, if the circulatory system is not intact, contributes significantly to serious hemorrhage. Erythrocyte stroma initiates intravascular hemolysis (Quick et al., 1954), whereas hemoglobinemia in the absence of erythrocyte stroma does not induce consumptive coagulopathy and appears to be relatively innocuous, at least in subhuman primates (Birndorf, Lopas, 1970).

Of 25 cases of septic abortion at Parkland Memorial Hospital in which the blood culture was positive for *Clostridium perfringens,* 5 of the 11 with intense hemolysis proved fatal, whereas none succumbed of the 13 in whom gross hemolysis did not develop. All women who exhibited overt intravascular hemolysis developed renal failure and, if they did not die very soon, were treated by dialysis. One woman with severe thrombocytopenia and azotemia, when heparinized for hemodialysis, bled from the gastrointestinal tract, with fatal results. Subsequent studies of renal function in those who survived demonstrated return of normal function.

Available evidence, scant as it is, would appear to support the use of whole blood to treat the hemorrhage and, to a degree, the coagulation defects. The intravascular compartment should be vigorously refilled without causing circulatory overload. The benefits, if any, from heparin administration have not been established. Corrigan (1977) carefully reviewed 222 cases of septic shock and disseminated intravascular coagulation from a variety of causes to determine if heparin therapy influenced the clinical course. He concluded that heparinization did not favorably affect the mortality rate. In our experience in women whose vasculature is not intact, heparin does one thing for certain, namely, aggravate the hemorrhage.

Severe disruption of the coagulation mechanism can develop with abortion complicated by gram-negative sepsis in the absence of intense intravascular hemolysis. A series of pathologic events induced especially by endotoxin that include activation of factor XII, other procoagulants, and plasminogen, as well as various kinins and components of complement, are thought to be involved in the genesis of the coagulation defects and shock associated with severe gram-negative sepsis (McCabe, 1973).

Prompt restoration and maintenance of circulation and appropriate steps to control the infection, including evacuation of infected products of conception, are most important for a successful outcome. There is no good evidence that routine hysterectomy, rather than prompt curettage to remove infected products of conception from an intact uterus, improves the outcome. Management is described further in Chapter 24 (p. 613).

COAGULATION DEFECTS POSSIBLY INDUCED BY HEMORRHAGE

Rarely, severe hemorrhage with overt disruption of the coagulation mechanism characteristic of consumptive coagulopathy may develop in a woman without evidence of any disease known to incite intravascular coagulation, as for example, an apparently uncomplicated repeated cesarean section. The experimental observations of Turpini and Stefanini (1959) support the thesis that severe hemorrhage of itself can induce consumptive coagulopathy. Animal studies by some other investigators, however, have not confirmed their observations (Herman et al., 1972; Karayalcin et al., 1973). Treatment with whole blood and lactated Ringer's solution with or without fibrinogen, or platelet packs as described earlier in this chapter, for placental abruption, has been effective in cases treated at Parkland Memorial Hospital.

OTHER COAGULATION DEFECTS

Coagulation defects caused by *eclampsia* or *severe preeclampsia* are discussed in Chapter 27. Rarely, a hemophilia-like state may be acquired during the postpartum period as the consequence of development of an antibody to Factor VIII. Hampton and Hauth (1980) have described such a case in which the woman was kept alive through treatment with massive amounts of blood and cryoprecipitate. Attempts at immunosuppression with corticosteroids and plasmapheresis to try to remove antibody to Factor VIII appeared to be of little benefit.

Coagulation defects that are coincidental with pregnancy are considered in Chapter 28.

REFERENCES

Adachi A, Spivack M, Wilson L: Intravascular hemolysis: a complication of midtrimester abortion. Obstet Gynecol 45:467, 1975

Alperin JB, Haggard ME, McGanity WJ: Folic acid, pregnancy, and abruptio placentae. Am J Clin Nutr 22:1354, 1969

Attwood HD: A histological study of experimental amniotic-fluid and meconium embolism in dogs. J Pathol Bacteriol 88:285, 1964

Bailey CD, Newman C, Ellinas SP, Anderson GG: Use of prostaglandin E₂ vaginal suppositories in intrauterine fetal death and missed abortion. Obstet Gynecol 45:110, 1975

Beischer NA, Brown JB, Macafee J: Urinary estriol excretion before severe placental abruption. Obstet Gynecol 36:697, 1970

Bill AH: The treatment of placenta previa by prophylactic blood transfusion and cesarean section. Am J Obstet Gynecol 14:523, 1927

Birndorf NI, Lopas H: Effects of red cell stroma-free hemoglobin solution on renal function in monkeys. J Appl Physiol 29:573, 1970

Bonnar J, McNicol GP, Douglas AS: The behavior of the coagulation and fibrinolytic mechanism in abruptio placentae. J Obstet Gynaecol Br Commonw 76:799, 1969

Bowie JD, Rochester D, Cadkin AV, Cooke WT, Kunzman A: Accuracy of placental localization by ultrasound. Radiology 128:177, 1978

Brame RG, Harbert GM Jr, McGaughey HS Jr, Thornton WN Jr: Maternal risk in abruption. Obstet Gynecol 31:224, 1968

Brenner WE, Edelman DA, Hendricks CH: Characteristics of patients with placenta previa and results of expectant management. Am J Obstet Gynecol 132:180, 1978

Burkman RT, Bell WR, Atienza MF, King TM: Coagulopathy with midtrimester induced abortion: Association with hyperosmolar urea administration. Am J Obstet Gynecol 127:533, 1977

Campbell S, Kohorn E: Placental localization by ultrasonic compound scanning. J Obstet Gynaecol Br Commonw 75:1007, 1968

Chung AF, Merkatz IR: Survival following amniotic fluid embolism with early heparinization. Obstet Gynecol 42:809, 1973

Corrigan JJ: Heparin therapy in bacterial septicemia. J Pediatr 91:695, 1977

Courtney LD, Allington M: Effect of amniotic fluid on blood coagulation. Br J Haematol 22:353, 1972

Czer LSC, Shoemaker WC: Optimal hematocrit value in critically ill postoperative patients. Surg Gynecol Obstet 147:363, 1978

Dehner LP: Advanced extrauterine pregnancy and the fetal death syndrome. Obstet Gynecol 40:525, 1972

Dikshit K, Vyden JK, Forrester JS, Chatterjee K, Prakosh R, Swan HJC: Renal and extrarenal hemodynamic effects of furosemide in congestive heart failure after acute myocardial infarction. New Engl J Med 288:1087, 1973

Donald I, Abdulla U: Placentography by sonar. J Obstet Gynaecol Br Commonw 75:993, 1968

Dunster GD, Rhys Davies E, Ross FGM, John AH: Placental localization: Comparison of isotopic and ultrasonic placentography. Br J Radiol 49:940, 1976

Edson JR, Blaese RM, White JG, Krivit W: Defibrination syndrome in an infant born after abruptio placentae. Pediatrics 72:342, 1968

Filshie GM: The use of prostaglandin E₂ in the management of intrauterine death, missed abortion and hydatidiform mole. J Obstet Gynaecol Br Commonw 78:87, 1971

Gibbs CE: Maternal deaths in Texas, 1969 to 1973. Am J Obstet Gynecol 126:687, 1976

Goldstein DP, Reid DE: Circulating fibrinolytic activity: a precursor of hypofibrinogenemia following fetal death *in utero*. Obstet Gynecol 22:174, 1963

Goldstein DP, Johnson JP, Reid DE: Management

of intrauterine fetal death. Obstet Gynecol 21:523, 1963

Gottesfeld KR, Thompson HE, Holmes JH, Taylor ES: Ultrasound placentography: a new method for placental localization. Am J Obstet Gynecol 96:538, 1966

Gregory MG, Clayton EM Jr: Amniotic fluid embolism. Obstet Gynecol 42:236, 1973

Grimes DA, Cates W Jr: Fatal amniotic fluid embolism during induced abortion. South Med J 70:1325, 1977

Halmagyi DF, Starzecki B, Shearman RP: Experimental amniotic fluid embolism: mechanism and treatment. Am J Obstet Gynecol 84:251, 1962

Hampton RM, Hauth JC: Factor VIII antibody associated with pregnancy. Submitted for publication.

Hanzlik PJ, Karsner HT: Anaphylactoid phenomena from the intravenous administration of various colloids, arsenicals and other agents. J Pharmacol Exp Ther 14:379, 1920; 23:173, 1924

Hastwell GB: Amniotic fluid thromboplastic activity as an index of fetal maturity: a preliminary report. Aust NZ J Obstet Gynaecol 14:196, 1974

Heinemann HO: Right-sided heart failure and the use of diuretics. Am J Med 64:367, 1978

Herman CM, Moquin RB, Horwitz DL: Coagulation changes of hemorrhagic shock in baboons. Ann Surg 175:197, 1972

Hibbard BM, Jeffcoate TNA: Abruptio placentae. Obstet Gynecol 27:155, 1966

Hughes EC (ed): Obstetric-Gynecologic Terminology. Philadelphia, Davis, 1972, p 417

Jansen RPS: Relative bradycardia: A sign of acute intraperitoneal bleeding. Aust NZ J Obstet Gynaecol 18:206, 1978

Jennison RF, Walker AC: Foetal death in utero with hypofibrinogenemia managed conservatively. Lancet 2:607, 1956

Jimenez JM, Pritchard JA: Pathogenesis and treatment of coagulation defects resulting from fetal death. Obstet Gynecol 32:449, 1968

Jimerson SD, Crosby WM: Maternal mortality in Oklahoma: Hemorrhage remains a problem. Okla State Med Assoc J 71:197, 1978

Johnson HW: The conservative management of some varieties of placenta previa. Am J Obstet Gynecol 50:248, 1945

Karayalcin G, Kim KY, Aballi AJ: Coagulation changes after acute blood loss. Pediatr Res 7:357, 1973

Kates RJ, Schifrin BS: Self-limited acute defibrina-

tion in pregnancy: Case report. Am J Obstet Gynecol 124:432, 1976

Kent DR, Goldstein AI: Prostaglandin E$_2$ induction of labor for fetal demise. Obstet Gynecol 48:475, 1976

King DL: Placental migration demonstrated by ultrasonography. Radiology 109:163, 1973

Kitay DZ: Folic acid deficiency in pregnancy. Am J Obstet Gynecol 104:1067, 1969

Knab DR: Abruptio placentae. Obstet Gynecol 52:625, 1978

Kobayashi M, Hellman L, Fillisti L: Placenta localization by ultrasound. Am J Obstet Gynecol 106:279, 1970

Krupp PJ Jr, Barclay DL, Roeling WM, Wegener G: Maternal mortality: a 20 year study of Tulane Department of Obstetrics and Gynecology at Charity Hospital. Obstet Gynecol 35:823, 1970

Lerner R, Margolin M, Slate WG: Heparin in the treatment of hypofibrinogenemia complicating fetal death in utero. Am J Obstet Gynecol 97:373, 1967

Levin J, Algazy KM: Hematologic disorders in pregnancy. In Burrow GN, Ferris TF (eds): Medical Complications of Pregnancy. Philadelphia, Saunders, 1975

Liggins GC: Treatment of missed abortion by high dosage syntocinon intravenous infusion. J Obstet Gynaecol Br Commonw 69:277, 1962

Macafee CHG: Placenta previa: a study of 174 cases. J Obstet Gynaecol Br Emp 52:313, 1945

McCabe WR: Serum complement levels in bacteremia due to gram-negative organisms. New Engl J Med 288:21, 1973

Menon MKK, Sengupta M, Ramaswamy N: Accidental haemorrhage and folic acid deficiency. J Obstet Gynaecol Br Commonw 73:49, 1966

Ness PM, Perkins HA: Cryoprecipitate as a reliable source of fibrinogen replacement. JAMA 241:1690, 1979

Newton M: Postpartum hemorrhage. Am J Obstet Gynecol 94:711, 1966

Nielsen NC: Coagulation and fibrinolysis in mothers and their newborn infants following premature separation of the placenta. Acta Obstet Gynecol Scand 49:77, 1970

Orr JW Jr, Huddleston JF, Goldenberg RL, Knox GE, Davis RO: Association of extrauterine fetal death with failure of prostaglandin E$_2$ suppositories. Obstet Gynecol (Suppl) 53:57, 1979

Page EW, Fulton LD, Glendening MB: Cause of blood coagulation defect following abruptio placentae. Am J Obstet Gynecol 61:1116, 1951

Paterson MEL: The aetiology and outcome of abruptio placentae. Acta Obstet Gynecol Scand 58:31, 1979

Patterson SP, White JH, Reaves EM: A maternal death associated with prostaglandin E₂. Obstet Gynecol 54:123, 1979

Peterson EP, Taylor HB: Amniotic fluid embolism: an analysis of 40 cases. Obstet Gynecol 35:787, 1970

Pfeffer RI: Hypofibrinogenemia in the dead fetus syndrome treated with amniocaproic acid. Am J Obstet Gynecol 95:1095, 1966

Phelan JP, Cephalo RC: A better approach to fetal demise—PGE₂ suppository. Contemp Ob/Gyn 11:93, 1978

Phillips LL: Homologous serum jaundice following fibrinogen administration. Surg Gynecol Obstet 121:551, 1965

Phillips LL, Davidson EC Jr: Procoagulant properties of aminotic fluid. Am J Obstet Gynecol 113:911, 1972

Pineo GF, Recoeczi E, Hatton MWC, Brain MC: The activation of coagulation by extracts of mucus: a possible pathway of intravascular coagulation accompanying adenocarcinomas. J Lab Clin Med 82:255, 1973

Pritchard JA: Fetal death in utero. Obstet Gynecol 14:573, 1959

Pritchard JA: Changes in the blood volume during pregnancy and delivery. Anesthesiology 26:393, 1965

Pritchard JA: Haematological problems associated with delivery, placental abruption, retained dead fetus, and amniotic fluid embolism. Clin Haematol 2:563, 1973

Pritchard JA, Brekken AL: Clinical and laboratory studies on severe abruptio placentae. Am J Obstet Gynecol 97:681, 1967

Pritchard JA, Dugan RJ: Presumed amniotic fluid embolism with recovery. Ohio State Med J 52:379, 1956

Pritchard JA, Ratnoff OD: Studies of fibrinogen and other hemostatic factors in women with intrauterine death and delayed delivery. Surg Gynecol Obstet 101:467, 1955

Pritchard JA, Whalley PJ: Abortion complicated by Clostridium perfringens infection. Am J Obstet Gynecol 11:484, 1971

Pritchard JA, Cunningham FG, Mason RA: Coagulation changes in eclampsia: their frequency and pathogenesis. Am J Obstet Gynecol 124:855, 1976

Pritchard JA, Baldwin RM, Dickey JC, Wiggins

KM: Blood volume changes in pregnancy and the puerperium: II. Red blood cell loss and changes in apparent blood volume during and following vaginal delivery, cesarean section, and cesarean section plus total hysterectomy. Am J Obstet Gynecol 84:1271, 1962

Pritchard JA, Mason R, Corley M, Pritchard S: Genesis of severe placental abruption. Am J Obstet Gynecol 108:22, 1970

Quick AJ, Georgatsos JG, Hussey CV: The clotting activity of human erythrocytes: theoretical and clinical implications. Am J Med Sci 228:207, 1954

Ratnoff OD, Pritchard JA, Colopy JE: Hemorrhagic status during pregnancy. New Engl J Med 253:63, 1955

Reid DE, Weiner AE, Roby CC: I. Intravascular clotting and afibrinogenemia, presumptive lethal factors in the syndrome of amniotic fluid embolism. Am J Obstet Gynecol 66:465, 1953

Resnik R, Swartz WH, Plumer MH, Benirshke K, Stratthaus, ME: Amniotic fluid embolism with survival. Obstet Gynecol 47:295, 1976

Rizos N, Doran TA, Miskin M, Benzie RJ, Ford JA: Natural history of placenta previa ascertained by diagnostic ultrasound. AM J Obstet Gynecol 133:287, 1979

Santos R, Jimenez J, Duenhoelter J: Unpublished observations, 1978

Schneider CL: "Fibrin embolism" (disseminated intravascular coagulation) with defibrination as one of end results during placenta abruptio. Surg Gynecol Obstet 92:27, 1951

Schneider CL: Obstetric shock: some interdependent problems of coagulation. Obstet Gynecol 4:273, 1954

Schneider CL: Coagulation defects in obstetric shock: meconium embolism and heparin; fibrin embolism and defibrination. Am J Obstet Gynecol 69:758, 1955

Schneider CL, Henry MM: Meconium embolism in vivo. Am J Obstet Gynecol 101:909, 1968

Schulman H, Saldana L, Lin C-C, Randolph G: Mechanism of failed labor after fetal death and its treatment with prostaglandin E₂. Am J Obstet Gynecol in press, 1979

Seski JC, Compton AA: Abruptio placentae following a negative oxytocin challenge test. Am J Obstet Gynecol 125:276, 1976

Sher G: Pathogenesis and management of uterine inertia complicating abruptio placentae with consumption coagulopathy. Am J Obstet Gynecol 129:164, 1977

Sher G: A rational basis for the management of

abruptio placentae. J Reprod Med 21:123, 1978

Sherman E, Middleton EH: The management of missed abortion with hypofibrinogenemia. Maryland State Med J 7:300, 1958

Spence MR, Mason KG: Experimental amniotic fluid embolism in rabbits. Am J Obstet Gynecol 119:1073, 1974

Stander RW, Flessa HC, Glueck HI, Kisker CT: Changes in maternal coagulation factors after intra-amniotic infection of hypertonic saline. Obstet Gynecol 37:660, 1970

Stolte L, Seelen J, Eskes T, Wagatsuma T: Failure to produce the syndrome of amniotic fluid embolism by infusion of amniotic fluid and meconium into monkeys. Am J Obstet Gynecol 98:694, 1967

Stone SR, Whalley PJ, Pritchard JA: Inferior vena cava and ovarian vein ligation during late pregnancy. Obstet Gynecol 32:267, 1968

Sunden B: Placentography by ultrasound. Acta Obstet Gynecol Scand 49:179, 1970

Tricomi V, Kohl SG: Fetal death in utero. Am J Obstet Gynecol 74:1092, 1957

Tuck CS: Amniotic fluid embolism. Proc Royal Soc Med 65:2, 1972

Turpini R, Stefanini M: The nature and mechanism of the hemostatic breakdown in the course of experimental hemorrhagic shock. J Clin Invest 38:53, 1959

Weiner AE, Reid DE, Roby CC, Diamond LK: Coagulation defects with intrauterine death from Rh sensitization. Am J Obstet Gynecol 60:1015, 1950

Wexler P, Gottesfeld KR: Second trimester placenta previa: an apparently normal placentation. Obstet Gynecol 50:706, 1977

Whalley PJ, Scott DE, Pritchard JA: Maternal folate deficiency and pregnancy wastage: I. Placental abruption. Am J Obstet Gynecol 105:670, 1969

Woodfield DG, Galloway RK, Smart GE: Coagulation defect associated with presumed amniotic fluid embolism in the mid-trimester of pregnancy. J Obstet Gynaecol Br Commonw 78:423, 1971

Woods WG, Luban NLC, Hilgartner MW, Miller DR: Disseminated intravascular coagulation in the newborn. JAMA 133:44, 1979

Young GB: The peripatetic placenta. Radiology 128:183, 1978

22

Ectopic Pregnancy

GENERAL CONSIDERATIONS

Definition. In a normal intrauterine pregnancy, the blastocyst implants in the endometrium which lines the uterine cavity. Implantation anywhere else is referred to as an ectopic pregnancy. Ectopic pregnancy is a broader term than extrauterine pregnancy, since it includes implantation in the interstitial portion of the oviduct that lies within the myometrium and implantation in the cervix, as well as pregnancy in the extrauterine portion of the oviduct, the ovary, the broad ligament, and elsewhere in the abdomen. Although more than 95 percent of ectopic pregnancies involve the fallopian tube, tubal pregnancy is not synonymous with, but rather a very common type of, ectopic gestation.

Etiology. The following have been implicated in the cause of ectopic pregnancy (Brenner et al., 1980):

A. Conditions that prevent or retard the passage of the fertilized ovum into the uterine cavity.
  1. *Salpingitis,* which causes agglutination of the arborescent folds of the tubal mucosa with narrowing of the lumen or formation of blind pockets.
  2. *Developmental abnormalities of the tube,* especially diverticula, accessory ostia, and hypoplasia.
  3. *Peritubal adhesions* subsequent to postabortal or puerperal infection, appendicitis, or endometriosis, which cause kinking of the tube and narrowing of the lumen.
  4. *Previous operations on the tube,* either to restore patency, or occasionally the failure of a deliberate attempt to disrupt continuity (tubal ligation, partial resection, or fulgeration).
  5. *Tumors that distort the tube,* such as uterine myomas and adnexal cysts.
  6. *External migration of the ovum.* There may be a slight increased risk of ectopic pregnancy for the woman with but one oviduct whenever she ovulates from the contralateral ovary. By delaying the transport of the fertilized ovum through the oviduct, external migration theoretically enhances the development of invasive properties of the blastocyst, while still within the tube. This is probably not an important factor in human ectopic gestation.
  7. *Menstrual reflux.* Delayed fertilization of the ovum with menstrual bleeding at the usual time theoretically could

either prevent the ovum from entering the uterus or flush it back into the tube. Little direct support for this concept is available.

B. Increase in the receptivity of the tubal mucosa to the fertilized ovum.

1. *Ectopic endometrial elements* in the tubal mucosa. Many observers have reported foci of endometriosis in fallopian tubes, yet it is an uncommon finding particularly among indigent black patients in whom tubal pregnancy is prevalent and endometriosis is very uncommon.

Tubal pregnancy may rarely follow hysterectomy. Niebyl (1974) reviewed 21 such cases. In most instances, a very recently fertilized ovum was trapped in the oviduct at the time of hysterectomy, where it implanted and grew for a variable period. More rarely, an ovum was fertilized in the oviduct long after hysterectomy. In such cases, a fistula sufficient for passage of sperm had developed between the vagina and the severed end of the oviduct.

Incidence. The frequency of ectopic pregnancies compared to intrauterine pregnancies varies appreciably at different institutions. For example, in some of the more recent reports listed in Table 22-1, the frequency ranged from one ectopic pregnancy per 84 deliveries to one per 230 deliveries.

A recent increase in ectopic pregnancies, compared to the number of intrauterine pregnancies, as reported by Kallanberger (1978), Kitchin (1979), and their associates, is logical for several reasons. The widespread practice of voluntary curtailment of family size by women of demonstrated fecundity has reduced the number of infants born and, simultaneously, some of the technics used to accomplish this do not necessarily prevent ectopic pregnancy anywhere nearly as effectively as they do intrauterine pregnancies. Common examples are elective abortion to interrupt early intrauterine pregnancies, pregnancies in the presence of intrauterine devices (see Chap. 40, p. 1026), and pregnancies after tubal sterilization (see Chap. 40, p. 1035). The apparent increase in gonorrhea, when accompanied by an increase in gonococcal salpingitis, also predisposes to tubal pregnancy.

Anatomic Considerations. The fertilized ovum may develop in any portion of the oviduct, giving rise to *ampullar, isthmic, and interstitial tubal pregnancies.* In rare instances, the fertilized ovum may be implanted on the fimbriated extremity and occasionally even on the fimbria ovarica. The ampulla is the most frequent site of implantation and the isthmus the next most common. Interstitial pregnancy is uncommon, occurring in only about 2.5 percent of all tubal gestations. From these primary types, certain secondary forms of tuboabdominal, tuboovarian, and broad ligament pregnancies occasionally develop.

TABLE 22-1.
THE RATIO OF ECTOPIC PREGNANCIES TO DELIVERIES AT
SEVERAL INSTITUTIONS

INSTITUTION	AUTHORS	RATIO OF ECTOPIC PREGNANCIES TO DELIVERIES
1. Freedman's Hospital	Clark & Jones (1975)	1:84
2. Grady Memorial Hospital	Franklin & Zeiderman (1973)	1:118
3. Wilford Hall Hospital	Gilstrap & Harris (1976)	1:124
4. University of Virginia Hospital	Kitchin et al. (1979)	1:126
5. University of Oklahoma Hospital	Kallenberger et al. (1978)	1:160
6. University of Kentucky Medical Center	Harralson et al. (1973)	1:230

MODE OF IMPLANTATION OF THE ZY-GOTE. The fertilized ovum may implant in columnar or intercolumnar fashion. In the former, which is rare, the zygote becomes attached to the tip or side of one of the folds of the tubal mucosa; in the second, implantation occurs in a depression between two mucosal folds. In neither situation does the fertilized ovum remain on the surface, but promptly burrows through the epithelium into the tissue just beneath it. At its periphery is a capsule of rapidly proliferating trophoblast, which invades and erodes the subjacent connective tissue and muscle of the tube. At the same time, maternal blood vessels are opened, and the blood pours out into spaces, of varying size, lying within the trophoblast or between it and the adjacent tissue.

In the usual intercolumnar implantation, as soon as the zygote penetrates the epithelium it comes to lie in the muscular wall, since the tube lacks a submucosa.

The tube does not normally form an extensive decidua, but decidual cells can usually be recognized and distinguished from trophoblast. The tubal wall in contact with the ovum offers but slight resistance to invasion by the trophoblast, which soon burrows through it, opening up maternal vessels. Often, direct penetration through the peritoneal surface or through the capsular membrane leads to intraperitoneal rupture and tubal abortion, respectively. In some instances, however, early rupture results from the sudden opening of an artery and disruption of the weakened tubal walls from the increased pressure from blood. There is usually a marked increase in the vascularity of the affected tube; the larger arteries and veins are greatly hypertrophied. There is hypertrophy of the muscle cells, but no remarkable increase in their number. Except at the placental site, the tubal wall is thickened and its cells are spread apart by edema. In many advanced cases, the exterior of the tube shows evidence of peritonitis and peritoneal adhesions. The embryo or fetus in ectopic pregnancy is often absent or stunted.

UTERINE CHANGES. In ectopic pregnancies, the uterus undergoes some of the changes associated with early normal intrauterine pregnancy, such as softening of the cervix and isthmus and some increase in size. *These changes do not, therefore, exclude an ectopic pregnancy.* The degree to which the endometrium is converted to decidua is variable. Although the finding of uterine decidua without trophoblast suggests ectopic pregnancy, it is by no means a positive indication. In 1954, Arias-Stella described, as had others before him, changes of the endometrial glands and epithelium that he thought were caused by chorionic gonadotropin. The epithelial cells are enlarged and their nuclei are hypertrophic, hyperchromatic, lobular, and irregularly shaped. There is a loss of polarity, and the abnormal nuclei tend to occupy the luminal portion of the cells. The cytoplasm may be vacuolated and foamy, and occasional mitoses may be found. These endometrial changes have been collectively referred to as the Arias-Stella phenomenon. The cellular changes in the Arias-Stella reaction are not specific for ectopic pregnancy but rather the blighting of the conceptus, either intrauterine or extrauterine (Fig. 22-1).

The external bleeding seen commonly in cases of tubal pregnancy is uterine in origin and associated with degeneration and sloughing of the uterine decidua. Soon after the death of the fetus, the decidua degenerates and is usually shed in small pieces, but occasionally it is cast off intact, as a *decidual cast* of the uterine cavity. The absence of decidual tissue, however, does not exclude an ectopic pregnancy; Romney and co-workers (1950) identified secretory endometrium in 40 percent of cases of ectopic pregnancy, proliferative in 30 percent, and menstrual in 6 percent while decidua was present in only 20 percent.

TYPES OF TUBAL PREGNANCY

Tubal Abortion. A common termination of tubal pregnancy is separation of the products of conception from the endosalpinx and extrusion of the abortus through the fim-

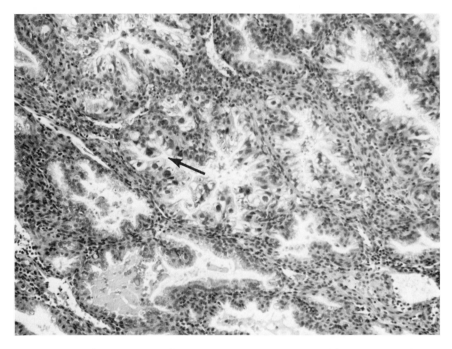

FIG. 22-1. Arias-Stella reaction. Some of the nuclei are enlarged (arrow), hyperchromatic, and irregularly shaped. Some of the cytoplasm is vacuolated and foamy. (Courtesy of Dr. Helen Graham)

briated end of the tube. The frequency of tubal abortion depends in great part upon the site of implantation of the zygote. In ampullary pregnancy, it is almost the rule, whereas intraperitoneal rupture is the usual outcome in isthmic pregnancy.

With regard to hemorrhage, tubal abortion does not differ from intraperitoneal rupture, except that in the former, bleeding occurs into the lumen of the tube, whereas in the latter it takes place directly into the peritoneal cavity. The immediate consequence of the hemorrhage with tubal abortion is the further loosening of the connection between the placenta and membranes and the tubal wall, and if separation is complete, the entire products may be extruded into the peritoneal cavity. At that point, hemorrhage may cease and symptoms disappear.

In complete tubal abortion, when the hemorrhage is moderate, the ovum may become infiltrated with blood and converted into a structure analogous to the blood mole observed in uterine abortion. Slight bleeding usually persists as long as the mole remains

in the tube, and the blood slowly trickles from the fimbriated extremity into the peritoneal cavity and pools in the rectouterine cul-de-sac. If the fimbriated extremity is occluded, the tube may gradually become distended by blood, forming a *hematosalpinx.*

After incomplete tubal abortion, pieces of the placenta or membranes may remain attached to the tubal wall and, after becoming surrounded by fibrin, give rise to a *placental polyp,* as may occur in the uterus after an incomplete uterine abortion.

Tubal Rupture. The invading, expanding products of conception may rupture the oviduct at any of several sites. Many of the cases of tubal pregnancy end during the first trimester by intraperitoneal rupture. As a rule, whenever tubal rupture occurs in the first few weeks, the pregnancy is situated in the isthmic portion of the tube a short distance from the cornu of the uterus. When the fertilized ovum is implanted well within the interstitial portion of the tube, rupture usually does not occur until later.

The immediate direct cause of rupture may be the trauma associated with coitus or a vigorous vaginal examination, although in the great majority of cases it occurs spontaneously. With intraperitoneal rupture, the entire products of conception may be extruded from the tube, or if the rent is small, profuse hemorrhage may occur without extrusion. In either event, commonly, the patient soon shows signs of collapse from hemorrhage and hypovolemia. If the woman is not operated upon and does not die from hemorrhage, the fate of the embryo or fetus will depend on the damage sustained by the products of conception and the duration of the gestation. If an early conceptus is expelled undamaged into the peritoneal cavity, it may reimplant almost anywhere, establish adequate circulation, and survive and grow, but this outcome is most unlikely because of the damage during the transition. The products of conception, if small, may be resorbed or, if larger, may remain in the cul-de-sac for years as an encapsulated mass or even become calcified to form a *lithopedion.*

If only the fetus is extruded at the time of rupture, however, the effect upon the pregnancy will vary depending on the extent of the injury sustained by the placenta. If it is very damaged, death of the fetus and termination of the pregnancy are inevitable, but if the greater portion of the placenta still retains its attachment to the tube, further development is possible. The fetus may then survive for some time, giving rise to a *secondary abdominal pregnancy.* In such cases, the tube may close down upon the placenta and form a sac in which it remains during the rest of the pregnancy; or while a portion of the placenta remains attached to the tubal wall, its growing periphery extends beyond the tube and establishes connections with the surrounding pelvic organs.

When the fetus escapes from the tube after rupture, it is nearly always surrounded by its membranes.

RUPTURE INTO THE BROAD LIGAMENT. When the original implantation of the ovum is toward the mesosalpinx, rupture

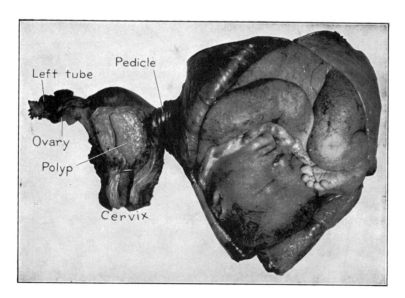

FIG. 22-2. Broad-ligament pregnancy at term. The sac has been opened to expose the fetus, thus hiding most of proximal and all of distal end of elongated right tube, which almost completely encircles the sac. In the region of the isthmus, the tube cannot be traced for some distance, as it merges with the wall of the sac. It is probably at this site that early rupture occurred. The torn distal end of the tube has been carried laterally by the growing fetus. In the photograph the right ovary and ruptured vessels are hidden on the undersurface of the sac near the cervix. (Courtesy of Dr. Thomas J. Sims.)

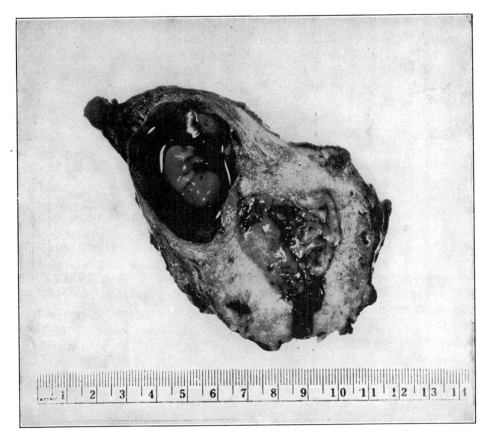

FIG. 22-3. Interstitial pregnancy with fetus in situ. Note thick decidua in empty uterus.

may occur at the portion of the tube not covered by peritoneum, so that the contents of the gestational sac are extruded into a space formed between the folds of the broad ligament. This condition is designated an intraligamentous or *broad ligament pregnancy* (Fig. 22-2). It may terminate either in the death of the embryo or fetus and the formation of a *broad ligament hematoma* or in the further development of the pregnancy. Occasionally, the broad ligament sac ruptures at a later period, and the fetus is extruded into the peritoneal cavity while the placenta retains its original position, forming a secondary abdominal pregnancy. The outcome depends largely upon the degree of completeness with which the placenta has separated.

Interstitial Pregnancy. When the fertilized ovum implants within the segment of the tube that penetrates the uterine wall, an especially grave form of tubal gestation, *interstitial pregnancy,* results (Figs. 22-3–22-5). Interstitial tubal pregnancy accounts for about 2.5 percent of all tubal gestations. Because of the site of implantation, no adnexal mass is palpable, but rather, there is variably asymmetry of the uterus that is often difficult to distinguish from an early intrauterine pregnancy. Hence, the early diagnosis is even more frequently overlooked than in other types of tubal implantation. Because of the greater distensibility of the myometrium compared with the tubal wall, rupture is likely to occur somewhat later, between the end of the second and the end of the fourth month. Because of the abundant blood supply from branches of both uterine and ovarian arteries immediately adjacent to the implantation site, the hemorrhage that attends the rupture may be rapidly fatal. In fact, tubal pregnancies in which death occurs before the

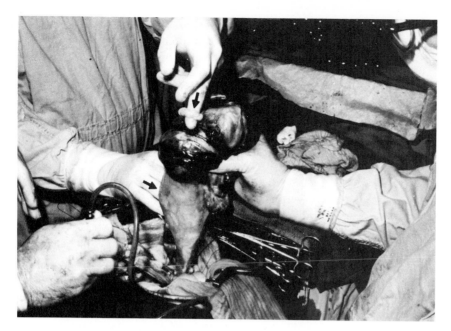

FIG. 22-4. Large ruptured interstitial pregnancy seen during hysterectomy. *Upper arrow* points to umbilical cord over the operator's finger. *Lower arrow* points to body of uterus.

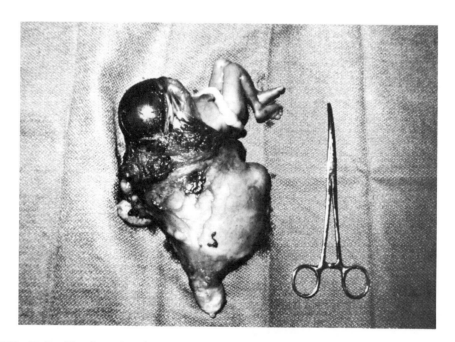

FIG. 22-5. The fetus has been removed from the large cavity that had developed in the interstitial portion of the tube and hypertrophied cornual region of the uterus before frank rupture.

woman can be brought to the hospital often fall into this group. Because of the large uterine defect, hysterectomy is commonly necessary. Very infrequently, an interstitial pregnancy may convert to a tubouterine pregnancy, as described below.

Combined and Multiple Pregnancies. In rare instances, tubal pregnancy may be complicated by a coexisting intrauterine gestation, a condition designated as *combined pregnancy*. Combined pregnancy is very often quite difficult to diagnose. Typically, laparotomy is performed because of a ruptured tubal pregnancy. At the same time, the uterus is congested, softened, and somewhat enlarged. Although these features are suggestive of intrauterine pregnancy, they are commonly induced by a tubal pregnancy alone. The incidence of combined pregnancy is about 1 in 30,000 births. Berger and Taymor (1972) described two cases of simultaneous intra-

uterine and tubal pregnancy that followed induction of ovulation with clomiphene therapy in one and menopausal gonadotropin treatment in the other. The ultimate in combined pregnancies may have been reported by Funderburk (1974), who described a woman with a fetus in the right tube, a fetus in the left tube, and a fetus in the uterus. Since he preserved both oviducts, the potential for still another record persists.

Twin tubal pregnancy, at the same stage of development, has been reported with both embryos in the same tube, as well as with one in each tube. Arey (1923) considered the subject in detail and concluded that single-ovum twins form a far greater proportion of tubal than of uterine pregnancies. He postulated that difficulties in implantation retard the growth of the zygote with the result that two embryonic areas develop rather than one. Simultaneous pregnancy in both tubes is the rarest form of double-ovum twin.

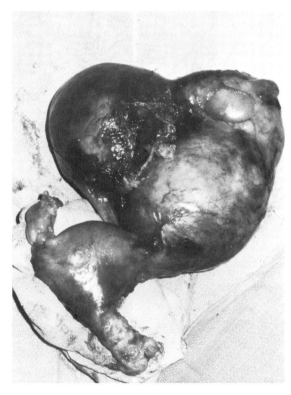

FIG. 22-6. The markedly dilated left fallopian tube contains a dead fetus weighing 1850 g.

Tubal pregnancy with death of the conceptus and without abortion or complete absorption may be followed subsequently by a tubal pregnancy in the same or opposite tube.

Tubouterine, Tuboabdominal, Tuboovarian Pregnancies. The so-called tubouterine pregnancy results from the gradual extension into the uterine cavity of products of conception that originally implanted in the interstitial portion of the tube. Tuboabdominal pregnancy is derived from a tubal pregnancy in which the zygote, originally implanted in the neighborhood of the fimbriated extremity, gradually extends into the peritoneal cavity. In such circumstances, the portion of the fetal sac projecting into the peritoneal cavity may form troublesome adhesions to the surrounding organs. As a result, removal of the sac is much more difficult. Both of these conditions are very uncommon.

The term tuboovarian pregnancy is employed when the fetal sac is adherent partly to tubal and partly to ovarian tissue. Such cases arise from the development of the zygote in a tuboovarian cyst or in a tube, the fimbriated extremity of which was adherent to the ovary at the time of fertilization (Fig. 22-6).

CLINICAL FEATURES OF TUBAL PREGNANCY

General Considerations. Before tubal rupture or abortion, the manifestations of a tubal pregnancy are diverse. Commonly, the woman (1) believes she is normally pregnant, or (2) believes she is "miscarrying" an intrauterine pregnancy, or (3) does not even suspect she is pregnant. Hence, the symptoms and signs of tubal pregnancy usually refer to the clinical picture encountered with tubal rupture or abortion, and these may be highly variable.

In the so-called textbook case of ruptured tubal pregnancy, normal menstruation is replaced by slight vaginal bleeding, which is

usually referred to as "spotting." Suddenly, the woman is stricken with severe lower abdominal pain, frequently described as sharp, stabbing, or tearing in character. Vasomotor disturbances develop, ranging from vertigo to syncope. Abdominal palpation discloses tenderness and vaginal examination, especially motion of the cervix, causes exquisite pain. The posterior fornix of the vagina may bulge because of blood in the cul-de-sac, or a tender, boggy mass may be felt to one side of the uterus. Symptoms of diaphragmatic irritation exist in perhaps 50 percent of cases. This is caused by blood in the peritoneum and is characterized by pain in the neck or shoulder, especially on inspiration. The patient may or may not be hypotensive while lying supine. If she is not hypotensive when supine, she may become so when placed in a sitting position.

Symptoms, Signs, Laboratory Studies. In cases of tubal pregnancy that present the aforementioned clinical picture, there can be little question as to the diagnosis, but ideally the diagnosis should be made earlier. Even though the symptoms and signs of ectopic pregnancy often range from indefinite to bizarre before rupture or abortion, increasing numbers of women are seeking medical care before the classic clinical picture develops. *The physician must make every reasonable effort to diagnose the condition before catastrophic events occur, but the task is seldom simple.* The following symptoms, signs, and laboratory studies must be carefully evaluated:

Pain may be unilateral or bilateral, in the lower abdomen or generalized, or just in the upper abdomen. In the presence of hemoperitoneum, pain from diaphragmatic irritation may be experienced. It has been generally assumed that the abdominal pain, often excruciating, associated with rupture of an ectopic pregnancy is caused by the escape of blood into the peritoneal cavity. Since there may be considerable pain in instances in which there is little hemorrhage, and little pain with considerable hemorrhage, it is obvious that blood is not the sole cause of the pain.

A relatively large amount of blood in the peritoneal cavity can, however, lead to a degree of peritoneal irritation and varying degrees of discomfort. Pritchard and Adams (1957) observed that the instillation of 500 ml, or somewhat more, of citrated whole blood into the peritoneal cavity more often than not caused abdominal tenderness, moderate intestinal distension, and especially pain in the top of the shoulder and the side of the neck from diaphragmatic irritation. The volume of blood, shed as a result of tubal rupture or abortion, required to cause this pain usually must be sizable for a significant amount to reach the diaphragm. This fact may account for the differences between the observations of Pritchard and Adams and those of Mengert and associates (1951), who noted that the intraperitoneal infusion of up to 300 ml of blood in adult women commonly produced only a feeling of fullness.

AMENORRHEA. *The absence of a missed menstrual period by no means rules out tubal pregnancy.* A history of amenorrhea is not obtained in a quarter or more of cases. One reason is that the women mistakes the uterine bleeding that frequently occurs with tubal pregnancy for a true menstrual period and so gives an erroneous date for the last menses. This important source of diagnostic error can be eliminated in many cases by a carefully obtained history. It is extremely important that the character of the last menstrual period be investigated in detail in respect to time of onset, duration, and amount of bleeding, and it is advisable to ask whether it impressed the patient as abnormal in any way.

VAGINAL SPOTTING OR BLEEDING. As long as placental endocrine function persists, uterine bleeding is usually absent but, when endocrine support of the decidua becomes inadequate, the uterine mucosa bleeds. The bleeding is usually scanty, dark brown, and maybe intermittent or continuous. Although profuse vaginal bleeding is suggestive of an incomplete intrauterine abortion rather than an ectopic gestation, such bleeding can occur with tubal gestations.

PREGNANCY TESTS. The placenta, in cases of ectopic pregnancy, commonly secretes less chorionic gonadotropin than does the placenta of a normal intrauterine pregnancy of the same gestational age. Therefore, the generally used immunologic tests, as well as earlier biologic tests, have been reported as positive in as few as 50 percent of ectopic pregnancies (Hallatt, 1975). When the sensitivity of the immunologic tests for chorionic gonadotropin is increased, the likelihood of a falsely positive result is also increased due to cross reaction with luteinizing hormone (see Chap. 10, p. 266). Radioimmunoassay for the β-subunit of chorionic gonadotropin is extremely sensitive, as well as specific for the pregnancy hormone. Lack of availability of the assay and the 24 hours or more to carry out the procedure have deterred its use. Modifications of the assay have been described that reduce the performance time to three hours without apparent loss of specificity, sensitivity, or precision (Rasor, Braunstein, 1977).

Because of the sensitivity of the assay for the β-subunit of chorionic gonadotropin, pregnancy may, at times, be confirmed so early that no macroscopic pathologic changes can be distinguished in the oviduct. Yaffe and associates (1979) described such a circumstance in which a tubal gestation was not appreciated at initial laparoscopy. The woman, after a missed period of 5 days, had developed pelvic pain. Chorionic gonadotropin was present in blood but no lesion was seen at laparoscopy. When laparoscopy was repeated 7 days later, because of persistent pain and vaginal bleeding, a mass was now visible in the ampulla of the tube.

BLOOD PRESSURE AND PULSE. The initial response to hemorrhage is either no change in pulse and blood pressure or occasionally the same as that witnessed during the controlled phlebotomy of blood donation, namely, a slight rise in blood pressure (see Fig. 21-2). In the otherwise healthy young woman with extrauterine pregnancy, only if bleeding continues at a rapid rate and hypovolemia becomes intense does the blood pressure fall and the pulse rate rise appreciably.

HYPOVOLEMIA. There are two simple means of detecting significant hypovolemia before the development of hypovolemic shock: (1) The blood pressure and pulse rates of the patient in the sitting and the supine positions are compared. A distinct decrease in blood pressure and rise in pulse rate in the sitting position are indicative most often of a sizable decrease in circulatory volume. (2) Urine flow should be monitored carefully, since hypovolemia (in the absence of potent diuretic treatment) causes oliguria before overt hypotension develops. The diagnosis and treatment of obstetric hemorrhage in general are considered in detail in Chapter 21, page 487.

ANEMIA. After hemorrhage, the depleted blood volume is restored towards normal by hemodilution over the course of a day or two. Even after a substantial hemorrhage, therefore, the hemoglobin level or hematocrit reading may at first show only a slight reduction. For the first few hours after an acute hemorrhage, a decrease in the hemoglobin or hematocrit level while the patient is under observation is a more valuable index of blood loss than is the initial reading, unless the initial reading is low and the anemia is normochromic, normocytic, and therefore characteristic of recent blood loss. If the bleeding stops and the shed erythrocytes are free in the peritoneal cavity, their absorption may help repair the anemia within several days. Hyperbilirubinemia usually does not develop (Pritchard, Adams, 1957).

PELVIC TENDERNESS. Exquisite tenderness on vaginal examination, especially on *motion of the cervix,* is demonstrable in over three quarters of women with ruptured or rupturing tubal pregnancies, but occasionally may be absent. Some degree of abdominal tenderness is present in about the same proportion of cases.

PELVIC MASS. A pelvic mass is palpable in about one half of the cases. The mass varies in size, consistency, and position, ranging as a rule between 5 and 15 cm in diameter, and is often soft and elastic. With extensive infiltration of the tubal wall with blood, however, it may be firm. It is almost always either posterior or lateral to the uterus.

UTERINE CHANGES. Because of the action of placental hormones, the uterus grows during the first three months of a tubal gestation to nearly the same size as it would in an intrauterine pregnancy. Its consistency, too, is similar as long as the fetus is alive. The uterus may be pushed to one side by the ectopic mass. In broad-ligament pregnancies, or when the broad ligament is filled with blood, the uterus may be greatly displaced. Uterine casts (decidual casts) are passed by a small minority of patients, possibly 5 or 10 percent.

TEMPERATURE. After acute hemorrhage, the temperature may be normal or even low. Temperatures up to 38C, and perhaps related to hemoperitoneum, may develop, but higher temperatures are rare in the absence of infection. Fever is important, therefore, in distinguishing ruptured tubal pregnancy from acute salpingitis, in which the temperature is commonly above 38C.

LEUKOCYTE COUNT. The leukocyte count varies considerably in ruptured ectopic pregnancy. In about half the cases, it is normal, but in the remainder, varying degrees of leukocytosis up to 30,000 may be encountered.

HEMOTHORAX. Right hemothorax has been identified with hemoperitoneum from ruptured ectopic pregnancy (Ganji, Vidrine, 1970; McNulty, 1960). A potential defect in the diaphragm has been postulated to account for the shift of blood into the pleural cavity.

CULLEN'S SIGN. A blue discoloration may, at times, be seen through the umbilical skin when there is extensive intraperitoneal hemorrhage. This rare sign is more likely to be discerned in thin women or those with an umbilical hernia.

PELVIC HEMATOCELE. In many cases of ruptured tubal pregnancy, there is gradual disintegration of the tubal wall followed by a slow leakage of blood into the tubal lumen, the peritoneal cavity, or both. Signs of active hemorrhage are absent, and even the mild symptoms may subside; but gradually the trickling blood collects in the pelvis, more or less walled off by adhesions, and a pelvic hematocele results. In some cases, the hematocele is eventually absorbed, and the patient recovers without operation. In others, it may rupture into the peritoneal cavity, or it may become infected and form an abscess. Most commonly, however, the hematocele causes continued discomfort and the physician is finally consulted weeks or even months after the original rupture. These cases present the most atypical manifestations.

Differential Diagnosis. Prompt diagnosis in ruptured tubal pregnancy is most important, yet there are few other disorders in the field of obstetrics and gynecology that present so many diagnostic pitfalls. The conditions most frequently confused with tubal pregnancy are (1) acute or chronic salpingitis, (2) threatened or incomplete abortion of an intrauterine pregnancy, (3) rupture of a corpus luteum or follicular cyst with intraperitoneal bleeding, (4) torsion of an ovarian cyst, (5) appendicitis, (6) gastroenteritis, and (7) discomforts from an intrauterine device.

SALPINGITIS. The disease most commonly mistaken for ruptured tubal pregnancy is salpingitis, in which there is often a history of similar attacks and usually no missed periods. With salpingitis, abnormal bleeding is not nearly so common as the spotting characteristic of tubal gestation. Pain and tenderness are more likely to be bilateral in salpingitis. A pelvic mass in tubal pregnancy, if palpable, is unilateral, whereas in salpingitis both fornices are likely to be equally resistant and tender. The temperature in acute salpingitis usually exceeds 38C. In either condition, a negative hormonal test for pregnancy may be obtained with most clinically available tests. Thus, a negative result will be of little diagnostic value.

ABORTION OF INTRAUTERINE PREGNANCY. In threatened or incomplete abortion of an intrauterine pregnancy, the uterine bleeding is usually more profuse. Shock from hypovolemia, when present, is usually in proportion to the extent of vaginal hemorrhage, but in tubal pregnancy hypovolemic shock is almost always far in excess of what might be expected from vaginal blood loss. The pain in uterine abortion is generally less severe, likely to be rhythmic, and located low in the midline of the abdomen, whereas in tubal pregnancy it is unilateral or generalized. If embryo or placenta is found in the vagina or at the external cervical os, the diagnosis of abortion of an intrauterine pregnancy is obvious, but it should be remembered that shed decidua may be abundant with an ectopic pregnancy. Moreover, combined extrauterine and intrauterine pregnancies may occur, albeit rarely. The marked histologic variations in the endometrium in cases of ectopic pregnancy are such that endometrial biopsy provides an often unreliable diagnostic criterion.

TWISTED CYST OR APPENDICITIS. In both torsion of an ovarian cyst and appendicitis, the signs and symptoms of pregnancy, including amenorrhea, are usually lacking and there is rarely a history of abnormal vaginal bleeding. The mass formed by a twisted ovarian cyst is more nearly discrete, whereas that of a tubal pregnancy is usually less well defined. With appendicitis, only rarely is there a mass found by vaginal examination, and pain on motion of the cervix is much less severe than in ruptured tubal pregnancy. The pain from appendicitis, furthermore, is often localized higher, over McBurney's point. If either appendicitis or a twisted ovarian cyst is mistaken for a tubal pregnancy, the error is not costly, since all three require prompt operation. Rupture of a follicle cyst or corpus luteum with bleeding into the peritoneal cavity may be extremely difficult, if not impossible, to distinguish from a ruptured tubal gestation.

GASTROINTESTINAL DISTURBANCES. In some women with a ruptured ectopic pregnancy, the prominent symptoms are diarrhea, nausea, and vomiting, along with abdominal pain. Inappropriate diagnosis and therapy have led to death.

INTRAUTERINE DEVICES.   Diagnosis of ectopic pregnancy is often more difficult in women who use an intrauterine device for contraception. The devices do not prevent ectopic pregnancies. Cramping pelvic pain and bleeding from the uterus, both common features of ectopic pregnancy, may be caused by an intrauterine device. Moreover, in some women the device predisposes to inflammation of the adnexa, which is typically unilateral.

Other Diagnostic Aids.   Because of the difficulties in diagnosis of ruptured tubal pregnancy, a variety of diagnostic aids other than tests for chorionic gonadotropin have been utilized. These include culdocentesis, curettage, colpotomy (culdotomy), culdoscopy, laparoscopy, and sonography.

SONOGRAPHY.   In more recent years, sonography has been applied to the diagnosis of tubal pregnancy. Identification of early products of conception in the fallopian tube by this means is difficult, but if the products of conception are clearly identified within the cavity of the uterus, it is extremely unlikely that an ectopic pregnancy coexists. Moreover, the absence of sonographic evidence of an intrauterine pregnancy but a positive pregnancy test and an abnormal pelvic mass almost always is tantamount to ectopic pregnancy.

CULDOCENTESIS.   The simplest technic for identifying hemoperitoneum is culdocentesis, since it can be performed without hospitalization. As the cervix is pulled toward the symphysis with a tenaculum, a long 16- or 18-gauge needle is inserted through the posterior vaginal fornix into the cul-de-sac, whence fluid can be aspirated. Failure to aspirate any fluid can be interpreted only as unsatisfactory entry into the cul-de-sac. Fluid containing fragments of old clots or bloody fluid that does not subsequently clot is compatible with the diagnosis of hemoperito-

neum resulting from an ectopic pregnancy. If the blood subsequently clots, it may have been obtained from an adjacent perforated blood vessel rather than from a bleeding ectopic pregnancy. The very important exception is brisk bleeding from the site of rupture in which case the blood may be aspirated from the cul-de-sac before it has had time to clot. With bleeding of such intensity, culdocentesis is rarely necessary to establish the diagnosis of an intra-abdominal catastrophe, one which demands immediate intravenous infusion of fluids, including whole blood, and prompt surgical intervention. Lucas and Hassim (1970) pointed out that culdocentesis is especially valuable for diagnosing ectopic pregnancy in populations of women in whom anemia and pelvic infection are common. Culdocentesis, however, is more likely to be unsatisfactory in women with previous salpingitis and pelvic peritonitis, since the cul-de-sac may have been obliterated.

CURETTAGE.   Differentiation between threatened or incomplete abortion of an intrauterine pregnancy and a tubal pregnancy may also be accomplished in many instances by curettage. If embryo, fetus, or placenta is identified, a simultaneous tubal pregnancy is extemely unlikely. When none of these structures is identified, tubal pregnancy is a probability. The identification of decidua alone in the uterine curettings strongly implies extrauterine pregnancy. Identification of secretory, proliferative, or menstrual type endometrium, however, does not exclude ectopic gestation.

COLPOTOMY (CULDOTOMY).   Direct visualization of the oviducts and ovaries can be accomplished by use of colpotomy unless pelvic inflammation, recent or remote, has obliterated the cul-de-sac, or the tubes are adherent to the broad ligaments or uterus to a degree that they cannot be mobilized sufficiently to be drawn into the field of vision. The procedure requires an experienced operator, a scrubbed and gowned associate, an operating room, and surgical anesthesia. Salpingectomy may at times be successfully performed through the colpotomy opening. This approach to definitive therapy, while championed by some, is not generally popular because of technical difficulties, especially if there are adhesions from chronic inflammation, and because of increased morbidity from infection.

LAPAROSCOPY. This technic has been reintroduced as a means of improving the accuracy of diagnosis of diseases of the pelvis, including ectopic pregnancy. Refined optic and electronic systems have overcome most of the objections that arose in the course of previous attempts to utilize transabdominal intraperitoneal lighted probes for visualization of organs. Nonetheless, successful and safe laparoscopy demands refined equipment, an experienced operator, an operating room, and, usually, surgical anesthesia. Complete visualization of the pelvis may be impossible in the presence of pelvic inflammation or recent or remote bleeding. At times, identification of an early unruptured tubal pregnancy may be difficult using the laparoscope, even though the tube is fully visualized. The tube may show little change in shape and minimal change in color if the pregnancy is early. Moreover, demonstration of tubal patency by the passage of dye through the tube does not exclude tubal pregnancy (Yaffe et al., 1976).

CULDOSCOPY. Visualization of pelvic organs through a culdoscope usually is more difficult than with a laparoscope. Culdoscopy, previously a much more popular procedure for visualizing the pelvic contents, requires entry through the cul-de-sac, with the patient in the knee-chest position.

LAPAROTOMY. If any doubt remains, laparotomy should be performed, since an unnecessary operation is far less tragic than death contributed to by indecision or delay. There is remarkably little morbidity associated with surgery which is limited to a carefully made and repaired suprapubic incision. At the same time, diagnosis is often enhanced appreciably by direct visualization and palpation of the pelvic organs that laparotomy al-lows. *It is imperative that laparotomy not be delayed while laparoscopy or colpotomy is performed on the woman with an obvious pelvic or abdominal catastrophe that requires immediate definitive treatment.*

Accuracy of Clinical Diagnosis. The clinical diagnosis of ectopic pregnancy is subject to both false positive and false negative errors. Perhaps 10 to 20 percent of patients operated upon with a diagnosis of ectopic pregnancy will have some other lesion. Conversely, a small percentage of all ectopic pregnancies will be found in patients subjected to laparotomy with a different preoperative diagnosis.

Mortality. Mortality rate from tubal ectopic pregnancies has been lowered. Reports covering a total of 2478 cases (Kostic, 1961; Malkasian et al., 1959; Riva et al., 1962; Sandmire, Randall, 1959; Schiffer, 1963; Torpin et al., 1961) include three deaths, or 1 in 826 ectopic pregnancies. Nonetheless, there is need for improvement. For example, Schneider et al. (1977) have reviewed 102 deaths from ectopic pregnancy recorded in Michigan between 1950 and 1974. Although some of these women presented too late for therapy to have been effective, many others had made a series of visits to physicians' offices, to emergency rooms, and even had been hospitalized and subsequently discharged without the diagnosis of ectopic pregnancy having been made. Schneider and associates (1977) emphasized that earlier diagnosis, adequate blood replacement, and aggressive surgical management could have saved at least 75 percent of all who died. May et al. (1978) reached essentially the same conclusion after carefully analyzing deaths from ectopic pregnancy in more recent years in North Carolina. They urged more intensive educational efforts be directed especially toward primary-care physicians.

Treatment. The treatment of tubal pregnancy most often has been salpingectomy, with or without ipsilateral oophorectomy. Simultaneous blood transfusion is, of course, a necessity if either hypovolemia or overt anemia is present. The response of most patients to the operation is dramatic.

SALPINGECTOMY. In removing the oviduct, it is advisable to excise as a wedge no more than the outer third of the interstitial portion (so-called cornual resection) and thereby minimize the rare recurrence of pregnancy in the tubal stump, yet not weaken the myometrium at that site. Resection so extensive as to reach the cavity of the uterus must be avoided, lest the defect created lead to uterine rupture in a subsequent pregnancy.

Since the tubal lesions that predispose to ectopic pregnancy are commonly bilateral, a substantial number of women treated by salpingectomy are likely either to be sterile after one ectopic gestation or to develop another extrauterine pregnancy in the remaining tube. Probably one-half or more of women who have had a tubal pregnancy fail to conceive again (Kitchin et al., 1979; Schenker et al., 1972); when they do, the risk of another ectopic pregnancy is substantial (13 of 56 pregnancies in the experience of Kitchin et al.). Tragically, infertility subsequent to an ectopic pregnancy is highest in nulliparous women.

CONSERVATION OF OVIDUCT. Because of the strong likelihood of infertility following tubal pregnancy treated by salpingectomy, an alternative to removing the oviduct should be considered. The cumulative experiences in 7 reports concerned with 352 women with ectopic pregnancies, on whom procedures to remove the pregnancy but preserve the tube had been performed, were that 119, or one-third, subsequently became pregnant in utero. Twenty-one, or 15 percent of those who conceived again, had a repeat ectopic pregnancy (Hallatt, 1975). The technics for conserving the oviduct basically involve either incising the tube longitudinally over the implantation site and shelling out the pregnancy products, or with more distal implantations, simply squeezing the tube so as to abort the products through the ampulla.

Such procedures do not guarantee patency of the tube; moreover, subsequent hemorrhage from the implantation site may necessitate reexploration and salpingectomy (Kelly et al., 1979).

IPSILATERAL OOPHORECTOMY. Removal of the adjacent ovary at the time of salpingectomy has been suggested as a possible means for both improving fertility and decreasing the likelihood of a subsequent ectopic pregnancy (Jeffcoate, 1967). Ovulation would thus always occur from the ovary immediately adjacent to the remaining oviduct. This should facilitate the pick-up of the ovum by that tube and avoid the possibility of external migration of the ovum and the ectopic pregnancy that might result from such a peripatetic egg. The importance of this phenomenon in the genesis of ectopic pregnancy is not clear, although Hallatt (1975) identified the corpus luteum on the opposite ovary and therefore, almost certainly, external migration of the ovum, in about one out of every five tubal pregnancies. Even so, removal of an otherwise normal appearing ovary on these grounds seems hardly justifiable. Most gynecologists leave the ovary when possible and, to minimize ovarian dysfunction and cyst formation, preserve all the blood supply possible by clamping the vessels in the mesosalpinx as close to the oviduct as possible.

STERILIZATION. It is important that before surgical exploration for a suspected ectopic pregnancy the woman be asked about her wishes for future pregnancies. If the woman has a reasonable number of children and the ectopic pregnancy is the consequence of failed contraception, the decision usually is in favor of sterilization. If so, and her condition is good, hysterectomy may be considered. Otherwise, tubal sterilization usually can be performed very quickly without increased risk. All organs possible should be conserved in the woman of low parity with a strong desire for future pregnancies in spite of the increased risk of a subsequent ectopic pregnancy.

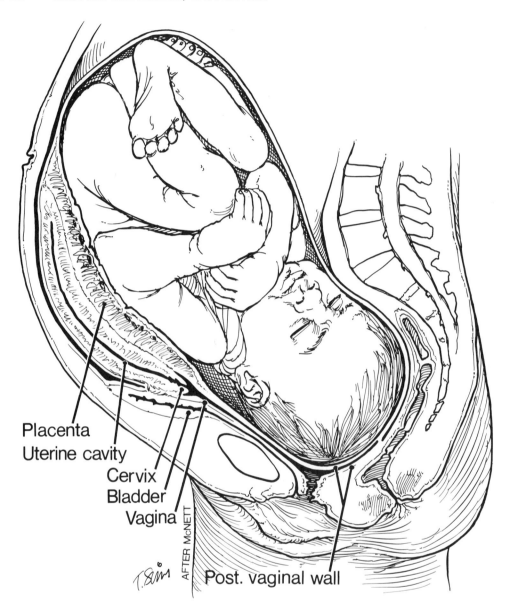

FIG. 22-7. Abdominal pregnancy at term. The placenta is implanted on the posterior wall of the uterus and broad ligament. The enlarged, flattened uterus is located just beneath the anterior abdominal wall. The cervix and vagina are dislodged anteriorly and superiorly by the large fetal head in the cul-de-sac.

AUTOTRANSFUSION. In the face of serious blood loss, retransfusion of blood collected in the abdomen has, at times, been advocated. Although this procedure is effective in an emergency, it is not advised as a routine because of the danger of reaction. Some workers, however, have recommended that if such blood is left in the abdomen, it will be of benefit to the patient. Pritchard and Adams (1957) demonstrated by means of suitably labeled erythrocytes that absorption of erythrocytes from the adult peritoneal cavity occurs over a period of days and is much too slow to be of significant help in combating either hypovolemia or anemia. Free blood in the peritoneal cavity at the completion of surgery makes it difficult to ascertain that hemostasis has been accomplished satisfactorily.

RH-NEGATIVE WOMEN.   If the woman is Rh-negative but not yet sensitized to Rho (D) antigen, and the potential for reproduction persists, Rho-immune globulin should be administered to protect against isoimmunization. Certainly, whenever Rh-positive blood is administered inadvertently to the previously unsensitized Rh-negative woman, sufficient immune globulin to protect her should be promptly administered.

ABDOMINAL PREGNANCY

Frequency.   The incidence of abdominal pregnancy is influenced by the frequency of ectopic gestation in the population being cared for, the ability to obtain care early in pregnancy, and the degree of suspicion of ectopic pregnancy exercised by those providing care. Almost all cases of abdominal pregnancy follow early rupture or abortion of a tubal pregnancy into the peritoneal cavity. An incidence for abdominal pregnancy of 1 in 3337 births at Charity Hospital in New Orleans was reported by Beacham and colleagues (1962), compared to 1 in 7931 births at Indiana University Hospital, noted by Strafford and Ragan (1977).

Etiology.   Typically, the trophoblast, after penetrating the wall of the oviduct, maintains to a degree its tubal attachment and gradually encroaches upon the neighboring peritoneum. Meanwhile, the fetus, usually but not always surrounded by amnion, continues to grow within the peritoneal cavity. In such circumstances, the placenta is found in the general region of the oviduct, which typically is no longer grossly identifiable as such, and over the posterior aspect of the broad ligament and uterus (Fig. 22-7). In much rarer instances, the conceptus appears to have escaped from the tube after rupture to reimplant elsewhere in the peritoneal cavity. Primary implantation of the ferti-lized ovum on the peritoneum is so rare that many authors have doubted its existence, as indicated in Cavanagh's (1958) extensive review. Conclusive proof of a primary abdominal pregnancy, however, was provided by Studdiford's (1942) well-documented case, which fulfills the following criteria upon which proof of such a pregnancy must rest: (1) normal tubes and ovaries with no evidence of recent or remote injury, (2) absence of any evidence of uteroplacental fistula, and (3) presence of a pregnancy related exclusively to the peritoneal surface and young enough to eliminate the possibility of secondary implantation following primary nidation in the tube.

King (1932) directed attention to a rare cause of abdominal pregnancy, namely, postoperative separation of the uterine wound of a previous cesarean section. In three of his four reported cases, the ovum had implanted upon omentum, over the uterine defect, whereas in the fourth it had become attached to the abdominal wall. He believed that in each case the fertilized ovum escaped through the defect in the uterine wall and implanted as a primary abdominal pregnancy.

Status of Fetus.   The condition of the fetus in abdominal pregnancy is exceedingly precarious and the great majority succumb. In a review of the world's literature, Ware (1948) cited a perinatal loss of 75.6 percent but that figure is probably falsely low because of the tendency to report cases with happy results. Beacham and co-workers (1962) are probably more nearly correct in reporting a fatal loss in their own series of about 95 percent. Some authors, moreover, report an incidence of congenital malformations in the infants as high as 50 percent, though others disagree.

If the fetus dies after reaching a size too large to be resorbed, it must undergo suppuration, mummification, calcification, or formation of adipocere (see below). Bacteria may gain access to a gestational sac, particularly when it is adherent to the intestines, with suppuration of its contents. Eventually, the abscess ruptures at the point of least resistance, and if the patient does not die from septicemia, fetal parts may be extruded through the abdominal wall or more commonly into the intestines or bladder. Mummification and the formation of a lithopedion occasionally ensue, and the calcified products of conception may be carried for years without producing symptoms until they cause dystocia in a subsequent pregnancy or symptoms from pressure. There are instances in which a period of 20 to 30 years elapsed before removal of a lithopedion at operation or autopsy. Much more rarely, the fetus is converted into a yellowish, greasy mass to which the term *adipocere* is applied. The various bizarre terminations of abdominal pregnancy have been well discussed, with illustrative cases, by King (1954).

Diagnosis. Since early rupture or abortion of a tubal pregnancy is the usual antecedent of an abdominal pregnancy, in retrospect, a history suggestive of the accident can usually be obtained. The abnormalities likely to be recalled include spotting or irregular bleeding and abdominal pain, which usually was most prominent in one or both lower quadrants. Unexplained transient anemia early in pregnancy may accompany the rupture or abortion.

In the one case of late abdominal pregnancy during the past 20 years cared for throughout most of her pregnancy at Parkland Memorial Hospital, anemia was identified when the woman was first evaluated near the end of the first trimester. The moderately severe normochromic, normocytic anemia was accompanied by reticulocytosis and modest hyperbilirubinemia, most of which was unconjugated. A careful evaluation uncovered no other abnormalities. Treatment of a presumed acquired hemolytic anemia with corticosteroids was followed by prompt correction and the discontinuation of the steroids. She remained asymptomatic until she developed severe preeclampsia at term. A somewhat growth-retarded, recently dead fetus was delivered by laparotomy. Quite recently, elsewhere in this same hospital an ectopic pregnancy caused similar hematologic changes that led to the misdiagnosis of an acquired hemolytic anemia until several weeks later when at laparotomy the true etiology was apparent.

SYMPTOMATOLOGY. Women with an abdominal pregnancy are likely to be uncomfortable but not sufficiently so to warrant thorough evaluation. Nausea, vomiting, flatulence, constipation, diarrhea, and abdominal pain may each be present in varying degrees. Multiparas may state that the pregnancy does not "feel right." Late in pregnancy, fetal movements may cause pain. Near term, the empty uterus has been alleged to go into spurious labor.

PHYSICAL EXAMINATION. By abdominal palpation, the abnormal position of the fetus, often a transverse or oblique lie can frequently be confirmed. Ease of palpation of the fetal parts however, is not a reliable sign, since they sometimes feel exceedingly close to the examining fingers in normal intrauterine pregnancies, especially in thin, multiparous women. *Massage of the abdomen over the pregnancy products does not stimulate the mass to become more firm, as it often does with advanced intrauterine pregnancy.* The cervix is usually displaced (Fig. 22-7), depending in part on the position of the fetus, and it may dilate somewhat, but appreciable effacement is lacking. The uterus may be outlined over the lower part of the pregnancy mass, especially if the placenta is attached to the broad ligament and in the cul-de-sac. By palpation of the fornices, small parts or the fetal head clearly outside the uterus may be identified occasionally.

OXYTOCIN STIMULATION. Cross and his collaborators (1951) emphasized that oxytocin can be a valuable aid in the diagnosis of abdominal pregnancy. If no evidence of uterine activity is detected using a sensitive strain gauge applied repeatedly to the maternal abdominal wall over the products of conception while oxytocin is infused intravenously in a sizeable dose, the pregnancy almost certainly is extrauterine. Hertz and co-workers (1977) could detect no uterine activity while infusing oxytocin in excess of 50 milliunits per minute. In their case the empty uterus lay inferior and posterior to the fetus. If the uterus were anterior, as in Figure

22-7, it might contract in response to oxytocin and possibly lead to the false conclusion of intrauterine pregnancy.

In a case described recently by Orr and associates (1979), before the diagnosis of abdominal pregnancy was made, not only did the uterus presumably contract in response to oxytocin, an oxytocin challenge test (see Chap. 14, p. 349) was interpreted as negative on two occasions. The 2000 g growth-retarded fetus expired undelivered one week later. The relationship between the abdominal wall, the uterus, and the extrauterine fetus was very similar to that depicted in Figure 22-7.

RADIOGRAPHIC EXAMINATION. A strong suspicion of abdominal pregnancy may be confirmed by x-ray examination with a probe or radiopaque material in the uterus. The fetus is then clearly shown to lie outside the uterine cavity. Unfortunately, such technics are not safe diagnostic procedures if the fetus is intrauterine, especially if alive.

ISOTOPE LOCALIZATION. These technics for localizing the placenta are likely to demonstrate only that the placenta is located in a region that is also appropriate for an intrauterine pregnancy. At times, gross discrepancy has been noted between the apparent location based on isotope studies and the actual implantation site. For example, in one case, the placenta was thought to be implanted adjacent to the liver but was subsequently removed with difficulty from the posterior cul-de-sac over the sigmoid colon.

SONOGRAPHY. In practice, sonographic findings with an abdominal pregnancy may not be so distinct as to allow an unequivocal diagnosis to be made. However, in some suspected cases, the sonographic findings may serve to identify the pregnancy as being definitely intrauterine.

Treatment. The operation for abdominal pregnancy may precipitate violent hemorrhage. Without massive blood transfusion, the outlook for many such patients is hopeless. Hence, it is mandatory that at least 2000

ml of compatible blood be immediately available in the operating room, with more readily available in the blood bank. Preoperatively, two intravenous infusion systems, each capable of delivering large volumes of fluid at a rapid rate, should be made operational. At the same time, systems for measuring central venous pressure and urine flow should be established to monitor the adequacy of the circulation as described in Chapter 21. Whenever time allows, the bowel should be prepared using both mechanical cleansing and antimicrobial agents, since the bowel is often intimately adherent to the placenta and membranes.

The massive hemorrhage that often occurs in the course of operations for abdominal pregnancy is related to the lack of constriction of the hypertrophied open vessels after placental separation. It has therefore been recommended that operation be deferred until the fetus is dead in anticipation of diminished vascularity of the placental site. Procrastination may be dangerous and undesirable, since partial separation of the placenta with hemorrhage occasionally occurs spontaneously in the interval of waiting. Moreover, even though the fetus may have been dead several weeks, bleeding may still be torrential. For these reasons, operation is indicated as soon as the diagnosis has been established and the appropriate steps preparative for surgery have been completed.

MANAGEMENT OF PLACENTA. Since removal of the placenta in abdominal pregnancy always carries the risk of hemorrhage, one should be sure that the blood vessels supplying the placenta can be effectively ligated before attempting removal of the organ. Partial separation can occur spontaneously or, more likely, in the course of the operation from manipulation while attempting to locate the exact site of attachment of the placenta. Since massive hemorrhage can occur, it is, for the most part, best to avoid unnecessary exploration of the surrounding organs. In general, the infant should be delivered, the cord severed close to the placenta, and the abdomen closed.

Unfortunately, the placenta, if left in the abdominal cavity, commonly causes complications in the form of infection, abscesses, adhesions, intestinal obstruction, and wound dehiscence. In one case, evidence of consumptive coagulopathy, including overt hypofibrinogenemia, developed two months following laparotomy for delivery of the fetus. The coagulation defects cleared spontaneously before the placenta was delivered surgically three weeks later. Removal of the placenta in that case was also prompted by right ureteral obstruction, which was relieved. Although the complications from leaving the placenta are troublesome and usually lead to subsequent laparotomy, they may be less grave than the hemorrhage that sometimes results from placental removal during the initial surgery.

Ware reported (1948) that when the placenta remained in situ, the test for chorionic gonadotropin may stay positive for as long as 35 days, an observation repeatedly confirmed by others.

Prognosis. As already mentioned, the perinatal loss from abdominal pregnancies is large. Ware (1948) found a maternal mortalilty rate of 14.5 percent in 249 cases collected from the world's literature from 1935 to 1948. As expected, with improvement in operative technic and especially with greater use of transfusion, Beacham's maternal mortality rate for a later period (1962) was 6 percent. Strafford and Ragan more recently (1977) also cite 6 percent for maternal mortality and 91 percent for perinatal mortality. Abdominal pregnancy is still one of the most formidable of obstetric complications.

OVARIAN PREGNANCY

In 1878, Spiegelberg formulated his criteria for diagnosis of ovarian pregnancy. He required that (1) the tube on the affected side be intact, (2) the fetal sac occupy the position of the ovary, (3) the ovary be connected to the uterus by the ovarian ligament, and (4) definite ovarian tissue be found in the sac

wall. The small number of authentic cases since 1878 attests to the rarity of true ovarian pregnancy, although Bobrow and Winkelstein (1956) were able to collect 154 cases from the literature and added one of their own that satisfied the criteria of Spiegelberg. Pratt-Thomas and associates (1974) have described ten cases, including one term pregnancy. It is not clear whether the use of an intrauterine contraceptive device predisposes to ovarian pregnancy as in Figure 22-8. Gray and Ruffolo (1978), for example, have described four instances of ovarian pregnancy in which each woman conceived with a Cu-7 intrauterine device in situ.

Although the ovary can accommodate itself more readily than the tube to the expand-

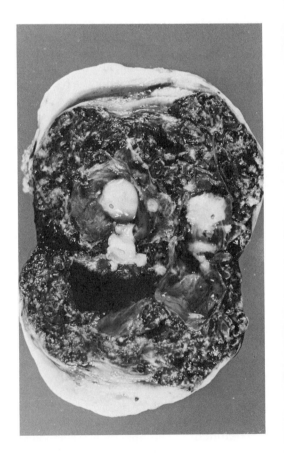

FIG. 22-8. Ovarian pregnancy in a woman using an intrauterine device. There are twin embryos each in a separate gestational sac. (From Kalfayan and Gunderson. *Obstet Gynecol* 55:25 suppl., 1980)

ing pregnancy, rupture at an early period is the usual termination. Nonetheless, there are recorded cases in which the ovarian pregnancy went to term, and a few produced living infants. The products of conception may degenerate early without rupture and give rise to a tumor of varying size, consisting of a capsule of ovarian tissue enclosing a mass of blood, placental tissue, and possibly membranes. The absence of a distinct decidua leads to direct invasion of the ovarian stroma by the trophoblast (Fig. 22-8).

The symptoms and physical findings are likely to mimic those of a tubal pregnancy or a bleeding corpus luteum.

At the time of operation early ovarian pregnancies are likely to be considered to be a corpus luteum cyst or bleeding corpus luteum (Rengachary et al., 1977). Early ovarian pregnancies should be treated when possible by wedge resection or cystectomy.

CERVICAL PREGNANCY

Cervical pregnancy is a rare form of ectopic gestation in which the ovum implants within the cervix at or below the internal os. Dees (1966) has estimated the incidence to be 1 in 18,000 pregnancies. The endocervix is eroded by the trophoblast and pregnancy proceeds to develop in the fibrous cervical wall, as illustrated in Figure 22-9.

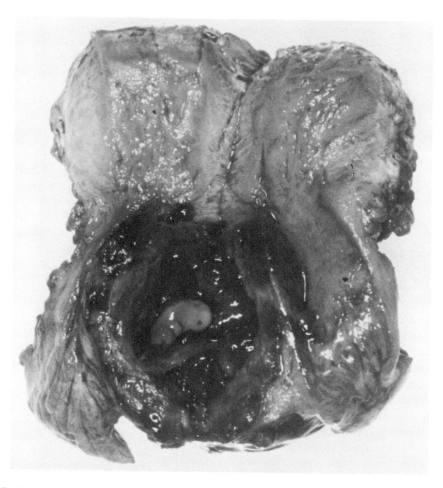

FIG. 22-9. Cervical pregnancy removed by hysterectomy nearly 3 months after last normal menstrual period and 1 month after onset of vaginal bleeding. (Courtesy of Drs. D. Rubell and A. Brekken.)

Usually, painless bleeding appearing shortly after nidation is the first sign. As pregnancy progresses, a distended thin-walled cervix with the external os partially dilated may be evident. Bleeding without pain is the common clinical characteristic. Above the cervical mass, a slightly enlarged uterine fundus may be palpated. Gabbe and co-workers (1975) reported two cases of cervical pregnancy with high fever that initially was erroneously attributed to septic intrauterine pregnancy.

Cervical pregnancy rarely goes beyond the 20th week of gestation and is usually terminated surgically because of bleeding. Since attempts at removal of the placenta vaginally may result in profuse hemorrhage and even death of the patient, there should be little hesitation in performing hysterectomy to control the bleeding. Only in nulliparas very anxious to maintain fertility should conservative procedures be attempted. Whittle (1976) describes one case in a primigravida from whom he dissected from the cervix a gestational sac 4 cm in diameter. The cervix was first clamped bilaterally and subsequently ligated at these sites. The friable, torn cervix was also sutured and the vagina firmly packed. One liter of blood was administered.

OTHER SITES OF ECTOPIC PREGNANCY

A primary *splenic pregnancy* has been vividly described by Mankodi and associates (1977). The symptoms and signs that led to laparotomy included pain in the epigastrium and left shoulder, hypotension, tachycardia, syncope, and tenderness in the vaginal fornices. At laparotomy considerable hemoperitoneum but normal pelvic organs were found. A rent in the hilar surface of the spleen prompted splenectomy. Microscopically, chorionic villi were identified invading otherwise normal splenic tissue at the site of the rent. A few cases of primary hepatic pregnancy have been described, including one with lithopedian formation (Luwuliza-Kirunda, 1978).

REFERENCES

Arey LB: The cause of tubal pregnancy and tubal twinning. Am J Obstet Gynecol 5:163, 1923

Arias-Stella J: Atypical endometrial changes associated with the presence of chorionic tissue. Arch Pathol 58:112, 1954

Beacham WD, Hernquist WC, Beacham DW, Webster HD: Abdominal pregnancy at Charity Hospital in New Orleans. Am J Obstet Gynecol 84:1257, 1962 (184 references cited)

Berger MJ, Taymor ML: Simultaneous intrauterine and tubal pregnancies following ovulation induction. Am J Obstet Gynecol 113:812, 1972

Bobrow ML, Winkelstein LB: Intrafollicular ovarian pregnancy. Am J Surg 91:991, 1956

Brenner PF, Roy S, Mishell DR Jr: Ectopic pregnancy: A study of 300 surgically treated cases. JAMA 243:673, 1980

Cavanagh D: Primary peritoneal pregnancy. Rationalization or established entity? Omental transference as an alternative explanation. Am J Obstet Gynecol 76:523, 1958

Clark JFJ, Jones SA: Advanced ectopic pregnancy. J Reprod Med 14:30, 1975

Cross JB, Lester WM, McCain J: The diagnosis and management of abdominal pregnancy with a review of 19 cases. Am J Obstet Gynecol 62:303, 1951

Dees HC: Cervical pregnancy associated with uterine leiomyomas. South Med J 59:900, 1966

Franklin EW, Zeiderman AM: Tubal ectopic pregnancy: etiology and obstetric and gynecologic sequelae. Am J Obstet Gynecol 117:220, 1973

Funderburk AG: Bilateral ectopic pregnancy with simultaneous intrauterine pregnancy. Am J Obstet Gynecol 119:274, 1974

Gabbe SG, Kitzmiller JL, Kosasa TS, Driscoll SG: Cervical pregnancy presenting as septic abortion. Am J Obstet Gynecol 123:212, 1975

Ganji H, Vidrine A Jr: Ectopic pregnancy presenting as hemothorax. Am J Surg 120:807,1970

Gilstrap LC, Harris RE: Ectopic pregnancy: A review of 122 cases. South Med J 69:604, 1976

Gray CL, Ruffolo EH: Ovarian pregnancy associated with intrauterine contraceptive devices. Am J Obstet Gynecol 132:134, 1978

Hallatt JG: Repeat ectopic pregnancy: A study of 123 consecutive cases. Am J Obstet Gynecol 122:520, 1975

Harralson JD, Van Nagell JR, Roddick JW Jr: Operative management of ruptured tubal pregnancy. Am J Obstet Gynecol 115:995, 1973

Hertz, RH, Timor-Tritch I, Sokol RJ, Zador I: Diagnostic studies and fetal assessment in advanced extrauterine pregnancy. Obstet Gynecol 50:63 (Suppl), 1977

Jeffcoate TNA: Principles of Gynaecology, 3d ed. New York, Appleton, 1967

Kallenberger DA, Ronk DA, Jimerson GJ: Ectopic pregnancy: A 15-year review of 160 cases. South Med J 171:758, 1978

Kelly RW, Martin SA, Strickler RC: Delayed hemorrhage in conservative surgery for ectopic pregnancy. 133:225, 1979

King EL: Postoperative separation of the cesarean section wound, with subsequent abdominal pregnancy. Am J Obstet Gynecol 24:421, 1932

King G: Advanced extrauterine pregnancy. Am J Obstet Gynecol 67:712, 1954

Kitchin JD III, Wein RM, Nunley WC Jr, Thiagarajah S, Thornton WN Jr: Ectopic pregnancy: Current clinical trends. Am J Obstet Gynecol 134:870, 1979

Kostic P: Cause of extrauterine pregnancy: analysis of clinical material of gynecologic hospital of the city of Belgrade. CR Soc Franc Gynecol 31:45, 1961

Lucas C, Hassim AM: Place of culdocentesis in the diagnosis of ectopic pregnancy. Br Med J 1:200, 1970

Luwuliza-Kirunda, JMM: Primary hepatic pregnancy. Brit J Obstet Gynaecol 85:311, 1978

McNulty JJ: Hemothorax as a presenting symptom in abdominal pregnancy. Obstet Gynecol 16:615, 1960

Malkasian GD, Hunter JS, Re Mine WH: Pregnancy in the tubal interstitium and tubal remnants. Am J Obstet Gynecol 77:1301, 1959

Mankodi RC, Sankari K, Bhatt SM: Primary splenic pregnancy. Br J Obstet Gynecol 84:634, 1977

May WJ, Miller JB, Greiss JC Jr: Maternal deaths from ectopic pregnancy in the South Atlantic region, 1960 through 1976. Am J Obstet Gynecol 132:140, 1978

Mengert WF, Cobb SW, Brown WW: Introduction of blood into the peritoneal cavity. JAMA 147:34, 1951

Niebyl JR: Pregnancy following total hysterectomy. Am J Obstet Gynecol 119:512, 1974

Orr JW Jr, Huddleston JF, Knox GE, Goldenberg RL, Davis RO: False negative oxytocin challenge test associated with abdominal pregnancy. Am J Obstet Gynecol 133:108, 1979

Pratt-Thomas HR, White L, Messer HH: Primary ovarian pregnancy: Presentation of ten cases, including one full-term pregnancy. South Med J 67:920, 1974

Pritchard JA, Adams RH: The fate of blood in the peritoneal cavity. Surg Obstet Gynecol 105:621, 1957

Rasor JL, Braunstein GD: A rapid modification of the Beta-h CG Radioimmunoassay: Use as an aid in the diagnosis of ectopic pregnancy. Obstet Gynecol 50:553, 1977

Rengachary D, Fayez JA, Jonas HS: Ovarian pregnancy. Obstet Gynecol 49:76 (suppl), 1977

Riva HL, Kammeraad LA, Andreson PS: Ectopic pregnancy: report of 132 cases and comments on the role of the culdoscope in diagnosis. Obstet Gynecol 20:189, 1962

Romney SL, Hertig AT, Reid DE: The endometria associated with ectopic pregnancy. Surg Obstet Gynecol 91:605, 1950

Sandmire HF, Randall JH: Ectopic pregnancy: review of 182 cases. Obstet Gynecol 14:227, 1959

Schenker JG, Eyal F, Polishuk WZ: Fertility after tubal pregnancy. Surg Gynecol Obstet 135:74, 1972

Schiffer M: A review of 268 ectopic pregnancies. Am J Obstet Gynecol 86:264, 1963

Schneider J, Berger CJ, Cattell C: Maternal mortality due to ectopic pregnancy: A review of 102 deaths. Obstet Gynecol 49:557, 1977

Spiegelberg O. Casuistry in ovarian pregnancy, Arch Gynaekol 13:73, 1878

Strafford JC, Ragan WD: Abdominal pregnancy: Review of current management. Obstet Gynecol 50:548, 1977

Studdiford WD: Primary peritoneal pregnancy. Am J Obstet Gynecol 44:487, 1942

Torpin R, Coleman J, Seifi M, Arshadi S: Ectopic pregnancy in Shiraz, Iran: study of 10 year record (154 cases). Am J Obstet Gynecol 82:456, 1961

Ware HH: Observations on thirteen cases of late extrauterine pregnancy. Am J Obstet Gynecol 55:561, 1948

Whittle MJ: Cervical pregnancy managed by local excision. Br Med J 2:795, 1976

Yaffe H, Navot D, Laufer N: Pitfalls in early detection of ectopic pregnancy. Lancet 1:277, 1979

Yaffe H, Sadovsky E, Beyth Y: Tubal pregnancy and tubal patency. Int J Gynaecol Obstet 14:265, 1976

23

Diseases and Abnormalities of the Placenta and Fetal Membranes

ABNORMALITIES OF PLACENTATION

Multiple Placentas in Single Pregnancies. Most frequently, the organ may be divided into two lobes. When the division is incomplete and the vessels extend from one lobe to the other before uniting to form the umbilical cord, the condition is termed *placenta bipartita* or bilobate placenta. The reported incidence of this placental anomaly varies widely, but in the experience of Fox (1978) it occurs in about 1 of 350 deliveries. If the two lobes are entirely separated, and the vessels remain distinct, not uniting until just before entering the cord, the condition is designated *placenta duplex.* Sometimes both features are present (Fig. 23-1) Occasionally, the organ may comprise three distinct lobes (placenta *triplex*). Rarely more than three lobes are present. Earn (1951) cited the report of a placenta which was formed of seven lobes.

Placenta Succenturiata. An important anomaly is the so-called *placenta succenturiata,* in which one or more small accessory lobes are developed in the membrane at a distance from the periphery of the main placenta, to which they ordinarily have vascular connection of fetal origin (see Chap. 6, Figs. 6-17 and 6-18). Placenta succenturiata is of considerable clinical importance because the accessory lobe is sometimes retained in the uterus after expulsion of the main placenta and may give rise to serious maternal hemorrhage. If, on examination of the placenta, defects in the membranes are noted a short distance from the placental margin, retention of a succenturiate lobe should be suspected. The suspicion is confirmed if vessels extend from the placenta to the margins of the tear. In such cases, even if there is no hemorrhage at the moment, the retained lobe should be removed manually. In most large series the incidence of accessory lobes is approximately 3 percent.

Ring-shaped Placenta. This is a very rare anomaly that occurs in less than 1 of 6000 deliveries. The placenta is annular in shape and sometimes a complete ring of placental tissue is present, but more commonly, because of atrophy of a portion of the tissue of the ring, a horseshoe shape is present. Fox (1978) considers this anomaly to be a variant

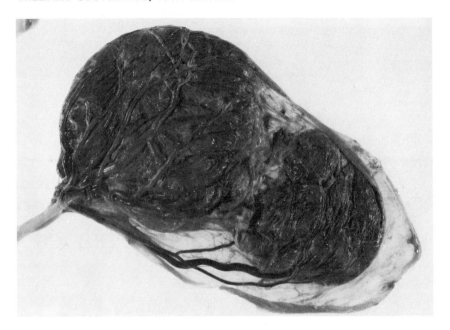

FIG. 23-1. Placenta with two lobes and velamentous insertion of cord.

of placenta membranacea. This placental abnormality appears to be associated with a greater likelihood of ante- and postpartum bleeding and fetal growth retardation.

Fenestrate Placenta.   This is an exceptionally rare anomaly of the placenta in which the central portion of a discoidal placenta is missing (Kleine, 1956). In some instances, there is an actual hole in the placenta but more often the defect involves villous tissue only, the chorionic plate being present. The clinical significance of this anomaly is that the abnormality may be mistakenly considered to represent a missing portion which is retained in the uterus.

Placenta Membranacea.   In rare circumstances, the entire fetal membranes are covered by functioning villi, and the placenta develops as a thin membranous structure occupying the entire periphery of the chorion (placenta membranacea). This abnormality does not appear to interfere with nutrition of the ovum but occasionally gives rise to serious hemorrhage. Bleeding often resembles that seen in central placenta previa, beginning in the second trimester and gradually increasing in severity to necessitate interrup-

tion of the pregnancy by hysterectomy or cesarean section. During the third stage of labor, the attenuated placenta does not readily separate from its area of attachment. Manual removal is sometimes very difficult in such cases.

Placenta Extrachorialis.   In these conditions, the chorionic plate of the placenta is smaller than the basal plate. If the fetal surface of such a placenta presents a central depression surrounded by a thickened, grayish-white ring, which is situated at a varying distance from the margin of the organ, the placenta is classed as a *cirumvallate placenta* (Fig. 23-2 and 23-3). When the ring coincides with the placental margin, the condition is sometimes described as a *marginate placenta.* Within the ring, the fetal surface presents the usual appearance, gives attachment to the umbilical cord, and shows the usual large vessels, which instead of coursing over the entire fetal surface terminate abruptly at the margin of the ring. In a circumvallate placenta, the ring is composed of a double fold of amnion and chorion with degenerated decidua and fibrin in between. In a marginate placenta, the chorion and amnion are raised at the margin by interposed decidua and fibrin, without folding of the membranes. These relations are illustrated in Figure 23-3. The cause of circumvallate and circummarginate placentation is not understood. Antepartum hemorrhage and prematurity are increased (Bernischke, 1974).

Large Placentas. While the normal term placenta without cord and membranes weighs on the average about 500 g, in certain diseases, such as syphilis, the placenta may weigh one-fourth, one-third, or even one-half as much as the fetus. The largest placentas are usually encountered in cases of erythroblastosis. In one such case, the fetus and placenta weighed 1140 and 1200 g, respectively, and in another, the placenta weighed over 2000 g.

Placental Polyp. Occasionally, parts of a normal placenta or a succenturiate lobe may be retained after delivery. These may form polyps consisting of villi in varying stages of degeneration and covered by regenerated endometrium. The clinical sequelae are often subinvolution of the uterus and late postpartum hemorrhage (see Chap. 36, p. 915).

Circulatory Disturbances

Infarcts. The most common lesions of the placenta, though of diverse origin, are referred to collectively as placental infarcts. Wallenburg (1971) has prepared an extensive and impressive monograph on the morphology and pathology of placental infarcts.

Overclassification of placental infarcts has led to unnecessary confusion. Minute subchorionic and marginal foci of degeneration are present in every placenta. These lesions are of clinical significance only when they are abundant, in which case they may interfere with the function of a sufficiently large portion of the placenta to hamper seriously the nutrition of the fetus and on occasion cause fetal death. In simplest terms, degenerative lesions of the placenta have two etiologic factors in common, namely, changes associated

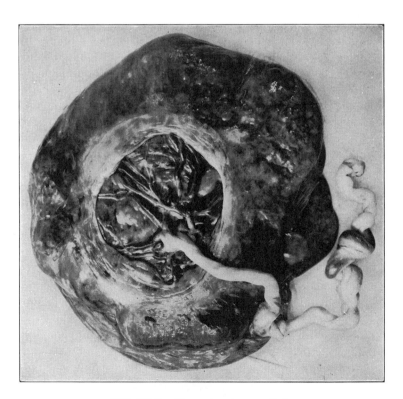

FIG. 23-2. Placenta circumvallata.

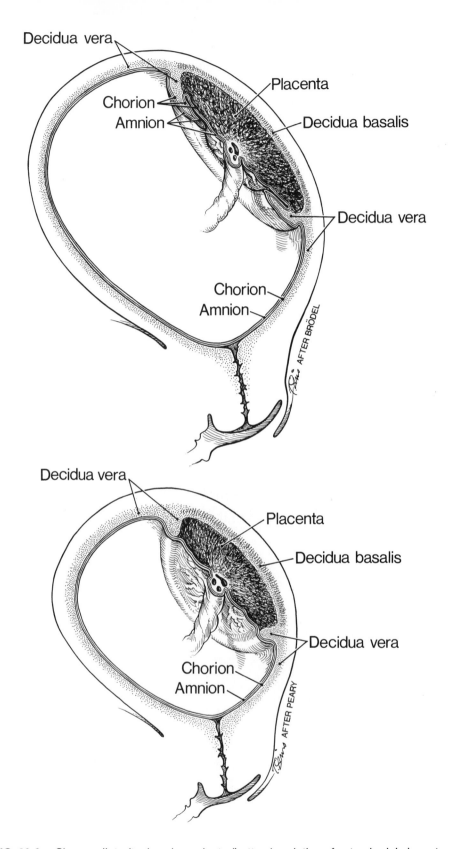

FIG. 23-3. Circumvallate (top) and marginate (bottom) varieties of extrachorial placentas.

554

with aging of the trophoblast and vascular changes in the uteroplacental circulation with their sequelae. The lesions are easy to explain on the basis that nutrition of the placental villi is derived essentially from the maternal rather than the fetal circulation. The principal histopathologic features include fibrinoid degeneration of the trophoblast, calcification, and ischemic infarction from occlusion of spiral arteries.

Although the placenta is by no means a dying organ at term (see Chap. 6, p. 121), there are morphologic indications of aging. During the latter half of pregnancy, syncytial degeneration begins and syncytial knots are formed. At the same time, the villous stroma usually undergoes hyalinization. The syncytium may then break away or float off, exposing the connective tissue directly to maternal blood. As a result, clotting occurs, and extensive propagation of the clot may result in the incorporation of other villi. Macroscopically, such a focus resembles closely an ordinary blood clot, but if not seen until it has become thoroughly organized, on section a firm, white island of tissue is revealed that looks like fibrinoid degeneration.

About the edge of nearly every term placenta there is a more or less dense yellowish-white fibrous ring representing a zone of degeneration, which is usually termed a *marginal infarct.* It may be quite superficial in places, but occasionally it extends a centimeter or two into the substance of the placenta. Underneath the chorionic plate, there are nearly always similar lesions, of more or less pyramidal shape, ranging from 0.2 cm to 2 or even 3 cm across the base, and extending downward with their apices in the intervillous space (subchorionic infarcts). Not infrequently, similar lesions are noted about the intercotyledonary septa, in which case the broadest portion rests upon the maternal surface and the apex points toward the chorionic plate. Occasionally, these lesions meet and form a column of cartilage-like material extending from the maternal to the fetal surfaces. Less frequently, round or oval islands of similar tissue occupy the central portions of the placenta (Fig. 23-4. A and B). By and

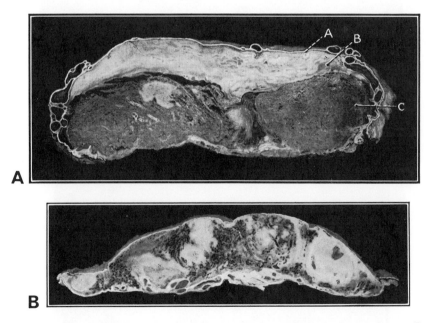

FIG. 23-4.A. Degeneration of the placenta. A. amnion and chorionic membrane. B. fibrinoid degeneration localized beneath the chorion. C. unchanged placental tissue. (In this instance, the infarct was unusually extensive, most likely contributing to the death of the fetus.) **B.** Degeneration of the placenta. Generalized fibrinoid deposition with little normal tissue remaining.

large, the lesions represent fibrinoid degeneration of trophoblastic elements. In early placentas, they may be identified as islands or knots of trophoblast, located principally on the maternal side of the chorionic plate and over the decidua, particularly in the vicinity of septa and at the margins of the placenta. Later, they may fuse to form large pale-staining masses and involve the tips of growing villi.

CALCIFICATION OF THE PLACENTA. Small calcareous nodules or plaques are observed frequently upon the maternal surface of the placenta and are occasionally so abundant that the organ feels like coarse sandpaper. In view of the widespread degenerative changes in the placenta, calcification is not surprising. In fact, the conditions for deposition of calcium in the aging placenta are almost ideal. Moderate degrees of calcification may be detected in at least half of all placentas examined roentgenologically. An extensive deposition of calcium is shown in Figure 23-5. Tindall and Scott (1965), in a study of the placentas of 3025 pregnancies, concluded that calcification in the placenta is a normal process.

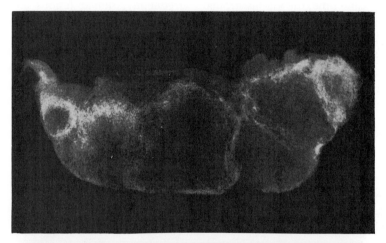

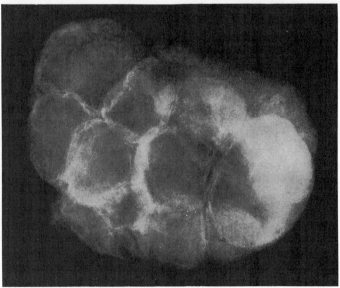

FIG. 23-5. Roentgenograms of the human placenta at term showing subchorionic and septal calcification. (Courtesy of Professor J. S. Scott)

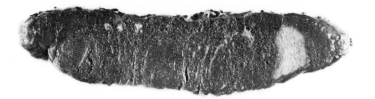

FIG. 23-6.   A localized area of pallor in a placenta which is due to fetal artery thrombosis. (From Fox. *Pathology of the Placenta,* Vol. 7. Philadelphia, Saunders, 1978, p. 131)

Clinical Significance of Degenerative Changes in the Placenta.   In general, "infarcts" of the placenta, caused either by local deposition of fibrin or by the more acute process of intervillous thrombosis, have little clinical significance, probably because of a relatively large margin of safety for most placental functions. Nonetheless, in certain maternal diseases, notably severe hypertension, the reduction in functioning placenta, especially when coupled with reduced blood flow to the uterus, may be sufficient to cause fetal death.

Villous (fetal) vessels may show endarteritic thickening and obliteration in association with fetal death. When the placental villi are excluded from their supply of maternal blood by fibrin deposits, hematomas, or direct blockage of the decidual circulation, they necessarily become infarcted and die. Histologically, the compromised villi are characterized by fibrosis, obliteration of fetal vessels, and gradual disappearance of the syncytium.

Fetal Artery Thrombosis.   Thrombosis of a fetal villous stem artery produces a sharply demarcated area of avascularity (Fig. 23-6). Fox (1978) found a single artery thrombosis in 4.5 percent of placentas from normal pregnancies and in 10 percent of placentas of pregnancies involving diabetic women. Benirschke and Driscoll (1974) observed an association between fetal artery thrombosis and anti-platelet antibodies in maternal serum. Fox (1978) has estimated that thrombosis of a single fetal stem artery will deprive only 5 percent of the villi of their blood supply. However, he also has observed a few placentas from fresh stillbirths in which 40 to 50 percent of the villi were deprived of their fetal blood supply.

Miscellaneous Abnormalities of the Placenta

Hypertrophic Lesions of the Chorionic Villi.   Striking enlargement of the chorionic villi is seen commonly in association with erythroblastosis of the hydropic variety (Fig. 38-8, p. 969). It has also been described in diabetes and occasionally in severe fetal disease, as, for example, in the case of congestive heart failure described by Gottschalk and Abramson (1957).

Abnormalities of the Placenta Detected By Microscopic Examination. Beginning after the 32nd week of gestation, clumps of syncytial nuclei are found that project into the intervillous space; these are called *syncytial knots.* By term up to 30 percent of villi may be involved; however, formation of knots by more than a third of villi is considered abnormal (Fox, 1965). In prolonged pregnancies there is a marked increase in the proportion of villi with syncytial knots, as there is in avascular villi resulting from fetal artery thrombosis. Generally increased numbers of syncytial knots are found in placentas in which reduced uteroplacental blood flow may have existed (maternal hypertension). However, fetal hypoperfusion of villi appears to be more important in the pathogenesis of this lesion.

It is well recognized that the number of *cytotrophoblastic cells* becomes progressively reduced as pregnancy advances. In a normal mature placenta, cytotrophoblastic cells are found in about 20 percent of the villi (Fox, 1964). However, at this stage of pregnancy such cells are few and inconspicuous. Numerous cytotrophoblastic cells are found in placentas of pregnancies of women with diabetes mellitus and Rho-isoimmunization with an affected fetus. More recently increased numbers of cytotrophoblasts have been observed in placentas of pregnancies complicated by pregnancy-induced hypertension and the number of cytotrophoblasts seems to increase progressively with the severity and duration of preeclampsia.

Inflammation of the Placenta. Changes that are now recognized as various forms of degeneration and necrosis were formerly described under the term placentitis. For example, small placental cysts with grumous contents were formerly thought to be abscesses. Nonetheless, especially in cases of prolonged rupture of the membranes, pyogenic bacteria do invade the fetal surface of the placenta and, after gaining access to the chorionic vessels, give rise to general infection of the fetus.

TROPHOBLASTIC DISEASES

There are three general categories of neoplastic trophoblastic disease:

1. *Hydatidiform Moles:* Hydatidiform moles of the complete variety are characterized by neoplastic proliferation of trophoblast, marked edema of the avascular villous stroma, and absence of a fetus and of amnion.
2. *Invasive Moles:* At times, the villi, with their proliferating neoplastic covering, invade and penetrate the uterus, or metastasize to distant organs, or both. Invasion or metastasis by such villi characterize an invasive mole. An invasive mole was formerly referred to as chorioadenoma destruens.
3. *Choriocarcinoma.* Neoplastic trophoblast without stroma may disseminate far and wide beyond the original site of implantation in the genital tract and proliferate profusely to cause death from extensive organ destruction and hemorrhage. Such behavior by trophoblast is called *choriocarcinoma.* It was formerly called chorionepithelioma.

Hydatidiform Moles

Complete (Classic) Hydatidiform Mole. The chorionic villi are converted into a mass of clear vesicles (Fig. 23-7). The vesicles vary in size from barely visible to a few centimeters in diameter and often hang in clusters from thin pedicles. The mass may grow large enough to fill the uterus to the size occupied by an advanced normal pregnancy.

The histologic structure is characterized by (1) hydropic degeneration and swelling of the villous stroma; (2) absence of blood

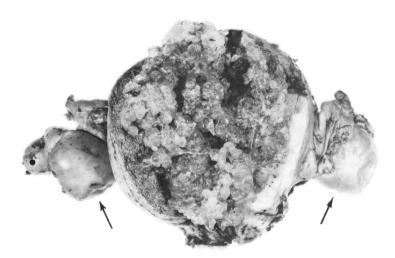

FIG. 23-7.   A complete hydatidiform mole. Note theca-lutein cysts in each ovary (arrows).

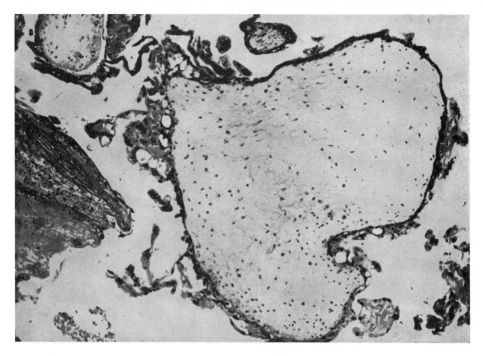

FIG. 23-8 Example of hydatidiform mole with slight to moderate trophoblastic hyperplasia, confined to the syncytium and considered as probably benign. (From Smalbraak. *Trophoblastic Growths*. Haarlem, Netherlands, Elsevier, 1957)

vessels in the swollen villi; (3) proliferation of the trophoblastic epithelium to a varying degree (Fig. 23-8), and (4) absence of a fetus and of amnion. The karyotype of a complete mole is 46, XX, which is now believed to be derived from a paternal haploid, X-carrying set of chromosomes that reaches the 46, XX status by its own duplication (Boué et al., 1976; Kajii and Ohama, 1977). Thus the moles are androgenetic in origin. (Androgenesis refers to the development of an ovum under the influence of a spermatozoan nucleus, the original nucleus of the ovum being either absent or inactivated.) Diploid androgenesis in these moles could be the consequence of fertilization by two X-carrying sperms (dispermy), or by a diploid sperm, or by a haploid X-carrying sperm followed by duplication of its chromosomes. The observations of Kajii and Ohama (1977) and Yamashita and co-workers (1979) serve to implicate the last mechanism.

The complete mole is the most common precursor of choriocarcinoma.

Partial (Incomplete) Hydatidiform Mole. When the hydatidiform changes are focal and less advanced, and there is a fetus or, at least, an amnionic sac, the condition has been classified as a partial hydatidiform mole (Szulman and Surti, 1978). There is slowly progressing hydatidiform swelling of some usually avascular villi while other vascular villi with a functioning fetal-placental circulation are spared (Fig. 23-9). Hyperplasia of the trophoblast is focal rather than generalized. The karyotype typically is triploid (Lawler and co-workers, 1979).

The likelihood of choriocarcinoma arising from a partial hydatidiform mole is debated. At the New England Trophoblastic Disease Center neither invasion nor metastases were observed in any of 21 partial moles (Berkowitz et al., 1979). However, Szulman and co-workers (1978) have reported a partial mole with demonstrated triploidy that required chemotherapy because of persistence of chorionic gonadotropin after evacuating the mole.

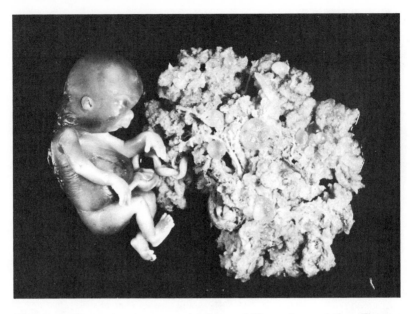

FIG. 23-9. Extensive molar change and a fetus of 20 weeks gestation. The pregnancy was complicated further by eclampsia. Before eclampsia developed, pregnancy-induced hypertension from molar pregnancy was not considered the cause of acute hypertension, since a fetal heart was heard.

Molar Degeneration. Difference of opinion remains as to when hydatid changes in the villi represent a hydatidiform mole and when they are merely a degenerative reaction, or molar degeneration. Hertig and Edmonds (1940) found that in two-thirds of the pathologic ova studied by them, there was early hydatid degeneration.

HISTOLOGIC DIAGNOSIS. Attempts to relate the histologic structure of individual hydatidiform moles to their subsequent malignant tendencies generally have been disappointing. Novak and Seah (1954), for example, were unable to establish precisely such a relation in 120 cases of hydatidiform mole or in the molar tissue submitted to them in 26 cases of choriocarcinoma following hydatidiform mole.

Ovarian Lutein Cysts. In many cases of hydatidiform mole, the ovaries contain multiple lutein cysts (Fig. 23-7), which may vary from microscopic size to 10 cm and more in diameter. The surfaces of the cysts are smooth, often yellowish, and lined with lutein cells. The incidence of obvious cysts in associ-

ation with a mole is reported to be from 25 percent to as high as 60 percent.

Lutein cysts of the ovaries are thought to result from overstimulation of lutein elements by large amounts of chorionic gonadotropin secreted by the proliferating trophoblasts. In general, extensive cystic change is usually associated with the larger hydatidiform moles and a long period of stimulation. Novak (1948) emphasized that most of the ovaries lacking gross cysts contain some microscopic cystic change and luteal hyperreaction often involving both thecal and granulosal elements. Moreover, lutein cysts are not limited to cases of hydatidiform mole. Girouard, Barclay, and Collins (1964) collected 15 cases of typical theca lutein cysts without hydatid mole or choriocarcinoma during pregnancy and added two of their own. The lutein cysts are especially interesting because eleven were associated with placental hypertrophy, six with fetal hydrops, and five with multiple pregnancies. The remainder were from apparently normal pregnancies. Oophorectomy should not be performed because of theca lutein cysts alone. After delivery of the mole, the cysts eventually regress and disappear. At times, after evacuation of a mole, paradoxically, the cystic ovaries enlarge before they regress.

Incidence. Hydatidiform mole occurs approximately once in about 1500 pregnancies in the United States and Europe but is much more frequent in some other parts of the world, especially in parts of Asia. The data of Wei and Ooyang (1963) are supportive of the conclusion that trophoblastic disease has been particularly prevalent in Taiwan, where the incidence of hydatidiform mole was one in 125 pregnancies. Marquez-Monter and co-workers (1963) reported a surprisingly high incidence of one in 200 in the General Hospital of Mexico and Martin (1978) has identified an incidence of one in 257 deliveries among native Alaskans.

PREVIOUS MOLE. Recurrence of hydatid mole is uncommon but is seen in about 2 percent of cases. Wu (1973) described a case of nine consecutive molar pregnancies!

AGE. Age has an important bearing on the incidence of hydatidiform mole, as indicated by the relatively high frequency among pregnancies toward the end of the childbearing period. The most pronounced effect of age is seen in women older than 45, when the relative frequency of the lesion is more than ten times greater than at ages 20 to 40. There are numerous authenticated cases of hydatidiform mole in women 50 years old and older, whereas normal pregnancy at such advanced ages is practically unknown (Jequier and Winterton, 1973).

Clinical Course. In the very early stages of development of the mole, there are few characteristics to distinguish it from normal pregnancy, but later in the first trimester and during the second trimester the following noteworthy changes are often evident:

BLEEDING. Uterine bleeding is the outstanding sign, occurring in 89 percent of 347 hydatidiform moles studied by Curry and associates (1975); this may vary from spotting

to profuse hemorrhage. It may occur just before abortion or, more often, it occurs intermittently for weeks or even months. As the consequence of such bleeding, anemia is rather common. Iron deficiency commonly and folate deficiency rarely may also play a role (Pritchard, 1965). At times, there may be considerable hemorrhage concealed within the uterus; moreover, a dilutional effect from appreciable hypervolemia has been demonstrated in some women with larger hydatidiform moles. Iron deficiency anemia is a common finding but occasionally megaloblastic erythropoiesis is evident, presumably due to poor dietary intake as the consequence of nausea and vomiting and to increased folate requirement imposed by rapidly proliferating trophoblast.

UTERINE SIZE. The growing uterus often enlarges more rapidly than usual, the size clearly exceeding that expected from the duration of gestation in about one-half of cases. Uterine size may be difficult to identify precisely by palpation in the nulliparous woman especially, because of the soft consistency of the uterus beneath a firm abdominal wall. At times ovaries appreciably enlarged by multiple lutein cysts may be difficult to distinguish from the enlarged uterus. The ovaries are likely to be tender to palpation.

FETAL ACTIVITY. Even though the uterus is enlarged sufficiently to lie well above the symphysis, typically no fetal heart action can be detected even with sensitive instruments that combine ultrasound and the Doppler principle. Rarely, there may be twin placentas with hydatidiform mole developing in one while the other placenta and its fetus appear normal. Also, very infrequently there may be extensive but incomplete molar change in the placenta accompanied by a living fetus (Fig. 23-9). Jones and Lauersen (1975) identified and described hydatidiform mole with a coexistent fetus 8 times in 175,000 pregnancies.

PREGNANCY-INDUCED HYPERTENSION. Of special importance is the frequent association of pregnancy-induced hypertension with molar pregnancies that persist well beyond the first trimester. Since the syndrome of pregnancy-induced hypertension is rarely seen before 24 weeks of gestation except in this circumstance, its appearance before 24 weeks strongly suggests hydatidiform mole, or at least extensive molar change.

EMBOLIZATION. Variable amounts of trophoblast with or without villous stroma escape from the uterus in the venous outflow. The volume may be such as to produce signs and symptoms of acute pulmonary embolism (Twiggs and associates, 1979), and even a fatal outcome in the absence of invasion of pulmonary tissue (Yelverton, 1972). Such fatalities are rare.

Much more often trophoblast with or without villous stroma will embolize to the lungs in volumes too small to produce overt block-

ade of the pulmonary vasculature, but subsequently they invade the pulmonary parenchyma to establish metastases which are evident roentgenographically. The lesions may consist of trophoblast alone (metastatic choriocarcinoma) or trophoblast with villous stroma (metastatic invasive mole). The subsequent course of such lesions is unpredictable. Some pulmonary lesions have been observed to disappear spontaneously either soon after evacuation of the uterus or even weeks to months later, while others proliferate and kill the woman unless she is actively treated.

DISTURBED THYROID FUNCTION. Plasma thyroxine levels may be elevated, but clinically apparent hyperthyroidism is uncommon. Curry and associates (1975) identified hyperthyroidism in 2 percent of cases. The elevation may be the effect primarily of estro-

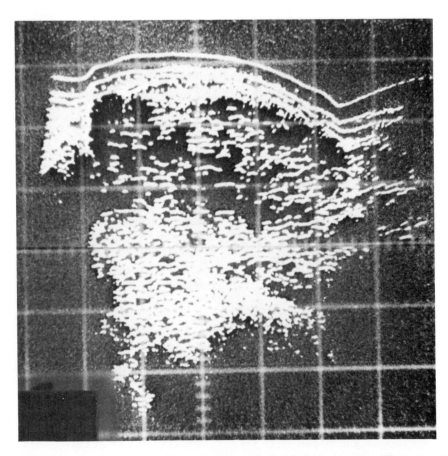

FIG. 23-10. A. Transverse B-mode sonogram made just below natural umbilicus showing diffuse pattern of intrauterine echoes characteristic of hydatidiform mole.

gen, as in normal pregnancy, in which case free thyroxine levels are not elevated, or the thyrotropinlike effect of chorionic gonadotropin in high concentration and possibly of a thyroid-stimulating hormone produced by trophoblast, in which case there is likely to be an appreciable elevation of circulating free thyroxine with signs and symptoms of hyperthyroidism.

SPONTANEOUS EXPULSION. Occasionally, hydatid vesicles, or "grapes," are passed before the mole is aborted spontaneously or removed by operation. Spontaneous expulsion is most likely to occur around the 4th month and is rarely delayed beyond the 7th month.

Diagnostic Features. Persistent bleeding and a uterus larger than the expected size arouse suspicion of a mole. Consideration must be given not only to possibilities of a normal placenta and single fetus, but also an error in menstrual data, or a pregnant uterus enlarged by myomas, hydramnios, or especially multiple fetuses.

SONOGRAPHY. The greatest diagnostic accuracy can be obtained from the characteristic ultrasonogram of hydatidiform mole (Fig. 23-10. A and B). The safety and precision of sonography make it the technic of choice whenever it is available. Kobayashi and co-workers (1972), and others, have emphasized that some other structures, especially when scanned with B-mode ultrasonography, may yield a sonogram similar to that of a hydatidiform mole. These include a tangential section of a normal placenta, uterine myoma with early pregnancy, and pregnancies with multiple fetuses. A careful review of the history, coupled with careful ultrasonic

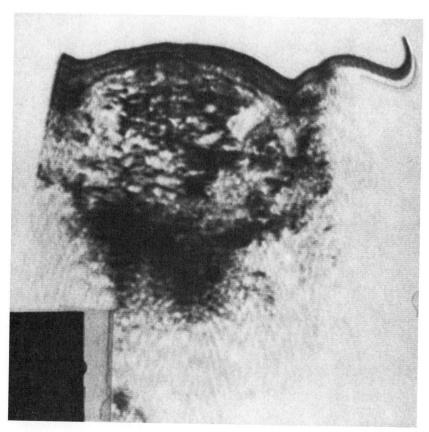

FIG. 23-10.B. Gray scale sonography at same level as in Figure 23-10.A.

scanning repeated in a week or two when necessary, should serve to avoid the incorrect diagnosis of hydatidiform mole when pregnancy products are actually normal. The development and application of gray scale sonography has provided even greater precision of diagnosis.

HYSTEROGRAM. Transabdominal intrauterine instillation of a radiopaque substance such as Hypaque produces a characteristic roentgenogram in cases of hydatidiform mole (Torres and Pelegrina, 1966; Zarou et al., 1970). The woman is prepared and the uterine cavity is penetrated with the needle as for amniocentesis (Chap. 14, p. 346). Then 20 ml of Hypaque is injected quickly and 5 to 10 minutes later an anteroposterior roentgenogram is made of the lower abdomen and pelvis. A characteristic honeycombed x-ray pattern is produced by contrast material surrounding the chorionic vesicles. There is a slight risk of abortion from the intra-amnionic injection of hypertonic radiocontrast material. With the widespread availability of sonography this technic is seldom used.

CHORIONIC GONADOTROPIN MEASUREMENTS. Tests for chorionic gonadotropin may be useful if a reliable quantitative method of assay is used and the considerable variation in gonadotropin secretion in normal pregnancy is appreciated, especially the elevated levels that sometimes accompany pregnancy with multiple fetuses (Chap. 7, p. 149). Assays performed on serum are subject to fewer variables than are measurements of urinary gonadotropin. Recently, a variety of immunoassays, including radioimmunoassay, have become popular. The result should be compared with the serum gonadotropin level for normal pregnancy at the stage in question. If it is far above the normal range for that stage of pregnancy, a presumptive diagnosis of mole may be made. It is clear from the remarkably variable gonadotropin values for normal pregnancy that no *single value* can be established as the borderline between normal and abnormal pregnancy. Very

high values in the first 2 or 3 months mean little, since they are encountered occasionally in normal pregnancy, especially with multiple fetuses. Beyond 100 days after the last menstrual period, however, there is in normal pregnancy a decline in chorionic gonadotropin, so that persistently high, and especially rising levels, after that time are strong evidence of abnormal growth of trophoblast (Delfs, 1975). If the slightest doubt remains, one or more assays repeated at intervals of a week should be performed in an attempt to observe the trend.

Tojo and associates (1974) studied the levels simultaneously of the glycoproteins chorionic gonadotropin and chorionic thyrotropin, as well as the protein placental lactogen, in serum of women with hydatidiform moles. Chorionic gonadotropin and thyrotropin levels most often were elevated while placental lactogen was lower than in normal pregnancies of the same gestational age. After molar evacuation, the time required for the disappearance of these hormones was longest for chorionic gonadotropin, shorter for chorionic thyrotropin, and very much shorter for placental lactogen.

In summary, the diagnostic features of hydatidiform mole are:

1. Continuous or intermittent bloody discharge evident by about the 12th week of pregnancy, usually not profuse, and often more nearly brown rather than red.
2. Enlargement of the uterus out of proportion to the duration of pregnancy in about one-half of the cases.
3. Absence of fetal parts on palpation or radiologic examination, even though the uterus may be enlarged to the level of the umbilicus or higher.
4. Characteristic ultrasonographic patterns.
5. A very high chorionic gonadotropin level in the serum (or less dependably in the urine) 100 days or more after the last menstrual period.
6. Preeclampsia-eclampsia earlier in pregnancy than usually found.

In differential diagnosis, great care must be taken to exclude a pregnancy with multiple fetuses, which may simulate hydatidiform mole in several respects.

Prognosis. In a collective review of 576 cases, Mathieu in 1939 found an immediate mortality rate of 1.4 percent, a figure that has been reduced practically to zero by more prompt diagnosis and appropriate therapy for hemorrhage (see Chap. 21 p. 490). Attempts in the past to deliver large moles vaginally sometimes led to uncontrollable and fatal hemorrhage.

About 10 percent of hydatidiform moles progress to invasive, potentially metastatic choriocarcinoma. Rarely, years may intervene between the occurrence of a hydatidiform mole and the development of choriocarcinoma. Natsume and Takada (1961) reported a case in which choriocarcinoma developed 9 years after a supravaginal hysterectomy for invasive mole (chorioadenoma destruens). From the subsequent course of 181 patients (Table 23-1) followed by Hertig and Sheldon (1947) before the use of chemotherapy it is evident that only a very small percentage of cases developed a lethal malignant tumor, although over a quarter did not initially have an entirely benign course. A sizable pro-

TABLE 23-1.
SUBSEQUENT COURSE OF 181 PATIENTS WITH HYDATIDIFORM MOLE AND NO CHEMOTHERAPY

	PERCENT
1. Initial spontaneous cure	73.5
2. Chorionepithelioma in situ*	3.5
3. Syncytial endometritis†	4.5
4. Chorioadenoma destruens	16.0
5. Choriocarcinoma	2.5
Total	100.0

* Chorionepithelioma in situ: a term introduced by Hertig and Sheldon to describe a small, discrete mass of superficially invasive, apparently malignant trophoblast without villi found in uterine curettings in association with pregnancy, usually of molar type.
† Syncytial endometritis: a term that most pathologists agree refers to an accentuation of the morphologic features of the placental site. Endometrium and myometrium are infiltrated by trophoblastic cells with varying degrees of inflammation, but the lesion is clinically benign (Hertig and Mansell).

portion regressed spontaneously or were cured by relatively simple procedures, such as dilatation and curettage. It is precisely this spectrum of lesions, ranging from completely benign to highly malignant, with a rather unpredictable intermediate group, that has produced dilemmas in diagnosis unmatched by any other tumor.

Curry and co-workers (1975) identified persistent chorionic gonadotropin-secreting trophoblast that was either malignant or had the potential to become malignant in 20 percent of 347 cases of hydatidiform mole. In 4 percent of these, metastatic disease was apparent. Goldstein (1974), and others, have noted a similar frequency of trophoblast that persisted for many weeks after evacuation of a mole until treatment with chemotherapy was carried out.

Treatment. The treatment of hydatidiform mole consists of two phases, the immediate evacuation of the mole and the later follow-up for detection of malignant change.

TERMINATION OF MOLAR PREGNANCY. Perhaps because of greater awareness, and certainly because of better technics for diagnosis, especially sonography, moles now are terminated more often under controlled circumstances rather than the chaos commonly associated with their spontaneous abortion. Usually there is time for adequate evaluation of the woman with a mole, who may be anemic, hypertensive, fluid-depleted, or show any combination of these.

PROPHYLACTIC CHEMOTHERAPY. Chemotherapy initiated before evacuating the mole has been recommended by some investigators but questioned by others. The merit of prophylactic chemotherapy, especially before evacuation, is questioned because of the complications that are induced by or that accompany evacuation of a mole. These include hemorrhage, uterine perforation, and infection. At times, evacuation initiated vaginally eventuates in hysterectomy. In these circumstances, the chemotherapeutic agents may contribute to morbidity and even mortality. It is much safer to withhold their use at least until after the immediate effects of any surgery have subsided.

Goldstein (1974) evaluated extensively the administration of actinomycin D, 12 µg per kg per day, started 2 to 3 days before evacuation usually by suction curettage. Trophoblastic disease persisted in only two of 100 women so treated, whereas 16 of a control group of 100 demonstrated persistent trophoblast. Nevertheless, Goldstein (1974) questioned the wisdom and necessity of administering a potent oncolytic agent to women who, in the great majority of instances, will have a benign course subsequent to evacuation. The minority of women with persistent trophoblast may then be treated chemotherapeutically quite successfully. Moreover, since there is failure of prophylactic chemotherapy, albeit infrequent, it is essential that women treated prophylactically be followed just as closely as if they had not been treated. Curry and associates (1975) concurred with Goldstein that the benefits from prophylactic chemotherapy so administered to women with hydatidiform moles do not justify the additional risks. They noted two deaths caused by toxicity from prophylactic chemotherapy.

VACUUM ASPIRATION. At least 2, and preferably 4, units of compatible whole blood are made ready and an intravenous infusion system is established suitable for rapid infusion of blood. Unless the cervix is long, very firm, and closed, which is very unlikely, dilatation can be safely accomplished under general anesthesia to a diameter sufficient to allow insertion of a large plastic suction curet. Anesthetic agents that relax the uterus, such as halothane (Fluothane), should be avoided. Throughout the procedure, oxytocin is infused intravenously to contract the body of the uterus. This decreases bleeding from the implantation site and, as the myometrium retracts, thickens the uterine wall, and thereby reduces the risk of perforating the uterus.

After the great bulk of the mole has been removed by aspiration and the myometrium has contracted and retracted, thorough *but gentle* curettage with a large sharp curet is usually performed. The tissue obtained by sharp curettage should be so labeled and submitted separately for careful histologic examination. This specimen may allow a better assessment of the malignant predisposition of the trophoblast and the subsequent biologic behavior of any tissue that persists in the uterus. Care must be taken neither to perforate the uterus nor to scrape so vigorously with the sharp curet as to invade deeply the myometrium and thereby weaken it. Facilities and personnel for immediate laparotomy are mandatory in case there is uncontrollable hemorrhage or serious trauma to the uterus.

OXYTOCIN, PROSTAGLANDIN, AND HYPERTONIC SALINE. Use of oxytocin without suction curettage to expel a large mole may prove unsatisfactory because either the uterus is not sufficiently stimulated to contract effectively, or, more likely, during the time that the cervix is dilating and the mole is being extruded, hemorrhage becomes profuse. Prostaglandin E₂ has been used rather than oxytocin (Filshie, 1971), but the same criticisms very likely apply to both agents. Intrauterine instillation of hypertonic saline is mentioned only to condemn its use.

HYSTEROTOMY. If suction curettage is not used to evacuate the large mole which is palpable well above the symphysis and the uterus is to be conserved, *hysterotomy* is the safest alternative. The incision should be large enough to evacuate the mole promptly but no larger. Oxytocin is infused and, after evacuating the mole, sharp curettage is performed through the incision.

HYSTERECTOMY. If the parity of the woman or her age is such that no further pregnancies are desired, *hysterectomy* may be preferred to suction curettage. Hysterectomy is a logical procedure in women of 40 or over, regardless of parity, and in women with three or more children, regardless of age, because of the frequency with which choriocarcinoma ensues in these age and parity groups. While hysterectomy does not eliminate metastatic trophoblastic disease, it does reduce appreciably the likelihood of such developing subsequently.

In 69 cases of hydatidiform mole, reported by Chun and her associates (1964), in which initial hysterectomy was performed because of advanced age or parity, two women developed choriocarcinoma 2½ to 3 years later, an incidence of 2.8 percent. In contrast, in 166 cases treated by evacuation of the molar tissue with conservation of the uterus, 14 women subsequently developed choriocarcinoma, a frequency of 8.4 percent. In any event, hysterectomy does not eliminate the necessity for careful follow-up. At laparotomy, it should be kept in mind that the ovaries often contain multiple theca-lutein cysts which need not be removed.

Follow-up Procedures. If the following extremely important procedures are not adhered to carefully, some women will die needlessly of choriocarcinoma. The prime objective of follow-up is prompt detection of any change suggestive of trophoblastic malignancy. To do so, it is necessary to rely on the chorionic gonadotropin values to detect persistent trophoblast. For this purpose, the test must be sufficiently sensitive and specific to detect very low levels of chorionic gonadotropin (Schreiber et al., 1976). Ordinary pregnancy tests are seldom satisfactory for this purpose.

Chorionic gonadotropin levels should fall progressively to undetectable levels; otherwise viable trophoblast probably persists. An increase signifies proliferation of trophoblast that is most likely malignant unless the woman is again pregnant. Estrogen-progestin contraceptives, therefore, have been used widely to prevent a subsequent pregnancy and to suppress pituitary luteinizing hormone that cross-reacts with many tests for chorionic gonadotropin. Stone and co-workers (1976), however, observed that the need for chemotherapy for trophoblastic tumor was increased significantly among women who took oral contraceptives starting shortly after evacuation of a hydatidiform mole. Moreover, oral contraceptives were found to delay the fall in chorionic gonadotropin excretion in women who did not require treatment with chemotherapy.

An initial roentgenogram of the chest should be obtained during the first examination of the woman to serve as a base line should future roentgenologic studies become necessary.

Although spontaneous disappearance of retained trophoblast is well known, the effectiveness of chemotherapeutic agents in the treatment of choriocarcinoma has led to the use of these drugs in women with retained molar trophoblast to preclude the development of choriocarcinoma and to hasten the disappearance of the retained trophoblast. Since chemotherapeutic agents, such as methotrexate, are highly toxic and potentially lethal, the risk of chemotherapy must be weighed carefully against the chances of spontaneous regression.

TREATMENT OF PERSISTENT TROPHOBLAST. If the level of circulating chorionic gonadotropin has plateaued or is rising, but there is no evidence of disease beyond the uterus, curettage, or hysterectomy, especially if the uterus is not important for future reproduction, will effect a cure in some cases, i.e., chorionic gonadotropin will disappear and the woman will remain well. If, however, the uterus is to be preserved or if there is roentgenographic evidence of lung lesions, chemotherapy is probably best started at this time with or without curettage. Therapy with methotrexate, and more recently actinomycin D, singly or in combination with other tumoricidal agents as described below, most often has been successful in these circumstances. Very small amounts of viable trophoblastic tumor can be detected by assaying for the β-subunit of chorionic gonadotropin. The observations of Jones, Lewis, and Lehr (1975) are strongly suggestive that once β-subunit activity disappears, therapy can be stopped safely without the likelihood of recurrence. Treatment is best carried out in centers by highly interested and experienced individuals with all facilities for monitoring precisely chorionic gonadotropin levels as well as bone marrow, hepatic, and renal function.

The general method of follow-up at the New England Trophoblastic Disease Center of women after evacuation of a hydatidiform mole is as follows:

1. Prevent pregnancy during the follow-up period.
2. Measure serum chorionic gonadotropin levels weekly using a specific radioimmunoassay.
3. Withhold therapy if the serum levels of chorionic gonadotropin continue to regress.
4. When the level is normal for 3 consecutive weeks, test monthly for 6 months.
5. Follow-up may be discontinued and pregnancy allowed after 6 months of no detectable chorionic gonadotropin.
6. Treatment for trophoblastic disease is instituted whenever the level of chorionic gonadotropin in serum plateaus for more than 2 consecutive weeks, or rises, or if metastases are detected.

During and after treatment the status of the trophoblastic disease is monitored as follows:

1. Prevent pregnancy until cure is established.
2. Measure serum or urine chorionic gonadotropin levels weekly using a specific radioimmunoassay.
3. After the first and any subsequent course of treatment withhold therapy as long as the level of chorionic gonadotropin regresses.
4. When the level is normal for 3 consecutive weeks, test monthly.
5. Follow-up may be discontinued after 12 consecutive months of normal chorionic gonadotropin levels and pregnancy is permissible thereafter.
6. Resume chemotherapy if the chorionic gonadotropin level plateaus for more than 2 weeks, or rises, or if metastases occur. Change the chemotherapy if the serum level plateaus after two consecutive courses or rises during or after a course. With these protocols, the duration of hospitalization, total dose of drug, and toxic side effects have been reduced substantially without loss of effectiveness of chemotherapy (Goldstein et al., 1975).

Walden and Bagshawe (1976) observed that women who develop trophoblastic tumors have, in general, a poor previous obstetric history which is not likely to be made worse by chemotherapy. Neither the trophoblastic neoplasia of itself nor its treatment with methotrexate and actinomycin D appears to exert an adverse effect on subsequent pregnancies (Lewis, 1980).

Choriocarcinoma

Etiology. Except for rare cases arising in teratomas, choriocarcinoma develops during or, very much more often, after some form of pregnancy. Approximately 40 percent of cases occur after hydatidiform mole, 40 percent after an abortion, and 20 percent after a pregnancy with a living fetus. Very rarely, it may coexist with an otherwise apparently normal pregnancy (Jones and Lauersen, 1975), but in most cases it appears to develop immediately afterward. Occasionally, choriocarcinoma subsequent to delivery seems to remain dormant for amazingly long periods before undergoing active growth, although many such reported cases may have resulted from an early unrecognized abortion in the interim.

Choriocarcinoma may result from an ectopic pregnancy as well as an intrauterine pregnancy. Govender and Goldstein (1977) have described the coexistence of an intrauterine pregnancy and a hydatidiform mole involving the oviduct, followed by pulmonary metastases. A similar phenomenon but with both pregnancies in utero has also been observed.

Choriocarcinoma in the mother which metastasized to the fetus has been described (Kruseman et al., 1977; Mercer, 1958). The hydropic stillborn fetus in the latter report appeared to have died as the consequence of severe fetal to maternal hemorrhage.

Pathology. This extremely malignant form of trophoblastic neoplasia may be considered a carcinoma of the chorionic epithelium, although in its growth and metastasis it often behaves like a sarcoma. The factors involved in malignant transformation of the chorion are unknown. In choriocarcinoma, the predisposition of normal trophoblast to invasive growth and erosion of blood vessels is greatly exaggerated. The characteristic gross picture is that of a rapidly growing mass invading both uterine muscle and blood vessels, causing hemorrhage and necrosis. The tumor is dark red or purple and ragged or friable. If it involves the endometrium, bleeding, sloughing, and infection of the surface usually occur early. Masses of tissue buried in the myometrium may extend outward, appearing on the uterus as dark, irregular nodules that eventually penetrate the peritoneum.

Microscopically, columns and sheets of trophoblast penetrate the muscle and blood vessels, sometimes in plexiform arrangement and at other times in complete disorganization, interspersed with clotted blood (Fig. 23-11). An important diagnostic feature of choriocarcinoma, in contrast to hydatid mole or invasive mole, is absence of a villous pattern. Both cytotrophoblast and syncytial elements are involved, although one or the other may predominate. Cellular anaplasia exists in varying and often marked degrees, but is less valuable as a criteron of trophoblastic malignancy than in other tumors. The difficulty of cytologic evaluation is one of the factors leading to error in the diagnosis of choriocarcinoma from examination of uterine curettings. Cells of normal trophoblast at the placental site have been diagnosed erroneously as choriocarcinoma.

Metastases often occur very early and generally are blood-borne because of the affinity of trophoblast for blood vessels. The most common site of metastasis is the lungs (over 75 percent); the second most common is the vagina (about 50 percent). The vulva, kidneys, liver, ovaries, and brain also contain metastases in many cases. Lutein cysts occur in over one-third of the cases.

Clinical History.   Choriocarcinoma may follow hydatid mole, abortion, ectopic pregnancy, or normal pregnancy. Except with moles, there is usually no evidence of malignancy immediately after the pregnancy. The

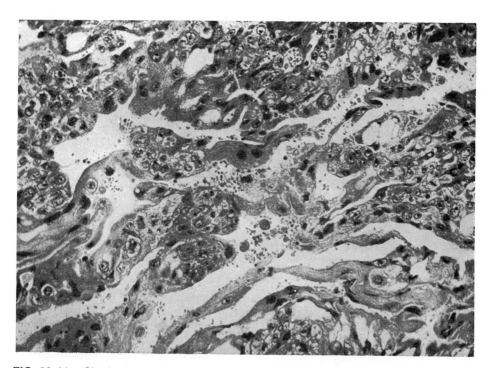

FIG. 23-11.   Choriocarcinoma. Numerous mitoses can be seen in Langhans' cells, mainly surrounded by syncytium, broad bands of which also border the tissue spaces. (From Smalbraak. *Trophoblastic Growths.* Haarlem, Netherlands, Elsevier, 1957)

most common, though not constant, sign is irregular bleeding after the immediate puerperium in assocation with uterine subinvolution. The bleeding may be continuous or intermittent, with sudden and sometimes massive hemorrhages. Perforation of the uterus by the growth may cause intraperitoneal hemorrhage. Extension into the parametrium may cause pain and fixation that is suggestive of inflammatory disease.

In many cases, the first indication of the condition may be the metastatic lesions. Vaginal or vulvar tumors may be found. The woman may complain of cough and may produce bloody sputum arising from pulmonary metastases. In a few cases, it has been impossible to find choriocarcinoma in the uterus or pelvis, the original lesion having disappeared, leaving only distant metastases growing actively.

If unmodified by treatment, the course of choriocarcinoma is rapidly progressive, death occurring usually within a few months to one year in the majority of cases. The most common cause of death is hemorrhage in various locations.

Diagnosis. Recognition of the possibility of the lesion is the most important factor in diagnosis. All cases of hydatidiform mole should be under suspicion and followed as described. Any case of unusual bleeding after term pregnancy or abortion should be investigated by curettage but especially by measurements of chorionic gonadotropin, since absolute reliance cannot be placed on the findings of examination of curettings. Malignant tissue may be buried within the myometrium, inaccessible to the curet.

Solitary or multiple nodules present in a chest x-ray that cannot be otherwise explained are suggestive of the possibility of choriocarcinoma and warrant an assay for chorionic gonadotropin. It should be kept in mind, however, that some nontrophoblastic tumors secrete small amounts of chorionic gonadotropin (Shane and Naftolin, 1975). Persistent or rising titers of gonadotropin in the absence of pregnancy are indicative of trophoblastic neoplasia. Assays, of course,

should be repeated before resorting to radical therapy.

Treatment. Current treatment of choriocarcinoma is radically different from, and more successful than, that of the past. Formerly, the only hope for cure was hysterectomy, or, even more remote, resection of a metastatic lesion. In 1955 Drs. M.C. Li and Roy Hertz successfully treated a woman with a metastatic gestational trophoblastic neoplasm by employing methotrexate (Li and coworkers, 1956). As described below, currently the therapy of choice is methotrexate (4-amino, ^{10}N-methylpteroylglutamic acid), alone or in combination with other agents, especially actinomycin D. Whereas all cells are affected by these drugs, embryonic cells, by virtue of their rapid cellular division and growth, are particularly sensitive. The overall cure rate in recent years for persistent gestational trophoblastic neoplasia of all severities has been about 90 percent (Lewis, 1980). Patients in a "low risk" category, and therefore having a good prognosis, have been cured virtually 100 percent of the time. "Low risk" category is identifed as excreting in urine less than 100,000 IU of hCG per 24 hours, duration of the disease of less than 4 months, and metastases limited to the lung or pelvis. Cure usually has been achieved for "low risk" patients following treatment with a single chemotherapeutic agent. Treatment with a single agent reduces serious treatment toxicity. Fortunately, in those instances in which single agent therapy proved ineffective, prompt treatment with combination chemotherapy most often did prove to be effective.

Patients who may be classified as "high risk" because of their poorer prognosis for cure have been identified. They excreted more than 100,000 IU of hCG per day, had their disease for more than 4 months, and had metastases other than in the lung or pelvis. In this group combination chemotherapy, in spite of increased toxicity, has produced the highest cure rate. Hammond and coworkers (1973) and Jones and Lewis (1974) achieved a complete remission rate of 70 percent and 80 percent in "high risk," or "poor prognosis," patients so treated.

In the past, cerebral metastases proved to be uniformly fatal. High-voltage irradiation, coupled with methotrexate and other chemotherapeutic agents may eradicate such lesions on occasion (Weed and Hammond, 1980). Gurwitt et al. (1975), for example, report an instance of intracranial hemorrhage late in an otherwise apparently normal pregnancy. Postpartum, a nidus of choriocarcinoma, with cerebral hemorrhage, was discovered during craniotomy, and a solitary tumor nodule was identified radiologically in the right lung. Treatment consisted of cerebral radiation and chemotherapy with methotrexate, actinomycin D, and chlorambucil. The woman was alive and apparently healthy 2 years later. The child appeared to be normal.

Invasive Mole

Invasive mole (chorioadenoma destruens) occupies an intermediate position between benign hydatidiform mole and highly malignant choriocarcinoma. The incidence of the condition, like that of choriocarcinoma, is very low.

Diagnosis. The distinguishing features of invasive mole, as compiled by Novak and Seah (1954) are (1) excessive trophoblastic overgrowth and (2) extensive penetration by the trophoblastic elements, including whole villi, into the depths of the myometrium, sometimes to involve the peritoneum or the adjacent parametrium or vaginal vault (Fig. 23-12). Such moles are locally invasive, though generally lacking the pronounced tendency to widespread metastasis that is characteristic of choriocarcinoma. As contrasted with the typically benign hydatidiform mole, in invasive mole, microscopically large fields of trophoblast are usually found, although even entirely benign appearing moles with very little trophoblastic hyperplasia may

exhibit extreme invasiveness, the other feature of this lesion.

Novak and Seah (1954) stressed the fact that invasive mole, in contrast to choriocarcinoma, has a well-preserved villous pattern. They emphasized repeatedly that even a few villi should militate against the diagnosis of choriocarcinoma. In this connection, Tow (1966) suggested new histopathologic terms that deemphasized the importance of the villous pattern or its absence. According to him, invasive mole may best be designated *villous choriocarcinoma,* and choriocarcinoma referred to specifically as *avillous choriocarcinoma.*

In some cases, invasive mole cannot be diagnosed until after hysterectomy, but in others it frequently can be recognized presumptively, or at least suspected, by the occurrence of intraabdominal hemorrhage or by the findings on palpation of parametrial invasion or the demonstration of vaginal extension.

Treatment. Chemotherapy with methotrexate even without hysterectomy usually has brought about a complete remission. However, treatment may require hysterectomy because of uterine perforation by the tumor and massive intraabdominal hemorrhage.

Other Tumors of the Placenta

Angioma of the Placenta. Various angiomatous tumors of the placenta ranging widely in size have been described and because of the resemblance of their components to the blood vessels and stroma of the chorionic villus, the term *chorioangioma* or *choriangioma* is the most appropriate designation. The tumors are most likely hamartomas of primitive chorionic mesenchyme. The small growths are essentially asymptomatic, but the larger tumors may be associated with hydramnios or antepartum hemorrhage. Fetal death and malformations are uncommon complications, although there may be a positive correlation with low birth weight. Severe iron deficiency anemia has been identified in the neonate as the consequence of chronic fetal to maternal hemorrhage associated with multiple small chorioangiomas

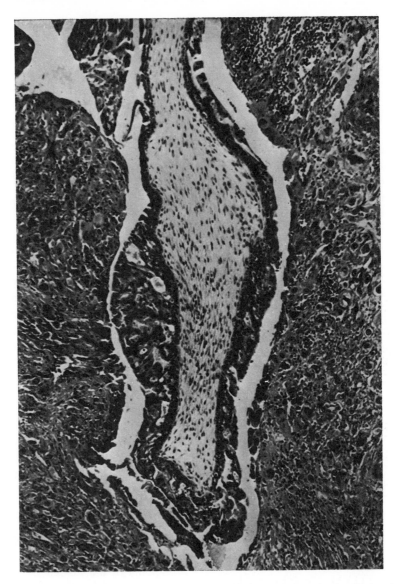

FIG. 23-12. Invasive hydatidiform mole (chorioadenoma destruens), showing molar villus with hyperplastic trophoblast penetrating deeply into myometrium. (Courtesty of Dr. Ralph M. Wynn)

(Cunningham, Pritchard, unpublished). Thrombocytopenia plus microangiopathic hemolytic anemia has been observed in a newborn infant in association with a large, partially infarcted placental chorioangioma (Bauer and associates, 1978).

Tumors Metastatic to the Placenta. Metastases of malignant tumors to the placenta are rare. (Freedman and MacMahon, 1960); (Horner, 1960). Malignant melanoma apparently is the most common, making up nearly one-third of the reported cases, but any tumor with hematogenous spread is theoretically a source of potential placental metastases.

Cysts of the Placenta. Cystic structures are frequently observed on the fetal surface and occasionally in the depths of the placenta. Small cysts a few millimeters in diameter were noted in 56 percent of the placentas studied by Kermauner (1900). Larger lesions, occasionally up to 8 to 10 cm in diameter, are much less common. They exert little or no effect on the course of the pregnancy.

Such cysts are derived from the chorionic membrane, as shown by the fact that the amnion can be stripped readily from them. Their contents are usually colorless and transparent, but sometimes they are bloody or grumous, and then they may be mistaken for abscesses. Histologically, the lining membrane consists of one or more layers of relatively large epithelial cells with round vesicular nuclei, in various stages of degeneration. Part of the wall may appear acellular after the trophoblastic elements, which presumably give rise to the cysts, have been obliterated by fibrinoid degeneration.

ABNORMALITIES OF THE UMBILICAL CORD

Achordia. Browne (1925) described two infants, one stillborn and the other liveborn, in whom the placenta seemed to be attached directly to the fetal abdominal wall.

Abnormalities in Cord Length. Umbilical cord length varies appreciably; the mean length is about 55 to 60 cm but normally may vary from 18 to 120 cm. Walker and Pye (1960) found that boy babies had a slightly longer cord than did girls and that the full cord length was attained by 28 weeks gestation. They also found that the cord was around the neck of the infant in 17 percent of newborns. Extremes in cord length in abnormal instances vary from apparently no cord (achordia) to lengths up to 300 cm. Eastman and Hellman (1961) considered cord length of less than 35 cm to be abnormal. Vascular occlusion by thrombi and true knots are more common in excessively long umbilical cords, and such long cords are more likely to prolapse during labor. Rarely excessively short umbilical cords may be instrumental in abruptio placenta, inversion of the uterus, or intrafunicular hemorrhage which has been described frequently as a cause of fetal death due to exsanguination.

Absence of One Umbilical Artery. Benirschke and Brown (1955) were principally responsible for drawing attention to the association between a single umbilical artery and its frequent association with fetal malformation. The absence of one umbilical artery, according to Benirschke and Dodds (1967), characterized 0.85 percent of all cords in singletons and 5 percent of the cords of at least one twin. A single umbilical artery was found in 2.5 percent of abortuses. About 30 percent of all infants with one umbilical artery missing had associated congenital anomalies.

Bryan and Kohler (1974) identified 143 umbilical cords, or 0.72 percent, to have a single artery out of nearly 20,000 examined. Among the 143 infants, the incidence of major malformations was 18 percent, retarded fetal growth, 34 percent, and prematurity, 17 percent. According to the studies of Froehlich and Fujikura (1973) mortality was high (14 percent) among infants with a single umbilical artery, but of those who survived infancy, serious anomalies were no more common than in the control group. However, Bryan and Kohler (1975) followed 98 infants with a single umbilical artery and found that previously unrecognized malformations became apparent in 10.

In the United States, Peckham and Yerushalmy (1965) clearly demonstrated that a single umbilical artery occurs twice as often in newborns of white women than it does in those of black women. It is also known that the incidence is considerably increased in newborns of women with diabetes mellitus. Based on the finding of an extraordinarily high incidence of fetal malformations when a single umbilical artery exists, it is essential that each umbilical cord be examined carefully in order to ascertain the number of umbilical arteries present.

Abnormalities of Cord Insertion. The umbilical cord usually, but not always, is inserted at or near the center of the fetal surface of the placenta.

MARGINAL INSERTION. Insertion of the cord at the margin of the placenta is sometimes referred to as a *battledore placenta.* Some have found that such insertion was common in instances of premature labor (Brody and Frenkel, 1953); others have not (Fox, 1978).

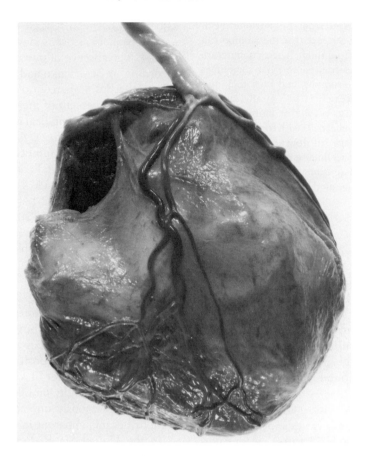

FIG. 23-13. Velamentous insertion of cord. The placenta (bottom) and membranes have been inverted to expose the amnion. Note the large fetal vessels within membranes (top) and their proximity to the site of rupture of the membranes.

VELAMENTOUS INSERTION OF CORD. The so-called velamentous insertion of the cord is of considerable practical importance (Fig. 23-13). In this condition, the vessels of the cord separate in the membranes at a distance from the placental margin, which they reach surrounded only by a fold of amnion. This mode of insertion is noted in a little over 1 percent of singleton deliveries but much more frequently with twins, and it is almost the rule with triplets. With velamentous insertion of the cord the likelihood of fetal anomalies is increased.

These variations of insertion of the cord may be determined at the time of implantation. The body stalk, which later becomes the umbilical cord, attaches the inner cell mass to the chorionic shell (see Fig. 5-20). Since the human zygote implants with the inner cell mass down toward the endometrium, the placenta and body stalk are adjacent. According to one theory, minor degrees of rotation give rise to the usual eccentric location of the cord. The more marked the rotation of the zygote, the farther the umbilical cord will be from the center of the placenta. In that way, progressive rotation produces marginal and velamentous insertions. The theory goes on to explain that when the zygote implants with the inner cell mass 180 degrees from the endometrium, the umbilical cord and placenta come to lie at opposite poles, and all the fetal vessels will be located in the membranes.

VASA PREVIA. When with velamentous insertion some of the fetal vessels in the membranes cross the region of the internal os and present ahead of the presenting part of the fetus, the condition is termed vasa previa. At times, the careful examiner will be able to palpate a tubular fetal vessel in the membranes overlying the presenting part. Compression of the vessels between the examining finger and the presenting part is likely to induce changes in the fetal heart rate. At times, they may be visualized directly by employing amnioscopy.

With vasa previa, there is considerable potential danger to the infant, for rupture of the membranes may be accompanied by rupture of a fetal vessel and lead to exsanguination of the infant (Fig. 23-14).

Whenever there is hemorrhage antepartum or intrapartum, the possibility of vasa previa and a ruptured fetal vessel exists. The rupture of the vessel may occur independent of rupture of the membranes (Carp et al., 1979). Unfortunately, the amount of fetal blood which can be shed without killing the fetus is relatively small compared to the volumes of blood that usually cause concern with antepartum or intrapartum hemorrhage of

maternal origin. Blood can be ascertained to be of fetal origin by demonstrating resistance of hemoglobin to denaturation with alkali or by identifying numerous nucleated red cells in a smear treated with Wright's stain.

Cord Abnormalities Capable of Impeding Blood Flow. Several mechanical and vascular abnormalities of the umbilical cord are capable of impairing fetal–placental blood flow.

KNOTS OF THE CORD. False knots, which result from kinking of the vessels to accommodate to the length of the cord, should be distinguished from true knots, which result from active movements of the fetus. In some 17,000 deliveries in The Collaborative Study on Cerebral Palsy, Spellacy and co-workers (1966) found an incidence of true knots of the umbilical cord of 1.1 percent with a perinatal loss of 6.1 percent in the presence of true knots. The incidence of true knots in the cord is unusually high in monoamnionic twins.

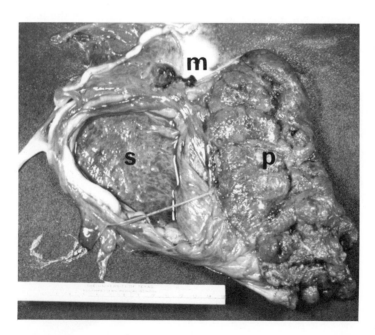

FIG. 23-14. Velamentous insertion of the umbilical cord and ruptured vasa previa with rapidly fatal fetal hemorrhage. Milk injected through the umbilical vein of the cord escaped at the site of the rupture (m = milk; p = maternal surface of placenta; s = site of rupture of fetal membranes through which the fetus was delivered).

LOOPS OF THE CORD. The cord frequently becomes coiled around portions of the fetus, usually the neck. In 1,000 consecutive deliveries studied by Kan and Eastman (1957), the incidence of coiling of the umbilical cord around the fetal neck ranged from one loop in 21 percent to three loops in 0.2 percent of deliveries. Coiling of the cord around the neck is an uncommon cause of fetal death. In monoamnionic twinning, however, a significant fraction of the high perinatal mortality rate is attributed to entwining of the umbilical cords (see Fig. 26-12, p. 653).

TORSION OF THE CORD. As a result of fetal movements, the cord normally becomes twisted. Occasionally, the torsion is so marked that the fetal circulation is compromised. Extreme degrees of torsion probably occur only after the death of the fetus.

STRICTURE OF THE CORD. Most, but not all, infants with cord stricture are stillborns, and it seems that the stricture plays a role in producing fetal death (Fig. 23-15). Cord stricture, for unknown reasons, is associated with an extreme focal deficiency in Wharton's jelly. Stricture is commonly associated, causally, with torsion.

HEMATOMA OF THE CORD. Hematomas occasionally result from the rupture of a varix with subsequent effusion of blood into the cord (Fig. 23-16). Dippel (1940) found hematomas of the cord once in every 5505 deliveries at or near term, and that hemorrhage usually results from rupture of the umbilical vein. He observed that about one-half of the fetuses with hematomas of the cord are stillborn. However, this does not establish a direct causal relationship.

CYSTS OF THE CORD. Cysts occasionally occur along the course of the cord and are designated true and false, according to their origin. True cysts are quite small and may be derived from remnants of the umbilical vesicle or of the allantois. False cysts which may attain considerable size result from liquefaction of Wharton's jelly.

EDEMA OF THE CORD. This condition rarely occurs by itself but is frequently associated with edema of the fetus. It is very common with macerated fetuses.

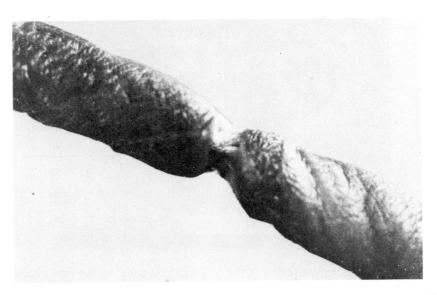

Fig. 23-15. A sharply localized stricture in a cord from a stillborn infant. (From Fox. *Pathology of the Placenta*, Vol. 7. p. 442 Philadelphia, Saunders, 1978)

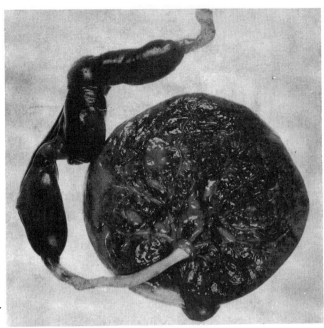

FIG. 23-16. Hematoma of the umbilical cord.

DISEASES OF THE AMNION

Meconium Staining. The brownish-green discoloration from meconium staining is characteristic. The amnion may be slippery from mucus discharged in the meconium. Meconium staining is relatively common; Benirschke (1974) identified it in 13 percent of 2000 consecutive placentas examined. He reported that in the majority of cases no other evidence of fetal distress was identified and the subsequent course of the newborn infant was normal. Fujikura and Klionsky (1975) identified meconium staining of the membranes or fetus in 10.3 percent of 43,000 live-born infants in the Collaborative Study of Cerebral Palsy and Other Disorders. The neonatal mortality rate was 3.3 percent in the stained group compared to 1.7 percent in the nonstained group.

Inflammation of the Amnion. Since amnionitis is a manifestation of an intrauterine infection, it is associated frequently with prolonged rupture of the membranes and long labors. When mononuclear and polymorphonuclear leukocytes infiltrate the chorion, the resulting lesion is properly designated *chorioamnionitis.* Organisms commonly found are those present in the vagina and in maternal feces.

Cysts of the Amnion. Small cysts lined by typical amnionic epithelium are formed occasionally. The common variety results from fusion of amnionic folds, with subsequent retention of fluid.

Amnion Nodosum. These nodules in the amnion are sometimes called *squamous metaplasia* of the amnion or *amnionic caruncles.* They occur most commonly in the amnion in contact with the chorionic plate, but they may also be seen elsewhere. They usually appear near the insertion of the cord as multiple, rounded or oval, opaque elevations that vary from less than 1 to 5 mm in diameter. Bartman and Driscoll (1968) reported an association between amnion nodosum and multiple congenital abnormalities, including hypoplastic kidneys. On the basis of ultrastructural studies, they pointed out the difficulty of deciding whether amnion nodosum arises from a primarily diseased amnion or from the incorporation of shed fetal ectodermal derivatives.

DISORDERS OF THE AMNIONIC FLUID

Hydramnios. Hydramnios, sometimes called *polyhydramnios,* is an excessive quantity of amnionic fluid. Normally, the volume of amnionic fluid increases to about 1 liter, or somewhat more, by 36 weeks, but decreases thereafter. Postterm, there may be only a few hundred ml. Somewhat arbitrarily, more than 2000 ml of amnionic fluid is considered excessive, or hydramnios. In rare instances, the uterus may contain an enormous quantity of fluid, with reports of as much as 15 liters on record. In most instances, the increase in amnionic fluid is gradual, or *chronic hydramnios.* When the volume increases very suddenly, the uterus may become distended immensely within a few days, or *acute hydramnios.* The fluid in hydramnios is usually similar in appearance and composition to the amnionic fluid in normal conditions.

Incidence. Minor degrees of hydramnios, 2 to 3 liters, are rather common, but the more marked grades are not. Because of the difficulty of complete collection of the amnionic fluid, the diagnosis is usually based on clinical impression only. Therefore, the frequency of the diagnosis varies appreciably with different observers. For this reason, the published data on incidence vary widely, ranging from 1 in 62 deliveries, to 1 in 754. Hydramnios sufficient to cause clinical symptoms (generally in excess of 3000 ml of amnionic fluid) probably occurs about once in a thousand pregnancies, exclusive of twins. Acute hydramnios is also rare, occurring once in every 3600 deliveries in the cases reviewed by Buckingham (1960), and once in every 6200 births in the cases studied by Mueller (1948). The incidence of hydramnios is especially high in pregnancies complicated by diabetes and in the hydropic variety of erythroblastosis. Excessive amnionic fluid in one of the amnionic sacs is common in twin pregnancies. Most investigators have observed that hydramnios is more frequent in monozygotic than in dizygotic twinning.

The incidence of hydramnios associated with fetal malformations, especially those of the central nervous system and gastrointestinal tract, is high. For example, hydramnios accompanies about half of cases of anencephalus and nearly all cases of atresia of the esophagus (Scott and Wilson, 1957).

Etiology. The volume of amnionic fluid undoubtedly is controlled in a number of ways. Early in pregnancy, the amnionic cavity is filled with fluid very similar in composition to extracellular fluid. During the first half of pregnancy, transfer of water and other small molecules takes place not only across the amnion but through the fetal skin. Lind and Hytten (1970) considered amnionic fluid to be an extension of the fetal extracellular fluid space during the first half of pregnancy.

During the second trimester, the fetus begins to urinate, to swallow, and to inspire amnionic fluid (Abramovich et al., 1979; Duenhoelter and Pritchard, 1976; Pritchard, 1966). These processes almost certainly have a significant modulating role in the control of amnionic fluid volume. Although the major source of amnionic fluid is assumed to be the amnionic epithelium, no histologic changes in the amnion or chemical changes in the amnionic fluid in cases of hydramnios have been found.

Since the fetus normally swallows amnionic fluid, it has been assumed that this mechanism is one of the ways by which the volume of the fluid is controlled. The theory gains validity by the almost constant presence of hydramnios when swallowing is inhibited as, for example, in cases of atresia of the esophagus. Fetal swallowing is by no means the only mechanism for preventing hydramnios, for both Pritchard (1966) and Abramovich (1970) have measured quantitatively amnionic fluid swallowing and found in some instances of gross hydramnios appreciable volumes of fluid being swallowed.

In cases of anencephalus and spina bifida, increased transudation of fluid from the exposed meninges into the amnionic cavity may be an etiologic factor. Another possible explanation of hydramnios in anencephalus when swallowing is not impaired is excessive urinary excretion brought about by either stimulation of cerebrospinal centers that have been deprived of their protective coverings or possibly the lack of antidiuretic hormone. The converse is well established that fetal defects that cause anuria nearly always are associated with oligohydramnios (Bain and Scott, 1960).

In hydramnios associated with monozygotic twin pregnancy, the hypothesis has been advanced that one fetus usurps the greater part of the circulation common to both twins and develops cardiac hypertrophy, which, in turn, results in increased urine. Naeye and Blanc (1972) have identified in this syndrome dilated renal tubules, enlarged bladder, and an increased urinary output in the early neonatal period, suggesting that increased fetal micturition is responsible for the hydramnios. Conversely, donor members of parabiotic transplacental transfusion pairs had contracted renal tubules with oligohydramnios.

The hydramnios that rather commonly develops with maternal diabetes remains unexplained. Wladimiroff and co-workers (1975) identified sonographically the rate of fetal urine formation in such a case to be in the normal range.

Naeye and Blanc (1972) have also identified hypoplastic lungs commonly in neonates with hydramnios and question their role in the genesis of the hydramnios. The observations of Duenhoelter and Pritchard (1976) on both monkey and human fetuses establish that normal fetal lungs have the potential, at least, for the exchange of relatively large volumes of fluid as the consequence of the inspiration of amnionic fluid. Hypoplastic lungs may conceivably compromise this pathway for removal of amnionic fluid.

The weight of the placenta tends to be high in some cases of hydramnios. The enlarged placenta may contribute to the increase in amnionic fluid. The concentration of prolactin in amnionic fluid is increased compared to that of maternal plasma (Tyson et al., 1974). A role for prolactin in the control of amnionic fluid volume has not yet been clearly established (Josimovich and Merisko, 1975).

Symptoms. The major symptoms accompanying hydramnios arise from purely mechanical causes and result chiefly from the pressure exerted by the overdistended uterus upon adjacent organs. The effects on maternal respiratory functions may be striking. When distension is excessive, the mother may suffer from severe dyspnea and in extreme cases she may be able to breathe only in the upright position. Edema, the consequence of compression of major venous systems by the very large uterus, is common, especially of the lower extremities, the vulva, and the abdominal wall. Rarely, severe oliguria may result from obstruction of the urinary tract by the very large uterus. When the accumulation of fluid takes place gradually, the patient may tolerate the excessive abdominal distension with relatively little discomfort. In acute hydramnios, however, the distension may lead to disturbances sufficiently serious to threaten the life of the mother. Acute hydramnios tends to occur earlier in pregnancy than does the chronic form, often as early as the fourth or fifth month, and it rapidly expands the uterus to enormous size. Pain may be intense and the dyspnea so severe that the patient is unable to lie flat. As a rule, acute hydramnios leads to labor before the 28th week, or the symptoms become so severe that intervention is mandatory. In the majority of cases of chronic hydramnios, the amnionic fluid pressure is not appreciably higher than in normal pregnancy.

Diagnosis. Usually, uterine enlargement in association with difficulty in palpating fetal small parts and in hearing fetal heart tones is the main diagnostic sign of hydramnios. In severe cases, the uterine wall may be so tense that it is impossible to palpate any part of the fetus (Fig. 23-17). Such findings call for immediate sonographic or roentgenologic examination, or both, of the abdo-

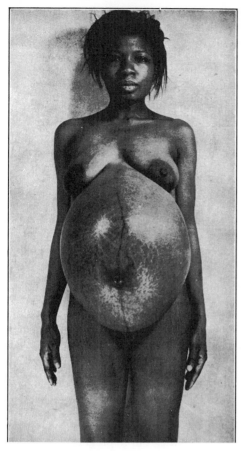

FIG. 23-17. Advanced degree of hydramnios; 5500 ml of amniotic fluid was measured at delivery.

men to identify multiple fetuses or fetal abnormalities. The differentiation between hydramnios, ascites, and a large ovarian cyst can usually be made without difficulty with sonography.

SONOGRAPHY. Large amounts of amnionic fluid can nearly always be readily demonstrated as an abnormally large echo-free space between the fetus and the uterine wall or placenta. At times, a fetal abnormality may also be demonstrated such as anencephaly or a dilated fetal stomach from simultaneous esophageal and duodenal atresia.

RADIOGRAPHY. A large radiolucent area around the fetal skeleton suggests hy-

dramnios, although a soft tissue mass such as a sacrococcygeal tumor may do the same. Most often, anencephaly and other gross skeletal defects are easily diagnosed. Amniography, using a contrast material such as Hypaque, helps identify excess amnionic fluid, soft tissue tumors projecting from the fetus, and the presence or absence of fetal swallowing.

Prognosis. In general, the more severe the hydramnios, the higher is the perinatal mortality rate, so that the outlook for the infant in major degrees of hydramnios is poor. Even though the sonogram and roentgenogram show an apparently normal fetus, the prognosis must be guarded. The incidence of fetal malformations is 20 percent (Queenan and Gadow, 1970). There is a further increase in perinatal mortality from prematurity, since the frequency of premature births in association with hydramnios is more than twice the overall rate. Erythroblastosis, the difficulties encountered by the infants of diabetic mothers, prolapse of the umbilical cord when the membranes rupture, and placental abruption as the uterus decreases in size add still further to the death rate.

The hazards imposed by hydramnios on the mother are significant but can usually be combated without serious threat to her life. The most frequent maternal complications are placental abruption, uterine dysfunction, and postpartum hemorrhage. Premature separation of the placenta sometimes follows escape of massive quantities of amnionic fluid because of the decrease in the area of the emptying uterus beneath the placenta. Uterine dysfunction and postpartum hemorrhage are the result of the uterine atony consequent upon overdistention. Abnormal presentations are more common and operative interference is more frequently required.

Treatment. Minor degrees of hydramnios rarely require treatment. Even moderate degrees of the complication, including cases in which there is some discomfort, can usually be managed without intervention until labor starts or until the membranes rupture spontaneously. If there is dyspnea or abdominal pain, or if ambulation is difficult, hospitalization becomes necessary. There is no satisfactory treatment for symptomatic hydramnios other than removal of some of the excessive amnionic fluid. Bed rest with sedation may make the situation endurable, but it rarely has any effect on the accumulation of fluid. Diuretics and restriction of water and salt are likewise ineffective and potentially dangerous.

AMNIOCENTESIS.   If the discomfort becomes acute as a result of the growing uterine mass, amniocentesis may be performed by abdominal paracentesis. The disadvantages inherent in rupture of the membranes through the cervix are the possibility of prolapse of the cord and of placental abruption. Very slow release of the fluid helps to obviate these dangers but is very difficult to accomplish through the cervical canal, since even a small nick in the membranes is usually quickly converted into a large rent. The slight dangers of abdominal amniocentesis in the presence of hydramnios are puncture of a fetal vessel and bacterial infection. Sonography is not only useful to identify hydramnios and associated fetal anomalies, but to locate the placenta and thereby perform amniocentesis such as to avoid puncturing the placenta. Without sonography, if the abdominal tap is performed slowly, an anterior placenta may possibly be recognized by the appearance of blood from the intervillous space before the chorionic plate has been punctured and a large fetal vessel is damaged. Careful aseptic technic should prevent infection.

The chief purpose of amniocentesis is relief of the mother's distress, and to that end it is eminently successful. At times, amniocentesis appears to initiate labor even though only a part of the fluid is removed; hence, relief of the patient's distress may not enable her to continue with the pregnancy. The volume of fluid removed at one time appears to be critical. Queenan (1970) and Pitkin (1976) have described cases of recurrent severe hydramnios treated by amniocentesis.

Whereas removal of a large volume of fluid at one time during the first pregnancy was soon followed by delivery of a very immature infant that succumbed, repeated amniocenteses with the frequent removal of smaller volumes during the next pregnancy was not, and therefore resulted in delivery of an infant sufficiently mature to survive.

TECHNIC OF AMNIOCENTESIS FOR HYDRAMNIOS.   To remove amnionic fluid from women with hydramnios, a commercially available plastic catheter that tightly covers an 18-gauge needle (Angiocath) may be inserted into the amnionic sac, the needle withdrawn, and an intravenous infusion set connected to the catheter hub. The opposite end of the tubing is dropped into a graduated cylinder placed on the floor, and the rate of flow of amnionic fluid is controlled with the screw clamp so that about 500 ml per hour is withdrawn. After about 1500 to 2000 ml has escaped, the uterus usually has decreased in size sufficiently so that the plastic catheter has pulled out of the amnionic sac and the flow stops. At the same time, maternal relief is dramatic and the danger of placental separation from decompression is very slight. Using strict aseptic technic, this procedure can be repeated as necessary to make the woman comfortable.

Oligohydramnios

In rare instances, the volume of amnionic fluid may fall far below the normal limits and occasionally be reduced to only a few ml of viscid fluid. The cause of this condition is not completely understood. Very small amounts of amnionic fluid may be found with prolonged gestation of several weeks duration. It is practically always present when there is either obstruction of the fetal urinary tract or renal agenesis (Bain and Scott, 1960). Therefore, anuria almost certainly has an etiologic role in such cases of oligohydramnios. A chronic leak from a defect in the membranes may reduce the volume of amnionic fluid somewhat but most often labor soon ensues.

When oligohydramnios occurs early in pregnancy, it is attended by serious consequences to the fetus, since adhesions between the amnion and parts of the fetus may cause serious deformities including amputation. Moreover, subjected to pressure from all sides, the fetus assumes a peculiar appearance, and musculoskeletal deformities, such as clubfoot, are frequently observed. Typically, in cases of oligohydramnios, the skin of the fetus appears dry, leathery, and wrinkled. When amnionic fluid is scant, pulmonary hypoplasia is very common (Bain and Scott, 1960). The possibilities to account for the hypoplasia are (1) an intrinsic lung defect with failure of the lung to excrete fluid essential to maintenance of amnionic fluid volume; (2) compression of the thorax by the uterus in the absence of amnionic fluid, which prevents chest wall excursion and lung expansion; and (3) lack of fluid to be inhaled into the terminal air sacs of the lung and, as a consequence, inhibition of lung growth. The appreciable volumes of amnionic fluid demonstrated by Duenhoelter and Pritchard (1976) to be inhaled by the fetus normally is suggestive of a role for the inspired fluid in expansion and, in turn, the growth of the lung.

REFERENCES

Abramovich DR: Fetal factors influencing the volume and composition of liquor amnii. J Obstet Gynaecol Br Commonw 77:865, 1970

Abramovich DR, Garden A, Jandial L, Page KR: Fetal swallowing and voiding in relation to hydramnios. Obstet Gynecol 54:15, 1979

Bain AD, Scott JS: Renal agenesis and severe urinary tract dysplasia. Br Med J 1:841, 1960

Bartman J, Driscoll SG: Amnion nodosum and hypoplastic cystic kidneys. Obstet Gynecol 32:700, 1968

Baver CR, Fojaco RM, Bancalari E, Fernandez-Rocha L: Microangiopathic hemolytic anemia and thrombocytopenia in a neonate associated with a large placental chorioangioma, Pediatr 62:574, 1978

Benirschke K: Diseases of the placenta. In Gluck L (ed): Modern Perinatal Medicine. Chicago, Year Book, 1974, p 99

Benirschke K, Brown WH: A vascular anomaly of the umbilical cord: the absence of one umbilical artery in the umbilical cords of normal and abnormal fetuses. Obstet Gynecol 6:399, 1955

Benirschke K, Dodds JP: Angiomyxoma of the umbilical cord with atrophy of an umbilical artery. Obstet Gynecol 30:99, 1967

Benirschke K, Driscoll SG (eds): The Pathology of the Human Placenta. New York, Springer-Verlag, 1974

Berkowitz RS, Goldstein DP, Bernstein M: Natural history of partial hydatidiform moles. Lancet 1:719, 1979

Boué J, Philippe E, Giroud A, Boué A: Phenotypic expression of lethal chromosomal anomalies in human abortuses. Teratology 14:3, 1976

Brody S, Frenkel DA: Marginal insertion of the cord and premature labor. Am J Obstet Gynecol 65:1305, 1953

Browne EJ: On the abnormalities of the umbilical cord which may cause antenatal death. J Obstet Gynaecol Br Emp 32:17, 1925

Bryan EM, Kohler HG: The missing umbilical artery. II. Paediatric follow-up. Arch Dis Child 50:714, 1975

Buckingham JC, McElin TW, Bowers VM, McVay J: A clinical study of hydramnios. Obstet Gynecol 15:652, 1960

Carp HJA, Mashiach S, Serr DM: Vasa previa: A major complication and its management. Obstet Gynecol 53:273, 1979

Chun D, Braga C, Chow C., Lok L: Clinical observations on some aspects of hydatidiform moles. Br J Obstet Gynaecol 71:180, 1964

Cunningham FG, Pritchard JA: Unpublished observations

Curry SL, Hammond CB, Tyrey L, Creasman WT, Parker RT: Hydatidiform mole: diagnosis, management, and long-time followup of 347 patients. Obstet Gynecol 45:1, 1975

Delfs E: Hydatidiform mole: an editorial. Obstet Gynecol 45:95, 1975

Dippel AL: Hematomas of the umbilical cord. Surg Gynecol Obstet 70:51, 1940

Donald I: Ultrasonic echo sounding in obstetrical and gynecological diagnosis. Am J Obstet Gynecol 93:935, 1965

Duenhoelter JH, Pritchard JA: Fetal respiration: Quantitative measurements of amnionic fluid inspired near term by human and rhesus fetuses. Am J Obstet Gynecol 125:306, 1976

Earn AA: The effect of a congenital abnormality of the umbilical cord and placenta on the newborn and mother. A survey of 5676 consecutive deliveries. J Obstet Gynaecol Br Emp 58:456, 1951

Eastman NJ, Hellman LM (eds): Williams Obstetrics, 12th ed. New York, Appleton, 1961

Filshie GM: The use of prostaglandin E$_2$ in the management of intrauterine death, missed abortion, and hydatidiform mole. Br J Obstet Gynaecol 78:87, 1971

Fox H: The villous cytotrophoblast as an index of placental ischaemia. Br J Obstet Gynaecol 71:885, 1964

Fox H: The significance of villous syncytial knots in the human placenta. Br J Obstet Gynaecol 72:345, 1965

Fox H: Pathology of the Placenta, Vol. 7, Monograph. Philadelphia, Saunders, 1978

Freedman WL, MacMahon FJ: Placental metastasis: review of the literature and report of a case of metastatic melanoma. Obstet Gynecol 16:550, 1960

Froehlich LA, Fujikura T: Follow-up of infants with single umbilical artery. Pediatrics 52:22, 1973

Fujikura T, Klionsky B: The significance of meconium staining. Am J Obstet Gynecol 121:45, 1975

Girouard DP, Barclay DL, Collins CG: Hyperreactio luteinalis: a review of the literature and report of two cases. Obstet Gynecol 23:513, 1964

Goldstein, DP: Prevention of gestational trophoblastic disease by use of actinomycin D in molar pregnancy. Obstet Gynecol 43:475, 1974

Goldstein DP, Pastorfide GB, Osathanondh R, Kosasa TS: A rapid solid-phase radioimmunoassay specific for human chorionic gonadotropin in gestational trophoblastic disease. Obstet Gynecol 45:527, 1975

Gottschalk W, Abramson D: Placental edema and fetal hydrops: a case of congenital cystic and adenomatoid malformation of the lung. Obstet Gynecol 10:626, 1957

Govender NSK, Goldstein DP: Metastatic tubal mole and coexisting intrauterine pregnancy. Obstet Gynecol 49:675, 1977

Gurwitt LJ, Long JM, Clark RE: Cerebral metastatic choriocarcinoma: a postpartum cause of "stroke." Obstet Gynecol 45:583, 1975

Hammond CB, Borchert LG, Tyrey L, Creasman WT, Parker RT: Treatment of metastatic trophoblastic disease: Good and poor prognosis. Am J Obstet Gynecol 115:451, 1973

Hertig AT, Edmonds HW: Genesis of hydatidiform mole. Arch Pathol 30:260, 1940

Hertig AT, Mansell H: Tumors of the Female Sex Organs: I. Hydatidiform Mole and Choriocarcinoma. Washington, D.C., Armed Forces Institute of Pathology, 1957

Hertig AT, Sheldon WH: Hydatidiform mole: a pathologico-clinical correlation of 200 cases. Am J Obstet Gynecol 53:1, 1947

Hertz R, Bergenstal DM, Lipsett MB, Price EB, Hilbish TF: Chemotherapy of choriocarcinoma and related trophoblastic tumors in women. JAMA 168:845, 1958

Horner EN: Placental metastases. Case report: maternal deaths from ovarian cancer. Obstet Gynecol 15:566, 1960

Jequier AM, Winterton WR: Diagnostic problems of trophoblastic disease in women age 50 or more. Obstet Gynecol 42:378, 1973

Jones WB, Lauersen NH: Hydatidiform mole with coexistent fetus. Am J Obstet Gynecol 122:267, 1975

Jones WB, Lewis JL Jr: Treatment of gestational trophoblastic disease. Am J Obstet Gynecol 120:14, 1974

Jones WB, Lewis JL Jr, Lehr M: Monitor of chemotherapy in gestational trophoblastic neoplasm by radioimmunoassay of the β-subunit of human chorionic gonadotropin. Am J Obstet Gynecol 121:669, 1975

Josimovich J, Merisko K: Prolactin-induced water shifts between amniotic fluid and fetal rhesus. Gynecol Invest 6:6, 1975

Kajii T, Ohama K: Androgenetic origin of hydatidiform mole. Nature 268:633, 1977

Kan PS, Eastman NJ: Coiling of the umbilical cord around the foetal neck. Br J Obstet Gynaecol 64:227, 1957

Kermauner F: Studies of the development of cysts and infarcts of the human placenta. Z Heilk 1:273, 1900

Kleine HO: Über seltene Plazentaformen: Gütelplazenta, Placenta biparita und Placenta fenestrata. Zentralblatt für Gynäkologie, 78:2029, 1956

Kobayashi M, Hellman LM, Cromb E: Atlas of Ultrasonography in Obstetrics and Gynecology. New York, Appleton, 1972

Kruseman AC, Lent MV, Blom AH, Lauw GP: Choriocarcinoma in mother and child, identified by immunoenzyme histochemistry. Am J Clin Pathol 67:279, 1977

Lawler SD, Pickthall VJ, Fisher RA, Povey S, Evans MW, Szulman AE: Genetic studies of complete and partial hydatidiform moles. Lancet 2:580, 1979

Lewis JL, Jr: Treatment of metastatic gestational trophoblastic neoplasms. Am J Obstet Gynecol 136:163, 1980

Lewis J Jr, Ketcham AS, Hertz R: Surgical intervention during chemotherapy of gestational trophoblastic neoplasms. Cancer 19:1517, 1966

Li MC, Hertz R, Spencer DB: Effect of methotrexate therapy upon choriocarcinoma and chorioadenoma. Proc Soc Biol Med 93:361, 1956

Lind T, Hytten FE: Relation of amniotic fluid volume to fetal weight in the first half of pregnancy. Lancet 1:1147, 1970

Marquez-Monter H, Alfaro de la Vega G, Robles M, Bolio-Cicero A: Epidemiology and pathology of hydatidiform mole in the General Hospital of Mexico. Am J Obstet Gynecol 85:856, 1963

Martin PM: II. High frequency of hydatidiform mole in native Alaskans. Int J Gynaecol Obstet 15:395, 1978

Mathieu A: Hydatidiform mole and chorio-epithelioma: collective review of literature for years 1935, 1936, and 1937. Int Abstr Surg 68:52, 181. 1939

Mercer RD, Lammert AC, Anderson R, Hazard JB: Choriocarcinoma in mother and child. JAMA 166:482, 1958

Mueller PF: Acute hydramnios. Am J Obstet Gynecol 56:1069, 1948

Naeye RL, Blanc WA: Fetal renal structure and the genesis of amniotic fluid disorders. Am J Pathol 67:95, 1972

Natsume M, Takada J: Choriocarcinoma: an unusual case recurring nine years after subtotal hysterectomy and followed by spontaneous regression of pulmonary metastases. Am J Obstet Gynecol 82:654, 1961

Novak E: Hydatidiform mole and chorioepithelioma. Am J Surg 76:352, 1948

Novak E, Seah CS: Benign trophoblastic lesions in Mathieu Chorioepithelioma Registry. Am J Obstet Gynecol 68:376, 1954

Novak E, Seah CS: Choriocarcinoma of the uterus. Am J Obstet Gynecol 67:933, 1954

Peckham CH, Yerushalmy J: Aplasia of one umbilical artery: incidence by race and certain obstetric factors. Obstet Gynecol 26:359, 1965

Pitkin RM: Acute polyhydramnios recurrent in successive pregnancies. Obstet Gynecol 48:425, 1976

Pritchard JA: Blood volume changes in pregnancy and the puerperium: IV. Anemia associated with hydatidiform mole. Am J Obstet Gynecol 91:621, 1965

Pritchard JA: Fetal swallowing and amniotic fluid volume. Obstet Gynecol 28:606, 1966

Queenan JT: Recurrent acute polyhydramnios. Am J Obstet Gynecol 106:625, 1970

Queenan JT, Gadow EC: Polyhydramnios: chronic versus acute. Am J Obstet Gynecol 108:349, 1970

Schreiber JR, Rebar RW, Chen H-C, Hodgen GD, Ross GT: Limitation of the specific serum radioimmunoassay for human chorionic gonadotropin in the management of trophoblastic neoplasms. Am J Obstet Gynecol 125:705, 1976

Scott JS, Wilson JK: Hydramnios as an early sign of oesophageal atresia. Lancet 2:569, 1957

Shane JM, Naftalin F: Abberant hormone activity by tumors of gynecologic importance. Am J Obstet Gynecol 121:133, 1975

Smalbraak H: Trophoblastic Growths. Haarlem, Netherlands, Elsevier, 1957

Spellacy WN, Gravem H, Fisch RO: The umbilical cord complications of true knots, nuchal coils and cords around the body. Am J Obstet Gynecol 94:1136, 1966

Stone M, Dent J, Kardana A, Bogshawe KD: Relationship of oral contraception to development of trophoblastic tumour after evacuation of a hydatidiform mole. Br J Obstet Gynaecol 83:913, 1976

Szulman AE, Surti U: The syndromes of hydatidiform mole. Am J Obstet Gynecol 131:665, 1978

Szulman AE, Surti U, Berman M: Patient with partial mole requiring chemotherapy. Lancet 2:1099, 1978

Tindall R, Scott JS: Placenta calcification: a study of 3025 singleton and multiple pregnancies. Br J Obstet Gynaecol 72:356, 1965

Tojo S, Mochizuki M, Kanazawa S: Comparative assay of HCG, HCT, and HCS in molar pregnancy. Acta Obstet Gynecol Scand 53:369, 1974

Torres AH, Pelegrina IA: Transabdominal intrauterine contrast medium injection. Am J Obstet Gynecol 94:936, 1966

Tow WSH: The classification of malignant growths of the chorion. Br J Obstet Gynaecol 73:1000, 1966

Tyson JE, Fielder AJ, Austin KL, Farinholt J: Placental lactogen and prolactin secretion in human pregnancy. In Moghissi KS, Hafez ESE (eds): The Placenta, Biological and Clinical Aspects. Springfield, Ill., Thomas, 1974

Twiggs LB, Morrow CP, Schlaerth JB: Acute pulmonary complications of molar pregnancy. Am J Obstet Gynecol 135:189, 1979

Walden PAM, Bagshawe KD: Reproductive performance of women succesfully treated for gestational trophoblastic tumors. Am J Obstet Gynecol 125:1108, 1976

Walker CW, Pye BG: The length of the human umbilical cord: a statistical report. Br Med J 1:546, 1960

Wallenburg HCS: On the Morphology and Pathogenesis òf Placental Infarcts. Groningen, Netherlands, Drukkerij Van Denderin, 1971

Weed JC Jr, Hammond CB: Cerebral metastatic choriocarcinoma: Intensive therapy and prognosis. Obstet Gynecol 55:89, 1980

Wei P-Y., Ouyang, P-C: Trophoblastic diseases in Taiwan. Am J Obstet Gynecol 85:844, 1963

Wladimiroff JW, Barentsen R, Wallenburg HCS, Drogendijk AC: Fetal urine production in a case of diabetes associated with polyhydramnios. Obstet Gynecol 46:100, 1975

Wu FY: Recurrent hydatidiform mole: a case report of nine consecutive molar pregnancies. Obstet Gynecol 41:200, 1973

Yamashita K, Wake N, Araki K, Makoto K: Human lymphocyte antigen expression in hydatidiform mole: Androgenesis following fertilization by a haploid sperm. Am J Obstet Gynecol 135:597, 1979

Yelverton RW: Maternal mortality due to trophoblastic emboli in benign trophoblastic disease. Report of a case and review of the literature. Presented at the Armed Forces District Meeting of the American College of Obstetricians and Gynecologists. Seattle, Washington, September 1972

Zarou DM, Imbleau Y, Zarou GS: The radiographic diagnosis of molar pregnancy. Obstet Gynecol 35:89, 1970

24

Abortion

Abortion is the termination of pregnancy by any means before the fetus is sufficiently developed to survive. When abortion occurs spontaneously, the term *miscarriage* has been applied by lay persons. Until the decision of the United States Supreme Court (Roe v Wade) in January, 1973, abortion in most states could be performed only to save the life of the mother and was referred to as *therapeutic abortion*. All nontherapeutic, induced abortions, therefore, were *criminal abortions*. Since the Supreme Court decision, *elective* or *voluntary abortion* performed at the request of the woman has emerged as the largest, by far, of the categories of abortion.

The Supreme Court decision voided the abortion statute of the State of Texas, but, nearly all state laws relative to abortion were affected. Moreover, the Court's decision went on explicitly to define the extent to which the States might regulate abortion:

(a) For the stage prior to approximately the end of the first trimester, the abortion decision and its effectuation must be left to the medical judgment of the pregnant woman's attending physician.

(b) For the stage subsequent to approximately the end of the first trimester, the State, in promoting its interest in the health of the mother, may, if it chooses, regulate the abortion procedures in ways that are reasonably related to maternal health.

(c) For the stage subsequent to viability the State, in promoting its interest in the potential of human life, may, if it chooses, regulate, and even proscribe, abortion except where necessary, in appropriate medical judgment, for the preservation of the life or health of the mother.

Viability. The term *viable* is widely used to identify a reasonable potential for subsequent survival if the fetus were to be removed from the uterus. Termination of pregnancy before term but after the fetus has achieved some potential for survival is referred to as preterm delivery of a premature infant. The gestational age at which the fetus upon delivery ceases to be an abortus and becomes an infant is most difficult to define. In many states, a birth certificate is prepared for any pregnancy at 20 weeks gestational age or more, or for any fetus that weighs 500 g or more.

The United States Supreme Court in its ruling on the legality of abortion used the term *viability* but did not define it. Moreover, the Court stated,

We need not resolve the difficult question of when life begins. When those trained in the respective disciplines of medicine, philosophy, and theology are unable to arrive at any consensus, the judiciary, at this point in the development of man's knowledge, is not in a position to speculate as to the answer.

The smallest surviving infant has been considered by some to be the one reported by Munro (1939). The infant was alleged to weigh about 400 g. The precision of measurement of the infant's weight on the village grocer's scales and the duration of gestation, which was said to be "two months premature," are suspect.

At Parkland Memorial Hospital during the course of 160,000 deliveries between 1956 and 1980, the smallest infant to survive weighed 580 g. That twin infant was severely growth retarded when delivered at 28 weeks gestational age because of severe pregnancy-induced hypertension. Of 121,000 pregnancy terminations at King's County Hospital between 1961 and 1972, two infants survived who weighed less than 700 g at birth (Kohl, 1975). The smaller survivor weighed but 540 g. The mother was hypertensive and most likely the infant was more mature than the birth weight suggests.

Infants that weigh 500 to 999 g are sometimes classified as *immature* rather than *premature,* although the degree of immaturity or prematurity ought to be based upon fetal age rather than weight. While weight can be determined quite precisely, the duration of gestation at times cannot. Nonetheless, the likelihood for extrauterine survival of a fetus correlates better with fetal age than with fetal weight. Prematurity and fetal growth retardation are considered especially in Chapter 37.

SPONTANEOUS ABORTION

Incidence. The incidence of spontaneous abortion has commonly been quoted as 10 percent of all pregnancies (Tietze, 1953; United Nations, 1954). This widely quoted figure has been derived from data that had at least two areas of instability, namely, failure to include early and therefore unrecognized abortions and the inclusion of illegally induced abortions that were claimed to be spontaneous.

The incidence of spontaneous abortion is difficult to determine precisely. First, agreement has to be reached as to when pregnancy actually begins. Does penetration of the ovum by a sperm constitute a pregnancy? Does cellular division of the fertilized ovum to form a blastocyst signal the onset of a pregnancy? Or does pregnancy begin with the invasion of the endometrium by the blastocyst? Second, the precision of the techniques that are used to identify a pregnancy are of obvious importance. For example, with the use of a test that can detect minute amounts of human chorionic gonadotropin (hCG), the frequency of abortion will be much higher than if the diagnosis is dependent upon histologic confirmation of shed trophoblast. Roberts and Lowe (1975) have provided cogent arguments to support their hypothesis that at least three fourths of very early pregnancies are aborted spontaneously, although most of the time the state of pregnancy is never identified.

Etiology. In the very early months of pregnancy, spontaneous expulsion of the ovum is nearly always preceded by death of the embryo or fetus. For this reason, etiologic considerations of early abortion involve ascertaining the cause of fetal death. In the subsequent months, on the contrary, the fetus frequently does not die in utero before expulsion and other explanations for its expulsion must be invoked. Fetal death may be caused by abnormalities in the ovum itself or in the generative tract, or by systemic disease of the mother and, rarely perhaps, of the father.

ABNORMAL DEVELOPMENT.   The most common morphologic finding in early spontaneous abortions is an abnormality of development of the embryo, the early fetus, or at times, the placenta. In an analysis of 1,000 spontaneous abortions, Hertig and Sheldon (1943) observed pathologic ("blighted") ova in which the embryo was degenerated

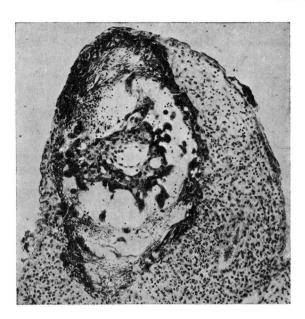

FIG. 24-1. Abnormal ovum. A cross section of a defective ovum showing an empty chorionic sac embedded within a polypoid mass of endometrium. (From Hertig and Rock. *Am J Obstet Gynecol* 47:149, 1944)

or absent in 49 percent (Fig. 24-1), embryos with visible localized anomalies in 3 percent, and placental abnormalities in 10 percent. Importantly, the incidence of morphologically abnormal products of conception among spontaneous abortions decreased remarkably as gestational age increased.

It is now appreciated that chromosomal abnormalities are common among embryos and early fetuses that are aborted spontaneously and account for much of early pregnancy wastage. From several studies it can be estimated that 50 to 60 percent of early spontaneous abortions are associated with a chromosomal anomaly of the conceptus (Boué and Boué, 1978).

Abnormalities in the number of chromosomes are much more common than are structural abnormalities of chromosomes. Structural abnormalities can be transmitted by one of the parents who is a balanced chromosome carrier or can arise de novo. The causes of the numerical errors include anomalous meiotic division of the gamete from either parent, dispermy at the time of fertilization, and abnormalities of early mitotic divisions. With

all of these numerical abnormalities in the chromosomes of the zygote, the parents most often have a normal chromosomal constitution.

Monosomies and trisomies are the most frequent abnormalities of number with most monosomic zygotes being 45, X. The missing chromosome in monosomic zygotes is rarely an autosome, but the extra chromosome in trisomic zygotes is nearly always an autosome. It is apparent from the use of banding technics that in early abortuses trisomies of all autosomes may be found which emphasizes the highly lethal nature of most autosomal trisomies.

Pregnancy destined to abort because of a chromosomally abnormal zygote may, on the one hand, go unrecognized because the products of conception are aborted with little or no delay in the onset of menstruation, or, on the other, may continue for some time after the embryo or early fetus has died. This latter phenomenon accounts for the markedly degenerated or absent embryo or early fetus commonly observed in the studies of Hertig and Sheldon and referred to above.

The age of the gametes, sperm and egg, may influence the spontaneous abortion rate. Guerrero and Rojas (1975) noted an increased incidence of abortion relative to successful pregnancies when insemination occurred 4 days before or 3 days after the time of shift in basal body temperature. They have concluded, therefore, that aging of the gametes within the female genital tract before fertilization increases the chance of abortion. Animal experiments have also shown that aging of spermatozoa and ova before fertilization is accompanied by an increased rate of abortion.

A suboptimal uterine environment, through its effects on implantation and early fetal nutrition, would be expected to lead to a defective conceptus. The appropriate hormonal control of tubal and uterine peristalsis, the multiple endocrine factors associated with appropriate maturation of the endometrium and formation of the decidua, the correct signal to and response of the blastocyst to implantation, and the cellular relation of trophoblast and endometrium must all be integrated to achieve nidation. It is perhaps remarkable that successful implantation occurs as often as it does. Immediately after implantation, furthermore, the trophoblast must obtain nutrition from the decidua and later tap maternal blood vessels, prior to the development of the villous circulation. If any of these mechanisms fail, survival of the ovum is jeopardized and abortion is likely to occur.

Many factors may affect both the intrauterine environment and the embryo. Some are well recognized, such as radiation, viruses, and chemicals. Because they can also produce malformations, these factors are called *teratogens.*

MATERNAL DISEASE. A variety of infectious diseases, chronic wasting diseases, endocrine abnormalities, deformity of the uterus or cervix, and trauma, emotional as well as physical, have been implicated in abortion, although the evidence for such correlations has not always been convincing.

INFECTIONS. Some chronic infections have been suspected of causing abortion. In particular, *Brucella abortus,* well known as a cause of chronic abortion in cattle, has been implicated. Many investigators, particularly Spink (1956), studied this organism and concluded that it has no significance in human abortion. According to some reports, *Listeria monocytogenes* (Rappaport et al., 1960), and Toxoplasma (Ruffolo et al., 1962) may be etiologic agents in abortion, although they appear to be less important in this country than in other parts of the world.

The isolation of *Mycoplasma hominis* and *Ureaplasma urealyticum* (formerly called T mycoplasmas) from the genital tract of some women who have aborted has led to the hypothesis that mycoplasma infections involving the genital tract may be abortifacient. McCormack (1979) has recently emphasized that there have been no properly controlled studies to test this hypothesis. Syphilis was formerly considered to be a common cause of abortion but syphilis rarely, if ever, causes abortion.

CHRONIC DEBILITATING DISEASES. In early pregnancy, chronic wasting diseases such as tuberculosis or carcinomatosis seldom have caused abortion; the patient often died undelivered. In later pregnancy, premature labor is not uncommonly associated with severe systemic maternal illness. Hypertension is seldom associated with abortion, but rather may lead to fetal death and to premature delivery.

ENDOCRINE DEFECTS. Abortion has often been attributed, perhaps without adequate reason, to deficient secretion of progesterone by first the corpus luteum and then the trophoblast. Since progesterone maintains the decidua, its relative deficiency would theoretically interfere with nutrition of the conceptus and thus contribute to its death. Other endocrine organs may possibly be involved in some cases of abortion.

LAPAROTOMY. The trauma of laparotomy may occasionally provoke abortion. In general, the nearer the site of surgery is to the pelvic organs, the more likely is abortion to occur. Ovarian cysts and pedunculated myomas may, however, be removed during pregnancy usually without interfering with the gestation. Peritonitis increases the likelihood of abortion. Postoperative sedation and the administration of progesterone or other progestational agents for the first week or 10 days after operation have been prescribed to diminish the probability of abortion, although the efficacy of these agents remains questionable.

ABNORMALITIES OF THE REPRODUCTIVE ORGANS. Local abnormalities and diseases of the generative tract are infrequent causes of abortion. Adnexal chronic inflammation and tumors of the uterus may result in sterility but rarely, if ever, cause abortion.

Even large and multiple *myomas* of the uterus do not necessarily cause abortion. The location of the myoma is more important in this regard than the size of the tumor. Submucous, but not intramural or subserous, myomas are likely to cause abortion. The only sure way to judge the behavior of a myoma in pregnancy is to allow a clinical test. An important lesion of the generative tract in contributing to abortion is the *incompetent cervix,* discussed further on page 598.

Uncomplicated displacements of the uterus should not cause abortion. Incarceration of *the uterus* in the pelvis, however, may culminate in late abortion unless the uterus is freed from the pelvis (see Chap. 25, p. 633).

PSYCHIC AND PHYSICAL TRAUMA. Both physicians and laymen are inclined to seek a simple explanation for commonplace medical phenomena. They may relate the abortion to a recent fall or blow or perhaps a fright. Multiple examples of trauma that failed to interrupt the pregnancy are forgotten. Only the particular event apparently related temporally to the abortion is remembered. Most spontaneous abortions, however, occur some time after death of the embryo or fetus. If abortion were caused by trauma, it would likely not be a very recent accident but an event that had occurred some weeks before the abortion, as a rule. That the traumatic factor is probably overemphasized is borne out by Hertig and Sheldon's analysis (1943) of 1000 cases of abortion; in only one instance were they willing to ascribe the cause to external trauma and psychic shock.

Pathology. Hemorrhage into the decidua basalis and necrotic changes in the tissues adjacent to the bleeding usually accompany abortion. The ovum becomes detached in part or whole and, presumably acting as a foreign body in the uterus, stimulates uterine contractions that result in expulsion. When the sac is opened, fluid is commonly found surrounding a small macerated fetus, or, alternatively, there may be no visible fetus in the sac, the so-called *blighted ovum.* Visualized through the dissecting microscope, the placental villi often appear thick and distended with fluid, the ends of the villous branches resembling little sausage-shaped sacs. Such fluid-filled villi are undergoing hydatid degeneration with the imbibition of tissue fluid (Chap. 23, p. 560).

Blood or carneous mole is an ovum that is surrounded by a capsule of clotted blood. The capsule is of varying thickness, with degenerated chorionic villi scattered through it. The small, fluid-containing cavity within appears compressed and distorted by the thick walls of old blood clot. This type of specimen is associated with an abortion that occurs rather slowly, so that blood is allowed to collect between the decidua and chorion and to coagulate and form layers.

Tuberous mole and tuberous subchorial hematoma of the decidua are names applied to the same lesion. The characteristic feature is a grossly nodular amnion resulting from its elevation by localized hematomas of varying size between the amnion and the chorionic membrane.

In late abortions occurring after the fetus has attained considerable size, several outcomes are possible. The retained fetus may undergo *maceration.* In such circumstances, the bones of the skull collapse, the abdomen becomes distended with a blood-stained fluid, and the entire fetus takes on a dull reddish color. At the same time, the skin softens and peels off at the slightest touch, leaving behind

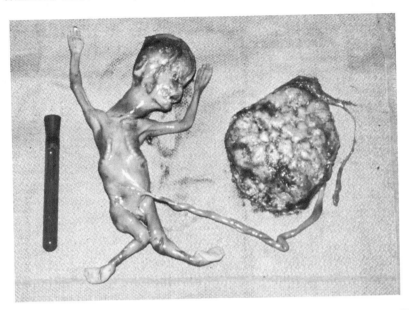

FIG. 24-2. Immature fetus retained dead in utero with placenta for many weeks. Characteristic thick, opaque amnionic fluid is contained in the stoppered tube.

the corium. The internal organs degenerate, becoming friable and losing their capacity for taking up the usual histologic stains. The amnionic fluid may be absorbed when the fetus becomes compressed upon itself and desiccated to form a *fetus compressus* (Fig. 24-2). Occasionally, the fetus becomes so dry and compressed that it resembles parchment, the so-called *fetus papyraceus.* This latter outcome is relatively frequent in twin pregnancy, if one fetus has died at an early period and the other has gone on to full development.

CATEGORIES OF SPONTANEOUS ABORTION

It is convenient to consider the clinical aspects of spontaneous abortion under five subgroups: threatened, inevitable, incomplete, missed, and habitual abortion.

Threatened Abortion. A threatened abortion is presumed when any bloody vaginal discharge or vaginal bleeding appears during the first half of pregnancy. A threatened abortion may or may not be accompanied by mild cramping pain resembling that of a menstrual period or by low backache. This definition of threatened abortion makes it an extremely commonplace occurrence, since one out of four or five pregnant women have vaginal spotting or heavier bleeding during the early months of gestation. Of those women who so bleed in early pregnancy, one-half or less actually abort. The bleeding of threatened abortion is frequently slight, but it may persist for days or weeks. Unfortunately, an increased risk of a suboptimal pregnancy outcome persists (Funderburk et al., 1980). When the discharge consists of old blood, the color is dark brown.

Some bleeding about the time of the expected menses may be physiologic, analogous to the *placental sign* described by Hartman (1929) in the rhesus monkey. In these animals, there is always at least microscopic bleeding. The blood apparently makes its way from ruptured paraplacental blood vessels and eroded uterine epithelium into the uterine cavity. Bleeding begins most commonly 17 days after conception, or about 4½ weeks after the last menses. In many of Hartman's animals, this bleeding could be observed grossly for several days. In the woman, furthermore, lesions of the cervix are likely to bleed in early pregnancy, especially postcoitum. Polyps presenting at the external cervical os as well as decidual reactions of the cervix tend to bleed in early gestation. Lower abdominal pain and persistent low backache usually do not accompany bleeding from these causes.

Since most physicians term all bleeding in early pregnancy threatened abortion, any treatment of so-called threatened abortion achieves a great likelihood of success. Most women who are in fact actually threatening to abort probably progress into the next stage of the process no matter what is done. If, however, the bleeding is attributable to one of the unrelated causes mentioned above, it is likely to disappear, regardless of treatment.

Inevitable Abortion. Inevitability of abortion is signaled by rupture of the membranes in the presence of cervical dilation. Under these conditions, abortion is almost certain. Rarely, a gush of fluid from the uterus occurs during the first half of pregnancy without serious consequence. The fluid may have previously collected between the amnion and chorion to escape with rupture of the chorion while the initial defect in the amnion has healed. Most often, however, either uterine contractions begin promptly, resulting in expulsion of the products of conception, or infection develops.

Incomplete Abortion. The fetus and placenta are likely to be expelled together in abortions occurring before the 10th week, but separately thereafter. When the placenta, in whole or in part, is retained in the uterus, bleeding ensues sooner or later, to produce the main sign of incomplete abortion. With abortions of pregnancies that are more advanced, bleeding is often profuse and may occasionally be massive to the point of producing profound hypovolemia. If the placenta is partly attached and partly separated, the splintlike action of the attached portion of placenta interferes with myometrial contraction in the immediate vicinity. The vessels in the denuded segment of the placental site,

deprived of the constriction by muscle fibers, bleed profusely.

Missed Abortion. A missed abortion refers to the prolonged retention of a fetus who died during the first half of pregnancy. A missed abortion has been defined as the retention of dead products of conception in utero for 8 weeks or more. The rationale for a time period of 8 weeks as the sine qua non for the diagnosis of a missed abortion is not clear. It certainly serves no useful clinical purpose. In the typical instance, early pregnancy is normal, with amenorrhea, nausea and vomiting, breast changes, and growth of the uterus. Upon death of the ovum there may or may not be vaginal bleeding or other symptoms denoting a threatened abortion. For a time, the uterus then seems to remain stationary in size but usually the mammary changes regress. The patient is likely to lose a few pounds in weight. Thereafter, from careful palpation and measurement of the uterus, it becomes apparent that it has not only ceased to enlarge but is becoming smaller, as a result of absorption of amnionic fluid and maceration of the fetus. Many patients have no symptoms during this period except persistent amenorrhea. If the missed abortion terminates spontaneously, and most do, the process of expulsion is quite the same as in any ordinary abortion. The product, if retained several weeks after fetal death, is a shriveled sac containing a greatly macerated embryo (Fig. 24-2).

Occasionally, after prolonged retention of the dead products of conception, serious coagulation defects develop. The patient may note troublesome bleeding from the nose or gums and especially from sites of slight trauma. The pathogenesis and treatment of the coagulation defects and any attendant hemorrhage in instances of prolonged retention of a dead fetus are considered in Chapter 21 (p. 515).

The reason why some abortions do not terminate after death of the fetus, while others do, is not clear. The use of the more potent progestational compounds to treat threatened abortion, however, may lead to missed abortion. For example, Piver and colleagues (1967) treated 57 women for threatened abortion with Depo-Provera (injectable medroxyprogesterone acetate); more than one-third of the women retained a dead fetus for more than 8 weeks. Moreover, Smith and co-workers (1978) observed that 73 percent of women who were given hormonal support because they threatened to abort did abort on the average 20 days later, whereas 67 percent of those who received no hormonal support aborted but on the average 5 days later. They concluded that the progestational agents did not improve the outcome in threatened abortion; instead, the hormones only prolonged the problem by delaying the inevitable.

Habitual Abortion. Repeated spontaneous abortion, its diagnosis, and possible treatment, are considered below.

TREATMENT

Threatened Abortions. Threatened abortions in women who desire the pregnancy will be divided into those with vaginal bleeding and no pain, and those with vaginal bleeding accompanied by pain.

EARLY PREGNANCY BLEEDING WITHOUT PAIN. A patient should be instructed to notify her physician immediately whenever vaginal bleeding occurs during pregnancy. If the bleeding is slight, and no cause is ascertained through careful inspection of the vagina and cervix, she should be so informed. If an intrauterine device is still present and the "string" is visible, the device should be removed for the reasons cited in Chapter 40 (p. 1026).

Although there is no convincing evidence that any treatment regimen favorably influences the course of threatened abortion, most obstetricians have found it wise to restrict the woman's physical activity. Prolonged bed rest is rarely indicated. Coitus should be interdicted during bleeding and perhaps for 2

weeks or so after the bleeding stops. If the bleeding persists, she must be reexamined and the hemoglobin concentration or hematocrit should be rechecked. If blood loss is sufficient to cause anemia, evacuation of the products of conception is generally indicated. If bleeding is so great as to cause hypovolemia, termination of the pregnancy is mandatory.

EARLY PREGNANCY BLEEDING WITH PAIN. Usually, the bleeding of abortion begins first, and cramping abdominal pain follows a few hours to several days later. The pain of abortion may be anterior and clearly rhythmic, simulating mild labor; it may be a persistent low backache, associated with a feeling of pelvic pressure; or it may be a dull, midline, suprasymphyseal discomfort, accompanied by tenderness over the uterus. Whichever form the pain takes, the prognosis for continuation of the pregnancy in the presence of bleeding and pain is poor. However, in some women with pain who threaten to abort the bleeding ceases, the pain resolves, and a normal pregnancy results. It may therefore be reasonable not to intervene to complete the abortion if the woman desires to continue the pregnancy. Little immediate harm should occur, but it is important to remember that the highest perinatal mortality rates are observed in women whose pregnancies were complicated early by threatened abortion.

Each woman should be examined thoroughly, for there is always the possibility that the cervix is already dilated and that abortion is inevitable, or that there is a serious complication such as extrauterine pregnancy or torsion of an unsuspected ovarian cyst. The patient may be kept at home in bed with mild sedation and codeine to relieve pain, but in general, if the symptoms are more severe, she should be hospitalized.

Sometimes women threatened with abortion are treated with progesterone intramuscularly or with a wide variety of synthetic progestational agents orally or intramuscularly. Some of the progestins, particularly those structurally related to testosterone, may result in virilization of the female fetus. Of greater importance is the lack of evidence of effectiveness of progestational agents in preventing most abortions and when "successful," the likelihood is a missed abortion as already described. Even in a group of habitual aborters who excreted low levels of pregnanediol, indicating impaired progesterone production, Goldzieher (1964), in a well-controlled study, could not demonstrate a beneficial effect of exogenous progestational agents.

Occasionally, in threatened abortion, slight hemorrhage may persist for weeks. It then becomes essential to decide whether there is any possibility of continuation of the pregnancy. If two consecutive analyses of blood or urine are negative for chorionic gonadotropin, the outlook is *almost* hopeless. Importantly, the presence of chorionic gonadotropin in blood or urine does not indicate whether the fetus is alive or dead. If the uterus, when accurately measured, does not increase in size, or becomes smaller, it is safe to conclude that the fetus is dead. An increase in uterine size indicates that the fetus is still alive or that a hydatidiform mole is present (see Chap. 23, p. 561).

The demonstration, by sonography, of a distinct, well-formed gestational ring with central echoes from the embryo implies that the products of conception are reasonably healthy. A gestational sac with no central echoes from an embryo or fetus implies, but does not prove, death of the conceptus (Fig. 24-3). When abortion is inevitable, the mean diameter of gestational sac is frequently smaller than appropriate for the gestational age. A single reading is insufficient, however, to determine the likelihood of abortion. Serial sonographic observations to document lack of fetal growth are essential (Kohorn and Kaufman, 1974). Once fetal death is definite, the uterus of 12 weeks size or less should be emptied by curettage as described on page 603. Some women may elect abortion before it is absolutely certain that the fetus is dead, rather than face further uncertainty and procrastination.

Whenever abortion appears imminent, it is wise to hospitalize the patient at once. If bleeding and pain persist unabated for 6 hours, it is probably best to face the inevitability of abortion and either perform a dilation and curettage during the first trimester of pregnancy, or, if more advanced, encourage its completion by injection of oxytocin intravenously in concentrations of 20 to 100 units per liter of lactated Ringer's solution or isotonic saline. Since oxytocin is likely to increase the pain, its administration often necessitates the administration of an effective analgesic. All tissue passed should be carefully studied to determine whether the abortion is complete and to try to ascertain whether the abortion is related to defective germ plasm or to some factor that has caused the uterus to empty itself of a normal ovum. Unless all of the fetus and placenta can be positively identified, curettage is indicated.

Inevitable Abortion. If in early pregnancy the sudden discharge of fluid, suggesting rupture of the membranes, occurs before any pain or bleeding, the patient may be put to bed and observed for further leakage of fluid, bleeding, cramping, or fever. If after 48 hours there has been no further escape of amnionic fluid, no bleeding or pain, and no fever, the patient may get up and, except for any form of vaginal penetration, continue her usual activities. If, however, the gush of fluid is accompanied or followed by bleeding and pain, or if fever ensues, abortion should be considered inevitable. The woman should be hospitalized, and the uterus emptied.

Incomplete Abortion. In instances of incomplete abortion, it is often unnecessary to dilate the cervix before curettage. In many cases, the retained placental tissue simply lies loose in the cervical canal and can be lifted from an exposed external os with ovum or ring forceps. The suction curettage technic, as described subsequently, is an acceptable alternative to sharp curettage for evacuating the uterus, especially if the procedure is to be performed with only local cervical anesthesia and moderate systemic analgesia such as meperidine. A patient with a more ad-

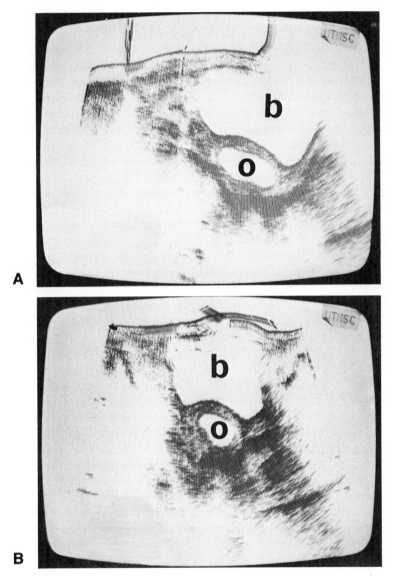

FIG. 24-3. Sonograms demonstrating empty intrauterine gestational sac 16 weeks after the last menstrual period. **A.** Longitudinal scan. **B.** Transverse scan. (O= blighted ovum; b= full bladder) Courtesy of Dr. R. Santos.

vanced pregnancy or who is actively bleeding should be hospitalized, blood-matched for transfusion, and the retained tissue removed without delay. Hemorrhage from incomplete abortion is occasionally severe but rarely fatal. Treatment of such hemorrhage is described in Chapter 21, page 490. Fever is not a contraindication to curettage once appropriate antibiotic treatment has been started (see Septic Abortion, p. 613).

Missed Abortion. Because of the risks involved in terminating by dilatation and curettage a missed abortion in which the fetus did not die until well after the first trimester, the treatment formerly was expectant. This method of management is emotionally trying for the woman and her relatives. Moreover, procrastination sometimes leads to coagulation defects (see Chap. 21, p. 515). Other technics for evacuating the fetus and placenta after the first trimester are described in Chapter 21 (p. 518) and below.

Habitual Spontaneous Abortion.

Habitual spontaneous abortion has been defined by various criteria of number and sequence, but probably the most generally accepted definition today refers to three or more consecutive spontaneous abortions.

ETIOLOGY. Repeated spontaneous abortion is more than likely a chance phenomenon in the majority of cases. Support for this view is provided by the observation that in the past the employment of any of a great variety of unrelated but presumed therapeutic modalities was followed by a successful pregnancy outcome 70 to 90 percent of the time.

It is important to try to differentiate spontaneous abortions that result from problems within the zygote from the much less common abortions that are due to maternal factors. Poland and Yuen (1978) have emphasized that in early abortions there is likely to be a usually nonrecurring cytogenetic abnormality of the conceptus which is responsible for the abortion whereas in late abortions fetal development is likely to have been normal with a maternal abnormality causing the abortion.

Boué and Boué (1978) have also pointed out that after the first trimester the frequency of fetal chromosomal anomalies is low for pregnancies that have aborted nonmalformed fetuses appropriate in size for the gestational age. These abortions most often are due to maternal causes, and there is an increased likelihood of a similar abortion, or premature birth, in a subsequent pregnancy. They have described the mean incidence of spontaneous abortion for all known pregnancies to be 15 percent. According to their observation, when the first pregnancy is a spontaneous abortion, the likelihood of the next pregnancy culminating in a spontaneous abortion is 15 percent, irrespective of the karyotype of the first abortus. If, however, the woman had previously given birth to a normal offspring, and with the next pregnancy expelled an abortus with an abnormal karyotype, the risk of spontaneous abortion with the subsequent pregnancy was only 7 percent, compared to a risk of 24 percent if the karyotype of the previous abortus was normal! The explanation for this somewhat unexpected observation is that chromosomal abnormalities in the aborted embryo or fetus were more likely to have been a chance, nonrecurring event due to abnormal meiosis, early mitosis, or dispermy, as described above. When the aborted fetus was chromosomally normal, however, the abortion was more likely to have been the consequence of an abnormality in the mother which was likely to persist into the next pregnancy, except for those women who had given birth to a normal child.

Boué and Boué (1978) recommend karyotyping the parents after they have experienced three spontaneous abortions; Luthy and colleagues (1979) suggest this be done after two spontaneous abortions. When karyotyping is performed, chromosomal banding technics should be applied. Mennuti and co-workers (1978), using banding technics, identified chromosomal balanced translocations in 5 partners from 34 couples studied because of two or more previous reproductive losses. They also identified the frequency of balanced translocation in one of the partners of couples who had suffered excessive pregnancy wastage to range from 6 percent (3 out of 50) to 25 percent (7 out of 28) and to average 10.4 percent (29 out of 278). However, Neu and co-workers (1979) identified but 1 of 32 women who had aborted three or more times to be a balanced translocation carrier and none of the 30 male partners to be so afflicted.

Some of the proposed, but not necessarily proven, maternal causes of spontaneous habitual abortion are considered below:

1. *Hormonal Abnormalities.* It has been suggested that there might be abnormal levels of one or more hormones to forecast abortion or even serve as therapeutic guides. Today, however, it is believed that even though the values may be low or may fail to rise, the levels of chorionic gonadotropin, placental lactogen, progesterone, es-

trogens, and thyroid hormone are not of great clinical utility in predicting the outcome of a particular pregnancy or of any value in determing hormonal replacement therapy. Reduced levels of these hormones usually are the consequence of irreversible damage to the fetoplacental unit.

2. *Nutritional Factors.* At this time, it appears most likely that only very severe general malnutrition predisposes to increased likelihood of abortion. There is no conclusive evidence, however, that dietary deficiency of any one nutrient or moderate deficiency of all nutrients is an important cause of abortion. The nausea and vomiting that develop rather commonly during early pregnancy, and any inanition so induced, rarely are followed by spontaneous abortion. In fact, the reverse is more likely to be true (see Chap. 13, p. 323).

3. *Infection.* Some chronic infections that involve the reproductive tract, the conceptus, or both, have been suspected of causing abortion, including those caused by species of *Mycoplasma, Brucella abortus, Listeria monocytogenes,* and *Toxoplasma gondii.* Their role, if any, in repeated abortion, has not been established.

4. *Incompatible Blood Groups.* Although maternal isoimmunization and subsequent fetal-maternal Rh incompatibility may cause stillbirth from erythroblastosis, these events only occasionally lead to late abortion. A statistical approach, in which the frequency of abortions and fetal deaths in each ABO mating group was recorded, has shown an increase, of questionable significance, in the frequency of abortions among ABO-incompatible matings.

5. *Psychiatric.* In a review of personality factors associated with habitual abortion, Tupper and Weil (1962) found that there were two types: the basically immature woman and the independent, frustrated woman. Results suggest that supportive therapy is as effective—or as ineffective—as anything else in preventing subsequent pregnancy loss.

6. *Anatomic Uterine Defects.* In a series of women studied at the Johns Hopkins Hospital, it appeared that about one of every four women with a double uterus would have serious reproductive problems (Jones and Jones, 1953). That 75 percent of women with a double uterus have no serious problem emphasizes the necessity for making certain that the anomaly was indeed the causative factor. The diagnosis and treatment of uterine anomalies are discussed in Chapter 25, page 629.

Uterine myomas can be regarded as the etiologic factor in abortion only if the remainder of the clinical investigation, including evaluation of the abortus, is negative and the hysterogram demonstrates a true deformity of the endometrial cavity. Myomectomy to remove an offending submucous myoma may weaken the uterus to the extent that rupture may ensue during a subsequent pregnancy, especially with labor.

7. *The Incompetent Cervix.* The term *incompetent cervix* is applied to a rather discrete obstetric entity characterized by painless dilatation of the cervix in the second trimester or early in the third trimester of pregnancy, followed by rupture of the membranes and subsequent expulsion of a fetus that is so immature that it almost always succumbs. This same sequence of events tends to repeat itself in each pregnancy. Thus the presumptive diagnosis can usually be made if a woman gives a history of spontaneous rupture of membranes not associated with pain very early in the third trimester or earlier in successive gestations.

Although the cause of cervical incompetence is obscure, previous trauma to the cervix, especially in the course of a dilatation and curettage, amputation, conization, or cauterization, appears to be a factor in many cases. In other instances, abnormal cervical development may play a role. However, the fact that the occurrence of cervical incompetence is rare in primigravidas who have had no cervical operations points strongly to trauma as the most common cause of this entity.

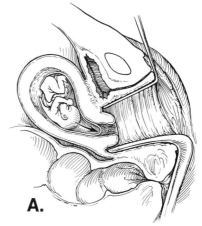

FIG. 24-4. Incompetent cervix treated by McDonald cerclage procedure. **A.** Somewhat dilated cervical canal and beginning prolapse of membranes (arrow). **B.** Start of the cerclage procedure with a suture of number 2 proline being placed superiorly in the body of the cervix very near the level of the internal os. **C.** Continuation of the placement of the suture in the body of the cervix so as to encircle the os *(Continued).*

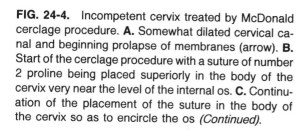

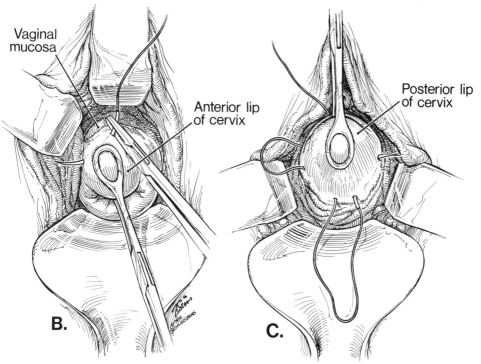

The cervical dilatation characteristic of this condition rarely becomes prominent before the 16th week, since before that time the products of conception are not sufficiently large to efface and dilate the cervix except when there are painful uterine contractions. Abortion from incompetence of the cervix is an entirely different and distinct entity from spontaneous abortion in the first trimester, since it results from different factors, presents a different clinical picture, and requires different management. Whereas spontaneous abortion in the first trimester is an extremely common complication of pregnancy, incompetence of the cervix is relatively rare.

Treatment of Incompetent Cervix. If other causes of habitual abortion in midpregnancy can be excluded, the treatment of the apparently incompetent cervix is surgical.

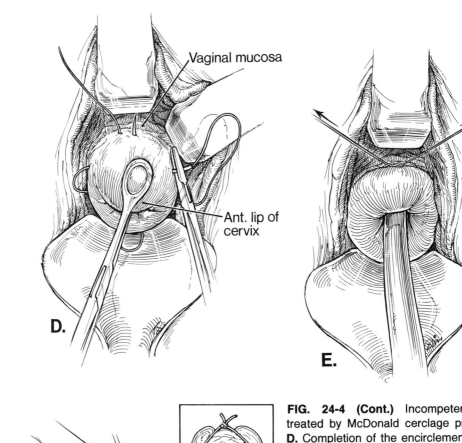

Vaginal mucosa

Ant. lip of cervix

D.

E.

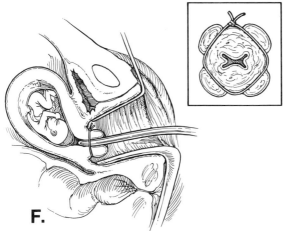

F.

FIG. 24-4 (Cont.) Incompetent cervix treated by McDonald cerclage procedure. **D.** Completion of the encirclement. **E.** The suture is tightened around the cervical canal sufficiently to reduce the diameter of the canal to a few mm and is then securely tied. In the illustration a *small* dilator has been placed just through the level of ligation to maintain patency of the canal when the suture is tied. **F.** The effect of the suture placement on the cervical canal is apparent.

The surgical treatment consists of reinforcing the weak cervix by some kind of pursestring suture. It is best performed after the first trimester but before a cervical dilatation of 4 cm is reached, if possible. Bleeding and uterine cramping are contraindications to surgery.

CERCLAGE PROCEDURES. Two main types of operation are in current use during pregnancy. One is a very simple procedure, as recommended by McDonald (1963) and illustrated in Figure 24-4. The other is the more complicated Shirodkar operation (1955). There is likely to be much less trauma and blood loss with the McDonald procedure during placement of the suture than with the Shirodkar procedure. Moreover, there is less scarring of the cervix and less likelihood of cervical dystocia with the McDonald procedure.

Success rates approaching 85 to 90 percent are being achieved with both the McDonald and the Shirodkar technics (Kuhn and Pepperell, 1977). In the event that the operation fails and signs of imminent abortion develop, it is urgent that the suture be released at once, since failure to do so promptly may result in grave sequelae. Rupture of the uterus or the cervix may be the consequence of vigorous uterine contractions with the ligature in place. If the membranes rupture in the absence of labor, the likelihood of serious infection in the fetus or the mother is increased appreciably if the suture is left in situ and delivery is delayed (Kuhn and Pepperell, 1977). Following the Shirodkar operation the suture can be left in place if it remains covered by mucosa, and cesarean section can be performed near term (a plan designed to prevent the necessity of repeating the procedure in subsequent pregnancies). Otherwise, the Shirodkar suture is released and vaginal delivery is permitted.

For the woman with a typical history of repeated abortions caused by an incompetent cervix, Lash and Lash (1950) devised an operation to be performed when she is not pregnant. The mucosa is dissected from the anterior lip of the cervix, and an elliptical incision is made in the anterior lip between the internal and external os. A small amount of tissue is removed and the defect closed with interrupted sutures. Subsequent infertility has been a complication of this procedure. We do not use the procedure.

Prognosis. With the exception of the incompetent cervix, the apparent cure rate after three abortions will range between 70 and 85 percent no matter what treatment is used, unless the treatment is abortifacient. In other words, the loss rate will be higher, but not a great deal higher, than that anticipated for pregnancies in general.

There is no evidence that the woman who has habitually aborted spontaneously is at greatly increased risk, when she finally carries her pregnancy to term, of having an abnormal child.

THERAPEUTIC ABORTION

A definition of therapeutic abortion that would appear to be acceptable to the majority of individuals, as well as being medically rational, follows: Therapeutic abortion is *the termination of pregnancy before the time of fetal viability for the purpose of safeguarding the health of the mother.*

Legal Aspects. Until the United States Supreme Court decision of 1973, only therapeutic abortions could be legally performed in most states. The most common legal definition of therapeutic abortion until then was termination of pregnancy before the period of fetal viability for the purpose of saving the *life* of the mother. Not too long before the Supreme Court decision, a few states extended the law to read "to prevent serious or permanent bodily injury to the mother" or "to preserve the life or health of the woman." A very few states allowed abortion if the pregnancy otherwise was likely to result in the birth of an infant with grave malformation.

Contrary to popular belief, the stringent abortion laws that were in effect were of fairly recent origin. Abortion before quickening (the term applied to the first definite perception of fetal movement, which most often occurs between 16 and 20 weeks of gestation), was either lawful or widely tolerated in both the United States and Great Britain until 1803. In that year, as part of a general restructuring of British criminal law, a basic criminal abortion statute was enacted that made abortion before quickening illegal. The Roman Catholic Church's traditional condemnation of abortion did not receive the ultimate sanction of universal law (excommunication) until 1869 (Pilpel and Norwick, 1969).

The British law of 1803 became the model for similar laws in the United States, but it was not until 1821 that Connecticut enacted the nation's first abortion law. Subsequently, throughout the nation abortion became illegal except to save the life of the mother. Since therapeutic abortion *to save the life of the woman* is rarely necessary or definable, it follows that the great majority of such operations previously performed in this country went beyond the letter of the law.

Indications.   Some of the indications for therapeutic abortion are discussed with the diseases that commonly have lead to the operation. A well-documented indication is heart disease in the wake of previous cardiac decompensation (p. 734). Another commonly accepted indication is advanced hypertensive vascular disease (p. 695). Still another is invasive carcinoma of the cervix (p. 626). While it is impossible to predict what the future acceptable indications for therapeutic abortion will be, the therapeutic abortion policy formerly established by the American College of Obstetricians and Gynecologists seems most rational:

Therapeutic abortion may be performed for the following medical indications:

1. When continuation of the pregnancy may threaten the life of the woman or seriously impair her health. In determining whether or not there is such risk to health, account may be taken of the woman's total environment, actual or reasonably foreseeable.
2. When pregnancy has resulted from rape or incest: In this case the same medical criteria should be employed in the evaluation of the patient.
3. When continuation of the pregnancy is likely to result in the birth of a child with grave physical deformities or mental retardation.

Public opinion will not likely tolerate disregard of women with unwanted pregnancies although the Right to Life movement is proving to be more vigorous than some had anticipated.

ELECTIVE (VOLUNTARY) ABORTION

Elective or voluntary abortion is the interruption of pregnancy before viability at the request of the woman but not for reasons of maternal health or fetal disease. The great majority of abortions now being done belong in this category. In 1977 1,300,000 elective abortions were performed in the United States (Table 24-1).

Counseling Before Elective Abortion.   Knowledge of the risks from abortion compared to the risks from allowing a pregnancy to continue is essential for appropriate counseling of the woman who desires an abortion. Unfortunately, all the risks, immediate and remote, imposed by the various technics for abortion in current use have not yet been appropriately quantified. Nonetheless, there are risks. Most every issue of every general medical journal, as well as obstetric and gynecologic journals, contains a report of yet another modification of technic for abortion, attesting thereby to the need for simpler, safer, and less expensive technics, especially for pregnancies beyond the first trimester.

In some instances, the pregnant woman may well want to avoid abortion and allow the pregnancy to continue if social and economic problems can be resolved. Especially in these circumstances, knowledgeable, compassionate counselors are of great value. In any event, because of the risks of abortion, both immediate and remote, counseling

TABLE 24-1.
ABORTIONS PERFORMED IN UNITED STATES, 1973–1977

	1973	1974	1975	1976	1977
No. of Abortions (millions)	0.74	0.90	1.0	1.2	1.3
% of all pregnancies	19	22	25	27	28
Rate of abortions per 1,000 women aged 15–44	17	20	22	25	26

From Forrest, Tietze, and Sullivan: *Fam Plan Perspect* 10:271, 1978.

should be an attempt to promote either early interruption of the pregnancy or the completion of the pregnancy, rather than procrastination until well beyond the first trimester and then abortion.

TECHNICS FOR ABORTION

The various technics for performing abortion currently in use are outlined and discussed below.

TECHNICS FOR ACCOMPLISHING ABORTION

I. *Surgical*
   A. Cervical dilatation and mechanical evacuation
      1. Curettage
      2. Vacuum aspiration (suction curettage)
   B. Laparotomy
      1. Hysterotomy
      2. Hysterectomy
II. *Medical*
   A. Oxytocin intravenously
   B. Intra-amnionic hyperosmotic fluids
      1. 20 percent saline
      2. 30 percent urea
      3. 50 percent dextrose
   C. Prostaglandins E_2, $F_{2\alpha}$, and derivatives
      1. Intra-amnionic injection
      2. Extraovular injection
      3. Vaginal insertions
      4. Parenteral injection
      5. Oral ingestion
   D. Various combinations of the above

Surgical

The products of conception may be removed surgically through an appropriately dilated cervix or transabdominally by either hysterotomy or hysterectomy.

Dilatation and Evacuation. Surgical abortion through the vagina is performed by first dilating the cervix and then evacuating the products of conception mechanically by curettage, or by the technic of vacuum aspiration (suction curettage), or both. The likelihood of uterine perforation, cervical laceration, hemorrhage, incomplete removal of the fetus and placenta, and infection increases after the 12th week from the last normal menstrual period, or 10 weeks after ovulation. For this reason, dilatation and curettage or vacuum aspiration is best performed before the duration of pregnancy has exceeded that limit. More recently, however, there have been several advocates of cervical dilatation and surgical evacuation through the vagina of the products of conception up to 16 weeks gestation, at least (Grimes and Cates, 1978; Hodari et al., 1977).

In the absence of disease, the pregnancies are commonly terminated by dilatation and evacuation without hospitalization. When an abortion is not performed in a hospital setting, it is imperative that the capabilities for effective cardiopulmonary resuscitation be immediately available and that hospitalization can be promptly facilitated whenever needed.

Mechanical dilatation of the cervix at the time of abortion is a potentially traumatic procedure. The risk of trauma can be minimized by inserting an agent into the cervical canal that will slowly swell and thus slowly dilate the cervix. Laminaria tents, illustrated in Figure 24-5, have long been used in Japan, and more recently in the United States and elsewhere, to help dilate the cervix for abortion. The tents are made from the stems of *Laminaria digitata* or *Laminaria japonica*, a brown seaweed obtained from northern ocean waters. The stems are cut, peeled, shaped, dried, sterilized, and packaged according to size (small, 3 to 5 mm in diameter; medium, 6 to 8 mm; and large, 8 to 10 mm).

The cleansed cervix is grasped anteriorly with a tenaculum. The cervical canal is carefully sounded, without rupturing the membranes, to identify the length of the canal so as to gain some impression as to its diameter and the resistance of the internal os. A laminaria tent of appropriate size is then inserted so that the tip passes just beyond the internal os using a uterine packing forceps or a radium capsule forceps (Fig. 24-5). Later,

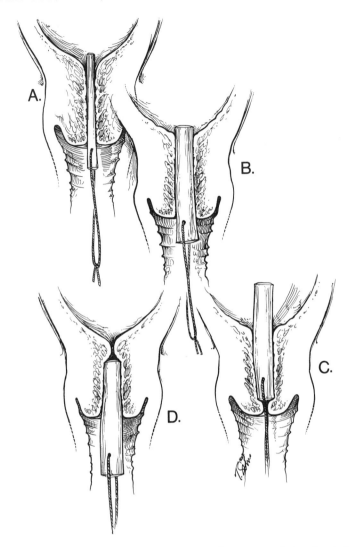

FIG. 24-5. Insertion of laminaria prior to dilatation and curettage. **A.** Laminaria immediately after being appropriately placed with its upper end just through the internal os. **B.** The swollen laminaria and dilated, softened cervix about 18 hours later. **C.** Laminaria inserted too far through the internal os; the laminaria may rupture the membranes. **D.** Laminaria not inserted far enough to dilate internal os.

usually after 8 to 24 hours, the tent will have swollen and thereby have dilated the cervix sufficiently to allow easier mechanical dilatation and curettage. The laminaria may cause cramping, which usually can be ameliorated with 0.6 g of aspirin or 60 mg of codeine orally every 3 to 4 hours.

At the time of abortion the laminaria is removed by grasping the attached thread, and the vulva, vagina, and cervix are cleansed.

The size and position of the uterus are carefully reevaluated through bimanual pelvic-abdominal examination. The anterior lip of the cervix is grasped with a multitoothed tenaculum and a local anesthetic is injected into the body of the cervix. Commonly, 5 ml of 1 or 2 percent solution of lidocaine is injected bilaterally. Alternatively, a paracervical block may be used (see Chap. 18, p. 446). The usual precautions for use of local anesthetics

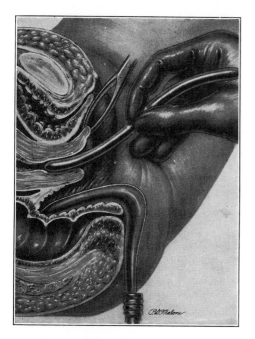

FIG. 24-6. Dilatation of cervix with Hegar dilator. Note that the fourth and fifth fingers rest against the perineum and buttocks, lateral to the vagina. This maneuver is a most important safety measure because if the cervix relaxes abruptly, these fingers prevent a sudden and uncontrolled thrust of the dilator, a common cause of perforation of the uterus.

must be observed since deaths have resulted from their use in abortion (Grimes and Cates, 1976).

The uterus is *carefully* sounded to identify the status of the internal os, and to confirm the size of the uterus and the attitude of the fundus. The cervix is further dilated with Hegar or Pratt dilators until a vacuum aspirator suction curet of appropriate diameter can be inserted. As shown in Figure 24-6, the fourth and fifth fingers of the hand introducing the dilator should rest on the woman's perineum and buttocks as the dilator is pushed through the internal os. This provides a further safeguard against uterine perforation.

Suction curettage is then used to aspirate most, if not all, of the pregnancy products. Two sizes of vacuum aspirators are illustrated in Figure 24-7. The vacuum aspirator is moved over the surface systematically so as to cover eventually all the uterine cavity.

Once this has been done and no more tissue is aspirated, the procedure is terminated. Gentle curettage with a sharp curet is then utilized if any placenta or fetal parts are thought possibly to remain in the uterus. A sharp curet is more efficacious and its dangers need not be greater than those of the dull instrument. Perforations of the uterus rarely occur on the downstroke of the curet, but they may occur when any instrument is introduced into the uterus. A curet, however, is a dangerous instrument if injudicious force is applied to it. As shown in Figure 24-8, the necessary manipulations should be carried out with the thumb and forefingers only.

It is reemphasized that morbidity, immediate and remote, will be kept to the minimum if (1) the cervix is adequately dilated without trauma before attempting to remove the products of conception, (2) the removal of the products of conception is accomplished without perforating the uterus, and (3) all of the products of conception (but not the decidua basalis) are removed.

MENSTRUAL EXTRACTION. Aspiration of the endometrial cavity using a small (6 mm) plastic suction curet within 1 to 3 weeks after failure to menstruate has been variously referred to as menstrual extraction, menstrual induction, instant period, atraumatic abortion, miniabortion, and lunch hour abortion (Wong and Schulman, 1974). Problems include the woman not being pregnant, the implanted ovum being missed by the suction curet, or uterine perforation.

PERFORATION. Accidental perforation of the uterus may occur during sounding of the uterus, dilatation, or curettage. The reported incidence of uterine perforation associated with elective abortion ranges from 1 in 111 abortions to 1 in 2,500 (Nathanson, 1972). Two important determinants of this complication are the skill of the physician and the position of the uterus, with a much greater likelihood of perforation if the physician is inexperienced and the uterus is retroverted.

Generally, the accident of uterine perfora-

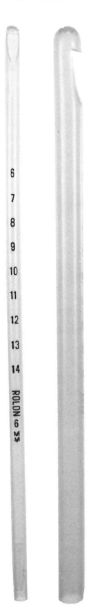

FIG. 24-7. Suction curets for vacuum aspiration of products of conception.

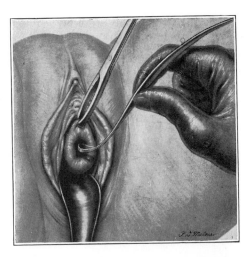

FIG. 24-8. Introduction of the sharp curet. Note that the instrument is held merely with the thumb and forefinger; in the upward movement of the curet, only the strength of these two fingers should be used. Moreover, just as soon as the curet has entered the cervical canal, the fourth and last fingers rest on the lateral perineum and the buttocks as further protection against uterine perforation.

foration of the uterus into the peritoneal cavity with a ring forceps or sharp curet, or a suction curet inserted unknowingly. In this circumstance, laparotomy to examine the bowel is the safest course of action. Laparoscopy to identify perforation has been suggested, but when this technic is employed bowel trauma may go unidentified.

SHARP VS. SUCTION CURETTAGE. The comprehensive study of Andolsek in Yugoslavia (1974) to identify and compare complications from abortion by sharp curettage with those performed by vacuum aspiration during the first trimester is the source of the following recommendations:

1. Vacuum aspiration is preferable to curettage for abortion since it is quicker, has a lower perforation rate, induces somewhat less blood loss at operation, and there are fewer infections afterward.
2. Vacuum aspiration should be performed within the first 10 weeks of gestation; in more advanced pregnancies, additional

tion is easy to recognize, as the instrument passes without hindrance farther than it could have had uterine perforation not occurred. Observation of the patient may be sufficient therapy if the rent in the uterus is small, as it may be if produced by a sound or dilator. Such small defects often heal readily without complication.

Considerable damage, especially to bowel, can be caused by manipulation through a per-

curettage as a second procedure may become necessary.

3. Treatment of Rh-negative women after abortion with anti-Rho (anti D) immunoglobulin is recommended, since about 5 percent of Rh-negative women sustaining abortion otherwise become immunized.

4. Some women will subsequently demonstrate cervical incompetence or uterine synechiae; the possibility of these complications should be explained to those contemplating abortion.

Hysterotomy and Hysterectomy. In few circumstances, abdominal hysterotomy or hysterectomy for abortion is preferable to either dilatation and curettage or medical induction. If uterine disease is present, hysterectomy often provides ideal treatment. If sterilization is to be performed, either hysterotomy with interruption of tubal continuity or hysterectomy may on occasion be more advisable than curettage or medical induction followed by partial resection of the oviducts (see Chap. 40, p. 1036). At times, hysterotomy or hysterectomy is necessary because of failure of medical induction during the second trimester.

The technics employed for hysterotomy are similar to those for cesarean section (see Chap. 43, p. 1085), except that the abdominal and uterine incisions are appreciably smaller. If further reproduction is anticipated, the smallest uterine incision that will allow removal of the fetus and placenta should be made away from the fundus, and the uterine wound carefully repaired.

Following abortion by abdominal hysterotomy, the potential for rupture during subsequent pregnancies is appreciable, especially during labor. Therefore, most obstetricians believe that in those women with previous hysterotomies, cesarean section is indicated for subsequent obstetric deliveries. After hysterotomy, Clow and Crompton (1973) identified 14 thin scars out of 31 evaluated in the subsequent pregnancy. Although Higginbottom (1973 believed that hysterotomy for abortion compared favorably with other methods of pregnancy termination, of the

242 cases reviewed by him, 12 required blood transfusion, three developed deep venous thrombosis, one had a pulmonary embolism, one had a repeat laparotomy for intestinal obstruction, and two subsequently required curettage for retained products of conception. Nottage and Liston (1975), based on a review of 700 hysterotomies, rightfully concluded that the operation is now outdated as a routine method for terminating pregnancy.

Medical Induction of Abortion

Very few effective, yet safe, abortifacient drugs have been discovered, although many naturally occurring substances have been utilized at some time by women desperate not to be pregnant. Serious systemic illness or even death, but not abortion, more often was the result.

Oxytocin. Intravenously administered oxytocin during the second trimester is seldom effective in terminating the intact pregnancy of a healthy woman. In circumstances of severe maternal disease, however, especially vascular disease or diseases complicated by maternal hypoxia, intravenous oxytocin is much more likely to effect uterine contractions that will evacuate the uterus. For example, at Parkland Memorial Hospital, termination of pregnancy with intravenous oxytocin was successful in five of eight primigravid eclamptic women pregnant with fetuses that weighed less than 1,000 g (Pritchard and Pritchard, 1975).

Once the cervix has undergone any degree of effacement and dilatation, either spontaneously or as the consequence of some other agent such as a prostaglandin, intravenously administered oxytocin is much more likely to prove effective for evacuating the products of conception.

There are complications from the use of oxytocin. If appreciable volumes of electrolyte-free solution are administered along with oxytocin, water intoxication may develop (see Chap. 17, p. 427). Rupture of the uterus from oxytocin infused during the first half of pregnancy has been documented in women of high parity (Peyser and Toaff, 1972), but is very unlikely. Rupture of the cervix or isthmus is well documented in instances in which oxytocin was given after intra-amnionic prostaglandin $F_{2\alpha}$ (p. 609). A bolus of oxytocin intravenously may produce troublesome hypotension (see Chap. 17, p. 427).

Intra-amnionic Hyperosmotic Solutions. In order to effect abortion during the second trimester, 50 percent dextrose solution, 20 to 25 percent saline, or 30 to 40 percent urea has been injected into the amnionic sac to stimulate uterine contractions and cervical dilatation. Use of hypertonic dextrose has been largely abandoned because of its relative ineffectiveness as well as the occasional occurrence of serious infection, including *Clostridium perfringens* sepsis.

MECHANISM OF ACTION. The mechanism of action of the hyperosmotic agents when placed in the amnionic sac is not clear. Most often the fetus is killed, but this does not explain their action nor does myometrial stretch from an increased intrauterine volume appear to be an important factor. Brunk and Gustavii (1973) suggested that decidual damage induced by the hyperosmotic material liberates prostaglandins which incite uterine contractions and cervical dilatation (see Chap. 15, p. 372).

HYPERTONIC SALINE. Intra-amnionically injected hypertonic saline was used as an abortifacient by the Japanese after World War II but later abandoned because of maternal morbidity and mortality. In spite of documented serious complications, hypertonic saline has become popular in the United States for midtrimester abortion once the pregnancy has advanced beyond the 15th week and the amnionic sac can be entered by transabdominal amniocentesis.

Kerenyi and co-workers (1973) reported 5000 consecutive abortions performed with hypertonic saline in 1 year using a uniform protocol. The duration of gestation was 16 to 24 weeks. Ultrasound was used to measure the biparietal diameter in cases thought to be 22 weeks gestation or more. Each woman was hospitalized throughout the procedure. Four gynecologists did all the saline instillations by first removing variable amounts of amnionic fluid and then infusing by slow drip 150 to 250 ml of 20 percent sterile saline solution. Four to six hours later an intravenous infusion of oxytocin was initiated and maintained at a rate of 50 milliunits per minute until one hour after abortion. Women with previous surgery involving incision of the myometrium were not accepted for saline abortion. Severe hypertensive, cardiac or renal disease, and severe anemia were the only other contraindications to saline abortion in this study. If, after 48 hours, little change had been produced in the cervix, the intra-amnionic saline instillation was repeated. If evacuation had not taken place after 2 more days, or if fever developed, the uterus was evacuated surgically. The frequencies of known complications for the last 1000 cases are presented in Table 24-2.

Although enthusiasm persists in the United States for abortion by injection of hypertonic saline, serious complications have been documented. Deaths have been caused

TABLE 24-2.
INCIDENCE OF COMPLICATIONS WITH
HYPERTONIC SALINE ABORTION

COMPLICATION	PERCENT
Retained placenta (4 hr)	12.9
Removed: digitally	(3.0)
instrumentally	(1.7)
by curettage	(8.2)
Estimated hemorrhage (over 500 ml)	2.3
Transfusion	0.5
Hypofibrinogenemia	0.3
Amniotic fluid embolism	0.1
Fever	2.3
Amnionitis	0.1
Cervical laceration	0.1
Perineal laceration	0.1
Required second saline instillation	1.4
Failure of inductions	0.4
Readmission for complications	0.5

From Kerenyi et al: *Am J Obstet Gynecol* 116:593, 1973.

by (1) hyperosmolar crisis following the entry of the hypertonic saline into the maternal circulation, (2) cardiac failure, (3) septic shock, (4) peritonitis, (5) hemorrhage, (6) disseminated intravascular coagulation, and (7) water intoxication (Lauersen and Birnbaum, 1975; Schiffer et al., 1973). Steinberg and associates (1972) identified fever in 18.5 percent of 302 women undergoing saline abortion; positive blood cultures were identified in 11 percent of 56 who were febrile. Myometrial necrosis has followed injection of hypertonic saline that apparently remained in contact with the myometrium (Wentz and King, 1972), and cervical and isthmic fistulas and lacerations have been described (Goodlin et al., 1972). Use of laminaria tents to prevent such cervical trauma has been recommended, but fistula formation has been documented following the use of such tents (Lischke and Gordon, 1974). Gross rupture of the body of the uterus from use of hypertonic saline plus oxytocin has been described (Horwitz, 1974). Serious disruption of the coagulation mechanism characterized by the changes of disseminated intravascular coagulation have been reported repeatedly with use of hypertonic saline for abortion (see Chap. 21, p. 521), and at least one death from intracranial hemorrhage has been described (Lemkin and Kattlove, 1973). Berger and colleagues (1975) have demonstrated abortion to occur more promptly when oxytocin was administered intravenously within 8 hours after instillation of hypertonic saline. The decrease in frequency of infection was accompanied by an increase in consumptive coagulopathy, however.

HYPEROSMOTIC UREA. Urea, 30 to 40 percent, dissolved in 5 percent dextrose solution, has been injected into the amnionic sac, followed by intravenous oxytocin, about 400 milliunits per minute. The hope that urea (plus oxytocin) would be at least as efficacious an abortifacient as hypertonic saline, but less toxic, has been fulfilled according to Weinberg and Shepard (1973). Burnett and coworkers (1975) have made similar observa-

tions for hyperosmotic intra-amnionic urea plus intravenous oxytocin.

Prostaglandins. Prostaglandin E_2, prostaglandin $F_{2\alpha}$, and derivatives of them have been investigated widely as abortifacients. They are administered orally, parenterally, into the amnionic sac, extraovularly, and as a vaginal suppository placed adjacent to the cervix. They are used alone, with intravenous oxytocin, with hypertonic solutions injected into the amnionic sac, with laminaria tents, and with curettage.

Certain major problems have evolved from their use that include: (1) troublesome adverse systemic effects; (2) delay in evacuation of products of conception; (3) incomplete evacuation of the products; (4) hemorrhage; (5) infection; and (6) cervical laceration and fistula formation. Consumptive coagulopathy, occasionally a complication of abortion with intra-amnionic saline, has been described with prostaglandins with fetal death of long duration.

INTRA-AMNIONIC   PROSTAGLANDIN $F_{2\alpha}$. The experiences at Parkland Memorial Hospital, which have been carefully evaluated by Duenhoelter and co-workers (1976), appear to be representative of those of others (Lowensohn and Ballard, 1974; Wentz et al., 1973). The technic that has been used for administration at Parkland Memorial Hospital is described below:

After scrubbing the lower abdomen and anesthetizing the puncture site with lidocaine, amniocentesis is performed using a 3½-inch long, 21-guage needle. When free-flowing amnionic fluid is demonstrated, 5 mg of prostaglandin $F_{2\alpha}$ is injected slowly. If, after 1 minute, the woman is asymptomatic and fluid can still be aspirated into the syringe, the rest of the 40 mg dose is injected. Immediately before or after the injection a laminaria tent of appropriate size is placed in the cervical canal as described on page 603.

If, after 24 hours, abortion is not thought to be imminent and the membranes remain intact, amniocentesis is repeated as described and 20 mg is now injected. A dilute solution of oxytocin is infused intravenously if membranes rupture without labor or if labor is not imminent 24 hours after the second injection. Moreover, in all cases, once the fetus is expelled, oxytocin is infused to aid in expulsion of the placenta and to minimize bleeding. If the placenta is not intact, suction curettage is carried out.

The cumulative abortion rate of 96 percent at Parkland Memorial Hospital during the first 48 hours after injection and use of laminaria is demonstrated in Figure 24-9. Complications, other than delay in evacuation, include (1) infection treated with antibiotics, 15 percent, which was usually associated with prolonged rupture of the membranes; (2) a lower hematocrit reading, i.e., 5 or more, 20 percent; (3) cervical laceration, 2 percent.

Grimes and Cates (1979) have compared 15 published reports concerned with the induction of abortion using the intra-amnionic injection of either prostaglandin $F_{2\alpha}$ or hypertonic saline. While abortion appeared to be quicker with prostaglandin $F_{2\alpha}$ unpleasant gastrointestinal side effects, hemorrhage, and incomplete abortion also were more common. Maternal mortality was about the same for both agents (23 per 100,000 for hyper-

tonic saline and 18 per 100,000 for prostaglandin $F_{2\alpha}$). A troublesome feature was the expulsion of a fetus with signs of life in up to 7 percent of prostaglandin-induced abortions compared to 1 percent or less with hypertonic saline. The legal implications associated with expulsion of a living abortus may be profound. Although the purpose of abortion is to destroy the fetus before viability—a right of every pregnant woman, according to the United States Supreme Court—statutes continue to be enacted to protect the abortus. For example, one recent law demands that an abortus with a heart beat or demonstrating any movement after expulsion from the mother be considered a living human child entitled to the same rights, powers, and privileges as a child born alive after the normal gestation period!

The intra-amnionic injection of prostaglandin plus hypertonic urea has been utilized by King and co-workers (1974) in an attempt to reduce the delay and increase the completeness of expulsion. They consider urea plus prostaglandin injected into the amnionic sac to be about as effective as urea plus continuous intravenous infusion of oxytocin.

Prostaglandin $F_{2\alpha}$ has been injected extraovularly to effect abortion late in the first

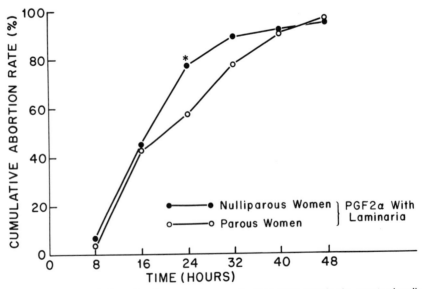

FIG. 24-9. The cumulative abortion rate (percent) after intra-amnionic prostaglandin $F_{2\alpha}$ plus laminaria. (From Duenhoelter and co-workers. *Obstet Gynecol* 47:469, 1976)

or early in the second trimester, when curettage for abortion is somewhat hazardous, but before 15 or 16 weeks, when transabdominal amniocentesis first becomes feasible: A Foley catheter is inserted through the cervix so that the balloon when inflated is just above the internal os. The drug in dilute solution is either injected at intervals or is continuously infused through the catheter by means of an infusion pump. Lauerson and Wilson (1974), as well as Dillon and associates (1974), have reported a higher success rate and possibly fewer side effects than when prostaglandin $F_{2\alpha}$ was injected into the amnionic sac. In the small series reported by Shapiro (1975), complications included incomplete evacuation, failure of evacuation, and infection, as well as nausea and vomiting, paralytic ileus, and substernal "pressure." Fraser and Brash (1974) witnessed severe bronchospasm in a few women to whom prostaglandin E_2 was administered extraovularly. They also expressed concern over the nursing time required to monitor women receiving the drug by this route.

Prostaglandins incorporated into a gel have been placed extraovularly in an attempt to avoid the necessity for continuous or repeated infusions (Lippert and Modley, 1973; Mackenzie et al., 1975).

Corson and Bolognese (1975) have been impressed by the abortifacient properties of prostaglandin E_2 during the first and second trimester when administered as a vaginal suppository, 20 mg every 4 hours. The great majority of patients aborted within 36 hours. Vomiting and diarrhea were common, as was fever, presumably induced by the drug.

Hillier and Embrey (1972) evaluated the intravenous administration of prostaglandin E_2 and $F_{2\alpha}$ in higher doses in an attempt to increase the success rate and shorten the time until abortion. Side effects were increased markedly. Coltart and Coe (1975) report a favorable outcome for a small group of late first-trimester and second-trimester abortions accomplished by giving prostaglandin E_2 plus oxytocin intravenously. No cervical damage or other serious morbidity was reported, but the series is quite small.

PROSTAGLANDIN ANALOGS. A series of prostaglandin analogs has been prepared and is being evaluated currently. One of these drugs, 15-methylprostaglandin E_2, when given intramuscularly, appears to have merit as an abortifacient during the second trimester (Dillon and coworkers, 1975; Sharma and associates, 1975). Unfortunately, nausea, vomiting, and diarrhea are common side effects. Antiemetic and antidiarrheal agents may reduce the frequency and intensity of these unpleasant side effects. The intramuscular route may prove to be especially advantageous for evacuating long dead products of conception in which amnionic fluid is likely to be very scant to absent.

LAMINARIA, PROSTAGLANDIN, UREA, AND OXYTOCIN. Perhaps the ultimate in the use of multiple abortifacients was reported by Strauss and co-workers (1979). They identified an average time for expulsion of the conceptus of 13 hours when first they inserted a laminaria tent into the cervical canal, then 4 hours later injected intra-amnionically 20 mg of prostaglandin $F_{2\alpha}$ plus 80 g of urea, and followed this with oxytocin infused intravenously at the rate of 333 milliunits per minute. Complications were troublesome but perhaps no more so than with medical inductions in general.

CONSEQUENCES OF ELECTIVE ABORTION

Maternal Mortality.   It is apparent that serious morbidity and even mortality have followed some elective abortions (Table 24-3). Nonetheless, legally induced abortion is a relatively safe surgical procedure, especially when performed during the first 2 months of pregnancy. The risk of death from abortion by dilatation and evacuation performed during the first 2 months is about 0.6 per 100,000 procedures. The relative risk of dying as the consequence of abortion is approximately doubled for each 2 weeks of delay after 8 weeks gestation (MMWR, 1979).

TABLE 24-3.
MORTALITY FROM ABORTION IN THE UNITED STATES,
1972–1977

	1972	1973	1974	1975	1976	1977
Legally Induced	24	25	25	29	11	15
Illegally Induced	39	19	6	4	2	4
Spontaneous	25	10	21	14	13	14
Total	88	54	52	43	26	33

From Forrest, Tietze, and Sullivan: *Fam Plan Perspect* 10:271, 1978.

Impact on Future Pregnancies. The effects of elective abortion on subsequent pregnancies continues to be disputed. For example, a World Health Organization Task Force on Sequelae of Abortion (1979) has reported a significantly higher risk of an adverse pregnancy outcome among women whose only previous pregnancy had been aborted when compared to the experiences of women who were either primigravid or whose only previous pregnancy had ended in live birth. The adverse pregnancy outcomes took the form of midtrimester spontaneous abortions, preterm deliveries, and low birth weight infants. These findings are similar to the previous findings of some investigators but are in conflict with those of about an equal number of investigators who detected no such adverse effects from a previous abortion. As an example of a study that yielded quite the opposite results, Daling and Emanuel (1977), using matched-pair analysis, identified no relationship between a previous induced abortion and low birth weight, premature delivery, stillbirth, neonatal death, spontaneous abortion, or congenital malformations in subsequent pregnancies. Cates (1979) who analyzed and tabulated 29 reports concerned with the apparent impact of previous abortions on subsequent pregnancies, concluded that data do not support firm conclusions about induced abortion either causing or not causing any of a variety of the complications alleged to be more common in pregnancies subsequent to induced abortion.

Clinical experiences in former years with the so-called incompetent cervix support the concept that this uncommon defect commonly followed induced abortion. Moreover, it seems likely that *forceful* dilatation of the cervix by surgical or medical technics sufficient to allow evacuation or expulsion of more advanced products of conception will continue to predispose to cervical incompetency.

Rupture of the uterus after hysterotomy, and less often after inadvertent uterine perforation at the time of abortion, may occur during a subsequent pregnancy with a disastrous outcome for the fetus, the mother, or both.

Adhesions that compromise the uterine cavity as the consequence of abortion and vigorous curettage or infection have resulted in infertility. Treatment has only been partially successful for this phenomenon of post-traumatic intrauterine adhesions, sometimes referred to as *Asherman's syndrome.* When infertility has been overcome, obstetric complications have been common. For example, in the experiences of Jewelewicz and associates (1976) only 18 of 36 women treated for Asherman's syndrome subsequently conceived. Moreover, of those 18, only 10 were delivered of infants who survived. There were 3 instances of placenta accreta and one of cervical pregnancy.

RESUMPTION OF OVULATION

Ovulation may occur as early as 2 weeks after an abortion. Lähteenmäki and Luukkainen (1978) detected a surge of luteinizing hormone (LH) 16 to 22 days after abortion in

15 of 18 women studied. Moreover, the plasma progesterone level, which had plummeted after the abortion, increased starting soon after the LH surge. These hormonal events are in excellent temporal agreement with the histologic changes observed in endometrial biopsies and the rise in basal body temperature after abortion, as described previously by Boyd and Holmstrom (1972). Therefore, it is important that effective contraception be initiated soon after abortion. The use of various contraceptive technics following abortion is discussed in Chapter 40.

SEPTIC ABORTION

Serious complications of abortion have been most often, but certainly not always, associated with criminal abortion. Severe hemorrhage, sepsis, acute renal failure, and bacterial shock have all developed in association with legal abortion but at a very much lower rate.

Abortal infection is most often caused by pathogenic organisms of the bowel and vaginal flora. Infection is most commonly confined to the uterus in the form of metritis, but parametritis, peritonitis (localized and general), and even septicemia are by no

TABLE 24-4.
BACTERIA PRESENT IN 76 CASES OF SEPTIC ABORTION WITH POSITIVE BLOOD CULTURES

ORGANISMS CULTURED	FREQUENCY (%)
Anaerobic	63
Peptostreptococcus (anaerobic streptococcus)	41
Bacteroides	9
Both	9
Clostridium perfringens	4
Aerobic	37
Escherichia coli	14
Pseudomonas	9
β-hemolytic streptococcus	4
Enterococcus	3
Combination	7

From Smith, Southern, and Lehmann: *Obstet Gynecol* 35:704, 1970.

means rare. Out of 300 cases of febrile abortions at Parkland Memorial Hospital shortly before the United States Supreme Court decision legalizing abortion, a positive blood culture was found in one-fourth. The organisms identified are listed in Table 24-4.

Treatment of the infection includes prompt evacuation of the products of conception. Although mild infections can be treated successfully with broad-spectrum antibiotics in the usual dosage, any serious infection should be attacked with great vigor from the very start. Daily doses of penicillin, 20 million units, and tetracycline, 2 g, both given intravenously, have, in general, yielded excellent results at Parkland Memorial Hospital, although this combination appears to be in conflict with the hypothesis of Jawetz and Gunnison (cited by Brumfitt). Their hypothesis, proposed more than 20 years ago, that bactericidal antibiotics given together often are synergistic, whereas a bactericidal and bacteriostatic antibiotic given in combination often are antagonistic, has proved to be more myth than valid hypothesis or substantiated observation (Brumfitt and Percival, 1971).

For septic abortion complicated by persistent, apparently resistant infection, or with evidence of overwhelming sepsis, as seen with bacterial shock, intravenous antibiotic therapy with similar doses of penicillin plus chloramphenicol, 3 to 4 g per day, has proved effective. Rather than chloramphenicol, clindamycin has been used in combination with kanamycin or gentamycin plus penicillin.

Bacterial Shock. Bacteremia, endotoxemia, and exotoxemia sometimes result in severe and even fatal shock. Such shock, which fortunately is now rare, was previously seen most often in connection with induced abortion, although it may occur as a result of infection in the genital or urinary tracts at any time during pregnancy or the puerperium. It is not peculiar to obstetrics, but is seen in a wide variety of postoperative infections, especially in urology patients.

Bacterial shock is much more resistant to treatment than shock from hypovolemia, and if intravenous therapy is continued for a long period of time despite lack of response, the patient may succumb from the complication of fluid excess while still hypotensive. The pathogenesis of bacterial shock is still not clearly understood.

An outline of therapy that has proved successful in most cases at Parkland Memorial Hospital is presented:

DIAGNOSIS AND TREATMENT OF BACTERIAL SHOCK

1. *Suspicion.* Whenever infection of the gravid uterus is suspected, blood pressure and urine flow should be closely monitored. Bacterial shock, as well as hypovolemic shock, should be considered whenever there is evidence of hypotension or oliguria.
2. *Recognition.* If hypotension and oliguria are not improved by the rapid administration of a liter of lactated Ringer's solution, the shock is more likely caused by bacterial products.
3. *Treatment*
   a. Control of infection
      (1) After obtaining anaerobic and aerobic cultures of blood and urine, as well as a smear for gram-stain

from the cervix or products of conception, intensive broad-spectrum antibiotic therapy is begun as described above. The kinds of organisms usually found in the blood are listed in Table 24-4. Cervical smears may be misleading except when there is an obvious abundance of pathogenic organisms, as, for example, *Clostridium perfringens,* demonstrated in Figure 24-10.

(2) Once antibiotic therapy has been started and the patient's condition has been stabilized, the infected products of conception are promptly removed by curettage. Hysterectomy is seldom indicated unless the uterus has been lacerated or the uterus is obviously intensely infected (Figs. 24-11A and B). Evidence is lacking that hysterectomy in the absence of gross trauma to the uterus, including that induced by infection, improves the prognosis (Hawkins et al., 1975; O'Neill et al., 1972; Pritchard and Whalley, 1971; Smith et al.,

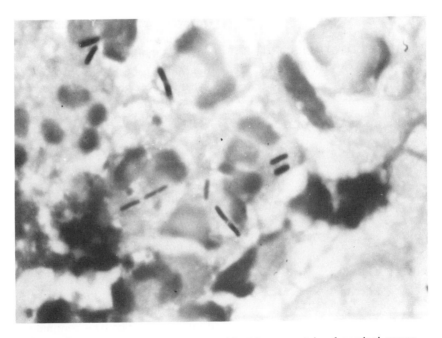

FIG. 24-10. *Clostridium perfringens* evident in gram stain of cervical smear.

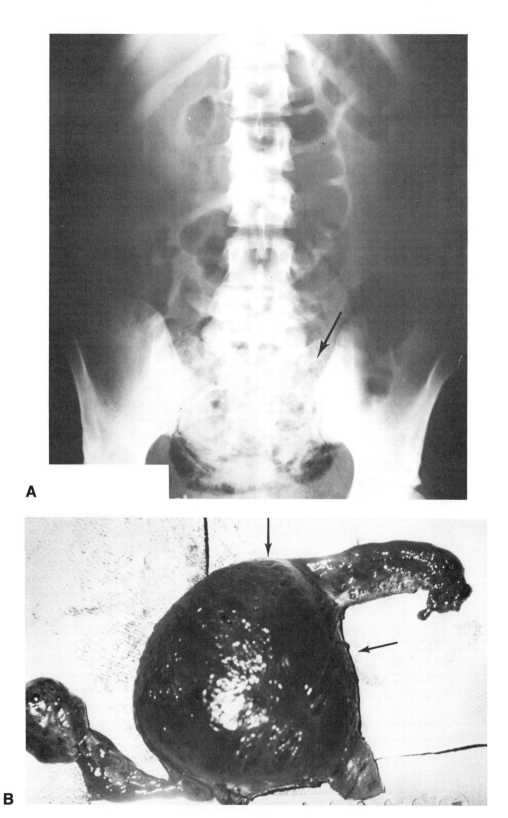

FIG. 24-11. A. The honeycombed pattern of gas in the pelvis (arrow) was caused by gas in the myometrium of a fatal case of postabortal *Clostridium perfringens* sepsis. **B.** The numerous rents in the serosa of the uterus (arrows) were the consequence of gas formation plus intensive necrosis from *Clostridium perfringens*.

1978). Since bacterial shock can develop hours after evacuation of the infected products from the uterus, careful monitoring must be continued.

b. Treatment of Shock. The primary goal is to establish effective perfusion of vital organs. The adequacy of the circulation may be ascertained by continuously monitoring urine flow and the central venous pressure.

(1) *Fluid therapy.* Whole blood is given in amounts that maintain the hematocrit at or slightly above 30. Electrolyte-containing fluids, such as lactated Ringer's solution, are given at a rate that maintains urinary flow at more than 0.5 ml, and preferably about 1.0 ml, per minute. Vigorous filling of the intravascular compartment is desirable, but circulatory overload with pulmonary edema must be avoided. Sodium bicarbonate solution may be of value in combating severe metabolic acidosis. *Central venous pressure* is monitored continuously as more fluids are given. If central venous pressure rises beyond normal, intravenous fluids must be restricted.

(2) *Adrenocortical steroids.* If control of the infection by antibiotics, and curettage and the infusion of blood and aqueous fluids do not result in prompt improvement, large doses of corticosteroids are probably indicated. Lillehei and associates (1958) have recommended 10g of hydrocortisone sodium succinate (Solu-Cortef) or its equivalent rapidly administered intravenously. We have used methylprednisolone-sodium succinate (Solu-Medrol), 500 mg given as a bolus intravenously. Steroid therapy need not be continued beyond the acute phase, and most often can be stopped abruptly.

(3) *Pressor agents.* These agents are not as popular as they were in the past, although selected ones, metaraminol and dopamine, may have some value when used in conjunction with the treatment modalities outlined above, especially appropriate filling of the intravascular compartment. Both have a powerful inotropic effect on the heart and are much less likely to cause necrosis than is levarterenol bitartrate (Levophed). A rise in blood pressure is sought that reestablishes urine flow, which, in turn, indicates effective organ perfusion.

(4) *Vasodilating agents.* Drugs such as isoproterenol have been recommended to relieve vasoconstriction (Du Toit, 1966). Their role in cases of septic abortion with endotoxic shock is questionable.

(5) *Oxygenation.* Vigorous respiratory support may be required in the form of oxygen administration, effective pulmonary toilet, and even mechanical ventilation. Adult respiratory distress syndrome is a serious complication.

(6) *Heparin.* The concept that intravascular coagulation occludes the microcirculation in endotoxic shock has led to the recommendation that heparin be used in these circumstances. To date, however, no adequate clinical trial has been reported that establishes the benefits from heparin to outweigh the risks. Moreover, animal studies of gram-negative sepsis point out that inhibition of intravascular coagulation by heparin does not necessarily lower mortality (Corrigan et al., 1974).

An illustrative case of septic abortion with intense but transient consumptive coagulopathy without gross hemolysis and not treated with heparin is summarized below and in Table 24-5.

Septic Abortion Without Gross Hemolysis. B.T., a 32-year-old multigravida, sought

TABLE 24-5.
HEMATOLOGIC DATA AND RENAL FUNCTION IN A CASE OF SEPTIC ABORTION WITH INTENSE INTRAVASCULAR COAGULATION BUT NO GROSS HEMOLYSIS

DATE AND TIME	FIBRINOGEN* (mg per dl)	SERUM FDP† (µg per ml)	THROMBIN TIME††	PLATELETS (mm³)	HEMATOCRIT	CREATININE CLEARANCE (ml per minute)	COMMENT
17 Jan							
1950	Large clot	8	—	—	35	—	
2300				curettage			
18 Jan							
0600	No clot	—	—	—	31	—	Generalized bleeding
0700	20	1,024	—	151 000	—	—	Hypotensive
1000	28	512	—	120 000	—	49	
1500	47	512	—	122 000	27	45	Afebrile
1930	67	512	—	158 000	—	36	Mild hypotension
19 Jan							
0900	172	128	18.7 (10.4)	118 000	27	14	
20 Jan	348	8	12.1 (10.2)	108 000	27	16	Normotensive
22 Jan	485	<4	12.2 (10.1)	129 000	31	20	
24 Jan	432	<4	13.0 (11.0)	172 000	27	35	
26 Jan	489	<4	11.4 (10.3)	336 000	28	50	
20 Feb	288	<4	12.0 (11.2)	—	37	119	

*Measured as thrombin clotable protein
†Fibrin degradation products measured by tanned erythrocyte agglutination inhibition technique
††Control value in brackets

617

help because of loss of amnionic fluid, cramping, and vaginal bleeding following 3½ months of amenorrhea. She was febrile and the pregnant uterus palpable above the symphysis was tender. An intravenous infusion of oxytocin soon accomplished expulsion of the fetus and placenta.

Four hours later her temperature rose to 40.5 C. Seven hours after evacuation of the products of conception brisk bleeding from the vagina and obvious oozing from previous venipuncture sites were documented by a physician. The blood pressure was 90/50 mm Hg, pulse 120, urine output 20 ml for the previous hour, hematocrit 31 percent compared to 35 percent initially, and the leukocyte count had fallen from 13,000 to 7000 mm³. Two ml of her blood added to a tube that contained 0.1 ml of thrombin yielded no visible clot.

Immediate treatment consisted of lactated Ringer's solution, 1 unit of whole blood and 2 units of thawed plasma, plus 2 units of packed erythrocytes. Urine flow was soon restored. Central venous pressure was monitored closely when the patient complained of a fullness in her chest and scattered rales were heard. Penicillin, kanamycin and clindomycin were administered. During the next 12 hours the bleeding first decreased appreciably and then stopped. Her subsequent clinical course was benign except for a transient rise in plasma creatinine to 4.4 mg per dl. She was discharged 11 days after admittance.

A variety of interesting observations made on the coagulation mechanism and on renal function are summarized in Table 24-5: Platelets were abundant and a morphologic study of the erythrocytes yielded normal results in a blood smear made when she was first seen in the emergency suite. A large, stable clot was present in the tube of blood that had been routinely drawn for crossmatch before evacuation of the products of conception. Serum removed later from that tube contained only 8 μg per ml of fibrin degradation products. Nine hours after admittance, she was bleeding excessively through the vagina and from sites of previous venipunctures. Severe hypofibrinogenemia was documented and the level of fibrin degradation products in serum had increased from 8 μg or less to 1024 μg per ml, yet the platelet count was only slightly below normal.

The plasma fibrinogen concentration then rose and the thrombin time and serum fibrin degradation products fell but at somewhat slower rates than usually observed with placental abruption. Erythrocyte deformity and some fragmentation of erythrocytes were observed to follow the consumptive coagulopathy.

Although severe oliguria did not persist after fluid therapy was started, the creatinine clearance fell to as low as 14 ml per minute 36 hours after the abortion had been completed. It then rose to 50 ml per minute 1 week later and to 119 ml per minute when next checked 4 weeks after the abortion. Recovery of renal function occurred without use of heparin even though the patient had chronic hypertension for which she had been subjected to thiazide therapy until the time of abortion and she was probably overtly hypotensive for several hours after the abortion before effective fluid therapy was instituted.

Acute Renal Failure. Persistent renal failure in abortion usually stems from multiple effects of infection. Less commonly, it has been induced by toxic compounds employed to produce abortion, such as soap, pHisoHex, or Lysol. Whereas very severe forms of bacterial shock are frequently associated with intense renal damage, the milder forms rarely lead to overt renal failure. Early recognition of this very serious complication is most important. The word "serious" is used advisedly in connection with acute renal failure in abortion, for the maternal mortality before the extensive use of dialysis exceeded 75 percent (Knapp and Hellman, 1959).

Renal failure is likely to be most intense when the cause of the sepsis includes *Clostridium perfringens* and the production of a very potent hemolytic exotoxin. Whenever intense hemoglobinemia complicates Clostridial infection, renal failure is the rule. At the outset, plans should be made to initiate effective dialysis early, before metabolic derangement becomes serious.

REFERENCES

Andolsek L: The Ljubljana abortion study 1971– 1973. Bethesda, Md, National Institute of Health Center for Population Research, 1974

Berger GS, Edelman DA, Kerenyi TD: Oxytocin administration, instillation to abortion time, and morbidity associated with saline instillation. Am J Obstet Gynecol 121:941, 1975

Berger GS, Tietze C, Pakter J, Katz SH: Maternal mortality associated with legal abortion in New York State: July 1, 1970–June 30, 1972. Obstet Gynecol 43:315, 1974

Boué A, Boué J: Chromosomal anomalies associated with fetal malformation. In Scrimgeour JB (ed): Towards the Prevention of Fetal Malformation. Edinburgh, Edinburgh University Press, 1978

Boyd EF Jr, Holmstrom EG: Ovulation following therapeutic abortion. Am J Obstet Gynecol 113:469, 1972

Brumfitt W, Percival A: Antibiotic combinations. Lancet 1:387, 1971

Brunk U, Gustavii B: Lability of human decidual cells: in vitro effects of autolysis and osmotic stress. Am J Obstet Gynecol 115:811, 1973

Burnett LS, King TM, Atienza MF, Bell WR: Intraamniotic urea as a midtrimester abortifacient: clinical results and serum and urinary changes. Am J Obstet Gynecol 121:7, 1975

Cates W Jr: Late effects of induced abortion. Hypothesis or knowledge? J Reprod Med 22:207, 1979

Clow WM, Crompton AC: The wounded uterus: pregnancy after hysterotomy. Br Med J 1:321, 1973

Coltart TM, Coe MJ: Intravenous prostaglandins and oxytocin for midtrimester abortion. Lancet 1:173, 1975

Corrigan JJ, Kiornat JF, Pagel CJ: Experimental gram negative sepsis: effect of heparin. Pediatr Res 8:399, 1974

Corson SL, Bolognese RJ: Vaginally administered prostaglandin E_2 as a first and second trimester abortifacient. J Reprod Med 14:43, 1975

Daling JR, Emanuel I: Induced abortion and subsequent outcome of pregnancy in a series of American women. N Engl J Med 297:1241, 1977

Dillon TF, Phillips LL, Risk A, Horiguchi T, Mootabar H: The efficacy of intramuscular 15 methyl prostaglandin E_2 in second trimester abortion. Am J Obstet Gynecol 121:584, 1975

Dillon TF, Phillips LL, Risk A, Horiguchi T, Mohajer-Shojai E, Mootabar H: The efficacy of intramuscular 15 methyl prostaglandin $F_{2\alpha}$ in second trimester abortion. Am J Obstet Gynecol 118:688, 1974

Duenhoelter JH, Gant NF, Jimenez J: Concurrent use of prostaglandin $F_{2\alpha}$ and laminaria for induction of midtrimester abortion. Obstet Gynecol 47:469, 1976

Du Toit HJ, Du Plessis JME, Dommisse J, Rorke MJ, Theron MS, DeVilliers VP: Treatment of endotoxic shock with isoprenaline. Lancet 2:143, 1966

Fraser IS, Brash J: Comparison of extra- and intraamniotic prostaglandins for therapeutic abortion. Obstet Gynecol 43:97, 1974

Funderburk SJ, Guthrie D, Meldrum D: Outcome of pregnancies complicated by early vaginal bleeding. Brit J Obstet Gynaecol 87:100, 1980

Goldzieher JW: Double-blind trial of a progestin in habitual abortion. JAMA 188:651, 1964

Goodlin R, Newell J, O'Hare J, Sturz H: Cervical fistula: a complication of midtrimester abortion. Obstet Gynecol 40:82, 1972

Grimes DA, Cates W Jr: Deaths from paracervical anesthesia used for first-trimester abortion. N Engl J Med 295:1397, 1976

Grimes DA, Cates W Jr: Gestational age limit of twelve weeks for abortion by curettage. Am J Obstet Gynecol 132:207, 1978

Grimes DA, Cates W Jr: The comparative efficacy and safety of intraamniotic prostaglandin $F_{2\alpha}$ and hypertonic saline for second-trimester abortion, J Reprod Med 22:248, 1979

Guerrero R, Rojas OI: Spontaneous abortion and aging of human ova and spermatozoa. N Engl J Med 293:573, 1975

Hartman CG: Uterine bleeding as an early sign of pregnancy in the monkey (Macaca rhesus), together with observations on fertile period of menstrual cycle. Bull Hopkins Hosp 44:155, 1929

Hawkins DF, Sevitt LH, Fairbrother PF, Tothill AU: Conservative management of septic chemical abortion with renal failure. N Engl J Med 292:722, 1975

Hertig AT, Sheldon WH: Minimal criteria required to prove prima facie case of traumatic abortion or miscarriage: An analysis of 1,000 spontaneous abortions. Ann Surg 117:596, 1943

Higginbottom J: Termination of pregnancy by abdominal hysterotomy. Lancet 1:937, 1973

Hillier K, Embrey MP: High-dose intravenous administration of prostaglandin E_2 and $F_{2\alpha}$ for the termination of midtrimester pregnancies. J Obstet Gynaecol Br Commonw 79:14, 1972

Hodari AA, Peralta J, Quiroga PJ, Gerbi EB: Dilatation and curettage for second trimester abortions. Am J Obstet Gynecol 127:850, 1977

Horwitz DA: Uterine rupture following attempted saline abortion with oxytocin in a grand multiparous patient. Obstet Gynecol 43:921, 1974

Jewelewicz R, Khalaf S, Neuwirth RS, Vande Wiele RL: Obstetric complications after treatment of intrauterine synechiae (Asherman's syndrome). Obstet Gynecol 47:701, 1976

Jones HW, Jones GES: Double uterus as an etiological factor in repeated abortion: indications for surgical repair. Am J Obstet Gynecol 65:325, 1953

Kerenyi TD, Mandelman N, Sherman DH: Five thousand consecutive saline inductions. Am J Obstet Gynecol 116:593, 1973

King TM, Atienza MF, Burkman RT, Burnett LS, Bell WR: The synergistic activity of intraamniotic prostaglandin F$_{2\alpha}$ and urea in the mid-trimester elective abortion. Am J Obstet Gynecol 120:704, 1974

Knapp RC, Hellman LM: Acute renal failure in pregnancy. Am J Obstet Gynecol 78:570, 1959

Kohl S: Testimony presented at trial of *Commonwealth of Massachusetts* v *Edelin,* Boston, January, 1975

Kohorn EI, Kaufman M: Sonar in the first trimester of pregnancy. Obstet Gynecol 44:473, 1974

Kuhn RPJ, Pepperell RJ: Cervical ligation: a review of 242 pregnancies. Aust NZ J Obstet Gynecol 17:79, 1977

Lähteenmäki P, Luukkainen T: Return of ovarian function after abortion. Clin Endocr 8:123, 1978

Lash AF, Lash SR: Habitual abortion: the incompetent internal os of the cervix. Am J Obstet Gynecol 59:68, 1950

Lauersen NH, Birnbaum SJ: Water intoxication associated with oxytocin administration during saline-induced abortion. Am J Obstet Gynecol 121:2, 1975

Lauersen NH, Wilson KH: Continuous extraovular injection of prostaglandin F$_{2\alpha}$ for mid-trimester abortion. Am J Obstet Gynecol 120:273, 1974

Lemkin SR, Kattlove HE: Maternal death due to DIC after saline abortion. Obstet Gynecol 42:233, 1973

Lillehei RC, MacLean LD: The intestinal factor in irreversible endotoxin shock. Ann Surg 148:513, 1958

Lippert TH, Modley T: Induction of abortion by the extra-amniotic administration of prostaglandin gels. J Obstet Gynaecol Br Commonw 80:1025, 1973

Lischke JH, Gordon HR: Cervicovaginal fistula complicating induced midtrimester abortion despite laminaria tent insertion. Am J Obstet Gynecol 120:852, 1974

Lowensohn R, Ballard CA: Cervicovaginal fistula: an apparent increased incidence with prostaglandin F$_{2\alpha}$. Am J Obstet Gynecol 119:1057, 1974

Luthy DA, Karp LE, Schulman JD: What part do chromosomes play in repeated reproductive failure? Contemporary Ob/Gyn 13:98, 1979

Mackenzie IZ, Hillier K, Embrey MP: Single extraamniotic injection of prostaglandin E$_2$ in viscous gel to introduce mid-trimester abortion. Br Med J 1:240, 1975

McCormack WM: Genital infections of perinatal importance. Clin Obstet Gynecol 22:313, 1979

McDonald IA: Incompetent cervix as a cause of recurrent abortion. J Obstet Gynaecol Br Commonw 70:105, 1963

Mennuti MT, Jingileski S, Schwarz RH, Mellman WJ: An evaluation of cytogenetic analysis as a primary tool in the assessment of recurrent pregnancy wastage. Obstet Gynecol 52:308, 1978

MMWR: Abortion-related mortality—United States, 1977. Center for Disease Control Morbidity and Mortality Weekly Report 28:301, 1979

Munro JS: Premature infant weighing less than one pound at birth who survived and developed normally. Can Med Assoc J 40:69, 1939

Nathanson BN: Management of uterine perforations suffered at elective abortion. Am J Obstet Gynecol 114:1054, 1972

Neu RL, Entes K, Bannerman RM: Chromosome analysis in cases with repeated spontaneous abortions. 53:373, 1979

Nottage BJ, Liston WA: A review of 700 hysterotomies. Br J Obstet Gynaecol 82:310, 1975

O'Neill JP, Niall JF, O'Sullivan EF: Severe postabortal *Clostridium welchii* infections: trends in management. Aust NZ J Obstet Gynaecol 12:157, 1972

Peyser MR, Toaff R: Rupture of uterus in the first trimester caused by high-concentration oxytocin drip. Obstet Gynecol 40:371, 1972

Pilpel HF, Norwick KP: When should abortion be legal? New York, Public Affairs Committee Inc, No 429, 1969

Piver MS, Bolognese RJ, Feldman JD: Long-acting progesterone as a cause of missed abortion. Am J Obstet Gynecol 97:579, 1967

Poland B, Yuen BH: Embryonic development in consecutive specimens from recurrent spontaneous abortions. Am J Obstet Gynecol 130:512, 1978

Pritchard JA, Pritchard SA: Standardized treatment of 154 consecutive cases of eclampsia. Am J Obstet Gynecol 123:543, 1975

Pritchard JA, Whalley PJ: Abortion complicated by *Clostridium perfringens* infection. Am J Obstet Gynecol 111:484, 1971

Rappaport F, Rubinovitz M, Toaff R, Krocheck N: Genital listerosis as a cause of repeated abortion. Lancet 1:1273, 1960

Roberts CJ, Lowe CR: Where have all the conceptions gone? Lancet 1:498, 1975

Ruffolo EH, Wilson RB, Weed LA: *Listeria monocytogenes* as a cause of pregnancy wastage. Obstet Gynecol 19:533, 1962

Schiffer MA, Pakter J, Clahr J: Mortality associated with hypertonic saline abortion. Obstet Gynecol 42:759, 1973

Shapiro AG: Extraovular prostaglandin $F_{2\alpha}$ for early midtrimester abortion. Am J Obstet Gynecol 121:333, 1975

Sharma SD, Hale RW, Sato NE: Intramuscular (15S)-methyl prostaglandin $F_{2\alpha}$ for midtrimester and missed abortions. Obstet Gynecol 46:468, 1975

Shirodkar VN: A new method of operative treatment for habitual abortions in the second trimester of pregnancy. Antiseptic 52:299, 1955

Smith C, Gregori CA, Breen JL: Ultrasonography in threatened abortion. Obstet Gynecol 51:173, 1978

Spink WW: The Nature of Brucellosis. Minneapolis, Univ of Minn Press, 1956

Steinberg CR, Berkowitz RL, Merkatz IR, Roberts RB: Fever and bacteremia associated with hypertonic saline abortion. Obstet Gynecol 39:673, 1972

Strauss JH, Wilson M, Caldwell D, Otterson W, Martin AO: Laminaria use in midtrimester abortions induced by intra-amniotic prostaglandin $F_{2\alpha}$ with urea and intravenous oxytocin. Am J Obstet Gynecol 134:260, 1979

Supreme Court of the United States Syllabus, *Roe et al.* v *Wade,* District Attorney of Dallas County, Jan 22, 1973

Tietze C: Introduction to the statistics of abortion. In Engle ET (ed): Pregnancy Wastage. Springfiled, Ill., Thomas, 1953, p 135

Tupper C, Weil RJ: The problem of spontaneous abortion. Am J Obstet Gynecol 83:421, 1962

United Nations, Department of Social Affairs. Foetal, Infant and Early Childhood Mortality: I. The Statistics. New York, United Nations, 1954

Weinberg PC, Shepard MK: Intra-amnionic urea for induction of mid-trimester abortion. Obstet Gynecol 41:451, 1973

Wentz AC, Burnett S, Atienza MF, King TM: Experience with intra-amniotic prostaglandin $F_{2\alpha}$ for abortion. Am J Obstet Gynecol 117:513, 1973

Wentz AC, King TM: Myometrial necrosis after therapeutic abortion. Obstet Gynecol 40:315, 1972

Wong T-C, Schulman H: Endometrial aspiration as a means of early abortion. Obstet Gynecol 44:845, 1974

World Health Organization Task Force on Sequelae to Abortion: Gestation, birthweight, and spontaneous abortion in pregnancy after induced abortion. Lancet 1:142, 1979

25

Diseases and Abnormalities of the Reproductive Tract

DISEASES OF THE VULVA AND VAGINA

Varices. Varicosities sometimes appear in the lower part of the vagina but are more common around the vulva. There they may attain considerable size and cause a sensation of weight and discomfort. Vulvar varices may rupture during labor or be torn or cut by lacerations or episiotomy. Unless so traumatized, the varicosities in most instances become asymptomatic and decrease remarkably, or even disappear, after delivery.

Inflammation of Bartholin's Glands. Gonococci or other pathogenic organisms may gain access to Bartholin's glands and form abscesses. The labium majus on the side affected becomes swollen and painful, at and surrounding the collection of pus. Aside from causing pain and discomfort, such abscesses may be the starting point of a puerperal infection. For these reasons, drainage must be established whenever an abscess develops during pregnancy. After the contents have escaped, the cut edge of the abscess cavity, if actively bleeding, is sutured with fine chromic catgut. A gauze wick or Word cath-

eter is inserted to keep the ostium open until granulation is complete. McCoy and Cunningham (1980) found in pus from Bartholin abscesses both aerobic and anaerobic bacteria in nearly 90 percent of cases. *Neisseria gonorrhoeae* was identified in only 4 of 35 cases. A broad-spectrum antibiotic to which *Neisseria gonorrhoeae* is sensitive should be administered for 7 to 10 days.

The treatment of asymptomatic *Bartholin's duct cysts,* which are frequently the sequelae of Bartholin's gland abscesses, is best postponed until after delivery. Rarely is a labial cyst of sufficient size to cause difficulty at delivery. If this should occur, aspiration with a syringe and small needle will suffice as a temporary measure. Definitive surgery, if necessary, should be postponed until later.

Urethral Diverticulae, Cysts, and Abscesses. Trauma to the urethra or infection of the periurethral glands may be followed by the formation of periurethral abscesses, cysts, and diverticulae. Abscesses usually drain spontaneously with, at times, cyst formation as a sequela. Most often, periurethral cysts are asymptomatic and are best not disturbed during pregnancy. A urethral diverticulum may fill with debris which empties intermittently through the urethra to give rise to proteinuria of obscure etiology until the diverticulum is recognized as the source. In general, an attempt at surgical excision should not be made during pregnancy.

Condylomas (Condylomata). Condylomata lata are small, flat excrescences that are highly infectious. *Treponema pallidum* is usually present on dark field examination. *Condylomata acuminata,* sometimes called *venereal warts,* however, are not caused by syphilis nor gonorrhea. *Condylomata acuminata* are found with about equal frequency in white and nonwhite women and there is a high incidence in young primigravidas. Growth of the warts is likely to be stimulated during pregnancy.

Treatment of venereal warts during pregnancy is not very satisfactory. Local washing of the external genitalia, plus cleansing of the vagina by gentle douching (see Chap. 13, p. 319), followed by thorough drying, performed at least daily, may inhibit proliferation of the warts, as well as minimize discomfort.

A 20 percent solution of podophyllin in tincture of benzoin applied to the lesions has long been used to try to eradicate venereal warts. Its use during pregnancy is not likely to be highly effective, and considerable local discomfort may ensue. Rarely, topical application of podophyllin has proved to be extremely toxic. Slater and co-workers (1978) describe intense systemic toxicity with coma after its cutaneous application; it resolved after charcoal hemoperfusion. They also cited previously reported fatalities, including death of the fetus, following topical application of podophyllin. Infrequently, these lesions attain enormous size (Fig. 25-1) and may necessitate cesarean section. If the woman is seen several weeks or more before the end of pregnancy, the large lesion sometimes can be removed by excision, fulguration, or both.

Cystocele and Rectocele. Attenuation of the fascial support that is normally interposed between the vagina and the bladder anteriorly and the rectum posteriorly leads to prolapse into the vagina of the bladder (cystocele) or the rectum (rectocele). In former years, vaginal delivery after a prolonged labor of a large infant without episiotomy, but with appreciable lacerations of the lower genital tract predisposed to the development of a cystocele and a rectocele. The more liberal use of cesarean section in cases of less than absolute cephalopelvic disproportion and of episiotomies for most vaginal deliveries, coupled with generally lower parity, have made large symptomatic cystoceles and rectoceles almost a rarity. Urinary stasis associated with a large cystocele predisposes to urinary tract infection. A large rectocele may fill with feces which, at times, can only be evacuated manually. Both lesions can block the normal descent of the fetus through the birth canal, unless they are emptied and pushed out of the way. Surgical repair of either should not be attempted during the antepartum or intrapartum periods. Rather, definitive repair, often with vaginal hysterectomy for associated uterine prolapse and sterilization, should be carried out after pregnancy-induced tissue hyperemia has completely subsided.

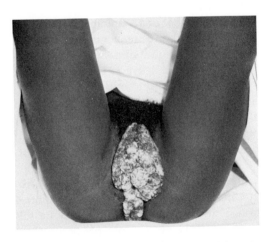

FIG. 25-1. Enormous confluent condylomata acuminata complicating pregnancy. The lesion attached to both labia majora by a relatively narrow base was excised and the defect easily closed with chromic suture. Subsequent vaginal delivery was uneventful.

Vaginal Tumors. Vaginal cysts, the

most frequent of benign vaginal tumors, may be discovered during pregnancy or sometimes not until the time of labor. Such cysts, usually embryologic rests (Gartner's or müllerian duct), may be of sufficient size to cause serious dystocia. Treatment depends upon the size and location of the cyst as well as the time at which it is first recognized. Drainage may be necessary. It is advisable to postpone surgical excision until after delivery and the puerperium.

CERVICAL NEOPLASIA

In the 1950s, the belief prevailed among indigent women of Dallas cared for at Parkland Memorial Hospital that "tying the tubes causes cancer." Women who were offered tubal sterilization at Parkland Memorial Hospital at that time were practically always indigent and of very high parity. Moreover, systematic cytologic screening for cervical neoplasia had not yet been established. Indeed, the association between tubal sterilization and malignancy noted by the women was epidemiologically sound! Invasive cancer of the cervix occurred most often in indigent women of high parity who were never previously screened for evidence of cervical neoplasia, the same population of women in whom most tubal sterilizations were then performed.

A vigorous program was instituted at that time using cervical cytology plus biopsy. Many cases of invasive cervical carcinoma and even more of preinvasive carcinoma were uncovered initially. It is gratifying that in more recent years invasive carcinoma has been found but rarely among the socioeconomically disadvantaged pregnant women cared for at Parkland Memorial Hospital.

Screening for Cervical Cancer. All pregnant women should undergo examination that includes evaluation of the cervix cytologically as well as by visual inspection and, unless actively bleeding and late in the second trimester or beyond, by palpation as described in Chapter 13, (p. 307). Any visible

fungating or ulcerating lesion should be evaluated by colposcopy or direct biopsy, since cytologic screening at times may fail to draw attention to a frankly invasive carcinoma.

Abnormal Cervical Cytology. Suspicious and positive findings in cervical smears is an indication for colposcopic evaluation to identify the responsible lesion. The cervix is examined and colposcopically directed biopsies made of any possibly malignant or premalignant lesion that is visualized. Colposcopy and directed biopsy during pregnancy has proved to be safe and reliable, thereby, in most cases, eliminating the need for conization (Benedet et al., 1977; DePetrillo et al., 1975; Ostergard and Nieberg, 1979).

If colposcopic examination is not available, multiple punch biopsies at the squamocolumnar junction should be obtained for evaluation by histologic techniques for carcinoma (Abitbol et al., 1973; Selim et al., 1973). Foci that do not stain with Lugol's solution should be preferentially biopsied. The multiple biopsies need not all be made on one occasion. Instead, the squamocolumnar junction can be "mapped" and biopsies obtained systematically over a period of time without hospitalization. Bleeding from biopsy sites can be controlled usually by a vaginal pack well-applied to the cervix for a few hours. Infrequently, the cervix during pregnancy may bleed to the extent that a suture about the biopsy site must be used to effect hemostasis.

Conization of the cervix is less satisfactory during pregnancy than in the absence of pregnancy for three reasons: (1) The epithelium and underlying stroma within the cervical canal cannot be so extensively excised because of the risk to the fetal membranes adjacent to the internal os. (2) Blood loss from the cervix during and after conization is appreciable in pregnant women and at times may be severe. (3) There is some increased risk of abortion or premature delivery. Fortunately, it has been the experience of most workers that either colposcopic directed biopsies or multiple punch biopsies of the squamocolumnar junction are an effective means of identifying invasive carcinoma, if present.

Dysplasia and Carcinoma in Situ.
These epithelial lesions need no immediate treatment when detected during pregnancy. The pregnancy should be allowed to continue and delivery accomplished without regard to the presence of either lesion (Boutselis, 1972; Parker, Addison, 1972). In general, the cervix should be reevaluated for neoplastic disease after the puerperium and appropriate therapy carried out that will range, depending upon the lesion that persists and the parity, from periodic reevaluation to hysterectomy. Cesarean hysterectomy to terminate the pregnancy and remove the affected cervix should be avoided unless there are other compelling indications for performing cesarean section. At times, it is difficult to be sure that all the cervix has been removed by cesarean hysterectomy.

For women who desire more children but have persistent severe dysplasia or carcinoma in situ after delivery, conization that includes the removal of all of the squamocolumnar junction, endocervical epithelium, and underlying stroma may be carried out and the specimen thoroughly studied histologically. Alternatively, the cervix may be carefully inspected with the colposcope and suspicious sites biopsied, followed by curettage of the endocervical canal. If endocervical dysplasia or neoplasia is found, conization is subsequently performed. If only dysplasia or carcinoma in situ of the squamocolumnar junction and exocervix is identified, cryotherapy can be applied. In the absence of stromal invasion, and with careful follow-up, pregnancy can be encouraged.

Invasive Carcinoma. Pregnancy coexisting with invasive carcinoma of the cervix complicates both diagnosis and treatment. Accurate identification of the extent of the cancer may be more difficult during pregnancy since induration of the base of the broad ligaments, which is characteristic in nonpregnant women of spread of tumor beyond the cervix, may be less prominent in the pregnant woman. Consequently, the extent of the tumor is more likely to be underestimated in the pregnant woman. Moreover, the decision for immediate interruption of the pregnancy versus allowing the fetus to achieve several more weeks of maturity before interruption almost always is difficult.

While few, if any, institutions have had great experience with the treatment of carcinoma of the cervix complicated by pregnancy, some generalizations can be made on the basis of some more recent reports, as well as the cumulative experiences at Parkland Memorial Hospital. Interestingly, the survival rate for invasive carcinoma of the cervix has not been profoundly different for pregnant and nonpregnant women within a given stage of disease. Moreover, the mode of delivery has not been shown to affect maternal survival significantly (Creasman et al., 1970). Nonetheless, when frankly invasive carcinoma is known to exist, most clinicians favor hysterotomy or cesarean section for terminating pregnancy, rather than labor and vaginal delivery.

Sufficient experience has accumulated to establish that for stage 1 invasive carcinoma complicated by pregnancy, extensive (radical) hysterectomy plus pelvic lymphadectomy is often the procedure of choice (Sall et al., 1974; Thompson et al., 1975). Dissection is facilitated by the softening of uterine supportive structures induced by the pregnancy, although blood loss is usually somewhat greater than in a nonpregnant woman.

For more extensive invasive cervical cancer, radiation therapy should be used. Early in pregnancy, external irradiation may be started without regard for the pregnancy products. They will be expelled spontaneously or, if not, they can be removed by curettage. Sources of radiation are subsequently applied in standard fashion to the cervix and adjacent parts. If the uterus is enlarged sufficiently to be easily palpated above the symphysis (beyond the first trimester), hysterotomy with the uterine incision remote from the cervix is performed to remove the pregnancy products. Care is taken to minimize adhesions, especially of bowel. After a week or so, external irradiation is started, followed by intracavitary application of radiation sources.

There are no data with which to establish, with any degree of confidence, the risk to the mother from delay in treatment of frankly invasive carcinoma for many weeks while the fetus matures. In general, unless the pregnancy has reached the third trimester, prompt treatment should be advised.

Carcinoma of the Endometrium. Adenocarcinoma of the endometrium with an intrauterine pregnancy is rare. Sandstrom and associates (1978) have described a case and reviewed the few instances reported previously by others. The most common lesion was adenoacanthoma.

DEVELOPMENTAL ABNORMALITIES OF THE GENITAL TRACT

Although developmental anomalies of the female genital tract are very uncommon in obstetric practice, some anomalies do contribute to serious fetal and maternal hazards.

Genesis. Because fusion of the two müllerian ducts to form a vagina, cervix, and uterine body in the human female takes place at three different levels at three different times, a variety of malformations can result. The three principal groups of deformities arising from three types of embryologic defects can be classified as follows:

1. The most common abnormality is the lack of or faulty midline fusion of the müllerian ducts. If there is complete lack of fusion, the result is the presence of two entirely separate uteri, cervices, and vaginas. With incomplete fusion, the defect may arise at the level of vagina, cervix, or uterus or in combinations of any of these two levels (Fig. 25-2).
2. There may be unilateral maturation of the müllerian duct with incomplete or absent development of the duct on the opposite side. The resulting defects are often associated with abnormalities of the upper urinary tract.
3. There may be defective canalization of the vagina, resulting in a transverse vaginal septum or, in the most extreme form, absence of the vagina.

Various classifications of these anomalies have been proposed, but none is completely satisfactory. The terminology is often so complicated and replete with Latin words that the relative obstetric significance of the disorders is obscured. A simplified classification is outlined below in which five types of uteri are recognized:

1. *Single.* The normal symmetric uterus, re-

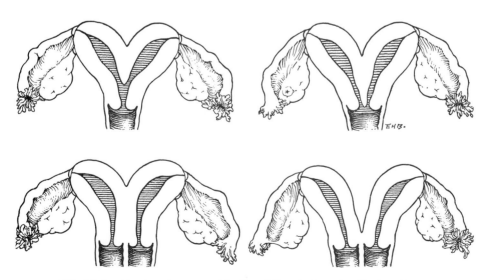

FIG. 25-2. Varying degrees of faulty midline fusion of müllerian ducts.

sulting from normal fusion of the müllerian ducts.

2. *Septate.* Essentially normal uterus externally, with little or no external notching of the fundus. Internally, a septum of varying thickness extends part or all the way from fundus to cervix, dividing the uterine cavity into two more or less distinct compartments.

3. *Bicornuate.* The Y-shaped, forked uterus occurs in a wide range of varieties. Externally it may have only a shallow notch, or it may be cleaved so deeply as to be called a "double uterus." The internal septum may be partial, or it may extend down to the cervix, creating two separate cavities. The distinguishing characteristic of this uterus, regardless of the extent of fundal notching, is the cervix. The term "bicornuate" is limited to a forked uterus having a single cervix, rather than one having a double cervix.

4. *Double.* This designation is reserved for those instances of failure of midline fusion of the müllerian ducts producing two hemiuteri, each having a distinct cervix. Complete reduplication of the uterus is sometimes referred to as *uterus didelphys.* At times, development of one of the hemiuteri may be further distorted to yield a rudimentary structure lacking a cervix, and therefore, without vaginal communication, or, less often, lacking even a uterine cavity.

5. *Single Hemiuterus.* There is maturation of but a single müllerian duct anlage with complete failure of the other. The uterus is further characterized by having only one oviduct attached.

There are four types of cervices:

1. *Single.* The normal cervix.

2. *Septate.* A cervix consisting of a single muscular ring partitioned by a septum. The septum may be confined to the cervix, or, more often, may be the downward continuation of a uterine septum or the upward extension of a vaginal septum.

3. *Double.* Two distinct cervices, each resulting from separate müllerian duct maturation. Both a septate and a true double cervix are frequently associated with a vaginal septum, the result being that many septate cervices are erroneously classified as double. The diagnosis depends on careful visual and digital examination of the cervix and is of clinical importance.

4. *Single Hemicervix.* Arises from unilateral müllerian maturation.

The vagina may be classified as follows:

1. *Single.* The normal vagina.

2. *Septate.* More or less complete longitudinal septum.

3. *Double.* It is often difficult to distinguish the double from the completely septate vagina. The true double vagina includes a double introitus and resembles a double-barreled shotgun, with each passage terminating in a distinct, separate cervix. At times with double vaginas one may end blindly.

4. *Transverse septum.* Transverse vaginal septa are of different developmental origin, resulting from faulty canalization of the united müllerian anlage, rather than faulty longitudinal fusion.

The obstetric significance of these defects can be anticipated. The various vaginal septa often are easily dilated, displaced, or surgically divided. The cervix, however, must undergo effacement and dilatation during labor. The septate cervix functions fairly well in these respects, but there is possible danger of rupture and consequent hemorrhage. The major obstetric difficulties arise from anomalies of the uterus. The uterus must dilate and hypertrophy sufficiently to permit enlargement during pregnancy adequate to accommodate a term-sized fetus in a proper longitudinal lie and at the appropriate time contract efficiently to expel the pregnancy products. The uterine defects resulting from maturation of only one müllerian duct or from complete lack of fusion often give rise to a hemiuterus that fails to dilate and hypertrophy appropriately and in turn to a host of possible

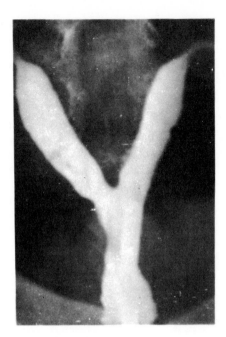

FIG. 25-3. Hysterogram of a bicornuate uterus. (Courtesy of Dr. Alvin Siegler.)

difficulties, including abortion, prematurity, pathologic lie, uterine dysfunction, and even uterine rupture. Since lesser defects of fusion lead to proportionately less serious obstetric difficulties, women with the relatively more common minor abnormalities such as arcuate or partially septate uteri may be expected to have relatively normal deliveries.

Diagnosis.   Some malformations are discovered by simple inspection, and others by bimanual examination. They are occasionally discovered first at cesarean section or during manual exploration of the uterine cavity after vaginal delivery. Fundal notching, palpated abdominally, most often is indicative of a malformed uterus. Without radiologic examination or direct visualization of the uterine cavity, it is difficult to distinguish the septate from the bicornuate uterus. *Hysterography* is of value to ascertain the configuration of the uterine cavity (Fig. 25-3).

A high index of suspicion is important for a high rate of detection of uterine malformations. Green and Harris (1976) identified 80 uterine developmental anomalies during the

course of 31,836 deliveries. They emphasized that detection was greatest during a period when one staff member was especially interested in the problem and espoused uterine exploration at delivery and, when an anomaly was suspected, suggested that hysterosalpingography be performed 6 to 8 weeks postpartum.

Sonography may be used to identify abnormal uterine development, although it often lacks the precision of diagnosis provided by hysterosalpingography. Especially during actual or suspected pregnancy, sonographic examination can be quite informative. In Figure 25-4, for example, 2 separate uterine cavities are seen. A gestational ring, probably abnormal, was first identified in the left cavity. It subsequently degenerated but tissue was not expelled. Ninety days later, a pregnancy ring was identified in the right uterine cavity. The correct interpretation was a missed abortion in the left uterine cavity and an apparently normal early pregnancy in the right. A healthy living infant was delivered subsequently (see Fig. 25-4).

UROLOGIC EVALUATION.   When asymmetrical development of the reproductive tract is found, urologic evaluation is indicated because of the frequent association of anomalies of the urinary tract. When there is uterine atresia on one side or one of double vaginas terminates blindly, an ipsilateral urologic anomaly is extremely common (Toaff, 1974; Wiersma et al., 1976; Woolf and Allen, 1953).

Prognosis.   With minor uterine defects, the prognosis is excellent. Most published reports include only obvious major defects. In these situations also, except for uterine rupture, the prognosis for the mother is generally good. Cesarean section is, of course, required more frequently. With uterine anomalies, the occurrence of low birth weight of the infant is at least three times the normal rate and consequently, perinatal loss is high. The abortion rate is also high. Among the 80 women with uterine developmental anomalies identified by Green and Harris

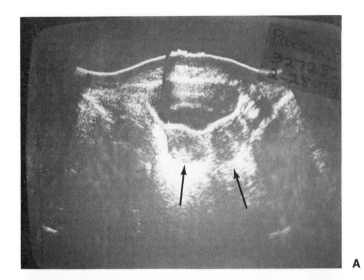

A

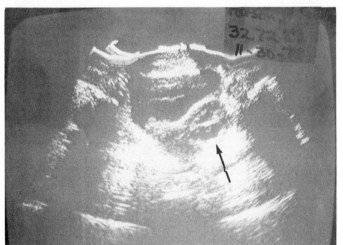

B

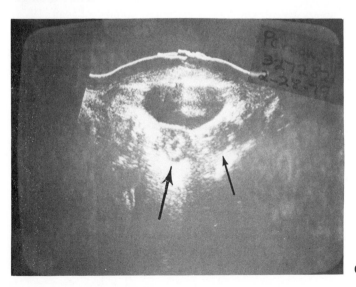

C

FIG. 25-4. In transverse sonogram **A,** two uterine cavities are apparent above arrows. In sonogram **B,** a pregnancy ring, probably abnormal, is seen in the *left* uterine cavity above arrow. In sonogram **C,** made 90 days later, a normal pregnancy ring is seen in the *right* uterine cavity above larger arrow but not in the left uterine cavity above smaller arrow. After 7 abortions, a 2900 g healthy infant was delivered as a double footling breech by cesarean section at 38 weeks gestation. Necrotic placental villi were expelled from the left uterus 2 days postpartum.

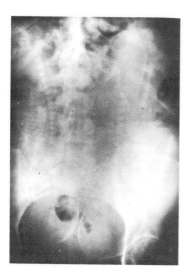

FIG. 25-5. Roentgenogram in a case of a double uterus with a near-term fetus in each. Each was delivered by cesarean section. (Courtesy of Dr. Jack Pearson.)

(1976), overall fetal wastage was 55 percent.

Treatment. Abnormal fetal presentations, which are common in abnormal uteri, are generally treated in the same way as when they occur in normal uteri. If uterine inertia occurs, it is generally unwise to stimulate these defective uteri with oxytocin. Cesarean section is the safer treatment but, unfortunately, the diagnosis is often unexpected.

Rarely, pregnancy occurs simultaneously in both hemiuteri (Fig. 25-5) or singly in a *rudimentary horn* (Fig. 25-6). Rolen and colleagues (1966) reviewed the histories of 70 pregnancies in rudimentary uterine horns. Although a few live births were reported, the duration of pregnancy before uterine rupture was usually 20 weeks or less. Intraperitoneal hemorrhage may be voluminous. Sometimes it is technically possible to remove only

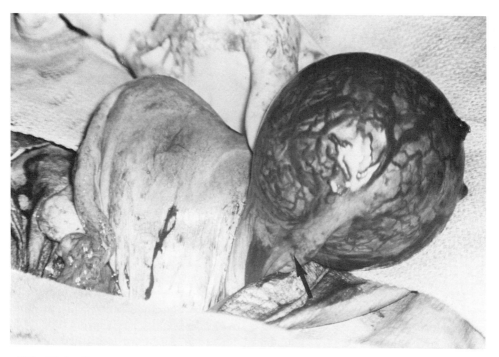

FIG. 25-6. Pregnancy of 15 weeks gestational age in left rudimentary hemiuterus as seen at laparotomy. The tense, vascular rudimentary uterus was bleeding from veins over its extremely vascular surface. The attached oviduct (arrow) was patent and the adjacent left ovary contained the corpus luteum of pregnancy. There was no cervix and no demonstrable communication with the right hemiuterus which did have a cervix and communicated with the vagina.

the damaged rudimentary horn, in which case the larger horn may be preserved.

Pregnancy in a rudimentary uterine horn 15 weeks after the last menstrual period is shown in Figure 25-6. There was no connection between the rudimentary horn and the opposite uterine horn or the vagina. The fertilizing sperm had to migrate out the oviduct attached to the patent uterine horn and cross transperitoneally to enter the oviduct attached to the rudimentary uterine horn. The woman complained of sudden, severe, cramping lower abdominal pain; she had missed three menstrual periods. A very tender mass was felt to the left of a somewhat enlarged uterus. Fetal heart action was identified in this mass with Doppler ultrasound. At laparotomy, about 200 ml of blood was free in the peritoneal cavity. A total hysterectomy and left salpingo-oophorectomy were performed. Her three previous pregnancies, all breech presentations, terminated in delivery of infants who weighed 750 g (expired), 1220 g, and 2815 g. The 2815 g infant was delivered by cesarean section. Although a rudimentary horn was identified at that time, tubal patency to that horn was not interrupted.

PLASTIC REPAIR.   When a patient presents with a uterine anomaly and a poor obstetric history with repeated abortions not ascribable to some other cause, plastic repair of the defect *(metroplasty)* may be justified. Musich and Behrman (1978), on the basis of obstetric outcomes before and after metroplasty in women cared for at the University of Michigan, concluded that women with septate or bicornuate anomalies and poor previous obstetric outcomes, are very likely to have good outcomes after repair.

UTERINE MALPOSITION

Anteflexion.   Exaggerated degrees of anteflexion are frequently observed in the early months of pregnancy, but are without significance. In the later months, particularly when the abdominal walls are very lax, the uterus may fall forward. The sagging occasionally is so exaggerated that the fundus lies considerably below the lower margin of the

symphysis pubis. Even in less striking instances of so-called *pendulous abdomen,* the pregnant woman may complain of various annoying symptoms, especially dragging pains in the back and lower abdomen. Amelioration of symptoms is frequently effected by wearing a properly fitted abdominal support.

Retrodisplacement.   Retroversion of the uterus is occasionally encountered during the first trimester, occurring in about 11 percent of women, according to Weekes and associates (1976). They noted not only a higher frequency of bleeding early in pregnancy in women with a retroverted uterus, but also an abortion rate of 16 percent, compared to 9 percent in women whose uterus was not retroverted. In their survey, perinatal mortality was slightly less, however, among women with a retroverted uterus. The biologic significance of these observations is not clear at this time. Most authorities, however, no longer regard the retroverted uterus per se to be a pathologic finding. Thus, it would need no treatment, except in the rare circumstance in which the growing retroverted uterus did not rise out of the pelvis by the end of the first trimester, but rather was incarcerated in the hollow of the sacrum, as shown in Figure 25-7. Women with a retroverted uterus should be evaluated frequently early in the second trimester, to make sure that the uterus is not incarcerated. If the uterus cannot be readily identified abdominally above the symphysis, pelvic examination is indicated. The woman with an incarcerated pregnant uterus otherwise is usually first seen complaining of abdominal discomfort and inability to void. As pressure from the full bladder increases, small amounts of urine are passed involuntarily, but the bladder never empties entirely *(paradoxical incontinence).* After the bladder has been emptied by catheterization, the uterus can usually be pushed out of the pelvis when the patient is placed in the knee-chest position; anesthesia is seldom necessary. A retention catheter should be left in place until bladder tone returns.

The urinary obstruction from an incarcerated gravid uterus can be so severe as to cause

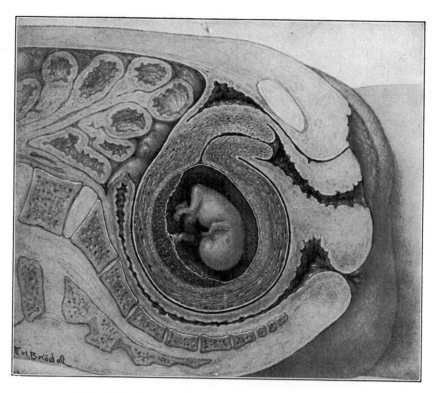

FIG. 25-7.   Incarceration of retroflexed pregnant uterus.

azotemia. With relief of the obstruction, there may be a marked diuresis with the loss of large amounts of sodium and potassium. Swartz and Komins (1977) have described such a case.

Sacculation of the Uterus.   Continuation of pregnancy in the presence of a gravid uterus persistently entrapped in the pelvis involves sacculation, i.e., extensive dilatation of the lower portion of the body of the uterus.

Rarely, the persistently entrapped retroverted uterus produces few symptoms, yet extensive dilatation of the lower portion of the body of the uterus, i.e., the lower uterine segment, takes place to accommodate the fetus. In a recent case at Parkland Memorial Hospital, at the time of cesarean section, the Foley catheter bulb in the bladder lay just below the level of the umbilicus. The cervix was at an equally high level. Most of the fetus, who was alive and weighed 2500 g, the amnionic fluid, and the fetal membranes were

contained in a remarkably thin sacculation of the anterior wall of the lower segment. The fetal head was entrapped in the most superior part of the sacculation, along with three loops of cord, by a constricting ring of myometrium. The fundus of the uterus and the placenta were contained in the true pelvis beneath a sharp sacral promontory. After delivery, the uterus soon contracted and retracted to assume a more normal shape. Weissberg and Gall (1972) reviewed the relatively few published reports of sacculation of the pregnant uterus.

Prolapse of the Pregnant Uterus.
Impregnation in a totally prolapsed uterus is very rare because of the difficulty of successful coitus, but impregnation when the uterus is only partially prolapsed is more common. In such cases, the cervix (Fig. 25-8), and occasionally a portion of the body of the uterus, may protrude to a variable extent from the vulva during the early months of

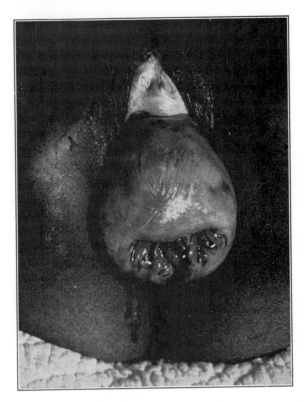

FIG. 25-8. Prolapse of cervix in pregnancy. Note extreme edema.

pregnancy. As pregnancy progresses, however, the body of the uterus usually rises gradually above the pelvis, and may draw the cervix up with it. If the uterus persists in its prolapsed position, symptoms of incarceration may appear during the third or fourth month of pregnancy.

For treatment of uterine prolapse during early pregnancy, the uterus should be replaced and held in position with a suitable pessary. If, however, the pelvic floor is too relaxed to permit retention of the pessary, the woman should be kept recumbent as long as possible until after the fourth month. When the cervix reaches or slightly protrudes from the vulva, scrupulous hygiene is mandatory. If much of the cervix persists outside the vulva and cannot be replaced, the pregnancy should be terminated.

When the vaginal outlet is markedly relaxed, the congested anterior or posterior vaginal walls sometimes prolapse during pregnancy, although the uterus may still retain its normal position. This condition may give rise to considerable discomfort and interfere with locomotion, and it is not amenable to treatment until after delivery. During labor, these structures may be forced down in front of the presenting part and interfere with its descent. In that event, they should be carefully cleansed and pushed back over the descending fetal presenting part.

MISCELLANEOUS CONDITIONS

Acute Edema of the Cervix. In very rare instances, the cervix, particularly its anterior lip, may become so acutely edematous and enlarged during pregnancy that it protrudes from the vulva. This condition, if not associated with preexisting hypertrophy, may disappear with bed rest almost as suddenly as it developed.

Enterocele. In rare instances, an enterocele of considerable size filled with loops of intestine may complicate pregnancy. If this condition occurs during pregnancy, the protrusion should be replaced and the woman kept in the recumbent position. During labor, the mass may interfere with the advance of the fetal head. In such cases, it should be pushed up or held out of the way as well as possible, to allow delivery of the head past the mass.

Torsion of the Pregnant Uterus. Torsion of the pregnant uterus of sufficient degree to arrest the uterine circulation and produce an acute abdominal catastrophe is one of the rarest accidents of human gestation.

Salpingitis and Tubo-Ovarian Abscess. Gonococcal salpingitis, salpingo-oophoritis, and pelvic peritonitis may develop during the first trimester of pregnancy by ascent of bacteria from the cervix to the endosalpinx. Once the chorion fuses with the decidua to obliterate completely the uterine cavity early in the second trimester, this pathway for ascending bacterial spread by way of the uterine mucosa is interrupted. Thereafter, primary acute inflammation of the tubes and ovaries is rarely, if ever, seen, although tubo-ovarian abscesses may form in previously infected structures. Presumably, the organisms reach the previously damaged oviduct and ovary through lymphatics or the bloodstream. Jafari and associates (1977) described the successful outcome of a term pregnancy complicated by a tubo-ovarian abscess, as well as the few experiences of others that have been reported.

In one of two instances of tubo-ovarian abscess complicating midpregnancy treated at Parkland Memorial Hospital during the past two decades, hysterectomy, as well as bilateral salpingo-oophorectomy, was carried out. The woman recovered after a very complicated postoperative course. In the other instance, the tubo-ovarian abscess was smaller and was mobilized intact. Therefore, only the affected tube and ovary were removed. The pregnancy subsequently proceeded normally, terminating in spontaneous vaginal delivery of a normal infant.

Even with extensive pelvic adhesions from previous pelvic infection, women usually suffer no adverse effects during pregnancy.

Pregnancy Complicated by Pelvic Tumors. Pregnancy is occasionally complicated by ovarian or uterine tumors. Although, as a rule, the tumors do not materially affect the course of pregnancy, they sometimes give rise both to erroneous estimates of gestational age and to serious dystocia. This problem is considered in detail in Chapter 32.

Hydrorrhea Gravidarum. Rarely, pregnant women may lose clear fluid from the uterus throughout much of pregnancy. The cause of this condition is not always obvious but may represent persistent *amniorrhea* following rupture of the membranes. Gregersen (1976) described a case with loss of fluid beginning about the 10th week of pregnancy and continuing until delivery at 31 weeks. Up to 200 ml of fluid per day was collected. The ruptured membranes may retract to such an extent that the fetus is no longer contained within the amnionic sac. Such an *extramembranous pregnancy* is demonstrated in Figure 25-9. Extramembranous pregnancy involving a twin has also been described (Panayiotis, Grunstein, 1979). The membranes were diamnionic and dichorionic with a single placenta in which there was appreciable circumvallate involvement on the side of the extramembranous fetus. The newborn quickly succumbed from anoxia. Pulmonary hypoplasia, presumably due to lack of amnionic fluid and thus the inability to inspire in utero was evident at autopsy. In an era of frequent amniocentesis, this rare complication, fortunately, does not appear to have increased.

Endometriosis. Since endometriosis is frequently associated with infertility, it is an uncommon complication of pregnancy. As emphasized in Scott's early report (1944), however, some women with endometriosis do become pregnant and, in the course of gestation, sometimes exhibit bizarre and vexing clinical pictures.

A rare complication of ovarian endome-

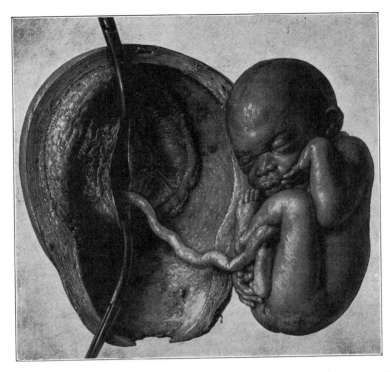

FIG. 25-9. Extramembranous pregnancy. Note collapsed fetal membranes held apart by clamps.

triosis in pregnancy is rupture of an endometrial cyst, with clinical features that are suggestive of acute appendicitis or tubal pregnancy. Another is an enlarging pelvic endometrioma that causes dystocia in labor. Many women with unrecognized endometriosis, however, doubtless go through pregnancy and labor without complications.

Of the 12 cases of *adenomyosis* associated with pregnancy that Scott (1944) was able to collect from a review of the literature, 5 were complicated by uterine rupture, 3 by postpartum hemorrhage, and 2 by dystocia resulting from the adenomyoma.

REFERENCES

Abitbol MM, Benjamin F, Castillo N: Management of cervical smear and carcinoma in situ of the cervix during pregnancy. Am J Obstet Gynecol 117:904, 1973

Benedet JL, Boyes DA, Nichols TM: Colposcopic evaluation of pregnant patients with abnormal cervical smears. Br J Obstet Gynaecol 84:517, 1977

Boutselis JG: Intraepithelial carcinoma of the cervix associated with pregnancy. Obstet Gynecol 40:657, 1972

Creasman WT, Rutledge FN, Fletcher GH: Carcinoma of the cervix associated with pregnancy. Obstet Gynecol 36:495, 1970

DePetrillo AD, Townsend DE, Morrow CP, Lickrish GM, DiSaia PJ, Roy M: Colposcopic evaluation of the abnormal Papanicolaou test in pregnancy. Am J Obstet Gynecol 121:441, 1975

Green LK, Harris RE: Uterine anomalies: frequency of diagnosis and associated obstetric complications. Obstet Gynecol 47:427, 1976

Gregersen E: Extramembranous pregnancy with amniorrhoea. Acta Obstet Gynecol Scand 55:69, 1976

Jafari K, Vilovic-Kos J, Webster A, Steptoe R: Tubo-ovarian abscess in pregnancy. Acta Obstet Gynecol Scand 56:1, 1977

McCoy C, Cunningham FG: Unpublished observations, 1980

Musich J Jr, Behrman SJ: Obstetric outcomes before and after metroplasty in women with uterine anomalies. Obstet Gynecol 52:63, 1978

Ostergard DR, Nieberg RK: Evaluation of abnormal cervical cytology during pregnancy with coloscopy. Am J Obstet Gynecol 134:756, 1979

Panayiotis G, Grunstein S: Extramembranous pregnancy in twin gestation. Obstet Gynecol (Suppl) 53:34S, 1979

Parker RT, Addison A: The surgical treatment of cervical neoplasia. South Med J 60:32, 1972

Rolen AC, Choquette AJ, Semmens JP: Rudimentary uterine horn: obstetric and gynecologic implications. Obstet Gynecol 27:806, 1966

Sall S, Rini S, Pineda A: Surgical management of invasive carcinoma of the cervix in pregnancy. Obstet Gynecol 118:1, 1974

Sandstrom RE, Welch WR, Green TH: Adenocarcinoma of the endometrium in pregnancy. Obstet Gynecol 53:73 suppl., 1979

Scott RB: Endometriosis and pregnancy. Am J Obstet Gynecol 47:608, 1944

Selim MA, So-Bosita JL, Blair OM, Little BA: Cervical biopsy versus conization. Obstet Gynecol 41:177, 1973

Slater GE, Rumack BH, Peterson RG: Podophyllin poisoning. Systemic toxicity following cutaneous application. Obstet Gynecol 52:94, 1978

Swartz EM, Komins JI: Postobstructive diuresis after reduction of an incarcerated gravid uterus. J Reprod Med 19:262, 1977

Toaff R: A major malformation—communicating uteri. Obstet Gynecol 43:221, 1974

Thompson JD, Caputo TA, Franklin EW III, Dale E: The surgical management of invasive cancer of the cervix in pregnancy. Am J Obstet Gynecol 121:853, 1975

Weekes ARL, Atlay RD, Brown VA, Jordan EC, Murray SM: The retroverted gravid uterus and its effect on the outcome of pregnancy. Br Med J 1:622, 1976

Weissberg SM, Gall SA: Sacculation of the pregnant uterus. Obstet Gynecol 39:691, 1972

Wiersma AF, Peterson LF, Justema EJ: Uterine anomalies associated with renal agenesis. Obstet Gynecol 47:654, 1976

Woolf RB, Allen WM: Concomitant malformations: frequent simultaneous occurrence of congenital malformations of the reproductive and urinary tracts. Obstet Gynecol 2:236, 1953

26

Multifetal Pregnancy

Morbidity and mortality are increased appreciably in pregnancies with multiple fetuses. It is not an overstatement, therefore, to consider a pregnancy with multiple fetuses to be a complicated pregnancy. Many of the complications that occur more commonly with multiple fetuses and are of obvious clinical significance are listed below:

1. Abortion
2. Perinatal mortality
3. Low birth weight
   Prematurity
   Growth retardation
4. Malformations
5. Fetal-fetal hemorrhage
   Hypovolemia and anemia
   Hypervolemia and hyperviscosity
6. Pregnancy-induced or
       aggravated hypertension
7. Maternal Anemia
   Acute blood loss
   Iron deficiency
   Folate deficiency
8. Maternal hemorrhage
   Uterine atony
9. Placental accidents
   Placental abruption
   Placenta previa
   Vasa previa
10. Hydramnios

11. Complicated labor
    Premature labor
    Prolonged labor
    Abnormal fetal presentation
    Cord prolapse

ETIOLOGY OF MULTIPLE FETUSES

Twin fetuses more commonly result from fertilization of two separate ova (*fraternal* or *dizygotic twins*). About one-third as often, twins arise from a single fertilized ovum that subsequently divides into two similar structures, each with the potential for developing into a separate individual (*identical* or *monozygotic twins*). Either or both processes may be involved in the formation of higher numbers of fetuses. Quadruplets, for example, may arise from one, two, three, or four ova.

Dizygotic twins are not in a strict sense true twins, since they result from the maturation and fertilization of two ova during a single ovulatory cycle. Newman (1923) wrote: "Strictly speaking, twaining is twining or two-ing—the division of an individual into two equivalent and more or less completely separate individuals." Also, monozygotic or identical twins are not always identical. As will be pointed out below, the process of division of one fertilized zygote into two does not necessarily result in equal sharing of protoplasmic materials. In fact, dizygotic, or fraternal twins of the same sex may *appear* more nearly identical at birth than do monozygotic twins; growth of monozygotic twin fetuses may be discordant and at times dramatically so.

Genesis of Monozygotic Twins. Valid hypotheses to explain single-ovum, or monozygotic twinning, are lacking. Monozygotic twins arise from division of the fertilized ovum at various early stages of development as follows:

1. If division occurs before the inner cell mass is formed and the outer layer of blastocyst is not yet committed to become chorion, i.e., within the first 72 hours after fertilization, two embryos, two amnions, and two chorions will develop. There will evolve a *diamnionic, dichorionic,* monozygotic twin pregnancy. The frequency of two chorions with monozygotic twinning in various reports has ranged from 18 to 36 percent (MacGillivray, 1978). There may be two distinct placentas or a single fused placenta, as depicted in A and B of Figure 26-1.

2. If division occurs between the fourth and eighth days, after the inner cell mass is formed and cells destined to become chorion have already differentiated, but those of the amnion have not, two embryos will develop, each in separate amnionic sacs. The two amnionic sacs will eventually be covered by a common chorion, thus giving rise to *diamnionic, monochorionic,* monozygotic twin pregnancy (Fig. 26-1. C).

3. If, however, the amnion has already become established, which occurs about 8 days after fertilization, division will result in two embryos within a common amnionic sac, or a *monoamnionic, monochorionic,* monozygotic twin pregnancy.

4. If division is initiated even later, i.e., after the embryonic disk is formed, cleavage is incomplete and conjoined twins are formed.

Frequency. The frequency of monozygotic twins appears to be relatively constant throughout the world at approximately one set of monozygotic twin infants per 250 births, and is largely independent of race, heredity, age, parity, and gonadotropin therapy for infertility. The incidence of delivery of dizygotic or fraternal twins is influenced remarkably by race, heredity, maternal age, parity, and, especially, "fertility drugs."

It is now apparent through the use of sonography early in pregnancy that the inci-

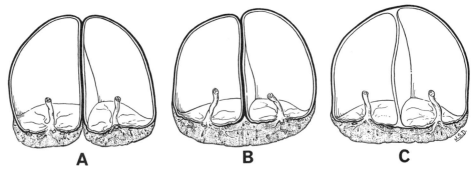

FIG. 26-1. A–C. Placenta and membranes in twin pregnancies: **A.** Two placentas, two amnions, two chorions (from either dizygotic twins or monozygotic twins with cleavage of zygote during first 3 days after fertilization). **B.** Single placenta, two amnions, and two chorions (from either dizygotic twins or monozygotic twins with cleavage of zygote during first 3 days). **C.** One placenta, one chorion, two amnions (monozygotic twins with cleavage of zygote from the fourth to the eighth day after fertilization).

dence of twin conceptions is much higher than indicated by figures based on the delivery of two fetuses. Robinson and Caines (1977), for example, by means of sonography performed during the first trimester, identified twin conceptions in 30 women, only 14 of whom eventually gave birth to two infants. Eleven of the 16 women who did not do so ultimately were delivered of a single fetus and a blighted ovum. Four more were diagnosed as having twin blighted ova, and one a blighted ovum and a missed abortion.

Multiple embryos and fetuses may rarely develop to varying degrees ectopically, i.e., outside the uterus. Such multiple ectopic pregnancies, as well as *combined pregnancies* in which there are one or more embryos or fetuses, extrauterine as well as one or more intrauterine, were considered in Chapter 22.

RACE. The frequency of birth of multiple fetuses varies significantly among different races. For example, Myrianthopoulos (1970) identified in the Collaborative Cerebral Palsy Study the birth of twins in one out of every 100 pregnancies among white women, compared to one out of 79 pregnancies for black women. In some areas of Africa the frequency of twinning is very high. Nylander (1969) in a survey of one rural community in Nigeria found that twinning occurred once in every 22 births! Twinning among Orientals is less common. In Japan, for example, among more than 10 million pregnancies analyzed, twinning was identified only once in every 155 births. These racial differences are the consequence of variations in the occurrence of dizygotic twinning.

HEREDITY. A partial answer to the question of the role of heredity in twinning has been provided by White and Wyshak (1964) in a study of 4000 records of the General Society of the Church of Jesus Christ of Latter-day Saints. They noted that women who themselves were dizygotic twins gave birth to twins at the rate of one set per 58 pregnancies whereas women whose husbands were dizygotic twins produced twins at the rate

of one set per 126 pregnancies. Bulmer's (1960) analysis of twins identified one out of 25 (4 percent) of their mothers to be a twin but only one out of 60 (1.7 percent) of their fathers to be twins. From these observations, it is apparent that as a determinant for twinning the genotype of the mother is much more important than that of the father.

MATERNAL AGE AND PARITY. The positive effects of increasing maternal age and parity on the incidence of twinning have been well demonstrated by Waterhouse (1950). For any increase in age up to about 40 or parity up to 7, the frequency of twinning increased. Twin pregnancies were less than one-third as common in women under 20 years of age with no previous children than in women 35 to 40 years of age with four or more previous children. More recently in Sweden, Pettersson and associates (1976) have confirmed the remarkable increase in multiple birth rate associated with increased parity. In first pregnancies, the frequency of multiple births was 1.27 percent, compared to 2.67 percent in the fourth birth order.

ENDOGENOUS GONADOTROPIN. Benirshke and Kim (1973) in their excellent review, "Multiple Pregnancy," present intriguing reasons for implicating elevated levels of endogenous follicle-stimulating hormone in the genesis of spontaneous dizygous twinning. A higher rate of dizygous twinning has been described for women who conceived within one month after stopping use of oral contraceptives, but not during subsequent months (Rothman, 1977). One possibility to account for the apparent increase is release of pituitary gonadotropin in amounts greater than usual during the first spontaneous cycle after stopping contraception. Another is simply increased fecundity among very recent users of oral contraceptives.

INFERTILITY AGENTS. The induction of ovulation by use of gonadotropins (follicle-stimulating hormone plus chorionic gonadotropin) or of clomiphene enhances remarkably the likelihood of ovulations of multiple ova. Multiple fetuses are common in pregnancies among patients in whom ovulation was induced by injections of gonadotropins (Gemzell et al., 1968). The incidence of multiple fetuses following gonadotropin therapy is 20 to 40 percent, and in one instance as many as 11 fetuses were aborted (Jewelewicz, Vande Wiele, 1975). Nonuplet pregnancy with spontaneous labor 27 weeks after induction of ovulation with human pituitary gonadotropin has been described by Garrett and associates (1976). None of the nine infants survived. Two of octuplets survived in Italy. Sextuplets after gonadotropin therapy have survived in South Africa as did five of the sextuplets born in Denver.

With clomiphene therapy, the likelihood of multiple fetuses is somewhat less than with human menopausal gonadotropin. Even so, among 2369 pregnancies following clomiphene 165 (6.9 percent) were known to be twin, 11 (0.5 percent) triplet, seven (0.3 percent) quadruplet, and three (0.13 percent) quintuplet (Merrell-National Laboratories Product Information Bulletin, 1972). Harlap (1976) identified in smaller groups in Israel the frequency of multiple fetuses following clomiphene treatment to be 13 percent.

RECENT TRENDS IN DIZYGOTIC TWINNING. In many countries for which data are available, including the United States, there apparently has been a decline in recent years in the frequency of dizygotic twinning (Editorial, Br Med J, 1976). The cause is not known. The decline seems too sharp to be ascribed solely to decreased parity.

Sex Ratios with Multiple Fetuses.

The percentage of male conceptuses in the human species decreases as the number of fetuses per pregnancy increases. Strandskov and co-workers (1946) found the sex ratio, or percentage of males, for 31 million singleton births in the United States to be 51.59 percent. For twins, it was 50.85 percent; for triplets, 49.54 percent; and for quadruplets, 46.48 percent. Two explanations have been offered: The differential fetal mortality between the sexes is well known, as it is for

the newborn infant, child, and adult. Survival is always in favor of the female and against the male. The "population pressure" with multiple fetuses in utero may exaggerate the biologic tendency noted in singleton pregnancies. A second possible explanation is that the female-producing zygote has a greater tendency to divide into twins, triplets, and quadruplets.

DETERMINATION OF ZYGOSITY

With the advent of organ transplantation, the zygosity of multiple fetuses from a single pregnancy has assumed more than theoretical importance.

Examination of Placenta. Appropriate

examination of the placenta and membranes often will serve to identify the zygosity of fetuses more firmly than will subsequent studies that yield less precise information at considerable inconvenience and expense. The following system for examination is recommended: As the first infant is delivered, one clamp is placed on the portion of the cord coming from the placenta. As the second infant is delivered two clamps are placed on the cord toward the placental side. Three clamps are used to mark the cord of a third infant, and so on as necessary. Until the delivery of the last fetus is completed, it is important that each segment of cord attached to the placenta remain clamped lest fetal hemorrhage occur through anastomosed fetal vessels in the placenta.

Delivery of the placenta should be accomplished with care to preserve the attachment of the membranes to the placenta since identification of the relationship of the membranes to each other is critical. With one common amnionic sac, which is a rare finding, or with juxtaposed amnions not separated by chorion arising between the fetuses, the infants are monozygotic. If adjacent amnions are separated by chorion, the fetuses may be monozygotic or more often dizygotic (Figs. 26-1–26-3). If the infants are of the same sex, blood group studies to identify zygosity may be ini-

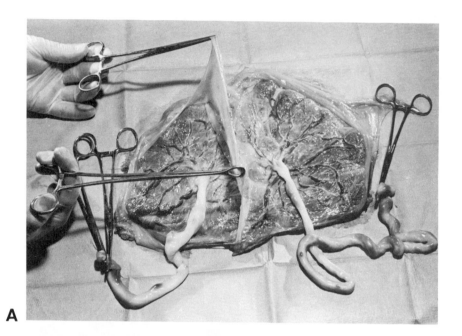

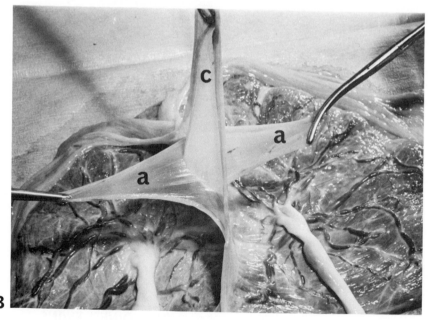

FIG. 26–2. A. The membrane partition that separated twin fetuses is elevated. **B.** The membrane partition consists of chorion (c) between two amnions (a).

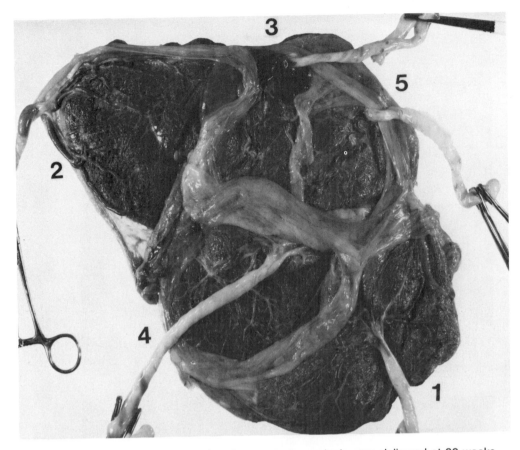

FIG. 26-3. Quintuplet placenta with five separate amnionic sacs delivered at 32 weeks gestation. Amnionic sacs no. 3 and 5 were not separated by chorion and therefore those infants are identical. Infant birth weights ranged from a high of 1530 g (no. 1) to 860 g (no. 5). All of the infants survived.

tiated at this time on samples of blood obtained from the umbilical cords. A difference in major blood groups is indicative of dizygosity. If these simple procedures fail to identify zygosity, more complicated technics, such as extensive blood group determinations of the twins and their parents, finger or footprints, and reciprocal skin grafts may have to be used to look for differences.

Sex. Although twins of opposite sex are almost always dizygotic, monozygotic twins rarely may be discordant for phenotypic sex. Schmidt and co-workers (1974), for example, described adolescent twins in whom concordance for 22 blood groups and other biochemical markers was demonstrated. The proband demonstrated classic features of Turner's syndrome, including a single sex chromosome (karyotype 45, XO), in tissue cultures from streak gonads. The karyotype of the other twin, a normal-appearing male, was 46, XY.

CONJOINED TWINS

In the United States, united or conjoined twins are commonly referred to as Siamese twins, after Chang and Eng Bunker of Siam, who were displayed worldwide by P. T. Barnum. If twinning is initiated after the embry-

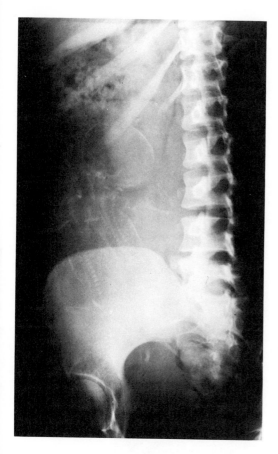

FIG. 26-4. Roentgenogram demonstrating twins of 22 weeks gestation that are joined at the thorax and upper abdomen.

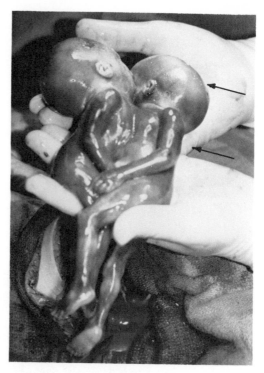

FIG. 26-5. Conjoined twins at delivery by hysterotomy. Their skeletons are demonstrated radiologically in Figure 26-4. The arrows indicate the approximate levels of the transverse sonograms depicted in Figure 26-6.

onic disc and the rudimentary amnionic sac have been formed, and if division of the embryonic disc is incomplete, conjoined twins result. When each of the joined twins is nearly complete, the commonly shared body site may be (1) anterior *(thoracopagus)*, (2) posterior *(pygopagus)*, (3) cephalic *(craniopagus)*, or (4) caudal *(ischiopagus)*. The majority are of the thoracopagus variety (Figs. 26-4–26-6). At Kandang Kerbau Hospital in Singapore, Tan and co-workers (1971) identified seven cases of conjoined twins among somewhat more than 400,000 deliveries (one in 70,000). Five sets were born alive but four died shortly thereafter. One of four sets of the thoracopagus variety survived beyond the neonatal period and the infants were sepa-

rated surgically at three months of age. The lone survivor at nine years of age appeared well, except for torticollis and a defect in the anterior wall of the chest.

When the bodies are only partly duplicated, the attachment is more often lateral. The incomplete division of the embryonic disc may begin at either or both poles and produce two heads; two, three, or four arms; three or four legs; or some combination thereof.

Vaginal delivery of conjoined twins may occur, since the union most often is somewhat pliable, although dystocia is common. Surgical separation of conjoined twins may be successful when organs essential for life are not intimately shared. The diagnosis of conjoined twins antepartum is demonstrated in Figures 26-4, 5, 6.

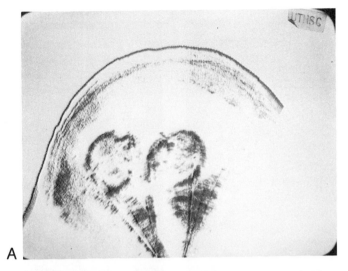

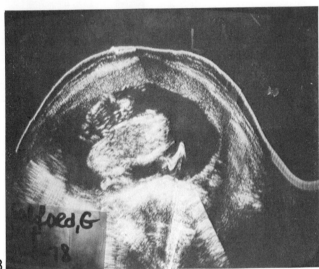

FIG. 26-6. Transverse sonograms of the conjoined twins shown in Figure 26-5. Two fetal heads are seen in sonogram **A.** In sonogram **B,** made parallel to A but 5 cm below, the fused thoraces are evident. Below the thoraces are extremities and above are the umbilical cords. (Courtesy of Dr. R. Santos)

HYDATIDIFORM MOLE

At times, twinning is expressed as a single fetus plus a hydatidiform mole. (The development of a hydatidiform mole is described in Chapter 23, p. 578.) Severe pregnancy-induced hypertension may develop at times before the 24th week, which is about as early as preeclampsia-eclampsia develops in the absence of a hydatidiform mole. The presence of a fetal heart and hypertension so early in pregnancy may cloud the etiology of the hy-

pertension until the unsuspected mole is identified either by sonography or at delivery (see Chap. 27, p. 666).

VASCULAR COMMUNICATIONS BETWEEN FETUSES

Frequently demonstrable in monochorionic placentas are vascular anastomoses, either artery to artery, artery to vein, or vein to vein, that allow gross admixture of blood between the fetuses. Shifts of blood between fetuses may lead to significant hypervolemia and hyperviscosity in the recipient and hypovolemia and anemia in the donor. Moreover, if the umbilical cord of the first infant is cut but the segment attached to the placenta is not adequately clamped, serious loss of blood from the second twin can soon take place.

Arteriovenous anastomoses may develop quite early in pregnancy and may vary appreciably in number and in size. As emphasized by Benirschke and Kim (1973), the arteriovenous communication often proceeds through the capillary bed of a placental cotyledon so that blood from one fetus enters the capillary bed of the cotyledon in the usual way but exits through the umbilical venous system of the other fetus.

The effects from the arteriovenous anastomoses can be profound. One monozygous or "identical" twin may be very much smaller than the other as the consequence of chronic intrauterine malnutrition. The anatomic changes described by Naeye (1965) in the underperfused twin resemble those found in growth-retarded singletons whose placentas were extensively infarcted. In monozygotic twins with anastomosed circulations, the hemoglobin concentration may be 8 g per dl or less in the hypoperfused twin and as much as 27 g per dl in the other. Hypotension, microcardia, and generalized runting characterize the overtly affected hypovolemic "identical" twin, in contrast to hypertension and cardiac hypertrophy in the hypertransfused twin. Hydramnios, perhaps the consequence of increased renal perfusion and, in turn, increased urine formation, may accompany the hypervolemia and polycythemia in the typically larger twin. At the same time, amnionic fluid may be scant to absent in the other sac, possibly as a result of marked oliguria in the underperfused twin.

Dangerous circulatory overload with heart failure may complicate the neonatal period if severe hypervolemia and blood hyperviscosity at birth are not promptly identified and treated by phlebotomy. Occlusive thrombosis is also much more likely to occur in this setting. Moreover, death of one monozygotic

fetus may precipitate in the other a serious degree of intravascular coagulation. Polycythemia may lead during the neonatal period to severe hyperbilirubinemia and, in turn, kernicterus (see Chap. 38, p. 972).

Viewed from the maternal side, one portion of the placenta often appears quite pale compared to the rest of the placenta when there is anemia in one twin and polycythemia in the other. The vascular anastomoses usually can be visualized directly after the overlying amnion is removed or by injecting milk into an umbilical artery.

Chimerism. A chimera is an individual with a mixture of genotypes from more than one ovum and sperm. Possible mechanisms include double fertilization of one ovum, and, in case of nonidentical fetuses, the transfer of genetic material from one across chorionic vascular anastomoses to the other. For example, the transfer of primitive blood cells from one dizygotic twin fetus through a vascular anastomosis to the other twin can lead to the production in the recipient of two populations of blood cells of quite dissimilar blood types, or *blood chimerism*. The "transfused" cells are not destroyed, since exposure of the recipient twin to the dissimilar antigens of the donor twin early in fetal development renders the recipient twin tolerant to the donor twin's tissues. Most commonly, blood chimerism has been discovered at the time of blood typing when discordant blood types are found (Benirschke, 1974).

Chimerism, in which cell lines are derived from different zygotes, is to be distinguished from *mosaicism,* in which two or more cell lines of different chromosomal composition arise from the same zygote as the consequence of nondisjunction during meiotic division.

Pulmonary Function. Surfactant production, as reflected by the lecithin-sphingomyelin (L/S) ratio in amnionic fluid, and pulmonary function after birth may differ markedly (Gluck, Kulovich, 1974). We have observed with quintuplets the L/S ratio in amnionic fluid to vary from less than 2 for the largest infant who weighed 1530 g at

32 weeks gestation, appropriate for his gestational age, to greater than 5 for the severely growth-retarded smallest infant, who weighed but 860 g. The largest infant developed appreciable respiratory distress, whereas the smallest infant did not.

DIAGNOSIS OF MULTIPLE FETUSES

It is unfortunate that twins rather commonly are not diagnosed before parturition. Powers (1973), in his analysis of complications and treatment in twin pregnancy, ascertained from various reports that from 5 percent to more than 50 percent of the time twins were not diagnosed before labor. The identification of pregnancy complicated by multiple fetuses is missed not so much because it is unusually difficult but because the examiner fails to keep the possibility in mind.

History and Physical Examination. A familial history of twins usually provides only a weak clue, but knowledge of recent administration of either clomiphene or pituitary gonadotropin provides a much stronger one. *During the second trimester, a discrepancy develops between gestational age determined from menstrual data and that from uterine size. The uterus that contains two or more fetuses clearly becomes larger than expected with a single fetus!* In the case of the uterus that appears large for gestational age the obstetrician must carefully consider the following possibilities: (1) inaccurate menstrual history, (2) multiple fetuses, (3) hydramnios, (4) hydatidiform mole, (5) uterine myomas or adenomyosis, (6) a closely attached adnexal mass, (7) the elevation of the uterus by a distended bladder, and (8) late in pregnancy fetal macrosomia.

Diagnostic Aids. A variety of technics are utilized to identify a multifetal pregnancy:

FETAL PARTS. Before the third trimester, it is difficult to diagnose twins by palpation of fetal parts. It is apparent in Figure 26-7 that even late in pregnancy it may not always be possible to identify twins by transabdominal palpation, especially if the woman is obese or hydramnios is present.

FETAL HEART. Late in the first trimester fetal heart action may be detected with generally available Doppler ultrasonic equipment (see Chap. 10, p. 262). Sometime thereafter it becomes possible to identify the separate contractions of two fetal hearts if their rates are clearly distinct from each other as well as from that of the mother. It is possible by careful examination to identify fetal heart sounds with the usual aural fetal stethoscopes at 18 to 20 weeks gestation. The presence of twins may be established electrocardiographically. Hon and Hess (1960) did so in 11 of 12 cases and Novotny and associates (1959), between the 20th and 27th weeks, diagnosed all 21 twin pregnancies this way. Other reporters, cited by Powers (1973), have not been so successful, especially in early pregnancy.

SONOGRAPHY. By careful sonographic examination, separate gestational sacs can be identified very early in twin pregnancy (between the 6th and 10th weeks of gestation) (Fig. 26-8). The gestational rings become less distinct after the 10th week, but multiple fetal heads, if present, usually can be identified and the biparietal diameter accurately measured after the 14th week of gestation (Fig. 26-9). The identification of each fetal head should be made in two perpendicular planes so as not to mistake a cross section of the fetal trunk for a second fetal head. A cross section of the fetal head remains round in both planes, whereas the trunk does not. Carefully performed sonographic scanning should detect practically all sets of twins.

As the number of fetuses increases, the accuracy of diagnosis, both as to the number of fetuses and to the biparietal diameter of each head, decreases. In the case of quintuplets, demonstrated in the roentgenogram in Figure 26-10, only four fetuses were identified with certainty either by sonography or by roentgenography. In the case of nonuplets studied by Kossoff and associates (1976), at

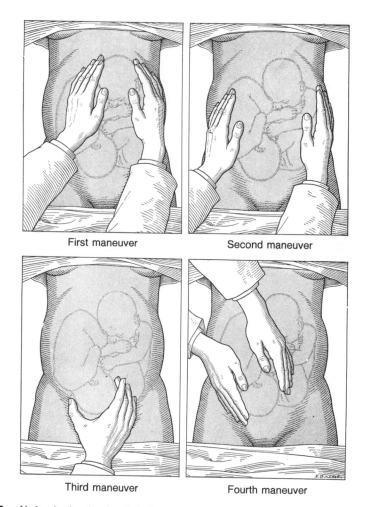

First maneuver

Second maneuver

Third maneuver

Fourth maneuver

FIG. 26-7.   Abdominal palpation in twin pregnancy. Cephalic presentation on the mother's right and frank breech on the left.

25 weeks gestational age only six of the nine fetuses were identified by sonography.

At times, conjoining of twins can be strongly suspected from sonographic observations. This was true in one pregnancy terminated at 22 weeks at Parkland Memorial Hospital (Figs. 26-5, 26-6). A roentgenogram was also supportive of the diagnosis of conjoined twin fetuses (Fig. 26-4). Vaughn and Powell (1979) describe conjoined twins diagnosed at 34 weeks gestation using a combination of sonography and amniography. The conjoined twins were delivered by cesarean section at 36 weeks.

In multifetal pregnancies, there is a general slowing of the rate of fetal growth compared to singleton pregnancies. Moreover, individual growth in the same multifetal gestation is commonly discordant. These variations in fetal growth typically are reflected by the biparietal diameter measured sonographically (Houlton, 1977).

RADIOGRAPHIC EXAMINATION. The indiscriminate use of x-ray should be avoided during pregnancy. Moreover, a roentgenogram of the maternal abdomen may not be useful in demonstrating multiple fetuses if taken during the first half of pregnancy, if the film is of poor quality, if the mother is obese, if there is excess amnionic fluid, or if one fetus moves during the exposure. Also,

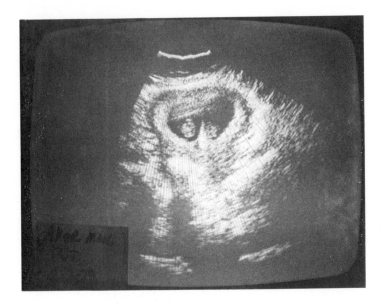

FIG. 26-8. Transverse sonogram demonstrating 2 gestational sacs each containing a fetus of 10 weeks menstrual age. (Courtesy of Dr. R. Santos)

a fetus may be excluded if the roentgenogram does not include the upper abdomen. There are times, however, when the importance of diagnosing the presence of multiple fetuses surely overrides the slight risk associated with a carefully obtained and interpreted roentgenogram (Fig. 26-10).

BIOCHEMICAL TESTS. The amounts of *chorionic gonadotropin* in plasma and in urine, on the average, are higher than those found with a singleton pregnancy but not so high as to allow a definite diagnosis (Thiery and co-workers, 1976). Neither are the amounts of chorionic gonadotropin so low as to differentiate clearly between a twin pregnancy and

a hydatidiform mole. *Placental lactogen* levels in maternal plasma average somewhat higher in twin pregnancy than in a singleton pregnancy. Measurement of placental lactogen at 29 to 30 weeks gestation to screen for twins has been proposed (Mägiste et al., 1976; Spellacy et al., 1978). Ideally, diagnosis of twins should be made somewhat before 29 to 30 weeks. Moreover, if the gestational age is known, clinical acumen alone should lead the obstetrician to suspect twins and to employ a technic for diagnosis that is far more precise than is the measurement of placental lactogen. The *alpha-fetoprotein level* in maternal plasma is commonly higher in pregnancies with twins than in those with a single

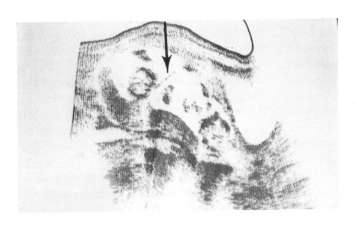

FIG. 26-9. Longitudinal gray scale sonogram of twins at 15 weeks gestation. The arrow points to membranes that divide the two amnionic sacs. The fetal trunk and an extremity are seen in the upper sac. A fetal head and extremities are apparent in the lower. (Courtesy Dr. R. Santos)

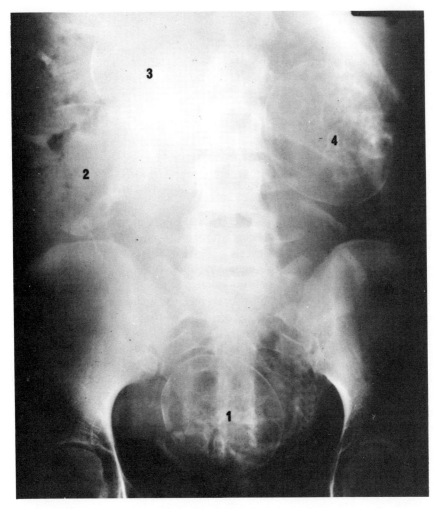

FIG. 26-10. Roentgenogram at 27 weeks' gestation that clearly demonstrates four fetal heads. A fifth fetus, not identifiable in this roentgenogram, weighed but 860 g when delivered 5 weeks later. (The placenta is demonstrated in Figure 26-3.)

fetus. Even though Keilani and co-workers (1978) found that in 40 percent of twin pregnancies the level was above the 95th percentile of the normal range for singleton gestations, the measurement provides little help in diagnosing twins over that provided by careful clinical evaluation. There are also somewhat higher maternal plasma levels on the average for *estrogens, alkaline phosphatase,* and *leucine aminopeptidase* ("oxytocinase"), and in urine for *estriol* and *pregnanediol.* So far, however, there is no biochemical test that will clearly differentiate in any individual case between the presence of one and more than one fetus.

PREGNANCY OUTCOME

Abortion. Abortion is more likely to occur with multiple fetuses than with a single fetus. The demonstration sonographically of two pregnancy rings with the subsequent disappearance of one or even both rings led Hellman and associates (1973) and Robinson and Caines (1977) to conclude that silent early abortion or resorption of one embryo is fairly common (p. 640). Both spontaneous abortion and surgically induced abortion have, on occasion, served to remove one fetus, yet the pregnancy continued until the birth of another fetus that survived.

RETAINED DEAD FETUS. On occasion, one fetus succumbs remote from term, yet the pregnancy continues with one living fetus. At delivery, the dead fetus with placenta and membranes may be readily identified but may be appreciably compressed (*fetus compressus*) or may be remarkably flattened through loss of fluid and most of the soft tissue except skin (*fetus papyraceous*). A striking example is presented in Figure 26-11 in which the papyraceous fetus died at midpregnancy while the other twin and its placenta thrived. Theoretically, at least, acquired coagulation defects (consumptive coagulopathy) could be triggered in the mother by the death of one of multiple fetuses. We have not observed dangerous hypofibrinogenemia in the mother. Death in utero of one twin may be followed by evidence of consumptive coagulopathy in the other.

Perinatal Mortality. The perinatal mortality rate for pregnancies complicated by twin fetuses is remarkably higher than for single fetuses. The increased risk of death in twins persists during the first year of life. It is not until the second year that mortality rates are the same for twins as for singletons (MacGillivray, 1978).

Perinatal loss with twins at many centers in the United States most commonly has ranged from 10 to 15 percent. For example, Kohl and Casey (1975) identified at several collaborative obstetric units in the United States a perinatal death rate of 10.9 percent (109 per 1,000) for twins who weighed at least 500 g at birth. For twins who weighed 1000 g or more, the perinatal death rate was 6.2 percent, or approximately three times that for singletons. Naeye and co-workers (1978), from data compiled through a prospective collaborative study in the United States, found that the perinatal death rate was 13.9 percent for twins compared to 3.3 percent for singletons. The perinatal death rate for monozygotic twins was 2.5 times that for dizygotic twins. There is an extremely high fetal death rate with the relatively rare variety of monozygous twinning in which both fe-

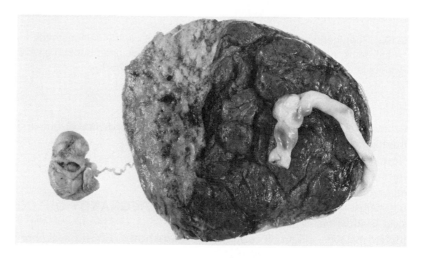

FIG. 26-11. To the left are a papyraceous fetus that died at midpregnancy, its cord, and its pale placenta. To the right are the normal placenta and cord of the healthy, 3200 g, twin.

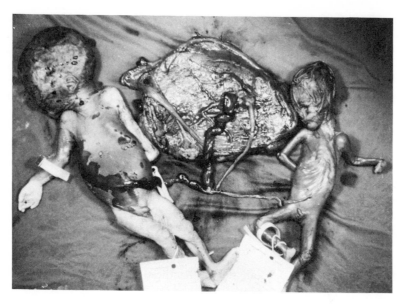

FIG. 26-12. Monozygotic twins in a single amnionic sac; the smaller fetus apparently died first and the second subsequently succumbed when the umbilical cords entwined.

tuses occupy the same amnionic sac. Death from intertwining of the umbilical cords is common (Fig. 26-12).

Duration of Gestation.   As the number of fetuses increases, the duration of gestation and birth weight decrease. McKeown and Record (1952) identified the mean duration of gestation for twins to be 260 days (37 weeks), and for triplets 247 days (35 weeks), compared to 281 days (40 weeks) for single fetuses. Caspi and associates (1976) ascertained precisely the time of ovulation for 111 pregnancies in women in whom ovulation was induced with pituitary plus chorionic gonadotropins. As shown in Table 26-1, the average duration of gestation decreased dramatically as the number of fetuses increased.

Birth Weight.   Powers (1973) noted the birth weight to be less than 2501 g in from 43 to 63 percent of twin infants in the many reports from the United States and Europe that he surveyed. Retarded fetal growth, as well as premature delivery, is important in the genesis of low birth weight in multifetal gestations. After the second trimester, growth of the multiple fetuses, as determined either by sonographic measurements or by birth weight, is likely to be impaired compared to that of the singleton fetus. In general, the larger the number of fetuses, the greater the degree of growth retardation. Moreover, when two or more fetuses are derived from a single ovum, the degree of growth retardation is likely to be much greater than when each fetus is derived from a different ovum. The differences in birth weight were quite dramatic in the Davis quintuplets presented in Figure 26-13. A. and B. When delivered at 32 weeks gestation, the three infants from separate ova weighed 1420 g, 1530 g, and 1440 g, whereas the two derived from the same ovum weighed 990 g and 860 g. Although the birth weights of the two monozygotic infants were nearly the same, remarkable differences have been observed. Even though gross differences in size are more common between monozygotic twins, marked discordance in size may complicate pregnancies in which each fetus arose from a separate ovum. For example, dizygotic twins, one of whom weighed 2300 g and the other 785 g, were delivered at Parkland

TABLE 26-1.
AVERAGE LENGTH OF GESTATION
FOR PREGNANCIES WITH KNOWN TIME
OF OVULATION AND
20 OR MORE WEEKS GESTATION

NO. OF FETUSES	NO. OF PREGNANCIES	WEEKS COMPLETED*
Singleton	82	39
Twins	21	35
Triplets	5	33
Quadruplets	3	29

* Calculated from 2 weeks before ovulation
From Caspi et al.: *Br J Obstet Gynaecol* 83:967, 1976

Memorial Hospital (Fig. 26-14). Both survived.

Malformations. Kohl and Casey (1975) identified major malformations in 2.12 percent of twin infants compared to 1.05 percent of singletons delivered during the same times and in the same institutions. The frequency of minor malformation was 4.13 percent in twins, compared to 2.45 percent in singletons. It appears, on the basis of the studies of Kohl and Casey, and others, that the frequency of malformations is nearly twice as great in twins as in singletons. Malformations are more common among monozygotic than dizygotic twins.

Subsequent Development. The pattern of subsequent development of the growth-retarded infant from a multifetal pregnancy varies. Babson and Phillips (1973), for example, reported that in monozygotic twins whose birth weights differed on the average by 36 percent, the twin who was smaller at birth remained so into adulthood. In their experience, height, weight, head circumference, and apparently intelligence often remained superior in the twin who weighed more at birth. Fujikura and Froelich (1974), however, failed to confirm a significant difference in mental and motor scores. Remarkable differences in size persist among the Davis quintuplets described above

(Fig. 26-13. A. and B.). At 3 years, 9 months of age, the largest infant at birth remains the largest and weighs 16.2 kg (36 pounds), while the smallest at birth remains the smallest and weighs 11.3 kg (25 pounds). Motor and intellectual development in all five, however, has been uniformly satisfactory.

It seems reasonable to summarize that each fetus involved in a multifetal pregnancy is at a disadvantage from the outset. His or her chance for survival is impaired remarkably compared to that of the fetus who is the sole occupant of the uterus. Those who do survive the newborn period are liable to suffer some form of physical, intellectual, or psychologic handicap, though in most instances their handicap will be minimal (MacGillivray et al., 1975).

Superfetation and Superfecundation. In superfetation, an interval as long or longer than an ovulatory cycle intervenes between fertilizations. Superfetation has not been unequivocally demonstrated in women, although it is theoretically possible until the uterine cavity is obliterated by the fusion of the decidua capsularis to the decidua vera. Thus, superfetation requires ovulation during the course of pregnancy, as yet unproven in humans, though known to occur in mares. Most authorities believe that the alleged cases of human superfetation result from marked inequality of growth and development of fetuses of the same gestational age, as described above.

Superfecundation refers to the fertilization of two ova within a short period of time, but not at the same coitus, nor necessarily by sperm from the same man. It may be that in many cases twin ova are not fertilized by sperm from the same ejaculate but the fact can be demonstrated only in exceptional circumstances. It is interesting that John Archer, the first physician to receive a medical degree in America, related in 1810 that a white woman after intercourse with both a white and a black man within a short period was delivered of twins, one of whom was white and the other mulatto. Terasaki and co-work-

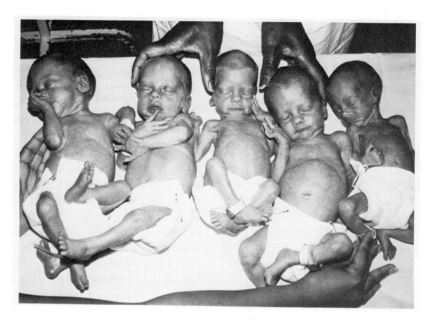

FIG. 26-13. A. Davis quintuplets at 3 weeks of age. The first, second, and fourth infants from the left each arose from separate ova while the third and fifth infants are from the same ovum.

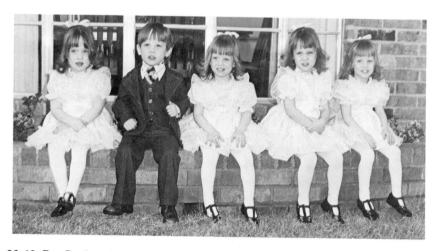

FIG. 26-13. B. Davis quintuplets at age three years, 9 months. They appear in the same order as in Figure 26-13.

ers (1978) have used tissue (HLA) typing to establish that dizygotic twins were sired by different fathers.

Maternal Adaptation.   In general, the degree of maternal physiologic change is greater with multiple fetuses than when there is a single fetus. For example, the average increase in maternal blood volume induced during pregnancy with twin fetuses is significantly larger (Pritchard, 1965; Rovinsky, Jaffin, 1966). Whereas the average increase in late pregnancy is about 40 to 50 percent with a single fetus, the mean increase amounts to about 50 to 60 percent with twins. Measurements in the same woman late in one preg-

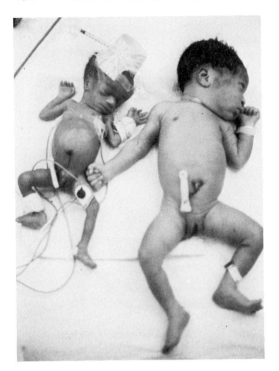

FIG. 26-14. Marked discordance in dizygotic twins. The larger infant weighed 2300 g, appropriate for gestational age. The markedly growth-retarded smaller infant weighed only 785 g. Both thrived.

nancy with a single fetus and at the same time in another pregnancy with twins are indicative that, typically, the maternal blood volume is about 500 ml greater with twins (Pritchard, Chase, unpublished). Interestingly, the average blood loss with vaginal delivery of 25 sets of twins averaged 935 ml, or nearly 500 ml more than with the delivery of a single fetus. Both the remarkable increase in maternal blood volume and the increased iron and folate requirements imposed by a second fetus predispose to a greater prevalence of maternal anemia.

The larger size of the uterus with multiple fetuses intensifies the variety of mechanical effects that occur during pregnancy. The uterus and its contents may achieve a volume of 10 liters or more and weigh in excess of 20 pounds! Especially with monozygotic twins, rapid accumulation of grossly excessive

amounts of amniotic fluid, i.e., *acute hydramnios,* may develop. In these circumstances, it is easy to envision appreciable compression and displacement of many of the abdominal viscera as well as the lungs by the elevated diaphragm. The size and weight of the very large uterus at times preclude more than a very sedentary existence by the woman pregnant with multiple fetuses.

At times, in pregnancies with multiple fetuses further complicated by hydramnios, maternal renal function may become seriously impaired, most likely as the consequence of obstructive uropathy. Quigley and Cruikshank (1977), for example, described two pregnancies with twin fetuses plus acute and severe hydramnios in which oliguria and azotemia developed. Maternal urine output and plasma creatinine levels promptly returned to normal after delivery. In case of gross hydramnios, transabdominal amniocentesis may be employed to provide relief for the mother and to allow the pregnancy to continue (see Chap. 23, p. 581).

The various stresses of pregnancy on the mother and the likelihood of serious maternal complications almost invariably will be greater with multiple fetuses than with a singleton. This should be taken into account, especially when counseling the woman whose health is compromised and who is recognized early in pregnancy to have multiple fetuses, or, for that matter, who is not pregnant but is considering treatment with agents used to induce ovulation.

MANAGEMENT OF PREGNANCIES WITH MULTIPLE FETUSES

To reduce perinatal mortality and morbidity significantly in pregnancies complicated by twins, it is imperative that (1) delivery of markedly premature infants be prevented, (2) fetal trauma during labor and delivery be eliminated, and (3) expert neonatal care be provided continuously from the time of birth. The first major step in fulfilling these goals is to identify early the pregnancy complicated by multiple fetuses. As soon as multiple fetuses (or embryos) are identified, meaningful efforts should be directed toward providing the fetuses with the best intrauterine environment possible. The availability of nutrients to the fetuses will depend upon (1) the concentrations of nutrients in maternal blood, (2) the rate of maternal blood flow through the placenta, (3) the rate of transfer of nutrients across the placenta to the fetal circulations, and (4) the adequacy of the fetal circulations.

Diet.   The requirements for calories, protein, minerals, vitamins, and essential fatty acids are further increased in women with multiple fetuses. The Recommended Dietary Allowances made by the Food and Nutrition Board of the National Research Council for uncomplicated pregnancy should not only be met but in most instances actually exceeded somewhat (see Chap. 13, p. 311). Therefore, consumption of energy sources should be increased by 300 kcal or more per day. Failure of the mother to gain weight equal at least to the weight of the pregnancy products, both fetal and maternal, is clear proof that the diet being consumed is inadequate. Iron supplementation is essential; 60 to 80 mg per day is recommended. Folic acid, 1 mg per day, may prove beneficial, although a diet adequate in protein provided from a variety of sources should supply adequate amounts of folate. Rigid sodium restriction is not beneficial to the fetuses.

Maternal Hypertension.   Pregnancy-induced and pregnancy-aggravated hypertension are much more likely to develop in pregnancies with multiple fetuses (see Chap. 27, p. 666). In general, parous women never previously hypertensive are "immune" to the development of hypertension during a subsequent pregnancy. This does not hold true, however, for a subsequent pregnancy complicated by multiple fetuses. The disorder not only occurs more often but tends to develop earlier and to be more severe. If women with

twins are hospitalized far in advance of term, as described below, the onset of hypertension may very likely be delayed and its severity reduced, although this has not been definitely established.

Bed Rest.   Several investigators, but not all, have proposed that bed rest is beneficial to twin fetuses presumably by increasing uterine perfusion and perhaps by reducing the physical forces that might act deleteriously on the cervix to hasten effacement and dilatation. Unfortunately, the benefits from bed rest are difficult to quantitate. Laursen (1973) concluded from his study of 315 pregnancies with twins that rest in the hospital will prolong pregnancy, increase birth weights significantly, and reduce perinatal mortality. When delivery occurred before the 35th week of gestation, the perinatal mortality rate was high and the perinatal deaths nearly always occurred in liveborn premature infants who soon succumbed from respiratory failure. After the 35th week, however, the perinatal mortality rate was remarkably lower, with stillbirths accounting for most of the deaths.

Komáromy and Lampé (1977), on the basis of a large study in Hungary, reached the same conclusion as Laursen. They identified the following differences between their hospitalized and nonhospitalized groups respectively: mean gestational age at delivery 37.4 weeks compared to 35.0 weeks; mean birth weight 2581 g compared to 1972 g; for birth weights below 2500 g, 43 percent compared to 77 percent. At any gestational age, the birth weights of twins whose mothers had been hospitalized averaged appreciably more than did the birth weights of those whose mothers were not hospitalized. Finally, perinatal mortality was 5.9 percent for twins in the hospitalized group compared to 21.7 percent in the nonhospitalized group.

In an interesting study in Malmö, Sweden, during a recent four-year period 88 percent of all twin pregnancies were identified by routinely scanning sonographically pregnant women during the second trimester. For those with twins, rest at home was prescribed until 29 weeks, at which time hospitalization was urged. The average hospital stay for the 86 women who participated was 55 days. If undelivered at 36 weeks, they were discharged from the hospital provided that the course of pregnancy was completely normal. With few exceptions, the pregnancies were not allowed to go beyond 38 weeks gestation. The perinatal mortality rate was 0.6 percent, the same as for singleton pregnancies, whereas for twin gestations not so managed the perinatal mortality rate was 10.5 percent (Persson et al., 1979).

The experiences of Jeffrey and co-workers (1974) in Denver were that bed rest promoted fetal growth but did not necessarily prolong gestation. In their experience, twin fetuses of mothers at bed rest weighed somewhat more than did fetuses of comparable gestational age whose mothers remained ambulatory. Weekes and co-workers (1977), have compared the outcomes of twin pregnancies treated by either bed rest or by cervical suture (cerclage), to those with no active treatment and found no remarkable differences in birth weights or gestational age at delivery. Perinatal mortality was 6.7 percent among those hospitalized and 5.6 percent for those not hospitalized.

Tamby Raja and co-workers (1978) have claimed lowered perinatal mortality, longer gestations, and higher birth weights for twin pregnancies in which the mothers were prophylactically given salbutamol orally compared to those treated with bed rest. Unfortunately, of the 50 pregnancies treated with salbutamol, six were excluded from analysis because of antepartum hemorrhage or severe preeclampsia and two because the fate of the pregnancy was unknown.

In recent years at Parkland Memorial Hospital, women with twins have been offered hospitalization on the High Risk Pregnancy Unit hopefully as early as the onset of the third trimester. Although women so hospitalized lead a very sedentary life, they are not strictly confined to bed. At a recent audit, 144 of 166 women so admitted stayed either until delivery or until they had completed 38 weeks gestations. The duration of stay was two weeks or more for 90 percent and four weeks or more for 68 percent. Perinatal mortality for the 288 fetuses was only 2.8 percent. Of the eight perinatal deaths, five were stillborn. Four of the five stillbirths were the consequence of fetal death at or very near 40 weeks gestation. The fifth dead fetus had expired remote from term before admittance to the hospital. Of the three neonatal deaths, only one was the consequence of prematurity. Another infant delivered at term died from a malformation incompatible with life (sirenomelia). The third infant born at 39 weeks died of intracranial hemorrhage and renal cortical necrosis. The co-twin had died in utero some time before delivery, which may have triggered the apparent consumptive coagulopathy.

The fetal outcome was much poorer in the 22 instances in which the undelivered mothers soon left the High Risk Pregnancy Unit. Seven of the 44 fetuses, or 15.9 percent, died.

It is our impression that, at least for the typically socioeconomically deprived women cared for at Parkland Memorial Hospital, the benefits to be derived from hospitalization during the third trimester of twin gestation include decreased frequency of premature labor, increased birth weight, decreased frequency of severe preeclampsia, and lowered perinatal mortality.

DELIVERY OF MULTIPLE FETUSES

Labor.   Many complications of labor and delivery, including premature labor, uterine dysfunction, abnormal presentations, prolapse of the umbilical cord, premature separation of the placenta, and immediate postpartum hemorrhage occur with appreciably greater frequency with multiple fetuses. Therefore, the conduct of labor and delivery with multiple fetuses is an excellent test of the acumen, skill, and judgment of the obstetric team who provides care for the woman and her fetuses.

So far, with the agents available in the United States, the capability is limited for arresting premature labor once labor is established. Bed rest, if not already being used, should be instituted. The problems of premature labor and attempts to arrest it and of lack of fetal lung maturity and its possible correction with corticosteroid therapy, are considered elsewhere (see Chap. 37, p. 932).

As soon as it is apparent that labor has been established, a number of steps are immediately taken to help assure a satisfactory outcome:

1. An appropriately trained obstetric attendant remains with the mother throughout labor. The fetal heart rates are monitored frequently, using any system of monitoring which, in that particular situation, will promptly identify significant changes in fetal heart rates. At times, continuous external electronic monitoring or, if the membranes are ruptured and the cervix dilated, evaluation of both fetuses by simultaneous internal and external electronic monitoring may prove quite satisfactory.
2. One liter of cross-matched whole blood (or its equivalent in blood fractions) are obtained.
3. A well-functioning intravenous infusion system capable of delivering fluid rapidly into the mother is established. (In the absence of hemorrhage or metabolic disturbance during labor, lactated Ringer's solution alternated with aqueous dextrose solution is infused at a rate of 60 to 120 ml per hour.)
4. Two obstetricians are immediately available and both are scrubbed and gowned at delivery. At least one should be skilled in intrauterine identification of fetal parts and intrauterine manipulation of the fetus.
5. An experienced anesthesiologist is immediately available in case intrauterine manipulation or cesarean section is necessary.
6. For *each* fetus, two people, one of whom is skilled in resuscitation and care of newborn infants, are appropriately informed of the case and remain immediately available.
7. The delivery area is immediately operational and provides adequate space for all members of the team to work effectively. Moreover, it is appropriately equipped to take care of all possible maternal problems plus resuscitation and maintenance of each infant.

Presentation and Position. With twins, all possible combinations of fetal positions occur. Either or both fetuses may present by the vertex, breech, or shoulder. Compound, face, brow, and footling breech presentation are relatively common, especially when the fetuses are quite small, there is excess anmionic fluid, or maternal parity is high. Prolapse of the cord is fairly common in these circumstances. Once labor has been established, if there is any confusion about the relationship of the twins to each other or to the maternal pelvis, a single anteroposterior roentgenogram of the abdomen often is very helpful.

Induction or Stimulation of Labor. Even though labor, in general, is shorter with twins, both rupture of the membranes without effective labor and prolonged, inefficient labor with or without previous rupture of the membranes do occur. These problems are often better handled by cesarean section unless there is little hope of salvaging the infants because of their gross immaturity. Occasionally, termination of pregnancy is desirable before the spontaneous onset of labor, as, for example, with severe pregnancy-induced hypertension. In these circumstances if the presenting part is well-fixed in the pelvis and the cervix dilated somewhat, amniotomy often will initiate labor and effect delivery. There is no reluctance by some obstetricians to give oxytocin by dilute intravenous infusion to initiate or to stimulate labor in pregnancies complicated by multiple fetuses. The risks compared to the benefits to mother and fetuses of oxytocin to initiate and maintain labor and delivery, compared with cesarean section, have not yet been adequately delineated in this circumstance.

Analgesia and Anesthesia. During labor and delivery of multiple fetuses, the decision as to what to use for analgesia and for anesthesia is unusually difficult because of the frequency of and, in turn, the problems imposed by (1) prematurity, (2) maternal hypertension, (3) desultory labor, (4) need for intrauterine manipulation, and (5) uterine atony and hemorrhage after delivery. There are undesirable effects from most forms of analgesia and anesthesia. Continuous epidural or caudal anesthesia in hypertensive women, or those who have hemorrhaged, may cause hypotension with inadequate perfusion of vital organs that is dangerous to both the mother and her fetuses. Moreover, conduction anesthesia may cause or further aggravate desultory or prolonged labor and is unlikely to provide adequate uterine relaxation for intrauterine manipulation when such is necessary. Use of narcotics, sedatives, and tranquilizers may lead to undue fetal depression if the fetuses are premature. Most forms of general anesthesia used for delivery will also depress the fetuses unless the anesthetic agents are carefully selected and skillfully administered, with little delay between induction of anesthesia and delivery. Paracervical block may cause transient fetal bradycardia.

The combination of thiopental, nitrous oxide plus oxygen, and succinylcholine, appropriately timed and in appropriate doses, has proved satisfactory at Parkland Hospital for cesarean section to deliver twins. For vaginal delivery, pudendal block skillfully administered along with nitrous oxide plus oxygen will provide appreciable relief of pain for spontaneous vaginal delivery. When intrauterine manipulation is necessary, as with internal podalic version, uterine relaxation is probably best accomplished with halothane. While halothane provides effective relaxation for intrauterine manipulation, it also commonly leads to an increase in blood loss during the third stage of labor until the uterus regains its ability to contract.

Vaginal Delivery.   More often, the presenting twin is the larger one. Typically, this twin bears the major brunt of dilating the cervix and the remaining soft tissues of the birth canal. Seldom with cephalic presentations are there unusual problems with delivery of the first infant. After appropriate episiotomy, spontaneous delivery or delivery assisted by use of outlet forceps usually proves to be quite satisfactory.

When the first fetus presents as a breech, major problems are most likely to develop if (1) the fetus is unusually large and the aftercoming head taxes the capacity of the birth canal, (2) the fetus is quite small so that the extremities and trunk are delivered through a cervix inadequately dilated for the head, or (3) the umbilical cord prolapses. When these problems are anticipated or identified, except in those instances in which the fetuses are so immature that they will not survive, cesarean section would often be the better way to effect delivery. Otherwise, breech delivery may be accomplished as described in Chapter 42, p. 1065.

The phenomenon of *locked twins* occurs rarely (once in 817 twin gestations, according to Cohen and co-workers, 1965). In order for locking to occur, the first fetus must present by the breech and the second by the vertex. With descent of the breech through the birth canal, the chin of the first fetus locks in the neck and chin of the second cephalic fetus. If unlocking cannot be effected, either cesarean section before the body is delivered or decapitation must be performed.

DELIVERY OF SECOND TWIN.   This demands experience that includes demonstrated intrauterine manual dexterity. As soon as the first twin has been delivered, the presenting part of the second twin, the size, and the relationship to the birth canal are quickly determined by careful combined abdominal, vaginal, and, at times, intrauterine examination. If the vertex or the breech is fixed in the birth canal, moderate fundal pressure is applied and the membranes are ruptured. Immediately afterward, the examination is repeated to identify prolapse of the cord or other abnormality. Labor is allowed to resume while the fetal heart rate is monitored closely. With reestablishment of labor there is no need to hasten delivery, unless there is deceleration of the fetal heart rate or persistent bradycardia, or bleeding from the uterus. Bleeding from the uterus indicates placental separation, which can be deleterious to both the fetus and the mother. If contractions do not resume within 10 minutes, dilute oxytocin may be used to stimulate appropriate myometrial activity that will lead to spontaneous delivery or delivery assisted by outlet forceps.

If the occiput or the breech presents immediately over the pelvic inlet but is not fixed in the birth canal, most often it can be guided into the pelvis with the vaginal hand while a hand on the uterine fundus exerts moderate pressure. Once the presenting part is fixed in the pelvic inlet, the membranes are ruptured and labor and delivery are conducted as described above.

If the occiput or the breech is not over the pelvic inlet and cannot be so positioned by gentle pressure on the presenting part, or if appreciable uterine bleeding develops, the problem of delivery of the second twin assumes serious dimensions. So as to take maximum advantage of the very recently dilated cervix before the uterus contracts and the cervix retracts, procrastination must be avoided. An obstetrician skilled in intrauterine manipulation of the fetus and an anesthesiologist skilled in providing anesthesia that will effectively relax the uterus are essential for vaginal delivery with a favorable outcome. If no one is present who is skilled in the performance of internal podalic version, or, if anesthesia that will provide effective uterine relaxation is not immediately available, prompt delivery of the second fetus by cesarean section is the better choice.

Internal Podalic Version. Through careful abdominal, vaginal, and intrauterine examinations, the various parts of the fetus are located. (Typically, if the buttocks and legs are on the left side of the mother, or right side of the obstetrician, a sterile intrauterine examining glove that covers the gown to above the elbow is drawn over the

right hand and arm.) The membranes are ruptured, both feet are accurately identified and grasped and only then are gently pulled into the birth canal. With the other hand applied to the abdomen, the vertex is simultaneously gently elevated toward the mother's sternum. An episiotomy is made or extended any time more room is needed for uterine and vaginal manipulation. The legs of the fetus are slowly drawn through the birth canal until the buttocks are visible anteriorly just beyond the maternal symphysis. A moist, warm towel is applied to the buttocks and gentle traction is continued until the lower thirds of both scapulas are visible. Next, the trunk is slowly rotated by gentle traction until the shoulder and arm on one side of the fetus are delivered. The rotation of the fetal trunk is now gently reversed to deliver the other arm and shoulder into the vagina. The aftercoming head may now be delivered either by simultaneous suprapubic external pressure to flex the head and gentle traction applied to the trunk, or by use of Piper forceps (see Chap. 42, p. 1070).

The cord is clamped promptly with two clamps on the placental side to identify it as the cord of the second infant. The placenta (or placentas) is immediately delivered by manual removal, if necessary. The uterus is explored for defects and for retained pregnancy products. As these steps are being carried out, the amount of anesthetic agent is decreased, and just as soon as uterine exploration has been completed, oxytocin is administered through the intravenous infusion system. Fundal massage, or preferably manual compression of the uterus with one hand in the vagina against the lower uterine segment and the other transabdominally over the uterine fundus, is applied to hasten and enhance myometrial contraction and retraction.

The cervix, vagina, periurethral region, vulva, and perineum are carefully inspected for lacerations likely to bleed which are repaired along with the episiotomy.

Cesarean Section. The recent trend in delivery of multiple fetuses at Parkland Memorial Hospital has been to use cesarean section much more often than in the past. For example, 44 percent of the twins cared for in the High Risk Pregnancy Unit, as cited previously, were delivered by cesarean section. The most common indication was presentation other than cephalic by one or both fetuses. Other major indications were rupture of membranes without labor, hypotonic uterine dysfunction, hypertension induced or aggravated by the pregnancy, fetal distress, gross discordance in the size of the fetuses with the smaller fetus the first candidate for vaginal delivery, and prolapsed cord. Liberal use of cesarean section, when one or both twins present as a breech or are in a transverse lie, has been espoused by others (Cetrulo et al., 1977; Taylor, 1976).

Twin fetuses create unusual problems. The mother may be even less tolerant of the supine position and therefore it may be necessary to rotate her position so as to move the uterus and its contents to one side (see Chap. 18, p. 448). A vertical incision in the lower uterine segment may be advantageous. If a fetus lies transversely and the arms are inadvertently delivered first, it is much easier and safer to extend upward the vertical uterine incision than to extend a transverse incision.

It is important that the uterus be well contracted during completion of the cesarean section and thereafter. Remarkable blood loss from the uterus may be concealed within the uterus and vagina and beneath the operating drapes during the time taken to close the incisions.

At times, attempts to deliver the second twin vaginally, after vaginal delivery of the first twin, may be not only unwise but even impossible, as for instance, when the second fetus is much larger than the first and in the breech position or in a transverse lie; or even more perplexing, when the cervix promptly contracts and thickens after delivery of the first infant and does not subsequently dilate. Prompt cesarean section may be performed in these circumstances and the infant possibly saved. Undoubtedly, maternal and perinatal morbidity and mortality would be appreciably less if cesarean section had been used at the outset.

Three or More Fetuses. All of the problems of twin gestation are intensified remarkably by the presence of even more fetuses. As emphasized by Jewelewicz and Vande Wiele (1975), with vaginal delivery the first infant is commonly born spontaneously or with little manipulation. However, subsequent infants are delivered according to the presenting part and may require complicated obstetric maneuvers, such as total breech extraction or internal podalic version, followed by breech extraction. Associated with malpositions is an increased incidence of cord prolapse and fetal collision. Moreover, reduced placental perfusion and hemorrhage from separating placentas are likely during the intrapartum period. Therefore, speed of delivery is very important. For these reasons, we believe that delivery of pregnancies complicated by the presence of three or more fetuses is probably better accomplished by cesarean section, reserving vaginal delivery for those circumstances in which the fetuses are markedly immature or maternal complications make cesarean section hazardous to the mother.

Itzkowic (1979) has reviewed 59 triplet pregnancies born in four major obstetric hospitals. Most deliveries were accomplished vaginally. The perinatal mortality rate was 232 per 1,000 (23.2 percent); 9 of the infants were stillborn while 32 who were born alive died during the neonatal period. Premature delivery and birth order were the most important identifiable factors in relation to neonatal death. Abnormal presentations frequently complicated the delivery of the second and especially the third fetus. The mortality rate for infants who were born last was double that for those who were born first and intermediate for those who were born second.

Postpartum. The kinds of puerperal complications are not different from those after birth of a single infant but their frequency and intensity, however, are often enhanced. The mother may be troubled by considerable physical fatigue and at times emotional depression from the increased work and responsibilities associated with the care of two or more infants.

Troublesome uterine bleeding later in the puerperium seems to be increased. Perhaps this is the consequence of impairment of involution and of reepithelialization of the larger placental implantation site. In general, supplemental iron should be continued for some weeks after delivery.

REFERENCES

Archer J: Observations showing that a white woman, by intercourse with a white man and a Negro man, may conceive twins, one of which shall be white and the other mulatto. Medical Repository, 3d Hexade 1:319, 1810

Babson SG, Phillips DS: Growth and development of twins dissimilar in size at birth. New Engl J Med 289:937, 1973

Benirschke K: Chimerism and mosaicism—Two different entities. In Wynn RM (ed): Obstetrics and Gynecology Annual. New York, Appleton, 1974, p 33

Benirschke K, Kim CK: Multiple pregnancy. New Engl J Med 288:1276; 1329, 1973

Bulmer MG: The familial incidence of twinning. Ann Hum Genet 24:1, 1960

Caspi E, Ronen J, Schreyer P, Goldberg MD: The outcome of pregnancy after gonadotropin therapy. Br J Obstet Gynaecol 83:967, 1976

Cetrulo CL, Freeman RK, Knuppel RA: Minimizing the risks of twin delivery. Contemp Ob/Gyn 9:47, 1977

Cohen M, Kohl SG, Rosenthal AH: Fetal interlocking complicating twin gestation. Am J Obstet Gynecol 91:407, 1965

Editorial: Worldwide decline in dizygotic twinning. Br Med J 2:1553, 1976

Fujikura T, Froelich LA: Mental and motor development in monozygotic co-twins with dissimilar birth weights. Pediatrics 53:884, 1974

Garrett WJ, Carey HM, Steven LM, Climie CR, Osborn RA: A case of nonuplet pregnancy. Austral N Zeal J Obstet Gynaecol 16:93, 1976

Gemzell CA, Roos P, Loeffler FE: Follicle stimulating hormone extracted from human pituitary. In Behrman S, Kistner RW (eds): Progress in Infertility. Boston, Little, Brown, 1968, pp 375–392

Gluck L, Kulovich MV: The evaluation of functional maturity in the human fetus. In Gluck L (ed): Modern Perinatal Medicine. Chicago, Year Book, 1974

Harlap S: Ovulation induction and congenital malformations. Lancet 2:961, 1976

Hellman LM, Kobayashi M, Cromb E: Ultrasonic diagnosis of embryonic malformations. Am J Obstet Gynecol 115:615, 1973

Hon EH, Hess OW: The clinical value of fetal electrocardiography. Am J Obstet Gynecol 79:1012, 1960

Houlton, MCC: Divergent biparietal diameter growth rates in twin pregnancies. Obstet Gynecol 49:542, 1977

Itzkowicz D: A survey of 59 triplet pregnancies. Br J Obstet Gynaecol 86:23, 1979

Jeffrey RL, Bowes WA Jr, Delaney JJ: Role of bed rest in twin gestation. Obstet Gynecol 43:822, 1974

Jewelewicz R, Vande Wiele, RL: Management of multifetal gestation. Contemp Ob/Gyn 6:59, 1975

Keilani Z, Clarke PC, Kitau MJ: The significance of raised maternal plasma alpha-fetoprotein in twin pregnancy. Br J Obstet Gynecol 85:510, 1978

Kohl SG, Casey G: Twin gestation. Mt Sinai J Med 42:523, 1975

Komáromy B, Lampé L: The value of bed rest in twin pregnancies. Int J Gynaecol Obstet 15:262, 1977

Kossoff G, Garrett WJ, Radovanovich G: Ultrasonic examination of a nonuplet pregnancy. Austral N Zeal J Obstet Gynaecol 16:203, 1976

Laursen B: Twin pregnancy: The value of prophylactic rest in bed and the risk involved. Acta Obstet Gynecol Scand 52:367, 1973

MacGillivray I: Twin Pregnancies. In Wynn RM (ed): Obstetrics and Gynecology Annual. New York, Appleton, 1978, p 135

MacGillivray I, Nylander PPS, Corney G: Human Multiple Reproduction. Philadelphia, Saunders, 1975

McKeown T, Record RG: Observations on foetal growth in multiple pregnancy in man. J Endocrinol 5:387, 1952

Mägiste M, Von Schenck H, Sjöberg NO, Thorell JI, Åberg A: Screening for detecting twins. Am J Obstet Gynecol 126:697, 1976

Myrianthopoulos NC: An epidemiologic survey of twins in a large prospectively studied population. Am J Hum Genet 22:611, 1970

Naeye RL: Organ abnormalities in a human parabiotic syndrome. Am J Pathol 46:829, 1965

Naeye RL, Tafari N, Judge D, Marboe CC: Twins: causes of perinatal death in 12 United States cities and one African city. Am J Obstet Gynecol 31:267, 1978

Newman HH: The Physiology of Twinning. Chicago, Chicago Press, 1923

Novotny CA, Haas WK, Callagan DA: Early diagnosis of multiple pregnancy: Use of electroencephalograph in prenatal examination. JAMA 171:880, 1959

Nylander PPS: The frequency of twinning in a rural community in Western Nigeria. Ann Hum Genet 33:41, 1969

Persson P-H, Grennert L, Gennser G, Kullander S: On improved outcome of twin pregnancies. Acta Obstet Gynecol Scand 58:3, 1979

Pettersson F, Smedby B, Lindmark G: Outcome of twin birth. Review of 1636 children born in twin birth. Act Paediat Scand 64:473, 1976

Potter EL: Pathology of the Fetus and Infant, 2nd ed. Chicago, Year Book, 1962, pp 1–50

Powers WF: Twin pregnancy: Complications and treatment. Obstet Gynecol 42:795, 1973

Pritchard JA: Changes in blood volume during pregnancy. Anesthesiology 26:393, 1965

Quigley MM, Cruikshank DP: Polyhydramnios and acute renal failure. J Reprod Med 19:92, 1977

Recommended Dietary Allowances, 9th rev ed. National Research Council, National Academy of Sciences, 1979

Robinson HP, Caines JS: Sonar evidence of early pregnancy failure in patients with twin conceptions. Br J Obstet Gynaecol 84:22, 1977

Rothman, KJ: Fetal loss, twinning and birthweight after oral-contraceptive use. New Engl J Med 297:468, 1977

Rovinsky JJ, Jaffin H: Cardiovascular hemodynamics in pregnancy: III. Cardiac rate, stroke volume, total peripheral resistance, and central blood volume in multiple pregnancy. Synthesis of results. Am J Obstet Gynecol 95:787, 1966

Schmidt, R, Nitowsky HM, Sobel EH: Monozygotic twins discordant for sex. Pediatr Research 8:395, 1974

Spellacy WN, Buhi WC, Birk SA: Human placental lactogen levels in multiple pregnancies. Obstet Gynecol 52:210, 1978

Strandskov HH, Edelen EW, Siemens GJ: Analysis of the sex ratios among single and plural births in the total "white" and "colored" U.S. populations. Am J Phys Anthrop 4:491, 1946

Tamby Raja RL, Atputharajah V, Salmon Y: Prevention of prematurity in twins. Austral N Zeal J Obstet Gynaecol 18:179, 1978

Tan KL, Goon SM, Salmon Y, Wee JH: Conjoined twins. Acta Obstet Gynecol Scand 50:373, 1971

Taylor, ES: Editorial. Obstet Gynecol Surv 31:535, 1976

Terasaki PI, Gjertson D, Bernoco D, et al.: Twins with two different fathers identified by HLA. New Engl J Med 299:590, 1978

Thiery M, Dhont M, Vandekerckhove D: Serum HCG and HPL in twin pregnancies. Acta Obstet Gynecol Scand 56:495, 1976

Vaughn TC, Powell LC: The obstetrical management of conjoined twins. Obstet Gynecol (Suppl) 53:67S, 1979

Waterhouse JAH: Twinning in twin pedigrees. Br J Soc Med 4:197, 1950

Weekes ARL, Menzies DN, DeBoer CH: The relative efficacy of bed rest, cervical suture, and no treatment in the management of twin pregnancy. Br J Obstet Gynaecol 84:161, 1977

White C, Wyshak G: Inheritance in human dizygotic twinning. New Engl J Med 271:1003, 1964

27

Hypertensive Disorders in Pregnancy

In some mysterious way, in certain women, the presence of chorionic villi, with or without a fetus, incites vasospasm and hypertension.

Pregnancy may induce hypertension in previously normotensive women or aggravate hypertension in women who are already hypertensive. Generalized edema, proteinuria, or both, often accompany hypertension induced or aggravated by pregnancy. Convulsions may develop in association with the hypertensive state, especially in women whose hypertension is ignored.

DEFINITIONS AND CLASSIFICATION

The unsatisfactory terms *toxemia of pregnancy* and *toxemias of pregnancy* have been applied variably to any or all disorders in which hypertension, proteinuria, or edema was present during pregnancy or the puerperium, and other disorders, as well. The Committee on Terminology of the American College of Obstetricians and Gynecologists suggested, instead, the following definitions and classification of hypertension that developed during pregnancy or the puerperium (Hughes, 1972): *Hypertension* is defined as a diastolic blood pressure of at least 90 mm Hg, or systolic pressure of at least 140 mm Hg, or a rise in the former of at least 15 mm Hg, or the latter of 30 mm Hg. The blood pressures cited must be manifest on at least two occasions 6 hours or more apart. *Proteinuria* is defined as more than 0.3 g per liter in a 24-hour collection, or greater than 1 g per liter in at least two random urine specimens collected 6 hours or more apart.

Preeclampsia is the development of hypertension with proteinuria, edema, or both, induced by pregnancy after the 20th week of gestation, and sometimes earlier when there is extensive hydatidiform changes in the chorionic villi. *Eclampsia* is the occurrence of convulsions, not caused by any coincidental neurologic disease such as epilepsy, in a woman whose condition also fulfills the criteria for preeclampsia. *Superimposed preeclampsia or eclampsia* is defined as the development of preeclampsia or eclampsia in a woman with chronic hypertensive vascular or renal disease. *Chronic hypertensive disease* is defined as the presence of persistent hypertension, of whatever cause, before the 20th week of gestation in the absence of neoplastic trophoblastic disease, or persistent hypertension beyond 6 weeks postpartum.

Gestational hypertension is defined as hypertension that develops during the latter half of pregnancy or during the first 24 hours after delivery. It is not accompanied by other evidence of preeclampsia or hypertensive vascular disease, and it disappears within 10 days following parturition. Gestational hypertension is most likely to be a variant of preeclampsia. *Gestational edema* is the generalized accumulation of fluid of greater than "one plus" pitting edema after 12 hours' bed rest or a weight gain of 5 pounds or more in a week. *Gestational proteinuria* is proteinuria during pregnancy in the absence of hypertension, edema, renal infection, or known renovascular disease; the existence of such an entity is questionable.

Significance. The hypertensive disorders in pregnancy are common complications of gestation and form one of the great triad of complications (hemorrhage, hypertension, and sepsis) that are responsible for the majority of maternal deaths. As a cause of perinatal death these disorders are even more important. The cause or causes of preeclampsia, eclampsia, and essential hypertension remain for the most part unknown, despite decades of intensive research, even though these disorders remain among the most important unsolved problems in obstetrics.

The large toll that may be taken by hypertension in pregnancy of maternal and infant lives is most often preventable. Good prenatal supervision, with the detection of signs and symptoms of incipient preeclampsia, followed by appropriate treatment, will ameliorate many cases sufficiently that the outcome for baby and mother is satisfactory.

Diagnosis. The syndrome of preeclampsia-eclampsia is unique to pregnant or puerperal women and has not been identified in animals to occur spontaneously nor has it been reproduced experimentally. Diagnosis is made on the basis of development of hypertension with proteinuria or edema, or both, plus convulsions in case of eclampsia, after 20 weeks gestation. These signs may appear a few weeks earlier with an advanced hydatidiform mole or with extensive molar change with yet enough appropriately functioning placenta persisting to maintain fetal life (see Fig. 23-9, p. 560), and very rarely with a normal-appearing placenta and fetus as described by Lindheimer and co-workers (1974). Preeclampsia and eclampsia occur most often in the first pregnancy. They may occur in later pregnancies, but in such instances there usually is a predisposing factor such as diabetes, multiple fetuses, fetal hydrops, hydatidiform mole, or underlying chronic vascular disease. In multiparas, the diagnosis should be suspect.

Preeclampsia generally is classified as "severe" if any of the following abnormalities develop:

1. Blood pressure of 160 mm Hg or more systolic, or 110 or more diastolic, that does not decrease when the woman is hospitalized and at bed rest.
2. Proteinuria of 5 g or more in 24 hours (3 or 4 plus on qualitative examination).
3. Oliguria (500 ml or less in 24 hours) and a rising plasma creatinine level.
4. Persisting cerebral or visual disturbances.
5. Epigastric or right upper quadrant pain.
6. Pulmonary edema or cyanosis.
7. Severe thrombocytopenia or overt intravascular hemolysis.
8. Hepatocellular damage.
9. Fetal growth retardation.

The differentiation between severe and mild preeclampsia is not wholly desirable, except in retrospect, since an apparently mild case can rapidly become severe. Blood pressure alone is not always a dependable indication of severity, for an adolescent woman with a pressure of 145/85 may develop convulsions, whereas some women with a blood pressure of 180/120 do not. Fortunately, most women suffering from preeclampsia do not have convulsions. In some, the process is inherently mild and hence does not advance to the eclamptic stage. In others, suitable treatment checks the process. In a third group, the termination of pregnancy, either spontaneously or operatively, forestalls the development of convulsions, and the woman returns to normal after delivery.

The diagnosis of chronic hypertension may be made from a history of or the finding of hypertension antedating pregnancy, the discovery of hypertension before the 20th week of pregnancy (with the exceptions noted above), or the persistence of hypertension long after delivery. The differentiation of chronic hypertension from preeclampsia may be difficult in women who are first seen during the latter half of gestation, since they may not know what their blood pressure values were before pregnancy. A source of further confusion is the fact that the blood pressure of the chronically hypertensive woman may decrease to the normal range during much of the second trimester as peripheral resistance falls, and then rise later in pregnancy to prepregnant hypertensive levels.

Women with antecedent hypertension, moreover, frequently react to pregnancy with the development of a syndrome that seems to be preeclampsia superimposed upon the underlying chronic disorder, or *chronic hypertension with superimposed preeclampsia.* The criteria for diagnosis of this condition are (1) evidence that the woman is suffering from chronic hypertension, and (2) evidence of the superimposition of an acute process, as demonstrated by an elevation of systolic pressure of 30 mm Hg or more, an elevation in diastolic pressure of 15 mm or more, and the development of a significant amount of proteinuria, usually with edema as well. Preeclampsia developing in chronically hypertensive women is likely to occur relatively early and may progress to eclampsia.

Hypertension alone that recurs late in subsequent pregnancies in the absence of a pregnancy event known to predispose very strongly to preeclampsia, as for example twins, is regarded by some as another episode of preeclampsia. Dieckmann (1952), who was probably correct, considered it to be a sign of latent essential hypertension or vasculorenal disease.

PATHOPHYSIOLOGY OF PREECLAMPSIA-ECLAMPSIA

Vasospasm. Vasospasm is basic to the disease process of preeclampsia-eclampsia. This concept, first advanced by Volhard (1918), is based upon direct observation of small blood vessels in the nail beds, ocular fundi, and bulbar conjunctivae, and it has been surmised from histologic changes that are seen in various affected organs. In preeclampsia, Hinselmann (1924), and later several others, noted alterations in the size of the arterioles in the nail bed, with evidence of segmental spasm that produced alternate regions of contraction and dilatation. Even more striking changes have been identified in the bulbar conjunctivae; Landesman and co-workers (1954) described marked arteriolar constriction, even to the extent that capillary circulation was intermittently abolished. Further evidence that vascular changes play an important role in preeclampsia-eclampsia is afforded by the frequency with which spasm of the retinal arterioles, commonly segmental, is found in this disorder.

The vascular constriction imposes a resistance to blood flow and accounts for the development of arterial hypertension. Vasospasm most likely exerts a noxious effect on the blood vessels themselves as well as the organs they supply. Circulation in the vasa vasorum is impaired, leading to damage of the vascular walls. Alternating segmental dilatation that commonly accompanies the segmental arteriolar spasm probably contributes further to the development of vascular damage, since endothelial integrity may be compromised by stretch in the dilated segments. Moreover, angiotensin II appears to have a direct action on endothelial cells causing them to contract. These events can create interendothelial leaks through which blood constituents, including platelets and fibrinogen, can pass and be deposited subendothelially (Brunner and Gavras, 1975). The vascular changes, together with local hypoxia of the surrounding tissues, presumably lead to hemorrhage, necrosis, and other disturbances that have been observed at times with severe pregnancy-induced hypertension. Deposition of fibrin is then likely to be prominent, as seen in fatal cases (McKay, 1965).

INCREASED PRESSOR RESPONSES. Normally, pregnant women develop refractoriness to the pressor effects of angiotensin II (Abdul-Karim and Assali, 1961). This refractoriness to angiotensin II is not a generalized phenomenon, however, since aldosterone secretion is strikingly increased in pregnant women and increased aldosterone secretion is modulated by the action of angiotensin II on the cells of the zona glomerulosa of the adrenal cortex. Based on the findings of a number of studies, Gant and co-workers (1973) concluded that the blunted response of pregnant women to the pressor effect of angiotensin II was brought about by a specific decrease in responsiveness of the vasculature. Refractoriness to angiotensin II pressor effects commences early in pregnancy (Fig. 27-

1) and in some women enormous amounts of angiotensin II are required to elicit a given pressor response. The refractoriness to angiotensin II appears to be mediated by the vascular tissue synthesis of a prostaglandin or prostaglandin-like substance (e.g., prostacyclin or prostaglandin E_2). Indeed, the refractoriness to the pressor effect of angiotensin II in pregnant women can be abolished by the administration of the prostaglandin synthetase enzyme inhibitors, indomethacin and aspirin (Everett et al., 1978). In some tissues angiotensin II action is mediated, at least in part, by promoting either the accelerated synthesis or the release of prostacyclin or of prostaglandins, or both. It is interesting to speculate that pregnancy brings about an increased capacity for prostaglandin formation in vascular tissue, normally with relatively greater synthesis of prostaglandins that induce vasodilatation than of prostaglandins, e.g., prostaglandin $F_2\alpha$, that promote vasoconstriction.

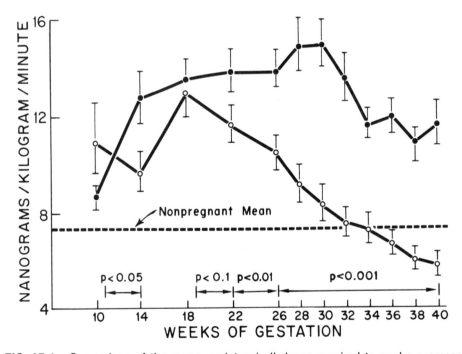

FIG. 27-1. Comparison of the mean angiotensin II doses required to evoke a pressor response in 120 primigravidas who remained normotensive (solid circles) and 72 primigravidas who later developed pregnancy-induced hypertension (open circles). (From Gant et al. *J Clin Invest* 52:2682, 1973)

Increased vascular reactivity to pressor hormones in women with early preeclampsia has been identified by Talledo, Chesley, and Zuspan (1968) using either angiotensin II or norepinephrine, and by Browne (1946) using vasopressin. More recently, Gant and co-workers (1973) demonstrated that in primigravidas increased vascular sensitivity to angiotensin II clearly preceded the development of pregnancy-induced hypertension. The primigravid women studied by them demonstrated, beginning early in pregnancy, progressively greater resistance to the pressor effect of infused angiotensin II (Fig. 27-1). However, those primigravid women destined to develop pregnancy-induced hypertension subsequently demonstrated a loss of the normal pregnancy resistance to angiotensin II some time before the onset of hypertension. Of all the normotensive women studied who at 28 to 32 weeks' gestation required more than 8 ng per kg per minute of angiotensin II to develop a standardized pressor response, 91 percent remained normotensive throughout the rest of the pregnancy. Conversely, among normotensive primigravid women requiring for a pressor response less than 8 ng per kg per minute at 28 to 32 weeks, 90 percent subsequently became overtly hypertensive.

A pressor response induced simply by the supine position, after lying in the lateral recumbent, has been demonstrated in some pregnant women by Gant and co-workers (1973). They found that the majority of nulliparous pregnant women who demonstrated at 28 to 32 weeks an increase in diastolic blood pressure of at least 20 mm Hg when turned from side to back later became overtly hypertensive; conversely, most women who did not demonstrate such a rise did not become hypertensive. Those women who demonstrated a supine pressor response were also abnormally sensitive to angiotensin II and vice versa. The mechanism by which the supine position may incite a rise in blood pressure is not clear, but it is another manifestation of intrinsic vascular hypersensitivity in women destined to develop pregnancy-induced hypertension.

Impaired Organ Function.   Changes in the function of a number of organs and systems, presumably in large part the consequence of vasospasm, have been identified in severe preeclampsia and eclampsia and are described below.

UTEROPLACENTAL CHANGES.   While precise measurements of uterine blood flow through the placenta are lacking, there is every reason to believe that placental perfusion by the mother is reduced in cases of pregnancy-induced hypertension. Everett and colleagues (1979) have presented evidence that is consistent with the view that the rate of clearance of dehydroisoandrosterone sulfate to estradiol-17β by the placenta is reflective of the level of maternal perfusion of the placenta. Normally, as pregnancy advances, the placental clearance of maternal plasma dehydroisoandrosterone sulfate through the formation of estradiol-17β by the placenta increases greatly. Moreover, in women destined to develop pregnancy-induced hypertension, the conversion of dehydroisoandrosterone sulfate to estradiol-17β before the onset of hypertension is even somewhat greater than that of the normal pregnant control group, an intriguing observation in itself. With the onset of pregnancy-induced hypertension, however, the conversion to estradiol-17β falls, as illustrated in Figure 27-2.

Browne and Veall (1953), Johnson and Clayton (1957), Dixon and associates (1963), and others measured the rate of disappearance of radiolabeled sodium from the uterus following its injection, presumably into the intervillous space or into the myometrium. The rate of clearance, very likely a reflection of uteroplacental blood flow, typically was prolonged in hypertensive pregnant women.

At the same time that uteroplacental blood flow is most likely to be compromised in women with pregnancy-induced hypertension, uterine activity—both spontaneous and in response to oxytocin—is increased, an observation of clinical importance. With all other conditions equal, the induction of labor

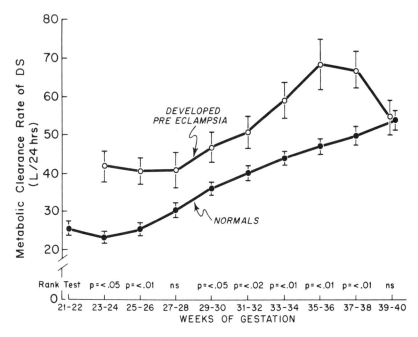

FIG. 27-2. Comparison of metabolic clearance rates of dehydroisoandrosterone sulfate (MCR_{DS}) in normal primigravidas as compared to those women in which preeclampsia ultimately developed. Note that the MCR_{DS} increased progressively throughout pregnancy in the 38 women who remained normal. In the 14 women who ultimately developed preeclampsia, initial values were higher and remained higher until 35 to 36 weeks' gestation (patients still clinically normal), at which time the values began to decrease. (From Gant et al. *Endocrinology,* International Congress Series, 273:1026, 1972)

with oxytocin in women with severe preeclampsia and eclampsia is more likely to be successful than in normal pregnant women. Simultaneously, the risk of uterine hyperstimulation with oxytocin is greater.

There are no studies specifically of placental function in pregnancy-induced hypertension but, with the fully developed syndrome, reduced placental function has been inferred from the presence at times of placental infarcts and retarded fetal growth. The latter, however, is very likely the consequence primarily of reduced maternal perfusion of the placenta rather than intrinsic placental debility.

From some observations, it can be implied that "hyperplacentosis," i.e., an excess of functioning placenta, is important in the genesis of preeclampsia-eclampsia. The syndrome is more likely to develop in pregnancies in which there is a superabundance of

trophoblast with chorionic villi, for example, hydatidiform mole and the large placentas that are characteristic of maternal diabetes, erythroblastosis fetalis, and multiple fetuses. Moreover, Gant and associates (1972), as mentioned, demonstrated a greater than normal metabolic clearance rate of maternal plasma dehydroisoandrosterone sulfate in primigravid women destined subsequently to develop pregnancy-induced hypertension.

Hertig in 1945 identified in preeclamptic pregnancies a lesion of the uteroplacental arteries characterized by prominent lipid-rich foam cells. Zeek and Assali in 1950 extended these observations and concluded that in preeclampsia there is a pathognomic lesion of the uteroplacental vessels which they termed acute atherosis. Most investigators are now in accord that a lesion occurs but they do not necessarily agree on the precise nature of the lesion. On the basis of the findings of electron microscopic studies of uteroplacental arteries obtained by biopsy of the placental implantation site, De Wolf and co-workers (1975) described the following: Early preeclamptic changes include endothelial damage, insudation of plasma constituents into the vessel wall, proliferation of myointimal cells, and medial necrosis. Lipid accumulates first in the myointimal cells and secondarily in macrophages. Kitzmiller and Benirschke (1973) identified by immunologic means fibrin, immune globulin, and components of complement in these lesions.

RENAL CHANGES. During normal pregnancy, renal blood flow and the glomerular filtration rate are increased significantly above nonpregnant levels (see Chap. 9, p. 241), but with the development of pregnancy-induced hypertension, renal perfusion, and glomerular filtration are reduced. Levels that are appreciably below normal nonpregnant levels, however, are found only with severe preeclampsia and eclampsia. Most often, therefore, the creatinine or urea concentration in plasma is not appreciably elevated above normal nonpregnant values. The plasma uric acid concentration is much more commonly elevated, especially in women with more severe disease. The elevation is a result primarily of decreased renal clearance of uric acid by the kidney, a decrease that exceeds the reduction in glomerular filtration rate and creatinine clearance (Chesley and Williams, 1945). Thiazide diuretics, as well as preeclampsia-eclampsia, cause an increase in uric acid in plasma. In our experience, measurements of plasma uric acid levels are of little value for diagnosis or prognosis.

The experience at Parkland Memorial Hospital has been that after delivery, in the absence of underlying chronic vascular disease, complete recovery of renal function can be anticipated. This would not be the case, of course, if *renal cortical necrosis*, an irreversible but rare lesion, had developed.

Histologic changes identifiable by light and electron microscopy are usually found in the kidney. Sheehan (1950) observed that the glomeruli were enlarged by about 20 percent, often pouting into the neck of the tubule. The capillary loops are variably dilated and contracted. The endothelial cells are swollen, and deposited within and beneath them are fibrils that have been mistaken for thickening and reduplication of the basement membrane.

Sheehan's interpretations have been confirmed by the findings of electron microscopic studies of renal biopsies taken from women with preeclampsia. Most (Farquhar, 1959; Mautner et al., 1962; Pollak and Nettles, 1960; and others), but not all (Ishikawa, 1961) of the electron microscopic studies are in agreement that the characteristic changes are glomerular capillary endothelial swelling, which Spargo and associates (1959) called "glomerular capillary endotheliosis," and subendothelial deposit of protein material. The endothelial cells are so swollen as to block partially, or even completely, the capillary lumens. Homogeneous deposits of an electrondense substance are found between the basal lamina and the endothelial cell and within the cells themselves (Figs. 27-3, 27-4). Vassalli and co-workers (1963), on the basis of immunofluorescent staining, have considered the material to be fibrinogen or a fibrinogen derivative and regard its presence as characteristic of preeclampsia. This observation, in part, has led to a theory that the renal lesions of preeclampsia-eclampsia are the result of intravascular coagulation initiated by something, presumably thromboplastin, released from the placenta (Page, 1972). Lichtig and co-workers (1975), however, were able to identify fibrinogen or its derivatives so deposited in but 13 of 30 renal biopsy specimens from women considered, for good reasons, to have preeclampsia, and in only 2 of the 30 was the amount of fibrin graded as more than a trace. An alternative explanation for the renal lesion has been proposed by Petrucco and colleagues (1974), who detected IgM and IgG, and sometimes complement, in the glomeruli of women with preeclampsia in proportion to the severity of the disease. They suggested that an immuno-

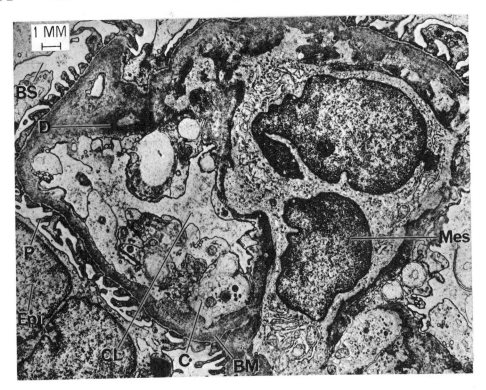

FIG. 27-3. The glomerular capillary lesion of preeclampsia. BS, Bowman's space; D, electrondense deposit, probably a derivative of fibrinogen; P, podocytes or foot processes of epithelial cell; Epi, nucleus of epithelial cell; CL, lumen of glomerular capillary; C, markedly swollen endothelia cytoplasm; BM, basement membrane (normal); MES, nucleus of mesothelial cell. From Chesley. *Hypertensive Disorders of Pregnancy.* New York, Appleton, 1978, p 70)

logic mechanism was active in the production of the glomerular lesion.

The renal changes identified by electron microscopy have been held out by some as being pathognomonic of preeclampsia, always present in that disease and specific for it. The uncertainties of clinical diagnosis are so great, however, as to preclude acceptance of such a one-to-one relation, except as an act of faith. The history of "pathognomonic" lesions in eclampsia engenders skepticism. One such lesion accepted in the past, but not now, was peripheral hemorrhagic necrosis of the hepatic lobules, as discussed below.

Renal tubular lesions are common in the kidneys of women with eclampsia, but what has been interpreted as degenerative changes may represent only an accumulation within the cells of protein reabsorbed from the glomerular filtrate. The collecting tubules may appear obstructed by casts from derivatives of protein, including, at times, hemoglobin.

In rare cases, the major portion of the cortex of both kidneys undergoes necrosis. *Renal cortical necrosis* is characterized clinically by oliguria or anuria and rapidly developing azotemia. The condition probably results from spasm of the renal arteries with resultant thrombosis of the intralobular arteries with extension from or into the glomerular capillaries. Although cortical necrosis of the kidney is known to have occurred in nonpregnant women and in men, in many institutions the lesion has been associated most often with pregnancy.

HEPATIC CHANGES. It is not clear whether hepatic blood flow increases during normal pregnancy and then decreases with the development of pregnancy-induced hypertension.

With severe preeclampsia and eclampsia, there are, at times, alterations in tests of hepatic function, including delayed excretion of bromosulfonphthalein and elevation of serum glutamic oxaloacetic transaminase levels (Combes and Adams, 1972). Hyperbilirubinemia is uncommon with preeclampsia-eclampsia. In our experience with 134 women, including 45 with eclampsia, only three had a serum bilirubin greater than 1.2 mg per dl, with 2.3 mg per dl as the highest value. An increase in serum alkaline phosphatase is usually in the form of heat-stable alkaline phosphatase, which most likely is of placental origin.

Hemorrhagic necrosis in the periphery of the liver lobule, identified commonly at autopsy, was long considered to be the characteristic lesion of eclampsia. However, the changes usually identified in fatal cases have seldom been demonstrated in liver biopsies of nonfatal cases (Combes and Adams, 1972; Ingerslev and Teilum, 1946). In our experience at Parkland Memorial Hospital, liver histology was normal in biopsies from six women with preeclampsia and twelve with otherwise uncomplicated eclampsia who were studied. Since the amount of tissue sampled by biopsy was small, some lesions may

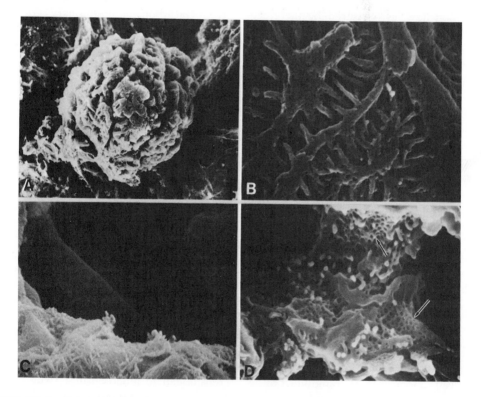

FIG. 27-4. Scanning electron micrographs. *A.* Enlarged, swollen glomerulus. × 500. *B.* Branching and interdigitation of terminal epithelial foot processes, usually normal in preeclampsia. × 20,000. *C.* Interior of a glomerular capillary. Endothelial fenestrae are not seen because of severe swelling of the cytoplasm. × 5,000. *D.* Normal glomerulus for comparison; note polygonal endothelial fenestrae (arrows). × 5,000. (Photographs by Ordóñoz, NG. From Lindheimer and Katz. *Renal Function and Disease in Pregnancy,* in press. Courtesy of Lea and Febiger)

be missed. Even so, the most characteristic feature of the hepatic lesion in eclampsia is it's variability in both extent and severity. It is agreed by most authorities, therefore, that periportal necrosis can be the result but not the cause of eclampsia.

In rare instances, subcapsular hemorrhage in the liver may become so extensive as to cause rupture of the capsule with massive hemorrhage into the peritoneal cavity. The mortality rate is high. Prompt surgical intervention with vigorous transfusion therapy can be life saving. One woman survived at Parkland Memorial Hospital after receiving blood and blood products from more than 200 donors!

BRAIN. McCall (1954) found that cerebral blood flow, as measured by the Kety-Schmidt nitrous oxide technic, was not reduced in women with pregnancy-induced hypertension; however, the possibility of focal hypoperfusion or hyperperfusion of the brain could not be excluded by this technic.

Nonspecific abnormalities in the electroencephalogram usually can be demonstrated for some time after eclamptic convulsions. An increased incidence of electroencephalographic abnormalities has been described for members of the families of women with eclampsia, a finding which is suggestive that some women who convulse as the consequence of pregnancy-induced hypertension are by inheritance predisposed to do so (Rosenbaum and Maltby, 1943).

The main postmortem lesions that have been described in the brain of women who died with eclampsia are edema, hyperemia, focal anemia, thrombosis, and hemorrhage. Sheehan (1950) examined the brains of 48 eclamptic women within about an hour after their death. Hemorrhages, ranging from petechiae to gross bleeding, were found in 56 percent of the cases. According to Sheehan, if the brain is examined within an hour after death, most often it is as firm as normal and there is no obvious edema. Govan (1961) investigated the cause of death in 110 fetal cases of eclampsia and concluded that cerebral hemorrhage was responsible in 39.

Forty-seven women died of cardiorespiratory failure; small hemorrhagic lesions were found in the brains of 85 percent of them. Govan described fibrinoid changes as a regular finding in the walls of the cerebral vessels. The lesions sometimes appear to have been present for some time, as judged from the surrounding leukocytic response and infiltration by pigmented macrophages, a finding that was suggestive that the prodromal neurologic symptoms and the convulsions may be related to the lesions.

CARDIO-PULMONARY CHANGES. After a convulsion, the respiratory rate most often is increased as the consequence of hypercarbia resulting from lactic acid production and, in turn, release of carbon dioxide from bicarbonate. Pulmonary edema has been found commonly at autopsy in fatal cases of preeclampsia-eclampsia. Its causes include heart failure, circulatory overload (which at times is iatrogenic), and aspiration of gastric contents while convulsing or afterward when the sensorium remains obtunded or a mask for oxygen is strapped to the face. If death does not follow the aspiration immediately, bronchopneumonia is a likely finding.

ENDOCRINE CHANGES. During normal pregnancy, plasma levels of renin, angiotensin II, and aldosterone are increased. Paradoxically, with pregnancy-induced hypertension, these substances commonly decrease toward the normal nonpregnant range (Weir et al., 1973). With the development of sodium retention, hypertension, or both, the rate of renin release by the juxtaglomerular apparatus decreases. Since renin is the enzyme that catalyzes the conversion of angiotensinogen to angiotensin I (which is then transformed to angiotensin II by converting enzyme in the lung) angiotensin II levels decline, and thence aldosterone secretion decreases. On the other hand, another potent mineralocorticosteroid, deoxycorticosterone (DOC), is strikingly increased in the plasma of women during the third trimester of pregnancy (see Chap. 9, p. 252). Importantly, the increase in DOC concentration does not appear to arise as the consequence of increased secretion of DOC by the maternal adrenal glands. Treatment of pregnant women with the potent glucocorticosteroid, dexamethasone, to reduce ACTH secretion, does not bring about a reduction in plasma levels of DOC and neither does ACTH treatment of near-term pregnant women cause an increase in plasma DOC levels. Since it has been shown that plasma progesterone is converted to DOC in nonadrenal tissues, it is reasonable to conclude that DOC formed in this manner is not subject to control by angiotensin II and thus the amount of DOC formed from plasma progesterone is not reduced by sodium retention or hypertension. Therefore, extra-adrenal DOC formation may play a crucial role in the pathogenesis or perpetuation of pregnancy-induced hypertension. Winkel and co-workers (1980) found that the fractional conversion of plasma progesterone to DOC varied widely among individuals (0.002 to 0.0022). This finding is very intriguing, since ordinarily, the fractional conversion of one steroid hormone to another is similar among normal persons. Thus, in near-term pregnant women producing 250 mg of progesterone per day, the amount of DOC produced from plasma progesterone could vary from 0.5 mg to 11 mg per 24 hours. Nonpregnant women produce, on average, 0.15 mg DOC per day. Given the progesterone produced in women with hyperplacentosis who are prone to develop preeclampsia, e.g., women with diabetes, multiple fetuses, fetal hydrops, and hydatidiform mole, the amount of DOC produced from plasma progesterone could be enormous.

The formation of DOC cannot be the only factor, however, in the development of pregnancy-induced hypertension. DOC levels were measured throughout pregnancy by Parker and colleagues (1979). They found that the concentrations of DOC in the plasma of a group of primigravid women who ultimately developed preeclampsia were no greater than the concentrations of DOC in primigravid women who remained normo-

tensive (see Figs. 27-5 and 9-16). Brown and co-workers (1972) had shown previously that the DOC levels in pregnant women who were already hypertensive were no greater than were those in normotensive gravidas. The possibility of a yet unidentified pressor hormone persists. Increased antidiuretic hormone activity to account for oliguria has been suggested but not proven.

Chorionic gonadotropin levels in plasma have been found inconstantly to be elevated; conversely, placental lactogen has been found inconstantly to be reduced.

Necrosis of the adrenal and the pituitary has been identified in some fatal cases of eclampsia (McKay, 1965). In our experience

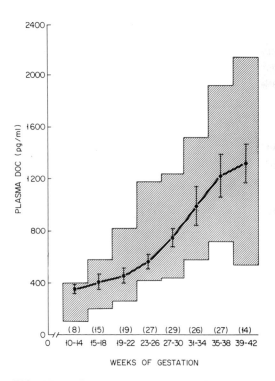

FIG. 27-5. Deoxycorticosterone (DOC) levels in primigravid women as a function of gestational age. The hatched area is the range of values in women who remained normotensive. The values represented by the solid circles and connected by the solid line are the values found in the plasma of women who ultimately developed preeclampsia. The vertical bars represent the extent of the standard error of the mean. (From Parker and colleagues, *Am J Obstet Gynecol,* in press, 1980)

with nonfatal cases, compromised adrenal or pituitary function is rare.

FLUID AND ELECTROLYTE CHANGES. Commonly, extracellular fluid in women with preeclampsia, and especially those with eclampsia, has accumulated beyond that of normal pregnancy. The mechanism responsible is not clear. Edema is evident at a time when, paradoxically, aldosterone levels are reduced compared to the remarkably elevated levels of normal pregnancy. As noted above, however, DOC levels in plasma remain elevated, but are not consistently greater than those in normotensive women. The electrolyte concentrations do not differ appreciably from those of normal pregnancy unless there has been vigorous diuretic therapy, dietary sodium restriction, or the administration of water with sufficient oxytocin to produce antidiuresis. Severe edema, by itself, is not indicative of a poor prognosis, nor does lack of appreciable edema guarantee a favorable outcome for pregnancies complicated by preeclampsia-eclampsia. After a convulsion, the bicarbonate concentration is lowered; carbon dioxide is generated from bicarbonate by the lactic acid produced and exhaled. The intensity of the acidosis will relate to the amount of lactic acid produced and its rate of metabolism, as well as the rate at which carbon dioxide is exhaled.

HEMATOLOGIC CHANGES. Important hematologic changes that have been identified at times in women with preeclampsia and eclampsia include (1) a decrease in, or actually an absence of, normal pregnancy hypervolemia; (2) alterations of the coagulation mechanism; and (3) evidence of increased erythrocyte destruction.

Hemoconcentration in women with eclampsia was emphasized by Dieckmann (1952) in his lengthy monograph, *The Toxemias of Pregnancy.* More recently Pritchard, Cunningham, and co-workers (unpublished observations) have systematically measured the degree of pregnancy hypervolemia in women with preeclampsia-eclampsia. Their findings are indicative that with eclampsia pregnancy hypervolemia most often is scant to absent, whereas with preeclampsia the blood volume is less likely to be so severely contracted. The woman of average size can be expected to have a blood volume near 5000 ml during the last several weeks of a normal pregnancy compared to about 3500 ml in the nonpregnant state. With eclampsia, however, much or all of the added 1500 ml of blood normally present late in pregnancy can be anticipated to be missing. Almost certainly, the lack of hypervolemia is the consequence of vasoconstriction, rather than the reverse. Hypoproteinemia has been considered by some to play a role in the reduced blood volume, but the concentrations of major plasma proteins commonly do not differ markedly from those of normal pregnancy.

It was taught by Dieckmann (1952), and more recently by others, that clinical improvement is characterized by hemodilution manifested by a fall in hematocrit, with the reverse true for an increase in hematocrit. In our experience, however, a significant fall in hematocrit occurs most often only with delivery. Moreover, rather than directly reflecting clinical improvement, the fall may reflect excessive blood loss at delivery or, rarely, markedly increased erythrocyte destruction, as described below, or both.

It is emphasized that in terms of capacity, in the absence of hemorrhage, the intravascular compartment in eclampsia is usually not underfilled. Vasospasm has contracted the space to be filled, a reduction that persists until after delivery when typically the vascular tree relaxes, the blood volume increases, and the hematocrit falls. The woman with eclampsia, therefore, is unduly sensitive both to blood loss at delivery and to vigorous fluid therapy administered in an attempt to expand the contracted blood volume to normal levels of pregnant women. Management of blood loss in these circumstances is considered in Chapter 21.

It has long been recognized that changes that imply intravascular coagulation and, less often pathologic erythrocyte destruction, may further complicate cases of pregnancy-induced hypertension, especially eclampsia

(Pritchard et al., 1954; Stahnke, 1922). In recent years, renewed interest in these changes have led to the concept by some investigators that not only is disseminated intravascular coagulation a characteristic feature of preeclampsia-eclampsia, but it has a dominant role in the pathogenesis of the syndrome. For example, Page (1972), as cited above, theorized that many of the changes of preeclampsia were the consequence of fibrin deposited in vital organs as a product of slow disseminated intravascular coagulation initiated by thromboplastin entering the maternal circulation from the placenta while rapid disseminated intravascular coagulation and fibrin so formed causes cerebral vascular occlusion and the convulsions of eclampsia.

Since our early reports (Pritchard et al., 1954), we have continued to search for evidence of coagulopathy in eclamptic women. The results of these studies are presented in Table 27-1. Thrombocytopenia, infrequently severe, was the most frequent finding. The platelet count was below 150,000 per mm³

in 24 of 91 cases (26 percent) but below 100,000 in only 14 women (15 percent). Importantly, thrombocytopenia has not been identified in the cord blood of the fetus (Pritchard and Cunningham, unpublished observations). Elevated levels of fibrin degradation products in serum were clearly identified in only 2 of 59 women (3 percent). Fibrin monomer was detected in plasma by the protamine paracoagulation test in only one of 15 cases evaluated. Unless some degree of placental abruption had developed, fibrinogen in maternal plasma did not differ remarkably from levels found late in normal pregnancy. Interestingly, the thrombin time was somewhat prolonged in one-third of the cases of eclampsia even when elevated levels of fibrin degradation products or fibrin monomer were not identified (Pritchard et al., 1976). The reason for this is not known. The various coagulation changes just described occur in our experience less frequently in women with preeclampsia.

Our observations on eclampsia, as well as

TABLE 27-1.

CHANGES IN COAGULATION FACTORS THAT IMPLY DISSEMINATED INTRAVASCULAR COAGULATION

	INTRAPARTUM PRIMIGRAVIDAS NORMALLY PREGNANT	MOST ABNORMAL VALUE FOR EACH CASE OF ECLAMPSIA
Platelets*		
Mean (cu mm)	278,000	206,000
−2 standard deviations	150,000	—
<150,000	0/20	24/91
<100,000	0/20	14/91
< 50,000	0/20	3/9
Serum Fibrin Degradation Products†:		
8 μg per ml or less	17/20	51/59
16 μg per ml	3/20	6/59
>16 μg per ml	0/20	2/59
Plasma Fibrinogen*		
Mean, mg per dl	415	413
−2 standard deviations	285	—
<285 mg per dl	0/20	7/89
Fibrin Monomer		
Positive	1/20	1/14

* Lowest value identified for each case of eclampsia.
† Highest value identified for each case of eclampsia.

those reported by Kitzmiller and associates (1974) for preeclampsia are most consistent with the concept that the coagulation changes are the sequelae of preeclampsia-eclampsia, or preeclampsia-eclampsia plus preexisting chronic vascular disease, rather than the cause. Very likely platelets aggregate and adhere to vessel walls whenever and wherever endothelial cells are discontinuous and promptly variable amounts of fibrin are deposited there. For reasons presented subsequently, treatment with heparin is not essential and may prove dangerous when such changes suggestive of disseminated intravascular coagulation are identified in women with preeclampsia-eclampsia.

Evidence of increased erythrocyte destruction ("microangiopathic hemolysis") in our studies of women with preeclampsia-eclampsia has ranged from those with no evidence to the very uncommon case with fulminant hemoglobinemia and hemoglobinuria, and to all degrees of alteration of erythrocyte morphology from most often no abnormality of shape to fragmented erythrocytes, basket cells, and, rarely, microspherocytes. Evidence of hemolysis, when present, promptly clears after delivery, in our experience.

Incidence of Preeclampsia-Eclampsia.

Preeclampsia-eclampsia most often affects nulliparas. Among them, the susceptibility is highest at each end of the age scale. The older nulliparas are increasingly likely to have chronic hypertension, which predisposes to the development of preeclampsia. Very young teen-age primigravidas are also at unusually high risk (Duenhoelter et al., 1975). Through ignorance, and at times shame, because of an illegitimate pregnancy, such girls may not seek prenatal care.

The incidence of preeclampsia is commonly stated to be about 5 percent, although remarkable variations are reported. At Parkland Memorial Hospital, for example, 30 percent of the black nulliparous pregnant women cared for demonstrate during pregnancy or the early puerperium diastolic blood pressures of at least 90 mm Hg on two or more occasions 6 or more hours apart. Most of these nulliparous women appear to have

pregnancy-induced hypertension rather than chronic hypertension. Socioeconomically more affluent white women develop hypertension during pregnancy less often, but when it does develop it may be just as severe and, if neglected, result in eclampsia.

Eclampsia is usually preventable and therefore should become rare as more and more women receive better prenatal care. The incidence throughout the country for all women is probably 1 in every 1000 to 1500 deliveries, but there are wide variations in different localities and countries. During the past 25 years and 170,000 deliveries, the incidence of eclampsia at Parkland Memorial Hospital had been close to one in 700; most of the emergency cases in Dallas and surrounding counties are brought to this hospital.

There is a familial tendency to preeclampsia-eclampsia. In a unique study of this question, Chesley, Annitto, and Cosgrove (1968) traced more than 96 percent of the grown daughters of women who had had eclampsia at the Margaret Hague Maternity Hospital. Among the 187 who carried pregnancies to viability, the incidence of preeclampsia in the first pregnancy was 26 percent. Moreover, four of the daughters, or 1 in 47, had eclampsia. A genetically determined predisposition has been implicated by Cooper and Liston (1979), as described below.

Theories as to Cause of Preeclampsia-Eclampsia.

Any satisfactory theory must take into account the following observations: Pregnancy-induced or aggravated hypertension is very much more likely to develop in the woman who (1) is exposed to chorionic villi for the first time, (2) is exposed to a superabundance of chorionic villi and covering trophoblast as with twins or hydatidiform mole, (3) has preexisting vascular disease, or (4) is genetically predisposed to the development of hypertension during pregnancy. While chorionic villi are essential, they need not support a fetus (hydatidiform mole), nor need they be located within the uterus (abdominal pregnancy).

The possibility that immunologic as well as endocrine and genetic mechanisms are involved in the genesis of pregnancy-induced hypertension is intriguing. The risk of pregnancy-induced hypertension is enhanced appreciably in circumstances where formation of blocking antibodies to antigenic sites on the placenta *might* be impaired such as during immunosuppressive therapy to protect a renal transplant during pregnancy (see Chap. 28, p. 711) or effective immunization by a previous pregnancy is lacking as in first pregnancies, or the number of antigenic sites provided by the placenta is unusually great compared to the amount of antibody as with the placentas of multiple fetuses.

As pointed out by Chesley (1971), everyone from allergist to zoologist has proposed a theory and suggested "rational therapy" based upon his theory, including mastectomy, oophorectomy, renal decapsulation, trephination, alignment of the woman with the earth's magnetic field with her head pointing to the North Pole, and all sorts of medical regimens. The interested reader is urged to examine the scholarly and entertaining review of various theories provided by Chesley in his elegant text, *Hypertensive Disorders in Pregnancy* (1978).

Recently Cooper and Liston (1979) explored the possibility that susceptibility to preeclampsia-eclampsia is dependent upon a single recessive gene. They calculated the frequencies to be expected in first pregnancies of daughters of women with eclampsia; daughters-in-law served as a control group. The frequencies calculated by them and those actually observed by Chesley and co-workers (1968) in daughters and daughters-in-law of women with eclampsia through his extensive long-term family studies are in remarkably close agreement.

Preeclampsia-eclampsia has its highest incidence among indigent women, but, according to Chesley (1974), this has not always been the case. In the early years of the present century, eclampsia was believed to be most common in middle- and upper-class women. Indeed, that observation led to the ready acceptance of the hypothesis that the dietary restriction of protein (meat) accounted for the reduction in the incidence of eclampsia in Germany during World War I.

Although there are suggestions that dietary deficiencies might cause preeclampsia-eclampsia, this hypothesis must be regarded as far from proved. Preeclampsia-eclampsia would be expected to be more common in multiparous women compared with nulliparous women if this thesis were correct. The opposite is true, however.

Carefully controlled epidemiologic studies of pregnancy have been conducted in Aberdeen, Scotland, where for many years the relevant data have been available for nearly all deliveries. Baird (1969) found that the incidence of preeclampsia did not differ significantly among the five social classes ranging from the professional and well-to-do (class I) through the unskilled laborers (class V), except for some slight increase in class III (skilled manual occupations).

CLINICAL ASPECTS OF PREECLAMPSIA

Clinical Course.   The two especially important signs of preeclampsia—hypertension and proteinuria—are changes of which the pregnant woman is usually unaware. By the time she has developed symptoms, such as headache, visual disturbances, or epigastric pain, the disorder is usually advanced. Hence, the importance of prenatal care in the early detection and management of this complication becomes obvious.

BLOOD PRESSURE.   The physiologic deviation of great importance in preeclampsia is vasospasm, especially of the arterioles. It is not surprising therefore that the most dependable warning sign of preeclampsia is a rise in blood pressure. The diastolic pressure is a more reliable prognostic sign than is the systolic, and any persisting diastolic pressure of 90 mm or more is abnormal.

WEIGHT GAIN.   Another sign of preeclampsia is sudden and excessive weight gain and in some women it is the first sign. Weight increments of about 1 pound per week may be regarded as normal, but when weight gain exceeds 2 pounds in any given week, or 6 pounds in a month, incipient preeclampsia must be suspected. Characteristic of preeclampsia is the suddenness of the excessive weight gain rather than an increase distributed throughout gestation. Sudden and excessive weight gain in gestation is attributable almost entirely to abnormal retention of fluid and is demonstrable, as a rule, before visible signs of edema such as swollen eyelids and puffiness of the fingers. In cases of fulminating preeclampsia or eclampsia, waterlogging may be extreme, and in such women a weight gain of 10 pounds or more in a week is not unusual.

PROTEINURIA.   Proteinuria   varies greatly not only from case to case but also in the same woman from hour to hour. The variability points to a functional (vasospasm) rather than an organic cause. In early preeclampsia, proteinuria may be minimal or entirely lacking. In the more severe forms proteinuria is usually demonstrable and may be as much as 10 g per liter. Proteinuria almost always develops later than the hypertension and usually later than excessive weight gain.

HEADACHE.   Headache is rare in milder cases but is increasingly frequent in the more severe grades. In women who develop eclampsia, severe headache is a frequent forerunner of the first convulsion. It is often frontal but may be occipital, and it is resistant to ordinary treatment with analgesics.

EPIGASTRIC PAIN.   Epigastric or right upper quadrant pain is another late symptom in preeclampsia and is indicative of imminent convulsions. It may be the result of stretching of the hepatic capsule possibly by hemorrhage, although it is thought by some to be of central nervous system origin.

VISUAL   DISTURBANCES.   Visual disturbances ranging from a slight blurring of vision to blindness may accompany preeclampsia. Although such disturbances are thought by some to be of central origin, they are most likely attributable to retinal arteriolar spasm, ischemia, edema, and in rare cases actual retinal detachment. In general, the prognosis for such detachments is good, the retina reattaching, as a rule, within a few weeks after delivery. Hemorrhages and exudates are extremely rare in preeclampsia and when present are indicative most often of underlying chronic hypertensive vascular disease.

Immediate Prognosis.   The immediate prognosis for the mother and fetus is dependent to a considerable extent on the gestational age of the fetus, whether improvement follows hospitalization, when and how delivery is accomplished, and whether eclampsia supervenes.

The perinatal mortality rate is variably increased in preeclampsia, as in the other hypertensive disorders, and it depends chiefly upon the time of onset and the severity of the disease. Much of the loss depends upon prematurity, either because of early spontaneous labor or because of therapeutic interruption necessitated by severe preeclampsia.

Prophylaxis.   Whether preeclampsia can be prevented is uncertain and, to some extent, is a matter of semantics. Since progression from mild preeclampsia to severe preeclampsia to eclampsia usually can be arrested, prenatal care must be credited with much of the marked reduction in the eclampsia mortality rate.

Because women seldom notice the signs of incipient preeclampsia, the early detection of the disease demands close antepartum observation, especially in women known to be predisposed to preeclampsia. The major predisposing factors are (1) nulliparity, (2) a familial history of eclampsia or preeclampsia, (3) multiple fetuses, (4) diabetes, (5) chronic vascular disease, (6) hydatidiform mole, and (7) fetal hydrops.

Rapid gain in weight any time during the latter half of pregnancy, or an upward trend in the diastolic blood pressure while still in the "normal" range, is a danger signal. Every woman should be examined by her obstetrician at least every week during the last month of pregnancy and every 2 weeks during the previous 2 months. At these visits, careful blood pressure recordings and weight checks of the woman are routine. Furthermore, all women should be advised verbally and, preferably, also by means of suitable printed instructions, to report immediately any of the well-known symptoms or signs of preeclampsia, such as headache, visual disturbances, and puffiness of hands or face. The reporting of any such symptoms, of course, calls for an immediate examination to confirm or exclude preeclampsia.

WEIGHT GAIN. Obstetricians often have attempted to limit weight gain to about 20 pounds, or even as little as 15 pounds, in the belief that preeclampsia can thereby be prevented. The total weight gained during pregnancy, however, probably has no relation to preeclampsia unless a large component of the gain is edema. Stringent restriction of weight gain is more likely to be detrimental rather than beneficial to both mother and fetus. The physician's scale, unfortunately, does not distinguish between the accumulation of edema fluid and the healthy deposition of fetal and maternal tissue.

DIURETICS AND SODIUM RESTRICTION. Natriuretic drugs, such as chlorothiazide and its congeners, have been severely overused. Although diuretics have been alleged to prevent the development of preeclampsia, the results of the studies of Kraus and co-workers (1966), and others, cast doubt on their real value. The women studied by Kraus and associates took either a placebo or 50 mg of hydrochlorothiazide daily during the last 16 weeks or more of gestation. The incidences of preeclampsia were identical (6.67 percent) in 195 primigravidas who took the diuretic and in 210 primigravidas who took the placebo. Similarly, the development of hypertension was unaffected in 565 multiparas. The failure of natriuretic drugs in the prevention of preeclampsia raises serious doubt about the efficacy of dietary restriction of sodium.

Thiazide diuretics and similar compounds are not so used on the Obstetrics Service at Parkland Memorial Hospital. While there is no clear evidence that they are of any value,

there is evidence that these agents can reduce renal perfusion as measured by creatinine clearance and more important, probably reduce uteroplacental perfusion (Gant et al., 1975). The thiazide diuretics can induce serious depletion of both sodium and potassium. Minkowitz and associates (1964) and Menzher and Prystowsky (1967) reported the findings of depletion of electrolytes and hemorrhagic pancreatitis in women who died following treatment of preeclampsia with chlorothiazide. Rodriguez and associates (1964), moreover, found severe thrombocytopenia in some newborns whose mothers had received thiazide diuretics.

Objectives of Treatment. The basic objectives of management of any pregnancy complicated by preeclampsia and eclampsia are (1) termination of the pregnancy with the least possible amount of trauma to the mother and the fetus; (2) birth of an infant who subsequently thrives; (3) complete restoration of the health of the mother.

In certain cases of preeclampsia, especially in women near term, all these objectives may be served equally well by the same treatment, namely careful induction of labor and delivery. It cannot be emphasized too strongly, therefore, that the most important information that the obstetrician can possess for the successful management of most pregnancies, and especially those that become complicated by hypertension, is precise knowledge of the age of the fetus (see Chap. 13, p. 306).

AMBULATORY TREATMENT. Ambulatory treatment has no place in the management of pregnancy-induced or pregnancy-aggravated hypertension. Excluding young nulliparas, some women whose systolic blood pressure does not exceed 135 mm Hg and whose diastolic pressure does not exceed 85 mm Hg, and in whom proteinuria is absent, may be managed tentatively at home pending the aggravation or abatement of signs and symptoms. Bed rest throughout the greater part of the day is essential. Moreover, these women should be examined twice a week rather than once, and be instructed in detail about the reporting of symptoms. With minor elevations of blood pressure, the response to this regimen is often immediate, but the woman must be cooperative and the obstetrician wary.

HOSPITAL MANAGEMENT. The indication for hospitalization of women with preeclampsia is a systolic blood pressure of 140 mm or above or a diastolic pressure of 90 mm or above. For an intelligent continuing appraisal of the severity of the case, upon admittance to the hospital a systematic method of study should be instituted that includes the following:

1. An appropriate history and general physical examination followed by daily search for the development of such signs and symptoms as headache, visual disturbances, epigastric pain, and rapid weight gain.
2. Weight obtained on admittance and every 2 days thereafter.
3. Blood pressure readings with an appropriate size cuff every 4 hours (except between midnight and morning, unless the midnight pressure has risen).
4. Frequent screening of the urine for protein.
5. Frequent measurements of plasma creatinine.
6. Frequent evaluation of fetal size by the same experienced examiner.

Remote from term, sonographic measurements of the biparietal diameter aid appreciably in the confirmation of fetal age and in the identification of fetal growth retardation (see Chap. 37, p. 944).

Bed rest throughout much of the day is essential and ample protein and calories should be included in the diet (Chap. 13, p. 311). Sodium and fluid intakes should be neither limited nor forced.

Phenobarbital has long been used for sedation in divided doses totaling 120 to 240 mg per day. The possibility of adverse effects on the fetus from phenobarbital should be considered, however. The combination of phenobarbital and phenytoin given to the woman with epilepsy has been demonstrated to cause a reduction in vitamin K-dependent coagulation factors in some fetuses. Moreover, phenobarbital has been reported to delay lung maturation, at least in the rabbit fetus (Karotokin et al., 1976).

The further management of a pregnancy complicated by preeclampsia will depend upon (1) its severity as demonstrated by the course in the hospital, (2) the duration of gestation, and (3) the condition of the cervix. Fortunately, many cases prove to be sufficiently mild and near enough to term that they can be managed conservatively until labor commences spontaneously or until the cervix becomes favorable for induction of labor. Complete abatement of all signs and symptoms, however, is uncommon until after delivery. *Almost certainly, the underlying disease never abates until after delivery!*

Occasionally preeclampsia is fulminating, as evidenced by blood pressure recordings in excess of 160/110, edema, and proteinuria. Headache, visual disturbances, or epigastric pain are indicative that convulsions are imminent; oliguria resulting from preeclampsia is another ominous sign. Such severe preeclampsia demands anticonvulsant and usually antihypertensive therapy followed by delivery. The prime objectives are to forestall convulsions, to prevent intracranial hemorrhage or serious damage to other vital organs, and to deliver an infant who survives and subsequently thrives.

In a more severe case of preeclampsia, as well as eclampsia, parenteral magnesium sulfate is a most valuable anticonvulsant agent, as attested by the experience of many clinics over many years. The magnesium sulfate may be given intramuscularly by intermittent injection or intravenously by continuous infusion. At Parkland Memorial Hospital, for preeclampsia, the dosage schedule for intramuscularly administered magnesium sulfate is the same as for eclampsia (p. 688). An initial intravenous loading dose is omitted, however, unless eclampsia is believed to be imminent and then the intravenous dose is also given. Since the period of labor and delivery is a more likely time for convulsions to develop, all women who have hypertension are treated at Parkland Memorial Hospital with intramuscular magnesium sulfate during labor and the early puerperium. Hydralazine (Apresoline), intermittently administered intravenously in appropriate doses, has proven to be an effective and safe antihypertensive agent; its use is discussed in more detail subsequently (p. 690).

TERMINATION OF PREGNANCY. The only specific treatment of preeclampsia is termination of the pregnancy. Because the baby may be premature, however, the tendency is widespread to temporize in many of these cases in the hope that a few more weeks of intrauterine life will give the infant a better chance. Such a policy is justified in milder cases. In severe preeclampsia, however, waiting may prove to be ill-advised, since the sequelae of preeclampsia itself may kill the fetus and, even in the lower weight brackets, the likelihood of fetal survival may be better in a well-operated neonatal intensive care unit than if left in the uterus.

Assessment of fetal and placental function has been attempted when there is hesitation to deliver the fetus because of prematurity. Serial measurements of plasma or urinary estriol, or of placental lactogen, heat-stable alkaline phosphatase, or cystine aminopeptidase in plasma, or the oxytocin challenge test, *may* show abnormal results when the fetoplacental unit is compromised (Chap. 14). So far, these tests have not been clearly demonstrated to provide valuable information otherwise unavailable for intelligent management of the pregnancy complicated by preeclampsia. Failure of the fetus to grow, as estimated clinically and by sonography, is a sign that the fetus is in jeopardy. Measurement of the L/S ratio in amnionic fluid may provide evidence of lung maturity, but it should be kept in mind during management of more severe cases that even when the L/S ratio is less than 2.0, respiratory distress may not develop and, if it does, most often it does not prove fatal (see Chap. 14, p. 335; Chap. 38, p. 957).

For a woman near term, with a soft, partially effaced cervix, even more mild degrees of preeclampsia probably carry more risk to the mother and her infant than does induction of labor by carefully monitored oxytocin stimulation. This is not the case, however, if the preeclampsia is mild but the cervix is firm and closed, indicating that abdominal delivery might be necessary if pregnancy is to be terminated. The hazard of cesarean section may be greater than that of allowing the pregnancy to continue under close observation in the hospital until the cervix is more suitable for induction.

With severe preeclampsia that does not improve after a few days of hospitalization as outlined above, termination of pregnancy is usually advisable for the welfare of both the mother and the fetus. Labor may be induced by administration of oxytocin. In severe cases, this procedure is often successful even when the cervix appears unfavorable. Whenever it appears that induction of labor almost certainly will not succeed, or attempts at induction of labor are not successful, cesarean section for the more severe cases is the procedure of choice. If cesarean section is to be performed, anesthesia with thiopental, nitrous oxide, and a muscle relaxant has many advantages (see Chap. 18, p. 440). With local infiltration for cesarean section, there is likely to be undue discomfort as well as danger of a convulsion. With subarachnoid or epidural block, hypotension detrimental to the fetus, as well as the mother, may occur (see Chap. 18, p. 452).

HIGH-RISK PREGNANCY UNIT. A high-risk pregnancy unit has been established at Parkland Memorial Hospital to provide care as just described. The results achieved have been remarkable as reported by Gilstrap, Cunningham, and Whalley (1978). Of 576 nulliparous women, usually teen-age and often black, admitted to the unit because of hypertension remote from term, 545 remained for care until the pregnancy was terminated; the perinatal mortality rate for this group was 0.9 percent. For the 31 who left the unit, although advised not to, the perinatal mortality was 13 percent! The mean birth weight of the infants whose mothers remained on the unit was 2974 g with 83 percent weighing 2500 g or more. As of 1980 more than 1500 women with mild to moderate preeclampsia have been so managed under the direction of Dr. Peggy Whalley and Dr. Kenneth Leveno with equally good results! The cost of providing the relatively simple physical facility, modest nursing care, no drugs other than an iron supplement, and the very few laboratory tests that are essential is slight compared to the cost of neonatal intensive care. Moreover, the quality of the infant is very likely better.

POSTPARTUM. After delivery there is usually rapid improvement, although, at times, the disease may transiently worsen. Eclampsia may develop any time during the first 24 hours after delivery but rarely thereafter. Therefore, all women with preeclampsia should be observed closely for at least the first 24 hours after delivery. At Parkland Memorial Hospital, except for the mild cases, magnesium sulfate therapy is continued for 24 hours postpartum with parenterally-administered hydralazine given intermittently as needed to lower a diastolic blood pressure of 110 mm Hg or higher.

The woman may be discharged even though still hypertensive if there is evidence that the hypertension is abating and she is otherwise well. Antihypertensive agents are not prescribed; instead she is reevaluated in 2 weeks. Most often, but not always, the hypertension of preeclampsia-eclampsia will have dissipated during this period. If so, the episode of pregnancy-induced hypertension does not mitigate against the use of oral contraceptives (see Chap. 40, p. 1018).

CLINICAL ASPECTS OF ECLAMPSIA

Eclampsia is an acute disorder characterized by clonic and tonic convulsions that are caused in some way by hypertension induced or aggravated by pregnancy. It is better to limit the diagnosis of eclampsia to convulsive cases, regarding fatal nonconvulsive cases of pregnancy-induced or aggravated hypertension as exceedingly severe preeclampsia.

CLINICAL COURSE. Depending on whether the convulsion first appears before labor, during labor, or in the puerperium, eclampsia is designated as antepartum, intrapartum, or postpartum. Eclampsia occurs most often in the last third of pregnancy and becomes increasingly frequent as term approaches. Nearly all cases of postpartum eclampsia appear within 24 hours after delivery. In rare instances, eclampsia is said to have begun as late as one week after delivery, but cases in which the first convulsion is observed more than 48 hours postpartum should be regarded with skepticism.

Almost without exception, preeclampsia precedes the onset of convulsions. Isolated cases are occasionally cited in which an eclamptic convulsion is said to have occurred without warning in women who were apparently in good health. Usually such a woman had not been examined by her physician for some days or weeks previously, and she had neglected to report symptoms of preeclampsia. Headache, visual disturbance, and epigastric or right upper quadrant pain are symptoms that should incite grave concern. Apprehension, excitability, and hyperreflexia often precede the convulsion, although a convulsion may occur in their absence. An aura usually does not precede the convulsion.

The convulsive movements usually begin about the mouth in the form of facial twitchings. After a few seconds the entire body becomes rigid in a generalized muscular contraction. The face is distorted, the eyes protrude, the arms are flexed, the hands are clenched, and the legs are inverted. All the muscles of the body are now in a state of tonic contraction. This phase may persist for 15 to 20 seconds. Suddenly the jaws begin to open and close violently, and forthwith the eyelids also. The other facial muscles and then all the muscles of the body alternately contract and relax in rapid succession. So forceful are the muscular movements that the woman may throw herself out of bed, and

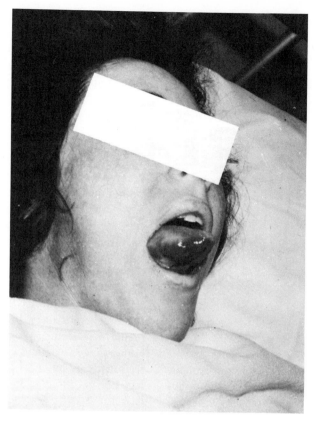

FIG. 27-6. Hematoma of tongue from laceration during eclamptic convulsion. Thrombocytopenia may have contributed to the bleeding.

almost invariably, unless protected, the tongue is bitten by the violent action of the jaws (Fig. 27-6). Foam, often blood-tinged, exudes from the mouth. The face is congested and the eyes are bloodshot. Few clinical pictures are so terrifying. This phase, in which the muscles alternately contract and relax, may last about a minute. Gradually, the muscular movements become smaller and less frequent, and finally the woman lies motionless. Throughout the seizure the diaphragm has been fixed, with respiration halted. For a few seconds the woman appears to be dying from respiratory arrest, but just when a fatal outcome seems almost inevitable, she takes a long, deep, stertorous inhalation, and breathing is resumed. Coma ensues. She will remember nothing of the convulsion or, in all probability, of events immediately before and afterward.

Most often the first convulsion is the fore-runner of other convulsions, which may vary in number from one or two in mild cases to ten to 20, or even 100 or more, in untreated severe cases. In rare instances, they follow one another so rapidly that the woman appears to be in a prolonged, almost continuous convulsion.

The duration of coma after a convulsion is variable. When the convulsions are infrequent, the woman usually recovers some degree of consciousness after each attack. As the woman arouses, a semiconscious combative state may ensue. In severe cases, the coma persists from one convulsion to another, and death may result before the mother awakens. In rare instances, a single convulsion may be followed by profound coma from which she never emerges, although, as a rule, death does not occur until after a frequent repetition of the convulsive attacks.

Respiration in eclampsia after a convulsion is usually increased in rate and may be stertorous. The rate may reach 50 or more per minute in response presumably to hypercarbia from lactic acidemia, as well as varying intensities of hypoxia. Cyanosis may be observed in severe cases. Temperatures of 39.5 C or more are of very grave prognostic import. The cause of the fever is probably central.

Proteinuria is almost always present and frequently is pronounced. The output of urine is likely to be diminished and occasionally is entirely suppressed. On microscopic examination, various types of casts are found in abundance. Hemoglobinuria and hemoglobinemia may rarely be observed.

Some degree of edema is probably present in all women with eclampsia. Often, the edema is pronounced and, at times, massive, but it may be occult.

After delivery, an increase in urinary output is usually an early sign of improvement. The proteinuria and edema ordinarily disappear within a week. In most cases, but certainly not all, the blood pressure returns to normal within 2 weeks after delivery. The longer the hypertension persists after delivery, the more likely the hypertension is chronic.

In antepartum eclampsia, labor may begin shortly thereafter and progress rapidly to completion, sometimes before the attendants are aware that the woman is having effective uterine contractions. If the attack occurs during labor, the contractions may increase in frequency and intensity and the duration of labor be shortened.

Occasionally, labor does not commence, convulsions cease, the coma disappears, and the woman becomes completely oriented. This improved state may continue for several days or longer, a condition known as *intercurrent eclampsia*. It has been claimed that such pregnancies may often return entirely to normal with complete subsidence of the hypertension and proteinuria, but such an event appears to have been rare. Although convulsions and coma may subside entirely and the

blood pressure and proteinuria may decrease somewhat, such women usually continue to show substantial evidence of disease. It is likely that they have merely returned to the preeclamptic state and after a few days of apparent improvement, are likely to convulse again. This second attack may be much more severe.

In fatal cases, pulmonary edema is common, especially during the terminal hours. Pulmonary edema also may be present in women who survive, but it is always a grave prognostic sign. Other signs of cardiac failure appear in the terminal stage of fatal eclampsia, especially cyanosis, a rising pulse rate, and a falling blood pressure.

In some women with eclampsia, death occurs suddenly, synchronously with or shortly after a convulsion, as the result of massive cerebral hemorrhage. In rare instances, hemiplegia may result from a sublethal cerebral hemorrhage. Eclampsia is followed very infrequently by psychosis in which the mother may become violent. The psychosis ordinarily lasts for 1 or 2 weeks. Chlorpromazine in carefully titrated doses has proved effective in the few cases of posteclampsia psychosis seen at Parkland Memorial Hospital. The prognosis in general is good, but occasionally there is preexisting mental illness.

Very infrequently, the woman finds herself blind as she begins to arouse from her coma. The disturbed vision, sometimes preceding the attack, is caused mainly by retinal edema, which usually disappears spontaneously. The blindness is sometimes central in origin, caused by a disturbance in the optic nerve or in the visual centers in the occipital lobe; the most logical explanation is edema of these structures. Rarely, detachment of the retina is observed. The blindness may persist for a few hours or for several weeks. Usually, however, the vision returns to normal within a week and the prognosis for sight is good.

Differential Diagnosis. Generally, one is much more likely to make a diagnosis of eclampsia too frequently than to overlook the disease, because epilepsy, encephalitis, men-

ingitis, cerebral tumor, acute porphyria, ruptured cerebral aneurysm, and even hysteria
may simulate it. Consequently, such conditions should be borne in mind whenever convulsions or coma occur during pregnancy,
labor, or the puerperium; and such conditions
must be excluded before a positive diagnosis
of eclampsia is made. Until eclampsia can be
excluded, however, all pregnant women with
convulsions must be suspect and kept under
close observation on the obstetric service of
the hospital.

TREATMENT OF ECLAMPSIA

The basic treatment of eclampsia consists of
control of convulsions and steps to effect delivery once the mother is free of convulsions
and hopefully conscious. It is emphasized that
once delivery is accomplished the pathologic
changes of eclampsia per se ameliorate re-

markably soon and subsequently are completely eradicated. This generalization holds
true for the dysfunction of the central nervous system, for the liver, for the kidneys,
and for any hematologic abnormalities, including thrombocytopenia and intense hemolysis!

Prognosis. The prognosis is always serious, for eclampsia is one of the most dangerous conditions with which the obstetrician
must deal, although the maternal mortality
rate in eclampsia has fallen notably in the
past three decades. The maternal mortality
rate reported since World War II for various
methods of treatment applied in several
countries is summarized in Table 27-2. In
these reports, the maternal mortality has
ranged from zero to as much as 10.3 percent.
At the same time the perinatal mortality rate
has ranged from 13 to 30 percent or more.
Precise comparisons of perinatal mortality

TABLE 27-2.
THE RESULTS IN SOME PUBLISHED REPORTS OF MATERNAL MORTALITY
FROM ECLAMPSIA

AUTHORS	TREATMENT	CASES (NO.)	MATERNAL DEATHS (PERCENT)
Dewar & Morris (1947)	Tribromethanol	44	4.5
Browne (1950)	Thiopental	26	7.6
Sheares (1957)	Lytic cocktail	124	8.8
Menon (1961)	Lytic cocktail*	402	2.2
Llewellyn-Jones (1961)	Lytic cocktail	150	6.6
Bryant and Fleming (1962)	Magnesium sulfate and veratrum alkaloids	253	1.6
Zuspan and Ward (1965)	Magnesium sulfate	59	3.4
Lopez-Llera (1967)	Lytic cocktail	107	10.3
Lean et al (1968)	Chlordiazepoxide or diazepam	90†	3.3
		60‡	5.0
Kawathekar et al. (1973)	Diazepam	16	6.3
Mojadidi and Thompson (1973)	Morphine and magnesium sulfate	30	6.7
Pritchard (1975)	Magnesium sulfate and standardized treatment regimen	154	0

* Chlorpromazine, Diethazine, and Meperidine.
† Includes postpartum eclampsia (up to 14 days).
‡ Excludes eclampsia that developed postpartum.

rates are difficult to make because of differences in the definition of stillbirth and neonatal deaths in different countries.

Historical Considerations. The maternal mortality rate of about 30 percent associated with immediate forced vaginal delivery or cesarean section late in the nineteenth century led to more conservative medical therapy. During the first quarter of the twentieth century, obstetricians were divided into "radicals" and "conservatives," with some following a "middle line." In the mid-1920s, reviews of the literature and comparison of the maternal mortality rates associated with radical and conservative managements indicated that the mortality rate was doubled by immediate cesarean section. Plass (1927), for instance, tabulated 4607 cases treated radically, with a maternal mortality rate of 21.7 percent; the mortality rate in 5976 cases managed conservatively was 11.1 percent. Holland (1921), in surveying the cesarean sections performed in Great Britain and Ireland, found that the mortality rate in eclampsia was 32 percent. In the late 1920s, the slogan became "Treat the eclampsia medically and ignore the pregnancy," and an overly conservative attitude prevailed. From this time, most every drug suspected of having a sedative effect, or hypotensive effect, or diuretic effect has been administered to the woman (and her fetus) with eclampsia. Usually several drugs have been employed simultaneously. Often the convulsions were controlled but the woman was rendered comatose by the medications rather than the disease. As the consequence of such empiric therapy, women with eclampsia have been treated in a most variable way, especially in institutions where eclampsia is uncommon.

Eclampsia Treatment at Parkland Memorial Hospital

Since 1955, standardized treatment applied uniformly to all cases of eclampsia at Parkland Memorial Hospital has consisted of (1) magnesium sulfate intravenously and intramuscularly to arrest convulsions and prevent their recurrence; (2) intravenous hydralazine intermittently as necessary to lower diastolic blood pressure of 110 mm Hg or higher; and (3) steps initiated to effect delivery once the woman had regained consciousness

(Pritchard and Pritchard, 1975). The dosage schedules to be described below for magnesium sulfate and hydralazine, while empiric, have been tested extensively for both efficacy and toxicity. Delivery in the majority of cases has been accomplished vaginally; conduction anesthesia has been avoided. Neither diuretics nor osmotic agents in the form of hypertonic glucose, mannitol, or albumin have been used to treat eclampsia. Heparin has never been used! Through December 1975, 162 consecutive cases of eclampsia were so treated with no maternal mortality. Moreover, all fetuses alive when treatment was initiated and who weighed 1800 g (4 lb) or more, survived.

The plan of management is presented in some detail:

CONTROL OF CONVULSIONS WITH MAGNESIUM SULFATE. As soon as eclampsia has been established as the probable diagnosis, magnesium sulfate ($MgSO_4 \cdot 7H_2O$ USP) is administered as follows:

1. 20 ml of 20 percent magnesium sulfate solution* (4 g) is injected intravenously in not less than 3 minutes, immediately followed by:
2. 20 ml of 50 percent magnesium sulfate solution, one-half (5 g) injected deeply in the upper outer quadrant of both buttocks through a 3-inch long, 20-gauge needle, in turn followed by:
3. *Every 4 hours* 10 ml of 50 percent magnesium sulfate solution (5 g) injected deeply in the upper outer quadrant in alternate buttocks but only after ascertaining that:
   (a) A knee jerk (patellar reflex) can be elicited
   (b) Urine flow has been 100 ml or more in the previous 4 hours
   (c) Respirations are not depressed

Magnesium sulfate so administered almost always promptly arrests the convulsions, but,

---

* 20 ml of 20 percent solution of magnesium sulfate can be made by mixing in a syringe 8 ml of 50 percent magnesium sulfate solution and 12 ml of sterile distilled water.

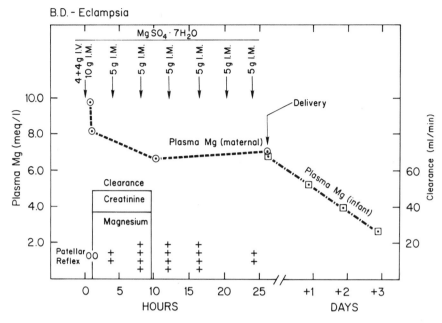

FIG. 27-7. Antepartum eclampsia in a 15-year-old primigravida treated with magnesium sulfate. She was atypical in that she convulsed again shortly after having received the intravenous loading dose of 4 g and intramuscular dose of 10 g of magnesium sulfate. Over 5 minutes, she received 4 g more of magnesium sulfate in a 20 percent solution intravenously and suffered no more convulsions. She then awoke, and her sensorium soon cleared. The patellar reflex was absent when the plasma level was 9.9 mEq per liter very soon after the initial injections but returned to levels of "2 plus" to "4 plus" with plasma levels of 6.5 mEq per liter. The clearance of magnesium by the kidney approached that of the creatinine clearance which was reduced until after delivery. The magnesium levels in maternal and cord plasma were the same; typically, the plasma level in the infant dropped slowly. (From Pritchard. *Semin Perinatol* 2:83, 1978)

very infrequently, another convulsion may soon appear. Experience has been that if the magnesium sulfate intravenous and intramuscular injections were completed within the 20 minutes before, the subsequent convulsion usually is brief and does not recur. If the interval is much longer than 20 minutes, or if the convulsion recurs, 10 ml more of 20 percent magnesium sulfate solution (2 g) if the woman was unusually small, otherwise 20 ml of 20 percent magnesium sulfate (4 g), are injected intravenously over no less than 3 minutes as illustrated in Figure 27-7. In the rare circumstance in which convulsions persist, sodium amobarbital (Sodium Amytal), up to 0.25 g, is slowly injected in-

travenously over a period of not less than 3 minutes.

Subsequent intramuscular injections of 10 ml of 50 percent solution of magnesium sulfate at 4-hour intervals depend upon the patellar reflex being elicited just before each injection. If absent, which is very unlikely, the reflex is rechecked at ½-hour intervals and the intramuscular dose of magnesium sulfate injected once the reflex is demonstrated. An active reflex ("hyperreflexia") is not an indication in our experience for increasing either the amount of magnesium sulfate injected or the frequency of the injection. The intramuscular injections are continued for 24 hours after delivery. In the conscious patient, to minimize local discomfort, 1 ml of 2 percent lidocaine is added to the magnesium sulfate solution before injecting intramuscularly.

During the first hour or so of the postictal period, the eclamptic woman before fully regaining consciousness may occasionally demonstrate physical agitation that can not be controlled by simple restraint. If this develops, to protect the mother from harming herself and her fetus, sodium amobarbital for sedation is injected intravenously in increments up to 0.25 g over not less than 3 minutes. Most often, however, the woman's confusion and agitation, as she regains consciousness, can be minimized by having an immediate member of the family at the bedside and by avoiding bright lights, loud noises, and numerous people in the room.

If respiratory depression were to develop, 10 ml of a 10 percent solution of calcium gluconate is given intravenously over 3 minutes. This proved effective in two cases of eclampsia in which it was used at Parkland Memorial Hospital. The pharmacology and toxicology of magnesium sulfate are considered in more detail below.

ANTIHYPERTENSIVE THERAPY. The intravenous injection of 4 g of magnesium sulfate produces a moderate lowering of blood pressure which most often is transient. Therefore, hydralazine is used to treat severe hypertension. Whenever the diastolic blood pressure reaches 110 mm Hg, hydralazine is administered as follows: A test dose of 5 mg is injected as a bolus intravenously and the blood pressure monitored every 5 minutes. If the diastolic pressure is not lowered to 90 to 100 mm Hg in 20 minutes, a 10-mg dose is similarly administered, and its effects monitored as described. This dose of hydralazine is repeated until the diastolic blood pressure is lowered to 90 to 100 mm Hg. The desired effect is most always achieved with from 5 mg to 20 mg of hydralazine. Hydralazine is next given whenever the diastolic blood pressure again reaches 110 mm Hg.

Diazoxide has not been used at Parkland Memorial Hospital, nor is it recommended.

The hypotensive response may be so great as to impair dangerously perfusion of vital organs including the placenta. Unfortunately, if diazoxide is used in close proximity to other antihypertensive agents that act by direct peripheral vasodilatation, profound and even fatal hypotension may ensue.

Metabolic derangements are commonly induced in the mother and the fetus, including edema from sodium and water retention, hyperglycemia, and hyperuricemia. Moreover, labor may be impaired by diazoxide, if not arrested (Physician's Desk Reference, 1979).

DIURETICS, HYPEROSMOTIC AGENTS, AND FLUID THERAPY. Urinary output is monitored hourly. Mannitol, hypertonic dextrose, and albumin are not used at Parkland Memorial Hospital to try to mobilize edema fluid, to try to increase urinary output or to expand the blood volume. Unless there is pulmonary congestion, diuretics are avoided, since oliguria reflects the intensity of the vasospastic disease, an intensification of the hypovolemia by blood loss at delivery, or both. However, if pulmonary edema were to develop, furosemide may be lifesaving.

In the absence of hemorrhage or hyponatremia, 5 percent glucose in lactated Ringer's solution is administered intravenously at a rate of 60 to 120 ml per hour.

LABORATORY STUDIES. Laboratory studies need not be extensive. Measurements of hemoglobin or hematocrit, leukocyte count, and platelet count, examination of a blood smear stained with Wright's stain, and careful visual inspection of plasma for abnormal amounts of bilirubin, hemoglobin, or other heme pigments are performed. Plasma electrolytes are measured, although they are unlikely to be abnormal unless the woman has previously been treated vigorously with diuretics or she has received oxytocin and appreciable volumes of aqueous glucose solution simultaneously. Hypocalcemia or hypercalcemia is rarely found. After a convulsion, the plasma bicarbonate concentration is variably reduced as the consequence of lactic acidemia and hyperventilation. The plasma creatinine concentration should be measured but is not likely to be elevated markedly unless vigorous diuretic therapy has been administered elsewhere, or the disease has been unusually severe, or there is underlying renal disease.

DELIVERY. Steps are taken to initiate labor and effect delivery once the woman regains consciousness to the extent that she can be oriented as to time and place. Immediately after a convulsion fetal bradycardia is common, most likely as the consequence of acidosis and hypoxia induced by the intense muscular activity. The generally favorable fetal outcomes at Parkland Memorial Hospital justify the policy of controlling the convulsions and providing oxygen, thereby allowing the mother and, in turn, the fetus to repair the metabolic derangement, rather than quickly performing a cesarean section. Once convulsions have been controlled and no other obstetric complications coexist or develop, there is no urgency for immediately effecting delivery, but neither is there reason for undue procrastination. Without obstetric contraindication to vaginal delivery, labor is induced with carefully administered intravenous oxytocin. Even when remote from term, the uterus often is responsive to oxytocin. Although very high plasma magnesium levels may impair myometrial contractility, the levels achieved with the dosage schedule described above do not. Labor has been induced successfully with oxytocin in 59 of 71 (83 percent) cases in which it was attempted at Parkland Memorial Hospital, including 7 of 10 cases in which fetal weight was less than 1000 g and all 20 in which the fetus weighed between 1000 and 2500 g (Pritchard, 1975). The frequency, duration, and apparent intensity of uterine contractions and the fetal heart rate are monitored closely. Hyperstimulation must be avoided.

Analgesia during labor is limited to 50 to 75 mg of meperidine and 25 mg of promethazine (Phenergan) given intravenously or intramuscularly, with the meperidene repeated at intervals of 2 hours or longer, and withholding administration during the 2 hours before delivery. If the fetus is premature, meperidine and similar agents are to be avoided.

If oxytocin induction fails, or if there are obstetric contraindications to the use of oxytocin, cesarean section is performed.

Blood loss at and after delivery is less well tolerated by women with eclampsia. The maternal blood volume typically is appreciably less than with normal pregnancy, thereby increasing the dangers from blood loss. *An abrupt fall in blood pressure at the completion of delivery or soon after most often indicates serious hypovolemia rather than immediate relief of the vasospastic disease!* The oliguria from severe hypovolemia following hemorrhage is treated with blood and lactated Ringer's solution and not with diuretics or hyperosmotic agents.

ANESTHESIA. Spinal, caudal, or lumbar epidural anesthesia is not used at Parkland Memorial Hospital for labor or delivery of the woman with eclampsia or preeclampsia because of the likelihood of hypotension from both regional sympathetic blockade and significant blood loss in the presence of an already shrunken blood volume (see Chap. 18, p. 452). For most forceps deliveries, and for cesarean sections, anesthesia consists of the administration of a small dose of sodium thiopental, followed by nitrous oxide plus oxygen, and succinylcholine. Anesthesia is begun only after the woman has received 30 ml of milk of magnesia orally and the obstetric team is fully prepared to deliver the fetus vaginally or to incise the abdominal wall. While the amount of succinylcholine necessary for appropriate muscle relaxation usually is less for the woman who has received magnesium sulfate, this does not contraindicate the simultaneous use of these two agents. Pudendal block or local perineal and vaginal infiltration, supplemented with nitrous oxide, often provides satisfactory pain relief for episiotomy and spontaneous vaginal delivery.

PERINATAL MORTALITY. With this treatment regime, the absolute perinatal mor-

TABLE 27-3.
ECLAMPSIA: FATE OF FETUSES
WEIGHING 1000 G OR MORE
(PARKLAND MEMORIAL HOSPITAL
1955–1975)

Total fetuses	122
Dead when eclampsia diagnosed	7
Alive when eclampsia diagnosed	115
Intrapartum death	1*
Born alive	114
Neonatal deaths	4†
Survived	110

* 1200 g.

† All less than 1800 g; the 100 fetuses weighing 1800 g (4 pounds) or more and alive when eclampsia was diagnosed all survived.

tality rate for 132 fetuses and newborns, including four sets of twins, of the 128 mothers with eclampsia before delivery was 15.9 percent, irrespective of fetal weight or duration of gestation, and including fetuses that were dead when the mother was brought to Parkland Memorial Hospital. Ten of the fetuses weighed less than 1000 g and two weighed less than 500 g. The outcomes for fetuses that weighed 1000 g or more at birth is considered in Table 27-3. Every one of the fetuses survived of the 100 who were alive when the diagnosis of eclampsia was made and who weighed 1800 g (4 pounds) or more at birth.

PHARMACOLOGY AND TOXICOLOGY OF MAGNESIUM SULFATE. Magnesium sulfate USP is $MgSO_4 \cdot 7H_2O$ and not $MgSO_4$. Magnesium sulfate administered as described will practically always arrest eclamptic convulsions and prevent their recurrence. The initial intravenous injection of 4 g is used to establish promptly a therapeutic level which is then maintained by the nearly simultaneous intramuscular administration of 10 g of the compound, followed by 5 g intramuscularly every 4 hours, as long as there is no evidence of potentially dangerous hypermagnesemia. With this dosage schedule, the plasma levels for magnesium that are achieved are therapeutically effective and range from 4 to 6 mEq per liter, compared to pretreatment plasma levels usually of less

than 2.0 mEq per liter (Chesley and Tepper, 1957; Stone and Pritchard, 1970). Magnesium sulfate injected deeply into the upper outer quadrant of the buttocks, as described above, has not resulted in erratic absorption and, in turn, erratic plasma levels; indeed, the reverse has been true.

The patellar reflex disappears by the time the plasma magnesium level reaches 10 mEq per liter, presumably as the consequence of a curariform action. This sign serves to warn of impending magnesium toxicity, since a further increase will lead to respiratory depression.

Parenterally injected magnesium is excreted rapidly through the maternal kidney; as the magnesium concentration in plasma increases, so does renal clearance. A fraction of the injected magnesium is deposited in bone.

In monkeys with angiotensin-induced hypertension late in pregnancy, Harbert and co-workers (1969) demonstrated slightly increased uterine blood flow in response to the infusion of magnesium sulfate. At the same time, arterial blood pressure decreased minimally.

Somjen and co-workers (1966) induced in themselves, by intravenous infusion, marked hypermagnesemia, achieving plasma levels to 15 mEq per liter. *Predictably, at such high plasma levels, respiratory depression developed that necessitated mechanical ventilation, yet there was little in the way of depression of the sensorium as long as hypoxia was prevented.*

The studies of Borges and Gücer (1978) provided convincing evidence that the magnesium ion has an effect on the central nervous system much more specific than generalized depression. They measured the effects of parenterally administered magnesium sulfate on epileptic neural activity induced in awake, undrugged subhuman primates. The infused magnesium sulfate suppressed neuronal burst firing and interictal electroencephalographic spike generation in neuronal populations rendered epileptic by topically applied penicillin G. The degree of cortical suppression increased as the plasma magnesium concentration increased and decreased as the magnesium level fell. Therefore, even though elevated concentrations of magnesium in plasma decrease acetylcholine release in response to motor nerve impulses, reduce motor end-plate sensitivity to acetylcholine, and decrease the motor end-plate potential, these actions do not account for, nor should they be implicated in, an explanation of the beneficial effects of magnesium sulfate in controlling the convulsions of eclampsia. Interestingly—indeed, amazingly—Donaldson (1978), and some other neurologists, for reasons that are hard to discern, have erroneously emphasized that magnesium sulfate is a "peripherally" acting anticonvulsant and therefore "bad medicine." They imply that the drug works only at concentrations which cause paralysis and, as the consequence, the woman with eclampsia so treated is "quiet on the outside but still convulsing on the inside." This conclusion could not have been based on direct experience with eclampsia and its control with parenterally administered magnesium! At the same time, Donaldson urges other forms of therapy but cites no data whatsoever to support his recommendations. Most other drugs that effectively arrest and prevent eclamptic convulsions do cause appreciable general depression of the central nervous system in both the mother and the newborn infant.

Magnesium ions in relatively high concentration will depress myometrial contractility both in vivo and in vitro. With the regime described above and the plasma levels that have resulted, no evidence of depression of myometrial function has been observed beyond a transient decrease in activity during and immediately after the initial intravenous loading dose. Typically, as the cutaneous flushing from the intravenous dose disappeared, uterine activity returned to preinjection intensity. Magnesium ions administered parenterally to the mother cross the placenta promptly to achieve equilibrium between mother and fetus. Magnesium sulfate, given as a single large dose intravenously, but not with smaller doses, may transiently cause a loss of beat-to-beat variability in the fetal heart rate (Pritchard, 1979).

The newborn infant may be depressed if severe hypermagnesemia exists at delivery. The kind of compromises that have been described by Lipsitz and English (1967) to develop at times in the newborn after maternal continuous intravenous therapy with magnesium sulfate have not been observed by us (Stone and Pritchard, 1970). The dosage schedule and route of administration described above, coupled with the safeguards observed before each injection, have effectively prevented worrisome adverse effects from hypermagnesemia in newborns at Parkland Memorial Hospital.

Indeed, Lipsitz (1971) agreed with our observations after further study in which he found that infants were unlikely to be compromised when the mother had received magnesium sulfate according to the protocol for the treatment of eclampsia described above. The use of magnesium sulfate in preeclampsia-eclampsia, its mechanisms of action, and its possible toxicity in mother and fetus-infant have been described in more detail elsewhere (Pritchard, 1979).

Other Treatment Agents. Some of the great variety of drugs that have been used in the treatment of eclampsia and severe preeclampsia are presented in Table 27-2. We have had little personal experience with most of them; for further information, the interested reader is referred to the various reports that are listed.

It should be pointed out that a tendency persists among some medical experts to group together for the purpose of treatment a variety of disease states that appear to have a common functional disturbance. So-called hypertensive encephalopathy is one that from time to time attracts interest and, in turn, incites recommendations for treatment broad in scope, without full appreciation of all of the problems created by the disease or evoked by the proposed treatment. Too often, when eclampsia is included under the category of hypertensive encephalopathy, lack of concern for the impact of the recommended therapy on the fetus is apparent. Moreover, it is not unusual for the recommendations to have been based on little or no data (Anonymous, 1979).

The recurrent recognition of thrombocytopenia occasionally and, less often, of other changes in the coagulation mechanism, with or without evidence of abnormal erythrocyte destruction (microangiopathic hemolysis) has led to the recommendation of treatment with heparin, fresh whole blood, fresh frozen plasma, platelets, fibrinogen, and other specific clotting factors as necessary (Beecham et al., 1974). To date, insufficient numbers of cases have been reported to evaluate the merits, if any, of such therapy. In two reports, it was concluded that heparin did not prove effective in ameliorating the clinical course of established preeclampsia (Bonnar et al., 1976; Howie et al., 1975). These experiences with heparin treatment appear similar to those reported by Butler and associates in 1950.

We continue to look for such hematologic changes in the relatively large numbers of women with eclampsia and preeclampsia cared for at Parkland Memorial Hospital but do not attempt treatment with heparin or with clotting factors other than those in blood bank blood used at times to treat blood loss from hemorrhage at delivery. We have never used heparin in these circumstances because of fear of enhancing intracranial hemorrhage on the one hand and an appreciation that correction of the defects occurs promptly after delivery on the other. The outcomes have been satisfactory, as already described. The safety of deliberate anticoagulation with heparin in the presence of severe hypertension is questionable and certainly cannot be recommended until much greater experience attesting to any benefits has been recorded.

SUBSEQUENT REPRODUCTIVE OUTCOMES. Because of the catastrophic implications of eclampsia, women so affected and their families often are quite concerned over the prognosis for future pregnancies. Moreover, gloomy accounts have repeatedly appeared in the obstetric literature; hypertension, for example, has been reported to occur in as high as 78 percent of women who previously had eclampsia.

Chesley and co-workers (1962), through meticulous, long-term follow-up studies of women with eclampsia at Margaret Hague Maternity Hospital between the years 1931 and 1952 have provided us with most useful information. For example, of 466 subsequent pregnancies in 189 of the eclamptic women, the fetal salvage was 76 percent but much of the loss was early abortion. Of the pregnancies that continued to 28 weeks or more, 93 percent resulted in infants that survived.

More recently, at Parkland Memorial Hospital the subsequent reproductive performance of black women with eclampsia during their first pregnancy has been ascertained. Of 101 pregnancies, 11 aborted and 91 infants weighing 500 g or more were delivered. Four of the 91 succumbed, 3 of whom weighed less than 1000 g.

Of the subsequent pregnancies, 25 percent were complicated by hypertension in the 189 previously eclamptic women observed by Chesley (1964). The hypertension, however, was severe in only 5 percent, while 2 percent were again eclamptic. Our experiences with previously eclamptic women are very similar.

Chesley emphasized that many of the recurrences of elevated blood pressure represent nothing more than chronic hypertension. Some women do have normal blood pressures between pregnancies and at follow-up; but in general, pregnancies following eclampsia are an excellent screening test for latent hypertensive disease. Nearly all women who develop recurrences of hypertension during subsequent pregnancies ultimately become hypertensive, whereas the prevalence of ultimate hypertension is extremely low in those who are normotensive in later pregnancies.

Chesley, Annitto, and Cosgrove (1976) traced to 1974 all but three of the 270 women surviving eclampsia at the Margaret Hague Maternity Hospital in the period 1931 through 1951. Women who had eclampsia in their first pregnancy carried to 28 weeks or more have shown no increase over the expected number of remote deaths.

by maternal treatment with phenobarbital. Am J Obstet Gynecol 124:529, 1976

Kitzmiller JL, Benirschke K: Immunofluorescent study of placental bed vessels in pre-eclampsia. Am J Obstet Gynecol 115:248, 1973

Kitzmiller JL, Lang JE, Yelonosky PF, Lucas WE: Hematologic assays in pre-eclampsia. Am J Obstet Gynecol 118:362, 1974

Kraus GW, Marchese JR, Yen SSC: Prophylactic use of hydrochlorothiazide in pregnancy. JAMA 198:1150, 1966

Landesman R, Douglas RG, Holze E: The bulbar conjunctival vascular bed in the toxemias of pregnancy. Am J Obstet Gynecol 68:170, 1954

Lichtig C, Luger AM, Spargo BH, Lindheimer MD: Renal immunofluorescence and ultrastructural findings in preeclampsia. Clin Res 23:368A, 1975

Lindheimer MD, Spargo BH, Katz AI: Eclampsia during the sixteenth week of gestation. JAMA 230:1006, 1974

Lipsitz PJ: The clinical and biochemical effects of excess magnesium in the newborn. Pediatrics 47:501, 1971

Lipsitz PJ, English IC: Hypermagnesemia in the newborn infant. Pediatrics 40:856, 1967

Llewellyn-Jones D: The treatment of eclampsia. Br J Obstet Gynaecol 68:33, 1961

Mautner W, Churg J, Grishman E, Dachs S: Pre-eclamptic nephropathy; an electron microscopic study. Lab Invest 11:518, 1962

McCall ML: Continuing vasodilator infusion therapy: utilization of a blend of 1-hydrazinophthalazine (Apresoline) and cryptenamine (Unitensin) in toxemia of pregnancy. Obstet Gynecol 4:403, 1954

McCartney CP: Pathological anatomy of acute hypertension of pregnancy. Circulation 30 (Suppl 2):37, 1964

McKay DG: Disseminated Intravascular Coagulation. New York, Harper & Row, 1965

Menzher D, Prystowsky H: Acute hemorrhagic pancreatitis during pregnancy and the puerperium associated with thiazide therapy. J Florida Med Assoc 54:564, 1967

Minkowitz S, Soloway HB, Hall JE, Yermakov V: Fatal hemorrhagic pancreatitis following chlorothiazide administration in pregnancy. Obstet Gynecol 24:337, 1964

Page EW: On the pathogenesis of pre-eclampsia and eclampsia. J Obstet Gynaecol Br Commonw 79:883, 1972

Parker CR, Everett RB, Quirk JG, Whalley PJ, Gant NF, MacDonald PC: Plasma concentrations of desoxycorticosterone (DOC) throughout pregnancy in normal women and in women who developed pregnancy-induced hypertension (PIH). Am J Obstet Gynecol, in press, 1980

Petrucco OM, Thomson NM, Lawrence JR, Weldon MW: Immunofluorescent studies in renal biopsies in pre-eclampsia. Br Med J 1:473, 1974

Plass ED: The conservative treatment of eclampsia. Med Herald Physiotherapist 46:153, 1927

Pollak VE, Nettles JB: The kidney in toxemia of pregnancy: a clinical and pathologic study based on renal biopsies. Medicine 39:469, 1960

Pritchard JA: The use of magnesium sulfate in preeclampsia-eclampsia. J Reprod Med 23:107, 1979

Pritchard JA, Cunningham FG, Mason RA: Coagulation changes in eclampsia: Their frequency and pathogenesis. Am J Obstet Gynecol 124:855, 1976

Pritchard JA, Pritchard SA: Standardized treatment of 154 cases of eclampsia. Am J Obstet Gynecol 123:543, 1975

Pritchard JA, Ratnoff OD, Weismann R Jr: Hemostatic defects and increased red cell destruction in preeclampsia and eclampsia. Obstet Gynecol 4:159, 1954

Pritchard JA, Weisman R Jr, Ratnoff OD, Vosburgh G: Intravascular hemolysis, thrombocytopenia and other hematologic abnormalities associated with severe toxemia of pregnancy. N Engl J Med 250:87, 1954

Rodriguez SU, Leikin SL, Hiller MC: Neonatal thrombocytopenia associated with antepartum administration of thiazide drugs. N Engl J Med 270:881, 1964

Rosenbaum M, Maltby G: Cerebral dysrhythmia in relation to eclampsia. Arch Neurol Psychiatr 49:204, 1943

Sheehan HL: Pathological lesions in the hypertensive toxaemias of pregnancy. In Hammond J, Browne FJ, Wolstenholme GEW (eds): Toxaemias of Pregnancy, Human and Veterinary. Philadelphia, Blakiston, 1950

Sims EAH: Pre-eclampsia and related complications of pregnancy. Am J Obstet Gynecol, 107:154, 1970

Somjen G, Hilmy M, Stephen CR: Failure to anesthetize human subjects by intravenous administration of magnesium sulfate. J Pharmacol Exp Ther 154:652, 1966

Spargo B, McCartney CP, Winemiller R: Glomerular capillary endotheliosis in toxemia of pregnancy. Arch Pathol 68:593, 1959

Stahnke E: Über das Verhalten der Blutplättchen bei Eklampsie. Zentralbl Gynaekol 46:391, 1922

Stone SR, Pritchard JA: Effect of maternally administered magnesium sulfate on the neonate. Obstet Gynecol 35:574, 1970

Talledo OE, Chesley LC, Zuspan FP: Renin-angiotensin system in normal and toxemic pregnancies. III. Differential sensitivity to angiotensin II and norepinephrine in toxemia of pregnancy. Am J Obstet Gynecol 100:218, 1968

Tillman AJB: The effect of normal and toxemic pregnancy on blood pressure. Am J Obstet Gynecol 70:589, 1955

Vassalli P, Morris RH, McCluskey RT: The pathogenic role of fibrin deposition in the glomerular lesions of toxemia of pregnancy. J Exp Med 118:467, 1963

Volhard F: Die Doppelseitigen Haematogenen Nierenerkrankungen. Berlin, Springer, 1918

Weir RJ, Fraser R, Lever AF, Morton JJ, Brown JJ, Kraszewski A, McIlevine GM, Robertson JIS, Tree M: Plasma renin, renin substrate, angiotensin II, and aldosterone in hypertensive disease of pregnancy. Lancet 1:291, 1973

Winkel CA, Milewich L, Parker CR Jr, Gant NF, Simpson ER, MacDonald PC: Conversion of plasma progesterone to deoxycorticosterone in men, nonpregnant and pregnant women, and adrenalectomized subjects: Evidence for steroid 21-hydroxylase activity in non-adrenal tissues. Presented before the 26th Meeting of the Society for Gynecologic Investigation, San Diego, March 21, 1979

Zeek PM, Assali NS: Vascular changes in decidua associated with eclamptogenic toxemia of pregnancy. Am J Clin Pathol 20:1099, 1950

Zuspan FP, Ward MC: Treatment of eclampsia. South Med J 57:954, 1964

28

Medical and Surgical Illnesses During Pregnancy and the Puerperium

Essentially all diseases that affect a woman when nonpregnant may be contracted during pregnancy. Moreover, the presence of the majority of diseases does not prevent conception.

For most systemic illnesses, the physiologic and anatomic changes inherent in normal pregnancy influence the symptoms, signs, and laboratory values to a considerable degree. As a consequence, the physician who is not aware of these changes induced by normal pregnancy may not be able to recognize a disease or may diagnose incorrectly some other disease, to the jeopardy of the mother and her fetus. Throughout this chapter, emphasis has been placed on the effects of interaction between the disease and the pregnancy as well as on the problems in diagnosis and treatment imposed by the gestational state. In practically all instances, the following questions are pertinent:

1. Is pregnancy likely to make the disease more serious, and if so, how?
2. Does the disease jeopardize the pregnancy, and if so, how and to what degree?
3. Should the pregnancy be terminated because of either gross risk to the mother or likelihood of grave damage to the fetus?
4. Should the pregnancy be allowed to continue under a very carefully defined regimen of therapy?
5. If the disease exists before pregnancy, is pregnancy contraindicated, and if so, what steps should be taken to protect the woman from pregnancy?

INFECTIONS OF THE URINARY SYSTEM

Although a urinary infection may involve only the bladder and thus represent true cystitis, infection of the renal calyces and pelvis is invariably accompanied by involvement of the renal parenchyma, a condition better described as pyelonephritis rather than pyelitis.

During pregnancy, active multiplication of bacteria within the bladder are identified most often when there has been recent instrumentation of the urinary tract or there is persistent asymptomatic bacteriuria. Since bacteria are normally found in the outer portion of the urethra, single catheterization or the use of an indwelling catheter is likely to introduce bacteria into the bladder, where the organisms encounter ideal conditions for multiplication, particularly during the puerperium. As was shown by Brumfitt and associates (1961), routine bladder catheterization before delivery initiates infection in approximately 9 percent of puerperal women. It follows that the number of puerperal urinary infections can be reduced appreciably by avoiding routine catheterization of the bladder at the time of delivery. When catheterization is unavoidable, prophylactic administration of antibacterial agents will usually prevent these infections.

Approximately 5 percent of pregnant women already have bacteriuria at the time of the first prenatal visit. As discussed below, however, prevalence varies considerably, being highest among socioeconomically deprived women of high parity, women who have had previous clinically apparent urinary tract infections, and women whose red cells sickle including those with sickle cell trait. Approximately 25 percent of women with *untreated asymptomatic bacteriuria* subsequently develop *symptomatic infection* of the urinary tract—cystitis or pyelonephritis—during the course of pregnancy.

Types of Infection

CYSTITIS.   Cystitis is inflammation of the bladder resulting most often from bacterial infection. Typically, it is characterized by dysuria, particularly at the end of urination, as well as urgency and frequency. There are few associated systemic findings. Usually, there is an abnormal number of leukocytes, as well as bacteria in the urine. Erythrocytes are commonly found in the urinary sediment, and occasionally even gross hematuria is seen. The term *cystitis* implies an infection confined to the bladder without involvement of the upper urinary tract. Although uncomplicated cystitis occurs, the upper urinary tract may soon be involved in an ascending infection.

ACUTE PYELONEPHRITIS.   This disease is the direct result of bacterial infection that may extend upward from the bladder or

through the blood vessels and lymphatics. The weight of clinical evidence indicates that the ascending route of infection is very much more common. Acute pyelonephritis is one of the most common medical complications of pregnancy.

The reported incidence of acute pyelonephritis complicating pregnancy and the puerperium approximates 2 percent and most often appears in the later part of pregnancy or in the early puerperium. The disease when unilateral is more frequently right sided.

The onset of signs and symptoms of the disease is usually rather abrupt. The woman who has previously been well or has complained of slight bladder irritation or hematuria suddenly develops fever, shaking chills, and aching pain in one or both lumbar regions. There may be anorexia, nausea, and vomiting. The body temperature most often is elevated but during the course of the disease may vary remarkably with hyperthermia to as high as 40C or more and hypothermia to as low as 34C. Tenderness can usually be elicited by firm palpation in one or both costovertebral angles. The urinary sediment contains many leukocytes, frequently in clumps, and the stained sediment, numerous gram-negative bacilli. *Escherichia coli* is the microorganism cultured commonly from the urine. Culture of the blood may, at times, demonstrate the same organism.

Pain in one or both lumbar regions and the characteristic urinary findings, as well as fever and costovertebral tenderness, should make the diagnosis clear. The condition may be mistaken, however, for labor, appendicitis, placental abruption, or infarction of a myoma, and, in the puerperium, for uterine infection.

Several factors predispose the pregnant woman to acute pyelonephritis. As a result of ureteral compression at the pelvic brim by the enlarging uterus, compression by the enlarged ovarian vein, and probably hormonal effects as well, there is a gradual dilatation of the renal calyces, pelves, and ureters, accompanied by a decrease in tone and peristalsis (see Chap. 9, p. 243). These changes cause stasis, a factor known to increase the susceptibility to renal infection.

In the early puerperium, the bladder commonly has a decreased sensitivity to intravesical fluid tension as the consequences of anesthesia, especially epidural or spinal, and after the anesthesia dissipates, from the overriding pelvic discomfort from a large episiotomy, lacerations, or hematomas. Moreover, starting immediately after delivery, oxytocin is commonly infused at rates which cause antidiuresis for an hour or so along with an appreciable volume of fluid. When the oxytocin is stopped there is likely to be a surge of urine which rapidly distends the bladder. Overdistention of the bladder, coupled with catherterization to provide relief, commonly leads to urinary tract infection!

ASYMPTOMATIC BACTERIURIA. The term *asymptomatic bacteriuria* is used to indicate actively multiplying bacteria within the urinary tract without symptoms of a urinary infection. The reported prevalence of bacteriuria during pregnancy varies from 2 to as great as 12 percent, depending on the parity, race, and socioeconomic status of the women surveyed. The highest incidence has been reported in black multiparas with sickle cell trait, and the lowest incidence has been found in white private patients of low parity.

Bacteriuria is typically present at the time of the first prenatal visit; after an initial negative culture of the urine, fewer than 1.5 percent acquire a urinary infection in the subsequent months until delivery (Whalley, 1967). The diagnosis of asymptomatic bacteriuria requires the demonstration of significant numbers of bacteria in the urine. In most instances, this can be accomplished by culturing clean voided specimens of urine without resorting to catheterization. A clean voided specimen of urine containing more than 100,000 organisms of the same species per ml of urine is most often evidence of infection. Smaller numbers of bacteria usually, but not always, represent contamination of the specimen during collection; with a high rate of urine formation, a lesser number of organisms of the same species is likely to represent infection rather than contamination.

Approximately 25 percent of women with asymptomatic bacteriuria during pregnancy subsequently develop an acute symptomatic urinary infection during that pregnancy. Moreover, eradication of bacteriuria with antimicrobial agents has been shown to be effective in the prevention of these infections.

Bacteriuria has been thought by some investigators to cause premature labor and, in turn, increased neonatal morbidity and mortality. In an early study by Kass (1962, 1965), the incidence of premature births, defined as a birth weight of 2500 g or less, among 95 women with bacteriuria who received only placebos during pregnancy was 27 percent, whereas among 84 women with bacteriuria who were treated with antimicrobial agents, the rate was only 7 percent. The corresponding rates of perinatal death were 14 and 0 percent, respectively. On the basis of an extensive study in Australia, Kincaid-Smith and Bullen (1965) also reported a relatively high proportion of infants of low birth weight among untreated bacteriuric women, but these investigators were unable to reduce significantly this proportion with antimicrobial therapy (21.5 percent compared with 17.3 percent). They concluded that bacteriuria in pregnancy is commonly a manifestation of underlying chronic renal disease, which accounts for the higher incidence of low-birth-weight infants and perinatal loss. Several other investigators have been unable to corroborate the alleged relation between bacteriuria and low birth weight (Table 28-1). Therefore, from the evidence currently available, it must be concluded that, although there may be a relation between bacteriuria and low birth weight, bacteriuria is not a prominent factor in the genesis of low birth weight or prematurity.

Even though bacteriuria plays a prominent role in the cause of acute pyelonephritis during pregnancy, the majority of women—perhaps three-fourths—with bacteriuria remain asymptomatic throughout pregnancy. Some of the women certainly have bacteriuria limited to the bladder without involvement of the kidney, but several studies clearly demonstrate that others have potentially serious renal disease. Postpartum urologic investigation of patients shown to have bacteriuria during pregnancy have substantiated that, in

TABLE 28-1.
INCIDENCES OF PREMATURE DELIVERIES IN WOMEN
WITH AND WITHOUT BACTERIURIA DURING
PREGNANCY

AUTHOR	BACTERIURIC PATIENTS*	NONBACTERIURIC PATIENTS*
Little (1966)	141 (9)	4,735 (8)
Norden (1965)	114 (15)	109 (13)
Sleigh (1964)	100 (7)	100 (7)
Whalley (1967)	176 (15)	176 (12)
Wilson (1966)	230 (11)	6,216 (10)

* Numbers in parentheses indicate percent.

many, bacteriuria persists after delivery. Moreover, in a significant number of these women, there is pyelographic evidence of chronic infection, obstructive lesions, or congenital abnormalities of the urinary tract (Kincaid-Smith and Bullen, 1965; Whalley et al., 1965, 1967).

On the basis of experiences at Parkland Memorial Hospital, screening routinely obstetric clinic patients is advised to detect bacteriuria, and, when positive cultures are obtained, to eradicate the infection. Women who do not respond to treatment, who subsequently become reinfected, or who relapse, should be thoroughly evaluated urologically after the puerperium (Fig. 28-1).

CHRONIC PYELONEPHRITIS. In contrast to acute pyelonephritis, chronic pyelonephritis may be associated with few or no symptoms referable to the urinary tract. In advanced cases, the major symptoms are those of renal insufficiency. There may or may not be a history of prior symptomatic infection of the urinary tract; in fact, in fewer than half of women with chronic pyelonephritis, is there a clear history of preceding cystitis or acute pyelonephritis. The pathogenesis of this disease is therefore obscure. As in all chronic progressive renal diseases, the maternal and fetal prognosis in a particular case depends on the extent of renal destruction. Women with hypertension or renal insufficiency have a poor prognosis, whereas those with adequate renal function may go through

pregnancy without serious complications. Regardless of the extent of renal destruction, chronic pyelonephritis complicated by pregnancy is associated with an increased risk of superimposed acute pyelonephritis, which, in turn, may lead to further deterioration of renal function. In that event, termination of pregnancy is justified.

Management of Infections of the Urinary Tract. A variety of drugs are now available for the treatment of urinary infections. Ideally, the choice of a particular antimicrobial agent should be based upon studies of the sensitivity of the infecting microorganism. In practice, however, most bacteria causing urinary tract infections in pregnancy are sensitive to the short-acting sulfonamides, nitrofurantoin (Macrodantin), and somewhat less often to ampicillin. Since sensitivity is predictable, treatment can be initiated with one of these three agents and changed if necessary, when the laboratory results are available.

Women with asymptomatic bacteriuria or symptoms confined to the lower urinary tract may be treated without being hospitalized. Treatment for 10 days with Macrodantin, 100 mg once a day, or with sulfisoxazole (Gantrisin), 1 g 4 times a day, has proved effective in the majority of cases so treated at Parkland Memorial Hospital.

In general, it is best for pregnant women with systemic manifestations of acute pyelonephritis to be hospitalized during the initiation of treatment and until clinical improvement is observed. During the first few days of therapy, patients with acute pyelonephritis should be watched carefully to detect signs or symptoms suggesting bacterial shock. Although this serious complication is quite uncommon, its gravity demands early recognition and prompt therapy. Urinary output should therefore be recorded carefully and blood pressure measured frequently during the initial stage of therapy in all patients with acute pyelonephritis. The levels of creatinine in plasma should be ascertained early in the

course of therapy. It is not generally appreciated that acute pyelonephritis in pregnancy may in some yet unexplained way cause a considerable reduction in glomerular filtration rate that is reversed, fortunately, by effective treatment of the infection (Fig. 28-2) (Whalley et al., 1975).

Antimicrobial agents used to treat infections of the urinary tract during pregnancy may, in certain circumstances, produce undesirable side effects, both maternal and fetal. Sulfonamides given to the mother before delivery will have crossed the placenta and may,

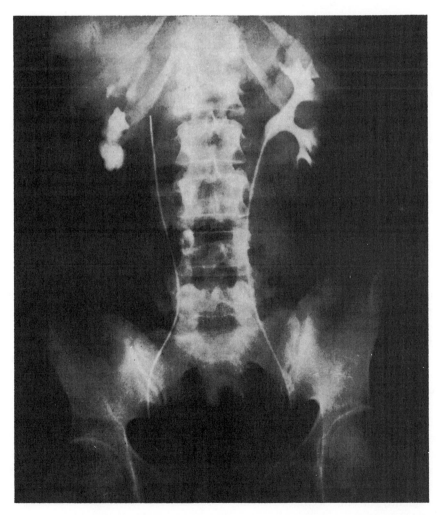

FIG. 28-1. Retrograde pyelogram obtained 3 months postpartum, showing marked destruction of the right calyceal system from long-standing asymptomatic infection. The patient, a multipara, had asymptomatic bacteriuria during pregnancy. There was no history of infection of the urinary tract. (Courtesy of Dr. P. J. Whalley)

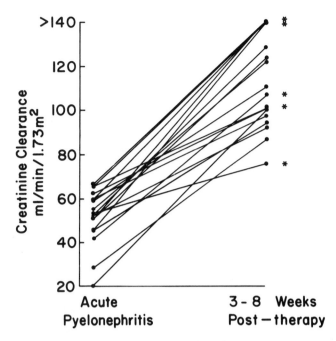

FIG. 28-2. Endogenous creatinine clearance values in 18 pregnant women during and 3 to 8 weeks after an attack of acute pyelonephritis; asterisk indicates patients reevaluated while still pregnant. (From Whalley, Cunningham, Martin. *Obstet Gynecol* 46:174, 1975)

in the presence of hyperbilirubinemia in the newborn, possibly increase the danger of kernicterus. These drugs cross the placenta and compete with unconjugated bilirubin for binding by albumin, and as a result there is an increase in unbound, free bilirubin. The sulfonamides, furthermore, may compete with bilirubin for glucuronyl transferase, which is required for conversion of free bilirubin to conjugated pigment. Nitrofurantoin may lead to hemolytic anemia in women whose erythrocytes are markedly deficient in glucose-6-phosphate dehydrogenase. Perhaps 2 percent of black women are homozygous for the X sex chromosome-linked enzyme deficiency and therefore are potential candidates for drug-induced hemolysis. Hemolysis develops rarely in our experience.

Tetracycline administered in the last trimester of pregnancy may lead to discoloration subsequently of the deciduous teeth. Therapy with large doses of tetracycline may precipitate in the woman a syndrome of azotemia, jaundice, and pancreatitis in preg-

nant women with impaired renal excretory function (Whalley et al., 1964).

Chloramphenicol may rarely produce serious and even fatal blood dyscrasias, such as aplastic anemia and thrombocytopenia. Streptomycin, kanamycin, and gentamicin (Garamycin) may be both ototoxic and nephrotoxic; moreover, streptomycin rapidly induces bacterial resistance.

Most urinary infections respond rapidly to adequate antimicrobial therapy. Clinical symptoms for the most part disappear during the first 2 days of therapy. Even though the symptoms promptly abate, therapy should be continued for at least 10 days. Cultures of urine usually become sterile within the first 24 hours if the microorganism is sensitive to the chosen drug. Since, however, the physiologic changes in the urinary tract are unaltered by treatment, a reinfection for the same reasons that caused the initial infection is always possible. If the subsequent culture of the urine is positive remote from the time of therapy, additional treatment is indicated using a drug to which the organism appears sensitive.

Prognosis. The prognosis for women with infections of the urinary tract in pregnancy is variable. Pyelonephritis during pregnancy must not be considered cured even though the symptoms subside completely and spontaneously, unless the urine remains sterile. The untreated woman harbors infection for a variable time after delivery. Although the majority of women who develop urinary infections during pregnancy may never have significant renal damage, some will eventually develop serious renal disease. It is therefore imperative to treat adequately all infections of the urinary tract during pregnancy. The responsibilities are not discharged until the physician is certain that the urine is free from organisms remote from the time of antibacterial therapy. Absence of pyuria is not in itself adequate evidence of cure. Finally, all patients who develop repeated infections of the urinary tract should be examined by intravenous pyelography after the puerperium.

Renal Tuberculosis. Tuberculosis of the kidney is a serious, but rare, complication of pregnancy. Renal tuberculosis is believed by some to pursue a rapidly unfavorable course, particularly during the later months of pregnancy. The question of the advisability of allowing the pregnancy to continue in any case of proved renal tuberculosis is therefore raised. A decision regarding termination of pregnancy should be based upon the individual findings in each case, however.

Whether the patient who has undergone nephrectomy for tuberculosis should be allowed to become pregnant is another question. The consensus is that pregnancy should be interdicted for about 2 years until absence of involvement and good function of the remaining kidney have been demonstrated.

Other Diseases of the Urinary System

URINARY CALCULI. Renal and ureteral lithiasis is an uncommon complication of pregnancy. Prather and Crabtree (1934) reported an incidence of 0.04 percent for renal stones and 0.08 percent for ureteral stones in 9823 deliveries; Harris and Dunnihoo (1967) reported a similar incidence. Since in many pregnant women there are some of the cardinal prerequisites for the formation of stones—namely, urinary stasis and infection—the incidence might be expected to be higher were it not for counteracting factors, one of which is undoubtedly the relatively short duration of pregnancy.

Women who have formed renal stones previously are generally at increased risk of doing so again. Coe and associates (1978), however, could find no evidence in such women that pregnancy increased that risk. Moreover, stone disease did not appear to have any prejudicial effect on pregnancy except for an increased frequency of urinary tract infections. They concluded that a woman with nephrolithiasis need not forego pregnancy as long as renal function is adequate.

The calculi during pregnancy seldom cause severe symptomatic obstruction. When calculi are discovered, the possibility of hyperparathyroidism should be considered.

Treatment depends on the symptoms and the duration of pregnancy. If the symptoms are severe surgical removal may be mandatory regardless of other considerations. During the latter half of pregnancy, the blood vessels supplying the kidney and ureter are remarkably enlarged; moreover, proper exposure of the lower ureter without emptying the uterus is often impossible. Most often, however, the stone passes spontaneously (Strong et al., 1978).

ACUTE GLOMERULONEPHRITIS. Acute poststreptococcal glomerulonephritis rarely develops during pregnancy. In reviewing the litarature, Nadler and co-workers (1969) were able to find reports of only 19 women with acute glomerulonephritis occurring between weeks 8 and 37 of pregnancy, and in only 3 of them was the diagnosis verified by biopsy. The diagnosis during pregnancy is based upon the history of a streptococcal infection 2 weeks before and supporting evidence is provided by an elevated antistreptolysin titer. Acute glomerulonephritis appearing during the last trimester of pregnancy may sometimes be clinically indistinguishable from pregnancy-induced hypertension, that is, preeclampsia and eclampsia. Prolonged hematuria or persistence of hematuria after delivery suggests acute hemorrhagic nephritis. In general, the treatment of acute glomerulonephritis is the same in the pregnant as in the nonpregnant patient.

There are insufficient data available to predict fetal or maternal prognosis. Some investigators have noted a high fetal loss from abortion, immaturity, or stillbirth; others have documented otherwise uneventful pregnancies. Since the clinical syndrome usually subsides within 2 weeks, a course of expectant observation is warranted. In particularly severe cases or when the disease persists longer than 2 weeks, interruption of the pregnancy may be advisable. In nonpregnant women, the mortality rate is less than 5 percent, death usually resulting from heart failure or unrelenting renal failure. Some patients never completely recover, lapsing gradually into chronic glomerulonephritis. Women with a history of acute hemorrhagic nephritis that has subsequently healed may undergo additional pregnancies without any appreciable increase in the incidence of complications, according to Felding's survey (1964, 1968).

CHRONIC GLOMERULONEPHRITIS. Chronic glomerulonephritis is characterized by the progressive destruction of renal glomeruli, eventually producing the so-called end-stage kidney. In most cases, the cause is unknown, although a few patients appear to develop the disease after a bout of acute glomerulonephritis that failed to heal.

The disease may present in one of six ways:

1. Some patients may remain asymptomatic for years, with proteinuria or an abnormal urinary sediment, or both, as the only indications of disease.

2. It may be discovered in some women during the course of evaluation for chronic hypertension.
3. The disease may first become manifest as the nephrotic syndrome.
4. It may present in an acute form quite similar to acute glomerulonephritis.
5. Renal failure may be the first manifestation.
6. The symptoms and signs of preeclampsia-eclampsia may precede discovery of chronic glomerulonephritis.

Regardless of the mode of onset, all patients with chronic glomerulonephritis eventually develop signs and symptoms of renal insufficiency and hypertensive cardiovascular disease.

The prognosis for the outcome of pregnancy in any given case is related to the level of the renal function and the presence or absence of hypertension. Except for an increased risk of superimposed preeclampsia, those women with relatively normal renal function and no hypertension may be carried successfully through pregnancy. Because of the likelihood of progression of the disease, however, the ultimate maternal prognosis is poor. Conversely, in women with extreme hypertension or azotemia, the outcome is poor for them and for the pregnancy, and therapeutic abortion often is advisable.

Because of the varying rates of renal destruction, it is difficult to evaluate the influence of pregnancy on the progress of the disease. Pregnancy in the absence of superimposed preeclampsia does not appear to accelerate appreciably deterioration in renal function. In some cases, the affected kidneys show the same pattern of response to pregnancy as do normal kidneys, with an increase in both glomerular filtration and renal plasma flow (Werkö and Bucht, 1956).

NEPHROSIS. The nephrotic syndrome, or nephrosis, is a disorder of multiple causes, characterized by massive proteinuria (in excess of 5 g per day), hypoalbuminemia, and hypercholesteremia, usually with hyperlipemia and edema. Diseases known to be associated with nephrotic syndrome include chronic glomerulonephritis, lupus erythematosus, diabetes mellitus, amyloidosis, syphilis, and thrombosis of the renal vein. In addition, the syndrome may result from poisoning by heavy metals, therapy with some drugs, and allergies to poison ivy or bee and wasp venom.

When the nephrotic syndrome complicates pregnancy, the maternal and fetal prognosis and the treatment depend on the underlying cause of the disease and the extent of renal insufficiency. Whenever possible, the specific cause should be ascertained and renal function assessed. In this regard, percutaneous renal biopsy may be of value. Serial studies of renal function in two of our patients with the nephrotic syndrome associated with chronic glomerulonephritis served to demonstrate the usual augmentation of renal function that characterizes pregnancy. Neither patient became hypertensive. A review of additional reported cases of nephrosis indicates that the majority of patients who are not hypertensive and do not have severe renal insufficiency may undergo a successful pregnancy, particularly since the advent of adrenocorticosteroid therapy (Studd and Blainey, 1969; Weisman et al., 1973). In certain cases, however, in which there is evidence of renal insufficiency or moderate to severe hypertension, or both, the prognosis for mother and fetus is poor, and interruption of the pregnancy is often indicated, particularly if renal function is deteriorating.

POLYCYSTIC DISEASE OF THE KIDNEY. This is a rare complication of pregnancy. The decision to allow pregnancy to continue depends almost entirely on the degree of renal involvement. If the disease has not progressed to the stage of hypertension, proteinuria, and azotemia, the outlook for the pregnancy is good. With mild hypertension and normal renal function, pregnancy carries the same risk as in women with other forms of chronic hypertension. With azotemia, the chance of a successful pregnancy is slight and the risk to the mother and fetus considerable

(Landesman and Scherr, 1956). Katz and associates (1979) have recorded a pregnancy in which the growth-retarded infant who was deliberately delivered remote from term survived, even though the mother was uremic from advanced polycystic kidney disease. Polycystic kidney disease is transmitted as an autosomal dominant trait.

PREGNANCY AFTER UNILATERAL NEPHRECTOMY. Because the excretory capacity of the kidneys is much in excess of ordinary needs, and because the surviving kidney usually undergoes hypertrophy with increased excretory capacity, women with one normal kidney most often have no difficulty in pregnancy. If the remaining kidney is chronically infected, however, further damage may result from the stasis induced by pregnancy, with the likelihood of more intense infection. Accordingly, before advising a woman with one kidney about the risk of future pregnancy, a thorough functional evaluation of the remaining organ is essential. Should it be found impaired, further childbearing is inadvisable. Even asymptomatic women should be carefully monitored to make certain that the single kidney is functioning satisfactorily.

ACUTE RENAL FAILURE. Acute renal failure associated with pregnancy has become much less common in recent years for a variety of reasons, including legalized abortion. Nonetheless, Harkins and associates (1974) reported a mortality rate of 22 percent for pregnant and puerperal women who did develop acute renal failure.

ACUTE TUBULAR NECROSIS. Acute tubular necrosis is the major category of acute renal failure during pregnancy. This lesion results apparently from ischemia related to acute and severe blood loss, severe sepsis, intrarenal vasospasm from a variety of causes, including preeclampsia-eclampsia, or a combination of these complications. The disease is therefore largely preventable by the following means: (1) prompt replacement of blood in instances of massive hemorrhage, as in abruptio placentae, placenta previa, rupture of the uterus, and post-partum uterine atony as described in Chapter 21; (2) careful observation for early signs of bacterial shock in patients with septic abortion, amnionitis, sepsis from other pelvic infections, or pyelonephritis; (3) prompt termination of pregnancies complicated by severe preeclampsia and eclampsia. The disease is not progressive; after healing has taken place, renal function usually returns to normal or near normal. Future pregnancies are therefore not necessarily contraindicated.

CORTICAL NECROSIS OF THE KIDNEY. Compared to acute tubular necrosis, bilateral necrosis of the renal cortex is very uncommon. However, when cortical necrosis has developed, it most often has been associated with pregnancy. For example, among 38 cases studied by Kleinknecht and co-workers (1973), 26 were obstetric in origin. Most of the reported cases in pregnant women have followed such complications as abruptio placentae, preeclampsia-eclampsia, or bacterial shock. The histologic lesion appears to result from thrombosis of segments of the renal vascular system. The lesion may be focal, patchy, confluent, or gross (Sheehan and Moore, 1953). Antecedent nephrosclerosis appears to increase the vulnerability of the kidney to this complication (Ober et al., 1956). Clinically, the disease follows the course of acute renal failure with oliguria or anuria, uremia, and generally death within 14 days unless dialysis is initiated. Differentiation from acute tubular necrosis during the early phase is possible only by renal biopsy. The prognosis depends on the extent of the necrosis, since recovery is a function of the amount of renal tissue spared. When the lesion is confluent, the mortality rate approaches 100 percent. The possible role of hemmorrhage and of intravascular coagulation in the genesis of renal cortical necrosis is considered in Chapter 21.

OBSTRUCTIVE RENAL FAILURE.   Rarely, the compression of the ureters by the preg-

nant uterus is greatly exaggerated causing ureteral obstruction and, in turn, severe oliguria and azotemia. O'Shaughnessy and co-workers (1980), as well as others have described this phenomenon as the consequence of a markedly overdistended gravid uterus. We have observed this phenomenon in one woman with gross hydramnios (9.4 liters) and an anencephalic fetus. Amniocentesis and removal of some of the amnionic fluid was followed promptly by a diuresis and a lowering of the plasma creatinine concentration.

POSTPARTUM ACUTE RENAL FAILURE. Wagoner and associates (1968) and Robson and associates (1968) described what they believed to be a new syndrome of acute irreversible renal failure occurring within the first 6 weeks postpartum. Pregnancy and delivery appeared to have been normal in the seven cases reported and none of the known causes of renal failure was present. The pathologic changes identified by renal biopsy were glomerular necrosis, glomerular endothelial proliferation, and necrosis, thrombosis, and intimal thickening of the arterioles. No vascular abnormalities were demonstrated in the other visceral organs in the four cases in which autopsy was performed. Morphologic changes in the erythrocytes consistent with microangiopathic hemolysis were present in the majority of cases. The cause of this rare syndrome is obscure; suggested factors in the pathogenesis included drug sensitivity (all seven patients had received an ergot preparation), consumptive coagulopathy, and a primary immunologic mechanism.

Other authors have described the same or a similar condition under the name of *postpartum hemolytic uremic syndrome* (Eisinger, 1972; Strauss and Alexander, 1976). According to Nissenson and co-workers (1979), 80 percent of affected women have died and only 5 percent have recovered, including a case described by them in which maintenance hemodialysis had been used for over a year.

The postpartum hemolytic uremic syndrome appears to be quite distinct from the syndrome of intravascular hemolysis and thrombocytopenia complicating severe pre-eclampsia or eclampsia (Pritchard et al., 1955). With the latter condition, among survivors there is relatively prompt recovery of renal function.

Postpartum acute renal failure has not been identified among the large number of women cared for on the Obstetric Service at Parkland Memorial Hospital. However, two puerperal women with idiopathic renal failure have been referred to the Renal Unit of Parkland Memorial Hospital where deformed and fragmented erythrocytes characteristic of microangiopathic hemolysis and evidence of consumptive coagulopathy were recognized, as well as severe azotemia. Therapy consisted of hemodialysis with and without prolonged heparinization. Initially, renal function improved somewhat in both, although neither was cured.

Hemodialysis During Pregnancy. Most often, failing renal function is accompanied by infertility. With chronic hemodialysis, however, fertility may be restored in a minority of cases (Perez et al., 1978). A few women have subsequently become pregnant and have been so managed throughout the pregnancy. Liveborn infants without evidence of severe growth retardation have been described. Trebbin (1979) has summarized several reported cases in which hemodialysis was used during pregnancy. He pointed out that pregnancy does not necessarily need to be terminated because the woman requires hemodialysis. In general, the prognosis must be assumed to be poor, however.

PREGNANCY AFTER RENAL TRANSPLANTATION

Murray and associates in 1963 reported two successful pregnancies in a woman who had a kidney transplanted from her identical twin sister. Since that time, there have been several reports of pregnancy in women who previously had received a kidney from immuno-logically nonidentical donors. Sciarra and colleagues (1975) summarized the Minnesota experiences of 17 pregnancies in 12 women, each of whom had received a renal transplant from other than an identical twin. All were maintained on immunosuppressive therapy with azathioprine and prednisone. Late-pregnancy hypertension ("toxemia of pregnancy") was the rule for the pregnancies that were allowed to continue. No other major obstetric problems were encountered. Bacterial and viral infections were common, however. One woman, after her third pregnancy, died of hepatitis. Two developed carcinoma-in-situ of the cervix. The development of a malignant condition among the immunosuppressed transplant recipients is now recognized as a further threat to their well-being.

Of the 12 liveborn infants in Sciarra's series, three were small for gestational age, seven were appropriate, and two were large. No malformations or other stigmata of the immunosuppressive therapy were identified in any of the infants.

Penn, Makowski, and Harris (1980) have described their extensive experiences with renal transplant and pregnancy. Fifty-six pregnancies in 37 women have culminated in 44 livebirths, including one set of twins; 3 more women were undelivered at the time of the report. Of 8 abortions, 1 was spontaneous and 7 were therapeutically performed because of impaired renal function, hypertension, or both; and one was a stillbirth (from maternal carbon monoxide poisoning).

Twenty of the 44 infants were born before 37 weeks gestational age; only 6 of the infants were small for gestational age. Four infants had congenital anomalies; 4 developed respiratory distress; 2 had adrenocortical insufficiency; 2 developed septicemia; and one newborn convulsed from an unknown cause. One infant with sepsis died at 10 days of age.

Four of the mothers have subsequently died. Two deaths occurred 30 and 50 months after pregnancy; both women refused to continue the immunosuppressive medications and died from graft rejection and uremia. Two died of overwhelming sepsis 9 months after a third pregnancy, and 82 months after a second pregnancy respectively.

Fifty-eight of 60 babies sired by fathers who had undergone renal transplant were normal. One infant was born with a meningomyelocele, hip dislocation, and talipes equinovarus. The other infant with congenital anomalies, including microcephaly and polycystic kidneys, died at birth.

Rudolph and associates (1979), by means of a questionnaire sent to most transplant centers in the United States, identified 440 pregnancies among renal transplant recipients. Therapeutic abortion was carried out 109 times. Stillbirths were low, but 20 percent of the infants were delivered prematurely. Rejection was a serious problem in 9 percent. Evidence of preeclampsia was common.

Eleven pregnant women have been cared for at Parkland Memorial hospital following renal transplant. All were taking prednisone and azathioprine for immunosuppression. Six infants, all of whom appeared healthy, were delivered at or near term and all have subsequently thrived. The adrenal response to ACTH when evaluated in two infants was found to be normal. One mother near the end of the second trimester became severely jaundiced. The pregnancy was further complicated by a large furuncle with staphylococcal bacteremia, partial placental abruption, and delivery of a stillborn infant at 26 weeks. On the basis of a liver biopsy and her clinical course, the jaundice was considered to be cholestatic in origin probably as the consequence of both pregnancy-induced changes and the immunosuppressive therapy with azathioprine. Therapeutic abortion was performed on three women and in one instance a missed abortion was terminated by curettage.

Five of the six mothers whose pregnancies continued into the third trimester became overtly hypertensive. The hypertension was accompanied by a decrease in creatinine clearance. In each instance, the hypertension cleared after delivery. The six deliveries were accomplished by cesarean section, after unsatisfactory induction of labor. In each instance the uterus was markedly levorotated, presumably as the consequence of the donor kidney having been placed in the right false pelvis, and the fetal head remained above the pelvic inlet.

ANEMIA AND OTHER DISEASES OF THE BLOOD

Definition of Anemia. The definition of anemia is complicated by the normal differences in the concentrations of hemoglobin between women and men, between white women and black women, between women who live at high altitude and those who live near sea level, between women who are pregnant and those who are not, and between pregnant women who receive iron supplements and those who do not. For reasons that follow, it can be said that anemia probably exists in women if the hemoglobin is less than 12.0 g per dl in the nonpregnant state, or is less than 10.0 g per dl during pregnancy or the puerperium (Pritchard and Scott, 1970; Scott and Pritchard, 1967). Both early in pregnancy and near term, the hemoglobin level of healthy women, however, is usually 11.0 g per dl or higher. During the puerperium, the hemoglobin concentration normally is not appreciably lower than before delivery. After delivery, the hemoglobin level commonly fluctuates to a moderate degree for a few days and then rises toward the nonpregnant level. The magnitude of the increase is to a considerable degree the resultant of the amount of hemoglobin added to the circulation during pregnancy and the amount shed during and after delivery.

Extensive hematologic measurements have been made in healthy women, none of whom were iron deficient, since each had histochemically proven iron stores. Nor were any of them overtly deficient in metabolically active forms of folic acid, since marrow erythropoiesis was normoblastic. Pertinent observations are presented in Table 28-2. The hemoglobin concentration of 85 healthy iron-sufficient nonpregnant women averaged 13.7 g per dl and ranged from 12.0 to 15.0 g for ± 2 standard deviations from the mean. In healthy iron-sufficient women who were 16 to 22 weeks pregnant, the mean hemoglobin was only 11.5 g per dl, and in 3 of the 81 evaluated it was 9.7 or 9.8 g per dl. The hemoglobin at or very near term averaged

TABLE 28-2.
HEMOGLOBIN CONCENTRATION IN HEALTHY WOMEN WITH
PROVEN IRON STORES

HEMOGLOBIN (g per dl)	STAGE OF PREGNANCY		
	Nonpregnant	Mid Pregnancy	Late Pregnancy
Mean	13.7	11.5	12.3
<12.0 Percent	1	72	36
<11.0 Percent	0	29	6
<10.0 Percent	0	4	1
Lowest	11.7	9.7	9.8

12.3 g per dl; in only 7 out of 95 was the hemoglobin less than 11.0 g per dl with the lowest value 9.8 g per dl.

The modest fall in hemoglobin levels observed during pregnancy in healthy women not deficient in iron or folate is caused by relatively greater expansion of the volume of plasma compared with the increase in hemoglobin mass and volume of erythrocytes. The disproportion between the rates at which plasma and erythrocytes are added to the maternal circulation normally is greatest during the second trimester. Later in pregnancy, plasma expansion ceases while erythrocyte production continues (see Chap. 9, p. 234).

Frequency. Although anemia is somewhat more common among indigent pregnant women, it is by no means restricted to them. The frequency of anemia during pregnancy varies considerably, depending primarily upon whether supplemental iron is taken during pregnancy. For example, at Parkland Memorial Hospital the hemoglobin levels at the time of delivery among women who took iron supplements averaged 12.4 g per dl whereas it was only 11.3 g per dl among those who received no iron. Moreover, in none of the group receiving iron supplements was the hemoglobin less than 10.0 g per dl, but it was below this level in 16 percent of the group who received no supplements (see Chap. 13, p. 313).

Etiology of Anemia. A classification based primarily on etiology and including most of the common causes of anemia in pregnant women is presented below:

Causes of Anemia During Pregnancy

Acquired
1. Iron-deficiency anemia
2. Anemia caused by acute blood loss
3. Anemia caused by infection
4. Megaloblastic anemia
5. Acquired hemolytic anemia
6. Aplastic or hypoplastic anemia

Hereditary
1. Thalassemia
2. Sickle-cell anemia
3. Sickle-cell–hemoglobin C disease
4. Sickle-cell–thalassemia disease
5. Homozygous hemoglobin C disease
6. Other hemoglobinopathies
7. Hereditary hemolytic anemia without hemoglobinopathy

Although laboratory error as a cause of apparent anemia has not been included in this table, the results from clinical laboratories may sometimes be grossly inaccurate. A common source of error during pregnancy stems from the rapid sedimentation rate of erythrocytes, which is induced by the hyperfibrinogenemia of pregnancy. If the specimen of blood is not thoroughly mixed *immediately* before sampling, the results are likely to be grossly inaccurate.

The observed differences between the hemoglobin levels in pregnant and nonpregnant women, coupled with the well-recognized phenomenon of hypervolemia induced by normal pregnancy, have led to the use by some of the term *physiologic anemia.* This poor term for describing a normal process is a source of confusion and should be discarded.

Screening for Anemia.   A limited but practical hematologic evaluation may be rather easily and promptly carried out at the time of the mother's visit to the clinic or office. The equipment and reagents required are simple and inexpensive. A few ml of venous blood are anticoagulated with Versenate. A centrifuge for performing microhematocrit measurements and a hematocrit reading device are employed to detect anemia. The plasma in the hematocrit tube is examined for icterus, and the thickness of the buffy coat is noted. If icterus is observed, studies to detect hemolytic disease or hepatic dysfunction are initiated. For black patients, a sickle-cell preparation is made using isotonic sodium metabisulfite; if positive, hemoglobin electrophoresis is usually indicated. Whenever the hematocrit approaches 30 or less, or when there is icterus, or when sickling is demonstrated, a blood smear with Wright's stain is used to evaluate the blood cells morphologically. These rather simple studies not only detect anemia but also provide important etiologic clues.

Acquired Anemias.   The two most common causes of anemia during pregnancy and the puerperium are iron deficiency and acute blood loss. Not infrequently the two are intimately related, since excessive blood loss with its concomitant loss of hemoglobin iron in one pregnancy can be an important cause of iron-deficiency anemia in the next pregnancy.

IRON-DEFICIENCY ANEMIA.   As discussed elsewhere (see Chap. 9, p. 234; see Chap. 13, p. 313) the iron requirements of pregnancy are considerable, but the majority of women undoubtedly have small stores of iron. In a typical gestation with a single fetus, the maternal need induced by pregnancy for iron averages close to 800 mg, of which nearly 300 mg go to the fetus and placenta whereas about 500 mg are used to expand the maternal hemoglobin mass. Approximately 200 mg more are lost through the gut, urine, and skin. This amount of iron usually exceeds considerably the iron stores available for such purposes. Unless the difference between the amount of stored iron available to the mother and the iron requirements of normal pregnancy is made up by absorption of iron from the gastrointestinal tract during pregnancy, iron-deficiency anemia develops.

With the rather rapid expansion of the blood volume during the second trimester, the lack of iron often manifests itself by an appreciable drop in the maternal hemoglobin concentration. Although the rate of expansion of the blood volume is not so great in the third trimester, the need for iron remains high because augmentation of the maternal hemoglobin mass continues and even more iron is transported at this time across the placenta from mother to fetus. Since the amount of iron diverted to the fetus from an iron-deficient mother is not much less than the amount normally transferred, the newborn infant of even a severely anemic mother does not suffer from iron-deficiency anemia.

Classic morphologic evidence of iron-deficiency anemia—erythrocyte hypochromia and microcytosis—is much less likely to be as prominent in the pregnant woman as in the nonpregnant woman with the same hemoglobin concentration. Iron-deficiency anemia during pregnancy, with a hemoglobin concentration of 9 to 11 g per dl, is usually not accompanied by obvious morphologic changes in the circulating erythrocytes. With this degree of anemia from iron deficiency, the serum iron is lower than normal, and there is no readily mobilizable stainable iron in the bone marrow. The serum iron-binding capacity is elevated but is in itself of little diagnositc value, since it is also elevated during normal pregnancy in the absence of iron deficiency. Moderate normoblastic hyperplasia of the bone marrow is also found to be similar to that in normal pregnancy.

The initial evaluation of a pregnant woman with moderate anemia should include measurements of hemoglobin, hematocrit, and cell indices, careful examination of a well-prepared smear of the peripheral blood, a sickle-cell preparation if the patient is black, and the measurement of the serum iron concentration. Examination of the bone marrow at this point is seldom done, although the demonstration of hemosiderin rules out iron deficiency. The diagnosis of iron deficiency in moderately anemic pregnant women is usually presumptive; it is based largely on the exclusion of other causes of anemia.

If the pregnant woman with iron-deficiency anemia of moderate degree receives adequate iron therapy, hematologic response can be detected first in a blood smear. New erythrocytes, normal or slightly larger than normal in size and polychromatophilic or basophilic, soon appear in the peripheral blood. Examination of a blood smear is simpler than a reticulocyte count and is probably a more accurate index of response in the moderately anemic patient. The rate of increase of the concentration of hemoglobin or of the hematocrit varies considerably but is usually somewhat slower than in nonpregnant women. The reason is related largely to the differences in blood volumes. During the latter half of pregnancy the newly formed hemoglobin is added to the characteristically much larger volume of blood. Moreover, the blood volume commonly continues to expand during the period of therapy, and as a consequence the production of a given amount of hemoglobin by the pregnant woman may not result in a rapid increase in hemoglobin concentration. There is little evidence, however, that normal pregnancy itself depresses erythropoiesis to any degree. Indeed, recently we were forced to perform repeated phlebotomies on an alloimmunized pregnant woman who had a very rare blood type. During the latter half of pregnancy 6 units (3000 ml) were removed without incident. Her hematocrit throughout the period of repeated phlebotomy ranged from 30 to 35; therapy was limited to iron.

In severe iron-deficiency anemia during pregnancy, the erythrocytes undergo the classic morphologic changes of hypochromia and microcytosis, and the diagnosis is usually made from the red cell indices and confirmed by examination of a well-prepared smear of the peripheral blood.

There has been some divergence of opinion regarding the best way to treat iron-deficiency anemia during pregnancy and the puerperium. The use of an effective parenteral iron medication guarantees that the expectant mother receives the iron. Oral preparations are preferred, however, if she understands the importance of taking the medication regularly. If she will not or, much less likely, cannot take the oral doses of iron, parenteral therapy is the alternative. Whatever treatment is employed, the objectives are reasonably prompt correction of the anemia and eventual restitution of iron stores. Both of these objectives can be accomplished with adequate doses of oral iron compounds supplying a daily dose of about 200 mg of *iron* (Table 28-3). To replenish iron stores, oral therapy should usually be continued for at least 3 months after the anemia has been

TABLE 28-3.
IRON CONTENT OF COMMONLY USED FERROUS COMPOUNDS

	EXSICCATED FERROUS SULFATE (FEOSOL PLAIN)	FERROUS GLUCONATE (FERGON)	FERROUS FUMARATE (IRCON)
Iron content (per g)	300 mg	110 mg	330 mg
Usual size of pill	0.2 g	0.3 g	0.2 g
No. of pills to supply about 200 mg iron	3	6	3

corrected (Pritchard and Mason, 1964). The major disadvantages of therapy with oral iron, therefore, are the possibility of failure of the woman to take the medication in adequate amounts and the danger of iron intoxication if young children should ingest large doses of the usually attractive tablets.

Whenever parenteral iron therapy is judged advisable during pregnancy, a satisfactory dose in most instances is one 5-ml ampule of iron-dextran providing 250 mg of iron for each 1.0 g per dl deficit in maternal hemoglobin concentration. Accordingly, if the hemoglobin level is 8.0 g per dl, the number of ampules to be injected is 13 minus 8, or 5 ampules. If the woman is unusually small, somewhat less iron-dextran is needed, and if quite large, the opposite is true. To provide sufficient iron for effective erythropoiesis, 250 mg of iron should be injected every 4 to 7 days. If, after the first few injections of iron-dextran, there is no evidence of hematologic response, it is important that the injections be stopped and the cause of the anemia reevaluated.

Folic acid may be given along with the iron as a safeguard against folate deficiency, although in our experience the response of pregnant women with iron-deficiency anemia treated with iron and folic acid is usually not appreciably better than when iron is given alone. There is no good evidence that the addition of cobalt, copper, molybdenum, or ascorbic acid to the iron tablet is advantageous. Ascorbic acid enhances iron absorption somewhat, so that less iron need be ingested to achieve a comparable level of absorption. The adverse effects of oral iron, however, relate primarily to the amount of iron absorbed rather than to the amount ingested. Most often, iron preparations that contain significant amounts of iron but are completely free of adverse effects are very poorly absorbed and consequently ineffective.

Iron-dextran administered intravenously has been evaluated extensively, especially in other countries. Although the frequency and intensity of adverse systemic reactions appear to be no greater than when given intramuscularly (Scott, unpublished), the United States

Food and Drug Administration has not yet approved the intravenous use of iron-dextran in amounts beyond 100 mg per day. The use of a single massive intravenous dose of iron dextran to provide instantaneously all of the iron that might be needed to correct anemia, provide for pregnancy, and to establish stores is irrational therapy!

Transfusions of whole blood or packed erythrocytes are seldom indicated for the treatment of iron-deficiency anemia unless hypovolemia from blood loss coexists or an operative procedure must be performed on a severely anemic woman. Whereas hypovolemia is commonly a prominent feature of anemia caused by acute blood loss, very severe anemia from failure of production of erythrocytes or their accelerated destruction may lead to some degree of cardiac insufficiency and pathologic hypervolemia. With acute blood loss and hypovolemia, it is essential to restore an adequate blood volume as well as to provide hemoglobin for oxygen transport; therefore, transfusions of whole blood are usually indicated. In case of severe anemia with compromised cardiac function and pathologic hypervolemia, however, the administration of whole blood, unless done with meticulous care, can lead to severe circulatory overloading, pulmonary edema, and death.

Exchange transfusion is an effective way to raise the hemoglobin concentration of severely anemic women without inducing or intensifying circulatory overload. A measured small volume of venous blood is withdrawn and immediately an equal volume of packed erythrocytes is injected; this sequence is repeated until the hemoglobin concentration is raised to a level adequate for supplying the oxygen needs of the mother and fetus. The use of the potent diuretic furosemide (Lasix) before transfusing packed erythrocytes is of value in reducing plasma volume and thereby allowing the intravascular compartment to accommodate the added erythrocytes without causing circulatory overload.

ANEMIA FROM ACUTE LOSS OF BLOOD. Anemia resulting from recent hemorrhage is more likely to be evident during the puerperium. Both abruptio placentae and placenta previa may be sources of serious blood loss and of anemia before as well as after delivery. Earlier in pregnancy, anemia caused by acute loss of blood commonly results from abortion, tubal pregnancy with rupture or abortion, and hydatidiform mole.

Acute hemorrhage may have no immediate effect on the hemoglobin concentration even though the hemorrhage leads to hypovolemia so severe as to cause overt collapse. Severe hemorrhage demands immediate blood replacement in amounts that restore and maintain adequate perfusion of vital organs (see Chap. 21, p. 490). Even though the amount of blood replaced commonly does not completely make up the deficit of hemoglobin created by the hemorrhage, in general, once dangerous hypovolemia has been overcome and hemostasis has been achieved, the residual anemia should be treated with iron. The moderately anemic woman who no longer faces the likelihood of further gross hemorrhage, who can ambulate without adverse symptoms, and who is not seriously febrile certainly is better treated with iron than with more blood transfusions.

ANEMIA ASSOCIATED WITH INFLAMMATION. A large variety of subacute and chronic infections may produce moderate and sometimes severe anemia, usually with normocytic or very slightly microcytic erythrocytes. The bone marrow is not markedly altered, but there may be hyperplasia of the leukocytic series that might be misinterpreted as a relative reduction in precursors of the erythrocytes, i.e., slight erythrocytic hypoplasia. The serum iron concentration is decreased, and the serum iron-binding capacity, although lower than in normal pregnancy, is not necessarily much below the normal nonpregnant range. The anemia appears to result, at least in part, from alterations in reticuloendothelial function and iron metabolism (Douglas and Adamson, 1975; Freireich et al., 1957). Iron released from the patient's senescent erythrocytes is retained rather than being returned promptly to the plasma to be reutilized by the bone marrow for production of hemoglobin. The fate of iron administered in therapeutic doses is similar. The life span of the erythrocyte, furthermore, is usually slightly shortened. The anemia, therefore, results from decreased erythropoiesis coupled with slightly increased destruction.

Chronic renal disease, suppuration, granulomatous infections, malignant conditions, and rheumatoid arthritis may also cause anemia, presumably by these same mechanisms. At least some cases of so-called *refractory anemia of pregnancy* probably are the consequence of one of these diseases that has gone unrecognized. The anemia of infection, chronic renal disease, and malignancy is refractory in the sense that it is not corrected by treatment with iron, folic acid, vitamin B_{12}, or any other known hematinic agent. Nonetheless, prophylaxis with iron and folic acid usually is desirable to offset any deficiency induced by pregnancy.

It also has been our experience that women with acute pyelonephritis and severe fever, but not with asymptomatic bacteriuria or mild clinical disease, often develop overt anemia. The genesis of the anemia appears to be increased red cell destruction at the onset, coupled with impairment of production that may persist for some weeks (Cunningham and Pritchard, unpublished).

MEGALOBLASTIC ANEMIA. The prevalence of megaloblastic anemia during pregnancy varies considerably throughout the world. In the United States, overt anemia with frankly megaloblastic erythropoiesis demonstrable in the bone marrow is a rare complication of pregnancy, but in some other parts of the world it is much more frequent. In this country, megaloblastic anemia beginning during pregnancy almost always results from folic acid deficiency. It is usually found in pregnant women who consume neither fresh vegetables, especially of the uncooked green leafy variety, nor foods with a high content of animal protein. Not infrequently, women with megaloblastic anemia develop troublesome nausea, vomiting, and anorexia during pregnancy. As the folate deficiency and anemia increases, the anorexia often be-

TABLE 28-4.

THE SEQUENCE OF CHANGES INDUCED BY DIETARY DEPRIVATION OF FOLIC ACID IN A NORMAL NONPREGNANT ADULT*

SEQUENCE OF CHANGES	WEEKS AFTER STARTING FOLATE-POOR DIET
1. Low concentration of serum folate	3
2. Hypersegmentation of neutrophils	7
3. Increased urinary formiminoglutamic acid	14
4. Low folate in erythrocytes	16
5. Erythrocytic macrocytosis	18
6. Megaloblastic marrow	19
7. Anemia	19

* Data from Herbert: *Trans Assoc Am Physicians* 75:307, 1962.

comes more intense, thus aggravating the dietary deficiency. In some instances of megaloblastic anemia ethanol ingestion is either the cause or contributes to its development. The cure is to eat well and stop drinking!

Deficiency of metabolically active forms of folic acid induces many biochemical and hematologic changes. Some of these changes are listed in Table 28-4 in the order that they have been observed to develop in experimentally induced folate deficiency in man. The sequence of changes resulting from folate deficiency is probably unaltered by pregnancy. In the peripheral blood, the earliest morphologic evidence of folic acid deficiency usually is hypersegmentation of some of the neutrophils during pregnancy. As anemia develops, the newly formed erythrocytes are produced in reduced numbers and are macrocytic, even if there has been previous iron deficiency with microcytosis. With preexisting iron deficiency, the more recently formed macrocytic erythrocytes would not be detected from the measurement of the mean corpuscular volume of the erythrocytes. Careful examination of a well-prepared smear of the peripheral blood, however, usually will reveal some macrocytes. As the anemia becomes more intense, an occasional nucleated erythrocyte appears in the peripheral blood. If smears of the buffy coat from peripheral blood are made in order to concentrate the nucleated erythrocytes, several such cells with the distinct features of megaloblasts are usually demonstrable (Goodall, 1957; Pritchard, 1962). At the same time, examination of the bone marrow reveals megaloblastic erythropoiesis. As the maternal folate defiency and, in turn, the anemia become severe, thrombocytopenia, leukopenia, or both may develop.

Herbert and co-workers (1962) estimated that in the normal nonpregnant women the daily folate requirements expressed as folic acid are in the range of 50 to 100 μg per day. During pregnancy, however, the requirements for metabolically active forms of folic acid are increased. The fetus and placenta extract folate from the maternal circulation so effectively that the fetus is not anemic even when the mother is severely anemic from folate deficiency. Cases have been recorded in which the newborn hemaglobin levels were 18.0 g or more per dl, while the maternal values were as low as 3.6 g per dl (Pritchard et al., 1970).

The treatment of megaloblastic anemia induced by pregnancy should include folic acid, a well-balanced diet, and usually iron. As little as 1 mg of folic acid administered orally once a day produces a striking hematologic response. Within 3 to 6 days after the beginning of treatment, the reticulocyte count is appreciably increased, and leukopenia and thrombocytopenia are promptly corrected. Sometimes the rate of increase in hemoglobin concentration or hematocrit is disappointing, especially when compared with the usual exuberant reticulocytosis that starts soon after therapy has been begun. Severe megaloblastic anemia during pregnancy is accompanied frequently by a smaller blood volume than that of a normal pregnancy, but soon after folic acid therapy has been started the blood volume usually increases considerably. Therefore, even though hemoglobin is being rapidly added to the circulation, the hemoglobin concentration does not precisely reflect the total amount of additional hemoglobin because of the simultaneous expansion of the blood volume (Lowenstein, Pick, and Philpott, 1955; Pritchard, 1962b).

Women who develop megaloblastic anemia during pregnancy commonly are also deficient in iron, although the lack of effective erythropoiesis resulting from the folate deficiency usually produces a considerable elevation of the plasma iron. With the onset of effective erythropoiesis, however, the concentration of iron in the plasma falls precipitously. Iron may then become the limiting factor in production of hemoglobin.

Megaloblastic anemia recurs rather often in subsequent pregnancies, very likely because of repeated dietary inadequacies but also perhaps in part because of a peculiarity in the absorption or utilization of folic acid.

During the past 15 years, a great deal of attention has been devoted to the frequency of maternal folate deficiency and megaloblastic anemia in pregnancy and the puerperium, the possible role of folate deficiency in various forms of reproductive failure, and the value of prophylactic administration of folic acid throughout pregnancy and perhaps the puerperium as well. The frequency with which maternal folate deficiency is detected will vary considerably, depending in large measure upon the intensity of the search and the criteria for diagnosis.

Markedly divergent views have been expressed concerning the value of the measurement of urinary formiminoglutamic acid (FIGLU) excretion after an oral load of histidine in the detection of folate deficiency during pregnancy. The Hibbards (1964), for instance, claimed that the FIGLU test provided a reliable index of defective folic acid metabolism. They reported an excellent correlation between evaluated FIGLU excretion and morphologic evidence of megaloblastic erythropoiesis in the marrow. Chanarin and associates (1963), however, as well as Chisholm and Sharp (1964), found that in any individual case, at least, the estimation of FIGLU excretion during pregnancy was of little value in ascertaining the cause of anemia and was not a substitute for biopsy of the bone marrow.

Hibbard, Hibbard, and co-workers (1964, 1969) maintained that faulty folate metabolism was an important cause of placental abruption, abortion, and fetal malformation. They concluded that the dangers of folate deficiency to mother and fetus were so great that early prophylaxis, even before conception, was advisable in any woman at increased risk unless facilities for regular assessment of folate status were available. These investigators, and some others, claimed a high frequency of folate deficiency in women who suffered any of several forms of pregnancy wastage and proposed a causal relation. Other investigators, however, have found maternal folate deficiency to be no more common among women who experienced some form of reproductive failure than in the general obstetric population. For example, in Dallas we found little difference in maternal plasma folate levels, neutrophil hypersegmentation, and pattern of marrow erythropoiesis in mothers with placental abruption, fetal malformation, or pregnancy-induced hypertension when compared with women whose pregnancies were not thus complicated (Pritchard et al., 1971; Scott et al., 1970; Whalley et al., 1969). Fleming and associates (1975), as well as others, determined the incidence of folate deficiency to be no greater among women whose pregnancies were complicated by hemorrhage, fetal malformation, or abortion than among those with normal pregnancies. Consequently, it appears very unlikely that intensive public health measures focused on providing folic acid supplementation to eradicate all suspicions of maternal folate deficiency would have a marked effect on reducing these various kinds of pregnancy wastage.

The actual folic acid requirements of pregnancy are not known, although 400 μg per day of folic acid orally sometimes produces a hematologic remission in the severely anemic pregnant woman who is consuming a diet poor in folate, and 1000 μg per day is quite effective (Pritchard et al., 1969). The studies of Hansen and Rybo (1967) in Sweden and of Chanarin and associates (1968) in England suggest that prophylaxis, if used, with 100 μg of folic acid daily probably is adequate for populations in which megaloblastic anemia is rarely found. If, however, the pregnant women are members of a population in which megaloblastic anemia develops rather commonly during pregnancy, this level of supplementation seems inadequate, according to the studies of Willoughby and Jewell (1968).

Whether to administer folic acid routinely to all pregnant women in the United States is debatable. If, however, prenatal vitamin supplements are prescribed, folic acid should be included, since there is more evidence that the pregnant woman might suffer from a deficiency of that vitamin than of the several others that are almost always included.

Megaloblastic anemia caused by lack of vitamin B_{12} during pregnancy is quite rare. *Addisonian pernicious anemia,* in which there is failure to absorb vitamin B_{12} because of lack of intrinsic factor, is extremely uncommon in women of reproductive age. Moreover, unless women with this disease are treated with vitamin B_{12}, infertility may be a complication (Ball and Giles, 1964). There is little reason for withholding folic acid during pregnancy simply out of fear of jeopardizing the neurologic integrity of women who might be pregnant and simultaneously have unrecognized, and therefore untreated, Addisonian pernicious anemia.

Breast-fed infants of mothers who suffer vitamin B_{12} deficiency, either as the consequence of lack of intrinsic factor or because of a strict vegetarian diet, may develop megaloblastic anemia during infancy (see Chap. 13, p. 316).

ACQUIRED HEMOLYTIC ANEMIA. Women with an acquired hemolytic anemia and in whom the results of a direct Coombs test are positive sometimes demonstrate marked acceleration of the rate of hemolysis during pregnancy. Prednisone and similar compounds seem to be nearly as effective as in the nonpregnant state. Associated thrombocytopenia may also be favorably affected by such steroid therapy. Pregnancy is not a contraindication to the use of the drugs, but since the underlying disease is usually chronic and progressive, repeated pregnancies are not advisable in women with acquired hemolytic anemia caused by autoimmune disease. Chaplin and associates (1973) provided a review of pregnancy complicated by idiopathic autoimmune hemolytic anemia.

Drug-induced hemolytic anemia is occasionally encountered during pregnancy. Infrequently, the hemolysis results from an antibody that, in the presence of a drug such as quinine, may cause lysis of erythrocytes.

Especially in black women, the hemolysis may much more often be related to an inherited specific enzymatic defect of the erythrocytes, the deficiency of glucose-6-phosphate dehydrogenase (G6PD) activity. There are very many variants of this enzyme. The erythrocytes of about 2 percent of black women are appreciably deficient in enzyme activity. In such instances, both X chromosomes are genetically deficient. The heterozygous state, with one deficient and one normal X chromosome, occurs in 10 to 15 percent of black women and results in a modest deficiency of enzyme activity. Several oxidant drugs may induce hemolysis in susceptible women.

Since young erythrocytes contain more G6PD activity than do older erythrocytes, the anemia ultimately becomes stabilized. In the absence of depression of the bone marrow, the anemia is rather promptly corrected after the drug is discontinued.

Intravascular hemolysis very infrequently complicates preeclampsia-eclampsia (Pritchard et al., 1976). The precise cause of the hemolysis is unknown (see Chap. 27, p. 678). Baker and Brain (1967) have suggested that the process of microangiopathic, or fragmentation, hemolysis may be responsible. The most fulminant acquired hemolytic anemia encountered during pregnancy is caused by the exotoxin of *Clostridium perfringens,* and this condition is often fatal (see Chap. 24, p. 614).

APLASTIC OR HYPOPLASTIC ANEMIA. Although rarely encountered during pregnancy, aplastic anemia is a grave complication. The diagnosis is readily made when anemia, usually with thrombocytopenia and leukopenia, and markedly hypocellular bone marrow are demonstrated. None of the erythropoietic agents that produce remission of the other anemias is effective. Corticosteroids such as prednisone may be of some value, and large doses of testosterone or other androgenic steroids are occasionally effective in treating aplastic anemia, especially in children. The effects from the administration of very large doses of testosterone or other potent androgens during pregnancy are unknown. A female fetus would likely develop the stigmata of androgen excess.

The two greatest risks to the woman with aplastic anemia during pregnancy are hemorrhage caused by thrombocytopenia and infection. Blood transfusion will combat, but not cure, aplastic anemia. A continuous search for infection should be made, and when it is found, specific antibiotic therapy should be started promptly.

When hypoplastic anemia antedates the pregnancy, marked improvement is unlikely after interrupting the pregnancy. When the disease develops during pregnancy, termination of the pregnancy may sometimes result in remission.

Delivery should be accomplished vaginally, if possible. If there are no large lacerations or incisions of the birth canal, and if the uterus is kept firmly contracted after delivery, an associated intense thrombocytopenia is not likely to cause fatal hemorrhage.

Severe red cell aplasia of unknown cause has been observed to develop during one pregnancy, followed by complete recovery after termination of the pregnancy, and without recurrence during the second pregnancy (Aggio et al., 1977).

Hemoglobinopathies. Sickle cell anemia (SS disease), sickle cell-hemoglobin C disease (SC disease), and sickle cell β-thalassemia disease (S-thalassemia disease) are the most common of the hemoglobinopathies. Maternal morbidity and mortality, abortion, and perinatal mortality are variably increased with each of these diseases (Cunningham and Pritchard, 1979; Fort et al., 1971; Pritchard et al., 1973).

SICKLE CELL ANEMIA. The inheritance of the gene for the production of sickle, or S, hemoglobin from each parent results in sickle cell anemia. In most communities, approximately one out of every 12 black individuals has the sickle cell trait, which results from inheritance of one gene for the production of S hemoglobin and one for normal

hemoglobin A. The theoretical incidence of sickle cell anemia among blacks is one out of every 576 ($1/12 \times 1/12 \times 1/4 = 1/576$), but the disease is not nearly so common in pregnant black women, perhaps only one-fourth to one-third of the theoretically calculated frequency. Undoubtedly, there are many deaths from this disease during childhood or early adulthood, and the fertility of women with sickle cell anemia is reduced.

Although usually made earlier, the diagnosis of sickle cell anemia is occasionally first made during pregnancy. Pregnancy is a serious burden to the woman with the disease, for the anemia often becomes more intense, the attacks of pain—the so-called pain crises—usually become more frequent, and infections and pulmonary dysfunction are more common. Fetal wastage is usually high; about one-half of all known pregnancies in women with sickle cell anemia have commonly terminated in abortion, stillbirth, or neonatal death (Fort et al., 1971; Pritchard et al., 1973).

Adequate care of women with sickle cell anemia or other sickle cell hemoglobinopathies in pregnancy necessitates close observation with careful evaluation of all symptoms, physical fingings, and laboratory studies. One rather common danger is that the woman may categorically be considered to be suffering from "sickle cell crises." As a result, ectopic pregnancy, placental abruption, pyelonephritis, and other serious obstetric problems that cause pain or anemia or both may be overlooked. The term *sickle cell crisis*, if used at all, is to be applied only after all other possible causes of pain or reduction in hemoglobin concentration have been excluded.

In our experience, in the absence of infection or nutritional deficiency, the hemoglobin concentration does not fall much below 7 g per dl, a level at or above which pregnant women with sickle cell anemia usually have no symptoms from the low level of hemoglobin. Since these women maintain their hemoglobin concentration by great augmentation of erythropoiesis to compensate for the markedly shortened life span of the erythrocytes, any factor that impairs erythropoiesis or increases destruction of erythrocytes results in aggravation of the anemia. The folic acid requirements during pregnancy complicated by sickle cell anemia are considerable. Since the dietary intake of folic acid may be inadequate, especially during episodes of pain, supplementary folic acid is usually indicated; 1 mg per day appears to be appropriate.

Labor with sickle cell disease should be managed essentially in the same way as with cardiac disease. The woman should be kept comfortable but not oversedated. In all cases, compatible blood should be readily available. If a difficult vaginal delivery or cesarean section is contemplated, the hemoglobin concentration should be raised by careful administration of packed erythrocytes. At the same time, care must be taken to prevent circulatory overload with heart failure and pulmonary edema. Continuous oxygen therapy, furthermore, should be insitituted during times of increased oxygen need.

According to Hendrickse and Watson-Williams (1966), acute sequestration of sickled erythrocytes is common late in pregnancy, during labor and delivery, and in the early puerperium. Dangerous anemia rapidly appears as a consequence and is accompanied by an increase in the size of the liver and of the spleen, unless the spleen has been destroyed previously by fibrosis. The acute sequestration is usually accompanied by intense bone pain and can be anticipated by frequently monitoring the hemoglobin concentration at the time of risk. Whenever the hemoglobin dropped below 6.0 g per dl or decreased at a rate of 2 g or more per 24 hours, Hendrickse and Watson-Williams recommended exchange transfusion with donor blood known to contain only hemoglobin A. The advantages derived from reducing the population of erythrocytes containing S hemoglobin through exchange transfusion, however, must be weighed against the dangers.

For some time, we administered transfusions of whole blood or of packed normal erythrocytes only to replace excessive blood loss or to augment circulating erythrocyte volume when anemia is very severe, that is, with a hemoglobin concentration of less than 7.0 g per dl. Before delivery, however, at least 1 liter of appropriately cross-matched blood was available, and a well-functioning intravenous infusion system was established. Excessive blood loss was promptly replaced with normal whole blood. We have managed in this manner a large number of pregnancies complicated by sickle cell anemia with no maternal deaths. Pregnancy wastage from either abortion or perinatal death approached 50 percent, however (Pritchard et al., 1973). The merits of transfusion of fresh erythrocytes that contain no hemoglobin S is being systematically investigated at Parkland Memorial Hospital. The results of these investigations are presented subsequently.

Hendrickse and Watson-Williams (1966) have advocated heparin therapy in patients with sickle cell anemia who developed severe bone pain during late pregnancy or the puerperium. The benefits derived from heparin administration, however, have not been firmly established. Dextran infusion was originally claimed to reduce bone pain and marrow infarction, but a well-controlled study subsequently failed to demonstrate any benefit over that provided by hydration with aqueous glucose solution (Barnes et al., 1965).

Because of the chronic debility from sickle cell anemia, the further complications caused by pregnancy, and the predictably shortened life span of these patients, sterilization, or at least a very effective means of contraception, is indicated, even in women of low parity. Oral contraceptives in the form of estrogen-progestin combinations probably are contraindicated in women with sickle cell anemia since erythrocyte sequestration and vascular occlusion inherent in the disease might be intensified.

SICKLE CELL-HEMOGLOBIN C DISEASE. Although about 1 out of 12 American blacks possesses the gene for production of hemoglobin S, only about 1 in 40 carries the gene for hemoglobin C. Therefore, the probability of this genetic combination in a black couple is about 1 in 600, and the probability of their child's inheriting the gene for hemoglobin S and an allelic gene for hemoglobin C is 1 in 4. As the consequence of these genetic frequencies, about 1 out of every 2,000 $(1/12 \times 1/40 \times 1/4)$ pregnant black women can be expected to have sickle cell-hemoglobin C disease, barring any significant mortality either before or during the years of reproductivity. We have found the disease to occur at this level of frequency among pregnant black women.

In nonpregnant women, the morbidity and mortality from the sickle cell-hemoglobin C disease are appreciably lower than those of sickle cell anemia. During pregnancy and the puerperium, however, the morbidity and mortality are increased greatly (Curtis, 1959; Fullerton et al., 1965; Pritchard et al., 1973). Attacks of severe bone pain and episodes of "pneumonitis" are fairly common during these times. The "pneumonitis" appears to be related to embolization of necrotic bone marrow. In an 18-year anterospective study at Parkland Memorial Hospital, the maternal mortality rate for a large series of pregnancies in women with sickle cell-hemoglobin C disease was close to 2 percent, and one out of eight pregnancies resulted in abortion, stillbirth, or neonatal death. Thus the perinatal mortality rate was somewhat greater than that of the general population but was nowhere nearly as great as with sickle cell anemia.

As in other pregnancies complicated by overt hemolytic anemia, the need for metabolically active forms of folic acid in women with sickle cell-hemoglobin C disease is increased, especially when anorexia is present. Iron deficiency is less common than in the general population of pregnant women, but it occasionally occurs, especially if the mother has not received transfusions previously. Therefore, supplementation with folic acid and in some instances with iron is of value. Whenever the hemoglobin concentration drops below 8.0 g per dl, a thorough search for the cause or causes is essential. The guidelines used for blood transfusion have been similar to those for sickle cell anemia.

Fullerton and co-workers (1962) in Africa urged that pregnant women with sickle cell-hemoglobin C disease receive iron and folic acid routinely, exchange transfusions with blood containing only hemoglobin A whenever a sudden decrease in hemoglobin concentration develops, and heparinization for severe bone pain to try to prevent embolization of necrotic marrow. They estimated the "natural" maternal mortality rate for pregnancy complicated by sickle cell-hemoglobin C disease in Africa to be 10 percent. They claimed the application of these several measures combined with good general medical care, including antimalarial therapy, to have been responsible for reducing their maternal mortality rate to 2.4 percent.

The frequent morbidity and relatively high mortality during pregnancy and the puerperium in women with sickle cell-hemoglobin C disease warrant limitation of family size. Erythrocyte transfusion studies in progress at Parkland Memorial Hospital are described below. To date, maternal morbidity, especially pain and "pneumonitis," has been appreciably less in women with sickle cell-hemoglobin C disease so transfused. Moreover, the fetal outcome has been rewarding.

SICKLE CELL-THALASSEMIA DISEASE. The inheritance of the gene for hemoglobin S from one parent and the allelic gene for β-thalassemia from the other results in sickle cell-β-thalassemia disease. Our experience with 37 pregnancies implies that the perinatal mortality and morbidity of this disease are similar to those of sickle cell-hemoglobin C disease (Pritchard et al., 1973). Maternal morbidity and mortality perhaps are somewhat less. Our recommendations for prenatal care, labor, and delivery, and the restriction on future pregnancies are the same in sickle cell-thalassemia, sickle cell-hemoglobin C disease, and sickle cell anemia.

Prophylactic Red Cell Transfusions in Pregnancies Complicated by Sickle Cell Hemoglobinopathies. As of the end of 1979 we had transfused prophylactically throughout pregnancy 40 women with sickle cell (SS) anemia, sickle cell-hemoglobin C (SC) disease, or sickle cell-beta thalassemia

(S-thal) disease. Once the diagnoses of pregnancy and of a sickle cell hemoglobinopathy were confirmed, recently collected packed red cells that contained no hemoglobin S were transfused in amounts and frequencies sufficient to reduce and maintain the percentage of red cells that would sickle after incubation in sodium metabisulfite solution to no more than 60 percent and to keep the hematocrit at 25 or higher. When the hematocrit was low, as was commonly the case with sickle cell anemia, most often simple transfusions of packed red cells were carefully administered after establishing a brisk diuresis by giving furosemide, 50 mg, intravenously. When the hematocrit was higher, as it commonly was with SC or S-thal disease, exchange transfusion was usually employed (Cunningham and Pritchard, 1979).

Maternal mortality was zero and maternal morbidity from the hemoglobinopathy was minimal among the 19 women with sickle cell anemia, 19 with SC disease, and 2 with S-thal disease. The degree of relief from debilitating sickle cell anemia provided one woman by transfusion with normal red cells during pregnancy is apparent in Figure 28-3.

Pregnancy wastage was limited to one spontaneous abortion and one stillborn out of 40 pregnancies. The stillbirth was associated with fulminant preeclampsia and severe heart failure in a woman with sickle cell anemia.

Although the perinatal mortality was remarkably low when compared to previous experiences, there was worrisome evidence of a compromised intrauterine environment in the form of fetal growth retardation, meconium staining of amnionic fluid, and during labor ominous decelerations in fetal heart rate. Moreover, morbidity from the transfusions, especially alloimmunization, has proved troublesome. Nonetheless, it has been concluded tentatively that both the mother with sickle cell hemoglobinopathy and her fetus are likely to benefit from prophylactic transfusions of normal donor red cells administered during one pregnancy according to the protocol employed in their

study. Sterilization has been encouraged after one such pregnancy with a successful outcome.

HEMOGLOBIN C AND C-THALASSEMIA DISEASES. Pregnancy and homozygous hemoglobin C disease or hemoglobin C-beta-thalassemia disease appear to be rather benign associations (Cunningham and Pritchard, unpublished; Smith and Krevans, 1959). The hemolytic anemia is usually but not always mild. If severe, it is likely to be the consequence of folic acid deficiency or some other superimposed cause. Supplementation routinely with folic acid and with iron, unless transfused, is likely to prove of value in pregnant women with any hemoglobinopathy.

SICKLE CELL TRAIT. The inheritance of the gene for the production of S hemoglobin from one parent and for A hemoglobin from the other results in sickle cell trait. In this circumstance, the amount of S hemoglobin produced is distinctly less than the amount of A hemoglobin. The frequency of red cell sickling among black individuals is about 8.5 percent (Schneider and co-workers, 1976).

Erythrocytes in smears of blood from women with sickle cell trait usually appear normal unless the blood has previously been markedly depleted of oxygen to produce sickled forms.

An extensive study with matched controls of the effect of sickle cell trait on pregnancy has been reported by Whalley (1963, 1964) and by Pritchard (1973) and their co-workers. Sickle cell trait did not influence unfavorably the frequency of abortion, perinatal mortality, low birth weight, or pregnancy-induced hypertension (Table 28-5). Infection of the urinary tract, however, was about twice as common in the group with sickle cell trait. Further investigations revealed that twice as many pregnant women with sickle cell trait had asymptomatic bacteriuria, as did black women whose erythrocytes did not sickle. One-third of the group with sickle trait and bacteriuria developed clinically evident pyelonephritis later in the antepartum period un-

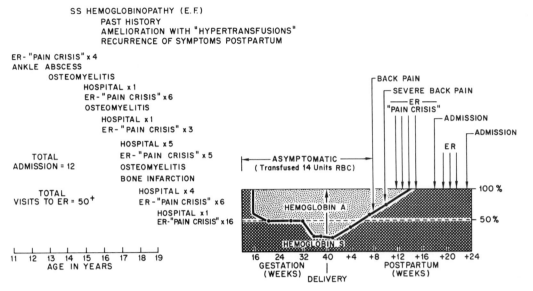

FIG. 28-3. E. F., sickle cell anemia. Debility before her first pregnancy is summarized on the left. To the right, the reduction in hemoglobin S level as the consequence of transfusion of 14 units of packed red cells, and the recurrence of severe pain 9 weeks after delivery are emphasized (ER = Emergency Room). (From Cunningham, Pritchard. *Am J Obstet Gynecol* 135:994, 1979)

less the bacteriuria was previously eradicated by appropriate therapy. Therefore, sickle cell trait should not be considered a deterrant to pregnancy on the basis of increased risks to the mother. However, the probability for a debilitating sickle cell hemoglobinopathy in her offspring is one in four whenever the father carries a gene for the production of an abnormal hemoglobin or for beta thalassemia.

HEMOGLOBIN C TRAIT. About 2.5 percent of the black population possesses the gene for producing hemoglobin C (Schneider et al., 1976). With hemoglobin C trait, the hemoglobin C fraction is less than hemoglobin A. In our experience, hemoglobin C trait does not predispose to pathologic pregnancies.

HEMOGLOBINOPATHY IN NEWBORN. The hemolytic anemia characteristic of these hemoglobinopathies is not operational in utero or at birth since most of the hemoglobin in the red cells is fetal (F) hemoglobin. After birth, as more and more newly synthesized

red cells contain more and more abnormal hemoglobin, the disease becomes clinically apparent. Kramer and colleagues (1979) have confirmed that newborn infants with sickle cell anemia, sickle cell hemoglobin C disease and homozygous hemoglobin C disease can be accurately identified at birth by hemoglobin electrophoresis done in uncontaminated cord blood using cellulose acetate support medium and buffer at pH 8.4 plus citrate agar gel and buffer at pH 6.2.

GENETIC COUNSELING. Identification of the more common hemoglobinopathies and their trait forms involves relatively simple laboratory procedures, and the genetic aspects of these diseases are straightforward. Therefore, genetic counseling can be readily provided. One out of every four children, on the average, will be afflicted with the disease whenever both parents have a trait form, as pointed out above. If one parent has the hemoglobinopathy and the other only the trait form, one-half of their children can be expected to inherit the hemoglobinopathy

TABLE 28-5.

PREGNANCY EXPERIENCES OF BLACK WOMEN WITH SICKLE CELL TRAIT COMPARED TO BLACK WOMEN WHOSE ERYTHROCYTES DO NOT SICKLE

| | BIRTH WEIGHT (G) | | PERINATAL DEATHS | APGAR SCORE (1 MINUTE) | | BACTERI-URIA* | PREG-NANCY HYPER-TENSION | HEMATO-CRIT |
	Mean	<2,501		Mean	<6			
1972								
Sickle trait	3,041	53/350	7/350	8.3	(6.1)	21/199	30/106	35.9
	(S.E.† 34.8)	(15.1)	(2.00)			(10.6)	(28.3)	
Sickle negative	3,041	60/379	8/379	8.2	(8.6)	10/198	35/105	36.6
	(S.E. 32.5)	(15.8)	(2.11)			(5.1)	(33.3)	
1960–1963								
Sickle trait	3,097‡	179/1,359	45/1,359	—	—	—	—	36.6
	(S.E. 17.1)	(13.2)	(3.31)					
Sickle negative	3,039‡	194/1,265	42/1,265	—	—	—	—	37.1
	(S.E. 17.6)	(15.3)	(3.32)					

From Pritchard, Scott, Whalley, Cunningham, and Mason: *Am J Obstet Gynecol* 117:662, 1973.
* 100,000 organisms per milliliter of urine
† S.E. = standard error
‡ P. = <0.05 and >0.01
Numbers in parentheses indicate percent.

and the other half the trait form. If both parents have a hemoglobinopathy, so will all their children.

The fetus genetically destined to demonstrate a sickle hemoglobinopathy may be identified if fetal erythrocytes can be obtained. Identification may also be made using restriction endonuclease technics applied to amniocytes (Phillips et al., 1980).

CONGENITAL SPHEROCYTOSIS. This abnormality is rarely encountered during pregnancy. If erythropoiesis is not impaired, the women have no major difficulties during pregnancy. In the case of congenital spherocytic anemia, splenectomy before pregnancy results in considerable reduction in the intensity of the hemolysis and, in turn, the anemia. The infant may inherit congenital spherocytosis and soon become anemic.

Thalassemias. All varieties of thalassemia are inherited as an autosomal recessive trait. Therefore, if both members of a couple are heterozygous for the same condition, the

probabilities are one in four that an offspring will be homozygous for that condition, two in four that he will be heterozygous, and one in four that he will not be affected. The genetically determined hematologic disorders that are classified as thalassemias are characterized by impaired production of one or more of the peptide chains that are normal components of globin. The impairment of globin peptide chain synthesis, coupled with the relative excess production of normal partner chains which precipitate within the red cell, is responsible for abnormalities in the red cells and the hemoglobin they contain, and for increased red cell destruction.

The various forms of thalassemia are classified according to the globin chain which is deficient in amount compared to its partner chain. The two major forms of thalassemia involve either impaired production of alpha peptide chains causing α-thalassemia, or of beta-chains to cause β-thalassemia. Detailed considerations of the molecular biology of hemoglobin production, including the thalassemia syndromes, have been provided by

Banks (1978), by Alger and co-workers (1979), and by Forget (1979).

α-THALASSEMIA. In the homozygous form of α-thalassemia, which genetically in white and Oriental individuals is the consequence of the deletion of four genes, no alpha chains are produced. The hemoglobin in the fetus consists chiefly of hemoglobin Barts, the globin of which is made up of four gamma peptide chains rather than two alpha and two gamma chains that characterize normal fetal hemoglobin (hemoglobin F). Hemoglobin Barts has an appreciably increased affinity for oxygen. The fetus dies in utero with the typical clinical features of hydrops fetalis.

The deletion of three genes may be compatible with extrauterine life; the condition is referred to as hemoglobin H disease. The abnormal red cells contain a mixture of hemoglobin H, the globin of which consists of four beta chains, and hemoglobin Barts. There is markedly increased red cell destruction presumably as the consequence of the spleen attempting to remove precipitated hemoglobin from the red cells.

A deletion of two genes results in α-thalassemia minor which is characterized by minimal to moderate hypochromic microcytic anemia.

The genetics of α-thalassemia in black individuals is less clear. Moreover, the disease is milder with α-thalassemia minor being a very mild disorder.

β-THALASSEMIA. In the homozygous state, which has been called thalassemia major, Cooley's anemia, or Mediterranean anemia, beta chain synthesis is markedly impaired. The great excess of alpha chains polymerize and precipitate within the markedly abnormal red cells. Severe hemolytic anemia characterizes the disease. The infant is little affected at birth since gamma chain production, and in turn the formation of hemoglobin F is not impaired. By 3 months of age, as production of hemoglobin F falls, the infant becomes severely anemic. He usually can survive thereafter only when trans-fused frequently. Girls who survive to adulthood often are infertile.

β-thalassemia minor, the heterozygous state, is characterized by mild to moderate hypochromic microcytic anemia. There seldom is any associated debility. The anemia of β-thalassemia minor is probably caused by impaired erythropoiesis coupled with slightly accelerated destruction of some erythrocytes. The hemoglobin concentration is typically 8 to 10 g per dl late in the second trimester, with an increase to between 9 and 11 g per dl near term, as compared with a hemoglobin level of 10 to 12 g per dl in the nonpregnant state (Alger et al., 1979; Freedman, 1969; Pritchard, 1962a). There is usually augmentation of erythropoiesis during pregnancy, as in normal women.

There is no specific therapy for β-thalassemia minor during pregnancy. Most often, the outcome for mother and fetus is satisfactory (Pritchard, 1962a; Smith et al., 1975). Blood transfusions are very seldom indicated except for hemorrhage. Iron and folic acid in prophylactic daily doses of about 30 mg and 1 mg, respectively, may be of value. Any disease that depresses the function of the bone marrow or increases destruction of erythrocytes naturally intensifies the anemia. Infections, therefore, should be promptly and adequately treated.

ANTENATAL DIAGNOSIS. Since the homozygous state for α-thalassemia is invariably fatal before or at the time of birth, the problem is not the same as for the offspring who is homozygous for β-thalassemia. Reticulocytes are capable of synthesizing the peptide chains of globin and the normal ratios for beta and gamma chain synthesis have been established for various gestational ages. β-thalassemia major is characterized by severe underproduction of beta chains. Fetal red cells may be obtained by technics described in Chapter 14 (p. 347). Alger and co-workers (1979), using such red cells, have reported considerable success in correctly identifying the presence or absence of the homozygous state. Obtaining the fetal red cells, however, has been accompanied by a fetal loss of about 10 percent.

Other Hematologic Disorders

Polycythemia. Polycythemia during pregnancy is usually related to hypoxia, most often resulting from congenital cardiac disease or a pulmonary disorder. If the polycythemia is severe, the probability of a successful outcome of the pregnancy is remote.

Polycythemia vera and pregnancy rarely coexist. Ruch and Klein (1964) described a case in which the hematocrit reading in the nonpregnant state was as high as 63. During each of two pregnancies, however, the hematocrit ranged from a low of about 35 during the second trimester to about 44 at term. Fetal loss seems to be high in women with polycythemia vera.

Thrombocytopenic Purpura. Thrombocytopenic purpura may appear clinically to be idiopathic or, more often, to be associated with aplastic anemia, acquired hemolytic anemia, eclampsia or severe preeclampsia, consumptive coagulopathy related to placental abruption or similar hyofibrinogenemic states, lupus erythematosus, megaloblastic anemia caused by severe folate deficiency, drugs, infections, allergies, or radiation.

A pregnant woman with idiopathic thrombocytopenic purpura should be under careful medical supervision. The thrombocytopenia is the consequence of an immune process and now is usually referred to as immune or autoimmune, rather than idiopathic, thrombocytopenia. Prednisone and similar corticosteroids have produced somewhat inconsistent results; they appear to be of value in correcting the abnormal capillary fragility, as well as often increasing the maternal platelet count. During a period of uncontrollable bleeding, or when major surgery is to be performed, transient improvement in platelet function may sometimes be achieved in the mother by transfusing platelets carefully collected from *ABO compatible*, very fresh blood.

Splenectomy during advanced pregnancy typically necessitates delivery of the fetus to provide adequate surgical exposure of the splenic pedicle.

Transfer of a platelet agglutinin from the mother to the fetus most often is the cause of passively acquired thrombocytopenia in the newborn infant (see Chap. 38, p. 977).

Territo and associates (1973) have recommended cesarean section if the maternal platelet count is less than 100,000, since the fetus is likely to be thrombocytopenic. It remains to be established that otherwise uncomplicated, orderly labor and minimally traumatic delivery lead to greater morbidity in the mother and the infant than does prophylactic cesarean section on a woman with thrombocytopenia (Laros and Sweet, 1975). Moreover, neither an acceptable maternal platelet count nor cesarean section provides absolute assurance that the fetus-infant will not hemorrhage as the consequence of severe throbocytopenia as exemplified by the infant in Figure 28-4 and described now:

The multiparous mother was troubled intermittently for many years by thrombocytopenia even though she had undergone splenectomy. A previous infant bled profusely following circumcision after which he was documented to be severely thrombocytopenic. The mother again became severely thrombocytopenic during her last pregnancy. The thrombocytopenia was corrected as long as she took prednisone. Her platelet count exceeded 100,000 at the time of delivery. Because of the possibility that the fetus might be thrombocytopenic and her desire for sterilization, it was elected to effect delivery by cesarean section. This was accomplished with no serious problems for the mother. However, the infant demonstrated cephalohematomas over the occipital bone and both parietal bones, the region of the infant's head which had been manipulated by the operator's hand to deliver the head from behind the maternal symphysis through the uterine and abdominal incisions. The platelet count was 17,000 in cord blood and dropped promptly to as low as 3000 per mm.[3] Treatment consisted of corticosteroids, platelet transfusions, and exchange transfusion in a desperate attempt to remove platelet antibody. The infant survived the hemorrhage and the treatment.

Ayromlooi (1978) and Scott et al. (1980) have recommended that once the cervix has dilated sufficiently during labor blood be obtained from the fetal scalp for a platelet count and, if the count is dangerously low, deliver the fetus by cesarean section. Otherwise allow labor to continue. Both the safety of early labor and safety of scalp sampling in the presence of severe thrombocytopenia need more careful evaluation before this approach can be generally accepted.

THROMBOTIC THROMBOCYTOPENIC PURPURA. This rare entity is characterized by thrombocytopenia, fever, neurologic abnormalities, renal impairment, and hemolytic anemia. Thrombotic thrombocytopenic purpura should not be confused with the uncommon case of preeclampsia-eclampsia complicated by thrombocytopenia and overt hemolysis (see Chap. 27, p. 677).

The classic histologic lesions of thrombotic thrombocytopenic purpura are thrombi consisting mostly of platelets and fibrin which can be found in the small vessels of virtually every tissue. Exchange transfusion, transfusion with plasma, and plasmapheris have improved remarkably the outcome of this once highly fatal disease. Lian and co-workers (1979) have presented evidence of a platelet aggregating factor in plasmas from three patients with thrombotic thrombocytopenic purpura, two of whom were pregnant and survived after transfusion with plasma. They suspect that there was a lack of a normal plasma inhibitor of the platelet aggregating factor in the diseased individuals.

The factor or factors responsible for thrombotic thrombocytopenic purpura do not appear to cross the placenta and incite comparable lesions in the fetus. At least Wurzel (1979) was unable to find such lesions in a fetus whose mother died of thrombotic thrombocytopenic purpura.

INHERITED COAGULATION DEFECTS. Obstetric hemorrhage is rarely caused by an inherited coagulation defect. The possibility of *von Willebrand's disease* probably has been

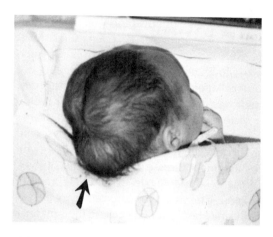

FIG. 28-4. Newborn infant with extensive cephalohematomas, especially over the occipital bone (arrow). The mother had chronic idiopathic (autoimmune) thrombocytopenic purpura which was treated with prednisone. Her platelet count at the time of cesarean section was 115,000 per mm^3; the infant's count was as low as 3000 per mm^3.

considered most often in women with bleeding suggestive of a chronic disorder of coagulation. The classic "autosomal dominant" form is usually symptomatic in the heterzygous state. A less common but clinically more severe "autosomal recessive" form is manifest when inherited from both parents each of whom demonstrates little or no disease. Von Willebrand's disease is characterized clinically by easy bruising, mucosal hemorrhage, and excessive bleeding with trauma, including surgery. Its laboratory features are a prolonged bleeding time, prolonged partial thromboplastin time, decreased factor VIII (immunologic activity as well as coagulation-promoting activity), and inability of platelets in plasma from an affected person to react to a variety of stimuli. Von Willebrand's disease is probably a heterogeneous syndrome with various underlying molecular defects (Zimmerman and co-workers, 1979).

Noller and associates (1973) summarized 17 cases, including four of their own, of pregnancy complicated by von Willebrand's disease. The hemostatic defects may improve during pregnancy. If factor VIII activity is very low, the administration of factor VIII-rich cryoprecipitate is recommended. Most persons with von Willibrand's disease are heterozygous and have only a mild bleeding disorder. When both parents have the disorder, their offspring may, if homozygous, develop a serious bleeding disorder. Fetoscopy has been used to obtain fetal blood which served to identify the fetus as not having severe von Willebrand's disease (Hoyer et al., 1979).

Classic hemophilia is exceedingly rare in women. The asymptomatic carrier of hemophilia may be identified because their plasmas contain a disproportionately high concentration of antihemophilic factor when measured immunologically compared to its coagulation-promoting activity. The mother who is a carrier of hemophilia has a gene defect on one of her X chromosomes and the male fetus who inherits that X chromosome will develop hemophilia. Identification of a female fetus excludes hemophilia except when the father has hemophilia *and* the mother is a carrier. The affected fetus may be identified at midpregnancy whenever fetal blood can be obtained employing fetoscopy (Mibashan et al., 1979).

Leukemia. In recent years some startling outcomes have been observed for women who have leukemia and conceived. Most of the cytotoxic drugs used in treatment cross the placenta, and therefore it was predicted generally that these agents would severely affect the fetus. To date this does not appear to be the case, at least during the second and third trimesters, although these agents may cause abortion or fetal abnormalities when given during the first trimester. Several cases of congenital leukemia in infants born of nonleukemic mothers have been recorded although no case of transmission of leukemia to the fetus has been authenticated. Levine and Collea (1979) have considered the problem of pregnancy complicated by chronic granulocytic leukemia and Lilleyman and associates (1977) and Bitran and Roth (1976) have done the same for acute leukemia.

Hodgkin's Disease. There are no convincing data that pregnancy adversely affects the disease. Holmes and Holmes (1978) have analyzed pregnancy outcomes when either the expectant mother or the father had the disease; the great majority of the outcomes for the 93 pregnancies were satisfactory.

Chapman and associates (1979) have observed ovarian failure to be a rather common accompaniment of chemotherapy for Hodgkin's disease. Twenty-five of 41 women were identified clinically and by endocrinologic studies to have ovarian failure.

DISEASES OF THE HEART

Heart disease is estimated to occur in approximately 1 percent of pregnancies. Rheumatic heart disease formerly accounted for the great majority of the cases but in recent years congenital heart disease has become more prevalent. Prophylaxis with antimicrobial agents has reduced the cardiac complications of rheumatic fever, and better medical management, together with a number of newer surgical technics, has enabled more girls with congenital heart disease to live into the childbearing age. Cardiac disease from hypertension contributes few cases of organic heart disease in pregnancy, whereas other varieties, such as coronary, thyroid, syphilitic, and kyphoscoliotic cardiac disease, cor pulmonale, contrictive pericarditis, various forms of heart block, and isolated myocarditis are even less common.

Heart disease may be a very serious complication of pregnancy leading to maternal death, but as will be pointed out, in the great majority of instances it need not be so.

Diagnosis. As discussed at some length in Chapter 9 (p. 238), many of the physiologic changes of normal pregnancy tend to make the diagnosis of heart disease much more difficult than it is in the nonpregnant state. For example, in normal pregnancy, systolic heart murmurs that are functional are quite common. Moreover, as the uterus enlarges and the diaphragm is elevated, the heart is elevated and rotated in such a way that the apex is moved laterally while the heart is somewhat closer to the anterior chest wall. Cardiac filling is increased, furthermore, accounting for the greater stroke volume during much of pregnancy. Respiratory effort in normal pregnancy is accentuated, at times suggesting dyspnea. Presumably, this change is brought about in large part by a stimulatory effect of progesterone on the respiratory center. Edema, a further source of confusion, is often prevalent in the lower extremities during the latter half of pregnancy. Therefore, systolic murmurs and edema, as well as changes that suggest cardiac enlargement and dyspnea, are commonplace in normal pregnancy. It becomes obvious that the physician must be quite careful not to diagnose heart disease during pregnancy when none exists, but not to fail to detect and treat appropriately heart disease when it does exist.

Burwell and Metcalfe (1958) list the following criteria, any one of which confirms the diagnosis of heart disease in pregnancy: (1) a diastolic, presystolic, or continuous heart murmur; (2) unequivocal cardiac enlargement; (3) a loud, harsh systolic murmur, especially if associated with a thrill; and (4) severe arrhythmia. Patients fulfilling none of these criteria rarely have heart disease. A history of rheumatic fever accompanied by the changes of normal pregnancy just summarized does not suffice for the diagnosis of valvular cardiac disease.

Prognosis. The likelihood of a favorable outcome for the mother with heart disease and her child-to-be depends upon (1) the functional capacity of her heart, (2) the likelihood of other complications that increase further the cardiac load during pregnancy and the puerperium, (3) the quality of medical care provided, and (4) the psychologic and socioeconomic capabilities of the expectant mother, her family, and the community. The last item may assume great importance, since a favorable outcome for the pregnancy is often achieved even in instances of markedly impaired cardiac function if the mother, her family, and the community will accept the need for, and provide an environment suitable for, a very sedentary life. For some women, these requirements may amount to hospitalization with complete bed rest throughout pregnancy and the puerperium.

The prognosis and recommended treatment of cardiac disease have been influenced inappropriately in some instances by certain physiologic measurements, the imprecise or incorrect interpretation of which led the authors to conclude that there was a peak maternal hemodynamic burden some weeks before term. Considerable emphasis has been placed, for example, on an apparent reduction in cardiac output after the thirty-second week of pregnancy (see Chap. 9, p. 238). The misconception persists that cardiac decompensation would seldom occur after this time, a belief not well supported by clinical observation. The decrease in maternal blood volume during the last weeks of pregnancy reported by some has been similarly considered to bring about a decrease in cardiac work. Most reported measurements, however, fail to identify a decrease in blood volume of any appreciable magnitude during the last several weeks. It is important that the physician understand that cardiac failure can develop during the last few weeks of the antepartum period, during labor, and during the puerperium. Indeed, of 542 women whose pregnancies were complicated by heart disease reported by Etheridge and Peperell (1977), 10 died with 8 of the deaths occuring during the puerperium.

Classification of Patients. There is no clinically applicable test for accurately measuring the functional capacity of the heart. In general, the best index is provided by the classification of the New York Heart Association, which is based on the patient's history of past and present disability and is uninfluenced by the presence or absence of physical signs:

Class I. Patients with cardiac disease and *no limitation of physical activity*. Patients in this class do not have symptoms of cardiac insufficiency, nor do they experience anginal pain.

Class II. Patients with cardiac disease and *slight limitation of physical activity*. These patients are comfortable at rest, but if ordinary physical activity is undertaken, discomfort results in the form of excessive fatigue, palpitation, dyspnea, or anginal pain.

Class III. Patients with cardiac disease and *marked limitation of physical activity*. These patients are comfortable at rest, but less than ordinary activity causes discomfort in the form of excessive fatigue, palpitation, dyspnea, or anginal pain.

Class IV. Patients with cardiac disease and *inability to perform any physical activity without discomfort*. Symptoms of cardiac insufficiency or of the anginal syndrome may occur even at rest, and if any physical activity is undertaken, discomfort is increased.

Hamilton and Thomson (1941) appropriately tabulated complications, previous or current, that point toward an unfavorable outcome for the pregnancy: (1) history of previous heart failure exclusive of failure at the time of acute rheumatic carditis; (2) prior heart disease and recent active rheumatic fever; (3) atrial fibrillation; (4) hemoptysis; (5) overt enlargement of any of the cardiac chambers; (6) aortic stenosis; (7) cardiac disease causing cyanosis.

General Management. The treatment of heart disease in pregnancy is dictated by the functional capacity of the heart. In all pregnant women, especially those with cardiac disease, excessive weight gain, *abnormal* retention of fluid, and anemia should be prevented. Increased bodily bulk increases the cardiac work, and anemia with its compensatory rise in cardiac output also predisposes to cardiac failure. The development of pregnancy-induced hypertension is hazardous, for

in this circumstance cardiac output can be maintained only by an increase in cardiac work commensurate with the increase in blood pressure. At the same time, hypotension is undesirable, especially in women with septal defects that allow shunting of blood.

MANAGEMENT OF CLASSES I AND II. With rare exceptions, women in class I and most in class II may be allowed to go through pregnancy. Throughout pregnancy and the puerperium, special attention should be directed toward the prevention and the early recognition of heart failure. A specific routine that assures adequate rest should be outlined for each patient. The recommendations of Hamilton and Thomson (1941) are still pertinent: The pregnant woman must rest in bed 10 hours each night and, in addition, must lie down for half an hour after each meal. Light housework and walking about on the level may be permitted. The patient should do no heavy housework or shopping. If possible, another person should remain in the house throughout the pregnancy to help with the housework. In essence, the pregnant woman must learn to spare herself all unnecessary effort and must rest as much as possible. Not infrequently, infection has proved to be an important factor in precipitating cardiac failure. Each woman should receive instructions to avoid contact with others who have respiratory infections, including the common cold, and to report at once any evidence of an infection.

The onset of congestive heart failure is often gradual and may be detected if attention is continually directed to certain particular signs. The first warning sign of cardiac failure is likely to be persistent rales at the base of the lungs, frequently with a cough. To be significant, the rales must still be audible after the patient has taken two or three deep breaths, for the rales that are sometimes heard in normal pregnant women disappear after one or two deep inspirations. A sudden diminution in the woman's ability to carry out her household duties, increasing dyspnea on exertion, attacks of smothering with cough, and hemoptysis are other signals warning of serious heart failure, as are progressive edema and tachycardia. Measurements appropriately made of the vital capacity at each visit are of value, for a sudden decrease may denote cardiac failure. Although the program outlined for the early detection of cardiac failure may seem scarcely applicable to patients in class I or class II, since they rarely decompensate during pregnancy, the interests of the mother and the fetus dictate that all cases of cardiac disease in pregnancy be regarded as at risk of possible decompensation.

Hospitalization before delivery of women with classes I and II cardiac disease is common practice. Delivery should be accomplished vaginally unless other obstetric complications require cesarean section. In spite of the physical effort inherent in labor and vaginal delivery, less morbidity and mortality have been recorded when delivery has been so accomplished.

Relief from pain and apprehension without undue depression of the infant or the mother is especially important during labor and delivery of women with cardiac disease. For the multiparous woman with a soft, effaced, somewhat dilated cervix, in whom little soft-tissue resistance is offered by the vagina and perineum, analgesics in moderate doses usually provide satisfactory pain relief. For women, especially nulliparas, in whom cervical dilatation, descent of the presenting part, and delivery will require greater force over a longer time, continuous epidural anesthesia often proves valuable for reducing pain and apprehension. The major danger of conduction anesthesia is maternal hypotension. Hypotension may be rapidly fatal in women with cardiac shunts, in whom flow may be reversed with blood passing from the right to the left side of the heart or the aorta, thereby bypassing the lungs. The technics of continuous conduction anesthesia are considered in Chapter 18.

For cesarean section, the combination of thiopental, succinylcholine, and nitrous oxide with at least 30 percent oxygen, with an endotracheal airway in place, has also proved quite satisfactory.

During labor, the patient should be kept in a semirecumbent position. Measurements of the pulse and respiratory rates should be made at least 4 times every hour during the first stage of labor, and every 10 minutes during the second stage. Increases in the pulse rate much above 100 per minute or in the respiratory rate above 24, particularly when associated with dyspnea, are signs of cardiac embarrassment that may progress to overt cardiac failure. With any evidence of cardiac embarrassment, intensive medical management must be instituted immediately. Only in the presence of the completely dilated cervix and an engaged presenting part may these changes be taken as indication for delivery. With the cervix only partially dilated and the mother showing obvious evidence of cardiac embarrassment, there is no method of delivery that will not intensify rather than relieve heart failure.

Immediate medical treatment calls for the use of morphine, oxygen, a rapidly acting digitalis preparation, a potent diuretic, and at times, rotating tourniquets. Morphine should be given intramuscularly in a dose usually of 10 to 15 mg. It will serve to allay apprehension, reduce the elevated respiratory rate, and in the second stage of labor reduce the voluntary muscular activity associated with uterine contractions. Oxygen is best given in the form of intermittent positive-pressure breathing to promote adequate oxygenation and to prevent or minimize pulmonary edema. Digitalis in the form of a rapidly acting glycoside should be given intravenously. Care must be exercised to avoid toxicity especially in the woman who is depleted of potassium as the consequence of previous diuretic therapy. The potent diuretic furosemide may be given intravenously in a dose of 40 to 80 mg.

Signs of cardiac embarrassment developing after complete dilatation of the cervix and engagement of the vertex are indications for prompt forceps delivery unless spontaneous birth is expected within a few minutes.

Women who have shown little or no evidence of cardiac distress during pregnancy, labor, or delivery sometimes decompensate after delivery. Therefore, it is important that the same meticulous care provided during the antepartum and intrapartum periods be continued into the puerperium. Postpartum hemorrhage, puerperal infection, and puerperal thromboembolism are much more serious complications of pregnancy in the woman with heart disease. If there was no evidence of cardiac embarrassment during labor, delivery, and the early puerperium, breast-feeding is usually not contraindicated. In general, if tubal sterilization is to be performed, it should be delayed until it is obvious that the patient is afebrile, not anemic, and capable of exercise without evidence of distress. Women who do not undergo tubal sterilization should be given detailed contraceptive advice, as should all puerperal women.

MANAGEMENT OF CLASS III. Women whose cardiac function is so diminished as to fall in class III present difficult problems that demand expert medical judgment and care. The important question is whether they should become pregnant. The rational answer is no, but many women will risk much for a baby. They and their families must understand the risk and be willing and able to cooperate to the fullest extent. To avoid cardiac decompensation, these women ideally should be kept in bed and observed very closely throughout all of pregnancy until after delivery. The method of delivery is vaginal, as in classes I and II, with cesarean section limited to strictly obstetric indications. A pregnant woman with a history of previous cardiac failure that was not associated with acute rheumatic carditis or whose cardiac lesion causing the failure has not been corrected surgically is best managed as class III, regardless of the current functional classification.

Should frank cardiac failure develop during the course of pregnancy, without exception the woman must remain in bed in the hospital throughout the remainder of pregnancy. With strict bed rest, digitalization, diuresis, and appropriate sodium restriction, the signs and symptoms of decompensation often disappear rapidly; but should the rule be broken, she will very likely return to the hospital in severe or even fatal cardiac failure.

Even though the woman has recently been in failure or is in failure at the time of labor, vaginal delivery, in general, is safer than cesarean section. Abundant evidence shows that these very sick women withstand major surgical procedures poorly and that heart disease itself is a contraindication rather than an indication for cesarean section.

The study of Bunim and Appel (1950) demonstrated that about one-third of class III cardiac patients will decompensate during pregnancy, unless preventive measures are taken. When such a woman is seen in the first trimester, a question of therapeutic abortion inevitably arises. Her desire for a child may be a determining factor, but class III cardiac disease is an urgent indication for therapeutic abortion unless the mother can be hospitalized for the duration of the pregnancy.

The experience of Gorenberg and Chesley (1958) at the Margaret Hague Maternity Hospital led them to conclude that any woman with heart disease seen early in gestation can be carried through pregnancy successfully if she and her family are willing to abide by certain strict rules. Their recommended regimen included bed rest in the hospital for the duration of pregnancy in any patient with class III disease. The application of this basic principle, together with good medical and obstetric care to well over 1000 patients in the cardiac clinic, reduced the maternal death rate to not much more than that of the general obstetric population. The extreme importance of rigid adherence to their rules is demonstrated clearly by the fact that cardiac disease was the leading cause of maternal death at the hospital, but those who died were not women attending their cardiac clinic.

Whereas it is well established that the woman with cardiac disease who receives appropriate care rarely dies during pregnancy or the puerperium, the possibility has been raised that pregnancy causes obscure deleterious effects that ultimately shorten her life span. In other words, it is suggested that pregnancy in some way might accelerate the rate of deterioration of cardiac function. The comprehensive studies by Chesley (1980) of a large number of pregnant women observed over a long period did not demonstrate or even suggest that pregnancy has a deleterious remote effect on the course of rheumatic heart disease.

Hospitalization for many months for the woman who has other children, or who perhaps is unmarried and does not desire the pregnancy, is a great price, psychologic as well as financial, for her, her family, and, in many instances, the community to pay. Moreover, the life expectancy of the woman with serious cardiac disease is appreciably shortened. Sometimes, therefore, the child will be motherless at a young age. Thus, even though therapeutic abortion is not mandatory to save the life of the mother when prolonged hospitalization and competent medical care can be provided, if these conditions are not available or are not acceptable to the woman, therapeutic abortion and sterilization, or at least effective contraception, is indicated. Therapeutic abortion demands the application of all of the safeguards discussed previously for safely accomplishing delivery, including vigorous treatment to correct cardiac decompensation before the procedure.

MANAGEMENT OF CLASS IV. The treatment of women with class IV heart disease is essentially that of cardiac failure in pregnancy, labor, and the puerperium. In the presence of cardiac failure, delivery by any known method carries a high maternal mortality rate. Accordingly, the treatment of heart failure in pregnancy is primarily medical rather than obstetric. The prime objective is to correct the decompensation, for only then will delivery be safe.

EFFECTS ON FETUS AND NEWBORN. In general, any disease complicated by severe maternal hypoxia is likely to lead to abortion, premature delivery, and intrauterine death. A relation of chronic hypoxia and the polycythemia it causes to the outcome of pregnancy has been demonstrated in studies on women with cyanotic heart disease. When hypoxia was so intense as to stimulate a rise in the hematocrit reading above 65 percent, all pregnancies ended in abortion. Whittemore et al. (1980) identified fetal wastage to be 36 percent in pregnancies of women with hypoxic congenital heart disease.

SURGICAL REPAIR. In recent years, to try to improve maternal cardiac function, several kinds of operations have been performed on the heart and large vessels, including open heart surgery with cardiopulmonary bypass (Koh et al., 1975). Schenker and Polishuk (1968) have analyzed the experiences of 182 women who conceived and delivered after *mitral valvotomy.* The procedure was performed on 30 women during pregnancy, with no deaths during or immediately after the operation, although three died later in the antepartum period. Apparently good clinical results after mitral valvotomy were not always followed by uncomplicated pregnancy and delivery. In fact, 10 of the 18 deaths after the operation were attributed to the effects of pregnancy and delivery. In 42 percent of all patients who had their first delivery after the operation, various stages of congestive heart failure were encountered. The puerperium was a particularly dangerous time. Wallace and co-workers (1971) reported similar experiences.

A number of women of reproductive age have received a *cardiac valvar prosthesis* to replace a severely damaged mitral or aortic valve. Continuous anticoagulant therapy is recommended by most authorities to prevent emboli. If the woman is not pregnant, warfarin is satisfactory, but this drug crosses the placenta and may cause hemorrhage and death in the fetus and newborn. Moreover warfarin during the first trimester may prove teratogenic. Heparin is the anticoagulant of choice antepartum. The pregnant woman can usually be instructed to inject heparin satisfactorily into the subcutaneous tissue (Bonnar, 1979). Just before delivery, the heparin is stopped. If delivery occurs while the anticoagulant is still effective and extensive bleeding is encountered, protamine sulfate should be given. Anticoagulant therapy with warfarin or heparin may be restarted the day after vaginal delivery, usually with no problems.

Lutz and co-workers (1978) and Harrison and associates (1978) have presented their experiences and reviewed those of others for women with heart valve prostheses. Some of the reported complications are cardiac failure, thromboembolism, fetal and maternal morbidity from anticoagulant therapy, and premature labor. Even though cardiac function may be adequate, the difficulties associated with prolonged administration of heparin to prevent arterial embolization tend to preclude repeated pregnancies. Therefore, in these women sterilization frequently has merit. Oral contraceptives containing estrogen and a progestin may be contraindicated. Bemiller and associates (1970) reported the successful outcome of pregnancy in a woman with an aortic valve prosthesis and congenital complete heart block.

Some patients with *patent ductus arteriosus* develop pulmonary hypertension, and, particularly if the systemic blood pressure falls, may have a reversal of blood flow from the pulmonary artery to the aorta with consequent cyanosis. Sudden drops in blood pressure at delivery, as with conduction anesthesia or hemorrhage, may lead to fatal collapse. Therefore, hypotension should be avoided whenever possible and treated vigorously if it occurs. Burwell and Metcalfe (1958) suggested that the ductus should not be ligated during pregnancy. In our own limited experience, however, the operation has proved to be relatively simple, and cardiac function improved dramatically.

Various operations have been performed on women with *tetralogy of Fallot* with variable results. The hematocrit reading often provides an index of the success of the procedure. As pointed out previously, if the hema-

tocrit reading is very high (greater than 65), spontaneous abortion occurs. With somewhat lesser degrees of polycythemia there is an increased incidence of abortion, premature delivery, and underweight infants. If signs of cardiac failure develop in early pregnancy and do not yield to medical treatment, therapeutic abortion is advisable.

The prognosis for a pregnancy complicated by *Eisenmenger's syndrome* is poor as it is with *pulmonary hypertension* of any cause. Both maternal and perinatal mortality rates for Eisenmenger's syndrome have been identified to be about 30 percent (Gleicher et al., 1979).

Coronary Thrombosis and Ischemic Heart Disease. These are rare complications of pregnancy. The treatment is quite similar to that for the nonpregnant patient. If anticoagulants are given, the likelihood of toxic effects of warfarin on the fetus must be considered. The advisability of a woman undertaking a pregnancy after a myocardial infarction is not clear. Since the underlying vascular disease is usually progressive, and since it frequently is associated with hypertension, pregnancy in general appears to be contraindicated. Cortis and Genseni (1977) advise coronary angiography and, if severe involvement is detected, pregnancy should be discouraged. These authors have reported 3 cases of myocardial infarction associated with pregnancy and reviewed 73 others described previously.

Postpartal and Peripartal Cardiomyopathy. A cardiomyopathy that develops before, during, or after delivery has been considered by some to be caused somehow by the pregnancy although the exact etiology is unknown (Burch, 1977). If the mother survives the episode of cardiac decompensation, she usually makes a complete recovery, although the disease has been reported to recur occasionally in a subsequent pregnancy. Even though the belief prevails that it is a unique syndrome induced in some way by pregnancy and characterized by congestive heart failure with cardiomegaly, pulmonary congestion, and electrocardiographic evidence of nonspecific myocardial damage, it is far from clear whether postpartum heart disease is a distinct clinical entity.

Kyphoscoliotic Heart Disease.

During pregnancy especially, severe degrees of kyphoscoliosis commonly cause serious cardiopulmonary problems, sometimes referred to as kyphoscoliotic heart disease. In these circumstances, some regions of the lungs in the markedly deformed thoracic cage may be quite emphysematous, while others are atelectatic, with both lesions contributing to an inadequate ventilatory capacity. In these circumstances, *cor pulmonale* is a frequent complication.

The increased oxygen demands and the cardiac work imposed by pregnancy and delivery must be taken into account in reaching a decision whether to allow the pregnancy to continue or to perform a therapeutic abortion. If pulmonary function studies indicate that the vital capacity is not reduced appreciably, the outcome most often is favorable. In women with marked degrees of kyphoscoliosis and markedly impaired pulmonary function, therapeutic abortion is indicated.

Frequently the bony pelvis is so distorted that cesarean section is necessary. The supine position during delivery may result in serious hypotension. The commonly used analgesics such as meperidine (Demerol) should be used carefully, since respiratory depression is very poorly tolerated. During and after delivery, meticulous care should be directed toward the prevention of further atelectasis, which could lead rapidly to severe hypoxia and death. Intermittent positive-pressure breathing using appropriate concentrations of oxygen with mucolytic agents is of value. Sterilization is often indicated. Kopenhager (1977) has provided an analysis of the obstetric and medical complications of 50 women with kyphoscoliosis.

Bacterial Endocarditis.

Bacterial endocarditis, acute or subacute, is rarely encountered during pregnancy and the puerperium. Treatment is the same as that for the nonpregnant woman.

PROPHYLAXIS. For women with any cardiovascular condition that predisposes to subacute or acute bacterial endocarditis there is always the remote possibility that bacteremia at delivery will prove to be dangerous. The Committee on the Prevention of Rheumatic Fever and Bacterial Endocarditis of the American Heart Association (AHA, 1977) has stated that "endocarditis following uncomplicated vaginal delivery is extremely rare; the necessity for antibiotic prophylaxis has not been firmly established. . . . However, since the person with a prosthetic valve appears to be at especially high risk, it may be wise to administer antibiotic prophylaxis with these procedures. This empiric recommendation is based more upon concern than definitive data."

An acceptable regimen for prophylaxis is 2 million units of aqueous procaine penicillin G plus 1 g of streptomycin intramuscularly at or shortly before delivery and repeated at 12-hour intervals for a total of 3 doses.

For all women who are treated for an infection during pregnancy and the puerperium and who have valvular heart lesions, blood cultures should be made for anaerobic as well aerobic organisms before antibiotic therapy is instituted.

Coarctation of the Aorta.

This is a relatively rare lesion. The collateral circulation arising above the level of the coarctation expands, often to a striking extent, to cause localized erosion of the margins of the ribs by the hypertrophied intercostal arteries. The typical findings on physical examination are hypertension in the upper extremities and normal to reduced arterial blood pressures in the lower extremities.

The major complications of coarctation of the aorta are congestive heart failure when there has been long-standing severe hypertension, bacterial endocarditis, and rupture of the aorta. The aortic ruptures are likely to occur late in pregnancy or early in the puerperium and are associated with changes in the media that are histologically similar to those characterizing Erdheim's idiopathic medial cystic necrosis. Congestive heart failure demands vigorous efforts to improve cardiac function and usually warrants interruption of the pregnancy. Bacterial endocarditis can be effectively treated by appropriate antibiotics. It has been recommended by some that resection of the coarctation be undertaken during pregnancy to protect against the possibility of dissecting aneurysm and rupture of the aorta. The operation, however, is not without significant risk, especially to the fetus, because all the collaterals must be clamped for variable periods of time during the procedure, possibly leading to serious fetal hypoxia. Some authorities have recommended that the woman with coarctation of the aorta be delivered by cesarean section lest the transient elevation of arterial blood pressure that commonly accompanies labor lead to rupture of either the aorta or a coexisting cerebral aneurysm. The available evidence, however, suggests that cesarean section should be limited to obstetric indications.

DISEASES OF THE RESPIRATORY SYSTEM

Pregnancy induces a number of changes in the respiratory system. Enlargement of the uterus causes the diaphragm to rise, the transverse thoracic diameter to increase, the vertical chest diameter to decrease, and the residual volume of air in the lungs to be reduced. The tidal volume is increased somewhat, and in response to the modest hyperventilation the plasma carbon dioxide is lowered slightly. During the latter part of pregnancy, the oxygen consumption is increased 15 to 25 percent above that of normal nonpregnant woman. (Chap. 9, p. 240).

Pneumonia. In general, pneumonitis causing an appreciable loss of ventilatory capacity is tolerated less well by women during pregnancy. This generalization seems to hold true irrespective of whether the cause of the pneumonia is bacterial, viral, or chemical. Moreover, as has been pointed out in the discussions of heart disease and of diabetes, hypoxia and acidosis are poorly tolerated by the fetus. Therefore, it is important to the pregnant woman and her fetus that pneumonia be diagnosed as soon as possible and that she be promptly hospitalized so that the disease can be most effectively treated.

Aspiration of gastric contents during anesthesia for delivery often results in severe chemical penumonitis, primarily as the consequence of the necrotizing effects of hydrochloric acid (Mendelson, 1946). Diagnosis and treatment of gastric aspiration are discussed in Chapter 18 (p. 440). The aspiration of gastric contents is not limited to anesthesia for delivery. Treatment of eclampsia with large doses of morphine or barbiturates, for example, has sometimes been followed by the aspiration of gastric contents.

Thromboembolism and Pulmonary Infarction. Both may be encountered during pregnancy, but they occur much more often during the puerperium. Diagnosis and treatment of these serious problems are discussed in Chapter 36 (p. 907).

Asthma. This is a rather common respiratory illness, which consequently is encountered relatively often in pregnant women. Pregnancy does not seem to exert any consistent predictable effect on bronchial asthma. In some pregnant women, asthma appears to be less of a problem; in others, it is more; and in still others, it remains about the same (Weinstein et al., 1979). The great majority of women with asthma can be safely carried through pregnancy, labor, and delivery. Respiratory infections and sometimes emotional stress may intensify the asthmatic attacks. Most drugs that have proved effective before pregnancy may be continued during pregnancy with one major exception: The use of medications that contain iodide must be avoided, for iodide is transported across the placenta to the fetus and concentrated in the fetal thyroid. When the mother ingests large doses of iodide over a prolonged period of time, the large amount of iodide reaching the fetus may induce a large goiter. Carswell and associates (1970) have reported several instances of congenital goiter and hypothyroidism caused by the maternal ingestion of iodides.

When severe attacks of asthma cannot be relieved by other types of medication, glucocorticoids may be given. Although there is evidence that cortisone is teratogenic when given to pregnant rabbits, rats, and some other animals, there is no strong evidence that it is teratogenic during human pregnancy. For example, Williams (1967) reported that of 33 infants whose mothers were receiving steroids for asthma at the onset of pregnancy, one had a serious anomaly. Therapeutic abortion might be indicated in the uncommon patient who, as the consequence of long-standing asthma, has reduced cardiopulmonary function. Since asthma is a chronic disease that in the adult predictably will persist for many years after the pregnancy, sterilization may have merit especially for the woman who desires no more children.

Pulmonary Resection. The effect of *pulmonary resection,* usually for bronchiectasis or tuberculosis, will depend upon the functional capacity of the remaining pulmonary tissue. In general, if function is equivalent to one normal lung and active pulmonary disease is not present, pregnancy is tolerated without undue risk to the mother and with a good likelihood of delivery of a healthy infant.

Tuberculosis. In recent years, the prognosis has improved remarkably for the woman with active pulmonary tuberculosis. Chemotherapy that has proved to be effective in the absence of pregnancy is also effective during pregnancy. Fortunately, several effective drugs do not appear to affect the fetus adversely. Scheinhorn and Angelillo (1977) discovered no increase in birth defects among children whose mothers during pregnancy

had been treated with isoniazid, ethambutol, or rifampin. Mild auditory and vestibular abnormalities were identified after streptomycin therapy.

Bowes (1975) has recommended that all women registering for prenatal care be screened for tuberculosis by appropriate skin testing. If the skin test is negative, no further evaluation is needed. If positive, a thorough history is obtained and a complete physical examination and chest roentgenogram are performed. If negative, no treatment is necessary until after delivery when generally isoniazid therapy is carried out for one year. However, very few clinics routinely screen all their obstetric patients in this way.

Evaluation of the degree of activity of the pulmonary disease roentgenographically at times may be difficult. As pregnancy advances and the diaphragm rises, the lungs undergo some degree of compression, which may mask the extent of the tuberculous lesion. In fact, this mechanical effect of pregnancy on the lung may conceal actual pulmonary cavitation. Therefore, treatment may have to be undertaken in the pregnant woman on less firm ground than if she were not pregnant.

In the absence of seriously impaired pulmonary function, analgesia and anesthesia for labor and delivery can usually be accomplished with any of the technics used for normal pregnancy. Tuberculosis is seldom an indication for therapeutic abortion unless there is disseminated tuberculosis or severely compromised cardiopulmonary function. Sterilization is warranted for women who desire no more children. Congenital tuberculosis is rare even when the mother has widespread disease. The newborn infant, however, is quite susceptible to tuberculosis. Therefore, the infant should be isolated immediately from the mother suspected of having active disease. Bowes (1975) has provided an informative review of tuberculosis in pregnancy.

Pelvic tuberculosis usually causes intractable sterility. According to Schaefer (1964), for example, only 31 term pregnancies have been reported in authenticated cases of genital tuberculosis. Other cases of pregnancy often terminate ectopically or in abortion and are sometimes followed by activation of the pelvic infection. Although treatment is still controversial, the consensus favors a combination of chemotherapy and surgical extirpation of the pelvic organs. In certain younger woman, however, more conservative therapy may be justified.

Sarcoidosis.   This disease is rarely identified in pregnant women. The available evidence implies that sarcoidosis seldom affects pregnancy adversely; some authors suggest that pregnancy may actually be beneficial (Dines and Banner, 1967). O'Leary (1968) noted that only women with extensive pulmonary involvement were at risk during pregnancy; the development of respiratory infection warrants hospitalization. Pregnancy is not a contraindication to the use of corticosteroids if they are needed.

DIABETES MELLITUS

Before the advent of insulin many women with diabetes were too ill to conceive. For example, Williams (1915), after 13 years as Chief of the Obstetrical Service of the Johns Hopkins Hospital, with a large consulting practice in addition, had encountered only one case of pregnancy complicated by recognized diabetes. The exact cause of the infertility in diabetic women during the preinsulin era is not clear, but amenorrhea was common, the incidence having been placed as high as 50 percent. Of the infrequent cases in which pregnancy occurred, about one-fourth of the mothers and about half of the fetuses and infants died.

Incidence.   The lack of agreement about the minimal requirements for the diagnosis of diabetes mellitus makes it difficult to acquire satisfactory figures for its prevalence. Even so, by diagnostic criteria acceptable to most workers, it is estimated that more than

5 percent of the population now have overt diabetes (Ganda and Soelder, 1977). The cause or causes for the remarkable increase in recent years are not known but environmental factors, as well as genetic predisposition, are implicated. Bases for incriminating environmental factors are provided by the following observations: For most young persons with insulin-dependent diabetes, there is no family history of diabetes. There is evidence to link viral infections to the development of some cases of diabetes. For example, a high incidence of diabetes has been found in young adults with congenital rubella. Moreover, antibodies to Coxsackie virus B4 were found much more often in sera from young diabetics than in controls (Rayfield and Seto, 1978). The concordance rate for diabetes in monozygous twins, rather than being nearly 100 percent if diabetes were solely genetic in origin, is actually less than 50 percent. The probability of interaction of environmental factors, especially viral, and of genetic predisposition, is supported by demonstrations of considerable variation in susceptibility to diabetes among different strains of mice and rats when injected with the same virus (Onodera et al., 1978). In human population studies an association has been found between the HLA system and some, but not all, forms of diabetes.

Classification.   Members of an international workshop, now called the National Diabetes Data Group, convened in 1978 to formulate, among other things, the following scheme for classifying diabetes mellitus, including diabetes apparent only during pregnancy (gestational diabetes).

I. Idiopathic diabetes mellitus
  1. Insulin-dependent
  2. Non-insulin-dependent
    a. Nonobese
    b. Obese
II. Gestational diabetes
III. Impaired glucose tolerance
IV. Previous abnormality of glucose tolerance

V. Potential abnormality of glucose tolerance
VI. Secondary diabetes mellitus

White (1978) has provided an update of her classification of pregnant women with diabetes which is presented in Table 28-6. Unfortunately, its increasing complexity may impair its usefulness.

Diagnosis during Pregnancy. The woman who presents with glucosuria, high plasma glucose levels, ketonemia, and ketonuria is no problem in diagnosis. The woman at the opposite end of the spectrum, with only minimal metabolic derangement caused by diabetes, is difficult to identify. The likelihood of impaired carbohydrate metabolism and related metabolic stigmata of diabetes is increased appreciably in women who have a strong familial history of diabetes, or have given birth to large infants, or demonstrate persistent glucosuria, or have unexplained fetal losses.

Reducing substances are commonly found in the urine of pregnant women, but their presence does not necessarily mean diabetes. Often the material is lactose, which should not be a source of needless concern if the urine is tested by a method that is specific for glucose. The commercially available testing substances, Tes-Tape and Clinistix, may be used to identify glucose in the urine while avoiding a positive reaction from lactose. Even when lactosuria is excluded, glycosuria caused by glucose is occasionally identified. Most often, the glucosuria does not reflect hyperglycemia from impaired glucose tolerance, but rather the lowered renal threshold for glucose induced by normal pregnancy, as discussed in Chapter 9 (p. 243). Nonetheless, the detection of glucosuria during pregnancy generally warrants further testing.

FASTING HYPERGLYCEMIA (OVERT DIABETES, CLASS B THROUGH T). The criterion for diagnosis of overt diabetes during pregnancy is the identification of fasting hyperglycemia on two or more occasions. Fast-

TABLE 28-6.
CLASSIFICATION OF DIABETES IN PREGNANT WOMEN

A	Chemical diabetes
B	Maturity onset (age over 20 years), duration under 10 years, no vascular lesions
C_1	Age 10 to 19 years at onset
C_2	10 to 19 years' duration
D_1	Under age 10 years at onset
D_2	Over 20 years' duration
D_3	Benign retinopathy
D_4	Calcified vessels of legs
D_5	Hypertension
E	No longer sought
F	Nephropathy
G	Many failures
H	Cardiopathy
R	Proliferating retinopathy
T	Renal transplant

ing hyperglycemia during pregnancy has been defined by the National Diabetes Data Group (1979) to be a *plasma* level of 105 mg per dl or higher (compared to 140 mg per dl or higher in nonpregnant individuals). The decision to establish a lower value during pregnancy was influenced, in part, by the fact that the plasma glucose level is lower during much of normal pregnancy than when nonpregnant.

ABNORMAL GLUCOSE TOLERANCE (CLASS A DIABETES). The diagnosis of Class A diabetes requires the use of an oral glucose tolerance test. On the days preceding the glucose tolerance test the woman should not have been fasting, but rather should have consumed at least 100 g of carbohydrate per day. As recommended by the National Diabetes Data Group (1979), after an overnight fast, blood is drawn and then 100 g of glucose in a 50 percent solution is ingested while continuing to otherwise fast. Further venous blood samples are obtained 1, 2, and 3 hours after ingesting the glucose. A diagnosis of Class A diabetes is made when 2 or more plasma glucose levels equal or exceed the following values: Fasting—105 mg per dl; 1 hour—190 mg per dl; 2 hours—165 mg per dl; 3 hours—145 mg per dl. If, however, two fasting plasma glucose levels exceed 105 mg per dl, the diabetes is classified as "overt" (at least Class B), rather than "chemical" (Class A). The values cited above as being critical levels for plasma glucose were derived originally on whole blood by O'Sullivan and Mahan (1964). The concentration of glucose in plasma is typically about 15 percent greater than that in whole blood.

It should be kept in mind that the pregnant woman with a normal fasting level for glucose but an abnormal glucose tolerance test early in pregnancy may occasionally develop overt diabetes late in pregnancy. Therefore, the plasma glucose levels while fasting should be checked periodically. Much more rarely, evidence of diabetes may ameliorate during pregnancy (Sheldon and Coleman, 1974).

The oral glucose tolerance test measures the balance between the absorption of glucose from the intestinal tract, its uptake by tissues, and its excretion in the urine, as well as stimulating the release from the gut of certain hormones that, in turn, augment the release of insulin from β-cells in the islets of Langerhans. In the absence of pregnancy, the oral test is preferred to the intravenous glucose tolerance test because of its greater sensitivity. The oral test during pregnancy suffers from greater variability in the rate of glucose absorption from the gut and, from a very practical standpoint, the likelihood of nausea and vomiting induced by the 100g of glucose to be ingested rapidly.

Effect of Pregnancy on Diabetes. The diabetogenic properties of pregnancy are borne out by the fact that some women who have no evidence of diabetes when not pregnant develop during pregnancy distinct abnormalities in glucose tolerance and, at times, clinically evident diabetes. Most often these changes are reversible. After delivery, the evidence of either the induction of or a worsening of diabetes usually disappears very rapidly, and the ability of the mother to metabolize carbohydrate returns to the prepregnancy status. As pointed out

in Chapter 9 (p. 230), pregnancy per se impairs insulin action. The insulin antagonism during pregnancy is the consequence of the actions of placental lactogen, which is abundant, and to lesser degrees those of estrogens and progesterone. Also, placental insulinase may contribute to the diabetogenic effects of pregnancy by accelerating insulin degradation (Steel et al., 1979).

During pregnancy, the control of diabetes may be made more difficult by a variety of complications. Nausea and vomiting may lead, on the one hand, to insulin shock in women who are receiving insulin and, on the other, to insulin resistance if the starvation is severe enough to cause ketosis. Infection during pregnancy commonly results in insulin resistance and ketoacidosis unless the infection is promptly recognized and both the infection and the diabetes are effectively treated. The vigorous muscular exertion of labor accompanied by the ingestion of little or no carbohydrate may result in troublesome hypoglycemia unless the amount of insulin given is reduced appropriately or an intravenous infusion of glucose is provided. After delivery, insulin requirements most often decrease at a rapid rate and to a considerable degree. Puerperal infection, however, may obtund this response or perhaps even increase the insulin requirements. Presumably, the rapid decrease in insulin requirements that is usually seen in the absence of other complications stems from the rapid disappearance of placental lactogen, estrogens, and progesterone following delivery of the placenta while levels of pituitary growth hormone remain low for a few days.

It was thought by some that the fetus ameliorates maternal diabetes by producing insulin, which is transferred in significant amounts across the placenta to the mother. There is no good evidence, however, that the fetal pancreas is capable of providing insulin to the mother in amounts sufficient to ameliorate her disease to any appreciable degree.

The pregnant woman, even in the absence of diabetes, is more prone to develop metabolic acidosis than when nonpregnant. Presumably, placental lactogen is responsible for this tendency by virtue of its carbohydrate-sparing and lipolytic actions. With diabetes, the likelihood of severe metabolic acidosis is increased appreciably.

Effects of Diabetes on Pregnancy. Diabetes is deleterious to pregnancy in a number of ways. The adverse maternal effects include the following:

1. The likelihood of preeclampsia-eclampsia is increased about fourfold; a considerable increase in preeclampsia-eclampsia is noted even in the absence of demonstrated preexisting vascular disease.
2. Infection occurs more often and is likely to be more severe in women with diabetes.
3. The fetus frequently is much larger and his size may lead to difficult delivery with injury to the birth canal.
4. Because of the tendency of the fetus to succumb before the onset of spontaneous labor, as well as the possibility of dystocia, cesarean section and the maternal risks that are imposed by this operation, are increased.
5. Hydramnios is common, and at times the large volume of amnionic fluid, coupled with fetal macrosomia, may cause cardio-respiratory symptoms in the mother.
6. Postpartum hemorrhage is more common than in the general obstetric population.

Maternal diabetes adversely affects the fetus and newborn infant in several ways:

1. In the absence of excellent management of the diabetes and the pregnancy the perinatal death rate is considerably elevated compared with that of the general population.
2. Morbidity is common in the newborn infant of a mother with diabetes. In some instances, the morbidity is the direct result of birth injury as the consequence of fetal macrosomia with disproportion between the size of the infant and the maternal pel-

vis. In others, it takes the form of severe respiratory distress and metabolic derangements that include hypoglycemia and hypocalcemia.
3. Anomalies have been identified more often in the fetuses of women with diabetes.
4. The infant may inherit at least a predisposition to diabetes.

Except for the brain, most organs of the fetus are affected by macrosomia that commonly, but not always, characterizes the fetus of the woman with diabetes (Fig. 28-5). At the same time, body fat is increased. The mechanisms responsible for the extra growth of the fetus are not clear. In several studies, however, the degree of fetal macrosomia appeared to correlate well with the degree of maternal hyperglycemia and lack of maternal vascular disease. Both favor the delivery of excessive amounts of glucose across the placenta to the fetus. This stimulates hyperinsulinism in the fetus and the hyperglycemia plus hyperinsulinism, in concert, enhances glycogen synthesis, lipogenesis, and protein synthesis in the fetus (Hill, 1978). There is abundant experimental evidence to support this concept. Mintz and co-workers (1972) injected the antibiotic streptozotocin into the circulation of the pregnant monkey to destroy the beta cells of the maternal islets of Langerhans. Maternal diabetes so produced was followed by fetal macrosomia. Cheek (1968) injected streptozotocin into the circulation of the monkey fetus to destroy the capacity of the fetus to make insulin. Fetal size was reduced appreciably. Moreover, marked fetal growth retardation with very poor development of striate muscle and near absence of adipose tissue has been observed in a newborn infant whose plasma and vestigial pancreas contained no insulin (Hill, 1978).

A fairly common finding at autopsy in the newborn infant of a diabetic mother is hypertrophy and hyperplasia of the islets of Langerhans. Although the changes are not specific, since they are also noted in erythroblastotic infants, they are sufficiently characteristic when found to suggest that the mother has

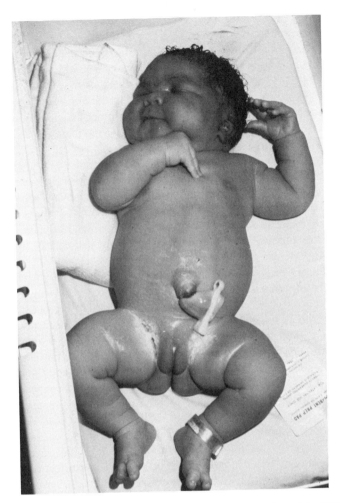

FIG. 28-5. Large baby of mildly diabetic mother. Birth weight 6050 g.

diabetes or prediabetes. This information may be useful in subsequent pregnancies. It has been suggested that maternal hyperglycemia and, in turn, fetal hyperglycemia are responsible for the striking increase in the size, and sometimes the number, of islets.

Management. It is readily apparent from the more recent experiences cited below, as well as other reports, that management which is based on a full appreciation of the following general principles will provide the best outcome for both the fetus-infant and his diabetic mother:

1. Abnormal carbohydrate metabolism should be detected and defined precisely.

2. Control of maternal glycemia is a very important factor in determining fetal outcome.

3. The pregnant woman with diabetes should be cared for throughout her pregnancy by experienced and skilled individuals.

4. The newborn infant of a mother with diabetes should be cared for from the time of birth by experienced and skilled individuals.

CLASS A DIABETES. Pregnant women without persistent fasting hyperglycemia, but with an abnormal oral glucose tolerance test (described above) are treated typically by diet alone and, in the absence of other indications, are delivered at term. In general, for women with gestational diabetes not requiring insulin there is no need to terminate the pregnancy early. In the usual circumstance an acceptable diet is that which is recommended by the American Diabetes Association in amounts that provide 30 to 35 calories per kg each day.

When carefully managed, perinatal mortality for pregnancies of women with Class A diabetes is no greater than that for the general obstetric population. Gabbe (1978) cites the figure 16 per 1000 for perinatal mortality in recent times. If the diabetes intensifies as pregnancy advances, however, the prognosis for the fetus-infant worsens. Therefore, throughout the remainder of pregnancy periodic checks of the plasma glucose concentration in the fasting state are essential to detect this event. During pregnancy perhaps 10 to 15 percent of women with Class A diabetes will develop overt diabetes.

OVERT DIABETES. The likelihood of successful outcomes for the fetus-infant and his overtly diabetic mother relate closely to the degree of control of diabetes that is achieved and the intensity of any maternal cardiovascular or renal disease.

In several series of overtly diabetic pregnancies published in recent years, perinatal mortality rates have not been much higher than those for the general population. The perinatal mortality rate reported by Gabbe and associates (1977) was 46 per 1000; by Kitzmiller and co-workers (1978), 36 per 1000; by Leveno and co-workers (1979), 45 per 1000; and by Schneider and associates (1980), 37 per 1000. Severe congenital malformations appeared to account for much of the increase in perinatal mortality over those values observed in the general population. There were no maternal deaths reported in these combined experiences which amounted to nearly 600 pregnancies.

The theme stressed uniformly in all of these reports was early diagnosis and meticulous management of the diabetes and of the pregnancy. All four reports serve to emphasize that, ideally, the maternal glucose level should be kept as close to normal as possible and the pregnancy should continue until the fetus is functionally mature unless the intrauterine environment is deteriorating. Then the fetus most often is better off being delivered even though premature. Interestingly and importantly, the specific technics emphasized by the several investigators to achieve good control of the diabetes and to monitor fetal well-being differed appreciably, as cited below, yet the perinatal outcomes were essentially identical!

The intelligent, well-coached, highly motivated pregnant woman with relatively stable diabetes, and who conscientiously follows her appropriate diet, which may have to be ingested in as many as five meals a day, and who takes multiple forms of insulin two or more times a day, has the best chance for achieving the euglycemic state. In actuality, many women who attempt such rigid control commonly run the risk of bouts of hypoglycemia that are dangerous not only to themselves but also to their fetuses. In any event, frequent measurements of plasma glucose, especially preprandially, and adjustment of insulin dosage and of diet on the basis of these measurements will help achieve the goal of avoiding serious hyperglycemia and hypoglycemia.

Important to a successful outcome for the fetus is precise knowledge of fetal age. A carefully obtained menstrual history and accurate measurements of uterine height during the second trimester provide useful information. Sonographic confirmation of fetal age often will prove of value. Sonographic evaluation later in pregnancy may serve to detect either fetal macrosomia, a common phenomenon, or growth-retardation, a complication seen especially when the mother has underlying vascular disease.

Effective counseling of the mother is an extremely important function of prenatal care. She must not only be seen often but also be instructed carefully as to how to recognize and deal with problems that arise in the interim. She must be encouraged to report immediately any of a variety of events to the physician who has accepted responsibility for her care. For example, respiratory or urinary infection, rather common occurrences during pregnancy, can rapidly precipitate ketoacidosis that is poorly tolerated by the fetus. The common complication of pregnancy—nausea and vomiting—may, if the mother does not eat appropriately, lead to the characteristic reaction of hyperinsulinism; and when more severe and prolonged, the starvation may lead to both serious acidosis and insulin resistance much sooner than if the woman were not pregnant.

The diabetic woman who is pregnant may have to be reeducated about the significance of glucosuria. Similar to the normal pregnant woman, she is likely to develop glucosuria as the consequence of the pregnancy-induced increase in glomerular filtration of glucose without increased tubular reabsorption. If she were to increase her insulin dosage to a level that avoids glucosuria, she may develop symptomatic hypoglycemia. In general, glucosuria is a signal to evaluate carefully the plasma glucose levels. Frank acetonuria most often means that the insulin dosage should be increased.

Tolbutamide (Orinase) and the other oral hypoglycemic agents should not be used during pregnancy, but instead insulin is given when indicated. Tolbutamide in large doses is teratogenic in some species, but there is no evidence that doses used clinically are necessarily teratogenic. Serious hypoglycemia has been observed, however, in the newborn infants of mothers treated with tolbutamide.

For many years, White (1965) administered an estrogen and a progestational agent to diabetic mothers throughout much of pregnancy. Compounds used included estradiol or stilbestrol with either progesterone or ethisterone, or a mixture of estradiol valerate and 17-hydroxyprogesterone caproate. These hormones are no longer used by White (1978). Elimination of these expensive drugs that may be teratogenic has not adversely affected the improved pregnancy salvage witnessed in more recent years.

Ideally, delivery of the overtly diabetic woman is accomplished close to term. At Parkland Memorial Hospital the women are requested to enter the hospital at 32 to 34 weeks gestation and to stay until delivered. Typically the L/S ratio in amnionic fluid is measured at 37 weeks and, if 2.0 or greater, delivery is effected during the 38th week of gestation. Until that time the fetus is considered not to be in serious jeopardy in utero as long as he is growing and there are no other complications, especially overt maternal hypertension or gross hydramnios. If either severe hypertension or acute hydramnios develops, delivery is carried out even though the L/S ratio is less than 2.0. Of 118 liveborn infants who were delivered according to this regimen, all survived except one who suffered from trisomy 18, incompatible with life. Of the four stillbirths, one who expired at 34 weeks might have been salvaged if delivery had been performed even earlier (Leveno et al., 1979).

Other groups who report comparable success rates have emphasized other plans of management in an effort to optimize the time selected for delivery. As well as hospitalizing the mothers at 34 weeks, Gabbe and associates (1977) have stressed the use, beginning at 30 to 32 weeks, of very frequent measurements of total urinary estriol or, more recently, the concentration of unconjugated plasma estriol (see Chap. 7, p. 159) plus the frequent use of the contraction stress test (see Chap. 14, p. 349). Interestingly, they believed that they were helped appreciably in their decision making by use of these technics whereas the group at Parkland Memorial Hospital did not find the tests to be essential.

Schneider and co-workers (1980), on the other hand, formulated and evaluated a method of management for pregnancies complicated by overt diabetes which emphasized ambulatory care throughout pregnancy until actual delivery. The expectant mother was taught self-measurement of blood glucose using a reflectance meter and, depending upon the results, either the alterations to make in insulin dosage and diet, or how to obtain expert advice immediately. They emphasized that an expert especially knowledgeable in obstetrics and diabetes, and who was intimately concerned with the mother's problems, was always available through electronic paging to provide such advice and to direct appropriate action whenever needed. As pointed out above, their low perinatal mortality rate is also meritorious. Schneider and co-workers have appropriately emphasized that without hospitalization costs for care were reduced. While they emphasized the virtue of reduced cost with ambulatory care, they also emphasized that they felt obligated to employ frequently a battery of tests similar to Gabbe and associates (1977) but not used by Leveno and co-workers (1979).

The measurement of 24-hour urinary estriol excretion, or of plasma unconjugated estriol concentration to monitor fetal well-being has received considerable attention from many other workers, as well as Gabbe, Schneider, and their associates. There is no doubt that unusually low excretion of estriol in urine or low concentration in plasma often, but not always, indicates that the fetus is in jeopardy. It remains to be proved, however, that the widespread application of measurements of urinary estriol to identify such a fetus will, of itself, reduce perinatal mortality significantly in diabetic pregnancies. To deliver a fetus thought to be in jeopardy of dying in utero, only to have him succumb from immaturity, accomplishes little, as emphasized by Barnes (1965). Studies have been carried out at several centers to evaluate the benefits that might be achieved from monitoring estriol excretion at close intervals during the latter half of the third trimester. As pointed out in Chapter 7 (p. 159), the bulk of evidence indicates that estriol measurements can be grossly misleading, being at times "abnormally low" when the immature fetus is not otherwise compromised, yet not be unusually low when the fetus is in serious jeopardy of death in utero. Goebelsmann and co-workers (1973) have emphasized that in diabetic women urinary estriol assays must be carried out and reported *daily* if obstetric management is to be based on estriol levels.

Glycosated hemoglobin A, commonly referred to as hemoglobin A_{1c} is likely to be elevated in diabetes and the magnitude of the elevation correlates inversely with the de-

gree of long-term control that has been achieved. Its measurement during pregnancy does not appear to have provided information of great clinical utility (Miller and co-workers, 1979).

DELIVERY. Cesarean section has been used commonly to avoid traumatic delivery of a large infant at or near term. Moreover, the reduced likelihood of effecting labor safely remote from term has also contributed appreciably to the use of cesarean section to effect delivery of the infant of a diabetic mother. In the four reports cited above with low perinatal mortality, the cesarean section rates were 55 percent in Los Angeles (Gabbe et al., 1977), 70 percent in a midwestern multicenter study (Schneider et al., 1980), 69 percent in Boston (Kitzmiller et al., 1978) and 81 percent in Dallas (Leveno et al., 1979).

Induction of labor may be attempted when the following criteria are met: (1) The fetus is not excessively large nor is the pelvis contracted. (2) Parity is not great. (3) The cervix is soft, appreciably effaced, and somewhat dilated. (4) The presenting part is the vertex and is fixed in the pelvis.

It is important to reduce considerably the dose of long-acting insulin given on the day of delivery. Regular insulin should be utilized to meet most or all of the insulin needs of the patient at this time, since the insulin requirements may drop markedly after delivery. During and after either cesarean section or labor and delivery, the mother should be adequately hydrated intravenously as well as supplied with glucose. Plasma glucose levels should be checked frequently and regular insulin administered accordingly. The urine, or preferably the plasma, should be checked for ketones. The insulin requirements may fluctuate markedly during the first few days after delivery. Starvation with resistance to insulin must be avoided and infection must be carefully searched for and promptly treated.

PERINATAL MORBIDITY. Even though perinatal mortality among infants of diabetic mothers has dropped remarkably in many centers in recent years, troublesome, but not necessarily serious, morbidity persists. This is clearly evident in the reports just cited. The most serious variety of morbidity is severe *congenital malformations* which fortunately are not greatly increased above that found in the general population (Simpson, 1979). *Hypoglycemia* is commonplace in the newborn infant presumably due in part, at least, to persistent hyperstimulation of the fetal beta islet cells by chronic hyperglycemia. *Hypocalcemia* and *hyperbilirubinemia* are also more common complications of the newborn period. Fortunately, the last three are readily treatable. *Idiopathic respiratory distress* may be somewhat more common among infants of diabetic mothers compared to infants in general of the same gestational age, although Gabbe (1977), Leveno (1979), and their coworkers did not find this to be a major problem. Possibly, increased insulin levels inhibit surfactant production (Neufeld et al., 1979).

It is extremely important that the robust appearance of the newly delivered infant not lead to inappropriate care. Although the infant may appear mature on the basis of his size, functionally he may be quite premature and must be so treated.

Contraception. The two most common forms of reversible contraception, estrogen-progestin oral contraceptives and the intrauterine device, may be contraindicated in women who have overt diabetes when nonpregnant. Oral contraceptives are likely to intensify the diabetes. Moreover, the vascular disease that rather often is associated with diabetes may potentiate the variety of hazards from vascular disease that have been described following use of oral contraceptives in the absence of diabetes (see Chap. 40, p. 1017). The risks from pelvic infection from an intrauterine device is very likely increased in the diabetic woman. Therefore, barrier methods seem the best choice for reversible contraception followed by sterilization once it is certain that the woman wants no more children.

DISEASES OF THE THYROID

It is difficult at times to differentiate changes of normal pregnancy from actual disease of the thyroid. Pregnancy normally induces changes that might be erroneously interpreted as indicating disease. The variations include modest diffuse enlargement of the gland, elevation of the level of circulating thyroxine and of thyroid-binding proteins, increased thyroid uptake of radioiodide, and decreased binding in vitro of triiodothyronine by resin (see Chap. 9, p. 250). It is reemphasized that in *normal* pregnancy and other hyperestrogenic states plasma thyroxine levels are compatible with hyperthyroidism while, simultaneously, the percentage uptake of triiodothyronine by resin is compatible with hypothyroidism!

Hyperthyroidism. Helpful signs for identifying hyperthyroidism during pregnancy are tachycardia (which exceeds that of normal pregnancy), including a high pulse rate while sleeping, exophthalmos, and failure to gain weight normally. In the great majority of cases of hyperthyroidism, the level of thyroxine in plasma is markedly elevated compared with normal values in the nonpregnant state. At the same time, in vitro binding tests fail to demonstrate the appreciably decreased uptake of triiodothyronine that is characteristic of normal pregnancy. Rarely, hyperthyroidism may be associated with normal plasma thyroxine values; instead, the triiodothyronine level is abnormally high (Martin et al., 1976). Measurement of radioiodine uptake by the thyroid is contraindicated during pregnancy. Once the test becomes generally available measurement of free thyroxine will prove to be most meaningful. However, it should be kept in mind that *careful* clinical evaluation, using those signs described above, is most important to a successful pregnancy outcome.

Treatment may be medical, or medical until such time as the mother is nearly euthyroid, and then surgical. Hyperthyroidism nearly always can be controlled by antithyroid drugs, so that the disease, if treated adequately, need not be a serious threat to the mother. Medical treatment, however, has the potential for causing severe fetal complications. Propylthiouracil and similarly acting compounds readily cross the placenta and may induce fetal hypothyroidism and goiter. Therefore, it became common practice to give propylthiouracil in doses that effectively suppressed maternal thyroid activity while the mother received thyroid hormone simultaneously allegedly to provide hormone to the fetus. Most likely, the hormone in doses so administered did not cross the placenta to the fetus in significant amounts. Actually, it served only to increase the maternal requirements for propylthiouracil and thereby increase, rather than decrease, the risk to the fetus. Goluboff and co-workers (1974) have emphasized that supplemental thyroid hormone may be undesirable because (1) it obscures laboratory indices of propylthiouracil overdosage, (2) it may increase the dosage of propylthiouracil required for control, and (3) it complicates recognition of remission which sometimes occurs during pregnancy. Moreover, in their experience, supplemental thyroid hormone did not always protect against the development of a goiter in the fetus. For these reasons, a regimen employing propylthiouracil or compounds with similar actions without administration of thyroid hormone has been followed in our clinic.

The dose of propylthiouracil should be increased until the woman appears clinically to be only minimally thyrotoxic and the level of thyroid hormone in the blood is reduced to the upper normal range for pregnancy. In case of severe hyperthyroidism, emergency treatment with large doses of propylthiouracil, combined with iodide, reserpine, or propanolol for a few days is not contraindicated by the pregnancy. Propanolol has also been used for long-term treatment of hyperthyroidism in pregnant women (Bullock et al., 1975; Langer et al., 1974). However, troublesome adverse effects have been described in newborn infants whose mothers were being treated with propanolol. The ad-

verse effects included fetal distress during labor, low Apgar scores, growth retardation, hypoglycemia, and hyperbilirubinemia (Habib and McCarthy, 1977).

Burrow and associates (1968) have carried out a long-term study of the intellectual and physical development, including thyroid function, of the children born to thyrotoxic mothers treated with propylthiouracil during pregnancy. Although the number of children studied was small, no adverse effects on subsequent growth and development were identified. The prolonged administration of iodide to the mother along with propylthiouracil appears to increase appreciably the likelihood of gross goiter in the fetus. Therefore, iodide should be used only preceding the time of thyroidectomy and *not* for long-term therapy.

Thyroidectomy may be carried out after the thyrotoxicosis has been brought under control. Opinions differ as to the wisdom of surgical treatment during the first trimester, a time when abortion is relatively common, or during the third trimester, when delivery may occur prematurely. From the beginning of the second trimester until early in the third trimester, however, for the woman who is incapable of adhering to an appropriate plan of medical treatment or for whom the drug proves toxic, subtotal thyroidectomy may be the treatment of choice after achieving control medically.

Breast-feeding is generally contraindicated when the mother is taking antithyroid drugs, since they are likely to be excreted in the milk in significant amounts.

Women with *Graves' disease,* even though they are no longer hyperthyroid, may give birth to infants with manifestations of thyrotoxicosis, including goiter and exophthalmos. Long-acting thyroid stimulator (LATS) and long-acting thyroid stimulator protector (LATSP), gamma globulins synthesized by the mother presumably as an autoimmune phenomenon, are transferred across the placenta to the fetus and can cause hyperthyroidism in the fetus and transiently in the newborn infant. The condition is suggested by a maternal history of thyrotoxicosis, identification of appreciable levels of LATS and LATSP in maternal serum, a history of a previously affected fetus-infant, and by persistent fetal tachycardia. Robinson and co-workers (1979) have reported a case in which the mother was given antithyroid medication to try to treat the fetus plus thyroxine to maintain euthyroidism in the mother. The endpoint used for establishing dosage of the antithyroid medication was the fetal heart rate. The newborn infant may require treatment for several weeks until the LATS and LATSP are ultimately metabolized.

Hypothyroidism. Overt hypothyroidism is often associated with infertility, and in women who do become pregnant the likelihood of abortion seems to be increased considerably. In general, hypothyroidism can be diagnosed if the expected rise during pregnancy in the level of circulating thyroxine fails to take place. Measurement of serum cholesterol is of little value, since normal pregnancy also induces an increase in the cholesterol concentration.

EFFECT ON FETUS AND INFANT. The infant of a mother with severe hypothyroidism may be a cretin. Hypothyroidism in infants following maternal radioactive iodine therapy is well documented (Green et al., 1971). Any infant whose mother was so treated during pregnancy and was not aborted must be carefully evaluated and perhaps treated prophylactically for hypothyroidism. Klein and co-workers (1974), and others, have pointed out that the clinical diagnosis of *congenital hypothyroidism* during the neonatal period is difficult and often missed. They recommended measurements on newborn blood to detect subclinical disease and, in turn, to provide effective treatment. If treatment of the affected infant is started early, mental retardation most often can be prevented. According to various reports based on mass screening of newborn infants, the frequency of congenital hypothyroidism so detected is one in 4000 to 7000 newborn infants (Varma, 1979).

Simple colloid goiter in the mother, if unassociated with hypothyroidism, has no influence on pregnancy.

Parathyroid Diseases

Hyperparathyroidism. This rarely complicates pregnancy, even though the disease is more common in women and has a peak incidence before the menopause. Whalley described four cases cared for at Parkland Memorial Hospital (1963). One case with parathyroid storm, characterized by hypercalcemia and convulsions, was especially interesting. The convulsions, coexistent with chronic pyelonephritis and chronic hypertension, might erroneously have been considered to have been caused by eclampsia.

Tetany has been noted occasionally in the newborn infants of mothers with hyperparathyroidism. At times it has led to a search that identified a maternal parathyroid adenoma (Hartenstein and Gardner, 1966). Pedersen and Permin (1975) have reviewed the published experiences concerning hyperparathyroidism and pregnancy.

Hypoparathyroidism. This is equally uncommon in pregnancy. Treatment with dihydrotachysterol or large doses of vitamin D, together with calcium gluconate or calcium lactate and a diet low in phosphates, usually prevents symptomatic hypocalcemia (O'Leary et al., 1966). The risk to the fetus from large doses of either dihydrotachysterol or vitamin D_2 has not been established. Whether these compounds cause cardiovascular and other anomalies is not clear.

OTHER ENDOCRINE DISORDERS

Diabetes Insipidus. The condition is a rare complication of pregnancy. Only two cases have been cared for in the last quarter of a century at Parkland Memorial Hospital, during which there were approximately 170,000 deliveries. As long as the women took vasopressin for replacement therapy, their pregnancies progressed without serious complication. This experience is similar to those reported by others. In a few instances, there appeared to have been an impairment of labor, possibly caused by lack of or reduced amounts of endogenous oxytocin (Hime and Richardson, 1978). Sende and associates (1975) were unable to detect oxytocin by radioimmunoassay in plasma of a pregnant woman with diabetes insipidus before labor, but during labor and the puerperium there was a surge of oxytocin. A woman described by Chau and associates (1969) lactated normally, with measured milk ejection pressures comparable to those of normal lactating women.

Diabetes insipidus without anterior pituitary deficiency has been described following massive hemorrhage and prolonged shock from placenta percreta (Collins et al., 1979).

Adrenal Dysfunction. Before 1953, only 50 published cases of *Addison's disease* in pregnancy had been identified, suggesting that untreated adrenal hypofunction caused sterility (Hunt and McConahey, 1953). With the advent of cortisone and related compounds, pregnancy has become much more common in women with adrenocortical hypofunction.

It is essential during pregnancy and the puerperium to observe the mother quite closely for evidence of either inadequate or excessive steroid replacement. Except at times of stress, replacement therapy need not be greater and sometimes may be less than in the nonpregnant state. There may be little or no need during pregnancy for compounds with potent mineralocorticoid action. During and after labor and delivery or after a surgical procedure, the amount of steroid replacement should be increased appreciably to approximate the normal response at that time in women with intact adrenals. It is important that shock from causes other than adrenocortical insufficiency be promptly recognized and treated, especially that caused by blood loss or bacterial infection.

Pregnancy associated with *Cushing's syndrome* is rare. The disease has been diagnosed during pregnancy and treated successfully at that time. In one instance an adrenocortical adenoma was resected (Grimes et al., 1973) and in another the pituitary-dependent adrenocortical hyperplasia was treated with pituitary irradiation during the pregnancy (Anderson and Walters, 1976); the infants were normal.

A few cases of *primary aldosteronism* in association with pregnancy have been reported. In view of the very high levels of aldosterone in normal pregnancies, it is not surprising that there may be amelioration of symptoms as well as electrolyte disturbances during pregnancy (Biglieri and Slaton, 1967). Although aldosterone is produced in large amounts during much of pregnancy, it is not essential for a successful outcome.

Development of *acromegaly* in a pregnant woman and in turn her fetus-infant has been described by Fisch and associates (1974). The mother was treated with x-irradiation to the pituitary fossa during the third trimester. The newborn infant presented a constellation of skeletal anomalies.

Pheochromocytoma. Pheochromocytoma is a rare complication of pregnancy; both the maternal and the fetal mortality rates have been extremely high (Schenker and Chowers, 1971). Favorable outcomes have been described more recently for individual cases in which the diagnosis was made late in pregnancy and the blood pressure was controlled pharmacologically during cesarean section and resection of the tumor (Burgess, 1979; Durham, 1977; Leak et al., 1977).

SEXUALLY TRANSMITTED DISEASES

The five classic sexually transmitted veneral diseases are syphilis, gonorrhea, chancroid, lymphogranuloma venereum, and granuloma inguinale. In more recent years the first two have increased remarkably in frequency while the last three have all but disappeared. Unfortunately, they have been replaced by other diseases that may be sexually transmitted, especially herpes infection of the genital tract.

Syphilis. During the past several years, there has been a disturbing increase in the incidence of syphilis. An unusually critical time to detect and treat syphilis is during pregnancy not only to protect the mother and her sexual partner from the numerous complications of syphilis but, especially important, to prevent the extensive pathologic changes that characterize congenital syphilis (see Chap. 38, p. 980). Fortunately, of the many congenital infections, syphilis is not only the most readily prevented, but it is also the most susceptible to therapy.

Following an incubation period of 10 to 90 days, primary syphilis appears. When infection is acquired during pregnancy, the primary lesion, or sometimes multiple lesions, involving the genital tract may be of such size or so located as to go unnoticed. In some instances, however, the lesion may be somewhat larger than usual, presumably because of the increased vascularity of the genitalia. The chancre lasts from 1 to 5 weeks and heals spontaneously. A nontender, solitary enlarged lymph node is often present.

Approximately 6 weeks after the appearance of the chancre, secondary syphilis may appear in the form of a highly variable skin rash. The lesions of secondary syphilis are often slight; they may be limited to the genitalia, where they appear usually as elevated areas, or condylomata lata, which occasionally cause ulceration of the vulva. Unfortunately, in many women no history of a local sore or rash can be elicited. The first suggestion of the disease is the delivery of an infant that may be either stillborn or liveborn but severely afflicted with congenital syphilis.

A suitable serologic screening test such as the Venereal Disease Research Laboratory (VDRL) slide test must be performed on blood obtained at the time of the first prenatal visit. Testing is required by law. Fortunately,

serologic tests for syphilis will almost always be positive by 4 to 6 weeks after contracting the disease. Because such reagin tests lack specificity, a treponemal test such as the Fluorescent Treponemal Antibody Absorption Test is used to confirm a positive result.

ANTIBIOTIC TREATMENT OF SYPHILIS. Penicillin remains the treatment of choice. The 1979 recommendations for treatment provided by the Center for Disease Control follow:

I. *Incubating Syphilis:* Patients exposed to infectious syphilis within the preceding 3 months, or of high risk based on epidemiologic grounds should be treated as for early syphilis as outlined under II. Where possible a diagnosis should be established. Women who are culture-positive for gonorrhea with no lesion and a nonreactive serology must also be considered at high risk. The aqueous procaine penicillin-G plus probenecid regimen for gonorrhea (described below) is also effective therapy for incubating syphilis. A reagin test for syphilis should be repeated three months after the initial therapy.

II. *Treatment for Syphilis of Less Than 1 Year's Duration*
   A. *Benzathine penicillin-G:* 2.4 million units total, half in each buttock, has the advantage of a single visit treatment. Aqueous procaine penicillin-G, 600,000 units per day for 8 days for a total of 4.8 million units, is effective, but requires multiple visits.
   B. For patients allergic to penicillin, two alternative regimens are recommended.
      1. Oral erythromycin stearate, ethyl succinate, or base, 2 g per day for 15 days, a total of 30 g.
      2. Oral tetracycline hydrochloride, 2 g per day for 15 days, a total of 30 g. Tetracycline is not recommended during pregnancy.

If during the year following treatment clinical signs recur or persist, a spinal fluid examination should be done and the patient retreated using the regimen described for syphilis acquired more than one year previously. The same retreatment regimen is used if the initial nonspecific antibody titer is greater than 1:8 or fails to decrease to negative or by fourfold within a 12-month period.

III. *Treatment of Syphilis of Indeterminate Length or More than 1 Year's Duration*

A. *Benzathine penicillin-G:* 2.4 million units intramuscularly weekly (1.2 million units in each buttock) for 3 successive weeks, a total of 7.2 million units. This is a regimen with good patient compliance. Alternatively, the patient can be given aqueous procaine penicillin-G, 600,000 units intramuscularly each day for 14 days, but the daily injections are a disadvantage. If the spinal fluid is positive, some investigators favor hospital admission and intravenous penicillin-G therapy, 2.4 million units given every 4 hours for 10 days.

B. For the patient allergic to penicillin, a spinal fluid examination must be performed prior to therapy. An alternative regimen during pregnancy is to use the oral forms of erythromycin (except the estolate) 500 mg, 4 times a day for 30 days, for a total of 60 g.

All patients with a positive spinal fluid should have spinal fluid testing at least every six months for three years.

IV. *Treatment of Syphilis in Pregnancy:* For pregnant patients not allergic to penicillin, treatment is the same as for the corresponding stage of syphilis in nonpregnant patients. For pregnant women who are allergic to penicillin, the only recommended therapy is erythromycin in the same form and dosage used in nonpregnant women for the same stage of disease.

The mother who has been treated successfully often remains susceptible to a subsequent syphilitic infection, as does her fetus. Therefore, it is very important during pregnancy to treat her sexual partner and to observe her closely for evidence of reinfection. When reinfection is detected, retreatment is necessary. Women who have been treated for syphilis during pregnancy should have monthly quantitative nontreponemal serologic tests for the remainder of the pregnancy. Women who show a rise in titer of 4 dilutions or greater should be treated.

V. *Treatment of Congenital Syphilis.* Every infant with suspected or proven congenital syphilis should have a cerebrospinal fluid examination prior to treatment, and should be followed at monthly intervals until the nontreponemal serologic tests are negative. Symptomatic infants or infants with a positive spinal fluid should be treated with aqueous penicillin-G, 500 units per kg intramuscularly or intravenously in two divided doses each day for a minimum of 10 days, or aqueous procaine penicillin-G, 50,000 units per kg intramuscularly each day for a minimum of 10 days.

Asymptomatic seropositive infants with a negative cerebrospinal fluid examination can be treated with a single dose of penicillin-G, 50,000 units per kg intramuscularly.

Infants born of mothers treated with erythromycin for syphilis during pregnancy should be managed as though they have congenital syphilis.

Gonorrhea. Infection in women caused by *Neisseria gonorrhoeae* may be limited to the lower genital tract, including the cervix, urethra, and periurethral and Bartholin's glands, or it may spread across the endometrium to involve the oviducts and the peritoneum. The organism also enters the bloodstream to cause arthritis uncommonly and endocarditis rarely.

Acute gonococcal salpingitis is not a problem in pregnancy after the 3rd month when the chorion laeve has fused with the decidua parietalis to obliterate the endometrial cavity between the cervix and oviduct. Rarely, a fallopian tube previously damaged by infection with *N. gonorrhoeae* may become reinfected during pregnancy with other organisms that reach the oviduct through the bloodstream or lymphatics.

The greatly increased prevalence of gonorrhea in recent years has not spared pregnant women; many obstetric clinics have noted gonococcal infections of the lower genitourinary tract quite commonly.

The pregnant woman may have asymptomatic local infection involving, singly or in combination, the lower genital tract, the lower urinary tract, and the rectum (Table 28-7). The infection may antedate the pregnancy; or the patient may have acquired the disease at the time of the insemination that resulted in pregnancy, in which case she is likely to develop symptomatic acute salpingitis; or she may have become infected locally after the uterine cavity was obliterated by fusion of chorion to decidua and a well-formed mucous plug had sealed the cervical canal. In any event, either no treatment or inadequate treatment with persistence of the infection allows her to infect her sexual partner, to suffer gonococcal arthritis or other disseminated disease, and to infect her infant at the time of delivery, thereby causing gonorrheal ophthalmia (see Chap. 20, p. 479), and to develop an ascending infection of the genital tract after delivery. Consequently, even asymptomatic disease during pregnancy should be identified and eradicated (see Chap. 13, p. 309).

TABLE 28-7.
FREQUENCY OF CULTURES POSITIVE FOR NEISSERIA GONORRHOEAE

SITE CULTURED	FIRST VISIT (PERCENT)	SECOND VISIT* (PERCENT)
Cervix	94	89
Vagina	78	82
Urethra	78	71
Rectum	49	57

From Schmale, Martin, and Domescik: *JAMA* 210:312, 1969.
* No treatment during interval from previous culture.

TREATMENT OF GONORRHEA. For uncomplicated gonococcal infections, the 1979 recommendations of the Center for Disease Control is aqueous procaine penicillin G, 4.8 million units intramuscularly divided into at least two doses but given at the same time, following 1 g of probenecid (Benemid) ingested just before the injections.

For pregnant women who are allergic to penicillin or probenecid, spectinomycin, erythromycin, or cefazolin are recommended for use as follows:

1. Erythromycin: 1.5 g orally followed by 0.5 g, 4 times a day for a total of 9.5 g. This regimen is safe for mother and fetus but not highly effective. The estolate forms of erythromycin is contraindicated because of liver toxicity.
2. Cefazolin: 2 g intramuscularly with probenecid 1 g orally. This regimen is probably effective but its safety for the fetus is not established.
3. Spectinomycin: 2 g intramuscularly. This regimen is effective but has not been established as safe for the fetus.

Follow-up cervical and anorectal cultures should be obtained 5 to 7 days after completion of therapy. At the present time spectinomycin is considered to be the drug of choice when treatment has failed using any of the other agents considered above. If treatment with spectinomycin fails, a test for penicillinase-producing organisms should be performed. Penicillinase-producing *Neisseria gonorrhoae* resistant to spectinomycin may be treated with cefoxitin 2.0 g in a simple intramuscular injection plus probenecid 1.0 g by mouth. Follow-up cultures should be obtained 1 to 2 weeks after completing treatment.

For disseminated gonococcal infection involving joints or skin the following treatment schedules with aqueous crystalline penicillin G are recommended:

1. Aqueous penicillin-G: 10 million units daily for 3 days or until there is significant clinical improvement. Follow with oral

ampicillin, 500 mg, 4 times a day, to complete 7 days of therapy.

2. Ampicillin: 3.5 g orally plus probenecid 1 g orally followed by ampicillin 500 mg, 4 times a day for a total of seven days therapy.

For pregnant women allergic to these drugs, erythromycin, 0.5 g intravenously every 6 hours for at least 3 days, may be used. Endocarditis and meningitis resulting from gonococcus require at least 10 million units of intravenous penicillin daily for 3 to 4 weeks for endocarditis and at least 10 days for meningitis.

The infant whose mother has gonorrhea requires treatment with aqueous penicillin G, 50,000 units for term-size infants and 20,000 units for those who are small (Center for Disease Control, 1979).

Herpes Simplex Virus Infections. Two types of herpes virus have been distinguished based on immunologic as well as clinical differences. Type I *Herpes hominis* is responsible for most nongenital herpetic lesions but much less commonly may also involve the genital tract. Type II *Herpes hominis* is recovered almost exclusively from the genital tract and probably is transmitted in the great majority of instances by sexual contact. The incidence of antibody specific for type II virus approaches 100 percent among prostitutes. In the absence of appropriate antibody, exposure to a sexual partner with herpetic lesions in the majority of instances results in clinical disease.

The prevalence of active herpes infection of the genital tract probably varies considerably among institutions. Perhaps 1 to 1.5 percent of pregnancies are complicated by genital herpes virus infections. The incubation period is 3 to 6 days for primary infection and 7 to 10 days for secondary infection. Symptoms and signs persist for 2 to 4 weeks. The vulvar and perineal vesicles are easily traumatized and commonly rupture and become secondarily infected. Vulvar lesions are likely to be extremely painful and may cause considerable debility, including urinary retention. There is no really effective treat-

ment. Severe secondary infection should respond to broad-spectrum antibiotic therapy. For severe discomfort, analgesics and topical anesthetics may provide appreciable relief.

Cervical involvement may take the form of a diffuse inflammation or discrete ulcers. However, involvement of the cervix and vagina is often asymptomatic. The virus may be shed from an infected cervix for months. Cervical smears usually, but not always, contain large multinucleate cells with eosinophilic inclusion bodies. They may be identified in a smear prepared for cervical cytologic study.

Maternal infection appears to be transmitted only rarely across the placenta or an intact chorioamnion to the embryo or fetus. Most often the fetus-infant becomes infected by virus that was shed from the cervix or lower genital tract invading the uterus following rupture of the membranes or the virus contacting the fetus as he descends through the cervix and the lower genital tract.

The infection in the newborn may take one of three forms: (1) disseminated, with involvement of major viscera; (2) localized with involvement confined to the central nervous system, eyes, skin, or mucosa; or (3) asymptomatic. Congenital and neonatal herpes simplex virus infections often prove lethal. Visintine and associates (1978) cite a mortality rate of 60 percent! Among survivors, serious ocular and central nervous system damage have been identified in at least one-half of survivors.

Attempts at treatment of the neonate, in general, have been disappointing. Vidarabine (adenine arabinoside) has been approved by the Food and Drug Administration for treatment of herpes simplex encephalitis but has not proved to be very effective. Therefore, considerable emphasis has been placed upon preventing contact with the virus during delivery.

Tejani and co-workers (1979) have investigated the prevalence of herpesvirus in the genital tract of 1094 expectant mothers at the time they were admitted in labor. The vulva and cervix were inspected for herpetic lesions and, when suspected, material for culture and for immunofluo-rescent staining was obtained. In the absence of suspicious lesions cultures only were obtained. The two women with active disease were correctly identified on the basis of physical findings. Both were delivered by cesarean section. Of the other 1092 women who were evaluated, virus was cultured from only one. That mother's complement fixation titer was 1:32, indicating previous infection. The infant, by coincidence delivered by cesarean section, was unaffected. Their observations serve to emphasize the value of careful examination of the vulva and cervix of all women early in labor.

The role of cesarean section to try to avoid acquisition of virus by the fetus-infant is not clear at this time. If lesions are present on the cervix, vagina, or vulva, and membranes are intact, cesarean section is probably indicated. The same is true when recent viral cultures from the genital tract are positive. Visintine and associates (1978) have emphasized the use of cervical cytology in emergency situations since herpesvirus cultures take 1 to 4 days to complete. Through use of the Papanicolaou smear technic and careful examination by an experienced cytologist, they have been able to identify about three-fourths of cases in which the culture proved positive.

Cesarean section has not been demonstrated to be of value in preventing serious infection in the infant when viral cultures are negative, or if membranes have been ruptured for more than a very few hours (Amstey and Monif, 1974; Light and Linnemann, 1974). Fortunately, proven genital herpes hominis infection late in pregnancy does not always condemn the infant who is delivered vaginally to serious viral infection (St. Geme et al., 1975).

The infant of a mother known or suspected of having genital herpes should be isolated in the nursery and cultured for herpes. In addition, liver function and spinal fluid should be monitored and the infant kept under close observation for up to 2 weeks.

It has been considered impractical and unnecessary by some neonatologists, but certainly not all, to separate a baby from his or her mother when the mother has herpetic lesions. Instead, she has been urged to wash her hands carefully and avoid any contact between her lesions, her hands, and the baby. Breast-feeding has been allowed under these conditions. It should be pointed out, however, that breast-feeding was implicated in one case of disseminated herpes simplex infection in a newborn infant (Dunkle et al., 1979). It has been recommended by some authorities (Kibrick, 1980) that parents and personnel with oral herpetic lesions be isolated from newborn infants, although Schriner and associates (1979) found that over 50 percent of 110 neonatal centers questioned did not isolate mothers with oral herpes from their infants.

Other Sexually Transmitted Diseases. These include *Trichamonad vaginitis* (see Chap. 13, p. 325), *Monilial vulvovaginitis* (see Chap. 13, p. 325). *Condyloma accuminata* (see Chap. 25, p. 624), *Chlamydia infections* (see Chap. 38, p. 980) and the now rare venereal diseases *Chancroid, Granuloma inguinale,* and *Lymphopathia venereum.*

In the pregnant woman, the lesions of *granuloma inguinale* tend to be multiple, large, quite foul-smelling ulcerations of the vulva, lower vagina, perineum, and cervix. The causative organism, *Donovania granulomatis,* at times disseminates to cause lesions remote from the lower genital tract, especially in bone. Diagnosis depends upon identification of Donovan bodies in large mononuclear cells in Giemsa-stained smears from the lesion. Tetracycline, 2 g per day, in divided doses for 15 to 20 days, is usually effective, although at times a vulvar lesion may heal incompletely or with gross deformity, ultimately requiring vulvectomy.

The primary genital infection of *Lymphopathia venereum* is transient and seldom recognized. Inguinal adenitis may follow and at times lead to suppuration. Ultimately, the lymphatics of the lower genital tract and the perirectal tissues may be involved in sclerosis and fibrosis, which cause vulvar elephantiasis and especially severe rectal stricture. Sometimes attention is first drawn to the disease in pregnant women when rectal examination is attempted. The Frei test is usually positive, as is the complement-fixation test. Sulfisoxazole (Gantrisin) has been the standard treatment of early disease; tetracycline is of value for treating draining buboes.

A careful vaginal examination is of utmost importance in deciding upon the method of delivery. If there is widespread pelvic scarring, cesarean section is indicated. Marked perirectal fibrosis with cicatricial changes in the rectovaginal septum is usually indicative of an extensive process that requires abdominal delivery. It is crucial to avoid difficult vaginal delivery, since most ruptures of the rectum have occurred in association with traumatic vaginal operations. Colostomy presents no special problems in abdominal or vaginal delivery. Although treatment with tetracycline may arrest the infection of lymphopathia venereum and clear up secondary infection, it fails to influence preexisting fibrotic changes.

Chancroid is usually a self-limiting disease that produces a painful, nonindurated ulcer, or "soft chancre," in the lower genital tract and painful inguinal lymphadenopathy. The causative organism, *Hemophilus ducreyi,* is sensitive to sulfisoxazole as well as several antibiotics.

DISEASES OF THE LIVER AND ALIMENTARY TRACT

Viral Hepatitis. Classification of viral hepatitis as either infectious hepatitis or serum hepatitis on the basis of a history of parenteral administration of blood or some blood products is no longer tenable. There are two distinct hepatitis viruses, now commonly referred to as hepatitis A and hepatitis B viruses that are capable of inducing hepatitis after ingestion or parenteral administration of infected material, and each causes hepatitis after a relatively well-defined period of incubation (Krugman and Giles, 1970). A "non-A, non-B" variety of hepatitis, referred to by some as hepatitis C, has been identified as the most common cause of hepatitis in recipients of multiple transfusions of blood or blood products (Krugman, 1975). Hepatitis B virus, as well as the A virus, may be transmitted by kissing and by various other forms of sexual contact (Fass, 1974; Szmuness et al., 1975; Villarejos et al., 1974). Most standard immune globulin preparations are of value for prophylaxis against Type A hepatitis and should be administered to pregnant women exposed to the disease or traveling in regions where the disease is epidemic.

Hepatitis B immune globulin preparations have proved to be effective in preventing clinical disease in spouses of individuals with active viral hepatitis and a positive test for hepatitis B surface antigen (Redeker et al., 1975). A vaccine for hepatitis B is currently being tested in homosexual males.

Hieber and co-workers (1977) reported on 50 instances of viral hepatitis complicating pregnancy at Parkland Memorial Hospital. All of the mothers survived and there was no excess pregnancy wastage, preterm deliveries, or evidence of fetal growth retardation. In 40 percent of the mothers the disease was due to type B virus. Two infants out of eight whose mothers developed type B hepatitis during the third trimester were found to be asymptomatic carriers of hepatitis B surface antigen and to have mild elevations of serum glutamic oxaloacetic transaminase for up to 45 months. These results are much more favorable than those reported previously by investigators in some countries. For example, D'Cruz and associates (1968) in Bombay, India, noted a mortality rate of 54 percent among 143 hospitalized pregnant or puerperal women compared with 26 percent in nonpregnant women. Malnutrition and the restriction of hospitalization to only the most seriously ill patients probably account for much of the difference in mortality rates.

It is important that the pregnant woman with hepatitis be diagnosed and so treated long before she becomes moribund. The physician must not ignore the possibility of hepatitis in any pregnant woman who complains of nausea and vomiting. Unfortunately, these symptoms are sometimes incorrectly ascribed to pregnancy itself rather than to hepatitis. As a result, supportive treatment may be ignored until the mother becomes gravely ill. Our regimen for the treatment of hepatitis in pregnancy consists basically of hospitalization, bed rest, and a good diet. Fluids, electrolytes, and calories are provided intravenously if vomiting is a problem.

Infants born to mothers with viral hepatitis are at risk of acquiring the virus in utero, or more likely during or subsequent to birth, especially when surface and e antigen titers are high (Papaevangelou et al., 1974).

Once the fetus or newborn infant is infected, there is a strong tendency for the infant to remain a chronic carrier. Long term effects of carrier status are not yet clear. Prompt prophylaxis in the newborn infant with immune globulin containing antibody appropriate for the virus may be effective (Kohler et al. 1974; Dosik and Jhaveri, 1978). Hepatitis B surface antigen has been detected in breast milk; hepatitis virus may also be present in serum exuding from excoriations of the nipples. Therefore, breast-feeding should be avoided (Krugman, 1975).

In the limited experiences with pregnancies complicated by chronic active hepatitis and cirrhosis at Parkland Memorial Hospital, the outcome has been favorable. Therapy consisted of prolonged hospitalization with a regular hospital diet and much rest.

Cirrhosis of the Liver. Women with cirrhosis are likely to be infertile. Cheng (1977) has reviewed the clinical features of pregnancy in women with hepatic cirrhosis and concluded that perinatal loss is high and the maternal prognosis is grave.

Acute Yellow Atrophy of the Liver. This rare complication of pregnancy occurs in two forms: (1) true acute yellow atrophy, a disease seen in pregnant as well as nonpregnant women and characterized by massive hepatocellular necrosis; and (2) "obstetric" acute yellow atrophy, or acute fatty metamorphosis of pregnancy, a disease characterized by fatty infiltration of the hepatic cells without necrosis. The association of true acute yellow atrophy with infectious hepatitis was shown conclusively by Lucké (1944). Similar cases were studied by Zondek and Bromberg (1947) in Israel in pregnant women during an epidemic of infectious hepatitis.

The belief that there is a type of fatty liver peculiar to pregnancy has received strong support from the studies of Sheehan (1961), as well as those of Ober and Le Compte (1955) and of Kahil and associates (1964). In the past this disease has often been fatal. Breen and associates (1972) described three cases of idiopathic fatty liver of pregnancy

with survival in which diagnostic studies include liver biopsy. Subsequent pregnancy in each instance was uncomplicated. A serious coagulopathy may accompany the condition (Moldin and Johannson, 1978).

The characteristic pathologic change is infiltration of all the hepatic cells by fine fatty droplets, without the necrosis that characterizes viral hepatitis. Although sporadic cases of acute fatty liver without obvious cause occur in pregnancy, indistinguishable cases resulting from toxicity of tetracycline have been reported in nonpregnant women by Schultz and associates (1963) and in similarly treated pregnant women with pyelonephritis by Whalley, Adams, and Combes (1964).

Liver Transplant and Pregnancy. Walcott and associates (1979) have described delivery of a normal infant at term after an uncomplicated prenatal course even though the mother had undergone a liver transplant because of hepatic necrosis from hepatic vein thrombosis 2 years before, was being treated continously with azathioprine and prednisone, and was not ovulating until treated with clomiphene citrate.

Obstetric Hepatosis. Described under a variety of names, including *recurrent jaundice of pregnancy, idiopathic cholestasis of pregnancy, cholestatic hepatosis,* and *icterus gravidarum,* this condition is characterized clinically by either icterus, pruritus, or both. The major lesion is intrahepatic cholestasis with centrolobular bile staining without inflammatory cells or proliferation of mesenchymal cells.

The modest hyperbilirubinemia results predominantly from conjugated pigment. Sulfobromophthalein excretion is impaired, and serum alkaline phosphatase may be elevated above the usual levels for pregnancy. Serum glutamic oxalacetic transaminase activity may be moderately elevated. These changes disappear after delivery but often recur in a subsequent pregnancy or when an oral contraceptive containing potent estrogen is employed.

Pruritus associated with obstetric hepatosis is caused by raised plasma levels of bile salts and may be quite troublesome. Cholestyramine has been reported to provide relief in most cases.

Reid and associates (1976) have observed appreciable pregnancy wastage among women with obstetric cholestasis: There were 5 stillbirths and 1 neonatal death among 56 pregnancies; intrapartum asphyxia was observed in 5 more pregnancies; 18 infants were delivered preterm; 5 of the mothers suffered postpartum hemorrhage. Johnston and Baskett (1979) observed much lower pregnancy wastage. However, they also found an abnormally high incidence of preterm births and postpartum hemorrhage.

Cholelithiasis and Cholecystitis.
There is a greater frequency (twice or three times as high) of cholelithiasis in women than in men. Acute attacks of gallbladder disease during pregnancy or the puerperium, in general, are managed the same way as for the nonpregnant woman. If cholecystectomy is to be performed, the second trimester is the optimal time since the risk of spontaneous abortion or delivery of an immature fetus is reduced and the uterus is not yet large enough to impinge on the field of operation. Even so, when surgery is thought to be indicated in the pregnant woman, procrastination should be avoided. Delay can only place the woman and her fetus in greater jeopardy. At times, just drainage of the gallbladder is the procedure of choice. Recent surgery does not complicate labor unduly.

Hill and associates (1975) described 20 instances of cholecystectomy during pregnancy at the Mayo Clinic. There was one spontaneous abortion at 10 weeks of gestation 42 days after the operation; maternal morbidity was low.

Gallbladder kinetics during pregnancy have been investigated by Braverman and associates (1980) using real-time sonography. After the first trimester, both gallbladder volume during fasting and residual volume after contracting in response to a test meal were twice as large as in nonpregnant subjects. Incomplete emptying may result in retention of cholesterol crystals, a prerequisite for cho-

lesterol gallstones. These findings are supportive, at least, of the view that pregnancy increases the risk of gallstones.

Although the use of contraceptive steroids has been implicated in increased frequency of gallbladder disease (Ch. 40, p. 1015), Braverman and associates did not identify increased gallbladder volume nor incomplete emptying in women who were taking them. Presumably, the very high progesterone levels that characterize the second and third trimesters of pregnancy are responsible for the diminished gallbladder activity. Progesterone has been shown to impair the gallbladder response to exogenously administered cholecystokinin in experimental animals.

Obesity. Marked obesity is a hazard to the pregnant woman and her fetus. For example, Tracy and Miller (1969), in the course of reviewing the pregnancies of 48 women whose weights averaged 284 pounds, noted that nearly two-thirds developed some obstetric complication. One of the five mothers diagnosed as having diabetes expired. Over half of the 48 were considered hypertensive, and pyelonephritis developed in five.

In our experience, a large variety of serious complications of pregnancy is more likely to develop in obese women, including hypertension, diabetes, aspiration of gastric contents during anesthesia, wound complications, and thromboembolism. The most extreme case of obesity we have encountered during pregnancy was in a young multipara who early in the third trimester weighed somewhat more than 500 pounds although she was only 62 inches tall. In spite of a multitude of complications, emotional as well as physical, six pregnancies have produced eight living children.

Management of obesity during pregnancy is a challenge. A program of weight reduction utilizing a diet restricted in calories but providing all essential nutrients has commonly been recommended for obese pregnant women. If such a regimen is to be used, it is mandatory that the quality of the diet be monitored closely and that ketosis not be allowed to develop.

JEJUNOILEAL BYPASS. The *small-intestinal bypass* operation performed to try to relieve obesity has been followed by pregnancy. Twenty-five children, including three sets of twins and one of triplets, have been born to 16 such women observed by Salmon (1975). Their birth weights averaged 3000 g, or 300 g less than did the children born to the women before the bypass operation. Two of the children had serious anomalies.

Seven pregnant women with a jejunoileal bypass have been cared for at Parkland Memorial Hospital. Six of the pregnancies were quite benign. All of the women received specifically supplemental iron, folic acid, vitamin B_{12}, plus a commercially available prenatal vitamin-mineral preparation. The six infants were appropriately grown and in good health. In one woman who had previously undergone bypass operation which excluded nearly all of the small intestine and utilized an end-to-end anastomosis, pregnancy created myriad problems: She lost appreciable weight while consuming between 6000 and 9000 calories per day. A growth-retarded infant was delivered by cesarean section which was necessitated by a prolapsed cord. He subsequently thrived. Postpartum, the mother developed severe hypoproteinemia, hypocalcemia with tetany, hypokalemia, hypomagnesemia, and vitamin K deficiency sufficiently intense to prolong appreciably the prothrombin time. She responded well to vitamin K, calcium gluconate, potassium chloride, and magnesium sulfate (given parenterally) and to a generous high-protein diet.

Woods and Brinkman (1978) in their review have considered further the problems imposed on pregnancy by jejunoileal bypass.

Hyperemesis Gravidarum. Nausea and vomiting of moderate intensity are especially common complaints from the second to the fourth month of gestation (see Chap. 13, p. 323). Fortunately, vomiting sufficiently pernicious to produce weight loss, dehydration, acidosis from starvation, alkalosis from loss of hydrochloric acid in vomitus, and hypokalemia has become quite rare.

Treatment of pernicious vomiting of pregnancy comprises correction of deficits of fluid and electrolytes and of acidosis or alkalosis. This requires appropriate amounts of sodium, potassium, chloride, lactate or bicarbonate, glucose, and water, which should be administered parenterally until the vomiting has been controlled. Appropriate steps should be taken to detect other diseases—for example, gastroenteritis, cholecystitis, hepatitis, peptic ulcer, and pyelonephritis. In many instances, social and psychologic factors contribute to the illness, as in the case of the young unwed mother who continues to live with her parents while they harass her because of her "sin." Commonly, in this circumstance, the woman improves remarkably while hospitalized, only to relapse after discharge. Positive assistance with psychologic and social problems often proves quite beneficial. Various antinausea medications commonly prescribed are likely to be toxic if ingested in large doses, especially by young children. For example, fatal overdosage from the ingestion of approximately 100 Bendectin tablets by a 3-year-old boy has been described (Bayley et al., 1975). Rarely is it necessary to interrupt the pregnancy. The subject of nausea and vomiting in pregnancy, including a number of bizarre theories, has been reviewed extensively by Fairweather (1968).

Appendicitis. Gestation does not predispose to appendicitis, but because of the general prevalence of the disease, there is an incidence of about 1 in every 2000 pregnancies, as shown in Black's extensive review (1960). Pregnancy often makes diagnosis more difficult. First, anorexia, nausea, and vomiting caused by pregnancy itself are fairly common. Second, as the uterus enlarges, the appendix commonly moves upward and outward toward the flank, so that pain and tenderness may not be prominent in the right lower quadrant (Fig. 28-6). Third, some degree of leukocytosis is the rule during normal pregnancy. Fourth, during pregnancy especially, other diseases may be readily confused with appendicitis, such as pyelonephritis, renal colic caused by a stone or kinking of a ureter, placental abruption, and red, or carneous, degeneration of a myoma.

Appendicitis increases the likelihood of

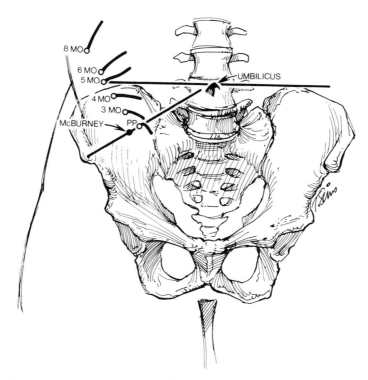

FIG 28-6. Changes in the position of the appendix as pregnancy advances. (mo. = calendar month; P.P. = postpartum). (Modified from Baer, Reis, and Arens. *JAMA* 98:1359, 1932)

abortion or premature labor, especially if peritonitis develops. The fetal loss rate, therefore, in most series is about 15 percent. As the appendix is pushed progressively higher by the growing uterus, walling off of the infection becomes increasingly unlikely and appendiceal rupture causes widespread peritonitis. Acute appendicitis in the last trimester, therefore, carries a much graver prognosis. Although antibiotics have reduced the mortality rate from acute appendicitis in pregnancy, the disease remains a serious complication of gestation.

The treatment, regardless of the stage of gestation, is immediate operation (Cunningham and McCubbin, 1975; Gomez and Wood, 1979). *Even though diagnostic errors sometimes lead to the removal of a normal appendix, it is better to operate unnecessarily than to postpone intervention until generalized peritonitis has developed.* The mortality rate of appendicitis today in the obstetric patient is essentially that associated with surgical delay.

It is important that during the operation and period of recovery both hypoxia and hypotension be avoided. If they are avoided and generalized peritonitis does not develop, the prognosis is quite good. Seldom, if ever, is cesarean section indicated at the time of appendectomy. Aside from local soreness, a recent abdominal incision should present no problem during labor and vaginal delivery.

Peptic Ulcer. An active peptic ulcer is rare during pregnancy, and complications such as perforation or hemorrhage are even rarer (Honiotes et al., 1970). Vasicka and co-workers (1957), however, have indicated that in a small proportion of cases, peptic ulcers become aggravated by pregnancy, and massive hemorrhage may occur. Taylor (1972) has observed hypopituitarism to develop following massive hemorrhage from a gastric ulcer late in pregnancy.

Pancreatitis. Pancreatitis during pregnancy is very uncommon. The diagnosis is complicated by a physiologic increase in serum amylase values during the second and third trimester; Kaiser and associates (1975) report values as high as 209 at midpregnancy, compared to 46 or less very early in pregnancy. The principles of therapy, in general, are the same as for nonpregnant patients. If the diagnosis is secure, treatment is medical rather than surgical exploration. Two commonly used drugs—tetracycline and thiazide diuretics—have been implicated in pancreatitis in pregnant women (Minkowitz et al., 1964; Whalley et al., 1964). Corlett and Mishell (1972) and Wilkinson (1973) have reviewed pancreatitis and pregnancy and stress the necessity for prompt medical management.

Intestinal Obstruction. This grave complication of pregnancy results most frequently from pressure of the growing uterus on intestinal adhesions resulting from previous abdominal operations. Of 10 cases reported by Bellingham, Mackey, and Winston (1949), there was a history of previous abdominal operation in nine. As emphasized by these authors, the mortality rate tends to be very high, chiefly because of error in diagnosis, late diagnosis, reluctance to operate on a pregnant woman, and inadequate preparation for surgery. The large pregnant uterus, furthermore, lying anterior to the intestinal obstruction, may mask the abdominal signs, thus contributing greatly to the difficulty of diagnosis.

Kohn, Briele, and Douglass (1944) have reported a remarkable case in which the same patient was operated upon for *volvulus* four times, three of the operations having been performed in the course of two pregnancies. In a review of the literature, they collected 79 cases of volvulus in pregnancy. In a third of the cases reported by Harer and Harer (1958), emptying the uterus by cesarean section was necessary to obtain proper exposure.

Carcinoma of the Bowel. Carcinoma of the rectum and colon is a rare complication of pregnancy, 65 cases having been reported in a review of the literature by Waters and Fenimore (1954).

Patients with *colostomies* usually go through pregnancy without difficulty. Intestinal obstruction caused by pressure of the enlarged uterus on the proximal loop of intestine concerned rarely occurs.

Ulcerative Colitis. In an analysis of one of the largest series of cases reported, Crohn and his associates (1956) found that colitis that is quiescent at the beginning of gestation is reactivated by pregnancy, usually in the first trimester, in about half the cases. If the colitis is already active at the time of conception, it is materially aggravated in three-quarters of the cases. They emphasize also the excessive and prolonged severity of postpartum recurrences. Felsen and Wolarsky (1948), in an analysis of the clinical course of 34 women with ulcerative colitis in 50 pregnancies, found that in one-third of the pregnancies the colitis was somewhat aggravated in the first trimester but was ameliorated in about one-half. When this disease becomes worse in gestation, the etiologic factor may be psychogenic, rather than related to any intrinsic effect of pregnancy. The patient's fear that pregnancy will aggravate her disease, for example, may precipitate an exacerbation. Reassurance is therefore an important part of management.

Regional Enteritis. Fieldring and Cooke (1970), in pregnancies complicated by Crohn's disease, found no evidence that pregnancy exerted adverse effects on the course of the disease or increased the mortality rate. Moreover, abortion, prematurity, and stillbirth were not increased. Sterility was the main problem encountered. Norton and Patterson (1972) have similarly concluded that pregnancy and regional enteritis do not affect each other adversely. Homan and Thorbjarnarson (1976), however, observed relapse in one-fourth of women with Crohn's disease after the pregnancy was completed.

Gingivitis. Rarely, the gums of pregnant women become inflamed and spongy, bleeding upon the slightest touch. In many cases, the condition clears almost immediately after delivery. It is best treated by a combination of oral hygiene and a well-balanced diet. An *epulis*, a focal, highly vascular swelling of the gingiva, is an occasional complication (see Fig. 9-15, p. 247).

Porphyria. Acute idiopathic porphyria is a rare metabolic dysfunction caused by an inborn error of porphyrin metabolism. It may present a wide range of symptoms often suggestive of diseases involving the gastrointestinal tract, pelvic organs, and nervous system. Brodie and co-workers (1977) have reviewed the pregnancy experiences of 39 women with this autosomally dominant disease. One woman died; total wastage was 13 percent. The diagnosis must be kept in mind whenever a pregnant woman describes bizarre acute abdominal pain.

OTHER VIRAL INFECTIONS

Various viruses have been recovered from the fetus, but only rubella virus, cytomegalovirus, herpesvirus hominis, and varicella-zoster virus are at all likely to be teratogenic. Others that may reach the fetus include the viruses causing measles (rubeola), smallpox (variola), vaccinia, poliomyelitis, hepatitis, Western equine encephalitis, mumps, and the Coxsackie B group.

About 5 percent of pregnancies are complicated by clinically apparent viral infections, according to the Collaborative Perinatal Research Study. When the common cold is excluded, the most frequent viral infections are influenza, flulike disease, herpesvirus infections, viral gastroenteritis, and viral infection of larynx, pharynx, and tonsils.

Rubella (German Measles). Rubella, a disease of minor importance in the absence of pregnancy, has been directly responsible for inestimable perinatal loss and serious malformations in the liveborn infant. The relation between maternal rubella and grave congenital malformations was first recognized by Gregg (1942), an Australian ophthalmologist.

DIAGNOSIS. The diagnosis of rubella is at times quite difficult. Not only are the clinical features of other illnesses quite similar, but subclinical cases with viremia and the capability of infecting the embryo and fetus do occur. Diagnosis of rubella, therefore, can be made with certainty only by isolation of the virus or by the more practical demonstration of a rising rubella antibody titer in the serum. Absence of rubella antibody indicates lack of immunity. The presence of antibody denotes an immune response to rubella viremia that may have been acquired anywhere from a very few weeks to many years earlier. If maternal rubella antibody is demonstrated at the time of exposure to rubella or sometime before, the mother can be assured that it is exceedingly unlikely that her fetus will be affected.

The nonimmune person who acquires rubella viremia demonstrates peak antibody titers 1 to 2 weeks after the onset of the rash, or 2 to 3 weeks after the onset of viremia, since the viremia precedes clinically evident disease by about 1 week (Cooper and Krugman, 1967). The promptness of the antibody response, therefore, may complicate serodiagnosis unless serum is collected initially within a very few days after the onset of the rash. If, for example, the first specimen was obtained 10 days after the rash, detection of antibodies would fail to differentiate between two possibilities: one, that the very recent disease was actually rubella and, two, that it was not rubella, but the person was already immune to rubella. The demonstration of specific IgM globulin in the pregnant woman indicates a primary infection within the previous month or so. Therefore, specific IgM estimations, if available, are useful for diagnosing recent rubella infection (Field and Murphy, 1972).

IMMUNIZATION. There is no known chemotherapeutic or antibiotic agent that will prevent viremia in nonimmune subjects exposed to rubella. The use of gamma globulin for this purpose is not recommended. Brody and co-workers (1965), during a rubella outbreak in an isolated community, gave relatively large doses of gamma globulin to boys but not to girls at the time of, or even before, exposure. The attack rate, measured by sero-conversion, among the boys was 44 percent and among the girls 85 percent. The group that received gamma globulin, therefore, was only partially protected. The data of Brody and associates also suggest that large doses of gamma globulin given at or before exposure to rubella may only minimize the clinical features of the disease. Viremia without clinically apparent disease can, of course, lead to fetal infection with disastrous consequences.

Even though women who are pregnant or who may conceive within the next 6 weeks or so should not be vaccinated, some states attempted to require women seeking marriage licenses either to have demonstrable immunity or to be immunized. In Colorado during 1971 and 1972, of those without immunity and about to enter wedlock, 21 percent were already pregnant! (Judson et al., 1974). Although the risk appears low (Hayden et al., 1980), rubella vaccine is contraindicated just before and during pregnancy.

The following program for immunizing women of childbearing age susceptible to rubella has proved satisfactory: (1) Identify susceptible women by means of the hemagglutination-inhibition antibody test. The majority of women will be immune to the rubella virus and can be so assured. (2) Nonimmune women are eligible for vaccination only if pregnancy can be avoided for at least 2 months after vaccination. Women least likely to become pregnant are those who have been delivered within the week before vaccination and those who take oral contraceptives in the approved way. Although there is laboratory evidence of prolonged fetal infection and tissue reaction, according to Brandling-Bennett (1974) and Modlin and associates (1976), no infant born alive to a woman vaccinated shortly before or after conception has provided clinical or laboratory evidence of rubella infection. Vaccinelike rubella virus has been recovered, however, from a fetus with histologic evidence of a cataract. The sero-negative mother had been immunized 7 weeks before conception. These observations suggest that attenuated rubella virus might be teratogenic when given to a woman early in pregnancy or up to at least 2 months before conception.

Mass vaccination programs in children have been undertaken. A very important question concerning the value of such immunization programs has yet to be answered: Will the antibody titers persist at levels sufficient to maintain immunity or will they fail to leave the woman vaccinated as a child susceptible to rubella?

EFFECTS OF NATURAL VIRUS. The numerous reports concerned with the frequency of major fetal developmental defects that are thought to be caused by rubella are difficult to interpret because of the lack of precision inherent previously in the diganosis of rubella. Forbes (1969) believed that the diagnosis of rubella may have been erroneous in as many as 50 percent of the cases. The frequency of congenital malformations, therefore, is probably higher than some reports have indicated. Rubella during the first month of pregnancy probably causes serious defects in up to 50 percent of the embryos and perhaps even more if those that abort spontaneously are considered. During the second month, the rate appears to be halved to about 25 percent, and during the third month, approximately halved again to about 15 percent.

It is now evident that many infants who are born alive suffer stigmata of continuing intrauterine and neonatal rubella infection. The syndrome of congenital rubella includes one or more of the following abnormalities:

1. Eye lesions, including cataracts, glaucoma, microphthalmia, and various other abnormalities.
2. Heart disease, including patent ductus arteriosus, septal defects, and pulmonary artery stenosis.
3. Auditory defects.
4. Central nervous system defects, including meningoencephalitis.

5. Retarded fetal growth.
6. Hematologic changes, including thrombocytopenia and anemia.
7. Hepatosplenomegaly and jaundice.
8. Chronic diffuse interstitial pneumonitis.
9. Osseous changes.
10. Chromosomal abnormalities.

Infants born with congenital rubella may shed the virus for many months and thus be a threat to other infants, as well as to susceptible adults who come in contact with the affected infants.

Although the likelihood of major malformations at birth from rubella is relatively slight if it is acquired after the first trimester, the infants whose mothers contracted the disease after the first trimester will not necessarily be healthy as demonstrated by the investigations of Hardy and associates (1969). Their long-term prospective epidemiologic inquiry to assess the impact of the extensive 1964 rubella epidemic in this country revealed 24 instances of serologic evidence of infection by rubella virus after the first trimester. Of the 22 liveborn infants, only 7 could be considered completely normal when followed for periods of up to 4 years. Townsend (1975) and Weil (1975) and their associates have reported progressive panencephalitis beginning in the second decade in children with congenital rubella infection. Even more recently, an unusually high incidence of juvenile diabetes has been identified among individuals who had congenital rubella (Rayfield and Seto, 1978).

An estimated 14 million children in the United States have not been vaccinated against rubella. Moreover, there is cause for concern regarding the duration of immunity following immunization. The possibility exists for a major rubella epidemic and its disastrous consequences for the affected fetus. Further consideration of the problems for the obstetrician posed by rubella are provided by Horstmann (1979).

Cytomegalovirus Disease. The virus responsible for cytomegalic inclusion disease may be harbored in the genital or urinary tract or both by a healthy mother and transmitted to the fetus across the placenta or during passage through the cervix and lower reproductive tract, or it may be harbored by the infant who ingests the virus in breast milk. Cytomegalovirus disease in the infant may cause hydrocephaly, microcephaly, microphthalmia, seizures, encephalitis, blindness, hepatosplenomegaly, and hematologic changes including thrombocytopenia and hemolytic anemia. At autopsy, cytomegalic inclusion bodies may be found in many organs of the body. The virus usually can be isolated in tissue culture of human cells. There are different antigenic types of the virus.

Although about 12 percent of women excrete the virus in urine or from the cervix during pregnancy and are likely to excrete the virus in their milk, few have offspring that are afflicted. Most often, a primary maternal infection seems necessary for the virus to be transmitted to and replicate in the fetus. Since primary infection is usually asymptomatic in the mother or, rarely, causes a mononucleosis-like syndrome, the disease is seldom suspected. Alford and co-workers (1974) emphasized that mental and auditory dysfunction occurs frequently enough to place this entity among the leaders of prenatal insults that induce developmental disability. No effective therapy for mother or infant is available. Cytomegalovirus disease seldom recurs in subsequent fetuses of the mother of one so afflicted.

Varicella. Varicella infections seem to be made worse by pregnancy. Varicella pneumonia, while very uncommon, is a grave illness during pregnancy, with high maternal mortality (Mendelow and Lewis, 1969; Pickard, 1968). Varicella may infect the embryo and fetus by transplacental passage of the virus. It may prove to be teratogenic when the embryo or fetus is infected (De Nicola and Hanshaw 1979). The virus may be acquired by the fetus in utero or during the course of delivery. Exposure to the virus just before delivery poses the greatest risk. If the baby is delivered before receiving varicella antibody from the mother, he may develop disseminated disease. Under these circumstances upwards to 30 percent will die unless they receive promptly zoster immune globulin if available. The immune globulin is not yet available for use in the mother.

Coxsackie Virus Disease. Coxsackie virus infection may be a serious complication of pregnancy, since it can be fatal to the fetus although causing only symptoms of a minor illness in the mother. Myocarditis and encephalomyelitis are the primary lesions. Whether maternal Coxsackie infection ever causes sublethal injuries of the embryo and fetus, thus producing congenital anomalies, is not known.

Mumps. This uncommon disease during pregnancy occasionally causes abortion or premature labor and may result in fetal death if infection occurs late in pregnancy (Blattner and Heys, 1961). Hyatt (1961) reviewed 90 published cases and noted that 16 percent of the infants were born with congenital defects. Manson and associates (1960), however, in 501 cases found that major fetal anomalies were not much more common than in the general population. Congenital mumps is very rare. Thus whether intrauterine mumps infection endangers the health of the fetus and infant in any way is not clear.

Measles (Rubeola). Most women are immune to rubeola, and therefore this disease is seldom encountered during pregnancy. Measles may cause premature labor but it is very unlikely that the infection causes congenital defects.

Influenza. In the great influenza pandemic of 1918, the disease, particularly the pneumonic type, was a serious complication of pregnancy. Harris (1919), in a statistical study based on 1350 cases, found a gross maternal mortality rate of 27 percent, which increased to 50 percent when pneumonia developed. The disease also had a most deleterious effect upon the pregnancy. The prognosis in uncomplicated epidemic influenza is excel-

lent, however, and in cases with the less serious complications, such as sinusitis, laryngitis, and bronchitis, the prognosis is also good. If pneumonia develops, the prognosis at once becomes serious. This complication should always be suspected when fever persists for more than 4 days. Although antibiotics are not effective against the virus of influenza, they are of value in the treatment of a secondary bacterial pneumonia.

The pandemic of so-called Asian influenza that swept the United States and other areas of the world in 1957 appeared to affect pregnant women with particular frequency and severity. In August and September of that year, for instance, 50 percent of the women in the childbearing age who died of influenza in Minnesota were pregnant (Freeman and Barno, 1959). In the same year, in that state, the leading cause of maternal death was influenza. Similarly, in New York City, the incidence in pregnant women was 50 percent higher than in nonpregnant controls, and the mortality rate also was higher (Bass and Molloshok, 1960). No convincing evidence has been derived that Asian influenza causes congenital malformations (Ebert, 1961; Saxen et al., 1960; Walker and McKee, 1959; Wilson et al., 1959). Vaccination against influenza is probably of value during pregnancy, especially when an epidemic is anticipated.

Common Cold. The pregnant woman appears to be slightly more susceptible to acute upper respiratory infections than the nonpregnant woman. Cases of pneumonia complicating pregnancy are often preceded by an acute cold. Hemolytic streptococcal puerperal infections may occur in patients who had acute respiratory infections at the time of delivery, and the incidence of hemolytic streptococci in the upper respiratory passages of such patients is much higher than it is in healthy women.

Poliomyelitis. Both the inactivated poliomyelitis vaccine (Salk) and the attenuated live vaccine (Sabin) are safe for immunization during pregnancy. With the widespread use of these vaccines, this disease is becoming a rarity in the United States. Siegel and Goldberg (1955), in a carefully controlled study in New York City, have shown that pregnant women not only are more susceptible to the disease, but have a higher death rate. The perinatal loss was about 33 percent; rarely, the fetus became infected. Cesarean section was not necessarily required even in the presence of extensive paralysis.

OTHER BACTERIAL INFECTIONS

Few bacterial infections in the mother are likely to spread to the fetus, at least before labor and delivery.

Scarlet Fever. Although the causative organism of scarlet fever, *Streptococcus pyogenes,* is sensitive to certain antibiotics, the disease in the early months of pregnancy has a tendency to cause abortion, presumably because of the high fever in the mother. Regardless of antibiotics, rigid isolation must be instituted and maintained in the treatment of a pregnant, parturient, or puerperal patient with scarlet fever. For no obvious reasons, scarlet fever has become very uncommon in recent years.

Erysipelas. Erysipelas is always a very serious disease, but is particularly dangerous in pregnant women because of the potential hazard of puerperal infection. The hemolytic streptococci associated with erysipelas may become more invasive, causing a septicemia and possibly producing fetal infection and even death. For the protection of other patients, strict isolation of women with erysipelas is absolutely essential. The disease should be actively treated with an appropriate antibiotic agent, which usually frees the patient of hemolytic streptococci in a relatively short time.

Typhoid Fever. According to Alimurung and Manahan (1952), pregnancy complicated by typhoid fever in former years re-

sulted in abortion or premature labor in 60 to 80 percent of cases, with a fetal mortality rate of 75 percent and a maternal mortality rate of 15 percent. The more recent experiences of Riggall and co-workers (1974) are much more favorable, however. Chloramphenicol or ampicillin is usually quite effective in arresting the disease. Antityphoid vaccines appear to exert no harmful effects when administered to pregnant women and should be given in an epidemic or when otherwise indicated.

Hansen's Disease. According to Maurus (1978), women with leprosy generally do well in pregnancy. Sulfones for treatment appear to be safe for use during pregnancy.

PROTOZOAL, PARASITIC, AND FUNGAL INFECTIONS

Toxoplasmosis. This protozoal infection is caused by *Toxoplasma gondii,* which is transmitted by eating infected raw or undercooked meat, through contact with infected cat feces, or it can be congenitally acquired after transfer from the infected mother across the placenta to the fetus. Infection with *Toxoplasma gondii* is thought to exist in a chronic asymptomatic form in perhaps 25 to 45 percent of women of reproductive age in the United States (Krick and Remington, 1978).

For congenital toxoplasmosis to occur, the mother must have acquired the infection during pregnancy. Alford and co-workers (1974) estimated that toxoplasmosis is acquired by the mother during one in every 150 to 700 pregnancies and infects the fetus late in pregnancy perhaps once in about 800 to 1400 pregnancies. Rarely, if ever, does a mother give birth to more than one child with congenital toxoplasmosis (Desmonts and Couvreur, 1974).

Fatigue, muscle pains, and sometimes lymphadenopathy are identified in the infected mother, but most often the maternal infection is subclinical. Infection early in pregnancy may lead to abortion, and later in pregnancy to a live-born infant with evidence of disease. However, most infants born with congenital toxoplasmosis do not manifest signs of clinical illness in the neonatal period. Those that do usually present evidence of generalized disease with low birth weight, hepatosplenomegaly, icterus, and anemia. Some infants will develop primarily neurologic disease with abnormal spinal fluid, convulsions, intracranial calcifications and hydrocephaly or microcephaly. Both groups of infants eventually develop chorioretinitis. Fortunately, among those infants who have been infected, most of them do not manifest serious clinical disease (Feldman, 1974).

Evidence of seroconversion or a significant increase in serially determined antibody titers may serve to detect recent infection. A combination of pyrimethamine and a sulfonamide or the antibiotic spiramycin has been reported to reduce the frequency of congenital infection (Krick and Remington, 1978).

Malaria. The incidence of abortion and premature labor is increased in malaria, although the likelihood of either relates to the severity of the disease and the promptness with which therapy is instituted. The increased fetal loss may be related to placental and fetal infection with malaria, but the evidence is somewhat contradictory, since parasites rarely cross the placenta to infect the fetus. Covell (1950), who studied this question extensively, cited an incidence of neonatal malaria in Africa of 0.03 percent. According to Jones (1950), parasites have an affinity for the decidual vessels and may involve the placenta extensively without affecting the fetus. There is a marked tendency toward recrudescence of the disease during pregnancy and the puerperium, just as after surgical operations.

Pregnancy does not contraindicate the administration of any of the commonly used antimalarial drugs. Some of the newer antimalarial agents have antifolic acid activity, however, and may contribute to the development of megaloblastic anemia (Chanarin, 1969). Lewis and associates (1973) suggest

prophylaxis with chloroquine, 500 mg orally once a week, starting before entering an epidemic area and continuing the treatment until 6 weeks postpartum.

Amebiasis. Dysentery caused by *Entamoeba histolytica,* especially with hepatic abscess, may be a quite serious illness during pregnancy. Therapy is similar to that for the nonpregnant woman.

Coccidioidomycosis. In the past, disseminated coccidioidomycosis during pregnancy commonly terminated in maternal death. In more recent years treatment with amphotericin B has been employed successfully in a number of cases (Harris, 1966); the drug is likely to be toxic.

COLLAGEN DISEASES

The collagen diseases, a group of disorders of connective tissue, appear to have as their common denominator an autoimmune response. Since these diseases are uncommon to rare, their effect on pregnancy, and vice versa, has been difficult to ascertain.

Systemic Lupus Erythematosus. As many as 1 in 400 women may have systemic lupus erythematosus. Attempts at correlating the clinical course of systemic lupus erythematosus and pregnancy often have been hindered by the protean nature of the disease, which predisposes to difficulty of uniform classification. Estes and Larson (1965), in a comprehensive study, reviewed the experience with systemic lupus erythematosus at the Columbia-Presbyterian Medical Center. To obtain a uniform sample, they included only patients with evidence of multiple system disease and a positive LE cell preparation. Of 213 women in whom the diagnosis of systemic lupus erythematosus was made, there were 36 who fulfilled the criteria and become pregnant during the course of their disease. Among this group of 36 there was a total of 25 pregnancies before the onset of the disease and 79 pregnancies afterward. The authors concluded that pregnancy did not alter the course of disease in the majority of women studied, a conclusion that has been reached subsequently by several other investigators (Grigor et al., 1977; Zurier et al., 1978). In general, women in remission at the beginning of pregnancy remained in remission throughout the pregnancy and in the puerperium. They were also of the opinion that, in the absence of lupus nephritis or hypertension, pregnancy imposes no undue maternal risk, although spontaneous abortions, especially, and fetal wastage, in general, were increased. The progression of renal involvement, and its accompanying high fetal loss, they concluded, was a contraindication to pregnancy in patients with lupus nephritis or hypertension.

Since the course of the disease is more favorable when pregnancy occurs during a period of clinical remission, women are best advised to await such remissions before attemtpting to become pregnant.

In general, administration of adrenocorticosteroids remains the treatment of choice during pregnancy. Azathioprine therapy has been continued throughout pregnancy in women with lupus erythematosus without teratogenic or other deleterious effects on the surviving infants (Devoe and Taylor, 1979; Sharon et al., 1974). Since a fall in maternal serum C3 complement levels may herald the onset of symptoms and provide a guide to therapy, Zurier and co-workers (1978) recommend serial measurements of C3 complement. Moreover, they emphasize that any increase in activity of the disease warrants vigorous treatment with corticosteroids which should be continued for 2 months or so postpartum to minimize the risk of exacerbation during that time.

Some, but not all, observers have noted a high rate of recrudescence of activity postpartum, possibly related to the release of deoxyribonucleic acid from the involuting uterus. Therefore, close observation should be continued during the puerperium.

The LE factor has been found in cord blood and transiently in the newborn's blood (Burman and Oliver, 1958). Transient hemolytic anemia, leukopenia, and thrombocytopenia have been described in the newborn as a result of transplacental passage of autoantibodies (Klippel et al., 1974). The fetus-infant whose mother has lupus is at risk of cardiac involvement including complete heart block. The heart disease may actually progress to severe heart failure and hydrops fetalis. Moreover, in some such pregnancies with fetal heart block the maternal disease has appeared as an undifferentiated collagen or vascular process which had *not yet* evolved to classical systemic lupus erythematosus (Kosmetatos et al., 1979; Reid et al., 1979).

Rheumatoid Arthritis (Rheumatoid Disease). In 1938, Hench reported marked improvement in the inflammatory component of rheumatoid arthritis during pregnancy. The pattern of improvement involved gradual amelioration of the signs and symptoms of the rheumatoid process, as occurs during a spontaneous remission. Apparently on the basis that corticosteroid levels in plasma were considered to be appreciably increased in pregnancy, Hench began to treat with cortisone individuals who had rheumatoid arthritis.

More recently, Neely and Persellin (1977) identified amelioration of activity of rheumatoid arthritis in 35 of 56 pregnancies (62 percent) but in 21 (38 percent) there was either no change in activity or the arthritis actually became worse. In four women the signs and symptoms of the disease first appeared during pregnancy. Thus in some women the course may occasionally worsen during pregnancy, and sometimes the disease may first appear at that time. Involvement of certain joints may interfere with delivery. For example, severe deformities of the hip may preclude vaginal delivery.

Dermatomyositis. Dermatomyositis is an uncommon acute, subacute, or chronic inflammatory disease of unknown cause involving skin and muscle. The disease may manifest itself as a severe generalized myositis with a cutaneous eruption and fever and a fatal outcome within a few days or weeks. It may also assume a chronic form, characterized by the gradual development of paresis with little, if any, cutaneous or systemic involvement.

About 20 percent of adults developing dermatomyositis are found to have an associated malignant tumor. The time of appearance of the two diseases, however, may be separated by several years. Extirpation of the malignant lesion is occasionally followed by a permanent remission of the dermatomyositis. The most common sites of the associated cancer are the breast, lung, stomach, and ovary. The uterus and cervix have also been reported as the primary sites.

There are so few reports of dermatomyositis in pregnancy that it is difficult to draw any definite conclusions about the effect of one upon the other. Tsai and associates (1973) have described a case of dermatomyositis which appeared during pregnancy and progressed rapidly. We have observed a case diagnosed and treated with prednisone before pregnancy in which during and after pregnancy the mother actually improved and the infant thrived.

Scleroderma. Scleroderma occurs mostly in young women of childbearing age, but its rarity prevents an accumulation of extensive data. Scleroderma was formerly considered to have a markedly deleterious effect upon pregnancy. Johnson and associates (1964) were more encouraging in their report of 36 pregnancies in a group of 337 women in whom scleroderma had developed before the age of 45. They concluded that pregnancy had little or no effect on the course of the disease and that scleroderma had a minimal effect on the pregnancy. In our limited experience, however, dysphagia seems to be aggravated by pregnancy.

Vaginal delivery may generally be anticipated, unless the changes wrought by scleroderma in the soft tissues produce dystocia requiring abdominal delivery. There is no evidence that babies born of mothers with scleroderma are harmed by the disease unless the mother is unable to eat appropriately.

Polyarteritis (Periarteritis) Nodosa. Polyarteritis nodosa is a rare disease with protean manifestations. The classic variety is a progressive illness characterized clinically by myalgia, neuropathy, gastrointestinal disorders, hypertension, and renal disease. Only a few documented cases of polyarteritis nodosa in association with pregnancy have been reported. The experience is too scant to draw any definitive conclusions about polyarteritis nodosa and pregnancy other than that the combination is associated with unfavorable maternal outcome (Siegler and Spain, 1965). Typically, the mother died postpartum with hypertension and renal involvement. The etiologic factor in polyarteritis nodosa apparently does not affect the fetus.

Glucocorticoids are used to treat polyarteritis nodosa. Although symptomatic relief may be dramatic, there is no evidence that such therapy leads to ultimate recovery.

Marfan's Syndrome. This disorder of connective tissue exhibits a mendelian autosomal pattern of inheritance that may be related to a dominant gene (McKusick, 1956). Both sexes are affected equally, and there appears to be no racial or ethnic basis for the syndrome. There are many mild cases in which the intrinsic lesion of the connective tissue affects neither well-being nor longevity and consequently escapes detection. In young adults, the syndrome may be a major cause of *dissecting aortic aneurysm,* which occurs much more commonly in pregnancy, as emphasized by Kitchen (1974).

Although the specific defect is still controversial, there is a degeneration of the elastic lamina in the media of the aorta. The cardiovascular lesion is the most serious abnormality, involving most often the ascending portion of the aorta, and predisposing to aortic dilatation or dissecting aneurysm. Early death in Marfan's syndrome is thus ultimately caused by either congestive heart failure or rupture of a dissecting aneurysm.

Marfan's syndrome alone is not an indication for abdominal delivery, for cesarean section does not protect against excessive stress on the aorta before the onset of labor. The role of cardiovascular surgery in Marfan's syndrome is poorly defined.

Rheumatic Fever. Identifiable rheumatic fever, manifested by carditis or arthritis, is rare in pregnancy. Differential diagnosis must include gonococcal arthritis and the sickle cell hemoglobinopathies.

DISEASES OF THE SKIN

Generally diseases of the skin occur with about the same frequency in pregnant as in nonpregnant women.

Herpes Gestationis. A serious dermatologic disease peculiar to pregnancy is herpes gestationis. This blistering disease of pregnancy usually presents as an extremely pruritic widespread eruption (Fig. 28-7). The lesions vary from erythematous and edematous papules to large, tense bullae. Common sites of involvement are the abdomen and the extremities.

Katz and co-workers (1976) have described a herpes gestationis serum factor which is a thermostable Ig G class protein. Immunofluorescence technics applied to a

skin biopsy are of value for confirming the diagnosis (Hertz et al., 1977). C3 complement is deposited along the basement membrane zone.

Prednisone in divided doses totaling 40 mg per day usually brings relief within a day or two and inhibits the formation of new lesions. The healed sites are not scarred but are usually hyperpigmented. The process may recur in subsequent pregnancies.

Lesions similar to those of the mother have been observed to develop in her newborn infant and then to clear spontaneously in a few weeks (Chorzelski et al., 1976). C3 complement deposited at the basement membrane of the infant's skin and the herpes gestationis factor in cord serum have been described by Katz and associates (1976).

Melanoma. Some benign nevi become malignant during pregnancy. The resulting melanoma may grow with unusual rapidity and may metastasize widely. The prognosis in pregnant women with melanoma is poor. Prophylactic removal of pigmented moles in pregnant women should be performed, according to Reynolds (1955), in the following circumstances: (1) moles on the trunk that are subjected to irritation; (2) moles on the genitals or feet, locations that are more likely

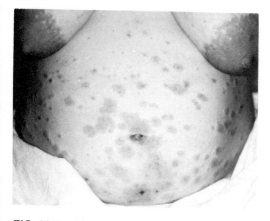
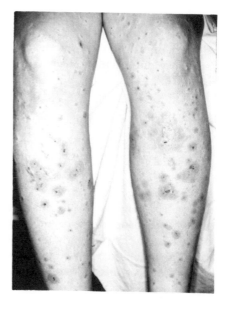

FIG. 28-7. Herpes gestationis at 30 weeks gestation. Subsequently, remarkable relief from the intense pruritis, as well as considerable decrease in the intensity of the skin reaction, was provided by glucocorticoid treatment.

to undergo malignant change; (3) moles that are smooth, blue, black, or dark brown; (4) moles that exhibit increased pigmentation, elevation of growth, enlargement in diameter, or association with ulceration, bleeding, or pain. Transplacental metastasis of a melanoma from mother to fetus has been reported by Holland (1949) and by others. Despite its rarity, melanoma is the most common tumor reported to metastasize to the placenta and fetus.

Pruritus.   Itching may occasionally be a distressing complication. It may extend over the greater part of the body or remain limited to the genitalia. It often gives rise to intense suffering, with itching sometimes so unrelenting that the woman is unable to sleep. Retention of bile salts induced presumably by estrogens may be the basis of the pruritis, at least in some cases (p. 758). Cholestyramine reduces the levels of bile salts and relieves pruritis (Herndon, 1972). The safety of use of cholestyramine during pregnancy has not been established.

Abnormalities of Pigmentation.   During pregnancy, increased pigmentation is frequently noted and may be particularly marked along the linea alba and about the breasts. In other cases, unsightly, more or less symmetric, brownish splotches (chloasma) appear upon the face. They are not amenable to treatment but usually disappear after childbirth. Oral contraceptives and stilbestrol may cause similar changes in pigmentation.

DISEASES OF THE NERVOUS SYSTEM

Epilepsy.   In general, epilepsy is not markedly affected by pregnancy, especially if allowances are made for appropriate ingestion of medication. During early pregnancy, nausea and vomiting may interfere with the ingestion of anticonvulsant medication, increasing the likelihood of seizures. Moreover, diphenylhydantoin and phenobarbital, the most commonly used drugs, are cleared more rapidly during pregnancy and as the consequence blood levels are likely to be lower than when nonpregnant (Lander et al., 1977). Furthermore, during labor, delivery, and the early puerperium, medication may be withheld deliberately or inadvertently, similarly increasing the likelihood of convulsions.

At times, it may be difficult to differentiate between eclampsia and epilepsy in the hypertensive pregnant woman. Magnesium sulfate parenterally administered will usually control the convulsions of epilepsy as well as those of eclampsia.

Idiopathic epilepsy to a degree appears to be a hereditable disorder. Epilepsy has been found to be about 4 times more frequent among children whose mothers have idiopathic epilepsy (Annegers et al., 1976). However, no increase was identified when the father had a convulsive disorder.

Bejerkedal and Bahna (1973) and others identified an excess of complications including congenital malformations, low birth weight, prematurity, and perinatal mortality attributable to anticonvulsant medications. Fedrick and others (1973) consider diphenylhydantoin (Dilantin) to be more likely than phenobarbital to produce congenital defects, but that if the two drugs are taken together, the effect is more pronounced than when either drug is used alone. Hanson and co-workers (1975, 1976) have described in children born to epileptic women treated with hydantoin anticonvulsants, a "fetal hydantoin syndrome" that includes craniofacial anomalies, and mental deficiency. Ten percent of infants studied were adversely affected. Trimethadione should not be used since it is one of the most potent of teratogens (Smith, 1977).

Several of the anticonvulsant drugs in common use tend to precipitate or aggravate a deficiency of folic acid, and megaloblastic anemia has been described in these circumstances (Chanarin, 1969).

At Parkland Memorial Hospital, maternal folate deficiency identified by low plasma folate levels is much more common than in the general obstetric population, although no cases of overt megaloblastic anemia have been identified among the pregnant women treated with anticonvulsant drugs (Pritchard et al., 1969). Folic acid has been claimed by some to increase the likelihood of convulsions (Strauss and Bernstein, 1974). Therefore, the benefits, if any, to be derived from folic acid supplements in these circumstances are not clear.

At Parkland Memorial Hospital, 77 pregnancies cared for in 43 women with epilepsy have been reviewed. The pregnancies were, for the most part, quite uncomplicated. The frequencies of spontaneous abortion, perinatal mortality, prematurity, and fetal malformation in this small series were similar to those in the general obstetric population. Each infant received 1 mg of vitamin K₁ (phytonadione) parenterally very soon after birth. None demonstrated abnormal bleeding, including the male infants who were circumcised. The newborn infant whose mother has been taking anticonvulsant medication may develop deficiencies of vitamin K-dependent coagulation factors (see Chap. 13, p. 322).

Intracranial Hemorrhage. Intracranial hemorrhage is a much more common cause of maternal death than is generally believed. Among 170 maternal deaths reported by Barnes and Abbott (1959), for example, 36 were caused by cerebral complications. Of these 36 deaths, 17, or about one-half, were the result of intracranial hemorrhage.

The main obstetric problem concerns the management of pregnancy and delivery in women who survive intracranial hemorrhage. Some, but certainly not all, authorities have favored cesarean section for delivery, and in cases in which the cerebral hemorrhage occurred shortly before or very early in pregnancy, some believe that therapeutic abortion is indicated (Gomberg, 1959; Mack et al., 1956). On the basis of a review of 142 cases of intracranial aneurysms that ruptured before or during pregnancy, Hunt and co-workers (1974) have concluded that there is little indication for elective cesarean section to replace vaginal delivery. Vaginal delivery following surgical correction of the aneurysm was well tolerated by the patients described by Minielly and co-workers (1979).

Paraplegia. Spinal cord lesions caused by trauma or tumor usually do not prevent conception. In women so affected, the pregnancy is likely to be complicated by urinary infections and pressure necrosis of the skin. Labor often is easy and comparatively painless. The second stage may be prolonged by an inability to increase intra-abdominal pressure, i.e., bear down.

Multiple Sclerosis. This disease is a rare complication of pregnancy, occurring about once in every 4000 gravidas, as reported by Sweeney (1953). In most cases, pregnancy has no effect on the course of multiple sclerosis. Although in some cases the condition seems to be aggravated in pregnancy, multiple sclerosis in pregnant women is often characterized by unexplained exacerbations and remissions.

Guillain-Barré Syndrome. Sudo and Weingold (1975) have described two instances of pregnancy complicated by this syndrome and reviewed 25 others previously reported. Respiratory insufficiency is a most serious problem as it is in the absence of pregnancy. The fetus does not appear to be affected neurologically. Ahlberg and Ahlmark (1978) have described a case in which the mother gave birth to twins during respirator treatment. All survived although the mother's respiratory paralysis persisted for several more weeks after delivery.

Myasthenia Gravis. With occasional exceptions, women with myasthenia gravis go through pregnancy and labor without difficulty; during the second stage of labor the woman may demonstrate impairment of voluntary expulsive efforts. Acetylcholine receptor antibodies have been detected in most myasthenic patients (Appel et al., 1975). These antibodies, most likely, can be transferred from the mother to her fetus.

Transient symptomatic myasthenia gravis

occurs in about 10 to 20 percent of the new-born infants of mothers with the disease. The neonatal myasthenia responds to minute doses of endophronium or similar drugs, sub-siding completely within 4 to 6 weeks. With-out prompt recognition and treatment, in-cluding good nursing care, the affected newborn infant may succumb to respiratory insufficiency caused by muscular weakness or the effects of aspiration. The fetus appears to be protected while in utero by a factor that inhibits the interaction between the receptors and antibody to the receptors (Abramsky and co-workers, 1979).

Any drug with a curarelike effect must be used with extreme caution. Such drugs in-clude magnesium sulfate and aminoglycoside antibiotics. Apparently, even the quinine in a gin-and-tonic may be harmful (Donaldson, 1978).

Huntington's Chorea. The obstetric importance of Huntington's chorea is chiefly eugenic, since this degenerative disease of the cerebral cortex and basal ganglia is inher-ited as a dominant autosomal trait. To attempt the elimination of this dread disease, thera-peutic abortion is justifiable.

Chorea Gravidarum. It is an extremely rare complication of gestation since rheu-matic fever has become so rare. Zegart and Schwarz (1968) identified only 1 case in the course of over 100,000 deliveries. Often the woman has previously suffered chorea which sooner or later abated spontaneously as it is likely to do during or after the pregnancy.

Migraine. The effects, if any, of preg-nancy on migraine are unpredictable. Ergota-mine-containing preparations should proba-bly be avoided during pregnancy, although ergotamine has nowhere near as potent an action on the myometrium as does ergono-vine.

Bell's Palsy. This idiopathic paralysis involving the facial nerve may be somewhat more common during pregnancy. Treatment and prognosis are the same as for nonpreg-nant women.

Carpal Tunnel Syndrome. The median nerve is vulnerable to compression within the carpal tunnel at the wrist. Typically, the woman awakes with a tingling in one or both hands. The fingers otherwise feel numb and useless. A splint applied to the very slightly flexed wrist and worn during sleep usually provides relief. The signs and symptoms most often regress after delivery.

Psychosis. Pregnancy and the puerpe-rium at times are sufficiently stressful to induce psychosis. The prognosis depends for the most part on the nature of the underlying psychiatric disorder that is almost always pres-ent.

Electroshock therapy has been used often in the past during pregnancy. One pregnant woman was transferred to Parkland Memo-rial Hospital when she convulsed spontane-ously with eclampsia during the course of electroshock therapy. The mother and infant survived.

Lithium carbonate, when used to treat manic-depressive pregnant women, appears to have teratogenic effects that are dose related. Therefore, if used, the smallest effective dose should be administered. The excretion of lithium by the kidney is increased in normal pregnancy but decreased by sodium-deplet-ing diuretics and sodium-poor diets (Gold-field and Weinstein, 1973; Schou et al., 1973). Lithium toxicity may be the conse-quence in both mother and fetus. The evi-dence appears strong for a teratogenic effect, especially on the heart, when lithium is ad-ministered during the first trimester (Wein-stein and Goldfield, 1975). Lithium is con-centrated in the milk; bottle-feeding probably is the better choice in this circumstance.

MISCELLANEOUS COMPLICATIONS

Carcinoma of the Breast. Pregnancy does not appear to exert much influence on the course of mammary cancer, and therapeu-tic abortion does not improve the prognosis for this disease. In the extensive investigation of Westberg (1946), based on 224 cases of breast carcinoma in pregnant and nursing women and a control series of 3000 nonpregnant women with mammary cancer, the difference in the survival rates was scarcely significant. Hochman and Schreiber (1953), and others since then, have contended that the 5-year survival rate in cancer of the breast coexisting with pregnancy is primarily dependent on the stage of the disease at the time of diagnosis, and that interruption of pregnancy has no bearing on the course. The results to be anticipated correspond with the expected survival rates when the same stage of the disease is not complicated by pregnancy. As Hochman and Schreiber (1953) pointed out, the increased vascularity of the breast during pregnancy, however, might result in rapid invasion of the lymph nodes and adjacent tissues and in distant hematogenous metastases. Provided that radical mastectomy was promptly performed, however, they maintained the increased vascularity has no effect on prognosis. Others since then similarly could find no evidence that pregnancy after mastectomy for cancer of the breast had an adverse effect on survival (Donegan, 1977; Zinns, 1979).

Diaphragmatic (Hiatal) Hernia. Rigler and Eneboe (1935) performed upper gastrointestinal radiologic examination on 195 unselected women in the last trimester of pregnancy. Among 116 multiparas, 21, or about 18 percent, had hiatal hernias, and among 79 primigravidas, 4 had hiatal hernias. Ten of these 25 patients were reexamined 1 to 18 months postpartum, and hernias were observed in only 3. Hiatal hernias seen during pregnancy may be produced by intermittent but prolonged increase in intra-abdominal pressure. These hernias are an occasional cause of vomiting, epigastric pain, and even bleeding from ulceration.

Separation of the Symphysis Pubis. Significant separations or ruptures of the symphysis pubis are associated with clinical symptoms in addition to roentgenologic findings. In general, only separations of more than 1.0 cm are symptomatic. Callahan (1953) reported an incidence of 1 to 2200 deliveries

at The New York Lying-In Hospital, whereas Waters (1953) cited a frequency of about only 1 to 20,000 at the Margaret Hague Maternity Hospital. The more recent experience at Parkland Memorial Hospital is closer to that of Waters, indicating that the complication is rare in this country today.

The symphysis may separate either during pregnancy or in the course of labor. If it occurs before labor, the separation may develop either spontaneously or after trauma. If the rupture takes place during labor, it is usually the result of a traumatic forceps delivery, but other cases have been attributed to forcible abduction of the patient's thighs during positioning for delivery.

The symptoms are symphyseal pain on motion, such as turning in bed, and tenderness over the symphysis or sacroiliac regions. Roentgenologic examination may reveal a slight separation or a widely gaping defect. Sacroiliac symptoms are noted in about one-third of the cases.

Treatment is orthopedic, current opinion favoring simple strapping in most cases. Recovery of function is usually complete, although some separation and motion of the joint may persist. Subsequent vaginal delivery without recurrence of the original symptoms may be anticipated.

REFERENCES

Abramsky O, Lisak RP, Brenner T, Zeidman A: Significance in neonatal myasthenia gravis of inhibitory effect of amniotic fluid on binding of antibodies to acetylcholine receptor. Lancet 2:1333, 1979

Aggio MC, Zunini C: Reversible pure red cell aplasia in pregnancy. N Engl J Med 2:222, 1977

AHA Committee Report: Prevention of bacterial endocarditis. Circulation 56:139A, 1977

Ahlberg G, Ahlmark G: The Landry-Guillain-Barré syndrome and pregnancy. Acta Obstet Gynecol Scand 57:377, 1978

Alford CA, Reynolds DW, Stagno S: Current concepts of chronic perinatal infections. In Gluck L (ed): Modern Perinatal Medicine. Chicago, Year Book, 1974

Alger LS, Golbus MS, Laros RK Jr: Thalassemia and pregnancy: Results of an antenatal screening program. Am J Obstet Gynecol 134:662, 1979

Alimurung MM, Manahan CP: Typhoid in pregnancy: report of a case treated with chloramphenicol and ACTH. J Philipp Med Assoc 28:388, 1952

Amstey MS, Monif GRG: Genital herpevirus infection in pregnancy. Obstet Gynecol 44:394, 1974

Anderson KJ, Walters WAW: Cushing's syndrome and pregnancy. Aust NZ J Obstet Gynaecol 16:225, 1976

Annegers JF, Hauser WA, Elveback LR, Anderson VE, Kurland LT: Seizure disorders in offspring of parents with a history of seizures—A maternal-paternal difference? Epilepsia 17:1, 1976

Appel SH, Almon RR, Levy N: Acetylcholine receptor antibodies in myasthenia gravis. N Eng J Med 293:760, 1975

Ayromlooi J: A new approach to the management of immunologic thrombocytopenic purpura in pregnancy. Am J Obstet Gynecol 130:235, 1978

Baker LRI, Brain MC: Heparin treatment of haemolytic anemia and thrombocytopenia in preeclampsia. Proc R Soc Med 60:477, 1967

Ball EW, Giles C: Folic acid and vitamin B_{12} levels in pregnancy and their relation to megaloblastic anemia. J Clin Pathol 17:165, 1964

Bank A: The thalassemia syndromes. Blood 51:369, 1978

Barnes JL, Abbott KH: Cerebral complications incurred during pregnancy and the puerperium. Calif Med 91:237, 1959

Barnes PM, Hendrickse JP deV, Watson-Williams EJ: Low-molecular weight dextran in treatment of bone-pain crises in sickle cell disease: a double blind trail. Lancet 2:1271, 1965

Bass MH, Molloshok RE: In Guttmacher AF, Rovinsky JJ (eds): Medical, Surgical and Gynecological Complications of Pregnancy. Baltimore, Williams & Wilkins, 1960, p 526

Bayley M, Walsh FM, Valaske MJ: Fatal overdosage from Bendectin. Clin Pediatr, 14:507, 1975

Bellingham F, Mackey R, Winston C: Pregnancy and intestinal obstruction: a dangerous combination. Med J Aust 2:318, 1949

Bemiller CR, Forker AD, Morgan JR: Complete heart block, prosthetic aortic valve, and successful pregnancy. JAMA 217:915, 1970

Benjamin F, Casper DJ: Comparative validity of oral and intravenous glucose tolerance tests in pregnancy. Am J Obstet Gynecol 97:488, 1967

Biglieri EG, Slaton PE Jr: Pregnancy and primary aldosteronism. J Clin Endocrinol 27:1628, 1967

Bitran JD, Roth DG: Acute leukemia during reproductive life; its course, complications and sequelae for fertility. J Reprod Med 17:225, 1976

Bjerkedal T, Bahna SL: The course and outcome of pregnancy in women with epilepsy. Acta Obstet Gynecol Scand 52:245, 1973

Black WP: Acute appendicitis in pregnancy. Br Med J 1:1938, 1960

Bonnar J: Venous thrombo-embolism and pregnancy. In Stallworthy J, Bourne G (eds): Recent Advances in Obstetrics and Gynecology No. 13. New York, Churchill Livingstone, 1979

Bowes WA Jr: Detection and treatment of tuberculosis. Contemp Ob/Gyn 6:43, 1975

Brandling-Bennett AD, Modlin JF, Herrmann K: The risk of rubella vaccination in pregnancy. Contemp Obstet Gynecol 4:77, 1974

Braverman DZ, Johnson ML, Kern F Jr: Effects of pregnancy and contraceptive steroids on gallbladder function. New Engl J Med 302:362, 1980

Brodie MJ, Moore MR, Thompson GG, Goldberg A, Low RAL: Pregnancy and acute porphyria. Br J Obstet Gynaecol 84:726, 1977

Brody JA, Sever JL, Schiff GM: Prevention of rubella by gamma globulin during an epidemic in Barrow, Alaska, in 1964. N Engl J Med 272:127, 1965

Brumfitt W, Davies BI, Rosser E: Urethral catheter as a cause of urinary-tract infection in pregnancy and puerperium. Lancet 2:1059, 1961

Bullock JL, Harris RE, Young R: Treatment of thyrotoxicosis during pregnancy with propranolol. Am J Obstet Gynecol 121:242, 1975

Bunim JJ, Appel SB: A principle for determining prognosis of pregnancy in rheumatic heart disease. JAMA 142:90, 1950

Burch GE: Heart disease and pregnancy. Am Heart J 93:104, 1977

Burgess GE: Alpha blockade and surgical intervention of pheochromocytoma in pregnancy. Obstet Gynecol 53:266, 1979

Burman D, Oliver RAM: Placental transfer of the lupus erythematosus factor. J Clin Pathol 11:43, 1958

Burwell CS, Metcalfe J: Heart Disease and Pregnancy. Boston, Little, Brown, 1958

Callahan JT: Separation of the symphysis pubis. Am J Obstet Gynecol 66:281, 1953

Carswell F, Kerr MM, Hutchinson JH: Congenital goitre and hypothyroidism produced by maternal ingestion of iodides. Lancet 1:1241, 1970

Center for Disease Control Recommended Treatment Schedules, 1979 (publication 97-796)

Chanarin I: The Megaloblastic Anaemias. Oxford and Edinburgh, Blackwell Scientific Publications. 1969

Chanarin I, Rothman D, Ward A, Perry J: Folate status and requirements in pregnancy. Br Med J 2:390, 1968

Chanarin I, Rothman D, Watson-Williams EJ: Normal formiminoglutamic acid excretion in megaloblastic anemia in pregnancy: studies on histidine metabolism in pregnancy. Lancet 1: 1068, 1963

Chaplin H Jr, Cohen R, Bloomberg G, Kaplan HJ, Moore JA, Dorner I: Pregnancy and idiopathic autoimmune haemolytic anemia. Br J Haematol 24:219, 1973

Chapman RA, Sutcliffe SB, Malpas JS: Cytotoxic-induced ovarian failure in Hodgkin's disease, II. Effects on sexual function. JAMA 242:1882, 1979

Chau SS, Fitzpatrick RJ, Jamieson B: Diabetes insipidus and parturition. Br J Obstet Gynaecol 76:444, 1969

Cheek DB (ed): Human Growth. Philadelphia, Lea and Febiger, 1968

Cheng Y-S: Pregnancy in liver cirrhosis and/or portal hypertension. Am J Obstet Gynecol 128:812, 1977

Chesley LC: Severe rheumatic cardiac disease and pregnancy: The ultimate prognosis. Am J Obstet Gynecol 136:552, 1980

Chisholm DM, Sharp AA: Formimino-glutamic acid excretion in anaemia of pregnancy. Br Med J 2:1366, 1964

Chorzelski TP, Jablonska S, Beutner EH, Maciejowska EWA, Jarzabek-Chorzelska M: Herpes gestationis with identical lesions in the newborn. Arch Dermatol 112:1129, 1976

Coe FL, Parks JH, Lindheimer MD: Nephrolithiasis during pregnancy. N Engl J Med 298:324, 1978

Collins ML, O'Brien P, Cline A: Diabetes insipidus following obstetric shock. Obstet Gynecol 53:175, 1979

Cooper LZ, Krugman S: Clinical manifestations of postnatal and congenital rubella. Arch Ophthalmol 71:434, 1967

Corlett RC Jr, Mishell DR Jr: Pancreatitis in pregnancy. Am J Obstet Gynecol 113:281, 1972

Cortis BS, Gensini GG: Can the risks of myocardial infarction in pregnancy be reduced? Bull Texas Heart Inst 4:49, 1977

Covell G: Congenital malaria. Trop Dis Bull 47:1147, 1950

Crohn BB, Yarnis H, Walter RI, Gabrilov JL, Crohn EB: Ulcerative colitis as affected by pregnancy. NY J Med 56:2651, 1956

Cunningham FG, McCubbin JH: Appendicitis complicating pregnancy. Obstet Gynecol 45:415, 1975

Cunningham FG, Pritchard JA: Pregnancy outcomes with sickle hemoglobinopathies: II. Evaluation of systematic transfusion. (Abstract) Gynecol Invest 7:81, 1976

Cunningham FG, Pritchard JA: Unpublished observations.

Cunningham FG, Pritchard JA: Prophylactic transfusions of normal red blood cells during pregnancies complicated by sickle cell hemoglobinopathies. Am J Obstet Gynecol 135:994, 1979

Curtis EM: Pregnancy in sickle cell anemia, sickle cell-hemoglobin C disease and variants thereof. Am J Obstet Gynecol 77:1312, 1959

D'Cruz IA, Balani SG, Iyer LS: Infectious hepatitis in pregnancy. Obstet Gynecol 31:449, 1968

DeLeeuw NKW, Lowenstein L, Hsieh Y: Iron deficiency and hydremia in normal pregnancy. Medicine 45:291, 1966

DeNicola LK, Hanshaw JB: Congenital and neonatal varicella. J Pediatr 94:175, 1979

Desmonts G, Couvreur J: Toxoplasmosis in pregnancy and its transmission to the fetus. Bull NY Acad Med 50:146, 1974

Devoe LD, Taylor RL: Systemic lupus erythematosus in pregnancy. Am J Obstet Gynecol 135:433, 1979

Dines DE, Banner EA: Sarcoidosis during pregnancy. JAMA 200:150, 1967

Donaldson JO: Neurology of Pregnancy. Philadelphia, Saunders, 1978

Donegan WL: Breast cancer and pregnancy. Obstet Gynecol 50:244, 1977

Dosik H, Jhaveri R: Prevention of neonatal hepatitis B infection by high-dose hepatitis B immune globulin. N Engl J Med 298:602, 1978

Douglas SW, Adamson JW: The anemia of chronic disorders: studies of marrow regulation and iron metabolism. Blood 45:55, 1975

Driscoll JJ, Gillespie L: Obstetrical considerations in diabetes in pregnancy. Med Clin North Am 49: 1025, 1965

Dunkle LM, Schmidt RR, O'Connor DM: Neonatal herpes simplex infection possibly acquired via maternal breast milk. Pediatrics 63:250, 1979

Durham JA: A noradrenaline secreting phaeochromoctoma complicating pregnancy. Aust NZ J Obstet Gynaecol 17:53, 1977

Ebert JD: First International Conference on Congenital Malformation. Summary and Evaluation. J Chron Dis 13:91, 1961

Eisinger AJ: The postpartum haemolytic uraemic syndrome. Br J Obstet Gynaecol 79:139, 1972

Estes D, Larson DL: Systemic lupus erythematosus and pregnancy. Clin Obstet Gynecol 8:307, 1965

Etheridge MJ, Pepperell RJ: Heart disease and pregnancy at the Royal Women's Hospital. Med J Aust 2:277, 1977

Fairweather D: Nausea and vomiting in pregnancy. Am J Obstet Gynecol 102:135, 1968

Fass RJ: Sexual transmission of viral hepatitis. JAMA 230:861, 1974

Fedrick J: Epilepsy and pregnancy: a report from the Oxford record linkage study. Br Med J 2:442, 1973

Felding C: Obstetric studies in women with renal disease in childhood. Acta Obstet Gynecol Scand 45:141, 1964

Felding C: The obstetric prognosis in chronic renal disease. Acta Obstet Gynecol Scand 47:166, 1968

Feldman HA: (Editorial) Congenital toxoplasmosis, at long last. N Engl J Med 290:1138, 1974

Felsen J, Wolarsky W: Chronic ulcerative colitis and pregnancy. Am J Obstet Gynecol 56:751, 1948

Field PR, Murphy AM: The role of specific IgM globulin estimations in the diagnosis of acquired rubella. Med J Aust: 2:1244, 1972

Fieldring JF, Cooke WT: Pregnancy and Crohn's disease. Br Med J 2:76, 1970

Fisch RO, Prem KA, Feinberg SB, Gehrz RC: Acromegaly in a gravida and her infant. Obstet Gynecol 43:861, 1974

Fleming AF: Hypoplastic anaemia in pregnancy. Br J Obstet Gynaecol 75:138, 1968

Fleming AF, Martin JD, Stenhouse NS: The relationship of maternal anaemia and folate deficiency to uterine haemorrhage during pregnancy and fetal malformation. Aust NZ Obstet Gynaecol 14:18, 1975

Forbes JA: International Conference on Rubella Immunization. I. Rubella as a Disease. Am J Dis Child 118:5, 1969

Forget BG: Molecular genetics of human hemoglobin synthesis. Ann Intern Med 91:605, 1979

Fort AT, Morrison JC, Berreras L, Diggs LW, Fish SA: Counseling the patient with sickle cell disease about reproduction: pregnancy outcome does not justify the maternal risk! Am J Obstet Gynecol 111:324, 1971

Fraser D, Turner JWA: Myasthenia gravis and pregnancy. Lancet 2:417, 1953

Freedman WL: Alpha and beta thalassemia and pregnancy. Clin Obstet Gynecol 12:115, 1969

Freeman DW, Barno A: Deaths from Asian influenza associated with pregnancy. Am J Obstet Gynecol 78:1172, 1959

Freireich EJ, Miller A, Emerson CP, Ross JF: The effect of inflammation on the utilization of erythrocyte and transferrin bound radioiron for red cell production. Blood 12:972, 1957

Fullerton WT, Turner AG: Exchange transfusion in treatment of severe anaemia in pregnancy. Lancet 1:75, 1962

Fullerton WT, Hendrickse JP deV, Watson-Williams EJ: Haemoglobin SC disease in pregnancy. In Jonxis JHP (ed): Abnormal Haemoglobins in Africa: a Symposium. Philadelphia, Davis, 1965

Gabbe SG: Application of scientific rationale to the management of the pregnant diabetic. Semin Perinat 2:361, 1978

Gabbe SG, Mestman JH, Freeman RK, Goebelsmann UT, Lowensohn RI, Nochimson D, Cetrulo C, Quilligan EJ: Management and outcome of diabetes mellitus, classes B-R. Am J Obstet Gynecol 129:723, 1977

Ganda OP, Soelder SS: Genetic, acquired and related factors in the etiology of diabetes mellitus. Arch Intern Med 137:461, 1977

Gleicher N, Midwall J, Hochberger D, Jaffin H: Eisenmenger's syndrome and pregnancy. Obstet Gynecol Survey 34:721, 1979

Gluck L, Kulovich MV: The evaluation of functional maturity in the human fetus. In Gluck L (ed): Modern Perinatal Medicine. Chicago, Year Book, 1974

Goebelsmann U, Freeman K, Mestman JH, Nakamura RM, Woodling BA: Estriol in pregnancy. II. Daily urinary estriol assays in the management of the pregnant diabetic women. Am J Obstet Gynecol 115:795, 1973

Goldfield MD, Weinstein MR: Lithium carbonate in obstetrics: guidelines for clinical use. Am J Obstet Gynecol 116:15, 1973

Goluboff LG, Sisson JC, Hamburger JI: Hyperthyroidism associated with pregnancy. Obstet Gynecol 44:107, 1974

Gomberg B: Spontaneous subarachnoid hemorrhage in pregnancy not complicated by toxemia. Am J Obstet Gynecol 77:430, 1959

Gomez A, Wood M: Acute appendicitis in pregnancy. Am J Surgery 137:180, 1979

Goodall HB: Microscopic examination of the "buffycoat" from the hematocrit in the investigation of anemia in pregnancy. J Clin Pathol 10:248, 1957

Gorenberg H, Chesley LC: Rheumatic heart disease in pregnancy: the remote prognosis in patients with "functionally severe" disease. Ann Intern Med 49:278, 1958

Green HG, Gareis FJ, Shepard TH, Kelley VC: Cretinism associated with maternal sodium iodide I[131] therapy during pregnancy. Am J Dis Child 122:247, 1971

Gregg NM: Congenital cataract following German measles in the mother. Trans Ophthalmol Soc Aust 3:35, 1942

Grigor RR, Shervington PC, Hughes GRV, Hawkins DF: Outcome of pregnancy in systemic lupus erythematosus. Proc Royal Soc Med 70:99, 1977

Grimes EM, Fayez JA, Miller GL: Cushing's syndrome and pregnancy. Obstet Gynecol 42:550, 1973

Habib A, McCarthy JS: Effects on the neonate of propanolol administered during pregnancy. J Pediatr 91:808, 1977

Hadley JA: Herpes gestationis: a report of a case. Br J Obstet Gynaecol 66:985, 1959

Hamilton BE, Thomson KJ: The Heart in Pregnancy and the Childbearing Age. Boston, Little, Brown, 1941

Hansen H, Rybo G: Folic acid dosage in prophylactic treatment during pregnancy. Acta Obstet Gynecol Scand 46 (Pt 7):107, 1967

Hanson JW, Myrianthopoulos NC, Harvey MAS, Smith DW: Risks of the offspring of women treated with hydantoins during pregnancy. Pediatr Res 10:449, 1976

Hanson JW, Smith DW: The fetal hydantoin syndrome. J Pediatr 87:285, 1975

Hardy JB, McCracken GH Jr, Gilkeson MR, Sever JL: Adverse fetal outcome following maternal rubella after the first trimester of pregnancy. JAMA 207:2414, 1969

Harer WB Jr, Harer WB Sr: Volvulus complicating pregnancy and the puerperium: a report of three cases and review of literature (37 references cited). Obstet Gynecol 12:399, 1958

Harkins JL, Wilson DR, Muggah HF: Acute renal failure in obstetrics. Am J Obstet Gynecol 118:331, 1974

Harris JW: Influenza occurring in pregnant women. JAMA 72:978, 1919

Harris RE: Coccidioidomycosis complicating pregnancy. Obstet Gynecol 28:401, 1966

Harris RE, Dunnihoo DR: The incidence and significance of urinary calculi in pregnancy. Am J Obstet Gynecol 99:237, 1967

Harrison EC, Roschke EJ, Ferenizi G, Mitani GH: Managing the pregnant patient with a heart valve prosthesis. Contemp Ob/Gyn 11:82, 1978

Harrison KA, Ajabor LN, Lawson JB: Ethacrynic acid and packed-blood cell transfusion in treatment of severe anaemia in pregnancy. Lancet 1:11, 1971

Hartenstein H, Gardner LI: Tetany of the newborn associated with maternal parathyroid adenoma. N Engl J Med 274:266, 1966

Hayden GF, Hermann KL, Weiss KE, Nieberg PI, Mitchell JE: Subclinical congenital rubella infection associated with maternal rubella vaccination in pregnancy. J Pediatr 96:869, 1980

Hench PG: Ameliorating effect of pregnancy on chronic atrophic (infectious rheumatoid) arthritis, fibrositis and intermittent hydrarthrosis. Proc Mayo Clin 13:161, 1938

Hendrickse JP deV, Watson-Williams EJ: The influence of hemoglobinopathies on reproduction. Am J Obstet Gynecol 94:739, 1966

Herbert V, Cunneen N, Jaskiel L, Kopff C: Minimal daily adult folate requirement. Arch Intern Med 110:649, 1962

Herndon JH Jr: Pathophysiology of pruritis associated with elevated bile acid levels in serum. Arch Intern Med 130:632, 1972

Hertz KC, Crawford PS, Chez RA, Katz SI: Herpes gestationis: An update. Obstet Gynecol 49:733, 1977

Hibbard BM: The role of folic acid in pregnancy. Br J Obstet Gynaecol 71:529, 1964

Hibbard ED: The FIGLU excretion test and defective folic-acid metabolism in pregnancy. Lancet 2:1146, 1964

Hieber JP, Dalton D, Shorey J, Combes B: Hepatitis and pregnancy. J Pediatr 91:545, 1977

Hill DE: Effect of insulin on fetal growth. Semin Perinat 2:319, 1978

Hill LM, Johnson CE, Lee RA: Cholecystectomy in pregnancy. Obstet Gynecol 46:291, 1975

Hime MC, Richardson JA: Diabetes insipidus and pregnancy. Case report, incidence, and review of literature. Obstet Gynecol Survey 33:375, 1978

Hochman A, Schreiber H: Pregnancy and cancer of the breast. Obstet Gynecol 2:268, 1953

Holland E: A case of transplacental metastasis of malignant melanoma from mother to foetus. Br J Obstet Gynaecol 56:529, 1949

Holmes GE, Holmes FF: Pregnancy outcomes of patients treated for Hodgkin's disease: a controlled study. Cancer 41:1317, 1978

Homan WP, Thorbjarnarson B: Crohn disease and pregnancy. Arch Surg 111:545, 1976

Honiotes G, Clark PJ, Cavanaugh D: Gastric ulcer perforation during pregnancy. Am J Obstet Gynecol 106:619, 1970

Horstmann DM: Rubella: Still a problem for the obstetrician. Contemp Ob/Gyn 13:67, 1979

Hoyer LW, Lindsten J, Blomäck M, Hagenfeldt L, Cordesius E, Strömberg P, Gustavii B: Prenatal evaluation of fetus at risk for severe von Willibrand's disease. Lancet 2:191, 1979

Hunt AB, McConahey WM: Pregnancy associated with disease of the adrenal glands. Am J Obstet Gynecol 66:970, 1953

Hunt HB, Schifrin BS, Suzuki K: Ruptured berry aneurysms and pregnancy. Obstet Gynecol 43:827, 1974

Johnson TR, Banner EA, Winkelmann RK: Scleroderma and pregnancy. Obstet Gynecol 23:467, 1964

Johnston WG, Baskett TF: Obstetric cholestasis. Am J Obstet Gynecol 133:299, 1979

Jones BS: Congenital malaria: 3 cases. Br Med J 2:439, 1950

Judson FN, Shaw BS, Vernon TM: Mandatory premarital rubella serologic testing in Colorado. JAMA 229:1200, 1974

Kahil ME, Fred HL, Brown H, Davis JS: Acute fatty liver of pregnancy: report of two cases. Arch Intern Med 113:63, 1964

Kaiser R, Berk JE, Fridhandler L: Serum amylase changes during pregnancy. Am J Obstet Gynecol 122:283, 1975

Kass EH: Pyelonephritis and bacteriuria. Ann Intern Med 56:46, 1962

Kass EH: Progress in Pyelonephritis. Philadelphia, Davis, 1965. (Contains six articles by various authors on bacteriuria in pregnancy.)

Katz M, Quagiorello J, Young BK: Severe polycystic kidney disease in pregnancy. Obstet Gynecol 53:119, 1979

Katz SI, Hertz KC, Yaoita H: Immunopathology and characterization of the HG factor. J Clin Invest 57:1434, 1976

Kibrick S: Herpes simplex infection at term. JAMA 243:157, 1980

Kincaid-Smith P, Bullen M: Bacteriuria in pregnancy. Lancet 1:395, 1965

Kitchen DH: Dissecting aneurysm of the aorta in pregnancy. Br J Obstet Gynaecol 81:410, 1974

Kitzmiller JL, Cloherty JP, Younger MD, Tabatabaii A, Rothchild SB, Sosenkol I, Epstein MF, Singh S, Neff RK: Diabetic pregnancy and perinatal outcome. Am J Obstet Gynecol 131:560, 1978

Klein AH, Agustin AV, Foley TP Jr: Successful laboratory screening for congenital hypothyroidism. Lancet 2:77, 1974

Kleinknecht D, Grünfeld J-P, Gomez PC, Moreau J-F, Garcia-Torres R: Diagnostic procedures and long-term prognosis in bilateral renal cortical necrosis. Kidney Intern 4:390, 1973

Klippel JH, Grimley PM, Decker JL: Lymphocyte inclusions in newborns of mothers with systemic lupus erythematosus. N Engl J Med 290:96, 1974

Koh KS, Friesen RM, Livingstone RA, Peddle LJ: Fetal monitoring during maternal cardiac surgery with cardiopulmonary bypass. Can Med Assn J 112:1102, 1975

Kohler PF, Dubois RS, Merrill DA, Bowes WA: Prevention of chronic neonatal hepatitis B virus infection with antibody to hepatitis B surface antigen. N Engl J Med 291:1378, 1974

Kohn SG, Briele HA, Douglass LH: Volvulus complicating pregnancy. Am J Obstet Gynecol 48: 398, 1944

Kopenhager T: A review of 50 pregnant patients with kyphoseoliosis. Br J Obstet Gynaecol 84:585, 1977

Kosmetatos N, Blackman MS, Elrad H, Aubry RH: Congenital, complete heart block in the infant of a woman with collagen vascular disease. J Reprod Med 22:213, 1979

Kramer MS, Rooks Y, Johnston D, Pearson HA: Accuracy of cord blood screening for sickle hemoglobinopathies. JAMA 241:485, 1979

Kreek MJ, Weser E, Sleisenger MH, Jeffries GH: Idiopathic cholestasis of pregnancy. N Engl J Med 277: 1391, 1967

Krick JA, Remington JS: Toxoplasmosis in the

adult—An overview. N Engl J Med 298:550, 1978

Krugman S: Hepatitis: current status of etiology and prevention. Hosp Prac 10:39, 1975

Krugman S, Giles JP: Viral hepatitis: new light on an old disease. JAMA 212:1019, 1970

Lander CM, Edwards VE, Eadie MJ, Tyrer JH: Plasma anticonvulsant concentrations during pregnancy. Neurology 27:128, 1977

Landesman R, Scherr L: Congenital polycystic kidney disease in pregnancy. Obstet Gynecol 8:673, 1956

Langer A, Hung CT, McA'Nulty JA, Harrigan JT, Washington E: Adrenergic blockade: a new approach to hyperthyroidism during pregnancy. Obstet Gynecol 44:181, 1974

Laros RK Jr, Sweet RL: Management of idopathic thrombocytopenic purpura during pregnancy. Am J Obstet Gynecol 122:182, 1975

Leak D, Carroll JJ, Robinson DC, Ashworth EJ: Management of pheochromocytoma during pregnancy. Can Med Assoc J 116:371, 1977

Lehman H, Huntsman RG: Man's Haemoglobins. Philadelphia, Lippincott, 1966

Levine AM, Collea JV: When pregnancy complicates chronic granulocytic leukemia. Contemp Ob/Gyn 13:47, 1979

Leveno KJ, Hauth JC, Gilstrap LC III, Whalley PJ: Appraisal of "rigid" blood glucose control during pregnancy in the overtly diabetic woman. Am J Obstet Gynecol 135:793, 1979

Lewis R, Lauersen NH, Birnbaum S: Malaria associated with pregnancy. Obstet Gynecol 42:696, 1973

Lian EC-Y, Harkness DR, Byrnes JJ, Wallach H, Nunez R: Presence of platelet aggregating factor in the plasma of patients with thrombotic thrombocytopenic purpura and its inhibition by normal plasma. Blood 53:333, 1979

Light IJ, Linnemann CC: Neonatal herpes simplex infection following delivery by cesarean section. Obstet Gynecol 44:496, 1974

Lilleyman JS, Hill AS, Anderton KJ: Consequences of acute myelogenous leukemia in early pregnancy. Obstet Gynecol Survey 33:393, 1978

Lindback T, Skjaeraasen J: Phospholipid concentrations in amniotic fluid from diabetic pregnant women. Pediatr Res 9:858, 1975

Little PJ: The incidence of urinary infection in 5000 pregnant women. Lancet 2:925, 1966

Lowenstein L, Pick C, Philpott N: Megaloblastic anemia of pregnancy and the puerperium. Am J Obstet Gynecol 70:1309, 1955

Lucké B: Pathology of fatal epidemic hepatitis. Am J Pathol 20:471, 1944

Lutz DS, Noller KL, Spittell JA Jr, Danielson GK, Fish CR: Pregnancy and its complications following cardiac valve prosthesis. Am J Obstet Gynecol 131:460, 1978

Mack HC, Schreiber F, Nielsen A, Huber PJ: Intracranial hemorrhage associated with pregnancy. Harper Hosp Bull 14:249, 1956

Martin DH, Montgomery DAD, Harley JMcDG: The occurrence of T_3 thyrotoxicosis in pregnancy. Irish J Med Sci 145:92, 1976

Maurus JN: Hansen's disease in pregnancy. Obstet Gynecol 52:22, 1978

Mendelow DA, Lewis GC Jr: Varicella pneumonia during pregnancy. Obstet Gynecol 33:98, 1969

Mendelson CL: Aspiration of stomach contents into the lungs during obstetric anesthesia. Am J Obstet Gynecol 52:191, 1946

Mibashan RS, Thumpston JK, Singer JD, Rodeck CH, Edwards RJ, White JM, Campbell S: Plasma assay of fetal factors VIIIC and IX for prenatal diagnosis of haemophilia. Lancet 1:1309, 1979

Miller JM Jr, Crenshaw C Jr, Selman I, Welt SI: Hemoglobin A_{1c} in normal and diabetic pregnancy. JAMA 242:2785, 1979

Minielly R, Yuzpe AA, Drake CG: Subarachnoid hemorrhage secondary to ruptured cerebral aneurysm in pregnancy. Obstet Gynecol 53:64, 1979

Minkowitz S, Soloway HB, Hall JE, Yermankou V: Fatal hemorrhagic pancreatitis following chlorothiazide administration in pregnancy. Obstet Gynecol 24:337, 1964

Mintz DH, Chez RA, Hutchinson DL: Subhuman primate pregnancy complicated by streptozotocin-induced diabetes mellitus. J Clin Invest 51:837, 1972

Modlin JF, Herrmann K, Brandling-Bennett AD, Eddins DL, Hayden GF: Risk of congenital abnormality after inadvertent rubella vaccination of pregnant women. N Engl J Med 294:972, 1976

Moldin P, Johansson O: Acute fatty liver of pregnancy with disseminated intravascular coagulation. Acta Obstet Gynecol Scand 57:179, 1978

Murray JE, Reid DE, Harrison JH, Merrill JP: Successful pregnancies after human renal transplantation. N Engl J Med 269:341, 1963

Nadler N, Salinas-Madrigal L, Charles AG, Pollak

VE: Acute glomerulonephritis during late pregnancy. Obstet Gynecol 34:277, 1969

National Diabetes Data Group: Classification of diabetes mellitus and other categories of glucose intolerance. Diabetes 28: (Dec), 1979

Neely NT, Persellin RH: Activity of rheumatoid arthritis during pregnancy. Texas Med 73:59, 1977

Neufeld ND, Sevanian A, Barrett CT, Kaplan SA: Inhibition of surfactant production by insulin in fetal rabbit lung slices. Pediatr Res 13:752, 1979

Nissenson AR, Krumlovsky FA, de Greco F: Postpartum hemolytic uremic syndrome. JAMA 242:173, 1979

Noller KL, Bowie EJW, Kempers RD, Owen CA Jr: Von Willebrand's disease in pregnancy. Obstet Gynecol 41:865, 1973

Norton RA, Patterson JF: Pregnancy and regional enteritis. Obstet Gynecol 40:711, 1972

Ober WB, Le Compte PM: Acute fatty metamorphosis of the liver associated with pregnancy: distinctive lesion. Am J Med 19:743, 1955

Ober WB, Reid DE, Romney SL, Merrill JP: Renal lesions and acute renal failure in pregnancy. Am J Med 21:781, 1956

O'Leary JA: A continuing study of sarcoidosis and pregnancy. Am J Obstet Gynecol 101:610, 1968

O'Leary JA, Klainer LM, Neuworth RS: The management of hypoparathyroidism in pregnancy. Am J Obstet Gynecol 94:1103, 1966

Onodera T, Yoon J-W, Brown KS, Notkins AL: Evidence for a single locus controlling susceptibility to virus-induced diabetes mellitus. Nature 274:693, 1978

O'Shaughnessy R, Weprin SA, Zuspan FP: Obstructive renal failure by an overdistended pregnant uterus. Obstet Gynecol 55:247, 1980

O'Sullivan JB, Mahan CM: Criteria for the oral glucose tolerance test in pregnancy. Diabetes 13:278, 1964

O'Sullivan JB, Charles D, Mahan CM, Dandrow RV: Gestational diabetes and perinatal mortality rate. Am J Obstet Gynecol 116:901, 1973

Papaevangelou G, Hoofnagle J, Kremastinou J: Transplacental transmission of hepatitis-B virus by symptom-free chronic carrier mothers. Lancet 2:746, 1974

Pedersen NT, Permin H: Hyperparathyroidism and pregnancy. Acta Obstet Gynecol Scand 54:281, 1975

Penn I, Makowski EL, Harris P: Parenthood following renal transplant. Kidney International (In press), 1980

Perez RJ, Lipner H, Abdulla N, Cicotto S, Abrams M: Menstrual dysfunction of patients undergoing chronic hemodialysis. Obstet Gynecol 51:552, 1978

Philips JA III, Kazazian HH III, Boehm CD, Scott AF, Panny SR, Smith KD: Prenatal diagnosis of sickle cell anemia: Value of linked γ-globin polymorphisms. Pediatr Res 14:526, 1980

Pickard RE: Varicella pneumonia in pregnancy. Am J Obstet Gynecol 101:504, 1968

Prather GC, Crabtree EG: The lone kidney in pregnancy. Trans Am Assoc Genitourin Surg 26:313, 1933

Pritchard JA: Hereditary hypochromic microcytic anemia in obstetrics and gynecology. Am J Obstet Gynecol 83:1193, 1962a

Pritchard JA: Megaloblastic anemia during pregnancy and the puerperium. Am J Obstet Gynecol 83:1004, 1962b

Pritchard JA: Anemias complicating pregnancy and the puerperium. In Maternal Nutrition and the Course of Pregnancy, Report of the Committee on Maternal Nutrition, Food and Nutrition Board, National Research Council. Washington, D.C., National Academy of Sciences, 1970

Pritchard JA, Mason RA: Iron stores of normal adults and replenishment with oral iron therapy. JAMA 190:897, 1964

Pritchard JA, Scott DE: Iron demands in pregnancy. In Hallberg L, Harwerth H-G, Vanotti A (eds): Iron Deficiency Pathogenesis, Clinical Aspects, Therapy. New York, Academic, 1970

Pritchard JA, Cunningham FG, Mason RA: Coagulation changes in eclampsia: Their frequency and pathogenesis. Am J Obstet Gynecol 124:855, 1976

Pritchard JA, Scott DE, Whalley PJ: Folic acid requirements in pregnancy-induced megaloblastic anemia. JAMA 208:1163, 1969

Pritchard JA, Scott DE, Whalley PJ: Maternal folate deficiency and pregnancy wastage: IV. Effects of folic acid supplements, anticonvulsants, and oral contraceptives. Am J Obstet Gynecol 110:375, 1971

Pritchard JA, Scott DE, Whalley PJ, Haling RF Jr: Infants of mothers with megaloblastic anemia due to folate deficiency. JAMA 211: 1982, 1970

Pritchard JA, Scott DE, Whalley PJ, Cunningham FG, Mason RA: The effects of maternal sickle cell hemoglobinopathies and sickle cell trait on reproductive performance. Am J Obstet Gynecol 117:662, 1973

Pritchard JA, Weisman R Jr, Ralnoff OD, Vosburgh GJ: Intravascular hemolysis, thrombocytopenia, and other hematologic abnormalities associated with severe toxemia of pregnancy. N Engl J Med 250:89, 1954

Rayfield EJ, Seto Y: Viruses and the pathogenesis of diabetes mellitus. Diabetes 27:1126, 1978

Redeker AG, Mosley JW, Gocke DJ, McKee AP, Pollack W: Hepatitis B immune globulin as a prophylactic measure for spouses exposed to acute type B hepatitis. N Engl J Med 293:1055, 1975

Reid R, Ivey KJ, Rencoret RH, Storey B: Fetal complications of obstetric cholestasis. Br Med J 1:870, 1976

Reid RL, Pancham SR, Kean WF, Ford PM: Maternal and neonatal implications of congenital complete heart block in the fetus. Obstet Gynecol 54:470, 1979

Reynolds AG: Placental metastasis from malignant melanoma. Obstet Gynecol 6:205, 1955

Riggall F, Salkind G, Spellacy W: Typhoid fever complicating pregnancy. Obstet Gynecol 44:117, 1974

Rigler LG, Eneboe JB: Incidence of hiatus hernia in pregnant women and its significance. J Thorac Surg 4:262, 1935

Robinson PL, O'Mullane NM, Alderman B: Prenatal treatment of fetal thyrotoxicosis. Br Med J 1:383, 1979

Robson JS, Martin AM, Ruckley VA, Macdonald MK: Irreversible postpartum renal failure. Q J Med 37:423, 1968

Ruch WA, Klein RL: Polycythemia vera and pregnancy. Obstet Gynecol 23:107, 1964

Rudolph JE, Schweizer RT, Bartus SA: Pregnancy in renal transplant patients. Transplantation 27:26, 1979

St Geme JW Jr, Bailey R, Koopman JS, Oh W, Hobel CJ, Imagawa DT: Neonatal risk following late gestational genital herpesvirus hominis infection. Am J Dis Child 129:342, 1975

Salmon PA: Pregnancies occurring in patients before and after bypass operation for weight loss. Personal communication, 1975

Saxen L, Hjelt L, Sjostedt JE, Hakosalo J, Hakosalo H: Asian influenza during pregnancy and congenital malformation. Acta Pathol Microbiol Scand 49:114, 1960

Schaefer G: Full term pregnancy following genital tuberculosis. Obstet Gynecol Survey 19:81, 1964 (112 references cited)

Scheinhorn DJ, Angelillo VA: Antituberculous therapy in pregnancy: Risks to the fetus. West J Med 127:195, 1977

Schenker JG, Chowers I: Pheochromocytoma and pregnancy. Review of 89 cases. Obstet Gynecol Survey 26:739, 1971

Schenker KG, Polishuk WZ: Pregnancy following mitral valvotomy. Obstet Gynecol 32:214, 1968

Schneider JM, Curet LB, Olson RW, Shay G: Ambulatory care of the pregnant diabetic. Obstet Gynecol (In press, 1980)

Schneider RG, Hightower B, Hasty TS, Ryder H, Tomlin G, Atkins R, Brimhall B, Jones RT: Abnormal hemoglobins in a quarter million people. Blood 48:629, 1976

Schou M, Goldfield MD, Weinstein MR, Villeneuve A: Lithium and pregnancy—I through III. Br Med J 2:135, 1973

Schriner RL, Kleiman MB, Gresham EL: Maternal oral herpes: Isolation policy. Pediatrics 63:247, 1979

Schultz JC, Adamson JS Jr, Workman WW, Norma TD: Fatal liver disease after intravenous administration of tetracycline in high dosage. N Engl J Med 269:999, 1963

Sciarra JJ, Toledo-Pereya LH, Bendel RB, Simmons RL: Pregnancy following renal transplantation. Am J Obstet Gynecol 123:411, 1975

Scott DE, Pritchard JA: Iron deficiency in healthy young college women. JAMA 199:147, 1967

Scott DE, Whalley PJ, Pritchard JA: Maternal folate deficiency and pregnancy wastage: II. Fetal malformation. Obstet Gynecol 36:26, 1970

Scott JR, Cruikshank DP, Kochenour NK, Pitkin RM, Warenski JC: Fetal platelet counts in the obstetric management of immunologic thrombocytopenic purpura. Am J Obstet Gynecol 136:495, 1980

Sende P, Pantelakis N, Suzuki K, Bashore R: Plasma oxytocin level in pregnancy with diabetes insipidus. Clin Res 23:242A, 1975

Sheehan HL: Jaundice in pregnancy. Am J Obstet Gynecol 81:427, 1961

Sheehan HL, Moore HC: Renal Cortical Necrosis and the Kidney of Concealed Accidental Haemorrhage. Springfield, Ill., Thomas, 1953

Sheldon J, Coleman T: Remission of diabetes mellitus during pregnancy. Br Med J 1:55, 1974

Siegel M, Goldberg M: Incidence of poliomyelitis in pregnancy. N Engl J Med 253:841, 1955

Siegler AM, Spain DM: Periarteritis nodosa in pregnancy. Clin Obstet Gynecol 8:280, 1965

Simpson JL: Genetics of diabetes mellitus and anomalies in offspring of diabetic mothers. Semin Perinat 2:383, 1978

Smith DW: Teratogenicity of anticonvulsant medications. Am J Dis Child 131:1337, 1977

Smith EW, Krevans JR: Clinical manifestations of hemoglobin C disorders. Bull Johns Hopkins Hosp 104:17, 1959

Smith MB, Whiteside MG, DeGaris CN: An investigation of the complications and outcome of pregnancy in heterozygous beta-thalassaemia. Aust NZ J Obstet Gynecol 15:26, 1975

Steel RB, Mosley JD, Smith CH: Insulin and placenta: Degradation and stabilization, binding to microvillous receptors, and amino acid uptake. Am J Obstet Gynecol 135:522, 1979

Strauss RG, Alexander RW: Postpartum hemolytic uremic syndrome. Obstet Gynecol 47:169, 1976

Strong DW, Murchison RJ, Lynch DF: The management of ureteral calculi during pregnancy. Surg Gynecol Obstet 146:604, 1978

Studd JWW, Blainey JD: Pregnancy and the nephrotic syndrome. Br Med J 1:276, 1969

Sudo, N, Weingold AB: Obstetric aspects of the Guillain-Barré syndrome. Obstet Gynecol 45:39, 1975

Sweeney WJ: Pregnancy and multiple sclerosis. Am J Obstet Gynecol 66:124, 1953

Szmuness W, Much MI, Prince AM, et al: The role of sexual behavior in the spread of hepatitis B infection. Ann Intern Med 83:489, 1975

Taylor DS: Massive gastric haemorrhage in late pregnancy followed by hypopituitarism. Br J Obstet Gynaecol 79:476, 1972

Tejani N, Klein SW, Kaplan M: Subclinical herpes simplex genitalis infections in the perinatal period. Am J Obstet Gynecol 135:547, 1979

Territo M, Finklestein J, Oh W, Hobel C, Kattlove H: Management of autoimmune thrombocytopenia in pregnancy and the neonate. Obstet Gynecol 41:57, 1973

Townsend JJ, Baringer JR, Wolinsky JS, Malamud N, Mednick JP, Panitch HS, Scott RAT, Oshiro LS, Cremer NE; Progressive rubella panencephalitis: late onset after congenital rubella. N Engl J Med 292:990, 1975

Tracy TA, Miller GL: Obstetric problems of the massively obese. Obstet Gynecol 33:204, 1969

Trebbin WM: Hemodialysis and pregnancy. JAMA 241:1811, 1979

Tsai A, Lindheimer MD, Lamberg SI: Dermato-myositis complicating pregnancy. Obstet Gynecol 41:570, 1973

Varma SK: Newborn screening for congenital hypothyroidism. Texas Med 75:57, 1979

Vasicka A, Lin TJ, Bright RH: Peptic ulcer and pregnancy: review of hormonal relationships and a report of one case of massive gastrointestinal hemorrhage. Obstet Gynecol Survey 12:1, 1957 (56 references cited)

Villarejos VM, Visona KA, Gutierrez D, Rodriquez A: Role of saliva, urine and feces in the transmission of type B hepatitis. N Engl J Med 291:1375, 1974

Visintine AM, Nahmias AJ, Josey WE: Genital herpes. Perinatal Care 2:32, 1978

Wagoner RD, Holley KE, Johnson WJ: Accelerated nephrosclerosis and postpartum acute renal failure in normotensive patients. Ann Intern Med 69:237, 1968

Walcott WO, Derick DE, Jolley JJ, Snyder DL, Schmid R: Successful pregnancy in a liver transplant patient. Am J Obstet Gynecol 132:340, 1978

Walker WM, McKee AP: Asian influenza in pregnancy: relationship to fetal anomalies. Obstet Gynecol 13:394, 1959

Wallace WA, Harken DE, Ellis LB: Pregnancy following closed mitral valvuloplasty. JAMA 217:297, 1971

Waters EG: Discussion of paper by JT Callahan: Separation of symphysis pubis. Am J Obstet Gynecol 66:292, 1953

Waters EG, Fenimore ED: Perforated carcinoma of the cecum in pregnancy. Obstet Gynecol 3:263, 1954

Weil ML, Itabashi HH, Cremer NE, Oshiro LS, Lennette EH, Carnay L: Chronic progressive panencephalitis due to rubella virus simulating subacute sclerosing panencephalitis. N Engl J Med 292:994, 1975

Weinstein AM, Dubin BD, Wojciech KP, Spector SL, Farr RS: Asthma and pregnancy. JAMA 241:1161, 1979

Weinstein MR, Goldfield MD: Cardiovascular malformations with lithium used during pregnancy. Am J Psychiatr 132:529, 1975

Weisman SA, Simon NA, Herdson PB, Franklin WA: Nephrotic syndrome in pregnancy. Am J Obstet Gynecol 117:867, 1973

Werkö L, Bucht H: Glomerular filtration rate and renal blood flow in patients with chronic diffuse glomerulonephritis during pregnancy. Acta Med Scand 153:177, 1956

Westberg SV: Prognosis of breast cancer for pregnant and nursing women. Acta Obstet Gynecol Scand (Suppl 4) 25:1, 1946

Whalley PJ: Hyperparathyroidism and pregnancy. Am J Obstet Gynecol 86:517, 1963

Whalley PJ: Bacteriuria of pregnancy. Am J Obstet Gynecol 97:723, 1967

Whalley PJ, Adams RH, Combes B: Tetracycline toxicity in pregnancy. JAMA 189:357, 1964

Whalley PJ, Cunningham FG, Martin FG: Transient renal dysfunction associated with acute pyelonephritis of pregnancy. Obstet Gynecol 46:174, 1975

Whalley PJ, Martin FG, Peters PC: Significance of asymptomatic bacteriuria detected during pregnancy. JAMA 198:879, 1965

Whalley PJ, Martin FG, Pritchard JA: Sickle cell trait and pregnancy. JAMA 189:903, 1964

Whalley PJ, Pritchard JA, Richards JR Jr: Sickle cell trait and pregnancy. JAMA 186:1132, 1963

Whalley PJ, Scott DE, Pritchard JA: Maternal folate deficiency and pregnancy wastage: I. Placental abruption. Am J Obstet Gynecol 105:670, 1969

White P: Classification of obstetric diabetes. Am J Obstet Gynecol 130:228, 1978

White P: Pregnancy and diabetes, medical aspects. Med Clin North Am 49:1015, 1965

Whittemore R, Wright MR, Leonard MF, Johnson M: Results of pregnancy in women with congenital heart defects. Pediatr Res 14:452, 1980

Wilkinson EJ: Acute pancreatitis in pregnancy: a review of 98 cases and a report of 8 new cases. Obstet Gynecol Survey 28:281, 1973

Williams DA: Asthma and pregnancy. Acta Allerg 22:311, 1967

Williams JW: The limitations and possibilities of prenatal care. JAMA 64:95, 1915

Willoughby MLN, Jewell FG: Folate status throughout pregnancy and in the postpartum period. Br Med J 4:356, 1968

Wilson MG, Heins HL, Imagawa DT, Adams JM: Teratogenic effects of Asian influenza. JAMA 171:638, 1959

Wilson MG, Hewitt WL, Monzon OT: Effect of bacteriuria on the fetus. N Engl J Med 274:115, 1966

Woods JR Jr, Brinkman CR III: The jejunoileal bypass and pregnancy. Obstet Gynecol Survey 33:697, 1978

Wurzel JM: TTP lesions in placenta but not fetus. N Engl J Med 301:503, 1979

Zegart KN, Schwarz RH: Chorea gravidarum. Obstet Gynecol 32:24, 1968

Zimmerman TS, Abildgaard CF, Meyer D: The factor VIII abnormality in severe von Willebrands disease. N Engl J Med 301:1307, 1979

Zinns JS: The association of pregnancy and breast cancer. J Reprod Med 22:297, 1979

Zondek B, Bromberg YM: Infectious hepatitis in pregnancy. J Mt Sinai Hosp 14:222, 1947

Zurier RB, Argyros TG, Urman JD, Warren J, Rothfield NF: Systemic lupus erythematosus: Management during pregnancy. Obstet Gynecol 51:178, 1978

29

Dystocia Caused by Anomalies
of the Expulsive Forces

Dystocia (literally difficult labor) is characterized by abnormally slow progress of labor. It is the consequence of four distinct abnormalities that may exist singly or in combination:

1. Uterine forces that are not sufficiently strong or appropriately coordinated to efface and dilate the cervix.
2. Forces generated by voluntary muscles during the second stage of labor that are inadequate to overcome the normal resistance of the bony birth canal and maternal soft parts.
3. Faulty presentation or abnormal development of the fetus of such a character that the fetus cannot be extruded by the vis a tergo (see Chap. 30).
4. Abnormalities of the birth canal that form an obstacle to the descent of the fetus (see Chap. 31).

Pelvic contraction is often accompanied by uterine dysfunction, and the two together constitute the most common cause of dystocia. Similarly, faulty presentation or unusual fetal size or shape may be accompanied by uterine dysfunction. *As a generalization, uterine dysfunction is common whenever there is disproportion between the presenting part of the fetus and the birth canal.*

UTERINE DYSFUNCTION

Normally, as described in Chapter 15 (p. 375), there is first *prodromal labor,* or a "latent phase," of several hours' duration during which, typically, the cervix becomes somewhat effaced but dilates only slightly. This period is characterized by mild contractions of variable frequency and short duration. Then follows *clinically apparent labor,* or the *active phase of labor.* During the active phase of labor, or perhaps better referred to simply as labor, the cervix dilates at a rate of 1 to 2 cm per hour and there is descent of the presenting part through the birth canal.

Failure of the cervix to dilate or of the presenting part to descend is cause for appreciable concern. Extension of either the first or second stage of labor may result in increased perinatal and maternal morbidity. Delay in cervical dilatation or prolongation of the second stage should alert the obstetrician to possible danger.

Uterine dysfunction in any phase of cervical dilatation is characterized by lack of progress, for one of the prime characteristics of normal labor is its progression. Friedman (1978), in an attempt at precision, defines prolongation of the latent phase as 20 hours in nulliparas and 14 hours in multiparas, while cervical dilatation of less than 1.2 cm per hour in nulliparas and 1.5 cm per hour in multiparas represents a protracted active phase. The diagnosis of uterine dysfunction in the so-called latent phase is difficult and sometimes can be made only in retrospect. One of the commonest errors is to treat women for uterine dysfunction who are not yet in active labor. Administration of an effective sedative usually curtails the troublesome discomforts of false labor while active labor will continue unabated.

There have been three significant advances in the treatment of uterine dysfunction: (1) the realization that undue prolongation of labor contributes to perinatal morbidity and mortality; (2) the use of very dilute intravenous infusion of oxytocin in the treatment of certain types of uterine dysfunction; and (3) the more frequent use of cesarean section to effect delivery rather than difficult midforceps delivery when oxytocin fails or its use is inappropriate.

Types. Reynolds and co-workers (1948) showed that the uterine contractions of labor are normally characterized by a gradient of myometrial activity, being greatest and lasting longest at the fundus (fundal dominance) and diminishing toward the cervix (see Chap. 15, p. 377). Caldeyro-Barcia and his colleagues in Montevideo (1950) advanced the work of Reynolds by inserting small balloons in the myometrium at various levels. With the balloons attached to strain-gauge transducers, they were able to show that there was, in addition to a gradient of activity, a time differential in the onset of the contractions in the fundus, midzone, and lower segment of the uterus. Larks (1960) described the exciting stimulus as starting in one cornu and then several milliseconds later in the

other, the excitation waves then joining and sweeping over the fundus and down the uterus.

The group in Montevideo made another significant contribution to the understanding of uterine dysfunction. By inserting a polyethylene catheter through the abdomen into the amnionic fluid, they ascertained that the lower limit of pressure of contractions required to dilate the cervix is at least 15 mm Hg, a figure in keeping with the findings of Hendricks and co-workers (1959), which also demonstrated that a normal spontaneous uterine contraction may exert a much higher pressure of about 60 mm Hg. From these observations, it is possible to define two types of uterine dysfunction. In one, *hypotonic uterine dysfunction,* there is no basal hypertonus and uterine contractions have a normal gradient pattern (synchronous), but the rise in pressure during a contraction is insufficient to dilate the cervix at a satisfactory rate (less than 15 mm Hg). In the other, *hypertonic uterine dysfunction,* or *incoordinate uterine function,* either basal tone is elevated or the pressure gradient is distorted, perhaps by contraction of the midsegment of the uterus with more force than the fundus or by complete asynchronism of the electrical impulses originating in each cornu, or both.

In the hypotonic variety of uterine dysfunction, contractions become less frequent and the uterus is easily indentable even at the acme of a contraction. Contractions of the "hypertonic" or incoordinate variety are typically much more painful although no more effective. As discussed below, hypotonic dysfunction often responds favorably to treatment with oxytocin. The opposite is most often true of the "hypertonic" variety, in which the abnormal pattern of uterine contractions is more likely to become accentuated and the tone of the uterine muscle increased. Exceptions have been documented, however, in which a misbehaving uterus with basal hypertonus and frequent, incoordinate contractions did convert to orderly physiologic contractions, apparently in response to intravenous oxytocin (Caldeyro-Barcia,

1957). In general, the likelihood of such a response is low while the risk of enhancing the hypertonus is considerable, in our experience.

Etiology. Pelvic contraction and fetal malposition are common causes of uterine dysfunction. That moderate degrees of pelvic contraction and fetal malposition may cause uterine inertia is of great clinical importance. Overdistension of the uterus, as with twins and with hydramnios, contribute to the condition. *However, in many instances—perhaps one-half—the cause of uterine dysfunction is unknown.* The main fault seldom lies within a cervix that is too rigid to dilate. In elderly primigravidas, and in women whose cervix is fibrosed from some cause, however, excessive rigidity of the cervix may be a factor in the production of dystocia.

Complications. Undue procrastination too often leads to an unfortunate outcome. Fetal and neonatal deaths are accompaniments of intrauterine infection, which commonly develops in prolonged dysfunctional labor. Although it may be wise for the mother's protection to treat these intrauterine infections with antibiotics, such therapy appears to be of little value in protecting the fetus. Maternal exhaustion may occur if labor is greatly prolonged; however, supportive therapy with adequate intravenous fluids should be initiated and delivery effected before these complications appear. Difficult labors and deliveries are more likely to leave psychologic scars on the mothers, as emphasized by Jeffcoate (1961), as well as Steer (1950). Both found that difficult labor exerted a definite deleterious effect upon future childbearing. These investigators showed that although more than two-thirds of their patients had further children after spontaneous delivery, only one-third did so after midforceps operations.

Treatment of Hypotonic Dysfunction. Two questions must be answered before a plan for treatment can be formulated:

(1) Has the woman actually been in active labor? If there has been rhythmic uterine activity sufficient in intensity to produce some discomfort, the cervix has been observed to undergo distinct changes in effacement *and* in dilatation to 3 cm at least, it is correct to conclude that there has been real, albeit abnormal, labor. (2) Is there cephalopelvic disproportion? Uterine inertia is often a protection against some degree of pelvic contraction or abnormalities of fetal size or presentation. Fortunately, the uterus does not typically persist in spontaneous activity that would lead to its own destruction, i.e., rupture. Instead, the usual forces of labor are replaced by hypotonic uterine dysfunction.

Most often, once the diagnosis of active labor followed by hypotonic uterine dysfunction has been made and the head is well fixed in the pelvis, the membranes, if intact, should be ruptured. Meconium staining of amnionic fluid is an ominous sign and makes close monitoring of the fetal heart even more vital. Close observation may be employed for a short period to see if the amniotomy will stimulate effective labor. Otherwise, a decision must be made whether to try to stimulate labor with oxytocin or to effect delivery by cesarean section.

OXYTOCIN STIMULATION. It should be ascertained that the birth canal is most likely adequate for the size of the fetal head and that the fetal head is well-flexed so as to utilize its smallest diameters to negotiate the birth canal (biparietal and suboccipitobregmatic diameters). A contracted pelvis is most unlikely when all the following criteria are met:

1. The diagonal conjugate is normal.
2. The pelvic sidewalls are nearly parallel.
3. The ischial spines are not prominent.
4. The sacrum is not flat.
5. The subpubic angle is not narrow.
6. The occiput is the presenting part for certain.
7. The fetal head descends through the pelvic inlet with fundal pressure.

If these criteria are not met, the alternatives are cesarean section, or possibly *careful* oxytocin stimulation. For the experienced obstetrician, x-ray pelvimetry usually provides little more information. For the less experienced clinician, x-ray pelvimetry may be an aid. If oxytocin is used, it is mandatory that the fetal heart rate and the frequency, intensity, and duration of the contractions be closely monitored. If the fetal heart is monitored discontinuously, it is imperative that it be checked at the minimum *immediately following* contractions rather than a minute or more afterward (see Chap. 14, p. 363).

TECHNIC FOR INTRAVENOUS OXYTOCIN. Ten units of oxytocin are thoroughly mixed with 1 liter of aqueous solution, usually 5 percent glucose in water or preferably a balanced salt solution. More dilute solutions can be prepared by doubling the amount of diluent or halving the amount of oxytocin. Although more dilute solutions have been found effective by numerous authors, the mixture (10 units per liter) is easy to prepare, safe, effective, and likely to cause least confusion. Since the solution contains 10 mU of oxytocin per ml, its rate of flow is easily calculated. The orifice in the drip chamber in commercially available intravenous sets is not well standardized, however. Although sets from individual manufacturers deliver drops of a fairly constant size, sets from each company should be tested. Use of a constant infusion pump enhances the precision of the dosage delivered, especially in the lower range, and is recommended.

The needle, *with the flow shut off*, is inserted into an arm vein, or preferably into an already well-functioning intravenous infusion line, and the flow started to deliver no more than 2 mU per minute. In true hypotonic dysfunction, this amount of oxytocin will not initiate tetanic uterine contractions, although one should be prepared to cut off the flow in case the uterus is overly sensitive to the drug. The flow can be very gradually increased to yield 20 mU per minute. It is rarely necessary to exceed this rate. Certainly, if a flow rate of 30 to 40 mU per minute fails to initiate satisfactory uterine contractions, greater rates of infusion are not likely to do so.

The mother should never be left alone while the infusion is running. The uterine contractions must be observed continually and the flow shut off immediately if they exceed 1 minute in duration or if the fetal heart rate decelerates significantly. When either occurs, immediate discontinuation of the flow nearly always corrects the disturbances, preventing harm to mother or fetus. The concentration in plasma rapidly falls; the mean half-life of oxytocin is of the order of about 3 minutes.

It must always be kept in mind that oxytocin possesses potent antidiuretic action. Whenever 20 mU per minute or more of oxytocin is infused, free water clearance by the kidney decreases appreciably. If aqueous fluids, especially dextrose in water, are infused in appreciable amounts along with the oxytocin, there exists the possibility of serious water intoxication that may lead to convulsions, coma, and even death (see Chap. 17, p. 427).

At Parkland Memorial Hospital, the following general precautions are exercised with the use of oxytocin to treat hypotonic uterine dysfunction:

1. The woman must have demonstrated true labor, not false or prodromal labor. The only valid evidence of labor is progressive effacement and dilatation of the cervix. Although the process has come to a standstill, it must have progressed to the extent of at least 3-cm dilatation. One of the most common mistakes in obstetrics is to try to stimulate labor in women who have not been in active labor.
2. There must be no other discernible evidence of mechanical obstruction to safe delivery.
3. Use of oxytocin is generally avoided in cases of overt uterine overdistension, such as gross hydramnios, a large singleton fetus, or multiple fetuses.

4. Women of high parity (more than 5), in general, are not given oxytocin because their uteri rupture more readily than those of women of lower parity. For the same reason, it usually is withheld from women over the age of 35 and especially those with a previous uterine scar.

5. The condition of the fetus must be good, as evidenced by normal heart rate and lack of heavy contamination of the amnionic fluid with meconium. A dead fetus is, of course, no contraindication to oxytocin unless there is overt fetopelvic disproportion.

6. The obstetrician must note the time of the first contraction after administration of the drug and be prepared to discontinue its use if a tetanic contraction occurs. It is imperative that hyperstimulation of the uterus be avoided. The frequency, intensity, and duration of contractions, and uterine tone between contractions must not exceed those of normal spontaneous labor.

Oxytocin is a powerful drug, and it has killed or maimed mothers through rupture of the uterus and even more babies through hypoxia from markedly hypertonic uterine contractions. The intravenous administration, however, as attested by many publications, has brought about a distinct advance in both its efficacy and safety. Failure to treat uterine dysfunction exposes the mother to the serious hazards of maternal exhaustion, intrapartum infection, and traumatic operative delivery. At the same time, failure to treat uterine dysfunction may expose the fetus to an appreciably higher risk of death, whereas the risk of intravenous oxytocin in dilute solutions should be negligible when used appropriately. Serious accidents, nevertheless, may accompany its use unless the precautions mentioned here are rigidly observed. The ruptured uterus illustrated in Figure 29-1 serves to emphasize the need for these precautions. In this case, oxytocin was administered to a multipara who was 38 years of age. Inasmuch as no other abnormalities were

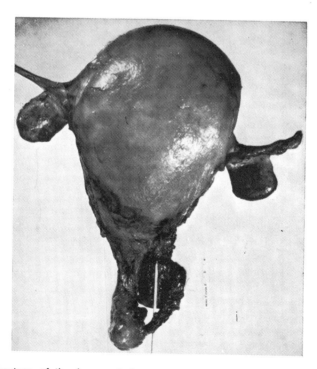

FIG. 29-1. Rupture of the lower uterine segment resulting from stimulation by dilute intravenous oxytocin in a 38-year-old multipara.

present, it must be assumed that the aging uterine muscle that had been repeatedly stretched previously could not stand the stimulation produced by the oxytocin.

One characterisitic of intravenous oxytocin is that when successful, it acts promptly, leading to noticeable progress with little delay. For any one rate of infusion the plasma level reaches a plateau after about 20 minutes as the rate of infusion and rate of destruction by oxytocinase achieve equilibrium. Therefore, the drug need not be used for an indefinite period of time to stimulate labor. It should be employed for no more than a few hours and then, if the cervix has not changed appreciably and if predictably easy vaginal delivery is not imminent, cesarean section should be performed. On the other hand, oxytocin should not be used to force cervical dilatation at a rate that exceeds normal. Ready resort to cesarean section in cases where oxytocin fails or in which there are contraindications to its use has served to diminish appreciably perinatal mortality and morbidity.

BUCCAL OXYTOCIN.   Oxytocin has been administered by placing tablets containing the drug against the buccal mucosa. Since transbuccal absorption is quite variable, either understimulation or overstimulation may occur. This technic has not been used at Parkland Memorial Hospital; rather, the drug is precisely administered intravenously with a calibrated infusion pump. Recently, transbuccal administration of oxytocin to induce or stimulate labor has been disapproved by the Food and Drug Administration.

PROSTAGLANDINS.   Prostaglandins $F_{2\alpha}$ and E_2 are potent uterotonic agents that are capable of inducing and augmenting labor although neither has been approved by the Food and Drug Administration for such use in this country. The possibility of uterine hypertonus following oral or intravenous administration is worrisome.

Considerable efficacy has been claimed for prostaglandin E_2 suppositories when used especially to ripen the unfavorable cervix of women in whom labor was to be induced. In the study of Shepherd and associates (1979), a suppository containing 3 mg of prostaglandin E_2 was inserted into the posterior vaginal fornix the evening before induction. If the cervix remained unfavorable, i.e., firm, minimally effaced and little dilated, the next morning a second "ripening" dose was inserted. Labor often followed the first or second suppository. If it did not, and the cervix was favorable (soft and somewhat effaced and dilated), amniotomy was performed or oxytocin was infused intravenously, or both. The cesarean section rate subsequent to the use of the prostaglandin E_2 suppositories among 502 women with a cervix considered at the outset to be unfavorable was only 2 percent. There was only one instance of uterine hypertonus described. The condition of the fetuses at birth as judged by Apgar scores was considered to be satisfactory.

Treatment of "Hypertonic" or Incoordinate Uterine Dysfunction.
Coming at the onset of labor, such dysfunction is characterized by uterine pain that appears to be out of proportion to the intensity of contractions and certainly out of proportion to their effectiveness in effacing and dilating the cervix. Because of the relative infrequency of this variety of dysfunctional labor, it has attracted little attention as a clinical entity, and thus its role in perinatal morbidity may be overlooked.

Oxytocin is rarely, if ever, indicated in the presence of uterine hypertonus with a living fetus. Cesarean section should be employed if the fetal heart rate should become abnormal. If the membranes are intact and there is no other evidence of fetopelvic disproportion, relief of pain and resting the mother by administering morphine may arrest the abnormal uterine activity. When she awakes, hopefully, more effective labor will be evident. It is important that such management does not lead to undue procrastination and unappreciated fetal distress, including the defecation of copious amounts of meconium into the amnionic fluid, and, in turn, serious meconium aspiration (see Chap. 38, p. 959). Tocolytic agents, such as ritodrine and salbutamol, have been used presumably with some success in other countries; these agents have not yet been widely used for this purpose in the United States.

INADEQUATE VOLUNTARY EXPULSIVE FORCE

With the achievement of full cervical dilatation the great majority of women cannot resist the urge to "bear down" or "push" each time that the uterus contracts. Typically, the laboring woman inhales deeply, closes her glottis, and contracts her abdominal musculature vigorously and repetitively to generate appreciable increases in intra-abdominal pressure throughout the time that the uterus is contracting. The combined force created by the contractions of the uterus and of the abdominal musculature propels the fetus down the vagina and, in the case of spontaneous delivery, through the vaginal outlet.

Causes. At times, the magnitude of the force created by the contraction of the abdominal musculature is sufficiently compromised to prevent spontaneous vaginal delivery. Iatrogenic factors that may cause impairment of such expulsive efforts include heavy sedation and various forms of anesthesia. Conduction anesthesia—lumbar epidural, caudal, or intrathecal—are likely to reduce the reflex urge for the woman to "push" and, at the same time, are likely to impair her ability to contract the abdominal muscles sufficiently to increase intra-abdominal pressure. General anesthesia, with loss of consciousness, certainly imposes these adverse effects.

In some instances, the inherent urge to "push" that develops in most women as the cervix becomes fully dilated is overridden by the intensification of pain that is created by bearing down. Rarely, insufficient expulsive efforts may be the consequence of long-standing paralysis of the abdominal musculature, as may occur after poliomyelitis or transection of the spinal cord.

Management. Careful selection of the kind of anesthesia and the timing of its administration are very important if compromise of voluntary expulsive efforts is to be avoided. With rare exception, intrathecal or general anesthesia should not be administered until all conditions for a safe low forceps delivery have been met, i.e., the fetal head is engaged, the sagittal suture is in the anteroposterior position, and the occiput distends the perineum and protrudes somewhat through the vaginal introitus with a contraction. With continuous epidural or caudal anesthesia, it may be necessary to allow the paralytic effects to wear off so that the mother in response to coaching can generate intra-abdominal pressure sufficient to move the fetal head into position appropriate for low forceps delivery. The alternatives—a possibly difficult midforceps vaginal delivery or cesarean section—are unsatisfactory choices in the absence of any evidence of fetal distress.

For the woman who cannot bear down appropriately with each contraction because of great discomfort, analgesia is likely to be of considerable benefit. Perhaps the safest for both fetus and mother is nitrous oxide, mixed with an equal volume of oxygen and provided during the time of each uterine contraction. At the same time, appropriate encouragement is most likely to be of benefit.

PRECIPITATE LABOR

Precipitate labor may result from an abnormally low resistance of the soft parts of the birth canal, from abnormally strong uterine and abdominal contractions, or very *rarely* from the absence of painful sensations and thus a lack of awareness of vigorous labor.

Maternal Effects. Precipitate labor and delivery are seldom accompanied by serious maternal complications if the cervix is appreciably effaced and easily dilated, the vagina has been previously stretched, and the perineum is relaxed. However, vigorous uterine contractions combined with a long, firm cervix, and a vagina, vulva, or perineum that resists stretch may lead to rupture of the uterus or troublesome lacerations of the cervix, vagina, vulva, or perineum. It is in these latter circumstances that the rare condition

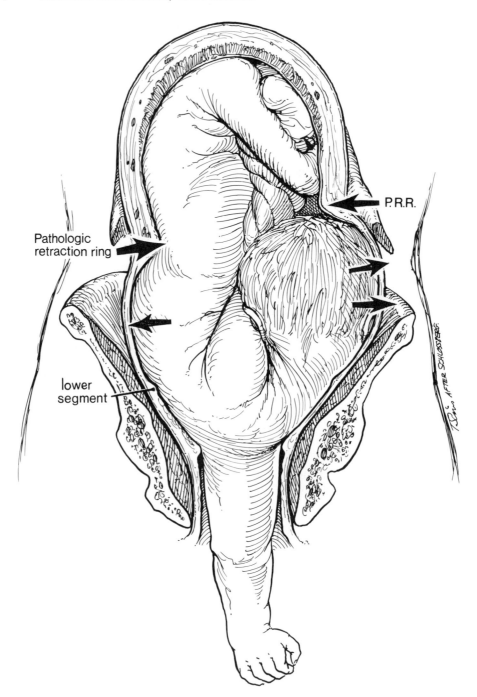

FIG. 29-2.   Neglected shoulder presentation. A thick muscular band to form a pathologic retraction ring has developed just above the very thin lower uterine segment. The force generated during a uterine contraction is directed centripetally at and above the level of the pathologic retraction ring. This serves to stretch further and possibly to rupture the very thin lower uterine segment below the retraction ring. (P.R.R. = pathologic retraction ring.)

amnionic fluid embolism is most likely to occur (see Chap. 21, p. 519). The uterus that contracts with unusual vigor before delivery is likely to be hypotonic after delivery with hemorrhage from the placental implantation site as the consequence (see Chap. 34, p. 878).

Effects on Fetus and Neonate. Perinatal mortality and morbidity from precipitate labor may be increased appreciably for several reasons. First, the tumultuous uterine contractions, often with negligible intervals of relaxation, prevent appropriate uterine blood flow and oxygenation of the fetal blood. Second, the resistance of the birth canal to descent of the head may cause intracranial trauma. Third, during an unattended birth, the infant may fall to the floor and be injured or may need resuscitation that is not immediately available.

Treatment. Unusually forceful spontaneous uterine contractions are not likely to be modified to a significant degree by the administration of analgesia. Importantly, if tried, the dose should be such that the infant at birth is not further depressed by the maternally administered analgesia. The use of general anesthesia with agents that impair uterine contractibility, such as halothane and ether, is often excessively heroic. Both epinephrine and magnesium sulfate parenterally administered have been claimed to be effective but the evidence that they are is weak. Certainly, any oxytocic agents being administered should be stopped immediately. Tocolytic agents, such as ritodrine and salbutamol, may prove effective but are not yet authorized for such use in the United States. It is indefensible to lock the mother's legs or hold the head back directly to try to delay delivery. Such maneuvers may damage the infant's brain.

LOCALIZED ABNORMALITIES OF UTERINE ACTION

Pathologic Retraction and Constriction Rings. Very rarely, localized rings or constrictions of the uterus occur in association with prolonged rupture of the membranes and protracted labors. The most common type is the so-called *pathologic retraction ring of Bandl* (Bandl, 1875), an exaggeration of the normal retraction ring described in Chapter 15, page 380, and often, but not always, the result of obstructed labor with marked stretching and thinning of the lower uterine segment. In such a situation, the ring may be clearly evident as an abdominal indentation and signifies impending rupture of the lower uterine segment (Fig. 29-2). Localized constrictions of the uterus are rarely seen today, since prolonged obstructed labors are no longer compatible with acceptable obstetric practice. They may, however, still occur occasionally as hourglass constrictions of the uterus following the birth of the first of twins. In such a situation, they can usually be relaxed and delivery effected with appropriate general anesthesia (see Chap. 26, p. 661).

Missed Labor. In rare instances, uterine contractions commence at or near term and, after continuing for a variable time, disappear without leading to the birth of the child. The fetus then dies and may be retained in utero for months or years undergoing mummification. This condition is known as missed labor. If uterine contractions disappear without leading to the birth of the child, and especially if the infant dies and is retained, abdominal pregnancy is a much more likely diagnosis than is missed labor. Management of prolonged retention of a fetus dead in utero is discussed in Chapter 21 (p. 515) and of extrauterine (abdominal) pregnancy in Chapter 22 (p. 542).

REFERENCES

Bandl L: Über Ruptur der Gebärmutter. Vienna, 1875

Caldeyro-Barcia R, Alvarez H, Reynolds SRM: A better understanding of uterine contractility through simultaneous recording with an internal and a seven channel external method. Surg Obstet Gynecol 91:641, 1950

Caldeyro-Barcia R: Oxytocin and pregnant human uterus. Proc. 4th Pan-American Cong. Endocrinol. Buenos Aires, 1957

Friedman EA: Labor: Clinical Evaluation and Management, 2nd edition. New York, Appleton, 1978

Hendricks CH, Quilligan EJ, Tyler AB, Tucker GJ: Pressure relationships between intervillous space and amniotic fluid in human term pregnancy. Am J Obstet Gynecol 77:1028, 1959

Jeffcoate TNA: Prolonged labour. Lancet 2:61, 1961

Larks SD: Electrohysterography. Springfield, Ill., Thomas, 1960

Reynolds SRM, Heard OO, Bruns P, Hellman LM: A multichannel strain-gauge tokodynamometer: An instrument for studying patterns of uterine contractions in pregnant women. Bull Hopkins Hosp 82:446, 1948

Shepherd J. Pearce JMF, Sims CD: Induction of labour using prostaglandin E_2 pessaries. Br Med J 2:108, 1979

Steer CM: Effect of type of delivery on future childbearing. Am J Obstet Gynecol 60:395, 1950

30

Dystocia Caused by Abnormalities in Presentation, Position, or Development of the Fetus

BREECH PRESENTATION

Incidence. Breech presentation is common remote from term as demonstrated in Table 30-1. Most often, however, sometime before the onset of labor the fetus will turn spontaneously to a vertex presentation so that breech presentation persists in only about 3 to 4 percent of singleton deliveries. For example, 3.2 percent of 33,562 infants delivered recently at Parkland Memorial Hospital presented as a breech.

Etiology. As term approaches, the uterine cavity, for reasons that are not totally clear, most often accommodates the fetus in a longitudinal lie with the vertex presenting. Breeches are much more common at the end of the second trimester of pregnancy than at or near term (Table 30-1). Factors other than prematurity that appear to predispose to breech presentation include uterine relaxation associated with great parity, multiple fetuses, hydramnios, oligohydramnios, hydrocephalus, anencephalus, previous breech delivery, uterine anomalies, and tumors.

Implantation of the placenta in either cornual-fundal region of the uterus has been suspected of predisposing to breech presentation. Recently, Fianu and Vaclavinkova (1978) have provided sonographic evidence of a very much higher prevalence of implantation of the placenta in the cornual-fundal region for breech presentations (73 percent) than for vertex presentations (5 percent). The frequency of breech presentation is also increased with placenta previa but only a small minority of cases of breech presentation are associated with placenta previa. Most recent studies do not show a strong positive correlation between breech presentation and contracted pelvis.

Significance. If labor occurs without prior conversion of the breech to a vertex presentation, an *increased* frequency of the following complications can be anticipated: (1) perinatal morbidity and mortality from difficult delivery; (2) low birth weight from prematurity, growth retardation, or both; (3) prolapsed cord; (4) placenta previa; (5) fetal anomalies and developmental abnormalities that appear after the newborn period; (6) uterine anomalies and tumors; (7) multiple

TABLE 30-1.
FETAL PRESENTATION AT VARIOUS GESTATIONAL
AGES DETERMINED SONOGRAPHICALLY

GESTATION (WEEKS INCLUSIVE)	TOTAL (NO.)	CEPHALIC (%)	BREECH (%)	OTHER (%)
21–24	264	54.6	33.3	12.1
25–28	367	61.9	27.8	10.4
29–32	443	78.1	14.0	7.9
33–36	638	88.7	8.8	2.5
37–40	463	91.5	6.7	1.7

Data from Scheer and Nubar: *Am J Obstet Gynecol* 125:269, 1976.

fetuses; and (8) operative intervention, especially cesarean section.

Diagnosis. The varying relations between the lower extremities and buttocks of the fetus in breech presentations form the categories of frank breech, complete breech, and incomplete breech presentations (Figs. 30-1–30-3). With a *frank breech* presentation, the lower extremities are flexed at the hips and extended at the knees and thus the feet lie in close proximity to the head. A *complete breech* presentation differs from a frank breech presentation in that one or both knees are flexed rather than both extended. With *incomplete breech* presentation, one or both hips are not flexed and one or both feet or knees lie below the breech, i.e., a foot or knee is lowermost in the birth canal. The frank breech appears most common when the diagnosis is established radiologically near term (Rovinsky et al., 1973).

ABDOMINAL EXAMINATION. Typically, the first maneuver identifies the hard, round, readily ballottable fetal head to occupy the fundus of the uterus (Fig. 30-4). The second maneuver indicates the back to be on one side of the abdomen and the small parts on the other. On the third maneuver, if engagement has not occurred, i.e., the intertrochanteric diameter of the fetal pelvis has not passed through the pelvic inlet, the breech is movable above the pelvic inlet. After engagement, the fourth maneuver shows the firm breech to be beneath the symphysis. The heart sounds of the fetus are usu-

ally heard loudest slightly above the umbilicus whereas with engagement of the fetal head the heart sounds are loudest below the umbilicus.

VAGINAL EXAMINATION. The diagnosis of a frank breech presentation is confirmed by palpating its characteristic components. Both ischial tuberosities, the sacrum, and the anus are usually palpable, and after further descent, the external genitalia may be distinguished.

Especially when labor is prolonged, the buttocks may become markedly swollen, rendering differentiation of face and breech very difficult; the anus may be mistaken for the mouth, and the ischial tuberosities for the malar eminences. Careful examination, however, should prevent that error, for the finger encounters muscular resistance with the anus, whereas firmer, less yielding jaws are felt through the mouth. Furthermore, the finger, upon removal from the anus, is sometimes stained with meconium. The most accurate information, however, is based on the location of the sacrum and its spinous processes, which establishes the diagnosis of position and variety.

In complete breech presentations, the feet may be felt alongside the buttocks, and in footling presentations, one or both feet are inferior to the buttocks (Fig. 30-5). In footlings, the foot can be readily identified as right or left on the basis of the relation of the great toe. When the breech has descended farther into the pelvic cavity, the genitalia may be felt; if not markedly edema-

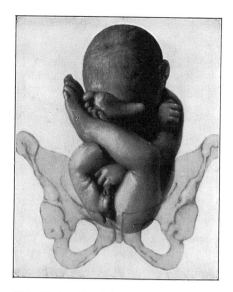

FIG. 30-1.   Frank breech presentation.

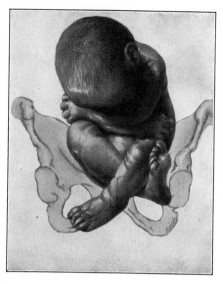

FIG. 30-3.   Incomplete breech presentation.

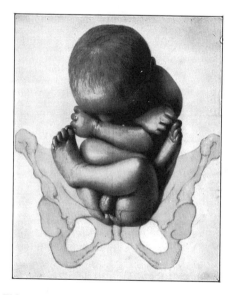

FIG. 30-2.   Complete breech presentation.

tous, they may permit identification of fetal sex.

X-RAY AND SONOGRAPHIC EXAMINATIONS.   Diagnosis may be facilitated by radiologic examination. Sonography used to identify a breech presentation usually does not identify the relationship of the lower extremities to the fetal pelvis as well as does x-ray. Fetal anomalies, however, are more likely to be detected with sonography.

Mechanisms of Labor.   There is a fundamental difference between delivery in cephalic and breech presentation. With a cephalic presentation, once the head is delivered, typically the rest of the body follows without difficulty. With a breech, however, successively larger or, in case of the head, very much less compressible parts of the fetus are born.

Spontaneous complete expulsion of the fetus who presents as a breech, as described below, is seldom successfully accomplished. As the rule, either cesarean section (see Chap. 43) or vaginal delivery that requires skilled participation by the obstetrician is essential for a favorable outcome (see Chap. 42).

Unless there is disproportion between the size of the fetus and the pelvis, engagement and descent of the breech in response to labor usually take place in one of the oblique diameters of the pelvis. The anterior hip usually descends more rapidly than the posterior hip, and when the resistance of the pelvic floor is met, internal rotation usually occurs, bringing the anterior hip toward the pubic arch and allowing the fetal bitrochanteric

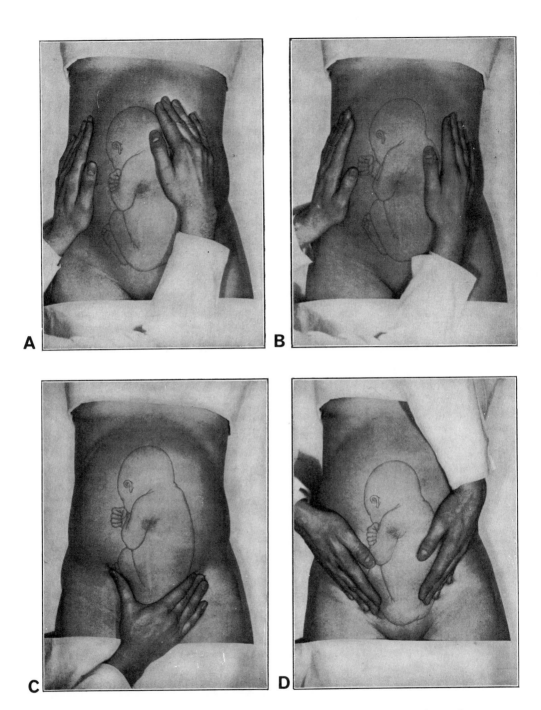

FIG. 30-4.   Palpation in left sacro-anterior position. **A.** First maneuver. **B.** Second maneuver. **C.** Third maneuver. **D.** Fourth maneuver.

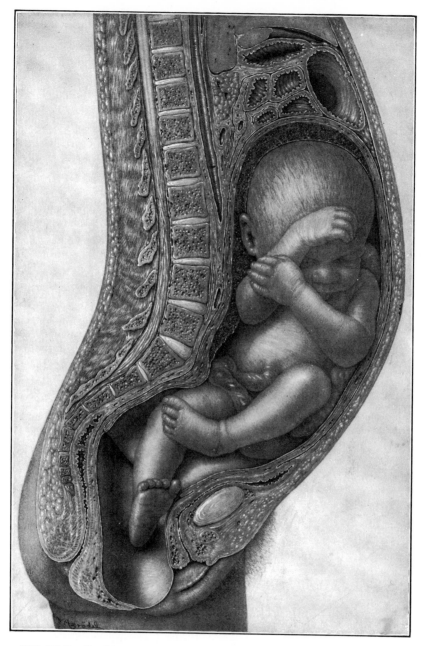

FIG. 30-5. Double-footling breech presentation. Second stage of labor.

diameter to occupy the anteroposterior diameter of the pelvic outlet. Rotation usually takes place through an arc of 45 degrees. If, however, the posterior extremity is prolapsed, it always rotates to the symphysis pubis, ordinarily through an arc of 135 degrees, but occasionally in the opposite direction past the sacrum and the opposite half of the pelvis through an arc of 225 degrees.

After rotation, descent continues until the perineum is distended by the advancing breech, while the anterior hip appears at the vulva and is stemmed against the pubic arch. By lateral flexion of the body, the posterior hip is then forced over the anterior margin of the perineum, which retracts over the buttocks, thus allowing the infant to straighten out when the anterior hip is born.

The legs and feet follow the breech and may be born spontaneously, although the aid of the obstetrician is usually required.

After the birth of the breech, there is slight external rotation, with the back turning anteriorly as the shoulders are brought into relation with one of the oblique diameters of the pelvis. The shoulders then descend rapidly and undergo internal rotation, with the bisacromial diameter occupying the anteroposterior diameter of the inferior strait. Immediately following the shoulders, the head, which is normally sharply flexed upon the thorax, enters the pelvis in one of the oblique diameters and then rotates in such a manner as to bring the posterior portion of the neck under the symphysis pubis. The head is then born in flexion, with the chin, mouth, nose, forehead, bregma (brow), and occiput appearing in succession over the perineum. Not infrequently, the breech engages in the transverse diameter of the pelvis, with the sacrum directed anteriorly or posteriorly. The mechanism of labor in the transverse position differs only in that internal rotation occurs through an arc of 90 degrees.

Infrequently, rotation occurs in such a manner that the back of the infant is directed toward the vertebral column instead of toward the abdomen of the mother. Such rotation should be prevented if possible. Although the head may be delivered by allowing the chin and face to pass beneath the symphysis, the slightest traction on the body may cause extension of the head. Extension, if uncorrected, increases the diameters of the head, which must pass through the pelvis (see Chap. 42, p. 1070).

Prognosis. With breech presentation, compared to cephalic presentation, both the mother and the fetus are at greater risk but to nowhere near the same degree.

MATERNAL. Because of the greater frequency of operative delivery, including cesarean section, there may be higher maternal morbidity and slightly higher mortality for pregnancies complicated by persistent breech presentation. Labor usually is not prolonged. Hall and Kohl (1956), in a large series of cases, showed the median duration of labor to be 9.2 hours for nulliparas and 6.1 hours for paras.

FETUS-INFANT.   *The prognosis for the fetus in a breech presentation is considerably worse than when in a vertex presentation.* Brenner and associates (1974) have provided a careful analysis of the characteristics and perils to the fetus from breech presentation. They determined the overall mortality rate for 1016 breech deliveries to be 25.4 percent compared to 2.6 percent for nonbreech deliveries at the University Hospitals of Cleveland. At every stage of gestation, they identified antepartum, intrapartum, and neonatal deaths to be significantly greater among breeches and the average Apgar scores to be lower for those who survived. During the latter half of pregnancy, the birth weight at any gestational age was somewhat less for breech infants than for nonbreech infants. Congenital abnormalities were identified in 6.3 percent of breech deliveries compared to 2.4 percent in nonbreech deliveries.

MATURE FETUS. Rovinsky and associates (1973), at Mount Sinai Hospital in New York City, looked especially at the risks associated with breech presentation for singleton fetuses who weighed 2500 g or more and were considered to be at or near term. The overall perinatal mortality rate for more than 2000 such infants was 3.17 percent compared to 0.84 percent for cephalic presentation at or near term. Major congenital anomalies were identified in 2.1 percent of those presenting as a breech versus 0.8 percent in those that were vertex. In one-third of the perinatal deaths, breech presentation or delivery, or both, were thought to be etiologic factors. Mortality and morbidity rates from trauma were understandably lowest in infants who weighed 2500 to 3000 g and highest among those who weighed 4000 g or more. Morbidity from trauma was progressively higher as the amount of obstetric manipulation to effect vaginal delivery increased. As might be expected, mortality and morbidity rates from trauma were higher when less experienced obstetricians delivered the breech.

In the Mount Sinai experiences, the incidence of overt prolapse of the cord among frank breeches at term was 3 times greater (1.7 percent) than for term vertex presentations; but for complete and footling breeches, cord prolapse was 20 times greater (10.9 percent). Moreover, the incidence of fetal distress of undetermined cause in term breeches was 6.4 percent, or 8 times greater than for term vertex presentations. No perinatal deaths were attributable to either breech presentation or delivery among the 425 (19.8 percent) that were delivered by cesarean section.

According to Rovinsky and associates, in retrospect it is likely that the deaths of 17 infants at term who succumbed as the consequence of labor and vaginal delivery, or about 1 percent of all term breech deliveries, would have been prevented by cesarean section. It is also pertinent that Brenner and co-workers identified in their study the perinatal mortality rate for fetuses of 32 weeks or greater gestational age and alive at the onset of labor to be 3.4 percent for those who were delivered vaginally while it was zero for those who were delivered by cesarean section.

With careful selection of cases and using cesarean section 58 percent of the time, Lyons and Papsin (1978) achieved zero perinatal mortality for both vaginal and abdominal breech deliveries of infants who weighed over 2500 g. Nonetheless, morbidity was evident in 5.6 percent of those who were delivered vaginally compared to 0.8 percent in those delivered by cesarean section.

Collea and colleagues (1978) have established an ongoing study to try to identify the optimal method of delivery of the fetus who presents as a frank breech at term. Of those women who were randomly selected as candidates for vaginal delivery, 50 percent were promptly excluded from further consideration because of possible fetopelvic disproportion based on x-ray pelvimetry. Of the 30 infants who were delivered vaginally all survived although two sustained injury to the brachial plexus.

PREMATURE FETUS. Vaginal delivery as a breech may be much more hazardous to the premature infant than previously thought. Ingemarsson and associates (1978) have compared neonatal mortality and the frequency of subsequent developmental abnormalities in 42 premature breech infants delivered by cesarean section with 48 premature infants who were delivered vaginally. For those delivered vaginally, six (14.6 percent) succumbed and developmental abnormalities were detected at 12 months in 10 (24 percent) of the survivors, compared to two deaths (4.8 percent) and one with developmental abnormalities (2.5 percent) among those who were delivered by cesarean section. In a paired controlled retrospective study at Parkland Memorial Hospital, of low birthweight infants (below 2500 g) who presented as a breech, Duenhoelter and co-workers (1979) identified mortality, as well as morbidity, to be much more common among those infants who were delivered vaginally. Seven of 44 who were delivered vaginally died (15.9 percent) compared to one of 44 (2.3 percent) delivered by cesarean section.

TRAUMA FROM BREECH DELIVERY. Tank and associates (1971) have examined the character of serious traumatic vaginal delivery. At autopsy, the organs most frequently found to be injured are in order of frequency the brain, spinal cord, liver, adrenal glands, and spleen. It is of interest that, in retrospective analysis of cases of "idiopathic" adrenal calcification, breech delivery was very common. Other sites of injuries from vaginal delivery include the brachial plexus; the pharynx, in the form of tears or pseudodiverticula from the obstetrician's finger in the mouth as part of the Mauriceau maneuver (see Chap. 42, p. 1071); and the bladder, which may rupture if distended. Traction may injure the sternomastoid muscle and, if not appropriately treated, lead to torticollis.

Prophylaxis. Whenever a breech presentation is recognized during the third trimester, some obstetricians, but not the majority, believe an attempt should be made by *external version* to substitute a vertex presentation (Chap. 42). External version is more readily accomplished in multiparous women with lax abdominal walls than in nulliparous women. Because of possible trauma, anesthesia should never be used.

External version, if properly and gently performed, carries little danger according to Ranney (1973), who reported his experiences with gentle attempts at external cephalic version in 860 instances of either breech presentation or, less often, transverse lie. The initial attempt was successful 781 times. Although many of the 781 fetuses reverted to an abnormal presentation, repeat attempts at conversion were usually successful. The failure rate during the third trimester increased as pregnancy advanced, with a marked rise after the 36th week. During the study, the overall frequency of breech delivery was only 0.6 percent, or about one-sixth the expected frequency. No trauma to the fetus was identified. There was no increase in the frequencies of placental abruption or of hemolytic disease in the newborn infants, although these have been reported by others. Ranney believes that successful external version relatively early in the third trimester, as well as lowering the risk associated with vaginal delivery, may reduce the likelihood of prematurity, which is more common with breech presentations.

Based on their experiences with 491 pregnancies in which the fetus presented other than cephalic, Ylikorkala and Hartikainen-Sorri (1977) have also concluded that a breech presentation any time during the third trimester warrants attempts at external version. These Finnish workers always used ultrasound to confirm the presentation of the fetus and location of the placenta. In some instances they administered spasmolytic, tocolytic, or analgesic drugs but never anesthesia. They were able to convert the presentation of the fetus to that of vertex in three-fourths of their attempts with no serious morbidity identified. The incidence of breech presentation decreased to 2.9 percent from the previous value of 4.5 percent. Thus they were unable to lower the incidence of breech delivery to the remarkable low level achieved by Ranney. Moreover, mean duration of pregnancy was no greater after successful external version than in those pregnancies in which attempts were unsuccessful.

Enthusiasm for external cephalic version is not shared by all. Bradley-Watson (1975), for example, seriously questioned the value of attempting external cephalic version. He attributed the following complications to external cephalic version: Antepartum hemorrhage (3 percent); premature labor (1.2 percent); fetal death (0.9 percent); and premature rupture of membranes (0.6 percent). Chapman and associates (1978) have described spinal cord transection in utero after an unsuccessful attempt at external cephalic version. Marcus and associates (1975) identified significant fetomaternal hemorrhage in six of 100 pregnancies in which external version was attempted. Therefore, immunoprophylaxis with anti-D globulin should be considered when the mother is Rh negative (see Chap. 38, p. 963).

Problems with Vaginal Delivery. Major problems do arise from vaginal delivery of a fetus in a breech presentation. Delivery of the breech draws the umbilicus and attached cord into the pelvis, which compresses the cord. Therefore, once the breech has passed beyond the vaginal introitus, the abdomen, the thorax, arms, and head must be delivered promptly. This entails the delivery of successively less readily compressible parts. With a mature fetus, some degree of molding of the fetal head may be essential for the head to negotiate the birth canal successfully. In this unfortunate circumstance, the alternatives with vaginal delivery are both unsatisfactory: Delivery may be delayed many minutes while the aftercoming head accommodates to the maternal pelvis, but hypoxia and acidosis become severe; or, delivery is forced causing trauma from compression, traction, or both, to the brain, spinal cord, skeleton, and abdominal viscera.

With a premature fetus, the disparity between the size of the head and the buttocks is even greater than with a larger fetus. At times, the buttocks and lower extremities of the premature fetus will pass through the cervix and be delivered, yet the cervix will not be delivered, yet the cervix will not be adequately dilated for the head to escape without trauma to the infant. In this circumstance, Dührssen's incisions of the cervix may be tried (see Chap. 41, p. 1060). Even so, trauma to the fetus and mother may be appreciable, and hypoxia in the fetus may prove disastrous. The frequency of prolapsed cord is considerable when the fetus is small or the breech is not of the frank variety.

Recommendations for Delivery. A diligent search for any other complication, actual or anticipated, that might further justify delivery by cesarean section has become a feature of many obstetricians' philosophy for managing delivery in breech presentations. To try to minimize infant mortality and morbidity, cesarean section is now commonly used in the following circumstances to deliver all but the very immature fetus whose potential for survival is negligible:

1. Breech presentation and a large fetus.
2. Breech presentation and any degree of contraction or unfavorable shape of the pelvis.
3. Breech presentation and a hyperextended head.
4. Breech presentation not in labor with maternal or fetal indications for delivery such as pregnancy-induced hypertension or rupture of the membranes for 12 hours or more.
5. Breech presentation and uterine dysfunction.
6. Footling breech presentation.
7. Breech presentation, an apparently healthy but premature fetus of more than 26 weeks gestation, and either active labor or need for delivery.
8. Breech presentation and previous perinatal death or children suffering from birth trauma.
9. Breech presentation and a firm request by the mother for sterilization.

LARGE FETUS. The experiences of Rovinsky and associates cited above, as well as others, have been that morbidity and mortality rates for the fetus at term increase with birth weight. Therefore, the fetus estimated to weigh 3500 g (8 pounds) or more would often benefit from delivery by cesarean section even though the mother's pelvis appears quite normal. This would allow for underestimation of fetal weight, a relatively common phenomenon when the fetus is large. With the head free in the uterine fundus, sonographic measurements of the biparietal diameter to estimate fetal size, unfortunately, are more likely to be erroneous than with a vertex presentation. Nonetheless, the obstetrician could feel much more secure about the estimate of fetal size if there was good agreement between the clinical and sonographic estimates.

UNFAVORABLE PELVIS. In contrast to labor with a cephalic presentation, there is no time for molding of the after-coming head. Therefore, a moderately contracted pelvis that previously proved no problem for delivery of an average size fetus who presented as a vertex might prove dangerous if the fetus were presenting as a breech. Rovinsky and colleagues (1973) urge not only accurate mensuration of pelvic dimensions but also precise evaluation of the pelvic architecture rather than reliance on pelvic indexes. Gynecoid (round) and anthropoid (elliptical) pelves are favorable configurations, but platypelloid (anteroposteriorly flat) and android (heart-shaped) pelves are not. The platypelloid pelvis typically is narrowed anteroposteriorly, which is unfavorable for the after-coming head. The android pelvis has a narrow forepelvis, which renders the inlet less favorable than the pelvic diameters would suggest.

HYPEREXTENSION OF FETAL HEAD. In perhaps 5 percent or less of cases of breech presentation at or near term, a roentgenogram shows the fetal head to be in extreme hyperextension (Fig. 30-6). Most often the cause of the hyperextension is not apparent

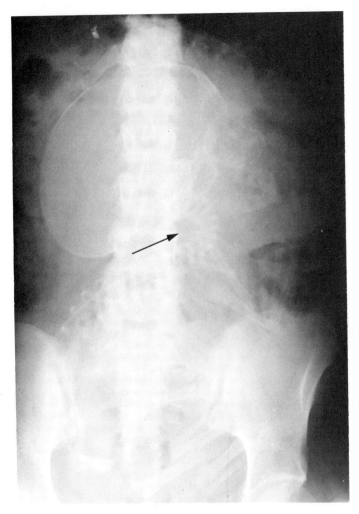

FIG. 30-6. Radiologic demonstration of a complete breech presentation with a markedly hyperextended cervical spine (arrow) and head. Delivery by cesarean section resulted in a normal newborn infant.

(Caterini et al., 1975). Vaginal delivery may result in considerable injury to the cervical spinal cord as reemphasized by Abroms and associates (1973), and Bhagwanani and associates (1973). In general, radiologic evidence of marked hyperextension of the fetal head after labor has been established as an indication for cesarean section.

NO LABOR OR UTERINE DYSFUNCTION. Induction of labor in women with a breech presentation is defended by some and condemned by others. Brenner and colleagues (1974) noted no significant differ-

ences in mortality rates and Apgar scores between cases with induced labor and those with spontaneous labor. In those instances in which oxytocin was used to augment labor, however, infant mortality rates were higher and Apgar scores were lower. The general policy at Parkland Memorial Hospital is to resort to cesarean section rather than oxytocin to induce or augment labor unless the fetus is very immature or has a severe anomaly.

FOOTLING BREECH PRESENTATION. The possibility of compression of a prolapsed cord or a cord entangled around the extremities as the breech fills the pelvis, if not before, is a threat to the fetus.

PREMATURE DELIVERY. If the fetus is premature, the aftercoming head may be trapped by a cervix that is sufficiently effaced and dilated to allow passage of the thorax but not the larger, less compressible head. The consequences of vaginal delivery in this circumstance all too often have been both hypoxia and physical trauma which are especially deleterious to the premature infant. Delivery of the apparently healthy, although premature, fetus by cesarean section reduces the risks of hypoxia, birth trauma, and their sequelae.

PREVIOUS PREGNANCY WASTAGE. The compelling desire to minimize any likelihood of trauma to the fetus may lead to the decision to perform cesarean section.

DESIRE FOR STERILIZATION. For the woman with a breech presentation and who desires sterilization, the risk of cesarean section to accomplish delivery and sterilization is probably not much greater than the summation of risks from vaginal breech delivery followed by celiotomy for sterilization.

VAGINAL DELIVERY. Vaginal delivery should be relatively safe for a frank breech presentation if (1) the pelvis is in no way contracted when examined by x-ray pelvimetry; (2) the fetus is judged not to be unusually large (less than 8 pounds) when examined independently by two or more trained examiners or when estimated sonographically; (3) spontaneous labor is demonstrated to effect orderly effacement and dilation of the cervix and descent of the breech through the birth canal; and (4) individuals skilled in breech delivery, in providing appropriate anesthesia, and in infant resuscitation are in immediate attendance. Even when every attempt is made to fulfill these criteria, the outcome for the infant is not always as good as when cesarean section is performed (Collea et al., 1978).

The physician who might naively champion any childbirth outside of a hospital setting is either not aware of the hazards of breech delivery in such a setting or is totally insensitive to the welfare of the fetus and the mother. The technics and precautions for vaginal delivery are detailed in Chapter 42, page 1065.

Cesarean Section. There is little question but that perinatal mortality and morbidity from trauma and hypoxia can be reduced by liberal use of cesarean section. Even for fetuses at term (2500 g or more), Rovinsky and associates (1973) have concluded from their analyses cited above that cesarean section improved the outcome for the fetus. During the 17 year period studied by them, the use of cesarean section for breech delivery increased dramatically.

This same trend in most training institutions towards delivery by cesarean section of the majority of fetuses that present as a breech means that one important criterion for safe vaginal breech delivery is becoming more and more difficult to fulfill: most resident training programs within the near future will not provide sufficient opportunity for acquisition of skills essential for successful vaginal breech delivery.

At Parkland Memorial Hospital, cesarean section is used very liberally for breech delivery. In recent years, nearly three-fourths of fetuses presenting by the breech have been delivered by cesarean section. This value is remarkably greater than, for example, the cesarean section rate of 10.7 percent reported for breech deliveries in 1956 by Hall and Kohl.

SUMMARY. The fetus in the breech position is likely to benefit from cesarean section carried out early in labor, if not before, but at the expense of an appreciable increase in maternal morbidity and a slight increase in maternal mortality. It is anticipated that the prevailing enthusiasm for offspring of the highest quality but of limited number will continue to stimulate frequent use of cesarean section for breech delivery. The technic of

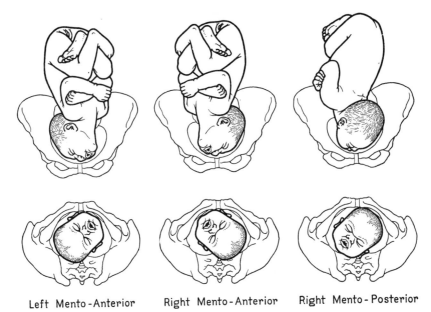

Left Mento-Anterior   Right Mento-Anterior   Right Mento-Posterior

FIG. 30-7. Left and right positions in face presentations.

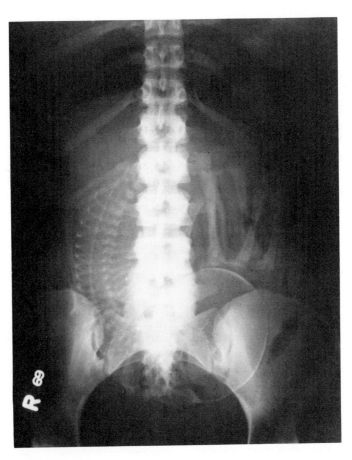

FIG. 30-8. Roentgenogram showing face presentation. Note spinal curvature of infant.

cesarean section is described in Chapter 43, page 1085.

FACE PRESENTATION

In face presentation, the head is hyperextended so that the occiput is in contact with the fetal back and the chin (mentum) is the presenting part.

Incidence. Cruikshank and White (1973) report an incidence of 1 in 600 or 0.17 percent; the Obstetrical Statistical Cooperative identified a similar frequency of 0.2 percent. Of 33,562 infants who were delivered recently at Parkland Memorial Hospital 0.3 percent presented as a face.

Diagnosis. Although abdominal findings may be suggestive, the clinical diagnosis of face presentation must rest on vaginal examination (Fig. 30-7). On vaginal palpation, the distinctive features of the face are the mouth and nose, the malar bones, and particularly the orbital ridges. It is possible to mistake a breech presentation for a face, since the anus may be mistaken for the mouth and the ischial tuberosities for the malar prominences. The fetal anus is always on a line with the ischial tuberosities, however, whereas the fetal mouth and malar prominences form the corners of a triangle. The roentgenographic demonstration of the hyperextended head with the facial bones at or below the pelvic inlet is quite characteristic (Fig. 30-8).

Etiology. The causes of face presentations are manifold, generally stemming from any factor that favors extension or prevents flexion of the head. Extended positions of the head, therefore, occur more frequently when the pelvis is contracted or the fetus is very large. In a series of 141 face presentations studied by Hellman and co-workers (1950), the incidence of inlet contraction was 39.4 percent. This high incidence of pelvic contraction, as well as large infants, is most important to consider in the successful management of face presentation.

In multiparous women, the pendulous abdomen is another factor that predisposes to face presentation. It permits the back of the fetus to sag forward or laterally often in the same direction in which the occiput points, thus promoting extension of the cervical and thoracic spine.

In exceptional instances, marked enlargement of the neck or coils of cord about the neck may cause extension. Anencephalic fetuses naturally present by the face because of faulty development of the cranium.

Mechanism. Face presentations are rarely observed above the pelvic inlet. The brow generally presents and is converted to a face presentation after further extension of the head during descent through the pelvis.

The mechanism of labor in these cases consists of the cardinal movements of descent, internal rotation, and flexion, and the accessory movements of extension and external rotation. Descent is brought about by the same factors as in vertex presentations. Extension results from the relation of the fetal body to the deflected head, which is converted into a two-armed lever, the longer arm of which extends from the occipital condyles to the occiput. When resistance is then encountered, the occiput must be pushed toward the back of the fetus while the chin descends (Fig. 30-9).

The object of internal rotation of the face is to bring the chin under the symphysis pubis. Unless the head is unusually small, natural delivery cannot otherwise be accomplished. Only in this way can the neck subtend the posterior surface of the symphysis pubis. If the chin rotates directly posteriorly, the relatively short neck cannot span the anterior surface of the sacrum, which measures about 12 cm in length (Fig. 30-9). Hence, the birth of the head is manifestly impossible unless the shoulders enter the pelvis at the same time, an event that is out of the question except when the fetus is markedly premature

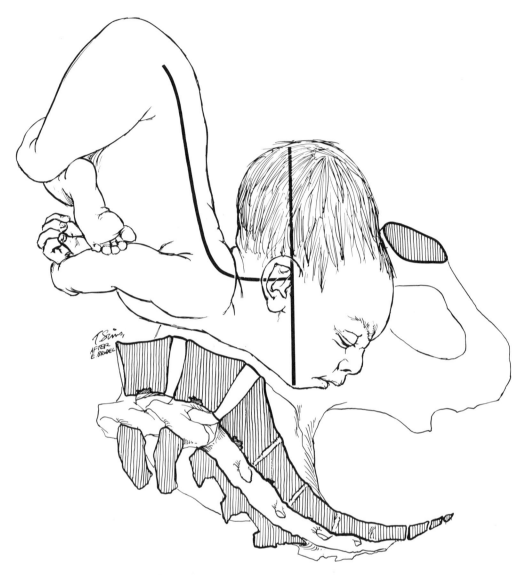

FIG. 30-9. Face presentation. The occiput is on the longer end of the head lever. The chin is directly posterior. Vaginal delivery is impossible unless the chin rotates anteriorly.

or macerated. Internal rotation in a face presentation results from the same factors as in vertex presentations.

After anterior rotation and descent, the chin and mouth appear at the vulva, the undersurface of the chin presses against the symphysis, and the head is delivered by flexion (Fig. 30-10). The nose, eyes, brow (bregma), and occiput then appear in succession over the anterior margin of the perineum. After the birth of the head, the occiput sags backward toward the anus. In a few moments, the chin rotates externally to the side toward which it was originally directed, and the shoulders are born as in vertex presentations.

Edema may sometimes distort the face sufficiently to obliterate the features and lead to erroneous diagnosis of breech presentation (Fig. 30-11). At the same time, the skull undergoes considerable molding, manifested by

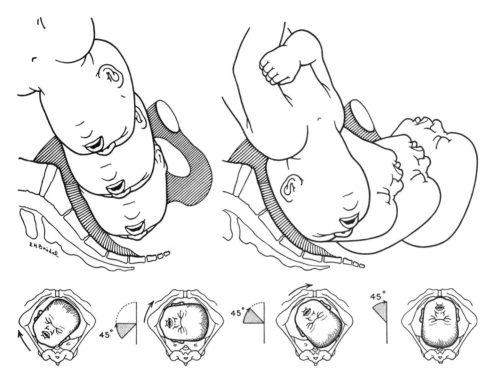

FIG. 30-10. Mechanism of labor for right mentoposterior position with subsequent rotation to mentum anterior and delivery.

increase in length of the occipitomental diameter of the head.

Treatment. In the absence of a contracted pelvis and the presence of effective spontaneous labor with no evidence of fetal distress, successful vaginal delivery will usually follow. As pointed out above, face presentations among term-size fetuses occur more commonly when there is some degree of contraction of the pelvic inlet. Therefore, cesarean section most often proves to be the best method for their delivery.

Other methods of management of face presentations are rarely, if ever, indicated in modern obstetrics. Outmoded are attempts to convert manually a face to a vertex presentation, manual or forceps rotation of a persistently posterior chin to a mentum anterior position, and internal podalic version and

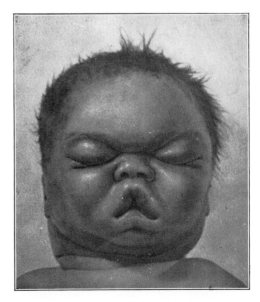

FIG. 30-11. Edema in face presentation.

extraction. All are likely to be unduly traumatic to both fetus and mother.

BROW PRESENTATION

With a brow presentation, that portion of the fetal head between the orbital ridge and the anterior fontanel presents at the pelvic inlet. The fetal head thus occupies a position midway between full flexion (occiput) and full extension (mentum or face). Except when the fetal head is small or the pelvis is unusually large, engagement of the fetal head and subsequent delivery cannot take place as long as the brow presentation persists.

Etiology. The causes of persistent brow presentation are essentially the same as those of face presentation. The brow presentation commonly is unstable and converts to a face or an occiput presentation. Cruikshank and White (1973), for example, observed either flexion to an occiput presentation or extension to a face presentation to take place in two-thirds of cases in which the presentation was initially that of the brow.

Diagnosis. The presentation may be recognized by abdominal palpation when both the occiput and chin can be easily pal-

pated, but vaginal examination is usually necessary. The frontal sutures, the large anterior fontanel, orbital ridges, eyes, and root of the nose can be felt on vaginal examination. Neither mouth nor chin is within reach however (Figs. 30-12, 30-13).

Mechanism. The mechanism of labor varies greatly with the size of the fetus. With a small fetus and a large pelvis, labor is generally easy. With larger fetuses, however, it is usually very difficult, since engagement is impossible until after marked molding that shortens the occipitomental diameter, or more commonly, either flexion to an occiput presentation or extension to a face presentation.

The considerable molding essential for delivery of the fetus where the brow presentation persists characteristically deforms the head. The caput succedaneum is over the forehead and may be so extensive that identification of the brow by palpation is impossible. In these instances, the forehead is prominent and squared, and the occipitomental diameter is diminished.

Prognosis. In the transient varieties of brow presentation, the prognosis depends upon the ultimate presentation. When the brow presentation persists, the prognosis is poor for vaginal delivery of an uncompro-

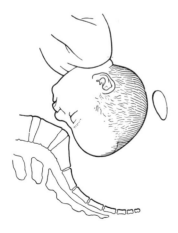

FIG. 30-12. Brow posterior presentation.

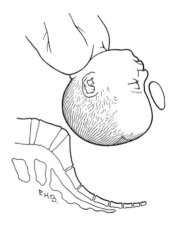

FIG. 30-13. Brow anterior presentation.

mised infant unless the fetus is small or the birth canal is huge.

Treatment. The principles underlying the treatment of brow presentations are much the same as those for a face presentation. If, by chance, spontaneous labor is progressing without any evidence of distress in the closely monitored fetus and without unduly vigorous uterine contractions, no interference is necessary. If labor becomes either unduly vigorous, or more likely ineffective, or if fetal distress is suspected, prompt cesarean section is indicated.

SHOULDER PRESENTATION

In this condition, the long axis of the fetus is approximately perpendicular to that of the mother, i.e., a *transverse lie.* When it forms an acute angle, an *oblique lie* results. An oblique lie is usually only transitory, however, for either a longitudinal or transverse lie commonly results when labor supervenes. For this reason, the oblique lie is termed *unstable lie* in Great Britain.

In transverse lies, the shoulder usually is over the pelvic inlet, with the head lying in one iliac fossa and the breech in the other. This condition is referred to as a *shoulder* or an *acromion presentation.* The side of the mother toward which the acromion is directed determines the designation of the lie as right or left acromial. Moreover, since in either position the back may be directed anteriorly or posteriorly, superiorly or inferiorly, it is customary to distinguish varieties as dorsoanterior and dorsoposterior.

Incidence. Transverse lie occurred once in 322 singleton deliveries (0.3 percent) both at the Mayo Clinic and the University of Iowa Hospitals (Cruikshank and White, 1973; Johnson, 1964). At Parkland Memorial Hospital the incidence was 0.4 percent among 33,562 infants delivered recently.

Etiology. The common causes of transverse lie are (1) unusual relaxation of the abdominal wall resulting from great multiparity, (2) prematurity, (3) placenta previa, and (4) contracted pelvis. The incidence of transverse lie increases with parity, occurring approximately 10 times more frequently in patients of parity of four or more than in nulliparous women. Relaxation of the abdominal wall with a pendulous abdomen allows the uterus to fall forward, deflecting the long axis of the fetus away from the axis of the birth canal into an oblique or transverse position. Placenta previa and pelvic contraction act similarly. A transverse or oblique lie occasionally develops in labor from an initial longitudinal presentation, the head or breech migrating to one of the iliac fossae.

Diagnosis. The diagnosis of a transverse lie is usually readily made, often by inspection alone. The abdomen is unusually wide from side to side, whereas the fundus of the uterus extends scarcely above the umbilicus.

On palpation, with the first maneuver no fetal pole is detected in the fundus. On the second maneuver, a ballottable head is found in one iliac fossa and the breech in the other. The third and fourth maneuvers are negative unless labor is well advanced and the shoulder has become impacted in the pelvis (Fig. 30-14, 30-15, 30-16). At the same time, the position of the back is readily identified. When the back is anterior, a hard resistant plane extends across the front of the abdomen; when it is posterior, irregular nodulations representing the small parts are felt in the same location (Fig. 30-14).

On vaginal examination, in the early stages of labor, the side of the thorax, if it can be reached, may be recognized by the "gridiron" feel of the ribs above the pelvic inlet. When dilatation is further advanced, the scapula and the clavicle are distinguished on opposite sides of the thorax. The position of the axilla indicates the side of the mother toward which the shoulder is directed. Later in labor, the shoulder becomes tightly

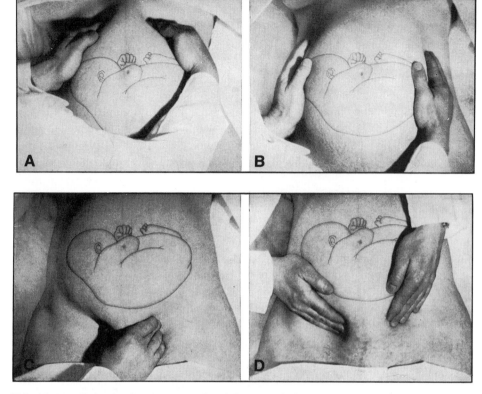

FIG. 30-14. Palpation in transverse lie, right acromiodorsoanterior position. **A.** First maneuver. **B.** Second maneuver. **C.** Third maneuver. **D.** Fourth maneuver.

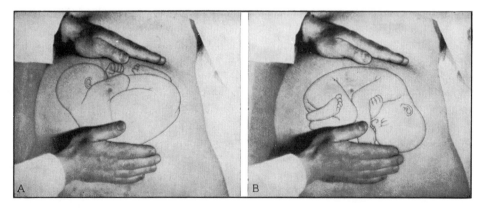

FIG. 30-15. Transverse lie, palpation of back in dorsoanterior **(A)** and in dorsoposterior **(B)** positions.

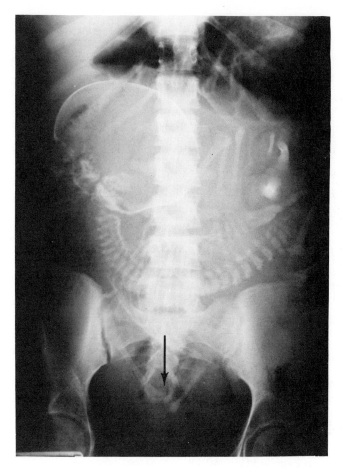

FIG. 30-16. Roentgenogram of a transverse lie which illustrates an elbow (arrow) at the level of the cervix.

wedged in the pelvic canal, and a hand and arm frequently prolapse into the vagina and through the vulva.

Course of Labor. The spontaneous birth of a fully developed infant is manifestly impossible in persistent transverse lies, since expulsion cannot be effected unless both the head and trunk of the fetus enter the pelvis at the same time. At term, therefore, both the fetus and the mother will die unless appropriate measures are instituted.

After the rupture of the membranes, if the mother is left to herself, the fetal shoulder is forced into the pelvis, and the corresponding arm frequently prolapses (Fig. 30-17). After some descent, the shoulder is arrested by the margins of the pelvic inlet, with the head in one iliac fossa and the breech in the other. As labor continues, the shoulder is firmly impacted in the upper part of the pelvis. The uterus then contracts vigorously in an unsuccessful attempt to overcome the obstacle. After a time, a retraction ring rises increasingly higher and becomes more marked. The situation is referred to as neglected transverse lie. If not vigorously and properly treated, the uterus eventually ruptures and the mother dies as well as the fetus.

If the fetus is quite small and the pelvis large, spontaneous delivery may eventuate despite persistence of the abnormal lie. In such cases, the fetus is compressed with the head forced against the abdomen. A portion

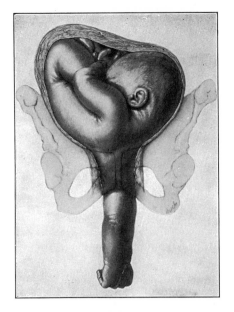

FIG. 30-17. Prolapse of an arm in transverse lie.

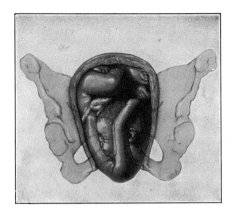

FIG. 30-18. Conduplicato corpore.

of the thoracic wall below the shoulder thus becomes the most dependent part, appearing at the vulva. The head and thorax then pass through the pelvic cavity at the same time, and the fetus, which is doubled upon itself *(conduplicato corpore),* is expelled (Fig. 30-18). Such a mechanism obviously is possible only in the case of very small infants and occasionally when the second fetus in a twin pregnancy is prematurely born.

Prognosis. Labor with shoulder presentations increases the maternal risk and adds tremendously to the fetal hazard. Most maternal deaths from this complication occur in neglected cases from spontaneous rupture of the uterus or traumatic rupture consequent upon late and ill-advised version and extraction. Even with the best of care, however, the chance of maternal death will be increased slightly for four reasons: (1) the frequent association of transverse lie with placenta previa, (2) the increased likelihood of cord accidents, (3) the almost inevitable necessity of major operative interference, and (4) the likelihood of sepsis after rupture of the membranes and extrusion of the arm through the vagina.

Management. In general, the onset of active labor in a woman with a transverse lie is indication for cesarean section. Attempts at conversion to a longitudinal lie by abdominal manipulation after labor is well established are not likely to be successful. Before labor or early in labor, with the membranes intact, attempts at external version are worthy of a trial in the absence of other obstetric complications that point toward cesarean section. If during early labor the fetal head can be maneuvered by abdominal manipulation into the pelvis, it should be held there during the next several contractions to try to fix the

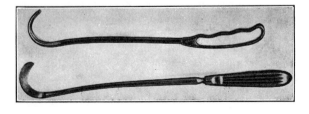

FIG. 30-19. Blunt hook, above. Sickle knife, below.

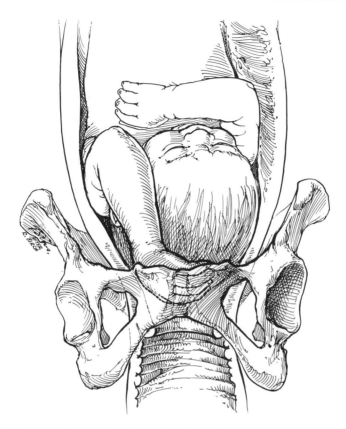

FIG. 30-20. Compound presentation. The right hand is lying in front of the vertex. With further labor, the hand and arm may retract from the birth canal and the head descend normally.

head in the pelvis. The fetal heart rate must be closely checked during this time. If these measures fail in the woman in labor, cesarean section should be performed promptly. Internal podalic version is indicated rarely, if ever (see Chap. 42, p. 1079).

Because neither the feet nor the vertex of the fetus occupies the lower uterine segment, a low transverse incision into the uterus may lead to difficulty in extraction of a fetus entrapped in the body of the uterus above the level of the incision. A vertical incision is therefore generally favored. The treatment of neglected transverse lie entails support in the form of antibiotics, fluid therapy, and transfusion if needed. Delivery may be accomplished abdominally by cesarean section or cesarean section-hysterectomy, as the situation demands (see Chap. 43, p. 1081).

If the cervix is fully dilated and the fetus is dead, decapitation by means of a blunt hook and scissors or sickle knife may permit vaginal delivery (Fig. 30-19). However, since destructive procedures may rupture the uterus, almost always cesarean section or cesarean hysterectomy is preferable, even with a dead baby.

COMPOUND PRESENTATION

In compound presentation, an extremity prolapses alongside the presenting part with both entering the pelvis simultaneously (Fig. 30-20).

Incidence. Goplerud and Eastman (1953) identified a hand or arm prolapsed alongside the head once in every 700 deliveries. Much less common was prolapse of one or both lower extremities alongside a vertex presentation or a hand alongside a breech presentation. More recently, Weissberg and O'Leary (1973) described compound presentations among infants that weigh 1500 g or more to occur once in 1600 deliveries.

Etiology. As expected, the causes of compound presentation are conditions that prevent complete occlusion of the pelvic inlet by the fetal head. In Goplerud and Eastman's series, the incidence of prematurity was twice the expected rate. Often, however, no cause is demonstrable.

Prognosis. Although the reported perinatal loss is above 25 percent, a major portion of the wastage is contributed by prematurity, prolapsed cord, and traumatic obstetric procedures.

Management. In most cases, the prolapsed part should be left alone, since most often it will not interfere with labor. In Goplerud and Eastman's series of 50 cases not associated with prolapse of the cord, 24, or approximately one-half, had no treatment. Normal delivery ensued in all with the loss of one infant. If the arm is prolapsed alongside the head, the condition should be observed closely to ascertain whether the arm rises out of the way with descent of the presenting part. If it fails to do so and if it appears to prevent descent of the head, the prolapsed arm should be gently pushed upward and the head simultaneously pushed downward by fundal pressure. Whenever fetal distress is detected, cesarean section is the treatment of choice.

PERSISTENT OCCIPUT POSTERIOR AND TRANSVERSE POSITIONS

Persistent Occiput Posterior Position.
Most often, occiput posterior positions undergo spontaneous anterior rotation followed by uncomplicated delivery. In 10 percent or less of cases, spontaneous rotation does not occur. Although the precise reasons for failure of spontaneous rotation are not known, transverse narrowing of the midpelvis undoubtedly plays a role.

The conduct of labor and delivery with the occiput posterior need not differ remarkably from that with the occiput anterior. The status of the fetus is readily monitored by frequently measuring the fetal heart rate during and especially immediately after a contraction. Progress of labor may be ascertained by checking the rate and extent of cervical dilatation and the descent of the fetal head through the birth canal. In most instances, delivery can usually be accomplished without difficulty once the head reaches the perineum, and during a contraction the fetal scalp protrudes through the vaginal introitus.

The possibilities for vaginal delivery are (1) await spontaneous delivery; (2) forceps delivery with the occiput directly posterior; (3) forceps rotation of the occiput to the anterior position and delivery; and (4) manual rotation to the anterior position followed by spontaneous or forceps delivery.

SPONTANEOUS DELIVERY. If the pelvic outlet is roomy and the vaginal outlet and perineum are somewhat relaxed from the previous vaginal deliveries, rapid spontaneous delivery will often take place. If the vaginal outlet is resistant to stretch and the perineum is firm, the second stage of labor may be prolonged appreciably before spontaneous delivery will occur. During each expulsive effort, with the occiput posterior the head is driven against the perineum to a much greater degree than when the occiput is anterior. Therefore forceps delivery after suitable episiotomy is often indicated.

FORCEPS DELIVERY AS AN OCCIPUT POSTERIOR. The need for more traction compared to forcep deliveries from the occiput anterior position can be minimized by making a larger episiotomy. In most instances, a mediolateral incision should be made to avoid lacerations into the anus and rectum. The use of forceps and a large episiotomy warrant more complete anesthesia than may be achieved with pudendal block and local perineal infiltration. The forceps are applied bilaterally along the occipitomental diameter as described in Chapter 41 (p. 1055).

It is important to identify the infrequent case in which the protrusion of fetal scalp through the introitus is the consequence of marked elongation of the fetal head from molding combined with the formation of a large caput. In this circumstance, the head may not even be engaged, i.e., the biparietal diameter has not yet passed through the pelvic inlet. Labor characteristically has been long in such a case and, in turn, descent of the head has been slow. Careful palpation above the symphysis discloses the fetal head to be present above the pelvic inlet. Prompt cesarean section is the appropriate method of delivery. It may be necessary at the time of operation to have an associate insert a sterile gloved hand into the vagina to dislodge the head upward.

FORCEPS ROTATION.   If the head is engaged, the cervix fully dilated, and the pelvis is adequate, forceps rotation may be attempted if the operator is sufficiently skilled to do so. These circumstances are most likely to prevail when expulsive efforts of the mother during the second stage are ineffective as, for example, with continuous regional anesthesia. Rotation by the so-called Scanzoni maneuver or with Kielland's forceps is described in Chapter 41, page 1056.

MANUAL ROTATION.   The requirements for forceps rotation must be met. When the hand is introduced to locate the posterior ear and thus confirm the posterior position, the occiput often rotates toward the anterior position. The head may be grasped with the fingers over the posterior ear and the thumb over the anterior ear and an attempt made to rotate the occiput to the anterior position (see Chap. 41, p. 1054).

Outcome.   Phillips and Freeman (1974) have reviewed the extensive experiences with occiput posterior positions at Grady Memorial Hospital, Atlanta, Georgia. Basic management of the persistent occiput posterior position was similar to that for the occiput anterior position, i.e., delivery without manual or forceps rotation. Compared to the occiput anterior position, labor was prolonged on the average 1 hour in parous women and 2 hours in nulliparous women. The perinatal mortality rate of 2.2 percent did not differ significantly from the 1.8 percent for the occiput anterior group. No significant rise in Apgar scores of less than 7 was found. Extension of the episiotomy, however, was increased appreciably. Phillips and Freeman comment that midline episiotomies are not acceptable for occiput posterior deliveries and, instead, adequate mediolateral incisions should be made.

At Parkland Memorial Hospital, either manual rotation to the anterior position followed by forceps delivery, or forceps delivery from the occiput posterior position is used to effect delivery. When neither can be done with relative ease, cesarean section is carried out.

Persistent Occiput Transverse Position.   In the absence of an abnormality of the pelvic architecture, the occiput transverse position is most likely a transitory one as the occiput rotates to the anterior position. If hypotonic uterine dysfunction, either spontaneous or the consequence of anesthesia, does not develop, spontaneous rotation is usually soon completed, which then allows the choice of spontaneous delivery or delivery with outlet forceps. If rotation ceases because of lack of uterine action and in the absence of pelvic contraction, vaginal delivery usually can be readily accomplished in a number of ways: The occiput may be manually rotated anteriorly or posteriorly and forceps delivery carried out from either the anterior or posterior position. Another approach recommended by some is to apply forceps of the Kielland type to the head in the occiput transverse position (see Chap. 41, p. 1056), then rotate the occiput to the anterior position, and now deliver the head with either the same forceps or with standard outlet forceps. If the failure of spontaneous rotation of the head is caused by hypotonic uterine dysfunction *without cephalopelvic disproportion,* dilute oxytocin may be infused while the fetal heart rate and the uterine contractions are closely monitored.

The genesis of the occiput transverse position is not always so simple nor is the treatment so benign. With the platypelloid (anteroposteriorly flat configuration) pelvis and the android (heart-shaped) pelvis, there may not be adequate room for rotation of the occiput to either the anterior or the posterior position. In case of the android pelvis especially, the head may not even be engaged yet the scalp be visible through the vaginal introitus as the consequence of considerable molding and caput formation. This situation, sometimes referred to as *deep transverse arrest,* is fraught with danger to both the fetus and the mother. If forceps are tried for delivery, it is imperative that undue force not be applied but, instead, delivery be accomplished by cesarean section.

FETAL MACROSOMIA

Birth weights rarely exceed 11 pounds (5000 g), although in 1979 the birth of an infant who weighed 16 pounds (7300 g) was widely reported in the United States. Postpartum, delayed glucose metabolism was detected in the mother. She had previously given birth to several infants who weighed 9 to 10 pounds. Certainly one of the largest infants on record weighed 23.75 pounds (10,800 g), as reported by Beach in 1879 (Barnes, 1957).

Several factors, alone or in combination, may be important in causing excessive fetal size. These include: (1) large size of the parents, especially the mother, (2) multiparity, (3) diabetes in the mother, and (4) some instances of prolonged gestation.

With large fetuses, dystocia may arise because the head becomes not only larger but harder and less malleable with increasing weight. Moreover, after the head has passed through the pelvic canal, dystocia may be caused by the arrest of even larger shoulders at either the pelvic brim or outlet (Fig. 30-21).

Incidence. It is common practice to designate all newborn infants weighing 4000 g or more as "excessive-sized." The incidence of these infants in more than 104,000 deliveries in the Obstetrical Statistical Cooperative was 5.3 percent, and the incidence of infants weighing 4500 g or more was 0.4 percent. Interestingly, among the often socioeconomically deprived, predominantly black population with a relatively low prevalence of diabetes cared for at Parkland Memorial Hospital, the frequency of birth weights of 4000 g or more among 20,000 recent deliveries was 5.1 percent.

Diagnosis. Serious dystocia may arise when an excessively large head attempts to pass through a normal pelvis, just as when a head of average size fetus is arrested by a definitely contracted pelvic inlet. At times, the head is delivered without great difficulty but the large shoulder girdle becomes entrapped. Dystocia from a large shoulder girdle is discussed subsequently. Inasmuch as the clinical estimation of the size of the fetus may be inaccurate, the diagnosis of excessive size is often not made until after fruitless attempts at delivery. Nevertheless, competent clinical examination should enable experienced examiners to arrive at a fairly accurate estimate. Sonographic evaluation of the dimensions of the head, thorax, and abdomen often enhances appreciably the confidence of the estimate.

Prognosis. Since excessive-sized infants are more often born to multiparous mothers and to women with diabetes, both the maternal and fetal risks are increased. In a report on 766 infants who weighed over 4500 g, Sack (1969) cited a perinatal loss of 7.2 percent. More distressing, 16 percent of the infants were severely depressed at birth, 11.4 percent had severe neurologic complications, and 4.5 percent of those who survived the

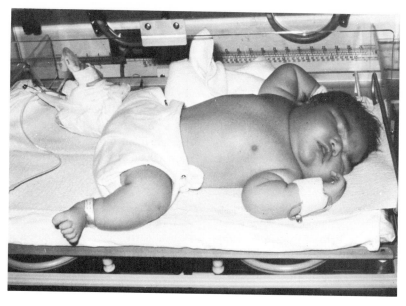

FIG. 30-21. This infant weighed 6065 g and was delivered by cesarean section. Delayed glucose metabolism ("gestational diabetes") was detected in the mother.

perinatal period were dead before the age of 7 years.

SHOULDER DYSTOCIA

Shoulder dystocia is a serious complication of delivery. The problem is that the head is delivered causing the cord to be drawn into the pelvis and compressed before it is realized that the shoulders cannot be delivered.

Incidence. Swartz' review (1960) of experiences with shoulder girdle dystocia indicated an incidence of 0.15 percent for all fetuses who weighed more than 2500 g, but an incidence in infants over 4000 g of 1.7 percent. A recent analysis of experiences at Los Angeles County-University of Southern California Medical Center has served to reemphasize the increased likelihood of shoulder dystocia following a prolonged second stage of labor managed by instrumental vaginal delivery of the head from the midpelvis (Benedetti, Gabbe, 1978). With a prolonged second stage and midpelvic delivery, the incidence of shoulder dystocia was 4.57 percent compared to 0.16 percent in the absence of a prolonged second stage of delivery.

Management. Reduction in the interval of time from delivery of the head to delivery of the body is of great importance to survival, but overly vigorous traction on the head or neck, or excessive rotation of the body, may cause serious damage to the infant. Infrequently, deliberate fracture of the clavicle may be necessary and life-saving to the infant. A large mediolateral episiotomy and adequate anesthesia are necessary.

The first step is to clear the infant's mouth and nose. Next, avoiding unnecessary force, the operator sweeps the posterior arm across the chest and delivers it. The shoulder girdle is then rotated into one of the oblique diameters of the pelvis. The anterior shoulder can usually be delivered at this point. Woods (1943) suggested another method, which utilizes the principle of a screw. The operator applies pressure to the infant's posterior scapula to rotate upward. The posterior shoulder then passes beneath the symphysis in a screw-like motion and is delivered as an anterior shoulder.

MALFORMATIONS OF THE FETUS AS A CAUSE OF DYSTOCIA

Hydrocephalus. Internal hydrocephalus, or excessive accumulation of cerebrospinal fluid in the ventricles of the brain with consequent enlargement of the cranium, occurs in about one in 2000 fetuses and accounts for about 12 percent of all severe malformations found at birth. Associated defects are common with spina bifida occurring in about one-third of the cases. Not infrequently, the circumference of the head exceeds 50 cm, and sometimes reaches 80 cm. The volume of fluid is usually between 500 and 1500 ml, but as much as 5 liters may accumulate. Breech presentation is found in about one-third of these cases. Whatever the presentation, gross cephalopelvic disproportion is the rule with serious dystocia as the usual consequence (Fig. 30-22, 30-23).

Diagnosis. Since the treatment of this complication of labor is usually straightforward, early diagnosis is the key to success.

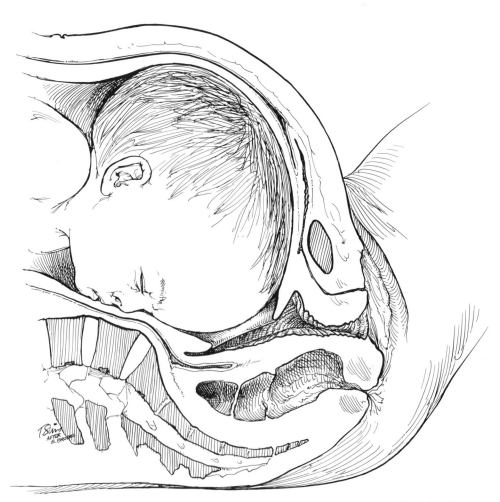

FIG. 30-22. Severe dystocia from hydrocephalus, cephalic presentation. Note the disparity between the small size of the face compared to the rest of the cranium.

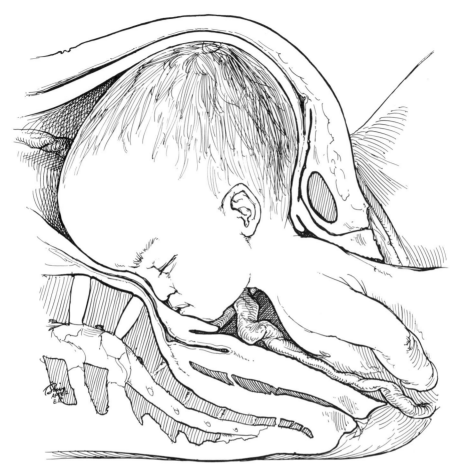

FIG. 30-23. Severe dystocia from hydrocephalus, breech presentation. Note the distension of the lower uterine segment.

In this condition particularly, an empty bladder facilitates both abdominal and vaginal examination. In cephalic presentations, a broad, firm mass above the symphysis is evident from abdominal examination. The thickness of the abdominal wall usually prevents detection of the thin, elastic, hydrocephalic cranium. The high head forces the body of the infant upward, with the result that the fetal heart is often loudest above the umbilicus, a circumstance leading to suspicion of a breech presentation. Vaginally, the broader dome of the head feels tense, but more careful palpation may disclose very large fontanels, wide suture lines, and an indentable, thin cranium characteristic of hydrocephalus. In cephalic presentations, roentgenography provides confirma-

tion by the demonstration of a large, globular head with a thin, sometimes scarcely visible cranial outline (Fig. 30-24).

Hydrocephalus is somewhat more difficult to diagnose with a breech presentation, since the roentgenographic outline of a normal fetal head often appears enlarged to a degree suggestive of hydrocephalus. This results from the fetal head lying more anterior than with a cephalic presentation and the divergence of x-rays inherent in diagnostic roentgenography. Therefore, in breech presentations hydrocephalus may not have been considered until it is found that the head cannot be extracted. The mistake may be avoided by particular attention to the following criteria: (1) the face of the hydrocephalic infant

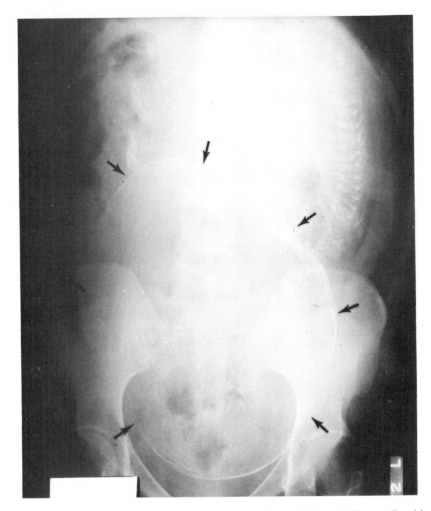

FIG. 30-24. Roentgenogram demonstrating huge hydrocephalus, further outlined by arrows; 2300 ml of cerebrospinal fluid was aspirated transvaginally (Figs. 30-26, 30-27).

is small in relation to the large head; (2) the hydrocephalic cranium tends to be globular, whereas the normal head is ovoid; and (3) the shadow of the hydrocephalic cranium is often very thin or scarcely visible.

Some of the difficulties inherent in radiologic diagnosis may be obviated by the use of sonography. The marked difference between the size of the hydrocephalic head and the thorax is apparent in the sonograms in Figure 30-25.

Prognosis. Rupture of the uterus is a danger and may occur before complete dilatation of the cervix. Hydrocephalus predis-

poses to rupture not only because of the obvious disproportion but also because the great transverse diameter of the cranium overdistends the lower uterine segment. When fetal hydrocephalus is overlooked, the maternal mortality rate is lamentably high.

Treatment. Most often, the size of the hydrocephalic head must be reduced to allow passage of the head through the birth canal. With a cephalic presentation, as soon as the cervix is dilated 3 cm or so, the huge ventricles may be tapped transvaginally with a needle. An 8-inch long, 17-gauge needle usually used for intrauterine transfusion has proved

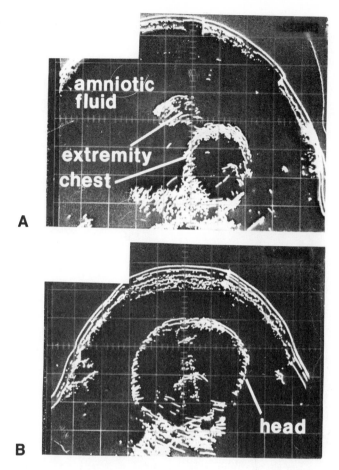

FIG. 30-25. Sonograms of a fetus with hydrocephalus and associated hydramnios. Visible in *A*, are the thorax, an extremity, and an excessive amount of amnionic fluid. In *B*, the head is remarkably enlarged compared to the thorax. (Courtesy of Dr. R. Santos)

quite satisfactory for promptly removing appreciable volumes of cerebrospinal fluid. In the case illustrated in Figures 30-26 and 30-27, 2300 ml of cerebrospinal fluid was removed. With cesarean section, it is also desirable at times to remove cerebrospinal fluid just before incising the uterus to circumvent dangerous extensions of a low transverse or vertical incision and to avoid deliberately creating a very long vertical incision in the uterus.

With a breech presentation, labor is allowed to progress and the breech and trunk are delivered. With the head over the inlet and the face toward the mother's back, the needle is inserted transvaginally just below the anterior vaginal wall and into the aftercoming head through the widened suture line. To protect the birth canal from the needle as it is passed toward the head, the more distal part of the needle, including the point, may be covered with a segment of sterile plastic tubing about 6 inches long cut from an intravenous infusion set.

If this transvaginal maneuver should fail, fluid may be withdrawn through a needle inserted transabdominally into the fetal head. After emptying the bladder and cleansing the skin, the needle is inserted in the midline somewhat below the maternal umbilicus and inferior to the top of the fetal skull. The transabdominal approach to remove cerebrospinal

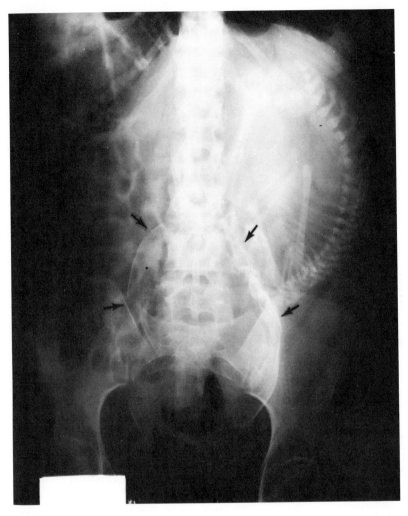

FIG. 30-26. Roentgenogram from same case as in Figure 30-24 after 2300 ml of cerebro-spinal fluid had been removed.

fluid might also be used in case of a cephalic presentation before trying to stimulate labor with oxytocin.

Feeney and Barry (1954) have shown that the infant mortality with congenital hydroce-phalus, including the mildest forms of the disorder, is 70 percent. Although cures have been reported, the prognosis for the child is exceedingly poor when hydrocephalus is so severe as to require drainage in order to accomplish vaginal delivery.

Enlargement of Fetal Abdomen. Enlargement of the fetal abdomen sufficient to cause grave dystocia is usually the result of a *greatly distended bladder* (Fig. 30-28), *ascites, or enlargements of the kidneys or liver.* Occasionally, the abdomen of a fetus affected with *edema* may attain such proportions that spontaneous delivery is impossible. Enlargement of the fetal abdomen may escape detection until fruitless attempts at delivery have demonstrated an obstruction. An enlarged abdomen and intra-abdominal accumulation of fluid can be diagnosed in utero by careful sonographic examination (Fig. 30-29, 30-30).

TREATMENT. If the abdominal enlargement is not discovered until the fetal head has been delivered, decompression of the fe-

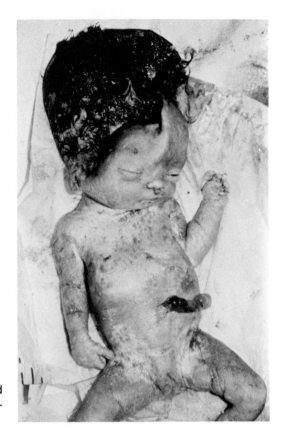

FIG. 30-27. Hydrocephalic infant delivered spontaneously after removal of 2300 ml of cerebrospinal fluid.

tal abdomen often becomes a necessity. The maternal bladder is emptied and the suprapubic area is cleansed. A large-gauge long needle as described for hydrocephalus, is inserted through the midline of the maternal abdomen into the fetal abdomen. Fluid in the fetal bladder or peritoneal cavity promptly escapes. The decompression may be aided by use of continuous suction. As the fetal abdomen approaches normal dimensions, the delivery is readily completed. At times, as with severe hydrops fetalis, ascites will be accompanied by such severe edema of the abdominal wall and so great an enlargement of the liver that removal of the peritoneal fluid provides insufficient decompression for easy delivery. Such cases, fortunately, are becoming extremely rare.

If the diagnosis of gross enlargement of the fetal abdomen is made before delivery, the decision must be made whether or not to perform a cesarean section. In general, the prognosis is very poor for the fetus with abdominal enlargement so marked as to cause dystocia, irrespective of route of delivery.

Incomplete Twinning. The embryologic bases of incomplete twinning is considered in Chapter 26. For practical purposes, three groups of double monsters may be distinguished: (1) incomplete double formations at the upper or lower half of the body (diprosopus dipagus); (2) twins that are united at the upper or lower end of the body (craniopagus, ischiopagus, or pygopagus); and (3) double monsters united at the trunk (thoracopagus and dicephalus).

Although twins may be known, conjoining is not usually identified until difficulty is encountered in attempting delivery. Since such pregnancies seldom go to term, conjoined twins may not exceed greatly the size of a normal fetus. Also, the connection between the halves is sometimes sufficiently flexible to allow vaginal delivery.

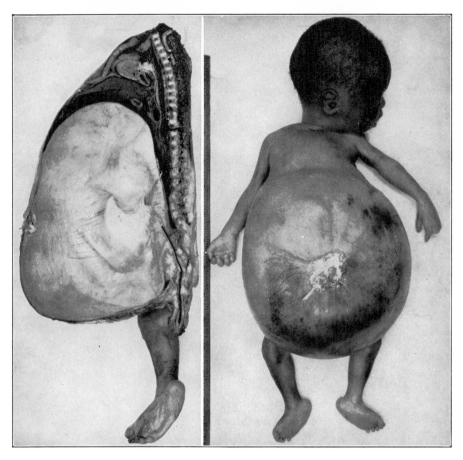

FIG. 30-28. Fetus at 28 weeks with immensely distended bladder. Delivery made possible by expression of fluid from bladder through perforation at umbilicus. Median sagittal section shows interior of bladder and compression of organs of abdominal and thoracic cavities. A black thread has been laid in the urethra. (From Savage. *Am J Obstet Gynecol* 29:276, 1935.)

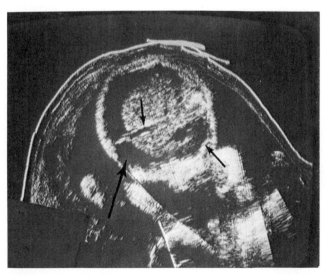

FIG. 30-29. Ascites demonstrated sonographically in a transverse scan of the fetal abdomen. The larger lower arrow points to the peritoneal cavity with ascites; the smaller upper arrow overlies the liver and points to the ductus venosus; the smaller arrow to the right is directed toward the stomach. (Courtesy of Dr. R. Santos)

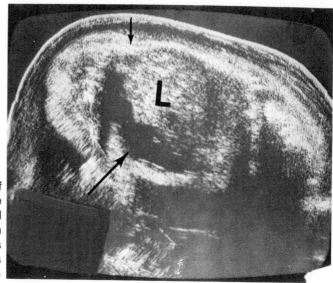

FIG. 30-30. A longitudinal scan of the fetal body in Figure 30-29. The larger lower arrow is directed toward the peritoneal cavity distended with fluid; the upper smaller arrow points to the spinal column; L indicates liver. (Courtesy of Dr. R. Santos.)

REFERENCES

Abroms IF, Bresnan MJ, Zuckerman JE, Fischer EG, Strand R: Cervical cord injuries secondary to hyperextension of the head in breech presentations. Obstet Gynecol 41:369, 1973

Barnes AC: An obstetric record from The Medical Record. Obstet Gynecol 9:237, 1957

Benedetti TJ, Gabbe SG: Shoulder dystocia. A complication of fetal macrosomia and prolonged second stage of labor with mid-pelvic delivery. Obstet Gynecol 52:526, 1978

Bhagwanani SG, Price HV, Laurence KM, Ginz B: Risks and prevention of cervical cord injury in the management of breech presentation with hyperextension of the fetal head. Am J Obstet Gynecol 115:1159, 1973

Bradley-Watson PJ: The decreasing value of external cephalic version in modern obstetric practice. Am J Obstet Gynecol 123:237, 1975

Brenner WE, Bruce RD, Hendricks CH: The characteristics and perils of breech presentation. Am J Obstet Gynecol 118:700, 1974

Caterini H, Langer A, Sama JC, Devanesan M, Pelosi MA: Fetal risk in hyperextension of the fetal head in breech presentation. Am J Obstet Gynecol 123:632, 1975

Chapman GP, Weller RO, Normand ICS, Gibbens D: Spinal cord transection in utero. Br Med J 2:398, 1978

Collea JV, Rabin SC, Weghörst GR, Quilligan EJ: The randomized management of term frank breech presentation: Vaginal delivery vs cesarean section. Am J Obstet Gynecol 131:186, 1978

Cruikshank DP, White CA: Obstetric malpresentations: Twenty years' experience. Am J Obstet Gynecol 116:1097, 1973

Duenhoelter JH, Wells CE, Reisch JS, Santos-Ramos R, Jimenez JM: A paired controlled study of vaginal and abdominal delivery of the low birthweight breech fetus. Obstet Gynecol 54:310, 1979

Feeney JK, Barry AP: Hydrocephaly as a cause of maternal mortality and morbidity: a clinical study of 304 cases. J Obstet Gynaecol Br Emp 61:652, 1954

Fianu S, Vaclavinkova V: The site of placental attachment as a factor in the aetiology of breech presentation. Acta Obstet Gynecol Scand 57:371, 1978

Goplerud J, Eastman NJ: Compound presentation: survey of 65 cases. Obstet Gynecol 1:59, 1953

Hall JE, Kohl SG: Breech presentation: a study of 1456 cases. Am J Obstet Gynecol 72:977, 1956

Hellman LM, Epperson JWW, Connally F: Face and brow presentation: The experience of the Johns Hopkins Hospital, 1896 to 1948. Am J Obstet Gynecol 59:831, 1950

Ingemarsson I, Westgren M, Svenningsen NW: Long-term follow-up of preterm infants in breech presentation delivered by cesarean section. Lancet 2:172, 1978

Johnson CE: Transverse presentation of the fetus. JAMA 187:642, 1964

Lyons ER, Papsin FR: Cesarean section in the management of breech presentation. Am J Obstet Gynecol 130:558, 1978

Marcus RG, Crewe-Brown H, Krawitz S, Katz J: Feto-maternal haemorrhage following successful and unsuccessful attempts at external cephalic version. Br J Obstet Gynaecol 82:578, 1975

Phillips RD, Freeman M: The management of the persistent occiput posterior position: A review of 552 consecutive cases. Obstet Gynecol 43:171, 1974

Ranney B: The gentle art of external cephalic version. Am J Obstet Gynecol 116:239, 1973

Rovinsky JJ, Miller JA, Kaplan S: Management of breech presentation at term. Am J Obstet Gynecol 115:497, 1973

Sack RA: The large infant: a study of maternal, obstetric and newborn characteristics; including a long-term pediatric follow-up. Am J Obstet Gynecol 104:195, 1969

Swartz DP: Shoulder girdle dystocia in vertex delivery; clinical study and review. Obstet Gynecol 15:194, 1960

Tank ES, Davis R, Holt JF, Morley GW: Mechanism of trauma during breech delivery. Obstet Gynecol 38:761, 1971

Weissberg SM, O'Leary JA: Compound presentation of the fetus. Obstet Gynecol 41:60, 1973

Woods CE: A principle of physics is applicable to shoulder delivery. Am J Obstet Gynecol 45:796, 1943

Ylikorkala O, Hartikainen-Sorri A: Value of external version in fetal malpresentation in combination with use of ultrasound. Acta Obstet Gynecol Scand 56:63, 1977

31

Dystocia Caused by
Pelvic Contraction

Any contraction of the pelvic diameters that diminishes the capacity of the pelvis can create dystocia during labor. Pelvic contractions may be classified as follows:

1. Contraction of the pelvic inlet
2. Contraction of the midpelvis
3. Contraction of the pelvic outlet
4. Combinations of inlet, midpelvic, and outlet contraction

CONTRACTED PELVIC INLET

Definition. The pelvic inlet is usually considered to be contracted if its shortest *anteroposterior diameter is less than 10.0 cm or if the greatest transverse diameter is less than 12.0 cm.* The anteroposterior diameter of the pelvis is commonly approximated by measuring manually the diagonal conjugate, which is about 1.5 cm greater. Therefore, inlet contraction is also usually defined as a *diagonal conjugate of less than 11.5 cm.* (The errors inherent in the use of this measurement are discussed in Chapter 11, p. 280).

Using clinical and at times x-ray pelvimetry, it is important to identify the shortest anteroposterior diameter through which the fetal head must pass. Occasionally, the body of the first sacral vertebra is displaced forward so that the shortest distance actually may be between this false promontory and the symphysis pubis.

The biparietal diameter of the fetal head at term has been identified by sonography before delivery to *average* from 9.5 to as much as 9.8 cm in different clinic populations, therefore, it might prove difficult or even impossible for some fetuses to pass through an inlet with an anteroposterior diameter of less than 10 cm. Mengert (1948) and Kaltreider (1952), employing x-ray pelvimetry, demonstrated that the incidence of difficult deliveries is increased to a similar degree when either the anteroposterior diameter is decreased below 10 cm or the transverse diameter is decreased below 12 cm. When both diameters are contracted, the incidence of obstetric difficulty is much greater than when only one diameter is contracted. The configuration of the pelvic inlet is also an important determinant of the adequacy of any pelvis, independent of actual measurements of the anteroposterior and transverse diameters and of calculated "areas."

Small women are likely to have a small pelvis, but at the same time, they are more likely to have small infants. Thoms (1937), in a study of 362 white primigravid women, found the average weight of the offspring to be significantly lower (278 g) in women with small pelves than in those with medium or large pelves. In veterinary obstetrics, it has been frequently observed that in most species maternal size rather than paternal size is the important determinant of fetal size.

Size of Fetal Head. Manual, radiologic, and ultrasonic technics are used with varying degrees of success to identify the size of the fetal head relative to that of the pelvic inlet.

CLINICAL ESTIMATION. Impression of the fetal head into the pelvis, as described by Müller (1880), may provide useful information. In an occiput presentation, the obstetrician grasps the brow and the suboccipital region through the abdominal wall with his fingers and makes firm pressure downward in the axis of the pelvic inlet. Pressure on the fundus by an assistant at the same time is usually helpful. The effect of the forces on the descent of the head can be evaluated by palpation with a sterile gloved hand in the vagina. If no disproportion exists, the head readily enters the pelvis and vaginal delivery can be predicted. Inability to push the head into the pelvis, however, does not necessarily indicate that vaginal delivery is impossible. A clear demonstration of the fetal head overriding the symphysis pubis is indicative of disproportion.

RADIOLOGIC ESTIMATION. In general, measurements of the diameters of the fetal head by roentgenographic techniques have been disappointing. The precision of roentgenocephalometry is much less than for x-ray pelvimetry.

SONOGRAPHIC MEASUREMENTS. Measurement of the fetal biparietal diameter by ultrasonic means allows precise measurement much more often than does x-ray (Figs. 31-1, 31-2). The freely floating fetal head, as in breech presentations, may, unfortunately, move sufficiently during sonographic examination to invalidate the measurement.

Presentation and Position of the Fetus. A contracted pelvic inlet plays an important part in the production of abnormal presentations. In normal nulliparous women, the presenting part frequently descends into the pelvic cavity before the onset of labor at term. When the pelvic inlet is considerably contracted, however, usually descent does not occur until after the onset of labor, if it occurs at all. Vertex presentations still predominate, but since the head floats freely over the pelvic inlet or rests more laterally in one of the iliac fossae, very slight influences may cause the fetus to assume other presentations. For example, face and shoulder presentations occur three times more frequently in women with contracted pelves, and prolapse of the cord and of the extremities four to six times more frequently.

Course of Labor. When the pelvic deformity is sufficiently pronounced to prevent the head from readily entering the inlet, the course of labor is prolonged.

ABNORMALITIES IN DILATATION OF THE CERVIX. Normally, dilatation of the cervix is facilitated by the hydrostatic action of the unruptured membranes or, after their rupture, by the direct application of the presenting part against the cervix. In contracted pelves, however, when the head is arrested at the pelvic inlet, the entire force exerted by the uterus acts directly upon the portion of membranes that overlie the dilating cervix. Consequently, early spontaneous rupture of the membranes is more likely to result.

After rupture of the membranes, the absence of pressure by the fetal head against the cervix and lower uterine segment predisposes to less effective uterine contractions. Hence, further dilatation of the cervix may proceed very slowly or not at all. Cibils and Hendricks (1965) have shown that the mechanical adaptation of the passenger to the bony passage plays an important part in determining the efficiency of uterine contractions. The better the adaptation, the more efficient are the contractions. Since adaptation is poor in the presence of a contracted pelvis, prolon-

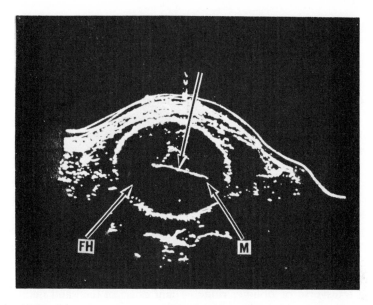

FIG. 31-1. Ultrasonic transverse scan of the fetal head, showing midline (B-mode cephalometry). The arrow is perpendicular to the linear midline structures of the fetal head. With this line as reference, the biparietal diameter of the head can be distinguished accurately. (FH, fetal head; M, midline of the fetal head.)

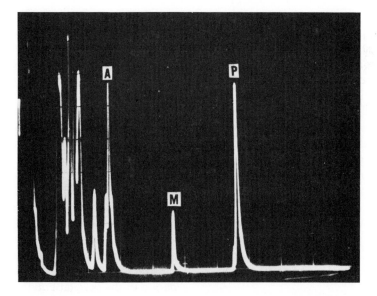

FIG. 31-2. Ultrasonic A-mode cephalometry. The probe is directed along the arrow shown in the B-mode presentation (Fig. 31-1). The anterior (A) and posterior (P) skull echoes are clearly seen with a midline echo (M) between them. The biparietal diameter of the fetal head is the distance between peaks A and P.

gation of labor often results. *With degrees of pelvic contractions incompatible with vaginal delivery, the cervix seldom dilates satisfactorily. Thus, the behavior of the cervix has a certain prognostic value in regard to the outcome of labor in women with inlet contraction.*

DANGER OF UTERINE RUPTURE. Abnormal thinning of the lower uterine segment creates a serious danger during a prolonged labor. When the disproportion between the head and the pelvis is so pronounced that engagement and descent do not occur, the lower uterine segment becomes increasingly stretched, and the danger of rupture becomes imminent. In such cases, a pathologic retraction ring may develop and can be felt as a transverse or oblique ridge extending across the uterus somewhere between the symphysis and the umbilicus. Whenever this condition is noted, prompt delivery is urgently indicated. Unless cesarean section is employed to terminate labor, there is the great danger of rupture of the uterus, as well as serious compromise of fetal well-being.

PRODUCTION OF FISTULAS. When the presenting part is firmly wedged into the pelvic inlet but does not advance for a considerable time, portions of the birth canal lying between it and the pelvic wall may be subjected to excessive pressure. As the circulation is impaired, the resulting necrosis may become manifest several days after delivery by the appearance of vesicovaginal, vesicocervical, or rectovaginal fistulas. Formerly, when operative delivery was deferred as long as possible, such complications were frequent, but today they are rarely seen except in neglected cases. In general, pressure necrosis follows a very prolonged second stage of labor.

INTRAPARTUM INFECTION. Infection is another serious danger to which the mother and the fetus are exposed in prolonged labors complicated by prolonged rupture of the membranes. The danger of infection is undoubtedly increased by repeated vaginal examinations and other intravaginal and intrauterine manipulations. If the amnionic fluid becomes infected, fever may or may not develop during labor.

Effects On The Fetus. Prolonged labor in itself is deleterious to the fetus. In women with labors of more than 20 hours or in women with a second stage of labor of more than three hours, Hellman and Prystowsky (1952) found a significant increase in perinatal mortality rates. If the pelvis is contracted and there is associated early rupture of membranes and intrauterine infection, the risk to the infant is compounded. Intrapartum infection as well as being a serious complication for the mother, is an important cause of fetal and neonatal death, since bacteria in amnionic fluid can make their way through the amnion and invade the walls of the chorionic vessels, thus giving rise to fetal bacteremia. Aspiration of infected amnionic fluid by the fetus causing pneumonia is another serious consequence.

CHANGES IN SCALP AND SKULL. A large *caput succedaneum* frequently develops on the most dependent part of the head during labor if the pelvis is contracted. The caput succedaneum may assume considerable proportions and lead to serious diagnostic errors. The caput may reach almost to the pelvic floor while the head is still not engaged, i.e., the biparietal diameter has not passed through the pelvic inlet. An inexperienced physician may make premature and unwise attempts at forceps delivery. The large caput disappears within a few days after birth.

Under the pressure of the strong uterine contractions, the bones of the skull overlap one another at the major sutures, a process referred to as *molding.* As a rule, the median margin of the parietal bone that is in contact with the sacral promontory is overlapped by that of its fellow; the same result occurs with the frontal bones. The occipital bone, however, is pushed under the parietal bones. These changes are frequently accomplished without obvious detriment to the child, although when the distortion is marked it may lead to tentorial tears and, when blood vessels are torn, to fatal intracranial hemorrhage. Such *molding* of the fetal head may produce diminution of 0.5 cm or so in the biparietal diameter without cerebral injury, but when greater degrees of molding occur, the likelihood of intracranial injury increases appreciably.

Coincident with the molding of the head, the parietal bone, which was in contact with the promontory, may show signs of having been subjected to marked pressure, sometimes becoming very much flattened. Accommodation is more readily accomplished when the bones of the head are imperfectly ossified. This important process may provide one explanation for the differences in the course of labor in two apparently similar cases in which the pelvis and the head present identical measurements. In one case, the head is softer and more readily molded, and spontaneous delivery results. In the other, the more resistant head retains its original shape and operative interference is required for its delivery.

Characteristic pressure marks may form upon the scalp covering the portion of the head that passes over the promontory of the sacrum. From their location, it is frequently possible to ascertain the movements that the head has undergone in passing through the pelvic inlet. Much more rarely, similar marks appear on the portion of the head that has been in contact with the symphysis pubis. Such marks usually disappear a few days after birth, although in exceptional instances severe pressure may lead to necrosis of the scalp.

Fractures of the skull are occasionally encountered, usually following forcible attempts at delivery, though sometimes they may occur with spontaneous delivery. The fractures are of two varieties, appearing either as a shallow groove or as a spoon-shaped depression just posterior to the coronal suture (Fig. 31-3). The former is relatively common but since it involves only the external plate of the bone, it is not very dangerous. The latter, however, if not operated upon, may lead to the death of the infant, since it extends through the entire thickness of the skull and gives rise upon its inner surface to projections that exert injurious pressure upon the brain and may cause hemorrhage. Accordingly, as

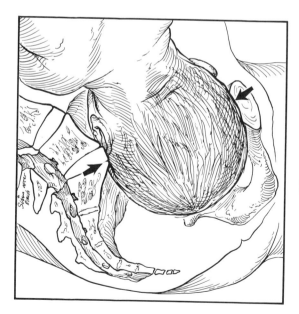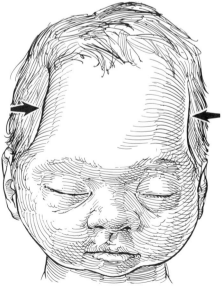

FIG. 31-3. Depression of skull (arrows) caused by labor with contracted pelvic inlet.

soon as feasible after delivery, it is advisable to elevate or remove the depressed portion of the skull.

PROLAPSE OF THE CORD. A serious complication for the fetus is prolapse of the cord, the occurrence of which is facilitated by imperfect adaptation between the presenting part and the pelvic inlet. Unless prompt delivery is accomplished, fetal death results from compression of the cord between the presenting part and the margin of the pelvic inlet.

Prognosis. The prognosis for successful vaginal delivery at term in cases of severe inlet contraction with an anteroposterior diameter of less than 9 cm can be stated as nearly hopeless. For the borderline group in which the anteroposterior diameter is only slightly below 10 cm, the prognosis for successful vaginal delivery is influenced significantly by a number of variables, as follows:

1. The presentation is of extreme importance with all but the occiput being unfavorable.
2. The size of the fetus is of obvious importance. Unfortunately, estimates of fetal size may be imprecise as discussed below.
3. Not only the diameters of the pelvic inlet, but also the configuration plays an important role. With an android configuration, for any given anteroposterior diameter of the inlet, there is less available space, especially in the forepelvis.
4. The frequency and intensity of spontaneous uterine contractions are informative. Uterine dysfunction, typically infrequent contractions of low intensity, is common with significant disproportion.
5. The behavior of the cervix in labor has great prognostic significance. In general, orderly spontaneous progression to full dilatation indicates that vaginal delivery most likely will be successful.
6. Extreme asynclitism is unfavorable, as is appreciable molding of the head without engagement.
7. Knowledge of the outcome of previous labor and delivery at term is helpful.
8. Finally, the prognosis for successful vagi-

nal delivery is altered by coincidental conditions that impair uteroplacental perfusion, for example, severe preeclampsia. In such circumstances, uterine contractions sufficient to dilate the cervix and propel the fetus through the birth canal are much more likely to compromise placental perfusion to such a degree that the fetus is distressed.

Treatment. The management of inlet contraction is determined principally by the prognosis for safe vaginal delivery. If, on the basis of the criteria reviewed, a delivery that is safe for both mother and child cannot be anticipated, cesarean section should be done. Today it is so rare to employ craniotomy that even dead fetuses are often delivered by cesarean section in cases of contraction of the pelvis. In a minority of instances, the prognosis in a given case can be reached before the onset of labor, and cesarean section can be done electively at an appointed time. A carefully managed trial of labor, however, is desirable in most instances. Women with inlet contraction are particularly likely to have both weak uterine contractions during the first stage of labor and a need for vigorous voluntary expulsive efforts during the second stage. Therefore, in general, the use of conduction anesthesia should be avoided. The course of labor should be monitored closely and the prognosis established as soon as reasonably possible. Although signs of impending uterine rupture should always be looked for if the contractions are strong, the danger of this accident is remote in primigravid women. With greater parity, however, the likelihood of rupture of the uterus increases. Finally, the administration of oxytocin in the presence of any form of pelvic contraction, unless the fetal head has unequivocally passed the point of obstruction, can be catastrophic for both the fetus and the mother.

CONTRACTION OF MIDPELVIS

Definition. The so-called plane of the obstetric midpelvis extends from the inferior margin of the symphysis pubis, through the ischial spines, and touches the sacrum near the junction of the fourth and fifth vertebrae. A transverse line drawn theoretically between the ischial spines divides the midpelvis into a fore portion and hind portion. The former is bounded anteriorly by the lower border of the symphysis pubis and laterally by the ischiopubic rami. The hind portion is bounded posteriorly by the sacrum and laterally by the sacrospinous ligament, forming the lower limits of the sacrosciatic notch. Average midpelvic measurements are as follows: transverse (interspinous), 10.5 cm; anteroposterior (from the lower border of the symphysis pubis to the junction of the fourth and fifth sacral vertebrae), 11.5 cm; and posterior sagittal (from the midpoint of the interspinous line to the same point on the sacrum), 5 cm. Although the definition of midpelvic contractions has not been established with the same precision possible in inlet contractions, the midpelvis should be considered contracted when the sum of the interischial spinous and posterior sagittal diameters of the midpelvis (normally, 10.5 cm plus 5 cm, or 15.5 cm) falls to 13.5 or below. There is reason to suspect that midpelvic contraction exists whenever the interischial spinous diameter is less than 10 cm. When it is smaller than 9 cm, the midpelvis is contracted. The preceding definition of midpelvic contraction does not, of course, imply that dystocia will necessarily occur in such a pelvis, but simply that it may develop, depending also upon the size and shape of the forepelvis, and the size of the fetal head, as well as the degree of midpelvic contraction.

Identification.   Although there is no satisfactory manual method of ascertaining midpelvic contraction, a suggestion of midpelvic contraction is sometimes obtainable by ascertaining on vaginal examination that the spines are prominent, that the pelvic side walls converge, or that the sacrosciatic notch is narrow. Eller and Mengert (1947), moreover, pointed out that the relation between the intertuberous and interspinous diameters of the ischium is sufficiently constant that narrowing

of the interspinous diameter can be anticipated when the intertuberous diameter is narrow. A normal intertuberous diameter, however, does not always exclude a narrow interspinous diameter.

Prognosis.   Midpelvic contraction is probably more common than inlet contraction and is frequently a cause of transverse arrest of the fetal head and, potentially, of difficult midforceps operations.

Treatment.   In the management of labor complicated by midpelvic contraction, the main injunction is to allow the natural forces of labor to push the biparietal diameter beyond the potential interspinous obstruction. Forceps operations may be very difficult when applied to a head the greatest diameter of which has not yet passed a contracted midpelvis. This difficulty may be explained on two grounds: (1) pulling on the head with forceps destroys flexion, whereas pressure from above increases it; (2) although the forceps blades occupy a space of only a few millimeters, this diminishes further the available space. Only when the head has been allowed to descend to such an extent that the perineum is bulging and the vertex is actually visible is it reasonably certain that the head has passed the obstruction. It is then usually safe to apply forceps. Strong suprafundal pressure should not be used to try to force the head past the obstruction.

The use of forceps to effect delivery in midpelvic contraction, usually undiagnosed, has been responsible for much of the stigma attached to the midforceps operation. Midforceps delivery is, therefore, contraindicated in any case of midpelvic contraction in which the biparietal diameter of the fetal head has not passed beyond the level of contraction. Otherwise, the perinatal mortality and morbidity rates associated with the operation are prohibitive.

The vacuum extractor (see Chap. 41, p. 1059) has been reported by some to be of advantage in some cases of midpelvic contraction *after the cervix has become fully dilated.* It need not cause deflection of the fetal head, nor does it occupy space, as do forceps. Oxytocin, of course, has no place in the treatment of dystocia caused by midpelvic contraction.

CONTRACTION OF THE PELVIC OUTLET

Definition. Contraction of the pelvic outlet is usually defined as diminution of the interischial tuberous diameter to 8 cm or less. The pelvic outlet may be likened roughly to two triangles (Figs. 31-4 and 31-6). The interischial tuberous diameter constitutes the base of both. The sides of the anterior triangle are the pubic rami, and its apex the inferior posterior surface of the symphysis pubis. The posterior triangle has no bony sides but

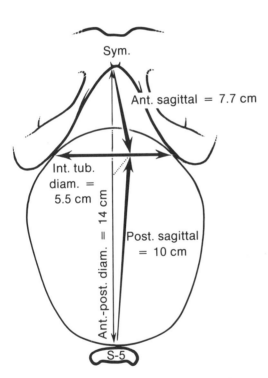

FIG. 31-4. Diagram of pelvic outlet of case shown in Figure 31-5. Even though the intertuberous diameter is quite narrow (5.5 cm), vaginal delivery is possible because of the long (10 cm) posterior sagittal diameter. (Int. tub. diam. = intertuberous diameter; Sym. = symphysis pubis; S-5 = fifth sacral vertebra)

is limited at its apex by the tip of the last sacral vertebra (not the tip of the coccyx).

Prognosis. It is apparent in Figure 31-4 that diminution in the intertuberous diameter with consequent narrowing of the anterior triangle must inevitably force the fetal head posteriorly. Whether delivery can take place, therefore, depends partly on the size of the posterior triangle or, more specifically, the interischial tuberous diameter and the posterior sagittal diameter of the outlet, as demonstrated in Figures 31-4 through 31-7. A contracted outlet may cause dystocia not so much by itself as through the often associated midpelvic contraction. *Outlet contraction without concomitant midplane contraction is rare.*

Even when the disproportion between the size of the fetal head and the pelvic outlet is not sufficiently great to give rise to serious dystocia, it may play an important part in the production of perineal tears. With increasing narrowing of the pubic arch, the occiput cannot emerge directly beneath the symphysis pubis but is forced increasingly farther down upon the ischiopubic rami. In extreme cases, the head must rotate around a line joining the ischial tuberosities. The perineum, consequently, must become increasingly distended and thus exposed to great danger of disruption. An extensive mediolateral episiotomy is usually indicated.

In view of potential significance of outlet contractions, palpation of the pubic arch should be part of the pelvic examination of the pregnant woman.

GENERALLY CONTRACTED PELVIS

Prognosis. Since the contraction involves all portions of the pelvic canal, labor is not rapidly completed after the fetal head has passed the pelvic inlet. The prolongation of labor is caused not only by the resistance offered by the pelvis but also in many instances by the faulty uterine contractions that frequently accompany diminution in the size of the pelvis and a fetus of average or larger size.

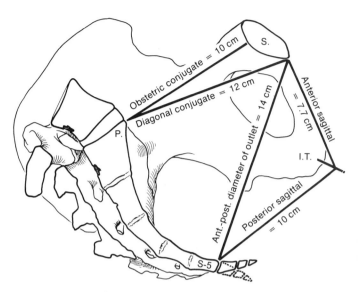

FIG. 31-5. Diagram of the lateral view of the same pelvis depicted in Figure 31-4. The long (10 cm) posterior sagittal diameter may allow the fetal head to negotiate the narrow (5.5 cm) intertuberous diameter (I.T. = ischial tuberosity; S. = symphysis pubis; P. = sacral promontory).

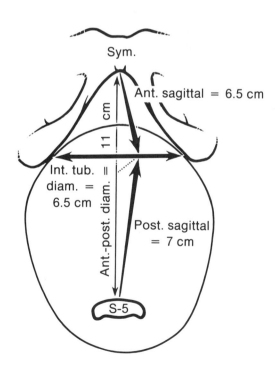

FIG. 31-6. Diagram of pelvic outlet in which the intertuberous diameter is narrow (6.5 cm) *and* the posterior sagittal diameter is quite short (7 cm), precluding vaginal delivery of most term-size fetuses. (Int. tub. diam. = intertuberous diameter; Sym. = symphysis pubis; S-5 = fifth sacral vertebra)

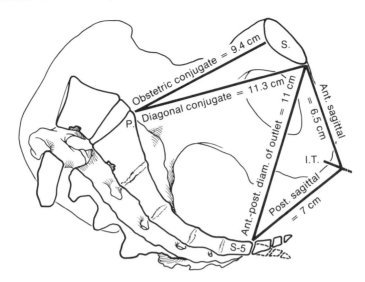

FIG. 31-7. Diagram of lateral view of the pelvis from the same case depicted in Figure 31-6. Note the short (7 cm) posterior sagittal diameter. (I. T. = ischial tuberosity; S. = symphysis pubis; S-5 = fifth sacral vertebra; P. = sacral promontory)

PELVIC FRACTURES AND PREGNANCY

Speer and Peltier (1972) reviewed their experiences and those of others with pelvic fractures and pregnancy. As expected, trauma from automobile collisions was the common cause of fracture. With bilateral fractures of the pubic rami, compromise of the capacity of the birth canal by callus formation or malunion was very common. The experiences at Parkland Memorial Hospital are that a history of previous fracture of the pelvis warrants careful radiologic evaluation of the pelvis later in pregnancy, unless cesarean section is to be performed for some other reason.

RARE PELVIC CONTRACTIONS*

Kyphotic Pelvis. Kyphosis, or humpback, when involving the lower portion of the vertebral column, is usually associated with a characteristically funnel-shaped distortion. The effect exerted

* Illustrations of several rare pelvic contractions appear in earlier editions of this textbook.

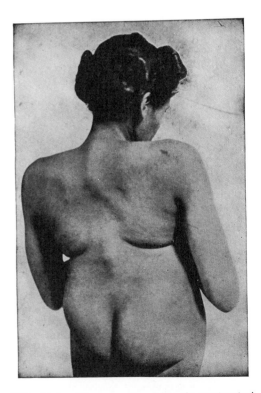

FIG. 31-8. Woman with obliquely contracted, kyphotic, funnel pelvis. Note presence of double gibbus. The lumbosacral deformity produced the funnel pelvis.

upon the pelvis by kyphosis differs according to its location. When the gibbus, or hump, is situated in the thoracic region, there is usually a compensatory pronounced lordosis beneath it, so that the pelvis itself is but little changed. When situated at the junction of the thoracic and lumbar portions of the vertical column, however, its effect upon the pelvis becomes manifest. It is further accentuated when the kyphosis is lower down and is most marked when it is at the lumbosacral junction (Fig. 31-8). If the vertebral defect is in the lumbosacral region, the upper arm of the gibbus may overlie the inlet.

DIAGNOSIS. The diagnosis is usually obvious, for the external deformity is readily visible and should at once suggest the possibility of a funnel pelvis. On palpation of the pubic arch, transverse narrowing of the pelvic outlet is observed, whereas by internal examination the lengthening of the obstetric conjugate is found. In lumbosacral kyphosis, there is no longer a promontory, and the bodies of the lower lumbar vertebrae overhang the superior strait. In this type of deformity, therefore, particular attention should be devoted to the length of the "pseudoconjugate," the distance from the upper margin of the symphysis pubis to the nearest portion of the vertebral column. Occasionally, the condition may be mistaken for spondylolisthesis.

EFFECT UPON LABOR. The mechanical conditions favor abnormal positions of the fetus. Generally when the distance between the tubera ischii is less than 8 cm, labor becomes difficult or impossible, according to the degree of transverse contraction of the outlet. In such cases, the dystocia is more pronounced than in typical funnel pelves presenting identical measurements, because the anterior displacement of the tip of the sacrum is inevitably associated with shortening of the posterior sagittal diameter.

EFFECT UPON THE HEART. In 50 fatal cases of kyphoscoliosis associated with pregnancy that were collected by Jensen (1938), at least 31 were caused by heart failure, far more than resulted from pelvic dystocia. Because of the collapse of the vertebral column, the volume of the thoracic cage in thoracic kyphoscoliosis is diminished, with consequent pressure exerted on the lungs and heart. As a result, the vital capacity is decreased to one-half the normal value, as shown by the

studies of Chapman and co-workers (1939). This reduction applies to both the absolute and relative vital capacities. In five patients with thoracic kyphoscoliosis studied by them, the vital capacity was from 35 to 53 percent of the total pulmonary volume, whereas in the normal women studied, the fraction was 57 to 69 percent of the total. The ratio of residual air to vital capacity was 1.3 in kyphoscoliotic patients and 0.6 in the normal subjects. In other words, in these deformed women, the usual mechanism of respiration is altered by the greater limitation of costal movement. The ribs move only ineffectively, and breathing is accomplished largely by movements of the diaphragm. Partial collapse and infection are but natural results of these poorly aerated lungs.

PROGNOSIS AND TREATMENT. The kyphoscoliotic patient is severely handicapped in childbearing. If the condition is entirely thoracic, cardiac complications are a threat; if the condition is entirely lumbar, midpelvic contraction is common, and if the condition is low down, contraction may be extreme. When the gibbus is thoracolumbar, both heart and pelvis may be sources of difficulty.

The prognosis here, as in all other types of contracted pelves, depends not only upon the dimensions of the pelvis but upon the progress of labor. If labor is prolonged with dimensions below the critical levels, delivery is best accomplished by cesarean section.

Kyphorachitic Pelvis. Kyphosis is nearly always of carious origin, but when caused by rachitis it is usually associated with scoliosis. In the rare cases of pure rachitis kyphosis, however, the pelvic changes are slight, for the effect of the kyphosis is counterbalanced to a great extent by that of the rachitis, the former leading to an elongation and the latter to a shortening of the conjugata vera. The kyphosis tends to narrow, and the rachitis to widen, the pelvic outlet. Thus it may happen that a woman presenting a markedly deformed vertebral column of this character may have a practically normal pelvis. The two processes, however, do not always counteract each other; and as a rule, when the kyphosis is high up, the pelvic changes are predominantly rachitic.

Scoliotic Pelvis. With scoliosis involving the upper portion of the vertebral column, there is usually a compensatory corresponding curvature in the opposite direction lower down, thus giving rise to a double, or S-shaped, curve. In such cases, the body weight is transmitted to the sacrum in the usual manner, so that the pelvis is not involved. When the scoliosis is lower down and involves the lumbar region, however, the sacrum takes part in the compensatory process and assumes an abnormal position, leading to slight asymmetry of the pelvis.

Kyphoscoliotic Pelvis. In this type of deformity, the distortion of the pelvis varies according to whether the kyphosis or the scoliosis is predominant. When the extent of the two deformities is approximately equal, however, the kyphotic changes in the pelvis predominate, although the influence of the scoliosis tends to counteract, to a certain extent, the transverse narrowing of the inferior strait.

Kyphoscoliorachitic Pelvis. Kyphosis resulting from rachitis is nearly always complicated by scoliosis, which usually predominates in the production of the pelvic deformity, because the kyphosis and the rachitis tend to counteract each other in their effect on the pelvis. The resulting pelvis, therefore, does not differ materially from that observed in scoliorachitis except that the tendency to anteroposterior flattening is partially counteracted by the action of the kyphotic vertebral column. Because of the scoliosis, the oblique deformity of the pelvic inlet is usually quite marked. Generally, however, this type of pelvis is more favorable, from an obstetric standpoint, than that resulting from scoliorachitis alone.

Extremely Rare Pelvic Contractions. In the past century and a half, descriptions of the seven following extremely rare contracted pelves have appeared in the obstetric literature. A busy obstetrician or even a large obstetric service in this country may in many years encounter none of them. Osteomalacia, for example, although seen in the Far East, is virtually absent from this country. For details, see *Williams Obstetrics,* 10th ed., 1950.

1. Robert pelvis
2. Split pelvis
3. Litzmann pelvis
4. Assimilation pelvis
5. Naegele pelvis
6. Osteomalacic pelvis
7. Spondylolisthetic pelvis

Pelvic Anomalies Resulting from Abnormal Forces Exerted by Femurs. Normally, when a woman stands erect, the upward and inward force exerted by the femurs is of equal intensity on either side and is transmitted to the pelvis through the acetabula. In walking or running, the entire body weight is transmitted alternately first to one and then to the other leg. In a person suffering from disease affecting one leg, the sound extremity must bear more than its share of the body weight; consequently, the upward and inward force exerted by the femur is generally greater upon that side of the pelvis. To these mechanical factors are attributed the changes in shape that accompany certain forms of lameness, provided the lesion appeared early in life.

Pelvic Deformities Caused by Unilateral Lameness. Coxitis occurring in early life nearly always gives rise to an obliquely contracted pelvis. If the disease appeared before the subject learned to walk, or if the child was obliged to keep to its bed for a prolonged period, there may have been imperfect development of the pelvis. The generally contracted type is produced, to which are added the mechanical effects and atrophic changes resulting from the unilateral disease (Fig. 31-9). They are manifested by imperfect development of the diseased side of the pelvis. The affected innominate bone is smaller than its fellow, and the iliopectineal line forming the arc of a circle has a smaller radius than that of the other side. At the same time, the sacral alae are more poorly developed on the affected side. The entire bone is somewhat rotated about its vertical axis, so that its anterior surface looks toward the normal side.

Oblique contraction of the pelvis may also develop when *unilateral luxation* of the femur occurs in early life, although it is usually less pronounced than that following coxitis. In such circumstances, the head of the bone is displaced backward and upward upon the outer surface of the ilium, where a new articular surface may occasionally be formed. The affected leg becomes considerably shortened, and a disproportionate share of the body weight is transmitted through the normal leg, forcing the healthy side of the pelvis upward, inward, and backward, and resulting in the same oblique contraction seen in coxalgia.

Unless the patient has had the benefit of proper orthopedic treatment in unilateral poliomyelitis, as well as in those cases in which disease at the knee or ankle or amputation early in life has caused shortening of one leg, similar changes occur in

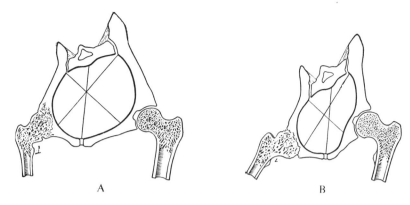

FIG. 31-9. Coxalgic pelvis before **(A)** and after **(B)** the subject has walked.

the pelvis, though they rarely assume the extreme obliquity that characterizes the coxalgic variety.

DIAGNOSIS. A limp at once suggests an obliquely contracted pelvis. When the condition has been present since early childhood, a pelvic deformity on the side corresponding to the unaffected leg is likely.

More accurate information can be obtained by careful examination of the unclothed patient, when the posture of the involved leg as well as the relative positions of the posterior or superior spines and the crests of the ilia may be ascertained. At the same time, the presence or absence of compensatory scoliosis may be noted in such cases.

EFFECT UPON LABOR. The effect of this type of pelvis upon labor varies with the extent and position of the deformity. If the affected side is so contracted that it prevents its being occupied by a portion of the presenting part, for all practical purposes a generally contracted pelvis exists. Engagement, if it can occur at all, will take place more readily when the biparietal diameter of the head is aligned with the long oblique diameter of the superior strait. All obstacles to labor have not yet been overcome, however, even after descent has occurred, since in many cases the inward projection of the ischium may lead to abnormalities in rotation. Generally, these pelves are not excessively contracted.

Coxarthrolisthetic Pelvis. Very exceptionally, as the result of localized softening near the acetabulum, the base of one or both acetabula yields to the pressure exerted by the head of the femur, projecting into the pelvic cavity and leading to a unilateral or bilateral transverse contrac-

tion. Eppinger (1903) designated such pelves as coxarthrolisthetic and attributed their production to delayed and deficient ossification of the base of the acetabulum. Breus and Kolisko (1912) stated that the deformity is usually related to gonorrheal coxitis, rather than to arthritis deformans or tuberculosis, as was formerly believed. Chiari (1911), however, described a specimen that he believed to have resulted from tabetic arthritis. Benda (1927) collected cases of this rare condition reported up to 1926 and critically considered their mode of production.

Pelvic Deformities Resulting from Bilateral Lameness. Children occasionally are born with *luxation of both femurs,* the heads of the bones lying, as a rule, upon the outer surfaces of the iliac bones, above and posterior to their usual location. In some cases, the acetabula are entirely absent, but more frequently they are rudimentary; new but imperfect substitutes then form higher up. The condition does not usually interfere seriously with learning to walk at the usual age, though the gait is more or less wobbly.

Because the upward and inward force exerted by the femurs is not applied in its usual direction through the acetabula, the pelvis becomes excessively wide and more or less flattened anteroposteriorly. The transverse widening is particularly marked at the inferior strait, while the flattening, as a rule, is not very pronounced. This pelvis, therefore, rarely offers any serious obstacle to labor and delivery.

Atypical Deformities of the Pelvis. The pelvis may rarely be deformed by bony outgrowths at various points and even less frequently by tumors. *Exotoses* are most frequently found on the posterior surface of the symphysis, in front of the sacroiliac joints, and on the anterior surface of the sacrum, although occasionally these may be formed along the course of the iliopectineal line.

Kilian (1854) indicated that such structures may form sharp, knifelike projections. He designated the condition *acanthopelyx* or *pelvis spinosa.* Such formations are rarely sufficiently large to present any obstacle to delivery, but because of their peculiar structure may cause considerable injury to the maternal soft parts.

Tumors of various kinds may arise from the walls of the false or true pelvis and so obstruct its cavity as to render labor impossible. Fibromas, osteomas, chondromas, carcinomas, and sarcomas of the pelvis have been described. These sometimes grow large and occasionally become cystic. Chondromas are the most common variety.

DWARF PELVIS. According to Breus and Kolisko (1900), several varieties of dwarfs must be distinguished: the "true," the hypoplastic, the chondrodystrophic, the cretin, and the rachitic dwarf.

In the *true dwarf,* there is a proportionate lack of general development in which epiphyses do not ossify but remain cartilaginous until an advanced age.

In the *hypoplastic dwarf,* the changes are quantitative rather than qualitative, the individual differing from the normal only in that she is miniature.

In the *chondrodystrophic dwarf,* the deformity results from chondrodystrophia fetalis or achondroplasia. It is characterized by changes in the epiphysial cartilage, which interfere with the normal apposition of bone, with the result that the shafts of the long bones are imperfectly developed. The individual therefore has a normally formed trunk, but the extremities are short and stumpy. The head is often brachycephalic, with a prominent forehead and saddle nose. Such dwarfs are fertile, in contrast to the cretins, in whom infertility is the rule.

In the *cretin dwarf,* the lack of development is general. The bony changes are allied to those observed in the true dwarf but are less marked.

The term *rachitic dwarf* should not be applied to people whose short stature results from skeletal deformities but should be restricted to those who would fall far below the normal height even if the deformities were straightened out.

Each of these varieties of dwarf has a characteristically shaped pelvis, which is more or less generally contracted.

TRUE DWARF (PELVIS NANA). This extremely rare variety of pelvis is generally contracted and tends toward the infantile type, but its most characteristic feature is the persistence of cartilage at all the epiphyses.

HYPOPLASTIC DWARF PELVIS. According to Breus and Kolisko (1904), this variety of pelvis is found in very small adults and is simply a normal pelvis in miniature. It differs significantly from that of the true dwarf in that it is completely ossified.

CHONDRODYSTROPHIC DWARF PELVIS. This variety of pelvis is characterized by an extreme anteroposterior flattening, which at first appears to resemble that of a rachitic pelvis. On closer examination, however, the flattening is seen to result from the imperfect development of the portion of the iliac bone entering into the formation of the iliopectineal line. As a result, the sacral articulation is brought much nearer the pubic bone than usual. In six pelves of this type described by Breus and Kolisko, the conjugata vera varied from 4 to 7 cm, whereas the transverse diameter of the superior strait was only slightly shortened, varying from 11 to 12 cm.

CRETIN DWARF PELVIS. This generally contracted pelvis is formed of imperfectly developed bones. Unlike that of the true dwarf, it does not present infantile characteristics but signs of a steady though imperfect growth throughout early life are seen. Unossified cartilage may be present focally in young subjects, but it disappears with advancing age and is never found in all the epiphyses as in the true dwarf pelvis.

RACHITIC DWARF PELVIS. True rachitic dwarfs are rare and possess generally contracted rachitic pelves, which do not differ, except by their small size, from other rachitic pelves.

REFERENCES*

Benda R: Contribution to the etiology and pathogenesis of coxitic protrusion of the acetabulum. Arch Gynaek 129:186, 1927

* In this chapter, several historical references are included. Further information may be found in earlier editions of this textbook.

Breus C, Kolisko A: Die pathologischen Becken-formen, Leipzig and Vienna, 1900. Vol. III:I. Teil Spondylolisthesis, pp. 17–159; Kypho-sen-Becken, pp. 163–307; Skoliosen-Becken, pp. 355–359

Breus C, Kolisko A: Die pathologischen Becken-formen. Leipzig and Vienna, 1904, Vol. I: Spaltbeken, pp 107–139; Assimilations-becken, pp 169–256; Zwegbecken, pp 259–366

Breus C, Kolisko A: Rachitis-Becken, Die patholo-gischen Beckenformen. Leipzig and Vienna, 1904, Vol I, part 2, p 435

Breus C, Kolisko A: Coxitis-Becken, Die patholo-gischen Beckenformen. Leipzig and Vienna, 1912, Vol III, pp 474–593

Chapman EM, Dill DB, Graybiel A: Decrease in functional capacity of lungs and heart resulting from deformities of chest: pulmonocardiac failure. Medicine 18:167, 1939

Chiari H: Spondylolisthesis. Bull Johns Hopkins Hosp 22:41, 1911

Cibils LA, Hendricks CH: Normal labor in vertex presentation. Am J Obstet Gynecol 91:385, 1965

Eller WC, Mengert WF: Recognition of mid-pel-vic contraction. Am J Obstet Gynecol 53:252, 1947

Eppinger: Pelvis-Chrobak (Coxarthrolisthesis-Becken). Beitrage, Geb Gyn Vienna 2:173, 1903

Hellman LM, Prystowsky H: Duration of the sec-ond stage of labor. Am J Obstet Gynecol 63:1223, 1952

Jensen J: The Heart in Pregnancy. St. Louis, Mosby, 1938, pp 333–341

Kaltreider DF: Criteria of midplane contraction. Am J Obstet Gynecol 63:392, 1952

Kilian HS: Das Stachelbecken (Acanthopelyx). Mannheim, Schilderungen neuer Beckenfor-men, 1854

Litzmann CCT: Die Formen des Beckens, nebst einem Anhang uber Osteomalacie. Berlin, 1861

Mengert WF: Estimation of pelvic capacity. JAMA 138:169, 1948

Muller: On the frequency and etiology of general pelvic contraction. Arch Gynaek 16:155, 1880

Naegele FC: Das schragverengte Becken. Mainz, 1839

Robert F: Beschreibung eines im hochsten Grade querverengten Beckens. Karlsruhe und Frei-burg, 1842

Speer DP, Peltier LF: Pelvic fractures and preg-nancy. J Trauma 12:474, 1972

Thoms H: The obstetrical significance of pelvic variations: a study of 450 primiparous women. Br Med J 2:210, 1937

32

Dystocia From Other Abnormalities of the Reproductive Tract

VULVAR ABNORMALITIES

Complete *atresia of the vulva* or the lower portion of the vagina is usually congenital and, unless corrected by operative measures, precludes conception. More frequently, vulvar atresia is incomplete, resulting from adhesions or scars following injury or infection. The defect may present a considerable obstacle to delivery but the resistance is usually overcome eventually by the continued pressure exerted by the fetal head, commonly at the cost of deep perineal tears.

Whenever the vulvovaginal outlet is small, rigid, and inelastic, dystocia and extensive lacerations are likely unless prevented by adequate episiotomy. Because of various factors, the vulva may become extremely edematous, but dystocia rarely results from edema alone. Thrombi and hematomas about the vulva, although more common during the puerperium, occasionally form late in pregnancy before or during labor and may give rise to difficulty (see Chap. 36, p. 915). Inflammatory lesions or tumors near the vulva may have a similar effect. Rarely, *condylomata acuminata* may be so extensive as to make vaginal delivery undesirable (see Chap. 25, p. 624), although it can usually be accomplished without extensive lacerations or hemorrhage. The danger of infection is increased, however. *Bartholin cysts* rarely become large enough to contribute to dystocia.

ABNORMALITIES OF THE VAGINA

Complete *vaginal atresia* is nearly always congenital and, unless corrected operatively, forms an effective bar to pregnancy. Incomplete atresia is either a manifestation of faulty development or results from postnatal accidents.

Occasionally, the vagina is divided by a *longitudinal septum,* which may be complete, extending from the vulva to the cervix, or more often incomplete, limited to either the upper or lower portion of the canal. Since such conditions are frequently associated with other abnormalities in development of the genital tract, their detection should always prompt careful examination to ascertain whether there is a coexistent uterine deformity (see Chap. 25, p. 627). A complete longitudinal septum usually does not cause dystocia, since the half of the vagina through which the fetus descends gradually dilates satisfactorily. An incomplete septum, however, occasionally interferes with descent of the head or breech over which the septum may become stretched as a band of varying thickness. Such structures are usually torn through spontaneously but occasionally are sufficiently resistant that either they must be divided or cesarean section must be performed.

Occasionally, the vagina may be obstructed by an *annular stricture* or band of congenital origin. These are unlikely to interfere seriously with delivery, however, since they usually yield before the oncoming head, requiring incision in only extreme cases.

Sometimes the upper portion of the vagina is separated from the rest of the canal by a *transverse septum* with a small opening. Such a stricture is occasionally mistaken for the upper limit of the vaginal vault and, at the time of labor, the opening in the septum is erroneously considered to be an undilated external os. On careful examination, however, the obstetrician can pass a finger through the opening and feel the cervix or on rectal examination can palpate the cervix through the anterior rectal wall above the level of the vaginal septum. After the external os has become completely dilated, the head impinges upon the septum and causes it to bulge downward. If the septum does not yield, slight pressure upon its opening will usually lead to further dilatation, but cruciate incisions may be required occasionally to permit delivery.

Atresia can result from scarring, the consequence of injury or inflammation. Following an infection in which much of the lining of the vagina sloughs, the vaginal lumen during healing may be almost entirely obliterated. Atresia may result from the corrosive action of abortifacients inserted into the vagina. Injuries that lead to extensive scarring, for example the trauma that may ensue during rape of a child by an adult male, may also cause vaginal atresia.

The effects of atresia vary greatly. In most cases, because of the softening of the tissues incident to pregnancy, the obstruction is gradually overcome by the pressure exerted by the presenting part; less often, manual or hydrostatic dilatation or incisions may become necessary. If, however, the structure is so resistant that spontaneous dilatation appears improbable, cesarean section should be performed at the onset of labor.

A *Gartner's duct cyst* may protrude into the vagina and even through the introitus and possibly be confused with a cystocele. A *cystocele* may be managed successfully by emptying the bladder, using a catheter and upward manual pressure on the prolapsed anterior vaginal wall. A Gartner's duct cyst may or may not slip above the presenting part. If not, the cyst may be aspirated aseptically.

Among the rare causes of serious dystocia are *neoplasms* such as *fibroma, carcinoma,* or *sarcoma* arising from the vaginal walls or adjacent structures.

Tetanic contraction of the levator ani, rarely, may seriously interfere with descent of the head. In that condition, analogous to vaginismus in nonpregnant women, a thick, ringlike structure completely encircles and markedly constricts the vagina about midway between the cervix and the vulva. Ordinarily, the obstruction yields under anesthesia.

ABNORMALITIES OF THE CERVIX

Atresia and Stenosis. Complete atresia of the cervix is incompatible with conception. In pregnancy, therefore, complete *cervical atresia* could only occur after conception.

Cicatrical *stenosis of the cervix* may follow extensive cauterization or difficult labor associated with infection and considerable destruction of tissue. For example, of the 10 cases of severe cervical dystocia following treatment of the cervix, reported by Gibbs and Moore (1968), previous conization was responsible in six. Cryotherapy is less likely to produce stenosis. Rarely, cervical stenosis is caused by extensive infiltration by carcinoma or by syphilitic ulceration and induration. Occasionally, it has resulted from corrosives, such as potassium permanganate tablets, used in an attempt to produce abortion. Amputation of the cervix with suturing to effect hemostasis and promote reepithelialization may lead to stenosis, although cervical incompetence is much more likely.

Ordinarily, because of the softening of the tissues during pregnancy, the stenosis gradually yields during labor. In rare instances, however, the stenosis may be so pronounced that dilatation appears improbable, and cesarean section should be employed to effect delivery.

In cases of *conglutination* of the cervical os, the cervical canal at the time of labor undergoes complete obliteration through effacement while the cervical os remains extremely small. Thus the presenting part is separated from the vagina by only a thin layer of cervical tissue. Ordinarily, complete dilatation promptly follows pressure with the fingertip, although in rare instances manual dilatation or cruciate incisions may be required.

Carcinoma of the Cervix. Dystocia may be a consequence of extensive infiltration of the cervix by carcinoma since dilatation is likely to be inadequate even when uterine contractions remain forceful. With lesser involvement, the cervix will usually dilate. The effects of carcinoma of the cervix upon pregnancy and vice versa, as well as appropriate treatment, are discussed in Chapter 25, (p. 626).

UTERINE DISPLACEMENTS

Anteflexion. Marked anteflexion of the enlarging pregnant uterus is usually associated with diastasis recti and a pendulous abdomen (see Chap. 25, p. 632). When the abnormal position of the uterus prevents the proper transmission of the force of the contractions to the cervix, cervical dilatation, as well as engagement of the presenting part, is impeded. Marked improvement may follow maintenance of the uterus in an approxi-

mately normal position by means of a properly fitting abdominal binder.

Retroflexion. As stated in Chapter 25, (p. 632), persistent retroflexion of the pregnant uterus is usually incompatible with advanced pregnancy. If spontaneous or artificial reposition does not occur, the woman either aborts or develops symptoms caused by incarceration of the uterus before the end of the fourth month. In very exceptional instances, however, pregnancy may proceed, in which event the adherent fundus remains applied to the floor of the pelvis, while the anterior wall stretches to accommodate the product of conception. In this condition, known as *sacculation,* the head of the fetus may occupy the displaced fundus, while the cervix is drawn up so high that the external os lies above the upper margin of the symphysis pubis. Consequently, during labor the contractions tend to force the infant through the most dependent portion of the uterus, while the cervix dilates only partially. Spontaneous delivery is thus impossible and rupture of the uterus may occur. For these reasons, cesarean section affords the best method of delivery and at the same time facilitates possible repositioning of the uterus.

PREVIOUS OPERATIVE CORRECTION. Fortunately, operative correction of the retroverted uterus has fallen into disrepute. The one indication may be to bring the retroflexed uterus into the anterior position as part of an operation for extensive pelvic endometriosis. Uterine suspension accomplished by shortening the round ligaments and plicating the uterosacral ligaments does not adversely affect subsequent labor. If, as part of the operation, the bladder was advanced on the anterior wall of the uterus, urinary frequency, as well as bladder discomfort, may be troublesome during pregnancy.

Pregnancy is contraindicated following the Watkins' interposition operation, an operation once performed by some to try to correct a cystocele. Pregnancy after fixation of the fundus of the uterus to the anterior abdominal wall to try to correct either uterine prolapse or uterine retroversion may be complicated by considerable discomfort as the pregnant uterus enlarges. Hopefully, both the Watkins' interposition operation and fixation of the uterus to the abdominal wall have been eliminated from contemporary gynecologic surgery.

Prolapse. Conception rarely occurs with complete uterine prolapse, and term pregnancy in a uterus completely outside the vulva is probably impossible. Naidu (1961), on the basis of a very large experience in India, reported eight cases of prolapse, one of which was complete and complicated by abortion at 22 weeks. Term pregnancy may occur with incomplete prolapse, although abortion is the more frequent outcome. With incomplete prolapse, the fundus after the first trimester occupies the usual position, while the hypertrophied and elongated cervix protrudes from the vagina. (see Chap. 25, p. 633). As a rule, the cervix retracts as pregnancy progresses, and perhaps if aided by a suitable pessary until near term, the danger of infection may be decreased. Occasionally, the cervix may be so edematous and hypertrophied that cesarean section is required for delivery.

OTHER PELVIC TUMORS

Uterine Myomas.   A myoma may be located immediately beneath the endometrial or decidual surface of the uterine cavity *(submucous myoma)*, immediately beneath the uterine serosa *(subserous myoma)*, or be confined to the myometrium *(intramural myoma)*. An intramural myoma, as it grows, may develop a significant subserous or submucous component, or both. Submucous and subserous myomas may, at times, be attached to the uterus by only a stalk *(pedunculated myoma)*.

Similar to the changes that occur in normal myometrium, myomas increase in size appre-

ciably as pregnancy advances and involute remarkably after delivery. Of the three varieties, submucous myomas of prominent size before conception are very likely to exert deleterious effects on the pregnancy. Implantation of the zygote in endometrium overlying a submucous myoma is seldom successful. Even when implantation occurs, subsequent growth and differentiation of a zygote implanted near a submucous myoma often leads to faulty placental implantation and abortion. Rarely, with a submucous myoma, pregnancy may progress to term and then the myoma prolapse through the cervix sometime before, during, or after delivery of the fetus or placenta.

As in the nonpregnant state, pedunculated subserous myomas may undergo torsion with necrosis to the extent that the myoma is detached from the uterus. At times, a subserous myoma may become parasitic, and much or all of its blood is supplied through highly vascularized omentum.

Myomas during pregnancy or the puerperium occasionally undergo "red," or "carneous degeneration" which, in actuality, is *hemorrhagic infarction.* The symptoms and signs of red degeneration are focal pain with tenderness on palpation and sometimes low-grade fever. Moderate leukocytosis is common. On occasion, the parietal peritoneum overlying the infarcted myoma becomes inflamed and a peritoneal "rub" develops. Red degeneration is difficult to differentiate at times from appendicitis, placental abruption, ureteral stone, or pyelonephritis. Treatment consists of analgesia such as codeine. Most often, the signs and symptoms abate within a few days.

Myomas may become infected during the course of puerperal metritis or septic abortion, and are especially likely to do so if the myoma is located immediately adjacent to the placental implantation site or if an instrument such as a sound or curet perforates the myoma. If the myoma is infarcted, the risk of infection is increased and the likelihood of cure of the infection, except by hysterectomy, is reduced.

PROGNOSIS. When compared to the number of women with uterine myomas who conceive, all these complications are quite infrequent. Most often myomas cause little difficulty except perhaps to make the uterus larger than expected from the menstrual history. Dysfunctional labor, entrapment of the placenta above a submucous myoma, and excessive bleeding from the placental implantation site after delivery have all been cited as worrisome complications. On the basis of our experiences at Parkland Memorial Hospital with a large population of black women in whom myomas are common, the complications just mentioned are very infrequent. Concern has been expressed at times about the huge size that might have to be achieved by the myomatous pregnant uterus and its contents. This is no more of a problem than exists when twins or hydramnios is a factor.

Myomas in the cervix or in the lower uterine segment may obstruct labor. Sonograms from such a case and a picture of the uterus are shown in Figure 32-1. A, B, and C. Although this did not occur in the case just described, myomas that lie within or contiguous to the birth canal earlier in pregnancy may be carried upward as the uterus enlarges with relief of obstruction to vaginal delivery. Thus the decision as to the method of delivery usually should not be made before the onset of labor.

MYOMECTOMY. This procedure should be limited to those tumors with discrete pedicles that can be easily clamped and ligated. Otherwise, myomas should not be dissected from the uterus, during pregnancy or delivery, for bleeding may be profuse and at times the uterus may have to be sacrificed. Typically, the myomas will undergo remarkable involution after delivery. In myomas resected during pregnancy or the puerperium there often are bizarre changes in the nuclei of the smooth-muscle cells, changes which may be confused with sarcoma.

The women who has previously undergone myomectomy and has subsequently conceived should be delivered by cesarean section, preferably before active labor has begun, if the myomectomy created a defect through or immediately adjacent to the endometrium.

Benign Ovarian Tumors. Ovarian tumors may be serious complications of pregnancy, may undergo torsion, and may pose insuperable obstacles to vaginal delivery. Moreover, even after spontaneous labor and delivery, they may give rise to disturbances during the puerperium.

Although all varieties of ovarian tumors may complicate pregnancy and labor, the most common are cystic (Fig. 32-2). Beischer and associates (1971) noted that of 164 ovarian tumors diagnosed during pregnancy, one-fourth were cystic teratomas, and one-fourth were mucinous cystadenomas. Four of the 164 (2.4 percent) were malignant. The most frequent and next most serious complication of ovarian cysts during pregnancy is torsion. The incidence of the accident was 12 percent in Booth's series (1963). Torsion is most common in the first trimester. The cyst may rupture and extrude its contents into the peritoneal cavity as the consequence of torsion, or during spontaneous labor, or during surgical removal. This event is not likely to be as devastating with serous cystomas as with dermoid cysts. Rupture of the latter may be followed by serious, even fatal, granulomatous peritonitis. When the tumor blocks the pelvis, it may lead to rupture of the uterus or the tumor may be forced into the vagina, the rectum, or the intervening rectovaginal septum. It seems surprising that spontaneous rupture of an ovarian cystoma is not more common.

An ovarian tumor complicating pregnancy is often entirely unsuspected. Careful examination of all pregnant women should eliminate a large proportion, but not all, of these errors. If an ovarian tumor does not occupy the pelvis, diagnosis through physical examination is especially difficult, since the abdominal enlargement may be attributed to a pregnancy more advanced than indicated by menstrual data, to multiple fetuses, or to hy-

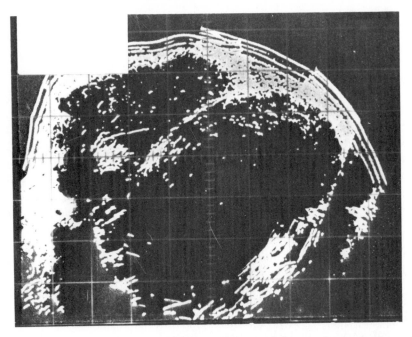

FIG. 32-1. A. Transverse B-scan sonogram of lower abdomen demonstrating a large nearly homogeneous mass which is the myoma shown in Figure 32-1. C. (Courtesy of Dr. R. Santos)

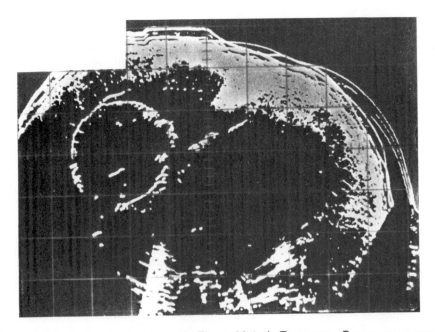

FIG. 32-1. B. Same case as shown in Figure 32-1. A. Transverse B-scan sonogram of upper abdomen demonstrating the fetus.

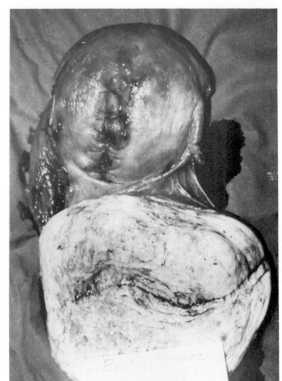

FIG. 32-1. C. Same case as shown in Figures 32-1. A. and B. Cesarean hysterectomy specimen. The upper mass is the body of the uterus that was just emptied by cesarean section. The lower mass is a huge myoma arising low in the uterus and now incised. The infant weighed 3250 g and the uterus with myoma weighed 2900 g. Red degeneration was not found. Delivery 2 years before had also been by cesarean section.

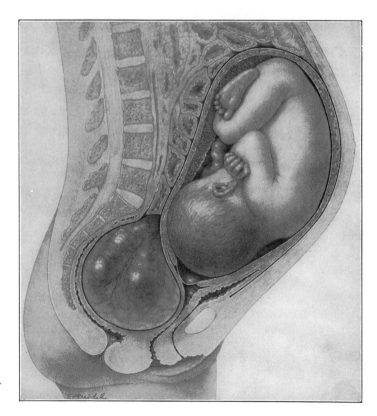

FIG. 32-2. Ovarian cyst producing dystocia.

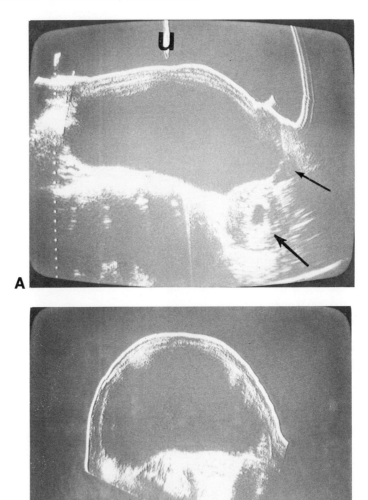

FIG. 32-3. Longitudinal **(A)** and transverse **(B)** sonograms demonstrate a huge cystic mass above the bladder (smaller arrow) and early pregnant uterus (larger arrow). The transverse scan was made at the level of the umbilicus (u). (**A** thru **E,** courtesy of Dr. R. Santos)

dramnios, and the true condition not recognized until after labor. Usually sonography can provide accurate differentiation between uterine enlargement and an extrauterine cystic mass. A dramatic instance is presented in Figure 32-3.

It must be kept in mind that early in pregnancy an ovary may be somewhat enlarged and thus create suspicion of neoplasm. En-

larged ovaries less than 6 cm in diameter are usually increased in size as the consequence of corpus luteum formation as demonstrated elsewhere (see also Fig. 26-8).

In view of the increased incidence of abortion during early pregnancy, the safest time to perform laparotomy is during the fourth month of gestation, provided operation can be postponed until that time. When the diag-

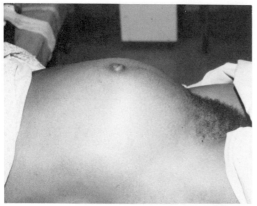

C

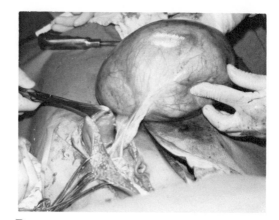

D

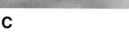

FIG. 32-3. (Cont.) The configuration of the abdomen **(C)** was suggestive of advanced gestation rather than the correct gestational age of 8 weeks. A 3500 g ovarian cyst **(D)** that arose from the tip of the left ovary and incorporated most of the oviduct was readily excised, along with the left tube and ovary, once the incision was extended to near the xiphoid. The external surface of the cyst was free of tumor excrescences. The cyst **(E)** was unilocular as evident in the sonograms.

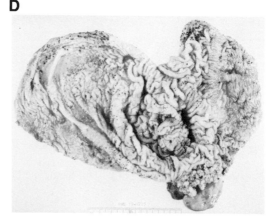

E

nosis is not made until late in pregnancy, it is usually advisable, except in the case of known or suspected malignant tumors, to delay laparotomy to try to avoid delivery of a premature infant. If the ovarian cyst is not impacted, it is preferable usually to permit spontaneous labor and remove the tumor later in the puerperium. If the tumor is impacted in the pelvis, cesarean section should be performed, followed by removal of the tumor if it can be mobilized from behind the uterus.

Carcinoma of the Ovary. Malignant ovarian neoplasms are rare in pregnancy. Only 41 cases were found in a literature survey by Valenti (1960), who along with Amico (1957), believed that the natural course of the disease is uninfluenced by pregnancy. If the tumor is discovered at the time of laparotomy or if the disease is widespread, the treatment should be the same as in the nonpregnant patient. In some circumstances it is justifiable to remove the tumor and allow the pregnancy to continue when a few more weeks would assure viability of the delivered infant. Even then, delivery should usually be by cesarean section, with decision regarding further surgery and chemotherapy based on the results of clinical and histologic examination.

Pelvic Masses of Other Origin. Labor may be obstructed by pelvic masses of various origins sufficiently large to render delivery difficult or even impossible. A *distended bladder,* with or without a cystocele, may obstruct delivery, as demonstrated in Figure 32-4. A large *cystocele* or *rectocele,* though occasionally offering slight obstacle to labor, can generally

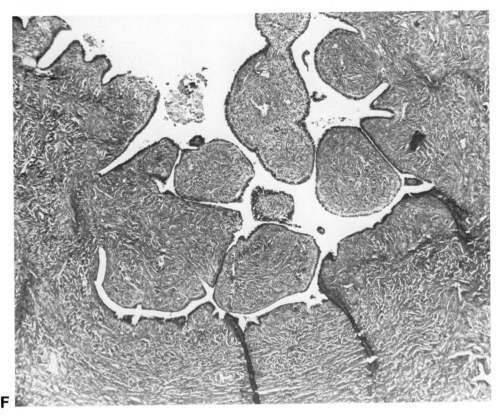

FIG. 32-3. (Cont.) The histologic diagnosis **(F)** was serous cystadenofibroma.

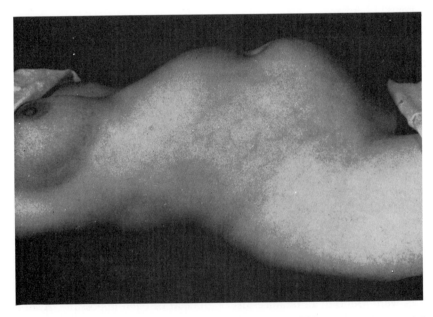

FIG. 32-4. Dystocia caused by distention of the bladder. This woman was sent to the hospital after 3 days of ineffectual labor at home. The cervix was thought to have been completely dilated for 24 hours. After catheterization of the greatly distended bladder, which yielded over 1000 ml of urine, the baby's head descended at once and delivery was accomplished easily.

be replaced during delivery. Tumors of the bladder may impede passage of the fetus though rarely seriously enough to require operative delivery. *Pelvic ectopic kidney* is a rare complication of pregnancy. Such a kidney may block the birth canal and sustain injury during passage of the fetus. Most of these women will deliver vaginally without hazard, but if the kidneys are entirely intrapelvic, abdominal delivery is safer.

In rare instances, an enlarged spleen may prolapse into the pelvic cavity and obstruct labor. Echinococcal cysts have been found in the pelvis. An old extrauterine gestation may obstruct the pelvic canal, interfering with the delivery of a subsequent intrauterine fetus. An *enterocele* rarely gives rise to dystocia. The herniated intestine can usually be replaced and the obstacle temporarily overcome, but when reduction is impossible, cesarean section is a safer procedure than is forcing the fetus over a large irreducible hernia. Tumors or inflammation arising from the lower part of the rectum or pelvic connective tissue also may give rise to dystocia.

REFERENCES

Amico JC: Pregnancy complicated by primary carcinoma of the ovary. Am J Obstet Gynecol 74:920, 1957

Beischer NA, Buttery BW, Fortune DW, Macafee CAJ: Growth and malignancy of ovarian tumours in pregnancy. Aust NZ J Obstet Gynaecol 11:208, 1971

Booth RT: Ovarian tumors in pregnancy. Obstet Gynecol 21:189, 1963

Gibbs CE, Moore SF: The scarred cervix in pregnancy and labor. Gen Pract 37:85, 1968

Naidu PM: Prolapse of the uterus complicating pregnancy and labour: A report of 8 cases. Br J Obstet Gynaecol 68:1041, 1961

Valenti C: On carcinoma of the ovary in pregnancy. Minerva Ginecol 9:4, 1960

33

Injuries to the Birth Canal

INJURIES TO THE PELVIC FLOOR AND VAGINA

Perineal Lacerations. All except the most superficial perineal lacerations are accompanied by varying degrees of injury to the lower portion of the vagina. Such tears may reach sufficient depth to involve the rectal sphincter and may extend to varying depths through the walls of the vagina. Bilateral lacerations into the vagina are usually unequal in length and separated by a tongue-shaped portion of vaginal mucosa (see Chap. 17, Figs. 17 and 19). Their repair should form part of every operation for the restoration of a lacerated perineum. Suturing of just the external integuments without approximation of underlying perineal and vaginal fascia and muscle will lead to relaxation of the vaginal outlet and may contribute to rectocele and cystocele formation, as well as uterine prolapse.

Vaginal Lacerations. Isolated lacerations involving the middle or upper third of the vagina but unassociated with lacerations of the perineum or cervix are less commonly observed. Vaginal lacerations in this location are usually longitudinal, resulting from injuries sustained during a forceps operation, though occasionally they accompany spontaneous delivery. Such lacerations frequently extend deeply into the underlying tissues and may give rise to copious hemorrhage, which, however, is usually readily controlled by appropriate suturing. They may be overlooked unless thorough inspection of the upper vagina is performed or at least careful attention is paid to bleeding from the genital tract in the presence of a firmly contracted uterus. *Bleeding while the uterus is firmly contracted is strong evidence of genital tract lacerations, retained placental fragments, or both.*

Lacerations of the anterior vaginal wall in close proximity to the urethra are relatively common. If superficial and not bleeding, repair is not indicated; otherwise, hemostasis necessitates their closure. If such lacerations are extensive, difficulty in voiding can be anticipated and an indwelling catheter placed.

Injuries to Levator Ani. Injuries to the levator ani as a result of overdistension of the birth canal may result in the separation of muscular fibers or in the diminution in their tonicity sufficient to interfere with the function of the pelvic diaphragm. In such cases, the woman eventually may develop pelvic relaxation. If these injuries involve the pubococcygeus muscle, urinary incontinence may supervene. The likelihood of such injuries is minimized by appropriate episiotomy.

INJURIES TO THE CERVIX

Etiology.   Traumatic lesions of the upper third of the vagina are uncommon by themselves but are often associated with extensions of deep cervical tears. In rare instances, however, the cervix may be entirely or partially avulsed from the vagina, with colporrhexis in the anterior, posterior, or lateral fornices. Such lesions usually follow difficult forceps deliveries performed through an incompletely dilated cervix and the forceps blades applied over the cervix. The cervical tears may extend to involve the lower uterine segment and uterine artery and its major branches, and even through the peritoneum. Fortunately, such extensive traumatic lesions are rare in modern obstetric practice. They may be totally unsuspected, but much more often they become manifest by excessive external hemorrhage or by the formation of a retroperitoneal hematoma. These extensive tears of the vaginal vault should be carefully explored. If there is the slightest question of perforation of the peritoneum, or of retroperitoneal or intraperitoneal hemorrhage, laparotomy should be performed. In the presence of damage of this severity, intrauterine exploration for possible rupture is, of course, also mandatory. Whereas formerly treatment of these lacerations by packing was recommended, *often with poor outcome,* surgical repair is much more satisfactory. Effective anesthesia, vigorous blood replacement, and capable assistance are mandatory for a satisfactory outcome.

Cervical lacerations up to 2 cm must be regarded as inevitable in childbirth. Such tears, however, heal rapidly and rarely are the source of any difficulty. In healing, they cause a significant change in the shape of the external os from round in shape before cervical effacement and dilatation to appreciably elongated laterally after delivery and recovery from effacement and dilatation.

In a minority of cases, the tears are much deeper, involving one or both sides of the cervix and possibly extending up to or beyond the vaginal junction. In rarer instances, the laceration may extend across the vaginal fornix or into the lower uterine segment or the broad ligament. Such extensive lesions frequently involve vessels of considerable size and are then associated with profuse hemorrhage.

Deep cervical tears occasionally occur during the course of spontaneous labor. In such circumstances, their genesis is not always clear. Such tears most often result, however, from traumatic deliveries through an incompletely dilated cervix.

Occasionally, during labor the edematous anterior lip of the cervix may be caught and compressed between the head and the symphysis pubis. If ischemia is severe, the cervical lip may undergo necrosis and separation. In still rarer instances, the entire vaginal portion may be avulsed from the rest of the cervix. Such *annular* or *circular detachment of the cervix* probably occurs only in neglected labors or in pregnant women receiving supraphysiologic doses of oxytocin.

In all traumatic lesions involving the cervix, there is usually no appreciable bleeding until after birth of the infant, when hemorrhage may be profuse. Slight cervical tears heal spontaneously. Extensive lacerations have a similar tendency, but perfect union rarely results. As the consequence of such tears, eversion of the cervix with exposure of the delicate mucus-producing endocervical glands is frequently the cause of persistent leukorrhea. If the leukorrhea persists after the puerperium, treatment with cautery or cryotherapy is usually beneficial. If a Papanicolaou smear has not been obtained during pregnancy, it should be obtained and the results reviewed before treatment is initiated.

Diagnosis.   A deep cervical tear should always be suspected in cases of profuse hem-

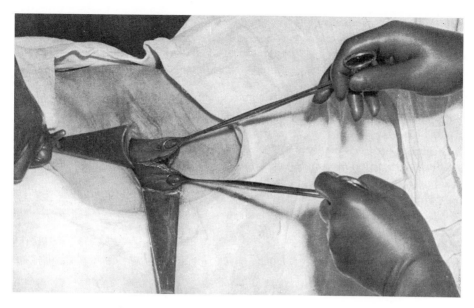

FIG. 33-1.   Cervical laceration exposed for repair.

orrhage during and after the third stage of labor, particularly if the uterus is firmly contracted. For a definitive diagnosis to be made, however, a thorough examination is necessary. Because of the flabbiness of the cervix immediately after delivery, digital examination alone is often unsatisfactory. The extent of the injury can be fully appreciated only after adequate exposure and visual inspection of the cervix.

In view of the frequency with which deep tears follow major operative procedures, the cervix should be inspected routinely at the conclusion of the third stage after all difficult deliveries, even if there is no bleeding. Annular detachment of the vaginal portion of the cervix should be suspected whenever an irregular mass of tissue with a circular central opening is cast off before or after birth of the infant.

Treatment.   Deep cervical tears should be repaired immediately. Treatment varies with the extent of the lesion. When the laceration is limited to the cervix, or even when it extends somewhat into the vaginal fornix, satisfactory results are obtained by suturing the cervix after bringing it into view at the vulva. Visualization is best accomplished when an *assistant* makes firm downward pressure on the uterus while the operator exerts traction on the lips of the cervix with fenestrated ovum or sponge forceps. The vaginal walls are held apart with retractors manipulated with aid of the assistant (Fig. 33-1). Since the hemorrhage usually comes from the upper angle of the wound, it is advisable to apply the first suture at the angle and suture outward. Interrupted chromic catgut sutures should be employed, since they do not have to be removed. The beginner is cautioned against overzealous suturing to try to restore the normal appearance of the cervix, for involution during the following few days may lead to stenosis.

RUPTURE OF THE UTERUS

Frequency.   It is apparent from the tabulations provided by Schrinsky and Benson (1978) that the incidence of rupture of the uterus varies appreciably among institutions, ranging from one in 100 deliveries to one in 11,000. While the frequency of uterine rupture from all causes probably has not decreased remarkably during the past several decades, the etiology of rupture has changed appreciably and the outcome has improved significantly.

Etiology. Currently, the most common cause of rupture is previous cesarean section and the next most common is probably stimulation of labor with oxytocin. Generally, the previously untraumatized, spontaneously laboring uterus will not persist in contracting so vigorously as to destroy itself.

An extensive classification of the etiology of rupture of the gravid uterus is presented below:

1. Uterine injury before current pregnancy
    Surgery involving myometrium
        Cesarean section or hysterotomy
        Repaired previous uterine rupture
        Myomectomy incision close to or through endometrium
        Deep cornual resection to remove interstitial oviduct
        Excision of uterine septum (metroplasty)
    Coincidental trauma to uterus
        Instrumented abortion (sounds, curets, or other devices)
        Sharp or blunt trauma (accidents, knives, bullets)
        Silent rupture during previous pregnancy
2. Uterine injury during current pregnancy
    Before delivery
        Persistent, intense, spontaneous contractions
        Oxytocin or prostaglandin administration
        Hypertonic solution injected intraamnionically
        Perforation by monitor catheter
        External trauma, sharp or blunt
        Marked uterine overdistention (multiple fetuses, hydramnios)
    During delivery
        Internal podalic version
        Difficult forceps delivery

        Breech extraction
        Fetal anomaly overdistending lower segment
        Vigorous fundal pressure
        Difficult manual removal of placenta
3. Uterine defects not necessarily related to trauma
    Congenital
        Pregnancy in incompletely developed uterus or uterine horn
    Acquired
        Placenta increta or percreta
        Invasive mole or choriocarcinoma
        Adenomyosis
        Sacculation of adherent retroverted uterus

Definitions. It is customary to distinguish between *complete* and *incomplete* rupture of the uterus, depending on whether the laceration communicates directly with the peritoneal cavity, or is separated from it by the visceral peritoneum over the uterus or that of the broad ligament. An incomplete rupture may, of course, become complete at any instant.

It is important to differentiate between *rupture of a cesarean section scar* and *dehiscence of a cesarean section scar.* Rupture refers, at the minimum, to separation of the old uterine incision throughout most of its length with rupture of the fetal membranes so that the uterine cavity and the peritoneal cavity communicate. In these circumstances, all or part of the fetus is usually extruded into the peritoneal cavity. In addition, there is usually bleeding, often massive, from the edges of the scar or from an extension of the rent into previously univolved uterine wall. Dehiscence of a cesarean section scar differs from rupture in that the fetal membranes are not ruptured and therefore the fetus is not extruded into the uterine cavity. Typically, with dehiscence the separation does not involve all of the previous uterine scar, and bleeding is absent or minimal. Dehiscence occurs gradually whereas ruptures are very likely to be symptomatic and, at times, fatal. With labor or intrauterine manipulations, a dehiscence may become a rupture.

Comparison of Classical and Lower-Segment Cesarean Section Scars.

The behavior of a classical scar, that is, a uterine incision through the body of the pregnant uterus rather than the lower uterine segment, in any subsequent pregnancy differs from that of a scar confined to the lower uterine segment. First, the probability of rupture of a classical scar is several times greater than that of a lower segment scar. Second, if a classical scar does rupture, the accident takes place before labor in about one-third of the cases. Rupture not infrequently takes place several weeks before term, before a cesarean section is ordinarily scheduled. In fact, Lazarus (1978) described disruption of a previous classical cesarean section scar at 12 weeks gestation with marked hemorrhage and hypovolemia. Therefore, delivery by subsequent cesarean section cannot prevent such ruptures. Lower-segment scars *that are confined to the noncontractile portion of the uterus rarely,* if ever, rupture before labor, and only infrequently do so during labor. Thus the policy of repeating cesarean sections very near term or early in labor would not be expected to lead to frequent uterine rupture.

The statistics available are insufficient to permit a precise calculation of the maternal mortality rate that attends rupture of a cesarean section scar. It is probably less than 5 percent, but the perinatal mortality rate is probably 50 percent or more.

Dehiscence of a lower-segment cesarean section scar is much more frequent than actual rupture, especially if the previous uterine incision was transverse. It is remarkable that these separated scars, covered only by the peritoneum, in many instances appear to cause no difficulty in labor or subsequently. Their frequency, however, and the possible associated risk, lend support to the dictum, "Once a cesarean, always a cesarean."

RUPTURE OF CESAREAN SECTION SCAR

Experiences at Parkland Memorial Hospital.

The experience at this institution has been that antepartum and during early labor separation of the low transverse uterine incision is almost always limited to dehiscence without an appreciable increase in maternal or perinatal morbidity. Separation of a vertical scar, however, is more likely to result in severe hemorrhage with an increased perinatal morbidity and mortality.

In one sample of 354 cases, in the great majority of which the previous uterine incision was of the low transverse variety, 211, or 60 percent, were considered to be in labor at the time of repeat cesarean section. There were two instances of uterine dehiscence and one of rupture of the scar. One dehiscence involved a previous low transverse uterine incision. The dehiscence was extended to effect delivery of the healthy infant and then the uterus was closed without much difficulty, using two layers of continuous chromic catgut. In the second case, the dehiscence of the low vertical incision was not repaired. Instead, cesarean hysterectomy was performed to comply with the woman's request for sterilization. In the one case of uterine rupture, a defect believed to be uterine was felt suprapubically during a uterine contraction. With her last two cesarean sections, a vertical uterine incision was made that apparently included some of the upper segment. At laparotomy, the separated vertical scar was covered by a hematoma of about 400 ml that was entrapped beneath the serosa and overlying adherent omentum. Blood had also infiltrated throughout the left broad ligament to the lateral wall of the pelvis. An infant who weighted 2950 g, with an Apgar score of 8 at 5 minutes, was delivered through the ruptured scar. Hysterectomy was performed with some difficulty because of dense adhesions (Fig. 33-2).

Another woman, in whom the cervix was fully dilated and the occiput at +2 station when she was admitted to the Labor-Delivery Unit, was promptly delivered using forceps, although she had previously undergone cesarean section. Immediate exploration of the uterus was conducted, as should be done in every case of previous cesarean section. Extensive separation of the vertical cesarean sec-

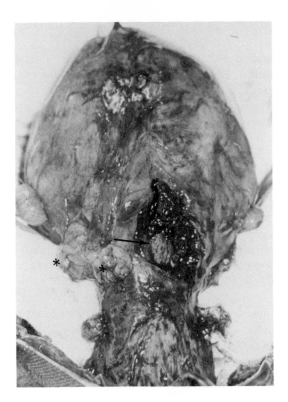

FIG. 33-2. Ruptured vertical cesarean section scar (arrow) identified at time of repeat cesarean section early in labor; asterisks indicate some of the sites of densely adherent omentum.

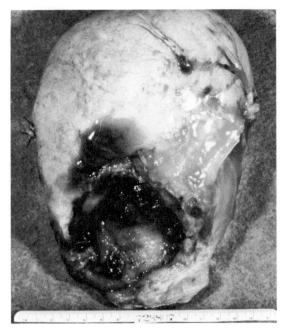

FIG. 33-3. Rupture of uterus identified immediately after vaginal delivery; the previous delivery was by cesarean section with a vertical uterine incision.

tion scar with appreciable hemorrhage was identified and the uterus was removed (Fig. 33-3). Both mother and infant survived.

Healing of the Cesarean Section Scar. Little information on this subject has been garnered from studies of cesarean section scars. Williams (1921) believed that the uterus heals by regeneration of the muscular fibers and not by scar tissue formation. He based his conclusion on the findings of histologic examination of the site of the incision

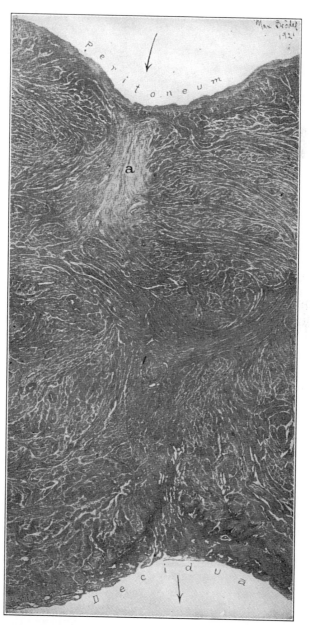

FIG. 33-4. Ideal healing of cesarean section scar. Scar tissue at a.

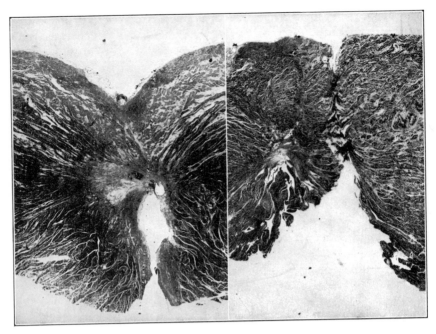

FIG. 33-5. Photomicrographs of two poorly healed cesarean section scars.

and on two principal observations: First, upon inspection of the unopened uterus at the time of repeated cesarean sections one usually finds no trace of the former incision or, at most, an almost invisible linear scar. Second, when the uterus is removed, often no scar is visible after fixation, or only a shallow vertical furrow in the external and internal surfaces of the anterior uterine wall is seen, with no trace of scar tissue between them. Schwarz and co-workers (1938), however, concluded that healing occurs mainly by the proliferation of fibroblasts. They studied the site of the incision in the human uterus some days after cesarean section, as well as in the uteri of guinea pigs, rabbits, and dogs, and they observed that as the scar shrinks, the proliferation of connective tissue becomes less obvious. Their conclusions appear to be justified by their histologic studies, particularly in cases of adequate approximation of the myometrial edges (Fig. 33-4). If the cut surfaces are closely apposed, the proliferation of connective tissue is minimal, and the normal relation of smooth muscle to connective tissue is gradually reestablished, accounting for the

occasional absence of even a trace of a former incision. Even when the healing is so poor that marked thinning has resulted, the remaining tissue is often entirely muscular (Fig. 33-5). The fundamental weakness appears to stem from failure to approximate the inner margins of the incision or from formation of a hematoma or abscess in the immediate vicinity.

Delivery Subsequent to a Cesarean Section. In most American clinics, previous cesarean section has been the most common indication for cesarean section. Recently, however, women often request and receive sterilization after delivery of their second infant and others are delivered vaginally even though previously delivered by cesarean section. As a consequence of this, the number of repeat cesarean sections relative to primary sections has decreased appreciably.

As will be pointed out in Chapter 43, in case of nonrecurrent cause for cesarean section, the general dictum "Once a cesarean section, always a cesarean" has been followed

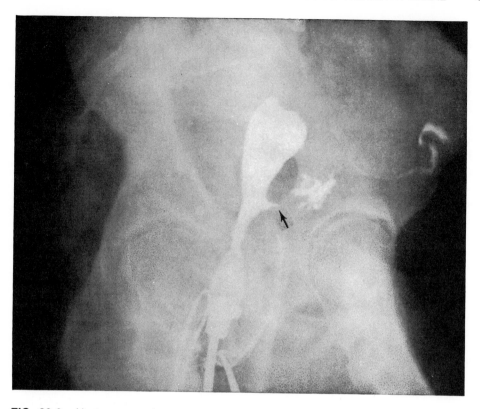

FIG. 33-6. Hysterogram showing defect in lower uterine segment following cesarean section.

by the majority of obstetricians in this country. The reverse appears to be true in several other countries, although Sir Norman Jeffcoate of the University of Liverpool, in delivering the Lloyd Roberts Lecture in Manchester, England, expressed increased concern about the reliability of the previous cesarean section scar. As the consequence of careful analyses of the fate of the scar in subsequent pregnancies, about two-thirds of such cases more recently were being delivered in his units by elective repeat cesarean section, compared to one-fifth earlier. He and his colleagues reemphasize that the quality of the scar *cannot* be forecast with any certainty from the presence or absence of puerperal morbidity postoperatively, or of pain and tenderness over the uterine scar before or during labor (Case et al., 1971).

Weaknesses of the scar may be detected sometimes by hysterography in the nonpreg-

nant state, as shown in Figure 33-6 and emphasized again by Beyth (1978). The accuracy of the procedure has not been established. We emphasize that neither radiologic examination nor any clinical findings, such as the women's course following the first operation, the location of the placenta in the present pregnancy, the type of previous operation or incision, the skill of the previous operator, or even the fact of an intervening vaginal delivery, provide incontrovertible proof of the integrity of a uterine scar under the stress of labor.

The difficulties inherent in formulating an inflexible policy concerning the mode of delivery after cesarean section are obvious. Although there is a greater tendency toward individualization in the United States today, most women with cesarean section scars are delivered again by cesarean section. If the previous cesarean section was performed because of pelvic contraction, cesarean section is repeated, of course, because the previous indication still exists. In general, gravidas who have undergone two or more previous sections of any type should also be delivered abdominally. Women with a previous classic cesarean section also should have the cesarean section repeated unless perhaps they go into labor at a time when the fetus is quite immature. The current concern for "fewer but better babies" leads to the avoidance of all unnecessary risks.

Merrill and Gibbs (1978) carefully analyzed the benefits and detriments from planned vaginal delivery following cesarean section among the women who were delivered at their large public institution. A trial of labor was allowed if the woman was known to have had previously a single low transverse cesarean section and if there were no recurring overt contraindications to labor or vaginal delivery. Oxytocin stimulation was used, if needed, as long as there were no other recognized contraindications to its use.

Of 634 women who had but one previous low transverse cesarean section, 526 (83 percent) were allowed a test of labor, 313 of

the 526 (60 percent) who labored were delivered vaginally. Few problems were encountered among the mothers and infants so delivered. One of the two ruptured uteri was removed; the other was repaired and tubal sterilization was performed. Hospital stay was reduced, compared to that of women who underwent scheduled repeat cesarean section.

Of the 213 women (40 percent) who labored unsuccessfully and then underwent cesarean section, one had a ruptured uterus. Because of the increased frequency and intensity of infection when cesarean section was performed after labor, postpartum stay commonly was prolonged, compared to that for women who underwent cesarean section without having labored. While Merrill and Gibbs concluded that there were economic benefits from this approach, they did not appear to have included in their cost accounting the extra staffing and intense monitoring that were provided during labor and delivery.

Figure 33-7 shows those factors that are considered at Parkland Memorial Hospital in deciding on the method of delivery of the woman whose previous pregnancy was terminated by cesarean section. A previous vertical incision is an indication for repeat cesarean section because almost always such an incision is made only when extra length is needed over that obtainable with a low transverse uterine incision. Thus the vertical incision most likely did extend well into the body of the uterus. If the previous transverse incision extended into the lateral large vessels, or if tearing or deliberate cutting resulted in a T-shaped or J-shaped incision, repeat cesarean section is performed. If sterilization is requested, the combined procedure of cesarean section and partial tubal resection is carried out. The great majority of women, according to this schema, qualify for repeat cesarean section.

An occult rupture discovered at a subsequent cesarean section does not require hysterectomy, for usually the edges of the scar may be reapproximated with good healing of the new wound.

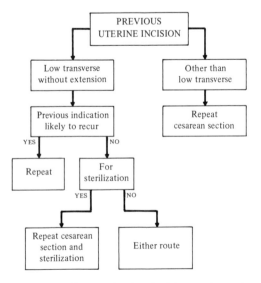

FIG. 33-7. Factors in the decision as to route of delivery following previous cesarean section.

RUPTURE OF THE UNSCARRED UTERUS

Traumatic Rupture. The uterus is surprisingly resistant to blunt trauma. Nonetheless, pregnant women sustaining blunt trauma to the abdomen should be watched carefully for signs of ruptured uterus, although the experiences at Parkland Memorial Hospital have been that rupture of the spleen or traumatic placental abruption, while rare, are relatively more common. Wounds that penetrate the abdomen are much more likely to involve the large pregnant uterus.

Unfortunately, administration of oxytocin in the first or second stage of labor has been a rather common cause of traumatic rupture, especially in women of high parity (Awais, Lebherz, 1970). In the past, traumatic rupture during delivery was produced most commonly by internal podalic version and extraction. Other causes of traumatic rupture include difficult forceps delivery, breech extraction (Figs. 33-8 and 33-9), and unusual fetal enlargement, such as hydrocephalus. Ruptured uterus caused by strong fundal pressure to try to accomplish vaginal delivery is particularly reprehensible.

Spontaneous Rupture of Uterus.

This catastrophe is more likely to occur in women of high parity. For this reason, oxytocin should rarely be given to undelivered women of high parity. Similarly, in women of high parity a trial of labor in the presence of cephalopelvic disproportion, or abnormal presentation such as a brow, may prove dangerous not only to the fetus but also to the mother.

PATHOLOGIC ANATOMY. The role in uterine rupture of excessive stretching of the lower uterine segment with the development of a pathologic retraction ring was stressed in Chapter 29 (p. 795). Rupture of the previously intact uterus at the time of labor most often involves the thinned-out lower uterine segment. The rent, when it is in the immediate vicinity of the cervix, frequently extends transversely or obliquely. Usually, the tear is longitudinal, however, when it occurs in the portion of the uterus adjacent to the broad ligament (Fig. 33-9). Although developing primarily in the lower uterine segment, it is not unusual for the laceration to extend farther upward into the body of the uterus or downward through the cervix into the vagina. At times, the bladder may also be lacerated. After complete rupture, the uterine contents escape into the peritoneal cavity, unless the presenting part is firmly engaged when only a portion of the fetus may escape.

Incomplete ruptures frequently extend into the broad ligament. In such circumstances, the hemorrhage tends to be less rapid than in the complete variety, the blood accumulating between the leaves with the formation of a large retroperitoneal hematoma that may involve sufficient blood loss to cause death. More frequently, fatal exsanguination supervenes after secondary rupture of the hematoma relieves the tamponading effect of the intact broad ligament. With incomplete rupture, the products of conception may remain within the uterus or assume a position between the leaves of the broad ligament.

Apparent spontaneous rupture of the uterus at times follows manipulations that may very well have caused unappreciated injury to the uterus. Two cases at Parkland Memorial Hospital fall in this category. In one, the previous pregnancy terminated with a septic abortion. At laparotomy following rupture of the uterus, omentum was adherent to the fundus at the site of uterine rupture, strongly suggesting that previous perforation of the uterus had occurred. In the other, vigorous curettage followed delivery of a hydatidiform mole and histologically myometrial fragments were identified. With this woman's next pregnancy, the uterus ruptured early in labor, the left uterine artery was severed, and rapid exsanguination followed. Taylor and Cummings (1979) described spontaneous rupture of the uterus of a primigravid woman before the onset of labor. The uterine fundus had been traumatized previously by a trocar inserted for laparoscopy.

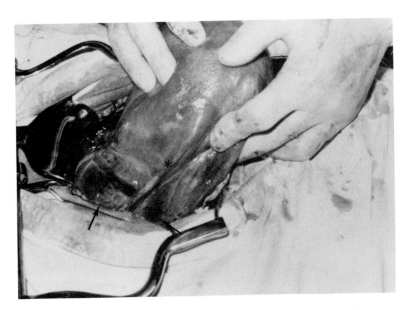

FIG. 33-8. A. Rupture of uterus with breech delivery; extensive bleeding beneath uterine serosa and bladder, and in left broad ligament (arrows). Asterisk identifies left round ligament.

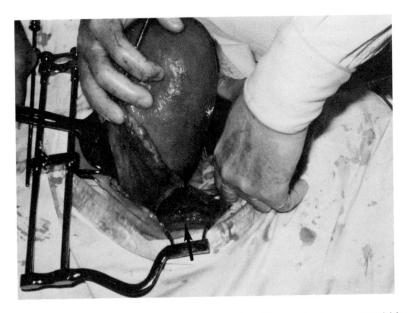

FIG. 33-8. B. The broad ligament has been opened and the ureter (upper arrow) identified medial to the iliac vessels (lower arrow).

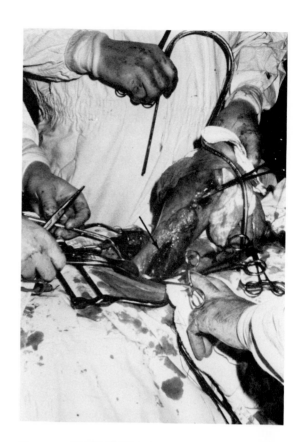

FIG. 33-8. C. Extent of rupture (arrow) of lateral wall of uterus is now apparent.

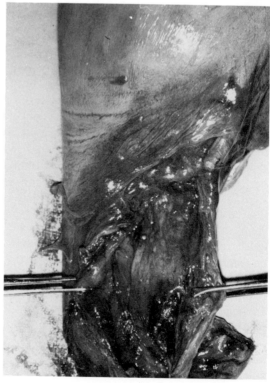

FIG. 33-9. Close-up view of resected uterus to show site of rupture observed in Figure 33-8.

Instances of uterine rupture have been observed in which hemorrhage was slight. The rupture did not involve large arteries and the emptied uterus contracted well after expulsion of the fetus and placenta into the peritoneal cavity. In very rare cases, the fetus may be extruded into the peritoneal cavity while the placenta remains functional within the uterus and the gestation continues as a *uteroabdominal pregnancy* (Badawy, 1962).

Clinical Course. Prior to circulatory collapse from hemorrhage, the symptoms and physical findings may appear bizarre unless the possibility of rupture of the uterus is kept in mind. As an example, a woman was recently transferred to Parkland Memorial Hospital near term with the diagnosis of pulmonary embolism. She stated that she had been treated for such following a previous pregnancy. She complained of pain on inspiration and shortness of breath, as well as abdominal pain thought to be labor. The symptoms directed to the chest were not the consequence of an embolus, however, but rather of hemoperitoneum from a ruptured uterus with blood irritating the diaphragm and causing the pain referred to the chest (see Chap. 22, p. 535).

If the accident occurs during labor, the woman, usually after a period of premonitory signs, at the acme of a uterine contraction, suddenly complains of a sharp, shooting pain in the abdomen and may cry out that "something ripped" or "something tore" inside her. Immediately after these symptoms and signs have appeared, there is cessation of uterine contractions, and the woman very recently in intense agony, suddenly experiences much relief. At the same time, there may be external hemorrhage, although it is often slight.

Since women who are in labor or who are being delivered are usually given analgesics, pain and tenderness may not be immediately evident, and the condition becomes manifest by the systemic effects of the hypovolemia.

If the fetus is partly or totally extrauterine, abdominal palpation or vaginal examination is helpful in identifying the presenting part which has moved away from the pelvic inlet. A firm, rounded body, the contracted uterus, may, at times, be felt alongside the fetus. Often fetal parts are more easily palpated than usual. On vaginal examination, sometimes a tear in the uterine wall can be palpated through which the fingers can be passed into the peritoneal cavity, where the viscera may be felt. *Failure to detect the tear by no means proves its absence.* In suspected cases, it is imperative that thorough examination be performed by an experienced examiner before the suspicion is abandoned. At times, either abdominal paracentesis in the flank or culdocentesis is indicated to identify hemoperitoneum. After delivery, culdocentesis can be performed through the posterior fornix into the cul-de-sac. The posterior lip of the cervix is grasped and a long 15-gauge needle is inserted beneath it through the fornix while the cervix is lifted anteriorly.

Prognosis. The chances for fetal survival are dismal; the mortality rates found in various studies ranged between 50 and 75 percent. However, if the fetus is alive at the time of the accident, the only chance of continued survival is afforded by immediate delivery, most often by laparotomy. Otherwise, hypoxia from both the separation of the placenta and maternal hypovolemia, is inevitable. If untreated, most of the women die from hemorrhage or less often later from infection, although spontaneous recovery has been noted in exceptional cases. Prompt diagnosis, immediate operation, the availability of large amounts of blood, and antibiotic therapy have improved greatly the prognosis for women with rupture of the pregnant uterus.

Immediate Treatment. The life of the woman will depend most often on the speed and efficiency with which hypovolemia can be corrected and hemorrhage controlled. Whenever rupture of the uterus is diagnosed, it is mandatory that immediately and simultaneously the following functions be carried out: (1) two effective intravenous infusion systems must be established, and lactated Ringer's solution or similar electrolyte-containing solutions are started; (2) compatible, or at least type-specific, whole blood, must be obtained in large quantities (3 liters to start), and it must be infused vigorously as soon as possible; (3) a surgical team, including an anesthesiologist, must be assembled. The hypovolemia may not be correctable until arterial bleeding has been brought under control surgically. Therefore, delay in operating is contraindicated. Instead, blood must be infused vigorously and the laparotomy is begun. In desperate cases, compression applied to the aorta may help to reduce the bleeding. Oxytocin administered intravenously may incite contraction of the myometrium and, in turn, vessel constriction, thereby reducing the bleeding. Clamping the ovarian vessels immediately adjacent to the uterus will help to conserve blood. Technics for monitoring the adequacy of the circulation, blood and blood-fraction replacement therapy, and the recognition and treatment of coagulation defects are considered in detail in Chapter 21.

HYSTERECTOMY VERSUS REPAIR. Hysterectomy is usually required, but in highly selected cases suture of the wound may be performed.

As part of the overall problem of rupture of the uterus, Mokgokong and Marivate (1976), based on a review of 335 cases treated in Durban, South Africa, considered the merits of hysterectomy compared to suture of the laceration. Maternal mortality was 7 percent and fetal mortality was 80 percent. Three-fourths of the cases involved women with previously unscarred uteri. Common specific causes of rupture of the previously unscarred uterus were cephalopelvic disproportion, fetal malpresentation, obstetric instrumentation, oxytocin stimulation, and internal podalic version. The uterine tears were usually longitudinal and lateral, often involving the uterine artery or its major branches.

They concluded that total hysterectomy, especially with longitudinal tears, is the surgical procedure of choice, although transverse lower segment lacerations may be dealt with adequately by repair of the rent. The frequency of subsequent successful pregnancies following repair of the rent was not provided.

Sheth (1968) reported the findings in a series of 66 cases in which repair of a uterine rupture was elected rather than hysterectomy. In 25 instances, the repair was accompanied by tubal sterilization. Thirteen of the 41 mothers who did not have tubal sterilization had a total of 21 subsequent pregnancies, but uterine rupture recurred in four instances.

In the presence of a large hematoma in the broad ligament, identification and ligation of the uterine vessels can be extremely difficult. In general, efforts to control hemorrhage by clamping indiscriminately at the site of rupture involving the lower segment, should be avoided. To do otherwise often leads to clamping and ligation of the ureter, bladder, or both. With uterine ruptures involving the lower segment, bleeding vessels must be visualized free of surrounding tissue and before clamping or the ureter and bladder must be demonstrated to be remote from the tissue that is clamped. Placement of clamps to control bleeding carries little risk when rupture involves the body of the uterus remote from the ureters and bladder. The broad ligament may be entered and the ascending uterine artery and veins safely clamped. Usually, the ovarian vessels should be promptly clamped adjacent to the uterus.

Ligation of the hypogastric arteries may reduce the hemorrhage appreciably. The ligation is accomplished by opening the peritoneum over the common iliac artery and dissecting down to the bifurcation of the external iliac and hypogastric arteries. The areolar sheath covering the hypogastric artery is incised longitudinally and a right-angle clamp is carefully passed just beneath the artery. Care must be taken not to perforate contiguous large veins. Suture, usually nonabsorbable, is then inserted into the open

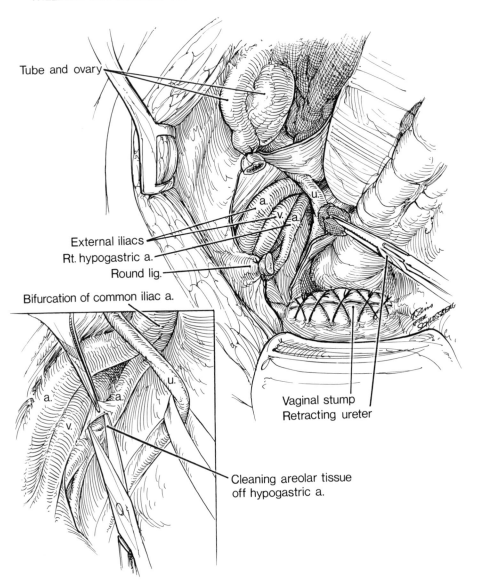

FIG. 33-10. Ligation of the right hypogastric artery. The areolar sheath covering the artery is being opened *(lower left)* (a. = artery, v. = vein, u. = ureter, lig. = ligament, rt. = right).

clamp, the jaws are locked, the suture is carried around the vessel, and the vessel is securely ligated (Figs. 33-10, 33-11). Pulsations in the external iliac artery, if present before tying the ligature, should be present afterward as well. If not, pulsations must be identified after arterial hypotension has been successfully combated in order to assure that the blood flow through the external iliac vessel has not been compromised. An important mechanism of action with hypogastric ligation, apparently, is reduction of pulse pressure in those arteries distal to the ligation. It is of interest that bilateral ligation of the hypogastric arteries per se does not appear to interfere seriously with subsequent reproduction. Mengert and associates (1969) documented successful pregnancies in five

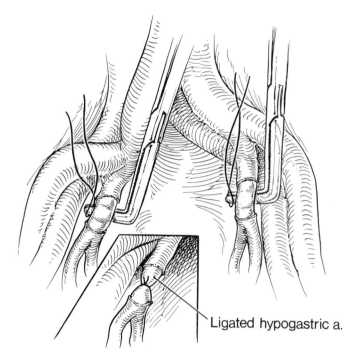

Ligated hypogastric a.

FIG. 33-11. Ligation of both hypogastric arteries. After the covering sheath has been opened and the artery has been carefully freed from the immediately adjacent veins, a ligature is carried beneath the artery with a right angle clamp and firmly tied (a. = artery).

women after bilateral hypogastric artery ligation. In three, the ovarian arteries were also ligated.

GENITAL TRACT FISTULAS FROM PARTURITION

In obstructed labor, the tissues of various parts of the genital tract may be compressed between the fetal head and the bony pelvis. If the pressure is brief, it is without significance, but if it is prolonged, necrosis results, followed in a few days by sloughing and perforation (Chap. 31, p. 834).

In most such cases, the perforation occurs between the vagina and the bladder, giving rise to a vesicovaginal fistula. Less frequently, the anterior lip of the cervix is compressed against the symphysis pubis, and an abnormal communication is eventually established between the cervical canal and the bladder, a vesicocervical fistula. If the woman has no infection, the fistula may heal spontaneously. More often it persists, requiring subsequent repair.

Rarely, the posterior wall of the uterus may be subjected to so much pressure against the promontory of the sacrum that necrosis results, and a fistula communicating with the cul-de-sac develops.

REFERENCES

Awais GM, Lebherz TB: Ruptured uterus, a complication of oxytocin induction and high parity. Obstet Gynecol 36:465, 1970

Badawy AH: Abdominal pregnancy in a previously ruptured uterus. Lancet 1:510, 1962

Beyth Y: Improved method for hysterographic evaluation of uterine scar. Acta Obstet Gynecol Scand 57:111, 1978

Case BD, Corcoran R, Jeffcoate N, Randle GH:

Ceasarean section and its place in modern obstetric practice. J Obstet Gynaecol Br Commonw 78:203, 1971

Lazarus, EJ: Early rupture of the gravid uterus. Am J Obstet Gynecol 132:224, 1978

Mengert WJ, Burchell RC, Blumstein RW, Daskal JL: Pregnancy after bilateral ligation of the internal iliac and ovarian arteries. Obstet Gynecol 34:664, 1969

Merrill BS, Gibbs CE: Planned vaginal delivery following cesarean section. Obstet Gynecol 52:50, 1978

Mokgokong ET, Marivate M: Treatment of the ruptured uterus. South Afr Med J 50:1621, 1976

Schrinsky DC, Benson, RC: Rupture of the pregnant uterus: A review. Obstet Gynecol Survey 33:217, 1978

Schwarz O, Paddock R, Bortnick AR: The cesarean scar: an experimental study. Am J Obstet Gynecol 36:962, 1938

Sheth SS: Results of treatment of rupture of the uterus by suturing. J Obstet Gynaecol Br Commonw 75:55, 1968

Taylor PJ, Cummings DC: Spontaneous rupture of a primigravid uterus. J Reproduct Med 22:169, 1979

Williams JW: A critical analysis of 21 years' experience with cesarean section. Bull Hopkins Hosp 32:173, 1921

34

Abnormalities of
the Third Stage of Labor

POSTPARTUM HEMORRHAGE

Definition. Postpartum hemorrhage has most often been defined as loss of blood in excess of 500 ml during the first 24 hours after birth of the infant. Through quantitative measurements of puerperal blood loss, however, the incongruity of this definition has been demonstrated clearly, since blood loss as the consequence of vaginal delivery *frequently* is somewhat more than 500 ml. Newton (1966), for example, measured the amount of hemoglobin shed by 105 women from the time of vaginal delivery through the next 24 hours and ascertained that the average blood loss was at least 546 ml. If appropriate allowance was made for the maternal blood discarded with the placenta, as well as that not measured because of incomplete recovery of shed hemoglobin, the blood loss during the first 24 hours averaged about 650 ml. Moreover, Pritchard and associates (1962) and DeLeeuw and co-workers (1968) demonstrated that erythrocytes equivalent to approximately 600 ml of blood are lost from the maternal circulation during vaginal delivery and the next several hours. Therefore, a blood loss somewhat in excess of 500 ml by accurate measurement is not necessarily

an abnormal event for vaginal delivery. Pritchard and associates noted that about 5 percent of women delivering vaginally lost more than 1000 ml of blood, according to measurements. At the same time, the results of their studies confirmed that the estimated blood loss commonly is only about one-half the actual loss. Moreover, based on an estimated blood loss greater than 500 ml, postpartum hemorrhage has been found in many hospitals to occur in about 5 percent of the deliveries. An estimated blood loss in excess of 500 ml in many institutions, therefore, may call attention to mothers who are bleeding excessively and warn the physician that dangerous hemorrhage is imminent. Hemorrhage after the first 24 hours is designated as *late postpartum hemorrhage* and is discussed under "Hemorrhages During the Puerperium" in Chapter 36, (p. 915).

Significance. Postpartum hemorrhage is the most common cause of serious blood loss in obstetrics. As a direct factor in maternal mortality, it is the cause of about one-quarter of the deaths from obstetric hemorrhage in the group that includes postpartum hemorrhage, low implanted placentas (placenta previa), placental abruption, ectopic pregnancy, hemorrhage from abortion, and rupture of the uterus.

Immediate Causes. The many factors of importance, singly or in combination, in the genesis of early postpartum hemorrhage are listed below:

1. Trauma to the genital tract
   Large episiotomy
   Lacerations of perineum, vagina, or cervix
   Rupture of uterus
2. Failure of compression of blood vessels at the implantation site
   Hypotonic myometrium
      General anesthesia (especially with halogenated compounds and ether)
      Poorly perfused myometrium (hypotension from hemorrhage or conduction anesthesia)
      Overdistended uterus (large fetus, multiple fetuses, hydramnios)
      After prolonged labor
      After very rapid labor
      After labor from vigorous oxytocin stimulation
      High parity
      Previous hemorrhage from uterine atony
      Uterine infection?
   Retention of placental tissue
      Abnormally adherent (placenta acreta, increta, and percreta)
      No abnormality of adherence (succenturiate lobe)
3. Coagulation defects
   Acquired ⎫ Intensify hemorrhage
   Congenital ⎭ from all of the above causes

Of all of these, the two most common causes of immediate postpartum hemorrhage are a hypotonic myometrium *(uterine atony)* and lacerations of the vagina and cervix. Retention of part or all of the placenta, a less common cause, may produce either immediate or delayed hemorrhage, or both. It is uncommon for an episiotomy alone to cause severe postpartum hemorrhage, although blood so lost averages about 200 ml and, at times, is much more (Odell, Seski, 1947).

Predisposing Causes. In the majority of cases, postpartum hemorrhage can be predicted well in advance of delivery. Examples in which trauma is likely to lead to postpartum hemorrhage include delivery of a large infant, midforceps delivery, forceps rotation, delivery through an incompletely dilated cervix or Dührssen's incisions of the cervix, any intrauterine manipulation, and vaginal delivery after cesarean section or other uterine incisions. Uterine atony causing hemorrhage can be anticipated whenever an anesthetic agent is to be used that will relax the uterus. Halothane and ether are prominent examples. The overdistended uterus is very likely to be hypotonic after delivery. Thus the woman with a large fetus, multiple fetuses, or hydramnios is prone to hemorrhage from uterine atony. Blood loss with the delivery of twins, for example, averages nearly 1000 ml, or nearly twice that associated with delivery of a singleton, and may be much greater (Pritchard, 1965). The woman whose labor is characterized by uterine activity that is either remarkably vigorous or barely effective is also likely to bleed excessively from uterine atony after delivery. Similarly, labor either initiated or augmented with oxytocin is more likely to be followed by postdelivery uterine atony and hemorrhage. The woman of high parity is at increased risk of hemorrhage from uterine atony. The risk is even greater if she has previously suffered a postpartum hemorrhage. Commonly, mismanagement of the third stage of labor involves an attempt to hasten delivery of the placenta short of manual removal. *Constant kneading and squeezing of the uterus that is already contracted are likely to impede the physiologic mechanism of placental detachment with incomplete placental separation and increased blood loss as the consequence.*

Clinical Characteristics. Postpartum hemorrhage before delivery of the placenta is called third-stage hemorrhage. Whether bleeding occurs before or after delivery of the placenta, or at both times, contrary to general opinion, there may be no sudden massive hemorrhage but rather a steady bleeding that at any instant appears to be moderate but persists until serious hypovolemia develops. Especially with hemorrhage after delivery of the placenta, the constant seepage may, over a period of a few hours, lead to enormous loss of blood. The effects of hemorrhage depend to a considerable degree upon the nonpregnant blood volume, the magnitude of pregnancy-induced hypervolemia, and the degree of anemia at the time of delivery. A treacherous feature of postpartum hemorrhage is the failure of the pulse and blood pressure to undergo more than moderate alterations until large amounts of blood have been lost, as emphasized in Chapter 21 (p. 490). The normotensive woman may actually become somewhat hypertensive in response to hemorrhage, at least initially. Moreover, the already hypertensive woman may be interpreted to be normotensive although remarkably hypovolemic. Tragically, the hypovolemia may not be recognized until very late.

In instances in which the fundus has not been adequately monitored after delivery, the blood may not escape vaginally but may collect instead within the uterus. The uterine cavity may thus become distended by 1000 ml or more of blood while an incompetent attendant fails to identify the large uterus or, having done so, erroneously massages a roll of abdominal fat. The care of the postpartum uterus must not, therefore, be left to an inexperienced person.

DIAGNOSIS. Except possibly when an intrauterine and intravaginal accumulation of blood is not recognized, the diagnosis of postpartum hemorrhage should be obvious. The differentiation between bleeding from uterine atony and from lacerations is tentatively made on the condition of the uterus. If bleeding persists despite a firm, well-contracted uterus, the cause of the hemorrhage most probably is lacerations. Bright red blood also suggests lacerations. To ascertain the role of lacerations as a cause of bleeding, careful inspection of the vagina, cervix, and uterus is

essential. Sometimes bleeding may occur from both atony and trauma, especially after major operative delivery. In general, inspection of the cervix and vagina should be performed after every delivery to prevent hemorrhage from cervical or vaginal lacerations. Anesthesia should be adequate to prevent discomfort to the mother during such an examination and there should have been no contamination of the lower genital tract or adjacent perineum. Examination of the uterine cavity, the cervix, and all of the vagina is essential after breech extraction and after internal podalic version, as well as when unusual bleeding occurs during the second stage of labor or immediately after birth of the infant.

PROGNOSIS. It should be possible to save the life of almost every woman with postpartum hemorrhage, even though hysterectomy may be required to do so in some instances. To obtain this objective, however, requires assiduous attention to all women immediately postpartum, an effective blood bank, and alert action by an experienced obstetric team. Although death from postpartum hemorrhage is rare in current obstetric practice in modern hospitals, it is common under less favorable conditions.

There are other hazards imposed by postpartum hemorrhage, not the least of which are transfusion reactions, including renal failure, and hepatitis.

SHEEHAN'S SYNDROME. Severe intrapartum or early postpartum hemorrage, furthermore, is on rare occasion followed by Sheehan's syndrome, which in the classic case, is characterized by failure of lactation, amenorrhea, atrophy of the breasts, loss of pubic and axillary hair, superinvolution of the uterus, hypothyroidism, and adrenal cortical insufficiency. The exact pathogenesis of Sheehan's syndrome is not well understood since such endocrine abnormalities in most women who hemorrhage severely are not evident. In some but not all instances of Sheehan's syndrome, varying degrees of necrosis of the anterior pituitary gland with impaired secretion of one or more of its trophic hormones account for the endocrine abnormalities. The anterior pituitary of some women who develop hypopituitarism after puerperal hemorrhage does respond to various releasing hormones, however, which implies, at least, impaired hypothalamic function rather than pituitary necrosis. Moreover, confirmatory histologic evidence of hypothalamic involvement has been provided by Whitehead (1963) who identified in some cases specific atrophic changes in the hypothalamic nuclei. Lactation after delivery usually, but not always, exludes extensive pituitary necrosis.

The incidence of Sheehan's syndrome was originally estimated to be one per 10,000 deliveries (Sheehan, Murdoch, 1938), and it appears to be equally rare today in continental United States, although 100 cases were identified in two decades in one hospital in Puerto Rico (Haddock et al., 1972). Perhaps the application of the many tests of hypothalamic and pituitary functions now available will identify milder forms of the syndrome to be much more prevalent. A schema of sequential stimulation tests for Sheehan's syndrome has been provided by DiZerega and co-workers (1978).

DIABETES INSIPIDUS. Severe hemorrhage at and immediately after delivery, as described on page 886, has been implicated in the development of diabetes insipidus without apparent anterior pituitary deficiency. The lesion is rare; in fact, Collins and associates (1979) claim to have reported the first case.

Management of Third-stage Bleeding.

Some bleeding is inevitable during the third stage of every labor as the result of transient partial separation of the placenta. As the placenta separates, the blood from the implantation site may escape into the vagina immediately ("Duncan mechanism") or may be concealed behind the placenta and membranes ("Schultze mechanism") until the placenta is delivered.

In the presence of any external hemorrhage during the third stage, the uterus should be massaged if it is not firmly contracted. If the signs of placental separation have appeared (see Chap. 17, p. 423), expression of the placenta should be attempted by pressure by the hand on the fundus of the uterus. Descent of the placenta is indicated by the cord becoming slack. If bleeding continues, manual removal of the placenta is mandatory.

TECHNIC OF MANUAL REMOVAL. When this operation is required, aseptic surgical technic should be employed. A sterile glove that covers the forearm to the elbow is recommended. After grasping the fundus of the uterus through the abdominal wall with one hand, the other hand with the long glove is introduced into the vagina and passed into the uterus, along the umbilical cord. As soon as the placenta is reached, its margin is located, and the ulnar border of the hand insinuated between it and the uterine wall (Fig. 34-1). Then with the back of the hand in contact with the uterus, the placenta is peeled off its uterine attachment by a motion similar to that employed in separating the leaves of a book. After its complete separation, the placenta should be grasped with the entire hand which is then gradually withdrawn. Membranes are removed at the same time by carefully teasing them from the decidua using ring forceps to grasp them as necessary. Some prefer to wipe out the uterine cavity with a sponge. If this is done, it is imperative that a sponge not be left in the uterus or vagina.

Management after Delivery of Placenta.

Irrespective of the method of delivery of the placenta, the fundus should always be palpated afterwards to make certain that the uterus is well contracted. If it is not firm, vigorous fundal massage is indicated. In some institutions, 0.2 mg of ergonovine (Ergotrate) or methylergonovine (Methergine) is administered routinely, either intravenously or intramuscularly. More commonly, because of the frequency of hypertension, these compounds are given only if there is excessive bleeding not controlled by an intravenous

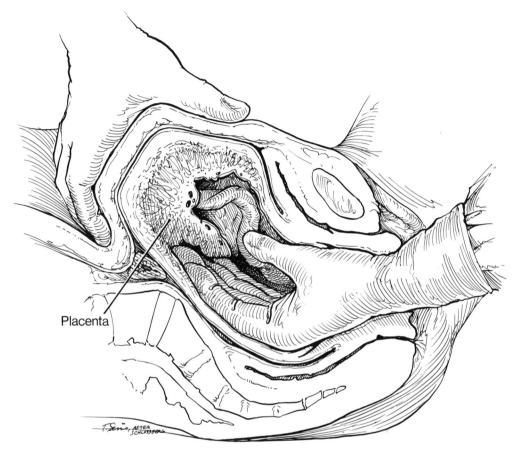

Placenta

FIG. 34-1.   Manual removal of placenta. The fingers are alternately abducted, adducted, and advanced until the placenta is completely detached.

infusion of oxytocin and uterine massage. Most often 20 units of oxytocin in 1000 ml of lactated Ringer's solution or normal saline proves effective when administered intravenously at a rate of 10 ml or so per minute simultaneous with effective massage of the uterus (see Chap. 17, p. 429). If such therapy does not prove effective, ergonovine (Ergotrate) or methylergonovine (Methergine), 0.2 mg administered intravenously, may stimulate the uterus to contract and retract sufficiently to control hemorrhage from the placental implantation site.

If bleeding persists despite these procedures, no time should be lost in haphazard efforts to control hemorrhage, but the following plan of management should be initiated immediately:

1. Employ bimanual uterine compression (Fig. 34-2). (This procedure will control most hemorrhage.)
2. Obtain help!
3. Begin transfusion of blood. The blood group of every obstetric patient should be known before labor, and cross-matched blood should be available for those in whom hemorrhage is anticipated. In emergency, type-specific whole blood is used.
4. Explore the uterine cavity manually for retained placental fragments or lacerations.
5. Thoroughly inspect the cervix and vagina after adequate exposure.

The technic of bimanual compression (Fig. 34-2) consists simply of massage of the poste-

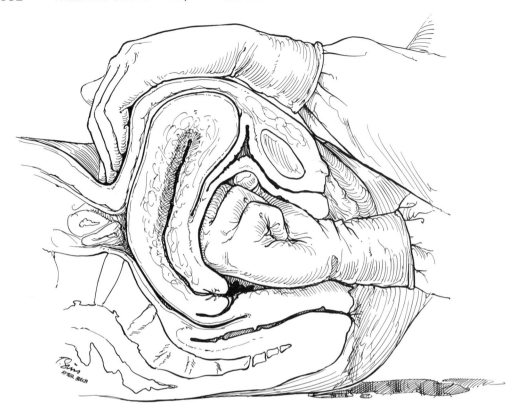

FIG. 34-2. Bimanual compression of the uterus and massage with the abdominal hand usually will effectively control hemorrhage from the uterine atony.

rior aspect of the uterus with the abdominal hand and massage through the vagina of the anterior uterine aspect with the other fist, the knuckles of which contact the uterine wall. Packing the uterus was an alternative procedure that formerly enjoyed greater popularity. *The late-pregnant uterus cannot be satisfactorily packed immediately after delivery since it dilates under the packing with further concealed hemorrhage that may be fatal.*

Blood transfusion should be initiated immediately in any case of postpartum hemorrhage in which abdominal massage of the uterus and oxytocic agents fail to control the bleeding. With transfusion and simultaneous manual compression of the uterus and oxytocin infused intravenously, additional measures are rarely required. If the operator's hand tires, an associate can relieve.

Prostaglandins have been tried to control hem-

orrhage after delivery of the placenta. Takagi and co-workers (1976) found that intravenously and intramuscularly injected prostaglandin $F_{2\alpha}$ was of little value in controlling uterine blood loss at delivery and adverse systemic effects were common. Corson and Bolognese (1977) described a case in which uterine atony following cesarean section appeared to respond to repeated intramuscular doses of prostaglandin $F_{2\alpha}$ after intravenously administered oxytocin and ergonovine were ineffective.

HEMORRHAGE FROM RETAINED PLACENTAL FRAGMENTS. Immediate postpartum hemorrhage is seldom caused by retained small placental fragments, but a remaining piece of placenta is a common cause of bleeding late in the puerperium. Inspection of the placenta after delivery must be routine. If a portion of placenta is missing, the uterus should be explored and the placental fragment removed, particularly in the face of continuing postpartum bleeding. Retention of a succenturiate lobe (see Chap. 6, Figs. 6-17 and 6-18) is an occasional cause of postpartum hemorrhage. The late bleeding that may result from a placental polyp is discussed in Chapter 36 (p. 915).

HEMORRHAGE FROM LACERATIONS. If rupture of the uterus is identified, laparotomy and, most often, hysterectomy, is mandatory for a favorable outcome (see Chap. 33, p. 873). Lacerations of the cervix and the vaginal vault somtimes cause profuse bleeding. Any time that bleeding persists in the presence of a firmly contracted intact uterus, hemorrhage from lacerations of the cervix or vagina should be suspected. In any case of protracted hemorrhage, moreover, even though the obstetrician is certain that uterine atony is the cause, inspection of the cervix and vagina is a necessary precaution to avoid overlooking a serious laceration. Proper exposure of the cervix and upper vagina to repair such lacerations usually requires an associate. Two retractors are inserted into the vagina, the walls of which are separated widely. Ring forceps are then placed on the anterior and posterior lips of the cervix, which is carefully inspected, especially laterally. Lacerations that are bleeding should be promptly repaired. Either interrupted single sutures or figure-of-eight sutures are employed, with the highest one placed slightly above the apex of the tear, because bleeding from cervical lacerations usually arises from a vessel at this point (see Chap. 33, p. 860).

HYSTERECTOMY. If rupture of the uterus is identified, hysterectomy is life-saving in most instances (see Chap. 33, p. 873). With an apparently intact uterus and when other measures to combat postpartum hemorrhage fail, the question of hysterectomy arises. If performed without initiating blood replacement on a woman who is profoundly hypovolemic, hysterectomy may hasten death. On the other hand, hysterectomy should not be delayed unduly. Vigorous transfusion therapy should be initiated and

surgery promptly begun. This approach will prevent deaths in cases in which all other measures to arrest hemorrhage fail. A technic is described in Chapter 43 (p. 1095).

INTRAUTERINE HOT LAVAGE. More than two decades ago treatment of postpartum hemorrhage by intrauterine lavage with hot saline was popular at Parkland Memorial Hospital. The results were stated to be good and morbidity was limited apparently to a very infrequent burn of the lower genital tract and perineum from overheated saline. Nonetheless, the frequency of its use decreased remarkably to where it is now rarely used. Interestingly, those individuals who earlier used the hot intrauterine douche in training with apparent enthusiasm have, for the most part, since abandoned it. The reasons for this are not clear. Fribourg and co-workers (1973) reviewed previous writings dealing with intrauterine hot lavage that proclaimed its efficacy for arresting hemorrhage from uterine atony. They traced the earlier enthusiasm for its use in the United States from W. F. Mengert most recently, back to E. J. Plass, and before that, to J. W. Williams. They also described excellent results in the treatment of postpartum hemorrhage from uterine atony in four women when hot saline was introduced into the uterus a few hours after delivery. In the one case so treated at Parkland Memorial Hospital in recent years, the results were far from dramatic. Indeed, hysterectomy finally had to be carried out to arrest the hemorrhage.

ABNORMALLY ADHERENT PLACENTA

In most instances, the placenta separates spontaneously from its implantation site during the first few minutes after delivery of the infant. The precise reason for delay in detachment beyond this time is not always obvious, but quite often it seems to be due to inadequate uterine contraction and retraction. Very infrequently, the placenta is unusually adherent to the implantation site with scanty or absent decidua, so that the physiologic line of cleavage through the spongy layer of decidua is lacking. As a consequence, one or more cotyledons of the placenta are firmly bound to the defective decidua basalis or even to the myometrium. When the placenta is densely anchored in this fashion, the condition is called placenta accreta.

Definitions. The term *placenta accreta* has come to be used to describe any implantation of the placenta in which there is abnormally firm adherence to the uterine wall. As the consequence of partial or total absence of the decidua basalis and imperfect development of the fibrinoid layer *(Nitabuch's layer),* the placental villi are attached to the myometrium *(placenta accreta),* (see Fig. 34-3) or actually invade the myometrium *(placenta increta),* or even penetrate through the myometrium *(placenta percreta)* (Fig. 34-4). The abnormal adherence may involve all of the cotyledons (total placenta accreta), a few to several cotyledons (partial placenta ac-

creta), or a single cotyledon (focal placenta accreta).

Significance. An abnormally adherent placenta, although an uncommon condition, assumes considerable significance clinically because of morbidity and, at times, mortality from severe hemorrhage, uterine perforation, and infection. The true frequencies of placenta accreta, increta, and percreta are unknown. Breen and associates (1977) for example, reviewed reports of this condition published since 1891. The incidence varied from one in 540 deliveries to one in 70,000 deliveries with an average incidence of approximately one in 7000.

Etiologic Factors. Abnormal adherence of the placenta is found most often in circumstances where decidual formation was likely to have been defective, for example, implantations in the lower uterine segment,

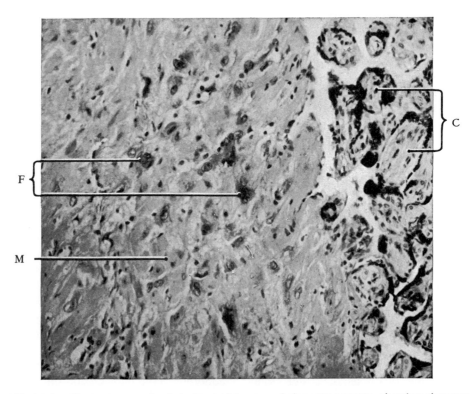

FIG. 34-3. Photomicrograph of uterine wall in case of placenta accreta, showing absence of decidua with chorionic villi in contact with myometrium. C. Chorionic villi. M. Myometrium. F. Trophoblastic giant cells.

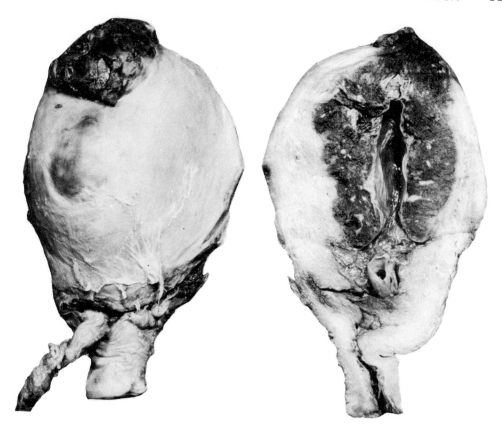

FIG. 34-4. Placenta percreta. On the left, the placenta is fungating through the fundus above the old classical cesarean section scar. In the opened specimen on the right the variable penetration of the fundus by the placenta is evident. (From Morrison. *Obstetrics and Gynecology Annual,* 1978, Appleton, p 113)

or over a previous cesarean section scar or other previous incisions into the uterine cavity, or after uterine curettage. Fox (1972), in his review of 622 reported cases of placenta accreta, noted the following characteristics: (1) placenta previa was identified in one-third of affected pregnancies; (2) one-fourth of the women had been delivered previously by cesarean section; (3) nearly one-fourth of the women had previously undergone curettage; (4) one-fourth of them were gravida six or more.

Clinical Course. Antepartum hemorrhage is common, but in the great majority of cases the antepartum bleeding is the consequence of a coexisting placenta previa. Invasion of the myometrium by placental villi at the site of a previous cesarean section scar may lead to rupture of the uterus during labor or even before. Labor is most likely to be normal, however, in the absence of placenta previa or an involved uterine scar.

The problems associated with delivery of the placenta and subsequent developments will vary appreciably depending upon the site of implantation, the depth of penetration into the myometrium, and the number of cotyledons involved. It is very likely that focal placenta accreta with implantation in the upper segment of the uterus occurs much more often than is recognized. The involved cotyledon is either pulled off the myometrium with perhaps somewhat excessive bleeding from that part of the implantation site, or the cotyledon is torn from the placenta and adheres to the implantation site with increased bleeding, immediately or later. This is probably the mechanism of formation of many so-called placental polyps (see Chap. 23, p. 553).

With more extensive involvement, however, hemorrhage becomes profuse as delivery of the placenta is attempted. Successful treatment demands immediate blood replacement therapy as described under "Obstetric Hemorrhage" in Chapter 21, and nearly always prompt hysterectomy.

With total involvement of the placenta (total placenta accreta), there may be very little or no bleeding from the uterus, at least until manual removal of the placenta is attempted. At times, traction on the umbilical cord will invert the uterus as described below. Moreover, usual attempts at manual removal of the placenta will not succeed, since a cleavage plane between the maternal surface of the placenta and the uterine wall cannot be developed. The safest treatment in this circumstance is prompt hysterectomy. Such a case is illustrated in Fig. 34-5A, B, and C.

Placenta percreta is more likely to be life-threatening than is placenta accreta or placenta increta, as exemplified by a case reported by Collins and associates (1978): During repeat cesarean section, severe hemorrhage began as the uterine serosa adjacent to the bladder was incised. The placenta had perforated the lower segment of the uterus and actually grown into the bladder. Removal of the placenta resulted in a 7-cm hole in the bladder. The massive hemorrhage was combatted with 11 liters of blood. The infant was anemic from blood loss consequent to incision of the placenta to effect delivery. The mother promptly developed diabetes insipidus without evidence of anterior pituitary dysfunction.

In the 622 published cases reviewed by Fox (1972), the most common form of "conservative" management was manual removal of as much placenta as possible and then packing of the uterus. One-fourth of the women died, or four times as many as when treatment consisted of immediate hysterectomy. He notes that "conservative" treatment of placenta accreta in at least four instances was followed by an apparently normal pregnancy.

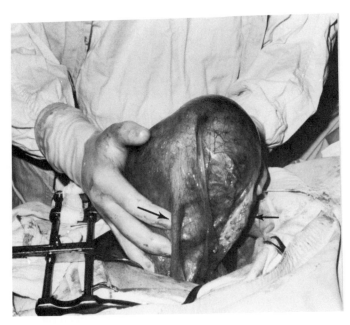

FIG. 34-5. A. Hysterectomy for placenta accreta. The uterine fundus contains the adherent placenta. Arrows point to round ligament (left) and ovary (right) separated by the oviduct.

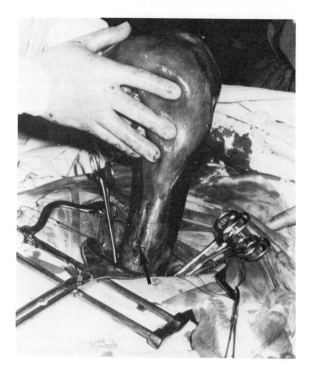

FIG. 34-5. B. The infundibulopelvic ligaments, broad ligaments, and cardinal ligaments have been resected. The incision in the lower segment (arrow) is used to palpate the margin of the cervix to identify where to enter the vagina.

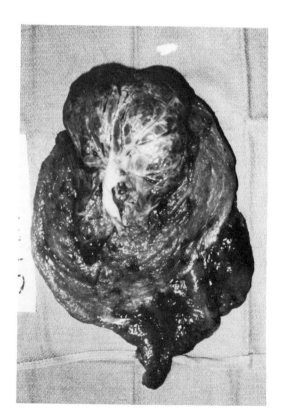

FIG. 34-5. C. The uterus has been opened anteriorly to show the adherent placenta (placenta accreta).

INVERSION OF THE UTERUS

Etiology. Complete inversion of the uterus after delivery of the infant almost always is the consequence of strong traction on an umbilical cord that is attached to a placenta implanted in the fundus of the uterus. Contributing to uterine inversion are a tough cord that does not readily break away from the placenta, combined with fundal pressure and a relaxed uterus including the lower segment and cervix. Placenta accreta may be implicated although uterine inversion can occur without the placenta being so firmly adherent. At times, the inversion may be incomplete (Fig. 34-6).

Clinical Course. Inversion of the uterus associated with the third stage of labor often is followed by circulatory collapse. Without prompt treatment, the woman may die (Fig. 34-7). It has been stated that shock tends to be disproportionate to blood loss (Greenhill, Friedman, 1974). Careful evaluation of the effects from transfusion of large volumes of blood in such cases does not support this concept, but, instead, makes it very apparent that blood loss in such circumstances often was massive but greatly underestimated. It is not unusual for even the woman who has received several units of blood because of hypotension to become anemic subsequently when isovolemic. Such outcomes are difficult to rec-

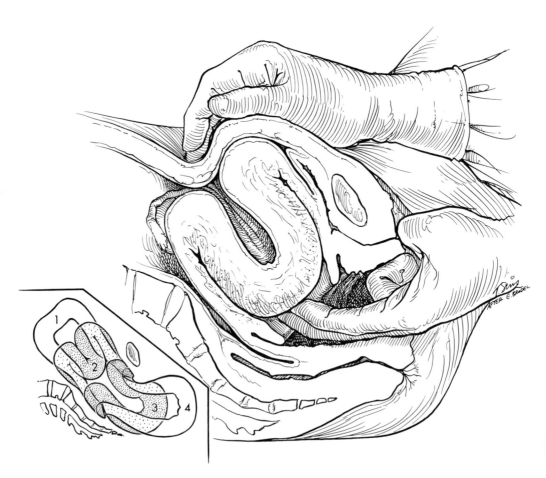

FIG. 34-6. Incomplete inversion of the uterus. Diagnosis by abdominal palpation of the craterlike depression and vaginal palpation of the fundal wall in the lower segment and cervix. Insert shows progressive degrees of inversion.

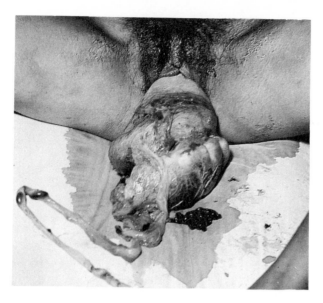

FIG. 34-7. A fatal case of inverted uterus following delivery at home. The placenta was firmly adherent to its implantation site in the fundus (placenta accreta).

oncile with the concept of shock out of proportion to blood loss (Watson et al., 1980).

Treatment. Delay in treatment increases the mortality rate appreciably. It is imperative that a number of steps be taken immediately and simultaneously:

1. Assistance, including an anesthesiologist, is summoned immediately.
2. The freshly inverted uterus with placenta already separated from it may often be replaced simply by immediately pushing on the fundus with the palm of the hand and fingers in the direction of the long axis of the vagina.
3. Preferably two intravenous infusion systems are made operational and lactated Ringer's solution and especially whole blood are given to refill the intravascular compartment and support cardiac output.
4. The placenta, if attached, is not removed until the infusion systems are operational, fluids are being given, and anesthesia, preferably halothane, has been administered. To do so before increases the hemorrhage. In the meantime, the inverted uterus, if prolapsed beyond the vagina, is replaced within the vagina.

5. After removing the placenta, the palm of the hand is placed on the center of the fundus with the fingers extended to identify the margins of the cervix. Pressure is then applied with the hand so as to push the fundus upward through the cervix.

As soon as the uterus is restored to its normal configuration, the anesthetic agent used to provide relaxation is stopped and simultaneously oxytocin is started to contract the uterus while the operator maintains the fundus in normal relationship. Initially, bimanual compression, as illustrated in Figure 34-2, will aid in the control of further hemorrhage until uterine tone is recovered. After the uterus is well contracted, the operator continues to monitor the uterus transvaginally for any evidence of subsequent inversion, although this occurrence is quite unlikely.

SURGICAL INTERVENTION. Most often, the inverted uterus can be restored to its normal position by the technics described above. For example, Kitchin and associates (1975) identified 11 "spontaneous" puerperal inversions among 25,000 deliveries and

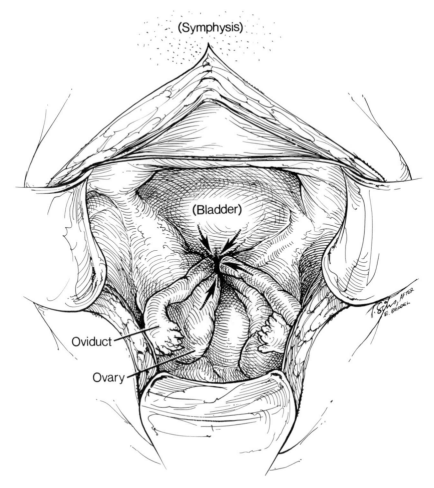

FIG. 34-8. Completely inverted uterus viewed from above.

in each instance the uterus was promptly replaced vaginally without significant morbidity other than hemorrhage from the uterus while in the inverted state. If the uterus cannot be reinverted by vaginal manipulation because of a dense constriction ring, as illustrated in Figure 34-8, laparotomy is imperative. The fundus may then be simultaneously pushed upward from below and pulled upward from above. A traction suture well placed in the inverted fundus may be of aid. If the constriction ring still prohibits reposition, it is carefully incised posteriorly to expose the fundus. After replacement of the fundus, the anesthetic agent used to relax the myometrium is stopped, oxytocin infusion is begun, and the uterine incision is repaired. The adjacent viscera are carefully examined for trauma.

REFERENCES

Breen JL, Neubecker R, Gregori CA, Franklin JE Jr: Placenta accreta, increta, and percreta. A survey of 40 cases. Obstet Gynecol 49:43, 1977

Collins ML, O'Brien P, Tabrah N: Placenta previa percreta with bladder invasion. JAMA 240:1749, 1978

Corson SL, Bolognese RJ: Postpartum uterine atony treated with prostaglandins. Am J Obstet Gynecol 129:918, 1977

DeLeeuw NKM, Lowenstein L, Tucker EC, Dayal

S: Correlation of red cell loss at delivery with changes in red cell mass. Am J Obstet Gynecol 84:1271, 1968

DiZerega G, Kletzky OA, Mishell DR Jr: Diagnosis of Sheehan's syndrome using a sequential stimulation test. Am J Obstet Gynecol 132:348, 1978

Fox H: Placenta accreta, 1945–1969. Obstet Gynecol Survey 27:475, 1972

Fribourg SRC, Rothman LA, Rovinsky JJ: Intrauterine lavage for control of uterine atony. Obstet Gynecol 41:876, 1973

Greenhill JP, Friedman EA: Biological Principles and Modern Practice of Obstetrics. Philadelphia, Saunders, 1974, p 687

Haddock L, Vega LA, Aguilo F, Rodriguez O: Adrenocortical, thyroidal and human growth hormone reserve in Sheehan's syndrome. Hopkins Med J 131:80, 1972

Kitchin JD III, Thiagarajah S, May HV Jr, Thornton WN Jr: Puerperal inversion of the uterus. Am J Obstet Gynecol 123:51, 1975

Newton M: Postpartum hemorrhage. Am J Obstet Gynecol 94:711, 1966

Odell LD, Seski A: Episiotomy blood loss. Am J Obstet Gynecol 54:51, 1947

Pritchard JA: Changes in the blood volume during pregnancy and delivery. Anesthesiology 26:393, 1965

Pritchard JA, Baldwin RM, Dickey JC, Wiggins KM: Blood volume changes in pregnancy and the puerperium: II. Red blood cell loss and changes in apparent blood volume during and following vaginal delivery, cesarean section, and cesarean section plus total hysterectomy. Am J Obstet Gynecol 84:1271, 1962

Sheehan HL, Murdoch R: Postpartum necrosis of the anterior pituitary: Pathological and clinical aspects. Br J Obstet Gynaecol 45:456, 1938

Takagi S, Yoshida T, Togo Y, Tochigi H, Abe M, Sakata H, Fujii TK, Takahashi H, Tochigi B: The effects of intramyometrial injection of prostaglandin $F_{2\alpha}$ on severe post-partum hemorrhage. Prostaglandins 12:565, 1976

Watson P, Besch N, Bowes WA Jr: Management acute and subacute puerperal inversion of the uterus. Obstet Gynecol 55:12, 1980

Whitehad R: The hypothalamus in post-partum hypopituitarism. J Pathol Bact 86:55, 1963

35

Puerperal Infection

Definition. Puerperal infection is infection of the genital tract after delivery. Previously used but less satisfactory synonyms are puerperal fever, puerperal sepsis, and childbed fever.

PUERPERAL MORBIDITY. Since most elevations of temperature in the puerperium are caused by puerperal infection, the incidence of fever after childbirth is a reliable index of the incidence of the disease. For this reason, it has been customary to group all puerperal fevers under the general term puerperal morbidity and to estimate the frequency of puerperal infection on this basis. Several definitions of puerperal morbidity have been established on the basis of the degree of pyrexia reached. The Joint Committee on Maternal Welfare has defined puerperal morbidity as a "temperature of 38.0 C (100.4 F) or higher, the temperature to occur on any two of the first 10 days postpartum, exclusive of the first 24 hours, and to be taken by mouth by a standard technic at least 4 times daily." This is probably the most commonly employed standard in the United States. This definition may suggest that all fevers in the puerperium are the consequence of puerperal infection. Elevations in temperature may, however, be the result of extraneous causes, such as pyelonephritis or upper respiratory infections. Unfortunately, the practical difficulties of differentiating extraneous causes of fever from puerperal infection are appreciable.

HISTORY. Puerperal infection is referred to in the works of Hippocrates and Galen. In the seventeenth century, Willis wrote on the subject of *febris puerperarum,* although the English term *puerperal fever* was probably first employed by Strother in 1716.

The ancients regarded the affection as the result of retention of the lochia, and for centuries this explanation was universally accepted. In the early part of the seventeenth century, metritis was thought to be the essential cause; the theory of "milk metastasis" of Puzos followed next. Until Semmelweis proved the identity of puerperal sepsis with wound infection and until Pasteur cultivated the streptococcus, and Lister demonstrated the value of antiseptic methods, many theories were suggested concerning the origin and nature of childbed fever. They are comprehensively discussed in the monographs of Eisenmann, Burtenshaw, and Peckham.

Although John Leake (1772) first made the suggestion of the contagiousness of puerperal infection, it remained for Alexander Hamilton to make the earliest positive statement on this subject in 1781. Alexander Gordon of Aberdeen clearly stated in a treatise on epidemic puerperal fever in 1795 the idea of the infectious and contagious nature of the disease, antedating the papers of

Holmes and Semmelweis by a half-century. Charles White (1773) of Manchester believed puerperal fever to be an absorption fever dependent on stagnation of the lochia. He advised the semirecumbent posture to facilitate drainage and insisted on rigorous cleanliness and ventilation of the lying-in room and complete isolation of infected patients. Although many other British observers had vague ideas upon the subject, it was not until the middle of the nineteenth century that such views were strongly urged. In 1843, Oliver Wendell Holmes read a paper before the Boston Society for Medical Improvement, entitled *The Contagiousness of Puerperal Fever,* in which he clearly showed that at least the epidemic forms of the infection could always be traced to the lack of proper precautions on the part of the physician or nurse. Four years later, Semmelweis, then an assistant in the Vienna Lying-In Hospital, began a careful inquiry into the causes of the frightful mortality rate attending labor in that institution, as compared with the relatively small number of women succumbing to puerperal infection when delivered in their own homes. As a result of his investigations, he concluded that the morbid process was essentially a wound infection caused by the introduction of septic material by the examining finger. Acting upon this idea, he issued stringent orders that the physicians, students, and midwives disinfect their hands with chlorine water, the forerunner of Dakin's solution, before examining parturient women. In spite of immediate surprising results, the mortality rate falling from over 10 to 1 percent, both his work and that of Holmes were scoffed at by many of the most prominent men of the time, and his discovery remained unappreciated until the influence of Lister's teachings and the development of bacteriology had brought about a revolution in the treatment of wounds.

PREDISPOSING CAUSES

In general, the longer the membranes have been ruptured before delivery, the greater the number of vaginal examinations, the more extensive the intrauterine manipulation for delivery of the fetus and placenta, the greater the size and number of incisions and lacerations, the greater is the likelihood of serious postpartum infection. The impression is widely held that puerperal infection is much more common in women from lower socioeconomic populations than in women who are private patients. The reasons for such difference need to be diligently investigated.

A variety of factors operative during pregnancy or delivery have been implicated in the genesis of puerperal infection:

ANTEPARTUM FACTORS. Although the evidence is mostly indirect, anemia, poor nutrition, and sexual intercourse have long been considered to predispose to puerperal sepsis. In spite of lack of strong direct evidence to implicate these three factors in the genesis of puerperal infection, anemia and poor nutrition should be prevented or appropriately corrected, and sexual intercourse should probably be avoided near term.

ANEMIA. The evidence is far from decisive that anemia per se increases the likelihood of infection (Buckley, 1975; Lukens, 1975). Animal experiments and in vitro studies have served to negate to a degree the established clinical impression that iron deficiency anemia predisposes to infection. For example, transferrin appears to have significant antibacterial action. Iron-deficiency anemia, of course, stimulates hypertransferrinemia. Moreover, growth of a variety of pathogenic bacteria is inhibited by lack of iron. Finally, some studies, at least, have failed to identify impairment of wound-healing in animals previously made iron-deficient.

NUTRITION. The role of nutrition in the genesis of infection is also not clear, although some recent studies indicate that cell-mediated immunity is likely to be impaired by malnutrition. Lymphocyte responses to antigens in vitro are depressed in iron-deficiency anemia as well as kwashiorkor according to Joynson and associates (1972). Kulapongs and co-workers (1974), however, found no such defect in studies of children with severe iron deficiency anemia.

SEXUAL INTERCOURSE. An increase in puerperal infection from sexual intercourse has not been clearly demonstrated. If, however, the membranes were ruptured at the time of coitus or were to rupture very soon after coitus, the infection rate most likely would be increased.

INTRAPARTUM FACTORS. During the intrapartum period, three factors have been traditionally implicated in the genesis of puerperal infection. They are iatrogenic introduction of pathogenic bacteria into the upper genital tract, trauma that devitalizes tissue, and hemorrhage. There is no doubt but what the first two are of considerable importance. It is very unlikely that any vaginal manipulation can be carried out with absolute asepsis. Therefore, every intravaginal and intrauterine examination must be carefully considered in terms of benefits to be achieved versus the risks of bacterial contamination. It is not so clear whether hemorrhage per se is of great significance. The trauma that led to hemorrhage and the manipulations associated with control of the hemorrhage and repair of the traumatized structures, however, certainly predispose to infection, as do the hematomas that often form in these circumstances.

BACTERIAL CONTAMINATION. The physician and others who care for the mother may carry infection to the parturient uterus in two ways. First, although the hands are covered with sterile gloves, bacteria already present on the pudenda and in the vagina may be carried into the uterine cavity during the course of examination or operative manipulation. Second, the gloves or instruments may be contaminated by virulent organisms as the result of droplet infection. The nose and mouth of all attendants in the delivery room should therefore be covered, and all persons with a respiratory infection should be excluded. Since the nasopharynx is the most common source of extraneous bacteria brought to the birth canal, all obstetric personnel in the delivery room must wear masks that cover the nose and mouth.

TRAUMA. Lacerations provide portals of entry and devitalized tissue an excellent cultural medium for pathogenic bacteria.

BLOOD LOSS. Hematomas easily infect and therefore enhance the likelihood of troublesome sepsis. Whether blood loss per se in the absence of trauma, reparative manipulations, or hematoma formation predisposes significantly to infection is not clear.

PATHOLOGY

After completion of the third stage of labor, the site of placental attachment is raw and elevated, dark red, and about 4 cm in diameter. Its surface is made nodular by the numerous veins that are normally occluded by thrombi. This site is an excellent culture medium for bacteria and a most likely portal of entry for pathogenic organisms. At this time, furthermore, the entire decidua is peculiarly susceptible to bacterial invasion, since it is less than 2 mm in thickness, is infiltrated with blood, and presents numerous small openings. Since the cervix rarely escapes some degree of laceration in labor, it is another ready site for bacterial invasion. Vulvar, vaginal, and perineal wounds provide additional portals of entry.

The lesions of puerperal infection, therefore, are basically wound infections. The inflammatory process may remain localized in these wounds or may extend through the blood or lymph vessels to tissues far beyond the initial lesion.

Lesions of the Perineum, Vulva, Vagina, and Cervix. A common puerperal lesion of the external genitalia is a localized infection of a repaired laceration or episiotomy wound. The apposing wound edges may become red, brawny, and swollen. The sutures often then cut through the edematous tissues, allowing the necrotic edges of the wound to gape, with the result that frank pus or sanguinopurulent material exudes from the wound. In this manner, complete breakdown of the site may occur. After traumatic operative delivery, wounds and contusions of the vulva are common. In extreme cases, the entire vulva may become edematous, ulcerated, and covered with exudate.

Lacerations of the vagina are common

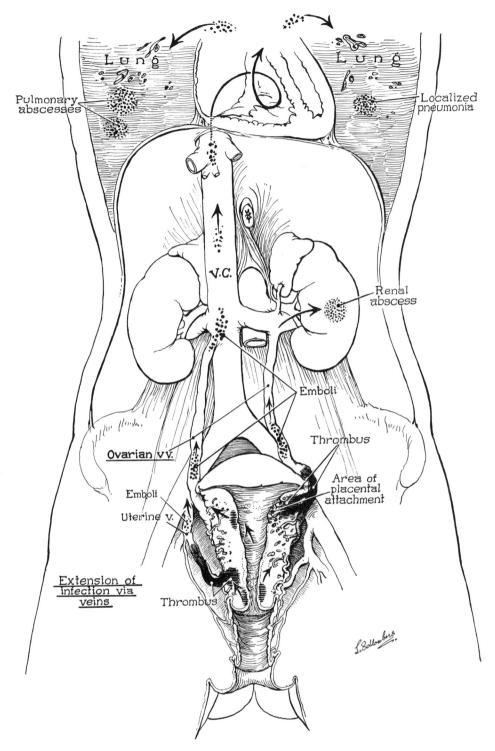

FIG. 35-1. Extension of puerperal infection in pelvic thrombophlebitis. (V.C. = inferior vena cava).

after operative delivery and may become infected directly or by extension from the perineum. The mucosa becomes swollen and hyperemic and may then become necrotic and slough. Extension may occur by infiltration, resulting in lymphangitis, but more likely the infection remains local.

Cervical infection is probably rather common, since lacerations are frequent and the cervix commonly harbors potentially pathogenic organisms. Moreover, since deep lacerations of the cervix often extend directly into the tissue at the base of the broad ligament, infection of such wounds may form the starting point for lymghangitis, parametritis, and bacteremia.

Metritis ("Endometritis"). The most common form of puerperal infection involves primarily the endometrium, or more exactly the decidua, and adjacent myometrium. During the first few hours to a few days after delivery, the bacteria successfully invade the decidua that remains, usually at the placental site. The infection spreads to involve the entire mucosa. If the infection is successfully confined near the surface, the necrotic infected mucosa is shed within a few days.

The appearance of the infected decidua varies widely. In some cases, the necrotic mucosa sloughs, the debris is abundant, and the discharge is foul, profuse, bloody, and sometimes frothy. In others, it is scant. Involution of the uterus may be retarded. Microscopic sections may show a superficial layer of necrotic material containing bacteria and a thick zone of leukocytic infiltration. The term *metritis* is more descriptive than endometritis, since the inflammatory response is almost certain to include to some degree the underlying myometrium.

Thrombophlebitis and Pyemia. One mode of extension of puerperal infection is along the veins, with resultant thrombophlebitis (Fig. 35-1). Halban and Kohler (1919), in autopsies of 163 women who died from puerperal infection before the era of antibiotics, found 82 instances of thrombophlebitis. In 36, it was the only mode of extension iden-

tified, whereas in 46 there was obvious coexisting lymphatic involvement. Thrombophlebitis results because the exposed placental site is a mass of thrombosed veins and because peptostreptococcus, bacteroides, and other anaerobic bacteria that frequently inhabit the vagina can thrive in the anaerobic medium provided by venous thrombi.

The veins most commonly involved in pelvic thrombophlebitis are the ovarian, since they drain the upper part of the uterus, which most often includes the veins of the placental site. The process is usually unilateral. Extension of the process into the left ovarian vein may reach its junction with the renal vein with involvement of that vessel and consequent renal complications. If the right ovarian vein is affected, the thrombosis may extend well into the inferior vena cava. At times, thrombosis of uterine veins extends to reach the common iliac veins.

Thrombosis of the infected vein may serve to limit the advance of the infection, and the thrombus may undergo organization. In other cases, the thrombus may suppurate, while the surrounding venous wall becomes edematous and necrotic. Very infrequently, large emboli may reach the pulmonary artery and cause sudden death. More often, small septic emboli reach the terminal branches of the pulmonary vessels and produce variable degrees of occlusion of the pulmonary microcirculation, and, in turn, cor pulmonale. At the same time, bacterial products released into the circulation may cause bacterial shock (see Chap. 24, p. 613). Pleurisy, pneumonia, and pulmonary infarcts, and abscesses may develop in this setting.

Peritonitis. Puerperal infection may extend by way of the lymphatics of the uterine wall to reach either the peritoneum or the loose tissue between the leaves of the broad ligaments. (Fig. 35-2), causing in the former instance peritonitis and in the latter parametritis (pelvic cellulitis).

Generalized peritonitis is a grave complication of childbearing. Typically, fibrinopurulent exudate binds loops of bowel to one another, and locules of pus may form be-

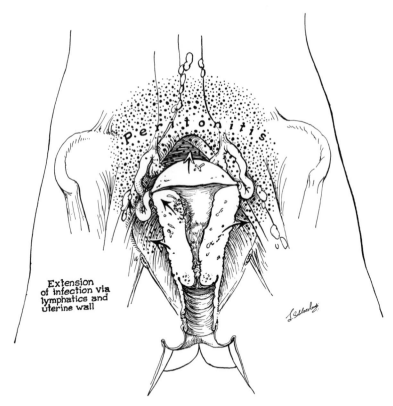

FIG. 35-2. Extension of puerperal infection in peritonitis.

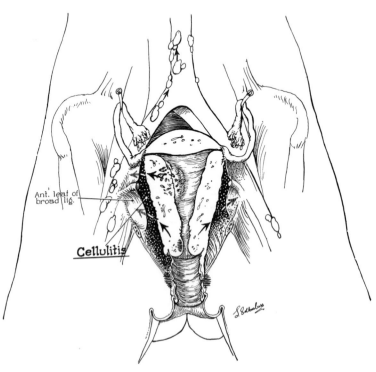

FIG. 35-3. Extension of puerperal infection in pelvic cellulitis (parametritis).

tween the loops. The cul-de-sac, the subdiaphragmatic space, and the folds between the infundibulopelvic and broad ligaments are common sites for abscess formation.

Pelvic Cellulitis (Parametritis). Infection of the retroperitoneal fibroareolar pelvic connective tissue may occur in three main ways:

1. It is caused by the lymphatic transmission of organisms from an infected cervical laceration, uterine incision for cesarean section, or a laceration of the uterus. Although lacerations of the perineum or vagina may be a cause of localized cellulitis, the process is usually limited to the paravaginal cellular tissue, rarely extending deeply into the pelvis (Fig. 35-3).
2. When cervical lacerations extend well into the connective tissue at the base of the broad ligaments, this tissue may be exposed to direct invasion by pathogenic organisms in the vagina. Similar results are frequently seen in cases of criminal abortion in which a sharp instrument has created a false passage into the paracervical connective tissue.
3. Pelvic cellulitis may be secondary to pelvic thrombophlebitis, which almost always is accompanied by some degree of cellulitis. If the thrombi become purulent, the venous wall may undergo necrosis and large numbers of organisms may be discharged into the surrounding connective tissue.

Pelvic cellulitis is more often unilateral but need not be so. The cellulitis may remain limited to the base of the broad ligament, but if the inflammatory reaction is more intense, the exudate may be forced along natural lines of cleavage. The most common form of extension is directly laterally, along the base of the broad ligament, with a tendency to extend to the lateral pelvic wall. As the mass increases in size, it distends the leaves of the broad ligament and, raising the anterior leaf upward, it may dissect its way forward to reach the abdominal wall just above Poupart's ligament. The uterus is pushed toward the opposite side and fixed. In other cases, high intraligamentous exudates spread from the region of the uterine cornua to the iliac fossae. Retrocervical exudates tend to involve the rectovaginal septum with the development of a firm mass posterior to the cervix. After cesarean section involvement of the connective tissue anterior to the cervix results in cellulitis of the space of Retzius with extension upward, beneath the anterior abdominal wall, as high as the umbilicus. Rarely, the process may extend out through the sciatic foramen into the thigh.

Cellulitis in the pelvic connective tissue follows an indolent course but ultimately undergoes either suppuration or, more commonly with appropriate antibiotic therapy, resolution. If suppuration occurs, one outcome is "pointing" above Poupart's ligament. The skin over the inguinal region becomes edematous, red, and tender; fluctuation indicates that the abcess is ready for incision. Another outcome is "pointing" in the posterior cul-de-sac. Either abscess, if not drained, may also rupture directly into the peritoneal cavity and cause fulminant putrid peritonitis.

BACTERIOLOGY

Organisms that invade the placental implantation site, and incisions, lacerations, and abrasions that are the consequence of labor and delivery may be normal inhabitants of the cervix and lower genital tract or may be introduced from exogenous sources. In modern obstetrics, an epidemic of serious puerperal sepsis rarely develops, as virulent bacteria are carried from person to person during labor, delivery, or early in the puerperium. Such an epidemic resulting from group A beta hemolytic streptococcus has been well documented (Jewett et al., 1968). Prompt administration of effective antibiotics and identification of the source of the infection prevented deaths and controlled the epidemic.

Common Pathogens. In the great majority of instances of puerperal infection, the bacteria responsible for the infection are those that normally flourish in the bowel and commonly inhabit the lower genital tract. Gorbach and co-workers (1973), for example, in 70 percent of cultures from the external cervix of healthy women, identified one or more potentially pathogenic anaerobic bacteria, as well as aerobic organisms. The anaerobic bacteria included species of *Bacteroides* (57 percent), *Peptostreptococcus* (33 percent), *Clostridium* (17 percent). Usually multiple species of bacteria were found. The pathogenicity of many of these bacteria is sufficiently great to cause, alone or in combination, extensive cellulitis (parametritis), abscesses, peritonitis, and suppurative thrombophlebitis.

Although the cervix and lower genital tract commonly harbor such bacteria, the uterine cavity is sterile before rupture of the amnionic sac. As the consequence of labor and delivery and associated manipulations, the uterus commonly becomes contaminated with anaerobic and aerobic bacteria. For example, Gilstrap and Cunningham (1979) in cultures of amnionic fluid obtained from the uterus at cesarean section performed on laboring women with membranes ruptured more than 6 hours identified the following bacteria: anaerobic and aerobic organisms in 63 percent; anaerobes alone in 30 percent, and aerobes alone in 7 percent. The anaerobic organisms were gram-positive cocci (species of *Peptostreptococcus* and *Peptococcus*) 45 percent; *Bacteroides* species, 9 percent; and *Clostridium* species, 3 percent. The aerobic organisms were various gram-positive cocci and *E. Coli*. An average of 2.5 different organisms per specimen were identified. These observations serve to reemphasize the polymicrobial nature of infections of the genital tract associated with delivery, especially cesarean section.

Bacterial Cultures. Precise identification of the bacteria responsible specifically for any given puerperal infection may be quite difficult. Even though satisfactory technics are employed for obtaining and culturing organisms from the uterine cavity, the results are difficult to interpret since potentially pathogenic bacteria are commonly found in cultures of the uterine cavity during the puerperium without clinical disease. Gibbs and associates (1975), as did Hite and coworkers (1947) three decades before, cultured one or more pathogens from swabbings of the uterine cavity in 70 percent or more of clinically healthy puerperal women. Appropriately performed anaerobic and aerobic blood cultures obtained before antibiotic treatment is begun may be more useful to identify at times the pathogens that actually cause the infection.

CLINICAL COURSE

Lesions of the Perineum, Vulva, Vagina, and Cervix. Local pain and dysuria, with or without urinary retention, are the common symptoms. Provided drainage is good, the reaction in these local conditions is seldom severe, the temperature remaining below 38.5C (101F). If, however, purulent material is dammed back by perineal or vaginal suture, the complication may be signaled by a chill and a sharp rise of fever.

Metritis. The clinical picture of puerperal metritis varies with the extent of the disease. When the infection is strictly confined to the endometrium (decidua), the cases are mild, with only slight elevation of temperature. More severe cases of metritis may be ushered in by a chill, high fever, and other evidence of a fulminating infection. Postpartum, the temperature begins to rise in a sawtooth fashion, to reach levels between 38.5C and 40C (101F and 103F). The pulse rate tends to follow the temperature curve. There is likely to be tenderness over the uterus, and after-pains tend to be bothersome. Even in the early stages there may be changes in the lochia. An offensive odor, long regarded as an important sign of uterine infection, results from invasion of the uterine cavity by anaerobic bacteria. Some infections, however, and notably with beta hemolytic streptococcus, are frequently associated with scanty, odorless lochia. Indeed, the gravity of a case of metritis may sometimes be in almost inverse proportion to the amount and putridity of the lochia. Leukocytosis may range from 15,000 to 30,000 cells per mm³, but in view of the physiologic leukocytosis of the early puerperium these figures are difficult to interpret. The symptoms are, however, quite variable. Some patients feel well, with no complaints. If the process is localized to the uterus, the temperature falls by lysis, and, even when untreated with antibiotics, by the end of a week the infection is usually over. Localized metritis may be misdiagnosed as a urinary tract infection or be attributed incorrectly to severe breast engorgement or pulmonary atelectasis.

Pelvic Cellulitis.   Pelvic cellulitis (parametritis) is the common cause of prolonged, sustained fever in the puerperium. Whenever steady elevations of temperature persist, the condition should be suspected. There is tenderness on one or both sides of the abdomen and tenderness on vaginal examination. As the process advances, other findings on vaginal examination may become more characteristic, such as fixation of the uterus by the parametrial exudate or induration in the fornices, and the development of a mass in the broad ligament. The exudate may extend upward and an area of resistance may be felt along the upper border of Poupart's ligament. Not infrequently it extends posteriorly into the lower part of the broad ligament along the sacrouterine folds and into the cellular tissue surrounding the uterus. In these cases, a rectal examination may be very helpful in diagnosis.

Absorption of the exudate occurs in the great majority of the cases, but it may require several weeks. In this process, the inflammatory process may become hard, and infrequently the final result may be dense scar tissue in the parametrium. Suppuration of the parametrial mass occurs in the remaining cases. Pointing of the abscess may not occur for weeks after the commencement of the illness. If the abscess can be adequately drained, recovery is usually prompt.

Peritonitis.   Puerperal peritonitis generally resembles surgical peritonitis except that abdominal rigidity is usually much less prominent. Pain may be severe. Marked bowel distension is a consequence of paralytic ileus. Rarely, in the course of pelvic cellulitis with abscess formation, a large abscess may rupture into the peritoneal cavity and produce catastrophic generalized peritonitis.

Septic Thrombophlebitis.   The clinical picture of septic thrombophlebitis is characterized by repeated chills, hectic temperature swings, a tendency toward distant spread (particularly in the lungs), and a prolonged course. Chills are a feature of the disease. The initial chill may be severe. The swings in temperature are often remarkable, with steep climbs from 96.0F to 105.0F, followed by a precipitous fall within an hour. Hypotension may develop as a direct consequence of bacterial products in the blood stream (bacterial shock), or hypoxia from impaired pulmonary perfusion, or both. Leukocytosis is often present, although leukopenia may develop very soon after escape of endotoxin into the bloodstream. Bacteria are present in the bloodstream during the chills; the offending organisms are commonly anaerobic and, therefore, more difficult to culture. The optimal time to take the blood is early in the chill or, if possible, just before the chill begins.

The typical case of pelvic thrombophlebitis formerly lasted for many weeks, often with a fatal outcome. With modern antimicrobial therapy, both the mortality rate and the duration of the disease have been reduced. The common cause of death was a pulmonary complication, usually a combination of vascular blockade by septic emboli, infarction, pneumonitis, and abscesses. With prompt, effective antibiotic therapy, and, at times, treatment with heparin or ligation of the inferior vena cava and ovarian veins, both mortality rate and the duration of the disease have been reduced appreciably.

Salpingitis.   Most often with pospartum sepsis the fallopian tubes are involved only with a perisalpingitis without subsequent tubal occlusion and sterility. Initial attacks of gonorrheal salpingitis during the puerperium are rare.

DIFFERENTIAL DIAGNOSIS

Most fevers occurring after childbirth are caused by infection of the genital tract, especially if the preceding labor has been attended by extensive vaginal or uterine manipulation or prolonged rupture of the membranes. In any event, every puerperal woman whose temperature rises to 100.4 F should be given a complete examination to rule out extrapelvic causes of fever and to establish the diagnosis of puerperal infection by exclusion in the absence of other findings.

The common extragenital causes of fever in the puerperium are *pyelonephritis, mastitis, respiratory infections,* and, in case of laparotomy, *wound abscess.* Pyelonephritis is a difficult problem in differential diagnosis. In the typical case, bacteriuria, pyuria, costovertebral angle tenderness, and spiking temperature point clearly to pyelonephritis. The clinical picture varies, however. Pyelonephritis should be confirmed by a urine culture that identifies quantitatively a significant number of a single species of bacteria. Mammary engorgement may occasionally give rise to a brief temperature rise during the first few days, which characteristically never lasts longer than 24 hours. The temperature curve of true mastitis is usually sustained and associated with mammary signs and symptoms that become overt by 24 hours. Meticulous inspection of the abdominal wound will usually disclose an abscess when present.

TREATMENT

Choice of Antibiotics. For many years, the combination of penicillin with a broad-spectrum antibiotic has been used, most often with success, to treat genital tract infections associated with delivery, even though *Bacteroides* species are resistant in vitro, at least, to most of the antibiotic combinations employed. Di Zerega and associates (1979) have compared the effectiveness of primary treatment of postcesarean section endomyometritis with penicillin plus gentamicin and with gentamicin plus clindamycin, an antibiotic to which *Bacteroides* is usually sensitive. The infection was effectively controlled by the antibiotic regimen in 95 percent of women who received clindamycin plus gentamicin compared to 71 percent of those who received penicillin plus gentamicin. Unfortunately, clindamycin may be quite toxic in some circumstances. Cunningham and co-workers (1978) observed that metritis and pelvic cellulitis following cesarean section responded satisfactorily to penicillin and an aminoglycoside about 70 percent of the time and to penicillin and tetracycline about 85 percent of the time.

For more than two decades at Parkland Memorial Hospital, the combination of tetracycline and large doses of penicillin G given intravenously has proved to be quite effective for the treatment of the great majority of puerperal infections as well as septic abortions (Pritchard and Whalley, 1971). At least until the safety of clindamycin has been more firmly established, or another antibiotic regimen is shown to be at least as effective and safe, the combination of penicillin and tetracycline continues to be used commonly in cases of puerperal infection treated at Parkland Memorial Hospital. With very severe infections involving the genital tract, such as those precipitating bacterial shock or producing intense hemolysis, more often, large doses of penicillin and chloramphenicol have been used, especially when there was impaired renal function. Less often, penicillin, clindamycin, and gentamicin have been employed.

Lesions of the Perineum, Vulva, and Vagina. These infected external wounds should be treated, like other infected surgical wounds, by establishing drainage. Stitches should be removed and the wound laid open.

Failure to do this may lead not only to infection of the paracervical and paravaginal connective tissue, but to a worse ultimate anatomic result. Relief of pain is afforded by effective analgesics. It is advisable to supplement these therapeutic measures with antibiotic therapy during the acute phase of the infection.

Metritis.   Mild cases without symptoms, with temperature under 38 C, and no chills, are best handled initially by simple measures. In this group, it is unnecessary to discontinue breast-feeding. In more severe cases, antibiotics are indicated. Breast-feeding is discontinued, not only because it exhausts the mother but also because it is usually futile in the presence of high fever.

Pelvic Cellulitis.   Antibiotics must be used. The physician should remain alert for signs of suppuration and abscess formation. The diagnosis of an abscess rests upon detection of a mass. The mass may be so tender that effective analgesia may be required to perform an adequate examination.

An abscess that forms in the broad ligament and "points" above Poupart's ligament may be surgically drained extraperitoneally, as illustrated in Figure 35-4. In modern obstetrics, this particular circumstance is rarely encountered. At times, an abscess may form in the posterior cul-de-sac. As the abscess begins to dissect the rectovaginal septum, drainage is established and maintained, as demonstrated in Figure 35-5.

Pelvic Thrombophlebitis.   Variable degrees of pelvic thrombophlebitis usually accompany parametritis and pelvic cellulitis. Treatment is customarily directed at the pelvic cellulitis rather than at pelvic thrombophlebitis alone. Anticoagulant drugs that are successfully used in femoral thrombophlebitis disease (see Chap. 36 p. 908) may be of less value in these cases, for the primary lesion is extravascular infection rather than thrombosis. Treatment with heparin is certainly indicated in cases of apparent or suspected pulmonary emboli. Ligation of the inferior vena cava and ovarian veins is life-saving when septic emboli continue to reach the lung in spite of heparinization. It is not yet clear, however, whether in suspected cases of pelvic septic thrombophlebitis *without* embolization the possible benefits from use of heparin outweigh the danger of bleeding. Josey and Staggers (1974) believe heparin to be of decided value in the treatment of such cases, as have others before them. The evidence presented so far is not decisive, however, that heparin administration is essential for a successful out-

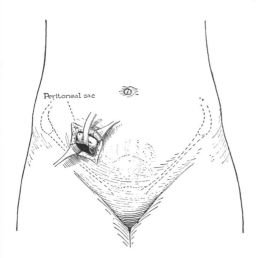

FIG. 35-4. Technic for opening localized collections of pus pointing above the inguinal ligament.

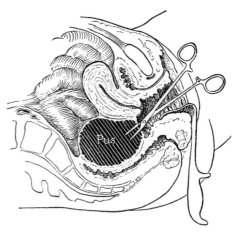

FIG. 35-5. Technic for opening collection of localized pus in the cul-de-sac of Douglas (posterior colpotomy).

come in the absence of any evidence of embolization. Pelvic venous thrombosis is considered further on page 909.

Generalized Peritonitis.   It is important to identify the cause of the generalized peritonitis. The treatment of peritonitis as the consequence of an infection that began in the uterus and extended to the peritoneum is medical in most instances. Conversely, peritonitis during the puerperium as the consequence of a lesion of the bowel or its appendages most often should be promptly treated surgically.

Antibiotic therapy should include those agents that are most likely to be effective against *Peptostreptococcus, Peptococcus, Bacteroides, Clostridia,* and aerobic coliform organisms. Clindamycin and gentamicin plus large doses of penicillin, should prove effective in most cases. Chloramphenicol, however, may prove to be less toxic than clindamycin plus gentamicin.

Appropriate fluid and electrolyte therapy is extremely important. With generalized peritonitis large amounts of fluid are often sequestered in the lumen and the wall of the gastrointestinal tract and, at times, in the peritoneal cavity. Vomiting, diarrhea, and fever also contribute appreciably to loss of fluid and electrolytes. The volumes of fluid and the amounts of electrolytes necessary to replace what is sequestered in the abdomen, aspirated from the gut, and lost through diaphoresis are usually quite large but must not be so massive as to produce circulatory overload.

Most often, paralytic ileus is a prominent feature of the disease process. The gastrointestinal tract should be decompressed by prompt, continuous nasogastric suction. Drugs to stimulate peristalsis are of no value. Oral feeding is withheld throughout the course of treatment until bowel function returns and flatus is expelled.

Procedures To Avoid.   Although countless local therapeutic measures have been recommended, such as intrauterine douches, swabbing of the endometrium with antiseptic solutions, continuous irrigation of the uterine cavity, instillations of glycerin, drainage with rubber tubes, and curettage, they have all been abandoned, since experience has shown them to be dangerous as well as futile. In the main, they tend to disseminate rather than halt the infection. Surgery is not indicated early in the course of the disease, although abscesses may form at various sites and need to be drained, and mechanical intestinal obstruction that has to be relieved may develop.

REFERENCES

Buckley RH: Iron deficiency anemia: Its relationship to infection susceptibility and host defense. J Pediatr 86:993, 1975

Burtenshaw: The fever of the puerperium. New York and Philadelphia Med J, June and July, 1904

Cunningham FG, Hauth JC, Strong JD, Kappus SS: Infectious morbidity following cesarean section. Comparison of two treatment regimens. Obstet Gynecol 52:656, 1978

De Zerega G, Yonekura L, Roy S, Nakamura RM, Ledger WJ: A comparison of clindamycin-gentamycin and penicillin-gentamycin in the treatment of post-cesarean section endomyometritis. Am J Obstet Gynecol 134:238, 1979

Eisenmann GE: Die Wundfieber und die Kindbettfieber, Erlangen, 1837

Gibbs RS, O'Dell TN, MacGregor RR, Schwarz RH, Morton H: Puerperal endometritis: A prospective microbiologic study. Am J Obstet Gynecol 121:919, 1975

Gilstrap LC III, Cunningham FG: The bacterial pathogenesis of infection following cesarean section. Obstet Gynecol 53:545, 1979

Gorbach SL, Menda KB, Thadepalli H, Keith L: Anaerobic microflora of the cervix in healthy women. Am J Obstet Gynecol 117:1053, 1973

Gordon A: A Treatise on Epidemic Puerperal Fever of Aberdeen. London, C G and J Robinson, 1795

Halban J, Köhler R: Die pathologische Anatomie des Puerperalprozesses. Vienna and Leipzig, 1919

Hamilton A: A Treatise on Midwifery, London, 1781

Hippocrates: Liber Prior de Muliebrum Morbis

Hite KE, Hesseltine HC, Goldstein L: A study of the bacterial flora of the normal and pathologic vagina and uterus. Am J Obstet Gynecol 53:233, 1947

Holmes OW: Puerperal Fever as a Private Pestilence. Boston, Ticknor & Fields, 1855

Jewett JF, Reid DE, Safon LE, Easterday CL: Child-bed fever: A continuing entity. JAMA 206:344, 1968

Josey WE, Staggers SR Jr: Heparin therapy in septic pelvic thrombophlebitis: A study of 46 cases. Am J Obstet Gynecol 120:228, 1974

Joynson DHM, Jacobs A, Walker DM, Dolby AE: Defect of cell-mediated immunity in patients with iron-deficiency anaemia. Lancet 2:1058, 1972

Kabins SA, Spira, TJ: Outbreak of clindmycin-associated colitis. Ann Intern Med 83:830, 1975

Kulapongs P, Suskind R, Vithayasai V, Olsen RE: Cell-mediated immunity and phagocytosis and killing function in children with severe iron-deficiency anaemia. Lancet 2:689, 1974

Leake J: Practical Observations on the Child-bed Fever; Also on the Nature and Treatment of Uterine Haemorrhages, Convulsions, and Such Other Acute Diseases, As Are Most Fatal to Women During the State of Pregnancy. London, J Walter, 1772

Lister J: On the antiseptic principle in the practice of surgery. Br Med J 2:246, 1867

Lukens JN: Iron deficiency and infection. Am J Dis Child 129:160, 1975

Peckham CH: A brief history of puerperal infection. Bull Int Hist Med 3:187, 1935

Pritchard JA, Whalley PJ: Abortion complicated by Clostridium perfrigens infection. Am J Obstet Gynecol 111:484, 1971

Puzos N: Première mémoire sur les depots laiteux, in Traites des accouchements, 1686, p 341

Strother: Critical Essay on Fevers. London, 1716

White C: Treatise on the management of pregnant and lying-in women and the means of curing but more especially of preventing the principal disorders to which they are liable. London, EC Dilly, 1773

Other Disorders of the Puerperium

THROMBOEMBOLIC DISEASE

Venous thromboembolic disease is considered under disorders of the puerperium because traditionally in obstetrics thromboembolism has been thought of primarily as a complication of the puerperium. Deep venous thrombosis and thromboembolism are not limited to just this period, however. In more recent years, there has been a decrease in the frequency of deep venous thrombosis and thromboembolism during the puerperium but perhaps an increase antepartum. Henderson, Lund, and Creasman (1972), for example, described 20 cases that developed antepartum among 29,770 pregnancies, but during the same period, only 16 were identified postpartum.

Undoubtedly, the frequency of venous thromboembolic disease during the puerperium decreased remarkably when early ambulation became widely practiced. Until as late as the 1950s, it had been common practice after delivery to prohibit ambulation for up to a week or more. **Stasis is probably the strongest single predisposer to deep vein thrombosis, and therefore should be kept to the minimum.** In more recent years, ante-cedent events that might possibly predispose to deep vein thrombosis during the antepartum period include possibly the use of oral contraceptives before conception and the greater prevalence of women working during pregnancy at jobs in which they sit for long periods of time.

Venous thrombosis traditionally has been classified as *thrombophlebitis* if an inflammatory response was apparent, or *phlebothrombosis* if such evidence was lacking. The inflammatory response presumably would anchor the clot more firmly and prevent embolism. Unfortunately, contiguous with and proximal to an adherent clot appreciable thrombus may form that is not adherent and therefore can easily break off to become an embolus. Thrombosis with a significant potential for generating pulmonary emboli may take place in the deep veins of the leg, thigh, or pelvis. Thrombosis that involves only the superficial veins of the leg or thigh is very unlikely to generate pulmonary emboli.

Superficial Venous Thrombosis. Antepartum or postpartum thrombosis limited strictly to the superficial veins of the saphenous system is treated with analgesia, elastic support, and rest. If it does not soon clear, or if deep venous involvement is suspected, heparin is given intravenously, as described below, until the process clears.

Deep Venous Thrombosis in the Leg. The signs and symptoms with deep venous thrombosis involving the lower extremity vary greatly depending in large measure on the degree of occlusion and the intensity of the inflammatory response. Diagnosing correctly deep venous thrombosis is not made easier by pregnancy, but rather the opposite is true.

POSTPARTUM DEEP VEIN THROMBOSIS. Classic puerperal thrombophlebitis involving the lower extremity, sometimes called *phlegmasia alba dolens* or *"milk leg,"* is abrupt in onset with severe pain and edema of the leg and thigh. The venous thrombosis typically involves much of the deep venous system from the foot to the iliofemoral region. Reflex arterial spasm sometimes causes a pale, cool extremity with diminished pulsations. Seldom is the reaction to deep venous thrombosis this intense, however. There may be appreciable volume of clot yet little reaction in the form of pain, heat, or swelling. Conversely, calf pain, either spontaneous or in response to squeezing, or to stretching the Achilles' tendon (Homan's sign), may be caused by a strained muscle or a contusion. The latter can be fairly common during the early puerperium as the consequence of inappropriate contact between the calf and the delivery table leg holders.

A variety of diagnostic procedures have been advocated. Probably the only accurate procedure is carefully performed and interpreted *phlebography* (Bonnar, 1979).

Treatment of deep venous thrombosis, in general, consists of heparin intravenously administered as described below, bed rest, and analgesia. Most agree that broad-spectrum antibiotic therapy is indicated if there is fever. Often the pain is soon relieved and the temperature returns to normal. Thrombectomy or sympathetic nerve block is not warranted in the great majority of cases. After the signs and symptoms have completely abated, graded ambulation should be started with the legs well wrapped in elastic bandages, or better, well-fitting elastic stockings, and the heparin continued. Recovery to this stage usually takes about a week.

For women who are *postpartum,* who are suffering their first attack, who have no obvious chronic vascular disease, and who are observed to be completely asymptomatic while fully ambulatory, anticoagulant therapy may be discontinued. Most often signs and symptoms of deep venous thrombosis do not recur. If, however, symptoms and signs do recur, therapy is promptly restarted but is not stopped when relief is obtained. Instead, prolonged anticoagulant therapy is continued on an outpatient basis. After discharge from the hospital, long-term treatment is maintained either with self-administered, subcutaneously injected heparin, or preferably with warfarin (Hull and coworkers, 1979).

ANTEPARTUM DEEP VEIN THROMBOSIS. Thrombosis antepartum involving the deep venous system is especially difficult to manage satisfactorily. When deep vein thrombosis involving a leg is not obvious but only suspected antepartum remote from term, it may be worthwhile to utilize phlebography while shielding the fetus from irradiation, to establish or exclude the diagnosis. (Bonnar, 1979). Otherwise, the woman will either have to undergo prolonged anticoagulation with its attendant risks, or run the risk of pulmonary embolism.

HEPARIN THERAPY. Therapy with intravenous heparin usually soon controls the disease, but the thrombosis, perhaps with embolization, is likely to recur antepartum, intrapartum, or postpartum unless anticoagulation is continued throughout these periods.

Administration of heparin on an outpatient basis is difficult to do safely. An indwelling venous catheter has been used by some for chronic intermittent intravenous administration (Pearson, 1972). The major risk from heparin to ambulatory patients who are anticoagulated with heparin in doses of 20,000 to 40,000 units per day is serious hemorrhage from trauma that otherwise would be minor. A safer, and now more popular, treatment regimen consists of the self-administration of heparin subcutaneously in doses of 5000 units 2 or 3 times a day (Bonnar, 1979). With so-called low dose heparin treatment that provides 10,000 to 15,000 units of heparin per day, there is some increase in the risk of recurrent thrombosis and possibly embolism compared to that with larger doses, but a much lower risk of hemorrhage. Asprin and other drugs that impair platelet function increase the risk of hemorrhage even with "low dose" heparin and therefore should be avoided. The heterogeneity of structure and of action of heparin has been recently summarized by Wessler and Gitel (1979).

WARFARIN (COUMADIN) THERAPY. Warfarin and related compounds that inhibit the synthesis of vitamin K-dependent coagulation factors cross the placenta and similarly impair the coagulation mechanism of the fetus. Moreover, there is evidence that warfarin may be teratogenic if used early in pregnancy. The administration of warfarin during the first 8 weeks of gestation may result in congenital malformations which include nasal hypoplasia, ophthalmologic abnormalities, and retarded development (Shaul and Hall, 1977). Whether the malformations are the consequence of microhemorrhages in embryonic cartilage or a more complex teratogenic action is not known.

It is recommended that, when anticoagulation is mandatory during the first trimester, heparin be used rather than warfarin or related compounds. Whenever warfarin is used, the dose must be carefully controlled so that the one-stage prothrombin time is kept below 30 percent but not less than 20 percent when compared to saline-diluted control plasma (or about 2 to 2½ times the prothrombin time of normal plasma). If this can be accomplished, the fetus is less likely to be in jeopardy of serious hemorrhage, at least until the onset of labor.

Because of the mechanical forces that develop during labor, the fetus is at increased risk of hemorrhage, especially intracranial hemorrhage, at this time. Therefore, if warfarin has been used as an anticoagulant during the antepartum period, the drug probably should be stopped some weeks before the anticipated time of delivery and anticoagulation with heparin started.

Pelvic Venous Thrombosis. During the puerperium, thrombi may form transiently in any of the dilated pelvic veins and probably do so relatively often. In general, pelvic venous thrombosis without thrombophlebitis is not likely to incite definitive signs or symptoms unless the thrombosis is extensive or pulmonary embolism occurs.

Ovarian vein thrombophlebitis causing clinically apparent illness is either a very uncommon complication of the puerperium or it resolves spontaneously, at times with the aid of antibiotics that were used to treat pelvic infection. Munsick and Gillanders (1980) identified the following clinical features from review of cases of ovarian vein thrombophlebitis reported by others and those that they had personally observed: *The cardinal symptom was pain* that developed typically on the second or third postpartum day with or without fever. Pain was present in the lower abdomen, the flank, or both. In some cases, but not all, a tender mass was palpable just beyond the uterine cornu. Always the thrombophlebitis involved the right ovarian vein; in a few instances it involved both the right and the left ovarian vein. Typical findings at laparotomy were a firm tumefaction of the ovarian vein overlaid by inflamed peritoneum. Peritoneal involvement may have spread to produce perisalpingo-oophoritis and periappendicitis. The thrombus may have extended into the inferior vena cava. If an intra-abdominal lesion that requires surgery, such as appendicitis, can be excluded without performing a laparotomy, treatment for ovarian vein thrombophlebitis recommended by them and others is heparin intravenously and broad-spectrum antibiotics.

Munsick and Gillanders (1980) considered the possible relationship of the direction of blood flow in the ovarian veins to the gene-

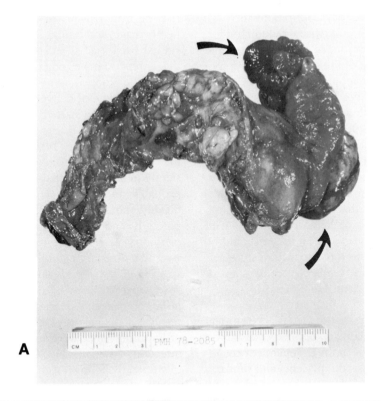

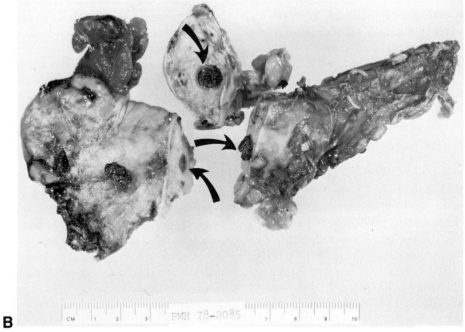

FIG. 36-1.   A. Resected thrombosed right ovarian vein plus right oviduct (upper arrow) and ovary (lower arrow). **B.** Same specimen after sectioning to demonstrate the thrombus (arrows).

sis of ovarian vein thrombophlebitis. From their radioangiographic studies performed during the puerperium, they suspect that in the upright position blood flow from the left ovarian vein is primarily retrograde to the uterus but antegrade from the uterus through the right ovarian vein. With such a flow pattern, bacterial contaminants would more likely ascend the right ovarian vein and provoke intimal damage and thrombophlebitis. They believe that such a mechanism would account for the great preponderance of involvement of the right, rather than the left, ovarian vein.

In the one case identified in recent years at Parkland Memorial Hospital laparotomy was performed because of the likelihood of a grave outcome if the suspected diagnosis of right ovarian vein thrombophlebitis proved to be appendicitis, instead. There was extensive inflammation, edema, and induration surrounding the enlarged thrombosed right ovarian vein, the right tube and ovary, and the appendix (Fig. 36-1). The vein was filled with firm clot that extended into the vena cava to just below the renal veins. Because of the extent of the disease, the right ovarian vein plus the clot that extended into the vena cava, and the appendix, right oviduct, and right ovary were resected. The inferior vena cava and uninvolved left ovarian vein were ligated; heparin therapy was started 48 hours after laparotomy; she soon recovered.

Suppurative pelvic thrombophlebitis and *septic emboli* that develop in association with bacterial infection are also discussed in Chapter 35, pages 897, 901, and 903.

Anticoagulation and Abortion. The treatment of deep venous thrombosis with heparin does not preclude termination of pregnancy by careful curettage. (see Chap. 24, p. 603). If all the products of conception are removed without trauma to the reproductive tract, heparin can be given in therapeutic doses at the termination of the procedure without undue risk. If abdominal hysterotomy is to be performed, those precautions

presented below for cesarean section are applicable. Experiences are lacking in which hypertonic saline or a prostaglandin has been used as an abortifacient in the presence of effective anticoagulation. The same is true for laparoscopic tubal sterilization. In both circumstances, it is anticipated that serious bleeding might be induced.

Anticoagulation and Delivery. The forces of labor and delivery may induce severe hemorrhage in the fetus if the mother has very recently been treated with warfarin. The effects of warfarin may be reversed by the slow intravenous administration of vitamin K_1 in a dose of 10 mg. The activities of the vitamin K-dependent clotting factors usually increase to safe levels within 8 hours in the mother but less rapidly in the fetus. Maternal transfusion of plasma or a plasma fraction rich in factors II, VII, IX, and X (Konyne) will correct the deficiency immediately in the mother but, unfortunately, not in the fetus. Hepatitis may be transmitted with this plasma fraction.

Most often, heparin should be started when warfarin is stopped. Heparin does not cross the placenta. The effects of heparin on blood loss at delivery will depend upon a number of variables, including the following: (1) the dose, route, and time of administration; (2) the magnitude of incisions and lacerations; (3) the intensity of myometrial contraction and retraction once the products of conception have been delivered; (4) the presence of other coagulation defects. The experiences at Parkland Memorial Hospital have been that measured blood loss is not greatly increased with vaginal delivery if the midline episiotomy is modest in depth, there are no lacerations of the genital tract, and the uterus promptly becomes firmly contracted and remains so after delivery of the placenta. Such ideal circumstances do not always prevail during and after vaginal delivery, however. Mueller and Lebherz (1969), for example, have described 10 women with antepartum thrombophlebitis treated with heparin. Three who continued to receive heparin during labor and delivery bled remarkably and developed severe postpartum hemorrhage with large hematomas. Blood replacement of 1500 ml, 2500 ml, and 4500 ml was essential, as was repeated drainage of the hematomas. Therefore, in general, heparin therapy should be stopped during the time of labor and delivery. If the uterus is well contracted and there has been negligible trauma to the lower genital tract, it can soon be restarted. Otherwise, a delay of 2 or 3 days may be prudent. Protamine sulfate administered intravenously most often will promptly and effectively reverse the effect of heparin but, of course, will be of no benefit for hematomas already formed. Protamine sulfate, if used, should not be given in excess of the amount needed to neutralize the heparin. Excess protamine has an anticoagulant effect.

Serious bleeding is likely when heparin in usual therapeutic doses is administered to someone who has undergone cesarean section within the previous 72 hours. After that, the risk of bleeding decreases with time so that by 1 week in the otherwise uncomplicated case there is slight risk. Again, preexisting defects in the hemostatic mechanism, such as thrombocytopenia, or impaired platelet function as induced by aspirin, enhance the likelihood of hemorrhage with heparin.

The woman who has very recently suffered a pulmonary embolism and who must be delivered by cesarean section presents a grave problem. Cesarean section and ligation of the inferior vena cava and the left ovarian vein near its insertion into the renal vein will usually yield the most favorable outcome. Nearly always in this situation tubal sterilization is also indicated.

Pulmonary Embolism. The greatest danger from venous thrombosis is pulmonary embolism. The reported incidence of pulmonary embolism associated with pregnancy has varied widely from 1 in 2700 deliveries (Stamm, 1960) to less than 1 in 7000 deliveries (Mengert, 1945).

Chest discomfort accompanied by shortness of breath, air hunger, tachypnea, or obvious apprehension, are strongly suggestive of pulmonary embolism during the puerperium. Bell and associates (1977) have carefully analyzed the clinical findings in a large number of individuals with angiographically identified pulmonary embolism. The most common abnormality was a respiratory rate of greater than 16 per minute. They emphasized that its frequency was so striking that a lower respiratory rate should rule against the diagnosis. Physical examination of the chest may or may not yield findings such as an accentuated pulmonic valve second sound, rales, or friction rub. Right axis deviation may or may not be evident in the electrocardiogram.

Even with massive pulmonary embolism, signs, symptoms, and laboratory data to support the diagnosis of pulmonary embolism may be deceivingly nonspecific, as borne out in a cooperative study sponsored by the National Heart and Lung Institute (Wenger et al., 1972). Ninety patients were identified by pulmonary angiography to have massive embolism. Although at least two lobar arteries were obstructed, the classic triad indicative of pulmonary embolism—hemoptysis, pleuritic chest pain, and dyspnea—was noted in only 20 percent of the subjects.

HEPARIN DOSAGE. In general, in either category of obstetric patients, therapy with heparin in appropriate doses is effective. Most often, 5000 to 7500 units given intravenously every 4 hours, depending primarily upon the size of the woman, soon accomplishes the stated goals.

Attempts to identify by laboratory testing whether the heparin dosage is adequate to inhibit further thrombosis yet not cause serious hemorrhage have been discouraging unless the laboratory has the capability of measuring heparin in plasma (Bonnar, 1979). Whole blood clotting times have long been used and more recently measurement of the plasma partial thromboplastin time has been recommended. The two tests often correlate poorly. An important test that tends to be forgotten is the frequent measurement of the hematocrit to detect significant but concealed hemorrhage. Careful clinical evaluation usually will provide the best information concerning adequacy of dosage. Clear evidence of clinical improvement with no evidence of hemorrhage is the desired goal.

It is important to remember that heparin is being administered whenever blood is to be drawn or medications are ordered to be given parenterally. Serious hemorrhage may occur especially when arterial blood is drawn for blood gas analyses just before or soon after the administration of heparin.

Therapy with heparin as described may be discontinued in the postpartum patient after 10 days to two weeks if the disease process has clearly abated and there is no evidence of underlying chronic vascular disease that would predispose to venous thrombosis and no evidence of underlying cardiopulmonary dysfunction. Wessler and Gitel (1979) recommend that treatment with heparin and oral anticoagulant overlap for 6 days after the prothrombin time has reached the therapeutic level. If, however, the woman is undelivered, there is real likelihood of recurrence of the venous thrombosis sometime during the subsequent antepartum, intrapartum, and postpartum periods. Therefore, anticoagulant therapy ought to be continued or possibly ligation of the inferior vena cava and ovarian veins be carried out as discussed below.

WARFARIN THERAPY. The problems associated with the use of heparin antepartum and intrapartum are considered above. If prolonged anticoagulation is desired for the postpartum woman, it may be used as described. Coagulation is not impaired in breastfed infants whose mothers are taking therapeutic doses of warfarin (DeSwiet and Lewis, 1977).

VENOUS LIGATION. In the very infrequent circumstances where heparin therapy fails to prevent recurrent pulmonary embolism, ligation of the vena cava below the level of the renal veins but above the entry of the right ovarian vein and of the left ovarian vein below its entry into the left renal vein is usually indicated. Serrated Teflon clips applied to the vena cava may be nearly as effective (Couch et al., 1975). In spite of previous

reports suggesting that obstruction of the vena cava causes placental abruption, there are several reports of successful ligation performed antepartum with favorable outcomes for the mother and usually the fetus (Stone et al., 1968). Caval and ovarian vein ligation for treatment of septic emboli from the pelvis is considered in Chapter 35, page 903.

The possibility of pulmonary embolism must always be kept in mind, especially during the puerperium. If the woman develops an embolus during her hospital stay, the diagnosis is more likely to be made and appropriate therapy started. Embolism may occur weeks after delivery, however, with no intervening symptoms. Under these circumstances, it is easy to ascribe the symptoms to some other cause, especially anxiety. A woman readmitted to Parkland Memorial Hospital provides an example:

A somewhat elderly, multiparous woman was admitted near term with total placental abruption and massive bleeding. Treatment included cesarean section and 15 units of whole blood. Eight days later, after a benign postpartum course, she was discharged. Three weeks after delivery she was awakened during the night by chest pain. In the morning she went to a physician who considered her to be "apprehensive and hyperventilating secondary to grief reaction." Rebreathing into a paper bag and diazepam were prescribed but gave no relief. The same day she came to Parkland Memorial Hospital where supporting evidence of pulmonary embolism was readily uncovered, including tachypnea, splinting of left side of chest on inspiration, abnormal chest x-ray, pulmonary perfusion defects demonstrated by lung scan in regions free of infiltrate, and, while breathing room air, an arterial blood P_{O_2} of 62 mm Hg and pH of 7.52. Treatment with heparin intravenously every 4 hours, was promptly started. At no time was there clinical evidence of thrombosis in the lower extremities and phlebograms were negative. Presumably the emboli came from the pelvis. She promptly recovered.

In general, whenever there is reasonable suspicion of pulmonary embolus, it is much safer to initiate an effective program of anticoagulation, as outlined in this chapter, rather than risk a second embolus, which may prove

TABLE 36-1.
EMERGENCY DIAGNOSTIC TESTS FOR PULMONARY EMBOLISM

TEST	FINDINGS SUGGESTIVE OF PULMONARY EMBOLISM	AIDS TO DIFFERENTIAL DIAGNOSIS	THERAPEUTIC IMPLICATION IF PULMONARY EMBOLISM IS PRESENT
ECG	Right axis shift (S1Q3T3) and right ventricular strain	To rule out acute myocardial infarction	Detection and treatment of arrhythmia
Chest roentgenogram	Enlargement of main pulmonary artery and right ventricle, infiltrate, pleural effusion, elevated diaphragm, or asymmetry of vasculature	To rule out pneumonia and congestive heart failure (may be secondary to pulmonary embolism)	Presence of acute right ventricular enlargement indicates life-threatening embolism
Arterial blood gases	Low P_{O_2} and P_{CO_2} are nearly constant findings in acute embolism	Normal P_{O_2} nearly excludes acute pulmonary embolism	Guide to oxygen therapy and guide to prognosis
Central venous pressure (CVP)	Elevated (if right ventricular failure is present)	If hypotension is present, low CVP nearly excludes pulmonary embolism as cause of hypotension	Central venous catheter provides route for administration of drugs or fluids and ready access to blood samples
Lung scan	Areas of oligemia (areas of the lung with a decreased concentration of radioactivity)	"Positive" scan can be caused by pneumonia, atelectasis, or other pulmonary lesions	Extent of avascular areas serves as a guide to severity of pulmonary embolism
Pulmonary angiography	Filling defects due to presence of emboli, cutoffs of pulmonary arteries, areas of decreased perfusion	Normal angiogram excludes large pulmonary embolus	Most accurate guide to extent of embolism

From Dalen and Dexter: *JAMA* 207:150, 1969
P_{O_2} indicates arterial oxygen tension

fatal. Dalen and Dexter (1969) have provided a succinct tabulation of emergency tests for pulmonary embolism (Table 36-1).

DISEASES AND ABNORMALITIES OF THE UTERUS

Subinvolution. Subinvolution is an arrest or retardation of involution, the process by which the puerperal uterus is normally restored to its original proportions. Subinvolution is accompanied by prolongation of the period of lochial discharge and sometimes by profuse hemorrhage. It may be followed by prolonged leukorrhea and irregular or excessive uterine bleeding. The diagnosis is established by bimanual examination. The uterus is larger and softer than normal for the particular period of the puerperium. Among the recognized causes of subinvolution are retention of placental fragments and pelvic infection. Since most cases of subinvolution result from local causes, they are usually amenable to early diagnosis and treatment. Ergonovine (Ergotrate) or methyl ergonovine (Methergine), 0.2 mg every 3 to 4 hours for 24 to 48 hours may lead to improvement. Metritis may be best managed by antibiotic therapy.

Postpartum Cervical Erosions. Cervical erosions, or eversions, are a complication of the late postpartum period. Shallow cauterization or cryotherapy can be used to remove persistent exuberant granulations, or the delicate exposed endocervical columnar epithelium, without causing stenosis of the endocervix.

Relaxation of the Vaginal Outlet and Prolapse of the Uterus. Extensive lacerations of the perineum during delivery, if not properly repaired, are commonly followed by relaxation of the vaginal outlet. Even when external lacerations are not visible, overstretching or submucosal tears may lead to marked relaxation. The changes in the pelvic supports during parturition predispose, moreover, to prolapse of the uterus and to urinary stress incontinence. These conditions may escape detection unless an examination is made at the end of the puerperium and unless the patients are subjected to long-term follow-up.

In general, operative correction should be postponed until the desired number of children has been achieved, unless, of course, serious disability, notably urinary stress incontinence, demands intervention.

HEMORRHAGES DURING THE PUERPERIUM

Occasionally, serious uterine hemorrhage develops in the latter part of the first week, or later in the puerperium. Hemorrhage most often is the result of abnormal involution of the placental site, but it may be caused also by retention of a portion of the placenta. Usually, the retained piece of placenta undergoes necrosis with deposition of fibrin, and may eventually form a so-called *placental polyp* (Fig. 36-2). As the scab of polyp detaches from the myometrium, hemorrhage may be brisk.

It has been generally accepted that with late postpartum hemorrhage from the uterus, prompt curettage is necessary. The experiences at Parkland Memorial Hospital, however, have been that curettage subsequent to late puerperal hemorrhage most often did not remove identifiable placental tissue. Hemorrhage was initiated by the separation of the retained products of conception which, in turn, were flushed out by the brisk hemorrhage. Curettage, rather than reducing hemorrhage, was more likely to traumatize the implantation site and incite more bleeding and, at times, to such a degree that hysterectomy had to be performed. Especially where there is good reason to want to preserve the uterus for future childbearing, treatment initially may best be directed at control of the bleeding with intravenous oxytocin, ergonovine, or methylergonovine. If the bleeding subsides, the woman is simply observed and if the bleeding stops, she is discharged. In general, curettage is carried out only if appreciable bleeding persists or recurs after such management.

Puerperal Hematomas. Blood may escape into the connective tissue beneath the skin covering the external genitalia or beneath the vaginal mucosa to form vulvar and vaginal hematomas. The condition usually follows injury to a blood vessel without laceration of the superficial tissues, and may occur with spontaneous, as well as operative, delivery. Occasionally, the hemorrhage is delayed perhaps as a result of sloughing of a vessel that had become necrotic from prolonged pressure.

Less frequently, the torn vessel lies above the pelvic fascia. In that event, the hematoma develops above it. In its early stages, the hematoma forms a rounded swelling that projects into the upper portion of the vaginal canal and may almost occlude its lumen. If the bleeding continues, it dissects retroperitoneally and thus may form a tumor palpable above Poupart's ligament, or it may dissect upward, eventually reaching the lower margin of the diaphragm.

Large vulvar hematomas (Fig. 36-3), particularly those that develop rapidly, may cause excruciating pain which often is the first symptom that is noticed. Hematomas of

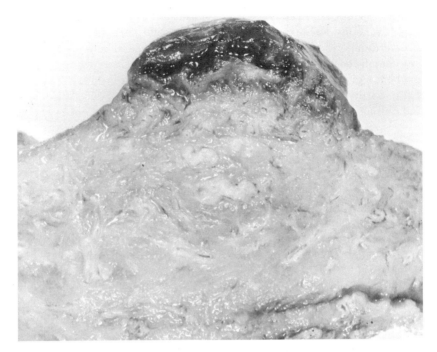

FIG. 36-2. Placental polyp. Hysterectomy was performed because of prolonged bleeding which resulted in severe anemia in a woman who wanted no more pregnancies.

moderate size may be absorbed spontaneously. The tissues overlying the hematoma may give way as a result of necrosis caused by pressure, and profuse hemorrhage may follow. In other cases, the contents of the

hematoma may be discharged in the form of large clots.

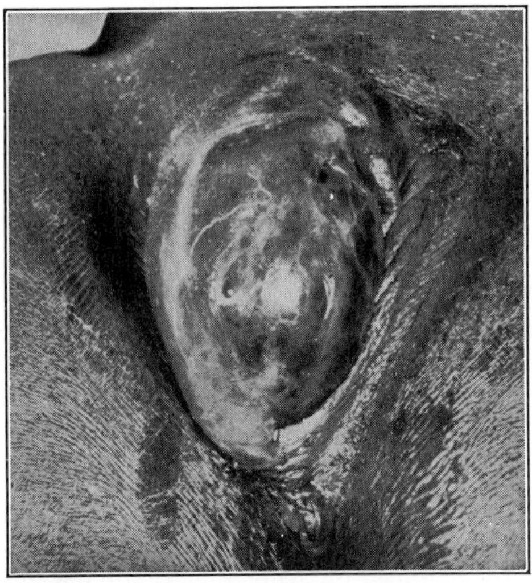

In the subperitoneal variety, the extravasation of blood beneath the peritoneum may be massive and occasionally fatal. Death may also follow secondary intraperitoneal rupture. Occasionally, rupture into the vagina leads to infection of the hematoma and potentially fatal sepsis.

A vulvar hematoma is readily diagnosed by severe perineal pain and the sudden appearance of a tense, fluctuant, and sensitive tumor of varying size covered by discolored skin. When the mass develops adjacent to the vagina, it may temporarily escape detection, but symptoms of pressure, if not pain, and inability to void should soon lead to a vaginal examination and the discovery of a round, fluctuant tumor encroaching on the lumen. When the hematoma extends upward between the folds of the broad ligament, it may escape detection unless a portion of the tumor can be felt on abdominal palpation or unless evidence of anemia or infection appear.

The prognosis is usually favorable, though

FIG. 36-3. Vulvar hematoma bulging into the right vaginal wall.

bleeding into very large hematomas has led to death.

TREATMENT. Smaller vulvar hematomas identified after leaving the delivery room may be treated expectantly. If, however, the pain is severe, or if they continue to enlarge, as they often do, the best treatment is prompt incision and evacuation of the blood with ligation of the bleeding points. The cavity can then be obliterated with mattress sutures. *With hematomas of the genital tract, blood loss is nearly always considerably more than the clinical estimate.* Hypovolemia and severe anemia should be prevented by adequate blood replacement. Broad-spectrum antibiotics are of value.

The subperitoneal and supravaginal varieties are more difficult to treat. They can be evacuated by incision of the perineum, but unless there is complete hemostasis, which is difficult to achieve by this route, laparotomy is advisable.

DISEASES OF THE URINARY TRACT

The puerperal bladder is not so sensitive to intravesical fluid tension as in the nonpregnant state. Moreover, it has become commonplace in modern obstetrics to establish an intravenous infusion system during labor in women. After delivery, the infusion system is then used to administer oxytocin during the first hour or so after delivery, if not longer. The oxytocin induces potent antidiuresis until the time the oxytocin is stopped, after which there is a prompt diuresis. The bladder then fills rapidly and may overdistend to a remarkable degree. General anesthesia, and especially conduction anesthesia with the temporarily disturbed neural control of the bladder, are important contributory factors. The woman in this circumstance may, in time, void small volumes of urine ("overflow incontinence") which mislead attendants into believing she is voiding normally. Inspection of the abdomen will disclose the uterine fundus to be much higher than it should be and beneath it there is a cystic mass, the distended bladder.

As stated above, trauma to the genital tract, especially with large hematoma formation, may cause urinary retention. Therefore, pelvic examination should be performed whenever urinary retention is identified.

The combination of residual urine and bacteriuria introduced by catheterization into a traumatized bladder present the optimal conditions for the development of infection of the urinary tract. The initial symptoms include dysuria, frequency, and urgency. Signs and symptoms of infection subsequently will vary, depending upon whether the infection is localized to the bladder or ascends to involve the upper urinary tract. After urine has been obtained for culture, treatment should consist of appropriate antibiotic or chemotherapeutic agents, as discussed in Chapter 28 (p. 704).

In case of overdistension of the bladder, it is usually best to leave an indwelling catheter in place for at least 24 hours so as to empty the bladder completely and prevent prompt recurrence, as well as to allow recovery of normal bladder tone and sensation. When the catheter is removed, it is necessary subsequently to demonstrate ability to void appropriately. If the woman cannot void after 4 hours, she should be catheterized and the volume of urine measured. If there is more than 200 ml of urine, it is apparent that the bladder is not functioning appropriately. The catheter should be left in again and the bladder drained for another day. If less than 200 ml of urine is obtained, the catheter can be removed and the bladder rechecked subsequently as just described. In general, the first time the woman voids spontaneously after removal of an indwelling catheter inserted because of previous inability to void and gross overdistention, she should be immediately catheterized for residual urine. If the volume exceeds 100 ml, constant drainage should be reinstituted and those steps in management just outlined should be resumed. There is evidence that antimicrobial therapy will reduce appreciably the likelihood of bacteriuria developing when bladder catheterization is limited to 4 days or less (Garibaldi et al., 1974).

DISORDERS OF THE BREAST

Engorgement of the Breasts. For the first 24 or 48 hours after the development of the lacteal secretion, it is not unusual for the breasts to become distended, firm, and nodular. This condition, commonly known as engorged breasts, or "caked breasts," often causes considerable pain and may be accompanied by a transient elevation of temperature. The disorder represents an exaggeration of the normal venous and lymphatic engorgement of the breasts, which is a regular precursor of lactation. It is not the result of overdistension of the lacteal system with milk.

Treatment consists of supporting the breasts with a binder or brassiere, applying an ice bag, and if necessary administering orally 60 mg of codeine sulfate or another analgesic. Pumping of the breast or manual expression of the milk may be necessary at first (Fig. 36-4), but in a few days the condition

is usually alleviated and the infant is able to nurse normally.

Suppression of Lactation. When, for a variety of reasons the infant is not to be breastfed, suppression of lactation becomes important. Perhaps the simplest method consists in support with a comfortable binder, ice bags, and mild analgesics for pain. Usually, all signs and symptoms will disappear in a few days if the breasts are not stimulated by pumping. Hormones, particularly estrogens, either alone or combined with testosterone, have been widely used for this purpose (Harrison, 1979). A single intramuscular injection of 4 ml of long-acting steroid esters in the form of estradiol valerate and testosterone enanthate (Deladumone), administered at the time of delivery, is claimed to be effective.

Several estrogens that have been used to try to suppress lactation have been shown to predispose to venous thrombosis and thromboembolism (Niebyl et al., 1979; Tindall, 1968, Turnbull, 1969). Moreover, their effect on lactation may be one of delay rather than effective suppresion. Niebyl and coworkers (1979) challenge their use on the

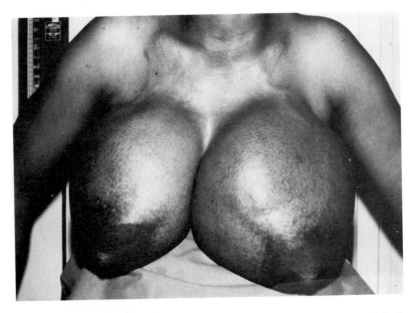

FIG. 36-4. Pathologic breast engorgement 3 days after delivery. Pumping of the breasts, uplift support, and analgesia provided relief. (Courtesy Dr. J. Duenhoelter)

bases of increased risk of thromboembolism and questionable benefit. These agents have not been used at Parkland Memorial Hospital even though the majority of mothers still do not breast feed their infants.

Bromocriptine, a dopamine agonist, stimulates the production of prolactin inhibitory factor which, in turn, causes a fall in plasma prolactin and the suppression of lactation. Nilsen and co-workers (1976) claimed bromocriptine to be superior to stilbestrol for suppressing lactation. The use of bromocriptine in the puerperium for this purpose has recently been approved by the Food and Drug Administration. Troublesome nausea has been associated with its use, and in the United Kingdom, at least, where it is approved for use, it is expensive.

Mastitis. Parenchymatous inflammation of the mammary glands is a rare complication of pregnancy but is occasionally observed during the puerperium and lactation.

The symptoms of suppurative mastitis seldom appear before the end of the first week of the puerperium and, as a rule, not until the 3rd or 4th week. Marked engorgement usually precedes the inflammation, the first sign of which is chills or actual rigor, which is soon followed by a considerable rise in temperature and an increase in pulse rate. The breast becomes hard and reddened, and the patient complains of pain. In some cases, the constitutional symptoms attending a mammary abscess are severe. Local manifestations may be so slight as to escape observation, however; such cases are usually mistaken for puerperal infection. In still another group of women, the infection pursues a subacute or almost chronic course. The breast is somewhat harder than usual and more or less painful, but constitutional symptoms are either lacking or very slight. In such circumstances, the first indication of the true diagnosis is often afforded by the detection of fluctuation.

ETIOLOGY. By far, the most common offending organism is *Staphylococcus aureus.* The immediate source of the staphylococci that cause this mastitis is nearly always the nursing infant's nose and throat. At the time of nursing, the organism enters the breast through the nipple at the site of a fissure or abrasion, which may be quite small. Whether the bacteria commonly cause mastitis simply by entering the lactiferous ducts of the breast with completely intact integument is not clear. In cases of true mastitis, the offending organism can nearly always be cultured from breast milk.

Suppurative mastitis among nursing mothers has at times reached epidemic levels. Such outbreaks most often coincide with the appearance of a new strain of antibiotic-resistant staphylococcus or the reappearance of one previously identified. Typically, the infant becomes infected in the nursery as he comes in contact with nursery personnel who carry the organism. The attendants' hands are the major source of contamination of the newborn. Especially in a crowded, understaffed nursery, it is a simple matter for the personnel inadvertently to transfer staphylococci from one colonized newborn infant to another. The colonization of staphylococci in the infant may be totally asymptomatic or may locally involve the umbilicus or the skin, but occasionally the organisms may cause a life-threatening, systemic infection.

PREVENTION. Safeguards to prevent colonization of the newborn with virulent strains of staphylococci necessitate exclusion from the care of the infant and mother of all personnel with a known or suspected staphylococcal lesion. Also, as a matter of daily routine, close inspection should be made of every infant, with prompt isolation of any who appear to be developing an infection of the cord or of the skin. Frequent use of soap or detergent for handscrubbing by personnel is essential. At the first sign of an outbreak, all personnel should be checked with appropriate cultures and phage-typing of swabbings from the posterior nares to identify carriers of more virulent strains of staphylococci.

At the time of an epidemic, the phenomenon of bacterial interference has been used successfully to prevent colonization of the newborn with highly virulent strains of *S.*

aureus (Light et al., 1967). As each newborn arrives at the nursery, the nares and umbilicus are directly inoculated with a strain of *S. aureus* known to be nonvirulent. This procedure usually blocks subsequent colonization by virulent strains.

The advent of antibiotics has markedly improved the prognosis in acute puerperal mastitis. Provided appropriate antibiotic therapy is started before suppuration begins, the infection can usually be aborted within 48 hours. Before initiating any antibiotic therapy, milk should be expressed from the affected breast onto a swab and promptly cultured. By so doing, the offending organism can be identified and its bacterial sensitivity ascertained. At the same time, the results of such cultures also provide information that is mandatory for a successful program of surveillance of nosocomial infections. The initial choice of antibiotic will undoubtedly be influenced to a considerable degree by the current experiences with staphylococcal infections at the institution in which the patient is receiving care. If, at the time, most staphylococcal infections are caused by organisms sensitive to penicillin, treatment with penicillin G is recommended. If the infection is caused by resistant, penicillinase-producing staphylococci, or if resistant organisms are suspected while awaiting the results of culture, a penicillinase-resistant compound should be used. It is important that treatment not be discontinued too soon. Even though clinical response may be prompt and striking, treatment should be continued for at least 10 days.

Nursing should be discontinued when a diagnosis of suppurative mastitis is made, for it may be quite painful and the milk is infected; moreover, the infant often harbors the organisms and can therefore cause reinfection. Since the infant almost always is colonized by the offending organism, he should be observed very closely for signs of infection. Once established, resistant staphylococcal infections tend to spread and recur among the family for protracted periods of time.

In the case of formation of frank abscesses, drainage in addition to antibiotic therapy is essential. The incision should be made radially, extending from near the areolar margin toward the periphery of the gland, to avoid injury to the lactiferous ducts. In early cases, a single incision over the most dependent portion of the area of fluctuation is usually sufficient, but multiple abscesses require several incisions. The operation should be done under general anesthesia, and a finger should be inserted to break up the walls of the locules. The resulting cavity is loosely packed with gauze, which should be replaced at the end of 24 hours by a smaller pack. If the pus has been thoroughly evacuated, the cavity of the abscess is obliterated and a complete cure is sometimes effected with great rapidity.

Galactocele.   Very exceptionally, as the result of the clogging of a duct by inspissated secretion, milk may accumulate in one or more lobes of the breast. The amount is ordinarily limited, but an excess may form a fluctuant mass that may give rise to pressure symptoms. They may resolve spontaneously or require aspiration.

Supernumerary Breasts.   One in every few hundred women has one or more accessory breasts *(polymastia)*. The supernumerary breasts may be so small as to be mistaken for pigmented moles, or, when without a nipple, for a lipoma. They rarely attain considerable size. They are likely to be situated in pairs on either side of the midline of the thoracic or abdominal walls, usually below the main breasts; they are also found in the axillae, and more rarely on other portions of the body such as the shoulder, flank, groin, or thigh. The number of supernumerary breasts varies greatly. When arranged symmetrically, two or four are most common, although ten have been described. A dramatic illustration of supernumerary breasts has been provided by Patnaik (1978).

Polymastia has no obstetric significance, although occasionally the enlargment of supernumerary breasts in the axillae may result in considerable discomfort. Frequently, a tongue of mammary tissue extends out into the axilla from the outer margin of a normal breast, whereas an isolated fragment is sometimes found in the same location. Such structures undergo hypertrophy during pregnancy. When lactation has been established, they may become swollen and painful. Ordinarily, they soon undergo regression and give no further trouble.

Abnormalities of the Nipples. The typical nipple is cylindric, projecting well beyond the general surface of the breast; its exterior is slightly nodular but not fissured. Variations, however, are not uncommon, some sufficiently pronounced to interfere seriously with suckling.

In some women, the lactiferous ducts open directly into a depression at the center of the areola. In marked cases of depressed nipple, nursing is out of the question. When the depression is not very deep, the breast may occasionally be made available by use of a breast pump.

More frequently, the nipple, although not depressed, is so greatly inverted that it cannot be used for nursing. In such a case, daily attempts should be made during the last few months of pregnancy to draw the nipple out, using traction with the fingers. Since the maneuver is rarely successful, however, if the nipples cannot be made available by the temporary use of an electric pump, suckling must be discontinued.

Nipples that are normal in shape and size may become fissured and therefore particularly susceptible to injury from the child's mouth during suckling. In such cases, the fissures almost inevitably render nursing painful, sometimes with a deleterious influence upon the secretory function. Moreover, such lesions provide a convenient portal of entry for pyogenic bacteria. For these reasons, every effort should be made to heal such fissures, particularly by protecting them from further injury with a nipple shield and topical medication. If such measures are of no avail, the child should not be permitted to nurse on the affected side. Instead, the breast should be emptied regularly with a suitable pump until the lesions are completely healed.

Abnormalities of Secretion. There are marked individual variations in the amount of milk secreted, many of which are dependent not upon the general health and appearance of the woman but upon the development of the glandular portions of the breasts. A woman with large breasts may produce only a small quantity of milk, whereas another with small, flat breasts may produce an abundant supply. Very rarely, there is complete lack of mammary secretion (agalactia). As a rule, it is possible to express a small amount from the nipple on the 3rd or 4th day of the puerperium. Occasionally, the mammary secretion is excessive (polygalactia).

Formerly, persistent lactation or galactorrhea (together with amenorrhea and signs of estrogen deficiency) was referred to as the Chiari-Frommel syndrome. It was believed that this disorder was a pregnancy-induced derangement in the hypothalmic-pituitary control of prolactin and gonadotropin secretion. A similar set of symptoms commencing independent of pregnancy was described by Ahumada (1932) and by Argonz and Del Castillo (1953). With the development of sensitive and accurate radioimmunoassays for prolactin and with the development of polytomography for evaluating the contents of the sella turcica, it has been demonstrated that microadenomas of the pituitary are the most common cause of galactorrhea, amenorrhea, and estrogen deficiency. Thus, the development of this triad should alert the physician to the likelihood of the existence of a microadenoma of the pituitary irrespective of whether the signs and symptoms begin in the puerperal period or remote from pregnancy.

DISORDERS OF THE NERVOUS SYSTEM

Obstetric Paralysis. Pressure on branches of the sacral plexus during labor is demonstrated by complaints of intense neuralgia or cramplike pains extending down one or both legs as soon as the head begins to descend into the pelvis. As a rule, the compression is rarely severe enough to give rise to grave lesions. In some instances, however, the pain continues after delivery and is accompanied by paralysis of the muscles supplied by the external popliteal nerve (the flexors of the ankles and the extensors of the toes). Occasionally, the gluteal muscles are affected to a lesser extent. In modern obstetrics, paralysis of this kind is rare. Footdrop resulting from improper positioning of patients in stirrups or leg holders is more common and should be prevented.

Separation of the symphysis pubis or one of the sacroiliac synchondroses during labor may be followed by pain and marked interference with locomotion.

Puerperal Psychoses. These conditions are discussed in Chapter 28.

REFERENCES

Ahumada JC, Del Castillo EB: (Amenorrhea and galactorrhea). Bol Soc Obstet Ginec (Buenos Aires) 11:64, 1932

Argonz J, Del Castillo EB: A syndrome characterized by estrogenic insufficiency, galactorrhea and decreased urinary gonadotropin. J Clin Endocrinol 13:79, 1953

Bell WR, Simon TL, DeMets DL: The clinical features of submassive and massive pulmonary emboli. Am J Med 62:355, 1977

Bonnar J: Venous thrombo-embolism and pregnancy. In Stallworthy J, Bourne G, (eds): Recent Advances in Obstetrics and Gynaecology. Edinburgh, Churchill-Livingstone, 13:173, 1979

Couch NP, Baldwin SS, Crane C: Mortality and morbidity rates after inferior vena caval clipping. Surgery 77:106, 1975

Dalen JE, Dexter L: Pulmonary embolism. JAMA 207:1505, 1969

DeSwiet M, Lewis PJ: Excretion of anticoagulants in human milk. N Engl J Med 297:1471, 1977

Garibaldi RA, Burke JP, Dickman ML, Smith CB: Bacteriuria during indwelling urethral catheterization. N Engl J Med 291:215, 1974

Harrison RG: Suppression of lactation. Seminars in Perinatology 3:287, 1979

Henderson SR, Lund CJ, Creasman WT: Antepartum pulmonary embolism. Am J Obstet Gynecol 112:476, 1972

Hull R, Delmore T, Genton E, Hirsh S, Gent M, Sackett D, McLoughlin D, Armstrong P:

Warfarin versus low-dose heparin in the long-term treatment of venous thrombosis. N Engl J Med 301:855, 1979

Light IJ, Walton RL, Sutherland JM, Shinefield HR, Brackvogel V: Use of bacterial interference to control a staphylococcal nursery outbreak. Am J Dis Child 113:291, 1967

Mengert WF: Venous ligation in obstetrics. Am J Obstet Gynecol 50:467, 1945

Mueller MJ, Lebherz TB: Antepartum thrombophlebitis. Obstet Gynecol 34:867, 1969

Munsick RA, Gillanders LA: A review of the syndrome of puerperal ovarian vein thrombophlebitis with some original observations on ovarian venous blood-flow postpartum. Obstet Gynecol Survey, submitted for publication

Niebyl JR, Bell WR, Schaaf ME, Blake DA, Dubin NH, King TM: The effect of chlorotrianisene as postpartum lactation suppression on blood coagulation factors. Am J Obstet Gynecol 134:518, 1979

Nilsen PA, Meling A-B, Abildgaard U: Study on the suppression of lactation and the influence on blood clotting with bromocriptine (CB 154) (Parlodel). Acta Obstet Gynecol Scand 55:39, 1976

Patnaik P: Axillary and vulval breasts associated with pregnancy. Br J Obstet Gynecol 85:156, 1978

Pearson JW: Discussion of report by Henderson, Lund, and Creasman. Am J Obstet Gynecol 112:485, 1972

Shaul WL, Hall JG: Multiple congenital anomalies associated with oral anticoagulants. Am J Obstet Gynecol 127:191, 1977

Stamm H: Obstetrical and gynecological mortality due to embolism in Central Europe and Scandinavia. Geburtshilfe Frauenheilkd 20:675, 1960

Stone SR, Whalley PJ, Pritchard JA: Inferior vena cava and ovarian vein ligation during late pregnancy. Obstet Gynecol 32:267, 1968

Tindall VR: Factors influencing puerperal thromboembolism. J Obstet Gynaecol Br Commonw 75:1324, 1968

Turnbull AC: Puerperal thromboembolism and the suppression of lactation. J Obstet Gynaecol Br Commonw 75:1321, 1968

Wenger NK, Stein PD, Willis PW, III: Massive acute pulmonary embolism: the deceivingly nonspecific manifestations. JAMA 220:843, 1972

Wessler S, Gitel SN: Heparin: New concepts relevant to clinical use. 53:525, 1979

37

Preterm and Postterm Pregnancies and Inappropriate Fetal Growth

A fetus or newborn infant whose weight is appreciably below normal is at increased risk of dying and, when he survives, at increased risk of being impaired physically and intellectually. The frequency of infants weighing less than 2500 g (5½ pounds) at birth has long served as one indicator of the overall quality of reproductive performance, especially for large populations. It is now fully appreciated, however, that there are two distinct mechanisms responsible for abnormally low birth weight. In one, the rate of growth is normal but for an unduly short period of time; in the other, the fetus fails to maintain a normal rate of growth. Thus, as has been emphasized throughout this book, a most important factor in the successful management of a pregnancy in which complications develop is precise knowledge of the gestational age of the fetus. Knowledge of gestational age is certainly essential to any correct decision concerned with the appropriateness of fetal growth. Unfortunately, for a variety of reasons, the gestational age may either be unknown, or worse, be in error. The error may arise as the consequence of the woman not obtaining prenatal care until very late in pregnancy and therefore long

after events important in identifying fetal age have passed or been forgotten, or the error may evolve from unrecognized delayed ovulation following menses induced by withdrawal of an oral contraceptive. At times, the error in gestational age may be caused or enhanced by confusion in terminology.

Definitions. Unfortunately, disagreement, and thus confusion, over terminology persists. Therefore, the following definitions are provided even though they may not have universal acceptance:

A *term pregnancy* is commonly defined as one in which at least 37 but less than 42 completed weeks have elapsed since the onset of the last menstrual period which, in turn, was followed about 2 weeks after its onset by ovulation and fertilization. Of course, the critical date for determining the age of the fetus is the date of ovulation or fertilization, which can differ from each other only by minutes to a day or so. *The time of onset of the last menstrual period has assumed clinical importance for determining fetal age only because it is usually known rather precisely, and, when spontaneous and previously quite regular, it most often is followed by ovulation about 2 weeks later.*

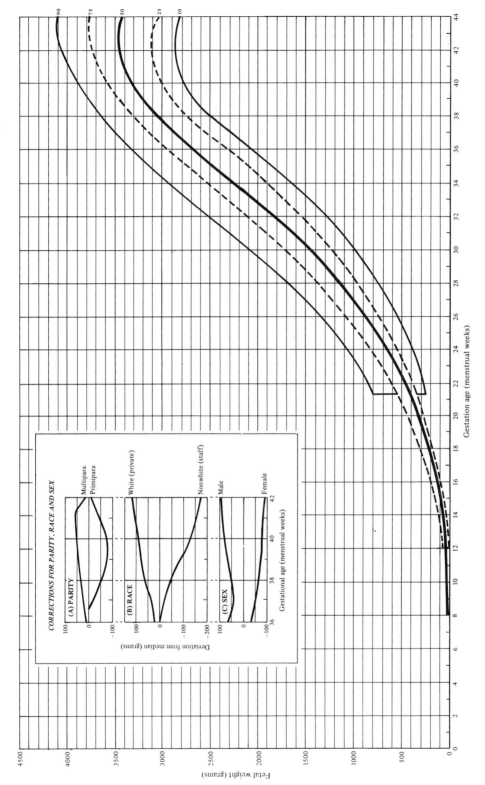

FIG. 37-1. Fetal weight. The 10th, 25th, 50th, 75th, and 90th percentiles of fetal weight in g throughout pregnancy and correction factors for parity, race (socioeconomic status) and sex are graphed. Data obtained from 31,202 prostaglandin-induced abortions and spontaneous deliveries. (Courtesy of Brenner and Hendricks. *Am J Obstet Gynecol* 126:555, 1976)

The fetus or newborn infant is referred to as a *fetus at term* or an *infant at term* during the interval from the 38th to the 42nd week after the onset of a menstrual period that was followed 2 weeks later by ovulation. Before the 38th week, *preterm* can be applied to categorize the fetus and the pregnancy; at 42 completed weeks *postterm* is appropriate. **Importantly, whenever possible, the gestational (menstrual) age should be cited in weeks rather than months or trimesters.**

Premature has long been used to designate the fetus or infant of less than 37 weeks gestational age. In some situations, at least, it might prove more informative not to use "premature" to describe the shortened gestational age of the fetus of infant, but rather use "premature" to describe function. For example, an infant at the time of birth may have achieved a gestational age of only 32 weeks and thus be chronologically premature, yet, from the standpoint of pulmonary function, demonstrate no difficulties in adapting to the external environment because pulmonary function was mature. To describe such a fetus or infant as *preterm* with mature pulmonary function, rather than premature with mature pulmonary function, might provide for greater clarity.

Postterm appropriately describes the fetus or newborn infant whose gestational age reaches 42 or more weeks. Again, it is highly desirous that the actual number of weeks of gestation be stated whenever possible. *Postdates* has more recently achieved considerable usage although the word seems to defy precise definition since the "dates" involved, other than the last menstrual period, are not clear. (Presumably, if the term *postdates* is acceptable, "predates" is eligible for incorporation into our medical vocabulary.)

A fetus or infant of low birth weight may be the consequence of an abnormally short gestational age but a normal rate of growth *(appropriately grown, preterm fetus or infant)*, or of a gestation of normal duration but with an impaired rate of growth *(growth-retarded, term fetus or infant)*, or of both a shortened gestation and an impaired rate of growth *(preterm, growth-retarded fetus or infant)*. The growth retarded fetus or infant is sometimes

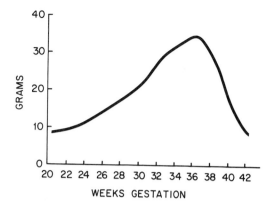

FIG. 37-2. Mean daily fetal growth (in g) during previous week of gestation. (Adapted from Hendricks. *Obstet Gynecol* 24:357, 1964)

described as *small for gestational age.* Especially in recent years, "small for gestational age" has been used to categorize an infant whose birth weight is clearly below average and usually below the 10th percentile for his gestational age, while an infant whose birth weight is above the 90th percentile has been categorized as *large for gestational age* (Fig. 37-1).

Typically, the fetus continues to grow after about 36 weeks gestation but at a slower rate (Fig. 37-2). When gestation is prolonged beyond term, some fetuses—perhaps the majority—continue to grow and may therefore achieve a remarkably large size. Those infants who did so have been referred to at times as *postmature* as well as postterm. Those who became undernourished and demonstrated evidence of suffering chronic distress in utero have often been classified as *dysmature.* Unfortunately, some obstetricians and pediatricians use "postmature" to designate all fetuses and infants in which the pregnancy is postterm, some apply it only to the large "overgrown" fetus or infant, while others designate only the undernourished, chronically distressed, newborn infant as postmature.

STANDARDS FOR NORMAL FETAL GROWTH AND DEVELOPMENT

The practice of equating fetal size with fetal age, which unfortunately has been firmly ingrained in obstetric and pediatric practices, by now should have been abandoned. For normal pregnancies, there is a strong correlation between the two, but at times the infant that is very small at birth may be chronologically and functionally quite mature. This phenomenon is observed perhaps most often when maternal vascular disease complicates the pregnancy. Conversely, the infant of normal term size may be dangerously preterm, as in some pregnancies complicated by diabetes. Not merely for nicety of diagnosis, but, importantly, for proper care of the infant, the preterm infant whose size is appropriate for his gestational age should be distinguished from the more mature infant who is growth-retarded, i.e., small for his gestational age.

Fetal Weights at Various Gestational Ages. It has proven difficult to obtain precise standards for gauging appropriate or inappropriate growth of the human fetus who is remote from term. In order to determine fetal weight precisely, the fetus must have been born, but the fetus of known gestational age who is born preterm is not the product of a normal pregnancy. For fetuses born preterm, Persson and co-workers (1978) have demonstrated that fetal growth rate, as reflected by the biparietal diameter measured sonographically, typically was somewhat retarded after the 26th week when compared to that for fetuses of normal pregnancies. The difference increased during the 3rd trimester to reach 3 to 4 mm at 36 weeks. Nonetheless, several investigators are to be congratulated for their laborious efforts to provide needed data even though the data might not be as precise as desired.

There is general agreement that the following factors influence birth weight, at least in term pregnancies: (1) *Sex:* Boys weigh more than girls. (2) *Parity:* Birth weight increases with parity at least through para 2. (3) *Race:* White babies at term weigh more than do black babies. In 1978, for example, the median birth weight for white infants was 3390 g and for black infants 3150 g.

In four different studies in the United States, the mean birth weights identified at 40 weeks gestation were in relatively close agreement for live-born infants (Brenner et al., 1976; Hoffman et al., 1974; Lubchenco et al., 1963; Naeye and Dixon, 1978). In these four studies, the mean birth weight at 40 weeks gestation was 3335 g and ranged from 3280 g to 3400 g. As gestational age decreased, however, the relative differences in mean birth weights increased more markedly, mostly because of the larger weights recorded by Hoffman compared to the other three groups. Fetal weights throughout pregnancy, including the 10th, 25th, 50th, 75th, and 90th percentiles and correction factors for parity, race, and sex, as determined by Brenner and co-workers (1976) are presented in Figure 37-1.

Estimating Gestational Age by Physical Examination. A reasonably precise estimation of gestational age may be quickly performed in the delivery room or nursery by evaluating the infant's development employing the sole creases, size of the breast nodule, scalp hair, earlobe, posture, and for the male infant, testes and scrotum (Fig. 37-3. A). A confirmatory neurologic examination can be carried out the day after delivery (Fig. 37-3. B).

THE PRETERM INFANT

The problems associated with preterm birth are deterrents to the achievement of the goal that all infants not only will be liveborn and survive, but will suffer neither physical nor psychologic impairment as the consequence of a hostile antepartum, intrapartum, or neonatal environment (Pritchard and Whalley, 1974). Any pregnancy in which there is a likelihood that this outcome will not be achieved must be considered high risk.* The

---

* High-risk pregnancy and fetal distress are two terms commonly used in pregnancy to incite or intensify special concern for the quality of the ultimate product of pregnancy, the newborn infant. Precise definition of fetal distress and of high-risk pregnancy is not simple and will continue to change as the science of perinatology provides new information.

CLINICAL ESTIMATION OF GESTATIONAL AGE
An Approximation Based on Published Data*

⬆ **Examination First Hours**

WEEKS GESTATION: 20 21 22 23 24 25 26 27 28 29 30 31 32 33 34 35 36 37 38 39 40 41 42 43 44 45 46 47 48

PHYSICAL FINDINGS

VERNIX
- APPEARS
- COVERS BODY, THICK LAYER
- ON BACK, SCALP, IN CREASES
- SCANT, IN CREASES
- NO VERNIX

BREAST TISSUE AND AREOLA
- AREOLA & NIPPLE BARELY VISIBLE NO PALPABLE BREAST TISSUE
- AREOLA RAISED
- 1-2 MM NODULE
- 3-5 MM
- 5-6 MM
- 7-10 MM
- 712 MM

EAR
- **FORM**: FLAT, SHAPELESS — BEGINNING INCURVING SUPERIOR — INCURVING UPPER 2/3 PINNAE — WELL-DEFINED INCURVING TO LOBE
- **CARTILAGE**: PINNA SOFT, STAYS FOLDED — CARTILAGE SCANT RETURNS SLOWLY FROM FOLDING — THIN CARTILAGE SPRINGS BACK FROM FOLDING — PINNA FIRM, REMAINS ERECT FROM HEAD

SOLE CREASES
- SMOOTH SOLES & CREASES
- 1-2 ANTERIOR CREASES
- 2-3 ANTERIOR CREASES
- CREASES ANTERIOR 2/3 SOLE
- CREASES INVOLVING HEEL
- DEEPER CREASES OVER ENTIRE SOLE

SKIN
- **THICKNESS & APPEARANCE**: THIN, TRANSLUCENT SKIN, PLETHORIC, VENULES OVER ABDOMEN EDEMA — SMOOTH THICKER NO EDEMA — PINK — SOME DESQUAMATION PALE PINK — FEW VESSELS — THICK, PALE, DESQUAMATION OVER ENTIRE BODY
- **NAIL PLATES**: AP. PEAR — NAILS TO FINGER TIPS — NAILS EXTEND WELL BEYOND FINGER TIPS

HAIR
- APPEARS ON HEAD
- EYE BROWS & LASHES
- FINE, WOOLLY, BUNCHES OUT FROM HEAD
- SILKY, SINGLE STRANDS LAYS FLAT
- PRECEDING HAIRLINE OR LOSS OF BABY HAIR SHORT, FINE UNDERNEATH

LANUGO
- AP. PEARS
- COVERS ENTIRE BODY
- VANISHES FROM FACE
- PRESENT ON SHOULDERS
- NO LANUGO

GENITALIA
- **TESTES**: TESTES PALPABLE IN INGUINAL CANAL — IN UPPER SCROTUM — IN LOWER SCROTUM
- **SCROTUM**: FEW RUGAE — RUGAE, ANTERIOR PORTION — RUGAE COVER — PENDULOUS
- **LABIA & CLITORIS**: PROMINENT CLITORIS LABIA MAJORA SMALL WIDELY SEPARATED — LABIA MAJORA LARGER NEARLY COVERED CLITORIS — LABIA MINORA & CLITORIS COVERED

SKULL FIRMNESS
- BONES ARE SOFT
- SOFT TO 1" FROM ANTERIOR FONTANELLE
- SPONGY AT EDGES OF FONTANELLE CENTER FIRM
- BONES HARD SUTURES EASILY DISPLACED
- BONES HARD, CANNOT BE DISPLACED

POSTURE
- **RESTING**: HYPOTONIC LATERAL DECUBITUS — HYPOTONIC — BEGINNING FLEXION THIGH — STRONGER HIP FLEXION — FROG-LIKE — FLEXION ALL LIMBS — HYPERTONIC — VERY HYPERTONIC

RECOIL - LEG
- NO RECOIL
- PARTIAL RECOIL
- PROMPT RECOIL

ARM
- NO RECOIL
- BEGIN FLEXION NO RECOIL
- PROMPT RECOIL MAY BE INHIBITED
- PROMPT RECOIL AFTER 30" INHIBITION

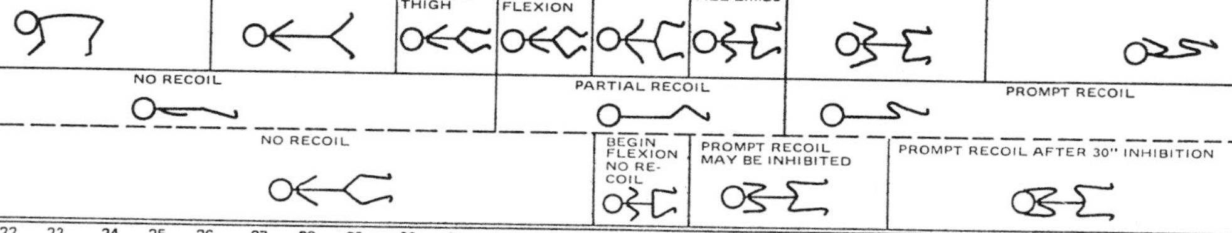

FIG. 37-3. A. Clinical estimation of gestational age.

927

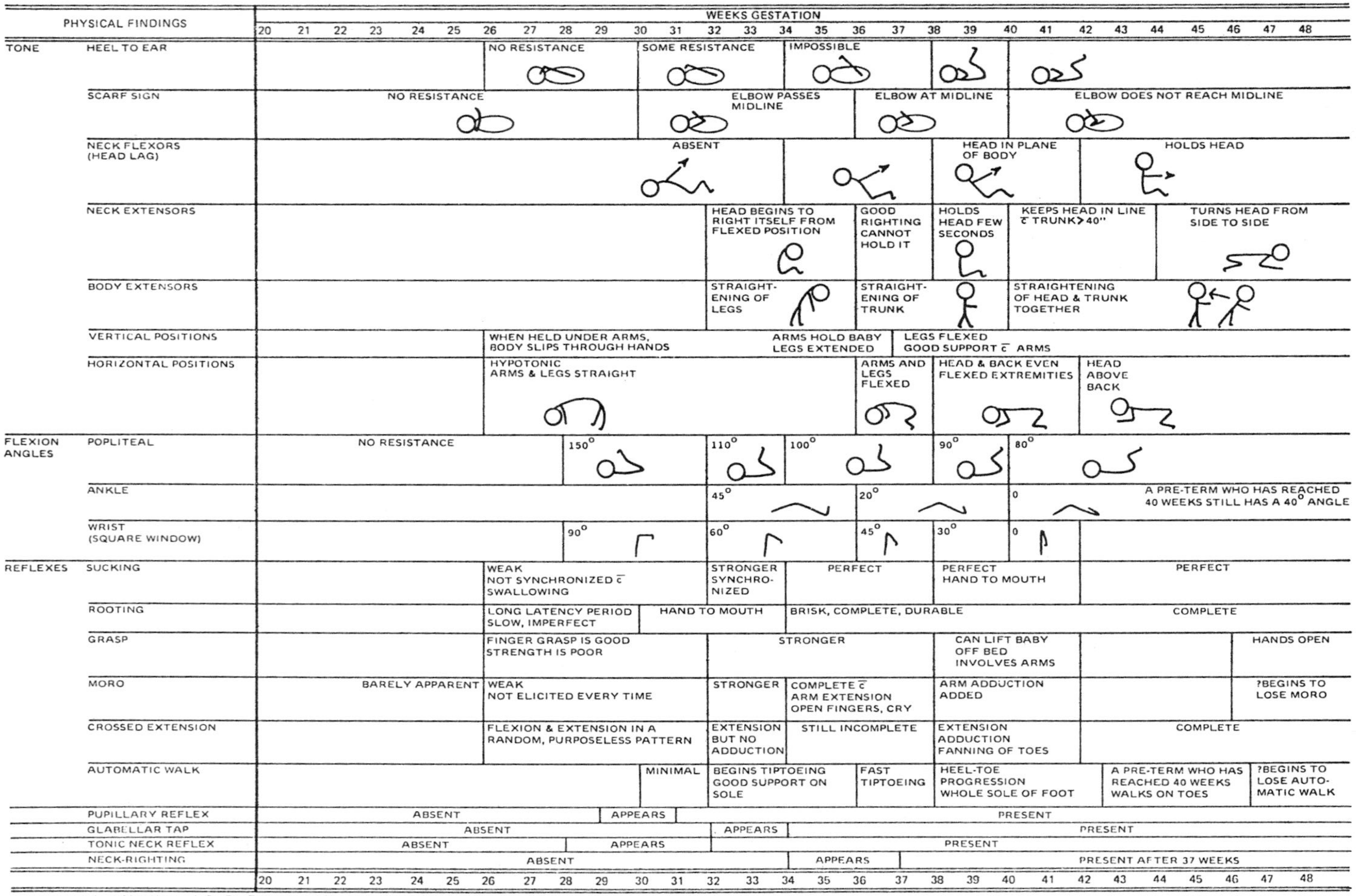

WEEKS GESTATION

Category	Physical Findings	Notes across 20–48 weeks
TONE	HEEL TO EAR	NO RESISTANCE → SOME RESISTANCE → IMPOSSIBLE
	SCARF SIGN	NO RESISTANCE → ELBOW PASSES MIDLINE → ELBOW AT MIDLINE → ELBOW DOES NOT REACH MIDLINE
	NECK FLEXORS (HEAD LAG)	ABSENT → HEAD IN PLANE OF BODY → HOLDS HEAD
	NECK EXTENSORS	HEAD BEGINS TO RIGHT ITSELF FROM FLEXED POSITION → GOOD RIGHTING CANNOT HOLD IT → HOLDS HEAD FEW SECONDS → KEEPS HEAD IN LINE c̄ TRUNK >40″ → TURNS HEAD FROM SIDE TO SIDE
	BODY EXTENSORS	STRAIGHTENING OF LEGS → STRAIGHTENING OF TRUNK → STRAIGHTENING OF HEAD & TRUNK TOGETHER
	VERTICAL POSITIONS	WHEN HELD UNDER ARMS, BODY SLIPS THROUGH HANDS → ARMS HOLD BABY LEGS EXTENDED → LEGS FLEXED GOOD SUPPORT c̄ ARMS
	HORIZONTAL POSITIONS	HYPOTONIC ARMS & LEGS STRAIGHT → ARMS AND LEGS FLEXED → HEAD & BACK EVEN FLEXED EXTREMITIES → HEAD ABOVE BACK
FLEXION ANGLES	POPLITEAL	150° → 110° → 100° → 90° → 80°
	ANKLE	45° → 20° → 90° → 0
	WRIST (SQUARE WINDOW)	90° → 60° → 45° → 30° → 0
REFLEXES	SUCKING	WEAK NOT SYNCHRONIZED c̄ SWALLOWING → STRONGER SYNCHRONIZED → PERFECT → PERFECT HAND TO MOUTH → PERFECT
	ROOTING	LONG LATENCY PERIOD SLOW, IMPERFECT → HAND TO MOUTH
	GRASP	FINGER GRASP IS GOOD STRENGTH IS POOR → STRONGER → CAN LIFT BABY OFF BED INVOLVES ARMS → COMPLETE
	MORO	BARELY APPARENT → WEAK NOT ELICITED EVERY TIME → STRONGER → COMPLETE c̄ ARM EXTENSION OPEN FINGERS, CRY → ARM ADDUCTION ADDED → HANDS OPEN → ?BEGINS TO LOSE MORO
	CROSSED EXTENSION	FLEXION & EXTENSION IN A RANDOM, PURPOSELESS PATTERN → EXTENSION BUT NO ADDUCTION → STILL INCOMPLETE → COMPLETE
	AUTOMATIC WALK	MINIMAL → BEGINS TIPTOEING GOOD SUPPORT ON SOLE → FAST TIPTOEING → HEEL-TOE PROGRESSION WHOLE SOLE OF FOOT
	PUPILLARY REFLEX	ABSENT → APPEARS → PRESENT
	GLABELLAR TAP	ABSENT → APPEARS → PRESENT
	TONIC NECK REFLEX	ABSENT → APPEARS → PRESENT AFTER 37 WEEKS
	NECK RIGHTING	ABSENT → APPEARS

Week scale: 20 21 22 23 24 25 26 27 28 29 30 31 32 33 34 35 36 37 38 39 40 41 42 43 44 45 46 47 48

Additional notations:
- A PRE-TERM WHO HAS REACHED 40 WEEKS STILL HAS A 40° ANGLE
- A PRE-TERM WHO HAS REACHED 40 WEEKS WALKS ON TOES
- ?BEGINS TO LOSE AUTOMATIC WALK

*Brazie, J.V., and Lubchenco, L.O.: The Estimation of Gestational Age Chart, in Kempe, Silver and O'Brien: Current Pediatric Diagnosis and Treatment, ed. 3, Los Altos, California, Lange Medical Publications, 1974, chapter 3.

Lit. 181, 12/74

FIG. 37-3. B. Confirmatory neurologic examination to be done after 24 hours.

TABLE 37-1.
NEONATAL SURVIVAL FOR INFANTS OF 34 WEEKS GESTATIONAL AGE OR LESS BORN DURING 1 YEAR AT PARKLAND MEMORIAL HOSPITAL

GESTATIONAL AGE (WKS)	LIVEBORN (NO.)	NEONATAL SURVIVAL (%)
25–26	8	0
27–28	19	74
29–30	25	88
31–32	41	95
33–34	85	100

great variety of maternal factors that may contribute to preterm birth and to fetal growth retardation are considered throughout this book. Some specific diseases of the newborn infant are discussed in Chapter 38, and birth injuries and malformations are considered in Chapter 39.

Fate of the Preterm Infant. The decrease in the neonatal death rate in the United States from 20.5 per 1000 live births in 1950 to 9.4 in 1978 has been due in large part to the fact that more preterm infants now survive. The availability of improved neonatal care has contributed remarkably to the reduction in neonatal mortality.

Neonatal mortality data for liveborn infants delivered remote from term at Parkland Memorial Hospital are presented in Table 37-1. There has been a remarkable improvement in recent years after the establishment of a functional neonatal intensive care unit. Comparable outcomes have been cited by Kopelman (1978).

A rightful concern has arisen from the prediction that, as the survival rate for very young and very small infants improved, there would be a drastic increase in the number of children who would be handicapped in some way. Wright and associates (1972), for example, carefully followed 70 infants who weighed 1500 g or less and compared their courses with normal-sized but otherwise presumably matched controls born between 1952 and 1956 at Chicago Lying-In Hospital.

Ten years later, they identified in the study group a remarkable excess of mortality, mental retardation, poor school performance, pyramidal tract disorders, and visual defects.

The more recent experiences of Stewart and co-workers (1977) are more favorable than those of Wright and associates. In Stewart's study, during the decade from 1965 to 1975, 32 percent of 148 liveborn preterm infants who weighed 1000 g or less at birth survived the neonatal period (28 days) when admitted to the Neonatal Unit of University College Hospital, London, England. Of those who weighed 751 g to 1000 g, 41 percent survived the neonatal period, whereas the survival rate for those who weighed 750 g or less was only 8 percent. Of all who survived the neonatal period, 9 died subsequently, leaving but 26 percent as long-term survivors. More girls than boys survived; more of the growth retarded infants survived than did those who were appropriately grown for their gestational age; more infants who were delivered by cesarean section survived; and more infants lived who were born during the last 5 years compared to the first 5 years.

In Stewart's study of 27 older children who weighed 648 g to 998 g at birth and whose gestational ages ranged from 24 to 35 weeks, 21 (78 percent) appeared normal, 2 (7 percent) had major handicaps, and 4 (15 percent) had lesser handicaps.

The experience of Jones and associates (1979) at Hammersmith Hospital, London, England, have not been so favorable. Over a 15-year-period, they have identified no significant improvement in neonatal mortality among infants whose very low birth weight was appropriate for gestational age, although there was some improvement among those who were small for gestational age. They identified no significant improvement in the proportion of handicapped children among the very low weight liveborn infants throughout the 15-year period, despite increasing complexity of care.

The populations evaluated by the two groups in London differed in that Jones' study population included all infants who showed any sign of life when born at Hammersmith

Hospital whereas Stewart's study population included a sizable number of very small infants who were born elsewhere and then transferred to their neonatal unit. The survival rate for infants who were transferred exceeded that of those who were born in the same hospital, which suggests, at least, that the infants who were selected for transfer were healthier and therefore more likely to survive.

Nonetheless, it seems fair to state that low-birth-weight infants who have no chromosomal abnormality or chronic fetal infection and who are appropriately cared for during and after birth most often will not be severely mentally retarded or otherwise grossly incapacitated. However, Zuelzer's statement of 1973 is still appropriate, namely, "There remains a marked discrepancy between the size of the problem and the size of the information."

Selection for Intensive Care. All hospitals that provide maternity care should, ideally, possess the facilities and the skilled personnel essential for effective intensive antepartum, intrapartum, and neonatal care. Lacking a sufficient number of such patients and the financial means for achieving this goal, a system should be developed for identifying high-risk pregnancies and for referral of the mother and her fetus to a regional center. Moreover, facilities for effecting rapid transport of the newborn infant in need of intensive care to such a center must be made generally available.

The recommendations made by the Wisconsin Perinatal Center, a pioneer in the conceptualization and implementation of regionalized intensive care, have been that for the following conditions strong consideration be given to transport of the mother and fetus or the newborn infant to a regional center:

1. Gestation of 34 weeks or less or birth weight below 2000 g
2. Maternal diabetes
3. Respiratory distress other than mild transient tachypnea
4. Neonatal seizures

5. Suspected infection of the fetus or infant
6. Meconium aspiration
7. Suspected congenital heart disease
8. Other anomalies requiring surgery
9. Early, severe, or persistent jaundice
10. Vomiting

Whether there is any gestational age or weight below which neonatal intensive care should not be instituted is a most difficult question, but from the standpoint of availability of facilities and economic necessity, it is one that cannot be avoided. Not only is such care restricted by limited personnel and facilities, it is proving to be very expensive. A most important consideration, therefore, in making any recommendation of so delicate a nature is, "What are the benefits that are likely to be achieved compared to those that would accrue to society from expenditure of the same money in other health care areas?" Physicians and other decision makers in the area of health care can no longer ignore this basic question. Hatwick (1973), in the course of discussing the economics of obstetric and newborn care, frankly stated: "While some find the economist's viewpoint repelling, its virtue stems from the fact that it recognizes what none of the other disciplines seem to recognize: Everything has its price. To ignore the cost is to make a decision to use resources in areas which may not be deserving of them." Indeed, the cost of prolonged neonatal intensive care is tremendous (Pomerance et al., 1978).

Graven (1973) commented that the extensive experiences with the neonatal intensive care facility in Wisconsin had been that infants who weighed less than 750 g, or who were less than 26 weeks' gestational age, were not a good investment of health care resources. He then recommended that physicians forego intensive care for this particular group of infants at least until the intensive care system is virtually unlimited. More recently, Stewart and co-workers (1977), on the basis of experiences cited above in some detail, concluded that intensive care during and after birth should be given to any infant whose gestational age is 24 weeks or more.

They emphasized that by so doing, mortality and potentially brain-damaging hazards to the survivors can be reduced. If, however, it becomes apparent that the infant has an abnormality, such as a large intraventricular hemorrhage that is virtually certain to cause a major handicap, they believe that, after consultation among all those involved, intensive care methods for sustaining life should be withdrawn.

PRETERM (PREMATURE) LABOR

Most often, it is advantageous physically, psychologically, and financially for the fetus to remain in utero until term but not unduly long thereafter. At times, however, he is better off being born even though preterm; an example is the severely growth retarded fetus in a persistently hostile intrauterine environment. Thus, a most important problem in obstetrics and perinatology is how best to identify precisely those circumstances in which the fetus is better off for being born even though he is preterm and may be functionally premature. Conflicting views and recommendations abound at this time but, appropriately, a great deal of interest currently exists regarding optimal timing of delivery, including the degree of interference that the obstetrician should bring to bear either to promote or to prevent delivery before term.

Causes of Preterm Labor. In the majority of instances, the precise cause or causes of labor before term are not known. Some conditions that predispose to labor before term are listed below:

1. Spontaneous rupture of membranes. Spontaneous labor remote from term not infrequently is preceded by spontaneous rupture of the membranes. Cause of the rupture is usually unknown.
2. Cervical incompetency. No doubt a small percentage of preterm labors and deliveries are the consequence of an incompetent cervix. Remote from term the incompetent cervix effaces and dilates appreciably not as the result of increased uterine activity but rather because of an intrinsic weakness in the cervix. Diagnosis and treatment of the incompetent cervix are discussed in Chapter 24, page 599.
3. Uterine anomalies. Very uncommonly, anomalies of the uterus are identified in cases of preterm labor and delivery. The greater the degree of reduplication of the uterus, i.e., the more extensive the septum and the more complete the separation of the uterus into two distinct horns, the greater the risk of premature labor. Diagnosis and management of this uncommon cause of preterm delivery are described in Chapter 25, page 629.
4. Overdistended uterus. Hydramnios, especially when acute and marked, or the presence of two or more fetuses, increases the risk of premature labor, presumably as the consequence of overdistension of the uterus inappropriate for the time in gestation.
5. Anomalies of the products of conception. Malformations of the fetus or of the placenta not only predispose to fetal growth retardation, but increase the likelihood of preterm labor as well.
6. Faulty placentation. Bleeding before the 3rd trimester, abruptio placentae, and placenta previa are likely to be associated with preterm labor.
7. Retained intrauterine device. The likelihood of preterm labor is appreciably increased when an intrauterine device persists in a pregnant uterus (see Chap. 40, p. 1026).
8. Fetal death. Death of the fetus remote from term commonly, but not always, is followed by spontaneous labor before term is reached.
9. Previous preterm delivery or late abortion. The woman who previously gave birth to a fetus remote from term is more likely to do so again even when no other predisposing factor is identified.
10. Serious maternal disease. Systemic disease in the mother, when it is severe, may cause premature labor and delivery. Serious hypoxia is a feature of some dis-

eases, for example, pneumonia, while high fever characterizes some others, for example, acute pyleonephritis. Neither acute pyelonephritis without marked fever nor asymptomatic bacteriuria has been commonly associated with premature delivery in our experience. Generalized peritonitis is likely to induce labor.

11. Elective induction of labor. Incorrect estimation of gestational age can create undue concern in the mind of the obstetrician over possible adverse effects on the fetus from presumed prolonged gestation or leads to considerable pressure from the mother-to-be or her family to intervene. However, induction of labor in some instances has been performed primarily for the convenience of the physician and a preterm infant delivered because of an erroneous estimation of gestational age. The use of oxytocin for *elective* induction of labor has been specifically disapproved by the Food and Drug Administration.

12. Unknown cause. Unfortunately, too many cases have to be so categorized.

Fedrick and Anderson (1976) have provided an extensive epidemiologic survey of factors associated with preterm birth.

Diagnosis of Preterm Labor. Early differentiation between true and false labor is often difficult before such a time that the uterus has contracted sufficiently to produce demonstrable effacement and dilatation of the cervix. Unfortunately, by this time, attempts to arrest labor may prove to be ineffective. Effective treatment with agents used so far appears to require early treatment. One result has been the inclusion of a number of cases of false labor which needed no treatment. In turn, the consequence has been confusion concerning the degree of effectiveness of most of the treatment regimens that have been proposed.

The following features, as outlined by Landesman (1972), are generally used to identify preterm labor: Uterine contractions

are occuring at least once every 10 min and last for 30 sec or more. If labor is soon obvious, treatment may be initiated. If not, uterine function is evaluated for 1 hour by means of external tocography to record the frequency and duration of contractions. Progressive dilatation of the cervix is, of course, indicative of labor.

Arrest of Preterm Labor. Before an attempt is made to arrest labor, the question must be asked and correctly answered, "Is further intrauterine stay more likely to be of benefit or of harm to the fetus?" In the past, the answer has been no more than academic, but highly effective agents for inhibiting labor most likely will sometime become generally available. Many neonatal deaths continue to be the direct consequence of marked prematurity, and the number of such deaths would undoubtedly be reduced by delaying delivery. Not all fetuses, however, would benefit from further intrauterine stay. This is born out by an annual stillbirth rate in the United States that nearly equals the neonatal death rate. Some of these stillborn fetuses would have lived if only the fetus had been delivered earlier. For example, retarded fetal growth is confused with prematurity, and the fetus, to his detriment, is left in a hostile intrauterine environment rather than a more favorable one provided by the nursery. Thus, the problem as to what is best for the fetus—not alone the mother—is not so simple that the obstetrician can automatically attempt to delay delivery in all cases of presumably preterm labor. The decision is made much easier if the gestational age is precisely known.

It is not surprising that great interest persists regarding effective treatment regimens for arresting spontaneous labor that develops long before term. Extensive reviews that emphasize pharmacologic attempts to arrest preterm labor have been provided by Barden (1977) and by Caritis and associates (1979).

TREATMENT REGIMENS FOR PRETERM LABOR. A number of treatment regimens that have been employed to try to arrest preterm labor are considered below:

1. BED REST. The treatment regimen that has been used most often is simply bed rest with the mother lying more comfortably on her side. In the relatively few controlled studies of the effect of various treatment modalities, the control group was placed at bed rest and, at times, given a placebo. Satisfactory results in the prevention or arrest of preterm labor may be so obtained. The success if attributable to bed rest and perhaps, in part, to the reassurance of the mother that she is being treated (Castrén et al., 1975; Hesseldahl, 1979).

2. PROGESTATIONAL AGENTS. Historically, with the recognition that parenterally administered progesterone would prolong pregnancy in rabbits, progesterone, and subsequently synthetic progestational agents, were employed to try to inhibit preterm labor. Most of the evidence to date is not very convincing that such agents are clinically effective, although Johnson and colleagues (1979) report preterm labor and low birth weight to have occurred less often in mothers who received weekly injections of 17α-hydroxyprogesterone caproate (Delalutin) prophylactically throughout pregnancy. Confirmation of their observations is needed.

3. ETHANOL. The use of intravenously administered ethanol to try to arrest preterm labor became popular somewhat more than a a decade ago following the favorable report by Fuchs and co-workers (1967). Initially, ethanol was thought to block the release of oxytocin from the neurohypophysis. There is now disagreement as to the role, if any, of endogenous oxytocin in human labor (see Chap. 15, p. 369). Ethanol may have a direct depressant action on the myometrium.

If ethanol is tried, the following regimen is suggested (Fuchs, 1979): A 10 percent solution of ethanol in 5 percent aqueous dextrose is infused at the rate of 7.5 ml per hour for each kg of body weight. After infusing

this loading dose for 2 hours, the rate of infusion is reduced from 7.5 ml to 1.5 ml per hour, which is then maintained for up to 12 hours. If contractions recur within 10 hours after stopping the infusion, the loading dose is reduced as follows:

Number of Hours Stopped × 10% of
Loading Dose

The maintenance dose remains the same.

If the cervix is more than 3 cm dilated or the membranes are ruptured, ethanol is not likely to be effective. Perhaps the strongest evidence to support the claim that ethanol is effective has been provided by Zlatnik and Fuchs (1972), who reported a delay of delivery for at least 72 hours in 17 of 21 women treated according to the dosage schedule just cited, compared to 8 of 21 who were managed the same way except that no ethanol was given. Lauersen and co-workers (1977), on the basis of a multicenter study, consider the β-adrenergic stimulator ritodrine (described below) to be more effective than ethanol for arresting preterm labor.

Ethanol infused as described can cause troublesome side effects in both the mother and the fetus-infant. Most women become overtly intoxicated and behave accordingly. Unless closely watched, they can become anesthetized with the attendant risks imposed by general anesthesia. Since nausea and vomiting are common, the possibility of severe—perhaps fatal—aspiration pneumonitis persists. Hypoglycemia and lactic acidemia may be induced by ethanol.

Ethanol rapidly crosses the placenta and distributes throughout the total body water of the fetus, as it does in the mother. The fetus becomes intoxicated as the mother becomes intoxicated and suffers metabolic derangement similar to the mother. The development of troublesome cardiovascular and metabolic abnormalities have been demonstrated in the fetal lamb (Kirkpatrick et al., 1976; Mann et al., 1975). Moreover, Fuchs and co-workers (1979) found respiratory distress to be more common in preterm infants whose mothers were treated with ethanol. They indicted the ethanol that persisted in the infant at birth as the culprit since the respiratory distress was concentrated in those infants who were born after failure of ethanol to arrest labor, even though the infusion was continued, and the ethanol levels were likely to have been higher at birth in these infants. Therefore, they urge that once it appears evident that ethanol is unable to arrest labor, the infusion of ethanol be stopped to permit the elimination of as much ethanol as possible before birth.

Since ethanol has been widely used and acclaimed to effectively arrest labor, it is not surprising that some obstetricians have encouraged its long-term consumption prophylactically by women considered to be at high risk of going into labor before term. Ethanol should not be so employed because of the likelihood of serious effects on the fetus from long-term use (see Chap. 13, p. 320).

4. MAGNESIUM SULFATE. It has long been recognized that ionic magnesium in a sufficiently high concentration can inhibit myometrial contractility in vivo as well as in vitro. The role of magnesium presumably is that of an antagonist of calcium.

Steer and Petrie (1977) have concluded that intravenously administered magnesium sulfate, 4 g as a loading dose followed by a continuous infusion of 2 g per hour, will usually arrest early labor. The design of their study, however, was far from ideal, and thus the validity of the conclusions that were drawn are suspect. Although magnesium sulfate is widely employed in obstetrics in the management of preeclampsia and eclampsia, the maintenance doses that are commonly used are usually less than 2 g per hour. Moreover, in our extensive experience with somewhat lower doses, there usually is little, if any, retardant effect on active labor. In any event, the mother must be monitored very closely for evidence of degrees of hypermagnesemia that are likely to prove toxic to her and to her fetus-infant since magnesium promptly crosses the placenta to produce concentrations in fetal plasma comparable to those in the mother. If magnesium intoxication is to be avoided, the patellar reflex should persist and certainly respirations should not be depressed. The pharmacology and toxicology of parenterally administered magnesium are considered in more detail in Chapter 27 (p. 692).

5. β-ADRENERGIC RECEPTOR STIMULANTS. Earlier in this century epinephrine in low doses was demonstrated to exert a depressant effect on the myometrium of the pregnant uterus. This observation led to epinephrine being considered an agent worthy of trial in the emergency treatment of the tetanically contracted uterus. However, its tocolytic effects proved to be rather weak, quite transient, and likely to be accompanied by troublesome cardiovascular effects. Moreover, in larger doses epinephrine may even enhance myometrial contractility.

In more recent years, a number of compounds capable of reacting predominantly with β-adrenergic receptors have been investigated. Some of these are now used extensively in the practice of obstetrics in other countries. Approval of one, ritodrine, for use in the treatment of preterm labor has been recommended by an Advisory Committee to the United States Food and Drug Administration.

The adrenergic receptors are located on the outer surface of the cell membrane where a specific agonist can couple with it. Adenylcyclase in the cell membrane of the smooth muscle cell is activated by the coupling of an agonist to the receptor. This enhances the conversion of adenosine triphosphate to cyclic adenosine monophosphate which, in turn, initiates a number of reactions that presumably reduce the intracellular concentration of calcium and thereby prevent activation of the contractile proteins, as described in Chapter 15 (p. 374).

There is now convincing evidence that there are two classes of β-adrenergic receptors and these are commonly referred to as β-1 and β-2 adrenergic receptors. The β-1 receptors are dominant in the heart and intestine while β-2 receptors are dominant in the myometrium, blood vessels, and bronchioles.

A number of compounds generally similar in structure to epinephrine have been evaluated in the search for an ideal one that would provide optimal stimulation of β-2 adrenergic receptors on myometrial cells and thus inhibit uterine contractions, but, at the same time, cause little or no adverse effects from stimulation of adrenergic receptors elsewhere. So far no compound has exhibited these utopian properties. Compounds that have been or are being employed to try to arrest labor include the following:

Isoxuprine was one of the first compounds to be extensively evaluated for tocolytic action. It does not appear to be remarkably effective, at least in doses that do not produce potentially dangerous side effects, especially marked tachycardia and hypotension.

Ritodrine in recent years has been widely used in other countries. In a multicenter study in the United States infants whose mothers were considered to be in labor preterm had a lower mortality rate, developed respiratory distress less often, and achieved a gestational age of 36 weeks or a birth weight of 2500 g, more often than did infants whose mothers were not so treated (Merkatz et al., 1980). Hesseldahl (1979), however, in a recent multicenter controlled study in Denmark, did not find any of several ritodrine treatment regimens tested to be more efficacious than "standard treatment" which consisted of bed rest and glucose infusion plus placebo tablets. Hesseldahl, perplexed by the discrepancy between his findings and those reported by some others earlier, did point out that possibly more women who received ritodrine in the Danish study were more predisposed to continue in labor than were those in the "standard treatment" group. Therefore, another trial is contemplated.

The adverse side effects identified in the mothers who received ritodrine in various doses during the same Danish multicenter trial, as reported by Osler (1979), included palpitations (9 to 13 percent), tachycardia (41 to 47 percent), and headache (7 to 23 percent). The blood pressure decreased seriously in three women, forcing discontinuation of the drug. Shortly after the intravenous administration of ritodrine there were increases in maternal plasma glucose, insulin, free fatty acids, glycerol, lactate and hydroxybutyrate. Serum iron, iron-binding capacity, and potassium were decreased.

Ritodrine treatment in the Danish multicenter study did not produce any recognized beneficial effects on the newborn infants when compared to those whose mothers received "standard treatment." On the contrary, according to Kristoffersen and Hansen (1979), the condition of the infants at birth tended to be worse in the ritodrine group.

Terbutaline is claimed to inhibit myometrial contractions effectively even when cervical dilatation is far advanced (Caritis et al., 1979). Its use to try to inhibit labor in twin gestation has been accompanied frequently by the development of maternal pulmonary edema (R. Creasy, personal communication).

Salbutamol has been acclaimed by some, similar to terbutaline, to be a very effective agent for arresting labor (Korda et al., 1974; Liggins and Vaughn, 1973; Rydén, 1977). However, Sims and co-workers (1978) and Reynolds (1978) found salbutamol to be no more effective than ethanol in arresting preterm labor. Adverse side effects were less marked with salbutamol than with ethanol.

Fenoterol structurally is very similar to ritodrine. It is not yet known whether fenoterol is any more or less effective, or causes more or less adverse reactions, than do the other beta mimetic agents currently being used in several countries. Epstein and associates (1979) observed sustained hypoglycemia accompanied by elevated insulin levels in most infants who were delivered within 2 days after the termination of fenoterol which had been administered to the mother to try to arrest labor.

The use of fenoterol has been extremely popular in West Germany. Kubli (1977) has commented that at least 1 million ampules and 6 million tablets of fenoterol have been used annually for a birth rate of about 6 million. However, no evidence has been presented that the use of so much of the compound has been accompanied by any remarkable decrease in the numbers of infants of low birth weight.

6. ANTIPROSTAGLANDINS. Such agents have been the subject of considerable interest once it was appreciated that prostaglandins are intimately involved in the myometrial contractions that characterize labor (see Chap. 15, p. 370). Antiprostaglandin agents may act by inhibiting the synthesis of prostaglandins or by blocking the action of prostaglandins on target organs.

A group of enzymes, collectively called prostaglandin synthetase, are responsible for the conversion of free arachidonic acid to prostaglandin. Several drugs are known to block the prostaglandin synthetase system, including aspirin and other salicylates, indomethacin, naproxen, and meclofenamic acid. Zuckerman and co-workers (1974), and others since, administered indomethacin to try to inhibit preterm labor and, in general, observed a favorable response.

Extensive investigations in humans of the use of prostaglandin synthetase inhibitors to try to inhibit labor preterm has been discouraged following recognition that such agents may adversely affect the fetus by inducing major cardiovascular changes, including premature closure of the ductus arteriosus. These changes have been recently reviewed by Levin (1980).

7. NARCOTICS AND SEDATIVES. Fear of arresting desirable labor by "too early" administration of narcotics, such as meperidine or morphine, and sedatives, such as secobarbital and pentobarbital, has long permeated the arena of clinical obstetrics. The evidence is weak, at best, that the fear is justified (see Chap. 18, p. 437). Certainly, there is no good evidence that they are effective in arresting preterm labor. There is good evidence, however, that narcotics and sedatives may dangerously depress the preterm infant when administered to the mother near the

time of delivery. Moreover, if they are employed in conjunction with ethanol, maternal depression may be profound. In fact, aspiration pneumonitis, with the death of both mother and fetus, has occurred in this circumstance.

8. DIAZOXIDE. This very potent antihypertensive agent can also inhibit contractions of the pregnant uterus. Side effects from diazoxide administration include maternal hypotension, tachycardia, increased cardiac output, hyperglycemia, hyperuricemia, and the retention of water, sodium, potassium, chloride, and bicarbonate. It appears likely that these multiple detrimental side effects will outweigh any favorable effect on labor. The drug is not approved for use for the treatment of threatened preterm labor.

9. OTHERS. *Oxytocin antagonists* are being evaluated as possible inhibitors of labor in spite of the debate that persists concerning the role, if any, of oxytocin in spontaneous human labor. However, to date, no clinical utility has been demonstrated. *Calcium antagonists* have also been tried experimentally. Ulmsten (1979) has reported that the calcium antagonist nifedipine in preliminary studies inhibited unterine contractions for up to 3 days in women in preterm labor, even though membranes were ruptured. Considering the ubiquitous nature of calcium and its importance in most biologic systems, it seems unlikely that a calcium antagonist will prove effective in stopping labor without producing a variety of adverse effects.

TENTATIVE CONCLUSION. The benefits to be derived from the use of these various agents that have been employed to try to arrest preterm labor do not appear to be profound. This tentative conclusion is reinforced to a degree by the analysis of previous results carried out by Hemminki and Starfield (1978) who evaluated the evidence provided in 16 published controlled clinical trials in which progestational agents, ethanol, or β-adrenergic drugs were employed. In but two of the therapeutic trials was the drug under study found to be more effective than a placebo in postponing delivery. In only one therapeutic trial was the drug found to affect favorably the outcome of the infant. They felt that additional clinical trials are needed urgently before the use of these drugs to try to inhibit labor is justifiable.

As things now stand, improvement in perinatal morbidity and mortality appear more likely to be achieved by concentrating on (1) identification of pregnancies in which preterm labor is very likely to develop, (2) early hospitalization, (3) optimal delivery, and (4) appropriate intensive neonatal care.

RUPTURE OF MEMBRANES BEFORE TERM

Rupture of the membranes at a time when gestational age might prove to be dangerously low is better referred to as *preterm rupture of the membranes* rather than *premature rupture of the membranes*. "Premature rupture of the membranes" has been applied most commonly to rupture of the membranes at any time before the onset of labor irrespective of whether the duration of gestation was 24 weeks or 44 weeks.

Rupture of the membranes long before term is a very important cause of perinatal morbidity and mortality and of maternal morbidity and even mortality. Most often, the rupture occurs spontaneously and for reasons unknown. At times, unfortunately, the cause is iatrogenic, as the consequence of an ill-timed attempt to induce labor. Technics for identification of rupture of the membranes are discussed elsewhere (see Chap. 17, p. 407).

There is far from unanimity of thought concerning optimal management of pregnancies complicated by rupture of the membranes remote from term. In the majority of cases, labor followed by delivery will ensue within a few days. Even so, it appears that for maternity services where the puerperal febrile morbidity rate is low, continued observation without vaginal manipulation may

prove to be of greater benefit to the preterm fetus than would steps to effect delivery. *Conversely, in those institutions in which puerperal febrile morbidity is common, the fetus, and the mother as well, may benefit from delivery within 24 hours.* The experiences at Parkland Memorial Hospital provide some verification of the latter attitude. The reason or reasons why infection of the fetus and mother following prolonged rupture of membranes is so common in many public institutions caring for socioeconomically less affluent women is not clear.

At Parkland Memorial Hospital, pregnancy complicated by rupture of the membranes remote from term has for some time been managed as follows:

1. Perform one sterile speculum examination to identify fluid coming from the cervix or pooled in the vagina. Demonstration of visible fluid or a positive nitrazine test is indicative of rupture of the membranes. The one sterile examination is concluded with the identification of the extent of cervical effacement and dilatation, confirmation of the presenting part, and exclusion of a prolapsed cord.

2. If the gestational age is no more than 32 weeks and there are no other maternal or fetal indications for delivery, the pregnancy is allowed to continue without prophylactic antibiotics under very close observation for signs of sepsis.

3. If the gestational age is greater than 32 weeks, and after 4 to 6 hours labor has not begun spontaneously, it is carefully induced with an intravenous infusion of dilute oxytocin, avoiding hyperstimulation. Breech presentation or transverse lie contraindicate induction. If induction fails, cesarean section is performed. At this and other institutions (Ritchie and McClure, 1979) neonatal mortality is now very low for infants born after 32 weeks gestation. Our results for the most recent year are presented in Table 37-1.

4. Labor and delivery are managed so as to minimize maternal hypotension and fetal hypoxia and acidosis, as well as infection,

since these events are known to increase the likelihood of fatal respiratory distress.

It has become common practice to give antibiotics prophylactically to the newborn infant born after prolonged (usually 24 hours) rupture of the membranes. If, in the experience of the institution, neonatal infection has proved to be common, antibiotic therapy may well be indicated; at the time of delivery a culture should probably be made of amnionic fluid, gastric aspirate, or a swabbing from the ear of the infant. Not all pediatricians agree to the advantages or the safety of antibiotic prophylaxis.

Accelerated Maturation of Pulmonary Function.

The infant who is born long before term is a candidate for the development of severe idiopathic respiratory distress syndrome (see Chap. 38, p. 957). The intense hypoxia and acidosis that ensues as the consequence of inadequate alveolar-capillary exchange of oxygen and carbon dioxide may prove fatal. Moreover, some infants who survive severe respiratory distress may suffer life-long physical or functional impairment. Since a major factor in the development of the respiratory distress syndrome is inappropriate production of pulmonary surfactant, intense interest persists concerning those phenomena involved in surfactant production (see Chap. 8, p. 187).

A variety of clinical events, some well-defined and others that are not, predispose to accelerated maturation of surfactant production sufficient to protect against the development of respiratory distress. Gluck (1979) contends that surfactant production is likely to be accelerated in pregnancies remote from term complicated by the following conditions: (1) *Maternal:* chronic renal or cardiovascular disease, long-standing pregnancy-induced hypertension, sickle cell disease, heroin addiction, or hyperthyroidism. (2) *Placenta and membranes:* placental infarction, chronic focal retroplacental hemorrhage, chorioamnionitis, or rupture of membranes. (3) *Fetal:* the anemic member of parabiotic twins or the smaller member of nonparabiotic twins.

PREMATURE RUPTURE OF THE MEMBRANES. Of those conditions listed above, rupture of the membranes remote from term is of exceptional importance not only because of its frequency but also because of the possibility that some delay in delivery may evoke lung maturation and thereby more than offset the risk of infection imposed by the delay. In some reports, but not all, a remarkable decrease in the incidence of respiratory distress has been claimed for the grossly preterm infant who was delivered more than 24 hours after gross rupture of the membranes. Yoon and Harper (1973), for example, in a retrospective study of infants whose birth weights were 1000 g to 2165 g, noted a frequency of respiratory distress of only 3.2 percent if membranes were ruptured more than 24 hours before delivery compared to 21.3 percent if ruptured less than 12 hours. There are reports by some other investigators that would appear to confirm their observations (Bauer et al., 1974; Sell and Harris, 1976). However, other reports have provided, at most, only partial confirmation (Berkowitz et al., 1977), while still other reports have failed to provide any confirmation whatsoever (Dluholucky et al., 1976; Jones et al., 1975; Liggins and Howie, 1974). Interestingly, removal of most of the amnionic fluid does not appear to accelerate pulmonary maturation in the fetal lamb.

Although it has been stated by some that antenatal infection provides a significant measure of protection against the development of respiratory distress and hyaline membrane disease, Dimmick and co-workers (1976) were unable to confirm such a protective action.

Therefore, in circumstances where delivery remote from term is considered to be in the best interests of the fetus, the mother, or both, the available evidence certainly is not supportive of a policy of deliberately rupturing the membranes and then delaying delivery for 24 hours or so to try to hasten lung maturation and thereby, hopefully, prevent respiratory distress. Moreover, in those situations where the fetus is in jeopardy of acquiring a serious infection as the consequence of spontaneous rupture of the mem-

TABLE 37-2.

RESPIRATORY DISTRESS SYNDROME (RDS) AND INTERVAL BETWEEN
COMPLETION OF BETAMETHASONE TREATMENT AND DELIVERY

TREATMENT-DELIVERY INTERVAL	BETA-METHASONE		CONTROL		P VALUE
	No.	% Rds	No.	% Rds	
< 24 hr	77	24.7	82	30.5	N.S.
1–7 days	182	8.8	156	23.7	0.001
7–20 days	33	21.2	28	7.1	N.S.
> 20 days	139	0.7	156	1.3	N.S.

From Howie and Liggins: Proceedings of the Fifth Study Group, Royal College of Obstetricians and Gynecologists, Oct. 1977, p. 281

TABLE 37-3.

RESPIRATORY DISTRESS SYNDROME AND GESTATIONAL AGE OF
INFANTS DELIVERED 1 TO 7 DAYS AFTER COMPLETION
OF BETAMETHASONE TREATMENT

GESTATIONAL AGE AT DELIVERY (WKS)	BETA-METHASONE		CONTROL		P VALUE
	No.	% Rds	No.	% Rds	
< 30	36	27.8	26	57.7	0.04
30–32	23	8.7	25	56.0	0.001
32–34	50	0.0	31	12.9	0.04
34 or more	73	5.5	74	5.4	N.S.

From Howie and Liggins: Proceedings of the Fifth Study Group, Royal College of Obstetricians and Gynecologists, Oct. 1977, p. 281

branes, the evidence that rupture of the membranes hastens lung maturation is not strong enough to risk delay of delivery.

GLUCOCORTICOID THERAPY. The observations of Liggins and Howie on the effects of glucocorticoids on lung maturation have rightfully received considerable attention (Howie and Liggins, 1977; Liggins and Howie, 1974). On the basis of their previous observations that corticosteroids administered to the ewe accelerated lung maturation in her preterm fetus, a well-designed study was initiated by them to evaluate the effects of maternally administered betamethasone acetate and phosphate on the prevention of respiratory distress in the subsequently delivered preterm newborn infant. A mixture of 6 mg of each compound was injected intramuscularly at the outset and again 24 hours

later. To try to delay birth, ethanol was administered very early in the study but later salbutamol was used and was considered to be superior. Their results demonstrated for infants born before 34 weeks of pregnancy a significant lowering of the incidence of respiratory distress and of neonatal mortality from hyaline membrane disease if birth was delayed for at least 24 hours and up to 7 days after completion of steroid therapy (Tables 37-2, 37-3). Numerous other investigators have made similar observations, including Ballard and associates (1979), Taeusch and associates (1979), Morrison and coworkers (1978), and Heinrichs and Storey (1980).

The mechanism by which betamethasone or other corticosteroids reduce the frequency of respiratory distress is not clear. Interestingly, the protective action is likely to be transient. Liggins and Howie (1974) noted that the frequency of respiratory distress increased when the infant was born more than 7 days after treatment with betamethasone, compared to that for infants delivered 1 to 7 days after completion of therapy. Moreover, Brown and associates (1979) observed in chronically catheterized fetal lambs that the increase in surfactant that followed dexamethasone administration was transient with surfactant levels falling to pretreatment values within 8 to 10 days. Therefore, if such compounds are used, retreatment must be considered whenever delivery has not occurred within 7 days of the initial treatment and the risk of early delivery persists.

In contrast to the generally favorable reports just cited, Quirk and co-workers (1979) in a retrospective analysis of 3 years experiences at Columbia-Presbyterian Medical Center identified no difference in fetal outcomes with and without the use of betamethasone. Of 84 markedly preterm infants whose mothers received betamethasone, 16.4 percent developed the respiratory distress syndrome compared to 14.1 percent of 84 infants whose mothers did not receive the steroid. Seventy-four (88 percent) of the treated group survived compared to 73 (87 percent) of the control group. They attributed the low incidence of respiratory distress in the control population to the avoidance of both compromised labor and trauamtic delivery.

The decision whether or not to use potent glucocorticoids to try to minimize the risk of severe respiratory distress in the infant born remote from term is a difficult one. Most evidence points to a reduction in the frequency of this serious pulmonary disorder but not to its complete eradication. At the same time, there are risks, immediate and remote, from the use of agents as potent as betamethasone. From the standpoint of the mother, the metabolic derangements that characterize diabetes are likely to be intensified, severe pregnancy-induced hypertension may be worsened, the risk of infection is increased, and wound healing may be impaired, especially so in case of transabdominal delivery. Moreover, the combination of a gluco-

corticoid to hasten lung maturation and a tocolytic agent to try to delay delivery may incite pulmonary edema. Pulmonary edema has developed during the course of therapy with betamethasone or dexamethasone plus the β-adrenergic stimulators terbutaline or ritodrine, the prostaglandin synthetase inhibitor indomethacin, and magnesium sulfate (Elliott et al., 1979; Rogge et al., 1979; Stubblefield, 1978; Tinga and Aarnoudse, 1979). Moreover, the combined use of betamethasone and ethanol has caused severe gastric hemorrhage necessitating transfusion (Gabert, 1974).

From the standpoint of the fetus-infant, as well as the potential for deterioration in utero as the consequence of the maternal complications just described, there is also increased immediate risk of sepsis from the use of the steroid and delayed delivery. Taeusch and associates (1979) identified serious infection in 13 percent of liveborn infants whose mothers had ruptured membranes and had received dexamethasone; 27 percent of the mothers became infected. By way of comparison, 6 percent of the infants were infected whose mothers had ruptured membranes but did not receive dexamethasone and 12 percent of the mothers became infected. While neonatal deaths due to respiratory distress were decreased in the steroid-treated group compared to the control group, the overall neonatal mortality in both groups was the same because of the increased number of deaths due to sepsis in the steroid treated group.

The long-term risks to the surviving infant from glucocorticoids so used are not yet known. However, the adverse effects that have been described following the administration of such steroids around the time of birth to experimental animals are discouraging. For example, in pregnant rats following betamethasone administration, the fetal death rate was increased and among survivors growth was impaired so that total body weight and weights of the brain, heart, liver, kidneys, and adrenals were reduced (Mosier et al., 1979). In the rhesus monkey fetus reduced fetal head circumference has been described (Johnson et al., 1979). However, Liggins (1976) found no gross difference with regard to intelligence quotient and social adjustment among children at 4 years of age whose mothers had received betamethasone according to the protocol described, and in the preliminary observations made by Brown and associates (1979) no delay in development was found following antenatal treatment with dexamethasone beyond that seen in infants not so exposed.

At Parkland Memorial Hospital glucocorticoids have not been employed remote from term to try to reduce the risk of respiratory distress for the following reasons:

1. Glucocorticoids have not been approved by the Food and Drug Administration for such use.
2. The long-term effects on the child exposed in utero are not yet known.
3. The incidence of maternal vascular disease at Parkland Memorial Hospital is high.
4. At this institution the likelihood of infection after rupture of the membranes is considerable, while fetal respiratory distress syndrome is uncommon.
5. Mortality among infants born remote from term is not sufficiently great to warrant the administration of glucocorticoids and attempting to delay delivery for 48 hours or more. For example, neonatal death rates during a recent 1-year period for infants born at 34 weeks gestational age or less are illustrated in Table 37-1. Of 85 infants who were delivered at 27 through 32 weeks gestational age, 88 percent survived, as did all of the 85 infants who were 33 or 34 weeks gestational age at birth.

Attention should continue to be directed toward the development of better ways to prevent the respiratory distress syndrome in infants who are delivered remote from term. Other modalities are being evaluated. One of these is thyroxine injected into the amnionic sac from which it is swallowed and then absorbed by the fetus. Preliminary studies are suggestive that the hormone so adminis-

tered can accelerate maturation of the human fetal lung (Mashiach et al., 1979). The degree of protection that can be achieved and the possible adverse effects on the fetus-infant remain to be determined.

MANAGEMENT OF PRETERM LABOR AND DELIVERY

In general, the more immature the fetus, the greater the risks from labor and delivery. This is now well established for breech delivery, which is a common presentation for the preterm fetus (see Chap. 30, p. 797), and undoubtedly is true to a degree for all immature fetuses regardless of presentation (Haesslein and Goodlin, 1979).

In case of contemplated vaginal delivery, labor, if induced, must not be unduly forceful (see Chap. 29, p. 790). Abnormalities of fetal heart rate and uterine contractions should be looked for preferably by continuous electronic monitoring. If the fetal heart is not monitored continuously, it must be evaluated at very close intervals by adequately trained attendants. Tachycardia is suggestive of sepsis while periodic decelerations imply cord compression or placental insufficiency. In either case, if a real attempt is going to be made to salvage the fetus, prompt cesarean section is advisable. It is imperative that the uterine incision be large enough to allow for a nontraumatic exit of the infant.

Even though fetopelvic disproportion is not a problem, except when there is a transverse lie, the resistance of the cervix and of the lower genital tract to dilatation by the presenting part of the fetus may be formidable, especially if the cervix is long, firm, and little dilated and the mother is nulliparous.

There is no question but that a liberal episiotomy for delivery is advantageous once the fetal head reaches the perineum. Argument persists as to the merits of spontaneous delivery versus forceps delivery to protect the more fragile preterm fetal head. It is doubtful whether use of forceps in most instances produces less trauma. The use of outlet forceps of appropriate size is of aid when induction anesthesia is used and voluntary expulsive efforts are obtunded. Forceps should not be employed to pull the fetus through a vagina that is resistant to dilatation or over a firm perineum.

At times, conduction anesthesia may be precluded by the maternal disease that led to premature delivery, for example, maternal hypertension, hemorrhage, or cyanotic heart disease. For the mother whose discomfort is too unpleasant, a mixture of nitrous oxide, 50 percent, and oxygen, administered during contractions, is likely to provide appreciable analgesia without depressing the fetus. The addition of pudendal or local nerve block provides for delivery (see Chap. 18, p. 445).

Importantly, just as the markedly preterm infant is to be afforded special care in the neonatal intensive care unit, the mother and fetus should be very closely observed in the labor and delivery unit. Furthermore, just as especially skilled physicians care for the markedly preterm infant after birth, especially skilled physicians should monitor the labor and personally effect the delivery of the markedly preterm fetus.

A physician proficient in resuscitative technics and who has been fully oriented as to the specific problems of the case should be present at delivery. The principles of resuscitation described in Chapter 20 are applicable, including prompt endotracheal intubation and ventilation.

THE GROWTH-RETARDED FETUS

Definition. Generally, a newborn infant is classified as *growth retarded,* or *small for gestational age,* if his birth weight falls below the 10th percentile for his particular gestational age. Mortality and severe morbidity are not greatly increased among fetuses and infants with lesser degrees of growth retardation and no serious malformations. For any gestational age, however, as weight decreases below the

10th percentile, the risk of fetal death increases remarkably.

Causes of Fetal Growth Retardation. The following conditions predispose to impairment of fetal size:

1. Small mother. Little women are more likely to give birth to small infants than are large women. About all that can be done to avoid potentially dangerous degrees of growth retardation is to take whatever steps possible to minimize growth retardation from the other causes listed below. In the case of a small woman, the birth of an infant whose weight is somewhat below the average for the whole population, is not necessarily an undesirable event. If the fetus were appreciably larger, he could experience difficulty in negotiating the typically small pelvis of the small mother.

2. Poor maternal weight gain. When the mother is of average size or smaller, lack of weight gain throughout pregnancy or arrested weight gain during the latter half of pregnancy, is more likely to result in a growth-retarded infant. If the mother is large and otherwise healthy, however, below average maternal weight gain is unlikely to be associated with appreciable fetal growth retardation. Even so, marked restriction of weight gain during pregnancy should not be attempted (see Chap. 13, p. 310).

3. Vascular disease. Chronic vascular disease, especially when further complicated by superimposed preeclampsia and proteinuria, commonly causes growth retardation. Pregnancy-induced hypertension occurring late in pregnancy without underlying chronic vascular or renal disease is much less likely to be accompanied by marked fetal growth retardation.

4. Chronic renal disease. Chronic renal disease with appreciably reduced renal clearance is commonly accompanied by retarded fetal growth.

5. Chronic hypoxia. Fetuses of women who

reside at high altitude are much more likely to weigh less than those of women who live at lower altitude. The same is true for fetuses of women with cyanotic heart disease or pulmonary insufficiency.

6. Maternal anemia. A low maternal hemoglobin concentration has been implicated in the genesis of fetal growth retardation. In our experience, however, growth retardation has been common only in the fetuses of women with sickle cell disease or with anemia associated with serious maternal disease.

7. Smoking. Tobacco smoking impairs fetal growth; the more cigarettes smoked, the greater the impairment.

8. Hard drugs. The use of heroin, and almost certainly other hard drugs, during pregnancy impairs fetal growth.

9. Alcoholism. The chronic consumption of appreciable amounts of alcohol by the mother during pregnancy results in growth retardation of the fetus often accompanied by physical malformation and subsequent intellectual impairment.

10. Abnormalities of placenta and cord. Placental lesions, including chronic focal placental abruption, intervillous thrombosis, extensive infarction, or a chorioangioma, are likely to cause retarded fetal growth which may be severe (Fig. 37-4. A and 4. B). A circumvallate placenta or a placenta previa may impair growth but usually the fetus is not markedly smaller than normal. Marginal insertion of the umbilical cord and especially velamentous insertion of the cord are more likely to be accompanied by a fetus who is growth retarded.

11. Multiple fetuses. The presence of two or more fetuses is likely to eventuate in appreciable growth retardation of one or both when compared to the normal singleton fetus (see Chap. 26, p. 653).

12. Previous birth of a growth retarded infant. Fetal growth retardation is likely to be repetitive even when no cause is identified. Moreover, the likelihood of fetal growth retardation is somewhat in-

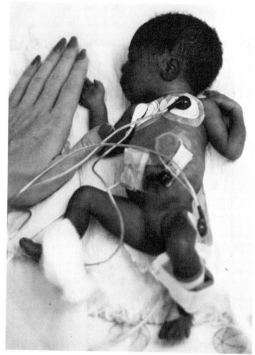

A

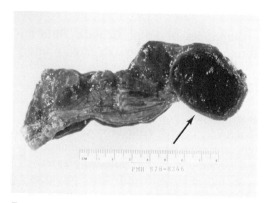

B

FIG. 37-4. A. The infant weighed but 650 g when delivered at 29 to 30 weeks gestation. The mother had become severely hypertensive. At delivery by cesarean section there was a subchorial hematoma of many days duration in the placenta (shown in Fig. 37-6. B), and the scant amnionic fluid was thick and green. The L/S ratio was 0.64. The infant thrived with no evidence of respiratory distress. B. Cross-sectional view of the subchorial hematoma (arrow) contained in the placenta of the severely growth-retarded, preterm infant illustrated in Figure 37-6. A.

creased among women whose sisters have had a growth retarded infant.

13. Fetal infections. Cytomegalic inclusion disease, rubella, and probably other chronic infections of the fetus can cause appreciable growth retardation.

14. Fetal malformations. In general, the more severe the malformation, the more likely the fetus is to be small for gestational age. This is especially evident in fetuses with chromosomal abnormalities or with serious cardiovascular malformations.

15. Prolonged pregnancy. The longer pregnancy endures beyond term the greater the likelihood of the fetus appearing undernourished and chronically distressed. During this time the fetus may not only fail to gain weight but may actually lose weight. Even so, the majority of fetuses probably continue to gain weight.

16. Extrauterine pregnancy. Commonly the fetus who is not housed in the uterus is growth retarded.

Diagnosis of Fetal Growth Retardation.
Identification through careful history taking of any of the factors listed above that predispose to retarded fetal growth should alert the obstetrician to the possibility of growth retardation in the current pregnancy. Moreover, careful estimation of gestational age and consistently careful evaluation of uterine size during the course of prenatal visits should serve to identify most instances of fetal growth retardation:

UTERINE FUNDAL HEIGHT. Belizán and co-workers (1978), as well as Jimenez and colleagues (1979) at our institution, have provided their observations concerned with the relationship between carefully measured uterine fundal height above the symphysis pubis and gestational age. The values for fundal heights at various gestational ages were nearly identical in the two studies. In the Dallas study the average fundal height was within 1 cm of gestational age throughout the period

from 18 to 30 weeks. Fetal growth retardation was strongly suspected when fundal height was compatible with the menstrual data early in pregnancy, but subsequently fundal height failed to keep pace with gestational age. Belizán and associates correctly identified 86 percent of fetuses whose birth weights fell below the 10th percentile while erroneously suspecting this degree of growth retardation in only 5 percent of pregnancies. Therefore, an appreciation of those circumstances in which fetal growth retardation is more likely to occur, coupled with meticulous clinical mensuration of fundal height, and in selected instances sonography, should serve to identify essentially all pregnancies in which a singleton fetus is demonstrating growth retardation. An appropriate technic for measuring uterine fundal height clinically is described in Chapter 13, page 308.

SONOGRAPHIC MEASUREMENTS. To evaluate correctly the results of sonographic measurements it must be appreciated that the fetus may demonstrate different patterns of growth retardation. In one form, sometimes referred to as symmetric, there is retarded growth that is generalized, and thus includes the head. With the other pattern of growth retardation, there is asymmetric growth with the head being spared. With symmetric growth retardation, the biparietal diameter, head circumference at the level of the third ventricle, and the abdominal circumference at the level of the umbilical vein or ductus venosus are comparably reduced. Therefore, these findings alone do not serve to differentiate between symmetrical fetal growth retardation and an erroneous gestational age. If, however, gestational age is certain from clinical data or from sonographic measurements made early in pregnancy, and microcephaly can be excluded, a small biparietal diameter and abdominal circumference are diagnostic of generalized growth retardation.

Measurement of the biparietal diameter and head circumference at the level of the third ventricle will not detect asymmetric growth retardation in which the head is

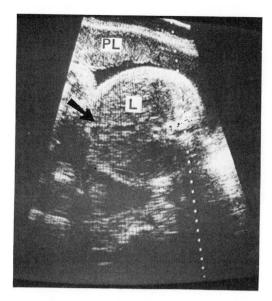

FIG. 37-5. Sonographic cross-sectional view of the fetal abdomen at the level of the ductus venosus (arrow). L = liver, PL = placenta. (Courtesy of Dr. R. Santos)

spared. Sonography performed so as to obtain a true cross-sectional view of the fetal abdomen at the level of the umbilical vein or ductus venosus allows the abdominal circumference to be measured rather precisely (Fig. 37-5). If the head circumference is large compared to the abdominal circumference, and hydrocephalus is excluded (see Chap. 30, p. 822), the fetus is asymmetrically growth retarded.

Normally, head circumference is greater than abdominal circumference measured at the level of the umbilical vein or ductus venosus until about 32 weeks gestation when they become about equal and remain so until about 36 weeks, after which the abdominal circumference normally exceeds head circumference. Campbell and Wilkin (1975) have further demonstrated that the abdominal circumference at the level of the umbilical vein correlates quite well with total body mass and therefore have used it to predict fetal weight and, in turn, to identify growth retardation. According to their studies, sonography performed so as to allow precise

measurement of the abdominal circumference at 32 weeks would serve to detect 87 percent of small for gestational age fetuses while a negligible number of false-positive diagnoses would be made. It is reemphasized that gestational age must be accurate if these measurements are to provide useful information.

Warshof and co-workers (1977) have provided a computer-derived table from which fetal weight can be readily predicted from the biparietal diameter and abdominal circumference measured sonographically. In their hands two standard deviations equaled 212 g per kg. They have found the table especially useful when there is head to body disproportion.

Management of the Growth-retarded Fetus. Unfortunately, in many instances of fetal growth retardation there is no specific treatment that will ameliorate the growth retardation while the pregnancy continues to term. Possible exceptions are inadequate maternal nutrition, heavy smoking, use of hard drugs, and possibly chronic alcoholism. Ideally, the use of tobacco, hard drugs, and alcohol can be curtailed. In case of maternal undernutrition, the ingestion of a diet adequate quantitatively and qualitatively should favorably influence fetal growth. Very sedentary living that approaches full-time bed rest may also favorably influence fetal growth and, at the same time, possibly reduce the risk of preterm labor.

FETAL GROWTH RETARDATION AT OR NEAR TERM. Prompt delivery is likely to afford the best outcome for the fetus who is suspected of being severely growth retarded at or near term (Fig. 37-6. A and 6. B).

Throughout labor, spontaneous or induced, those fetuses who are suspected of being growth retarded should be very closely monitored for evidence of distress, including abnormalities of fetal heart rate and the presence of copious amounts of meconium in the amnionic fluid. The likelihood of severe fetal

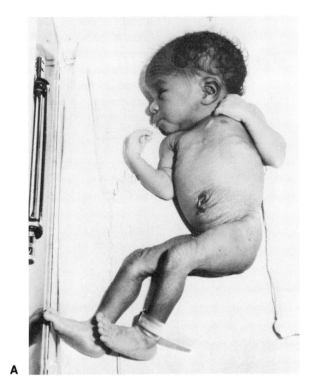

FIG. 37-6. A. Severely growth-retarded infant of 38 weeks gestational age but birth weight of only 1800 g. Delivery was by cesarean section. The chronically hypertensive mother had suffered two previous stillbirths. *(Continued)*

distress during labor is considerably increased since fetal growth retardation commonly is the result of inadequate placental transfer as the consequence of either faulty maternal perfusion, or ablation of functional placenta, or both. These conditions are likely to be aggravated by vigorous labor. Consequently, the capabilities for immediate cesarean section should be available. Moreover, it can be anticipated that the infant at birth may need expert assistance in making a successful transition to air breathing. He is at risk of being born hypoxic and of aspirating meconium into the lungs, thus compromising his chances of successful ventilation. As soon as the head is delivered from the vagina or from the uterus in case of cesarean section, the mouth pharynx and nares should be quickly aspirated by the obstetrician. Moreover, it is essential that care for the newborn

immediately after birth be provided by someone who can skillfully clear the airway below the vocal cords of noxious material, especially meconium, and ventilate the infant as needed. The severely growth retarded newborn infant is unusually susceptible to hypothermia and may also soon develop other metabolic derangements, especially serious hypoglycemia. Polycythemia and blood hyperviscosity occasionally cause serious difficulty unless effectively treated by limited exchange transfusion with plasma (Jones and Battaglia, 1977).

FETAL GROWTH RETARDATION BEFORE TERM. At times, the overtly growth retarded fetus is in serious jeopardy irrespective of whether he remains in utero or is delivered. For the fetus who is severely growth retarded but remote from term, the

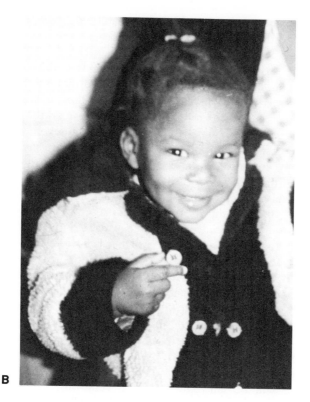

FIG. 37-6 B. (Cont.) The same infant at 13 months of age. Physical and intellectual development was normal at that time.

decision to proceed with delivery becomes a matter of trying to ascertain the degree of risk from further stay in utero compared to the risks from preterm delivery. Fortunately, the "stress" associated with severe fetal growth retardation appears commonly to accelerate lung maturation to a sufficient degree that respiratory distress and hyaline membrane disease do not develop. Identification of a lecithin-sphingomyelin (L/S) ratio of 2 or more, or identification of phosphatidylglycerol in amnionic fluid serves to identify those infants who are extremely unlikely to develop serious respiratory distress (see Chap. 14, p. 334). Generally, when lung maturity is assured, delivery of a fetus under the condition outlined above, rather than procrastination with further fetal deterioration, offers the best chance for survival.

There remains a troublesome group of growth-retarded fetuses for whom the causes of growth retardation are not reversible and measurements of surfactant components in amnionic fluid do not provide assurance that respiratory distress will not be a problem. For pregnancies thus complicated, a variety of antepartum tests have been proposed to try to identify the fetus for whom further confinement in utero is likely to be intolerable, yet do so before he has become so badly compromised that he does not survive after delivery. Procedures that have received considerable attention, and are discussed in more detail in Chapter 14, include the following: (1) Functional tests to identify the presence or absence of late decelerations of the fetal heart rate in response to uterine contractions (the contraction stress test or oxytocin challenge test) or the presence or absence of accelerations of the fetal heart rate in response to fetal movement (the nonstress test). (2) The concentration of estriol circulating in plasma or the amount of estriol excreted in the urine per 24 hours. (3) the level of placental lactogen (hPL) in maternal plasma.

Hobbins and associates (1978) in their considerations of management of the growth-retarded fetus, have displayed minimal to, at most, modest enthusiasm for any of the above tests, with the exception of the nonstress test. In general, if the fetal heart accelerates in response to fetal movement, the fetus is not likely to die in utero during the next several days *unless* there is an acute event that produces severe hypoxia. One such event that is of concern, especially when growth retardation is associated with maternal vascular disease, is placental abruption. If the heart rate does not respond to fetal movement (a nonreactive nonstress test) correct interpretation is difficult. The experiences of Schifrin (1979), not limited only to growth-retarded fetuses, have been that 80 to 90 percent of the time the outcome will be satisfactory. Thus, a nonreactive pattern by itself is not a sensitive predictor of fetal outcome.

In spite of the shortcomings inherent in these tests, Hobbins and associates (1978), Cetrulo and Freeman (1977), Tejani and Mann (1977), and others, describe the use of frequent measurements of 24-hour urinary estriol excretion and stress and nonstress tests to attempt further evaluation of fetal well-being or lack of same.

These tests are seldom used antepartum at Parkland Memorial Hospital. Instead, whenever severe intractable growth retardation is identified by careful clinical and sonographic measurements, the plan of management has generally been not to procrastinate but to effect delivery. By the time in gestation that fetal growth retardation has become severe, the fetus is usually mature enough to survive if (1) he is delivered promptly rather than allowing the risk of further compromise from a longer stay in utero; (2) he is closely monitored during labor to avoid further compromise or delivery is accomplished by cesarean section; and (3) he receives excellent neonatal care beginning immediately after delivery.

The presence of maternal disease which is worsening as the consequence of the pregnancy, and thereby threatens the well-being of the mother as well as the fetus, should certainly bear on the decision as to whether to deliver the severely growth-retarded fetus or to wait. Most any maternal disease falls into this category when the disease is characterized by vascular disease, renal disease, or both, and superimposed preeclampsia (pregnancy aggravated hypertension) supervenes (see Chap. 27, p. 696). Fortunately, in many such instances severe respiratory distress does not develop even when delivery is effected remote from term. In any event, with prompt delivery, fetal and neonatal salvage are likely to be improved compared to salvage when delivery is unduly delayed, even though the L/S ratio is less than two (Fig. 37–4. A). At the same time, with prompt delivery maternal deterioration is likely to subside.

Several observations that have been provided by Creasy (1979) are supportive of the general policy of prompt delivery of the fetus who is believed to be severely growth retarded (below the 10th percentile) even when remote from term. In their experience, as ours, respiratory distress syndrome has been an uncommon complication in the preterm newborn infant who was severely growth retarded. Moreover, when respiratory distress did occur, it was unlikely to prove lethal. In the more recent experiences at the University of California at San Francisco, 85 percent of infants with respiratory distress who weighed only 1000 to 1250 g at birth survived (see Chap. 38, p. 958). Furthermore, from extensive analyses of growth-retarded stillborn infants of various gestational ages, it was apparent that when fetal weight was below the 10th percentile and remained static, additional time in utero did not decrease mortality.

Labor and Delivery. From the outset, labor, spontaneous or induced with oxytocin, must be closely monitored to detect as soon as possible any adverse effects on the fetus. The general plan of management for the preterm growth-retarded fetus is the same as that outlined above for the preterm, appropriately grown fetus (p. 941). It is emphasized that the growth-retarded fetus is even more likely to become overtly distressed during labor since the growth retardation commonly is related to compromised placental transfer.

Subsequent Development of the Growth-retarded Infant.

Subsequent growth of the individual newborn infant who is growth retarded cannot be reliably predicted from his measurements at birth (Philip, 1978). The infant who is small for gestational age may demonstrate any of a variety of growth patterns during infancy and childhood. For example, in one study, after excluding those infants with obvious causes of growth retardation that persisted such as congenital infections, gross anomalies, and chromosomal abnormalities, the *average* weight and height of 96 infants increased from below the 10th percentile at birth to between the 10th and 25th percentile at 6 months of age (Fitzhardinge and Steven, 1972). Lubchenco (1976) has found that if the newborn infant was retarded in weight alone, he would most likely demonstrate subsequent normal growth, whereas, if he was also short at birth, he would more likely remain so. Fancourt and colleagues (1976) have observed that when fetal growth retardation, identified by small head growth sonographically, was detected before the 34th week of gestation, growth of the child was commonly slow, at least through the first 4 years. Therefore, prolonged symmetrical, or generalized, growth retardation in utero is likely to be followed by slow growth after birth, whereas the asymmetrically growth retarded fetus is more likely to "catch up" after birth (Fig. 37–6. B).

The subsequent neurologic and intellectual capabilities of the infant who was growth retarded in utero are not known precisely. Fancourt and associates found that in children for whom there was sonographic evidence of delayed head growth starting before the 3rd trimester, subsequent neurologic and intellectual development was also delayed.

POSTTERM PREGNANCIES

A postterm pregnancy is one that persists for 42 weeks or more from the onset of a menstrual period that was followed by ovulation about 2 weeks later. Although such a definition would include perhaps 10 percent, or even more, of pregnancies, some may not be actual postterm pregnancies but rather the result of an error in the estimation of gestational age. Again, the value of precise knowledge of the duration of gestation is evident for, in general, the longer the truly postterm fetus stays in utero, the greater the risk of a severely compromised fetus and newborn infant.

Causes. Some more rare conditions in which there often is failure of the fetus to be delivered at the usual time include anencephaly, placental sulfatase deficiency, and extrauterine pregnancy. Women who have experienced prolonged gestation with one pregnancy appear to be at increased risk of the same in a subsequent pregnancy. However, until the mechanisms involved in the spontaneous onset and maintenance of normal labor are precisely known, there is little likelihood that the precise cause or causes of prolonged gestation will be identified.

Effects on the Fetus-Infant. The fetus postterm may continue to gain weight in utero and thus be an unusually large infant at birth. The fact that he did grow serves as an indicator of uncompromised placental function and suggests, at least, that he should be able to tolerate the rigors of normal labor. However, his continued growth may have created a worrisome degree of fetopelvic disproportion and as the consequence labor may not be benign.

At the other extreme, the intrauterine environment may be so hostile to that fetus that further growth in utero is arrested. He may appear at birth actually to have lost considerable weight, especially from loss of subcutaneous fat and muscle mass. In the extreme case, the limbs appear long and very thin, there is severe desquamation of the epidermis and the nails and the amnion are commonly bile-stained. The infant whose gestational age is beyond 42 weeks and who presents this dystrophic appearance has been called "postmature" by some. However, the term "postmature" might best be applied to the postterm fetus who has continued to grow in utero and thus has achieved a size comparable to that of a normal infant who was conceived at the same time, but was born at term and thrived after birth. Since "postmature" has been applied in so variable a fashion, perhaps its use ought to be discarded to avoid further confusion. Other commonly used descriptions are "postmature and dysmature," "postdates and postmature," "postdates and dysmature," and "postterm and dysmature." We favor *postterm and dysmature,* to describe the obviously undernourished fetus-infant whose gestational age is more than 42 weeks.

Importantly, the fetus-infant need not be postterm to have developed the characteristic features of dysmaturity described above, for compromised placental function somewhat earlier in pregnancy may also lead to a similar appearance as is evident in the dystrophic newborn infant of 38 weeks gestational age who is illustrated in Figure 37–6. A.

Management of Postterm Pregnancy.

There remains little doubt that, even in the absence of any recognizable maternal complication, some fetuses who stay in utero much beyond 42 weeks are in progressively greater danger of suffering serious morbidity or even dying in utero or soon after birth. Therefore, it would be advantageous to those fetuses to deliver them by 42 weeks. However, at least five difficult problems persist that serve to discourage a policy of delivering all fetuses whose gestational age is suspected to be at least 42 weeks:

1. Gestational age is not always precisely known and thus the fetus may actually be appreciably less mature than thought.
2. It is very difficult to identify with precision those fetuses who are likely to die or to develop serious morbidity if left in utero.
3. The majority of fetuses fare rather well.
4. Induction of labor is not always successful.
5. Delivery by cesarean section increases appreciably the risk of serious maternal morbidity not only in this pregnancy, but in subsequent ones.

PARKLAND MANAGEMENT. The general plan of management at Parkland Memorial Hospital of pregnancies believed to be postterm, i.e., beyond 42 weeks gestation, is as follows:

1. POSTTERM AND FAVORABLE FOR INDUCTION OF LABOR. If the fetal head is well-fixed in the pelvis and well-applied to the cervix, and the cervix is soft, somewhat effaced, and at least 2 cm dilated, induction of labor is attempted with intravenous oxytocin (see Chap. 29, p. 790). When so selected, the great majority of women will soon go into labor. If the attempt to induce labor is unsuccessful, and the membranes have not ruptured, the women is allowed to go home if no abnormalities of fetal heart rate were detected by external electronic monitoring and there are no maternal complications, such as hypertension. If one week hence she has not gone into labor, the procedure is repeated.

2. POSTTERM BUT UNFAVORABLE FOR INDUCING LABOR. If at 42 and 43 weeks of gestation, conditions are considered to be unfavorable for inducing labor, no intervention is attempted as long as there are no maternal complications, the fetus is considered by the mother to be active, and amnionic fluid is thought to be present. Otherwise, an attempt at induction of labor is made with intravenous oxytocin. Management then is the same as described above. If still undelivered at 44 weeks gestation, delivery is accom-

plished. Generally intravenous oxytocin is infused to try to induce labor. If unsuccessful or contraindicated, cesarean section is performed.

3. POSSIBLY POSTTERM. In the absence of any identified complication of pregnancy, the woman is seen weekly and reassured that the risks that accrue from active intervention to effect delivery very likely exceed the potential risks from a possibly prolonged gestation.

In our experience the onset of labor may be a particularly dangerous time for the postterm fetus. Therefore, it is important that women whose pregnancies are known or suspected to be postterm come to the hospital as soon as they suspect that they are in labor. Upon arrival, while being observed for possible labor, they should be observed very closely for fetal heart changes that imply fetal distress.

Another particularly dangerous time for the postterm fetus is delivery. Aspiration of meconium should be minimized by effective suctioning of the pharynx as soon as the head is delivered, but before the thorax is delivered. If meconium is identified, the trachea should be aspirated as soon as possible after delivery by someone skilled in this technic (see Chap. 38, p. 959). Immediately thereafter, the infant should be effectively ventilated as needed. At times, the continued growth of the fetus postterm will eventuate in shoulder dystocia following delivery of the head. Therefore, an obstetrician who is experienced in managing this problem should be immediately available to effect delivery (see Chap. 30, p. 821).

In general, electronic monitoring of the fetal heart rate and of uterine contractions throughout all of labor is advantageous, and especially so whenever personnel appropriately skilled in the detection of fetal distress by auscultation and palpation (Haverkamp et al., 1979) cannot remain continually in attendance.

The question, "When should the membranes be ruptured?" is difficult to answer.

Loss of amnionic fluid following amniotomy may enhance the possibility of cord compression and perhaps also impair placental function. On the other hand, amniotomy is likely to identify the presence of thick meconium which can be dangerous to the fetus. Moreover, once the membranes are ruptured, a scalp electrode and intrauterine pressure catheter can then be placed, the use of which usually provides more precise data concerning fetal heart rate and uterine contractions than does external electronic monitoring. Importantly, with internal monitoring the woman is more likely to lie on her side which should favor placental perfusion, whereas, while balancing external monitoring equipment on her abdomen, she most often is inclined to stay on her back.

Identification of *thick* meconium in amnionic fluid is particularly worrisome. It is evidence of fairly recent fetal distress that may or may not persist. Of great importance, aspiration of meconium may cause severe pulmonary dysfunction and death during the newborn period (see Chap. 38, p. 959). The likelihood of successful vaginal delivery is reduced appreciably for the nulliparous woman who is in early labor with thick meconium in the amnionic fluid. Strong consideration is given to prompt cesarean section, especially when cephalopelvic disproportion is suspected or either hypotonic or hypertonic dysfunctional labor is evident.

OTHER PLANS OF MANAGEMENT. It has now become common practice in the management of the postterm pregnancy to apply a variety of procedures that have been championed as tests of fetal well-being. Most often these tests have included measurements two to seven times per week of either the amount of estriol excreted in the urine per 24 hours or its concentrations in plasma, the measurement one or more times per week of placental lactogen (hPL) in maternal plasma, and the evaluation one or more times each week of changes in fetal heart rate either in response to fetal movement (nonstress test) or in response to uterine contractions usually induced with oxytocin (contraction stress test), or both. As long as these tests remained normal, the fetus has been considered to be in little jeopardy from further stay in the uterus.

The major problems that have arisen with the use of these tests, aside from costs and inconvenience, are frequencies of false-positive and false-negative results that are unacceptable, at least to some obstetricians. Moreover, careful analyses of published reports concerned with posttern pregnancies provide no convincing evidence that their use has produced better results than has the preceding plan of management. Unfortunately, as emphasized by Kirschbaum (1979) in the course of discussing the problems associated with prolonged pregnancy, several technics now commonly employed to attempt fetal appraisal have been incorporated into clinical practice without vigorous objective proof of value as measured by their predictive strength and the prevention of perinatal morbidity and death. For example, Schneider and co-workers (1978), in their study of postterm pregnancies, found measurements of 24-hour urinary estriol excretion carried out every Monday, Wednesday, and Friday to be of little value in their hands. In no instance did a falling estriol correlate with a positive oxytocin challenge test. Eaton (1979), moreover, has described two instances of fetal death within 36 hours after a normal oxytocin challenge test that was performed because the pregnancy was prolonged. Berkowitz and Hobbins (1977) have been unable to confirm the earlier claim from their institution that measurements of hPL were of value in identifying the postterm fetus who is being compromised by his prolonged stay in utero.

The use of transabdominal amniocentesis has also been suggested to try to identify meconium in amnionic fluid and thereby possibly identify postterm fetuses who are likely to be in jeopardy. Indeed, serially performed amniocenteses identified meconium in amnionic fluid in 22 percent of cases of prolonged pregnancy studied by Knox and associates (1979). Although meconium was significantly associated with abnormal pro-

gression of labor, intrapartum fetal distress, and low Apgar scores, induction of labor after discovery of meconium, when compared to the results achieved with nonintervention, did not improve perinatal outcome. They concluded that a search for meconium through repeated antepartum transabdominal amniocenteses followed by induction of labor is of little value in the management of prolonged pregnancy.

REFERENCES

Ballard RA, Ballard PL, Granberg JP, Sniderman S: Prenatal administration of beta-methasone for prevention of respiratory distress syndrome. J Pediatr 94:97, 1979

Barden TP: Labor. In Pitkin Roy (ed): Year Book of Obstet Gynecol. Chicago, 1977, p 109

Bauer CR, Stern L, Colle E: Prolonged rupture of membranes associated with a decreased incidence of respiratory distress syndrome. Pediatrics 53:7, 1974

Belizán JM, Villar J, Nardin JC, Malamud J, De Vicuña LS: Diagnosis of intrauterine growth retardation by a simple clinical method: Measurement of uterine height. Am J Obstet Gynecol 131:643, 1978

Berkowitz RL, Hobbins JC: A reevaluation of the value of hCS determination in the management of prolonged pregnancy. Obstet Gynecol 49:156, 1977

Brenner WE, Edelman DA, Hendricks CH: A standard of fetal growth for the United States of America. Am J Obstet Gynecol 126:555, 1976

Brown ER, Nielsen H, Torday JS, Tauesch HW: Reversible induction of surfactant production in fetal lambs treated with glucocorticoids. Pediatr Res 13:491, 1979

Campbell S, Wilkin D: Ultrasonic measurement of fetal abdomen circumference in the estimation of fetal weight. Br J Obstet Gynaecol 82:689, 1975

Caritis SN, Edelstone DI, Mueller-Heubach E: Pharmacologic inhibition of preterm labor. Am J Obstet Gynecol 133:557, 1979

Castrén O, Gummerus M, Saarikoski S: Treatment of imminent premature labour. Acta Obstet Gynecol Scand 54:95, 1975

Cetrulo CL, Freeman R: Bioelectric evaluation in

intrauterine growth retardation. Clin Obstet Gynecol 20:979, 1977

Creasy RK: Intrauterine growth retardation: Optimal delivery time. Presented at the Seventy-Eighth Ross Conference on Pediatric Research (Obstetrical Decisions and Neonatal Outcome), San Diego, May 30, 1979

Dimmick J, Mahmood K, Altshuler G: Antenatal infection: Adequate protection against hyaline membrane disease? Obstet Gynecol 47:57, 1976

Dluholucky S, Babic J, Taufer I: Reduction of incidence and mortality of respiratory distress syndrome by administration of hydrocortisone to mother. Arch Dis Child 51:420, 1976

Eaton CJ: Discussion of paper by Knox GE, Huddleston JF, Flowers CE: Management of prolonged pregnancy: Result of a prospective randomized trial. Am J Obstet Gynecol 134:376, 1979

Elliott JP, O'Keeffe DF, Greenberg P, Freeman RK: Pulmonary edema associated with magnesium sulfate and betamethasone administration. Am J Obstet Gynecol 134:717, 1979

Epstein MF, Nicholls E, Stubblefield PG: Neonatal hypoglycemia after beta-sympathomimetic tocolytic therapy. J Pediatr 94:449, 1979

Fancourt R, Campbell S, Harvey D, Norman AP: Follow-up studies of small-for-dates babies. Br Med J 1:1435, 1976

Fedrick J, Anderson ABM: Factors associated with spontaneous pre-term birth. Br J Obstet Gynaecol 83:342, 1976

Fitzhardinge PM, Steven EM: The small-for-date infant. 1. Later growth patterns. Pediatrics 49:671, 1972

Fuchs F, Fuchs A-R, Lauersen NH, Zervoudakis IA: Treatment of pre-term labour with ethanol. Danish Med Bull 26:123, 1979

Fuchs F, Fuchs A-R, Poblete V, Resk A: Effect of alcohol on threatened premature labor. Am J Obstet Gynecol 99:627, 1967

Gabert H: Personal communication, 1974

Gluck L: Fetal Lung Maturity. Presented at the Seventy-Eighth Ross Conference on Pediatric Research, San Diego, May 30, 1979

Graven SN: Ethical Dilemmas in Current Obstetric and Newborn Care. Report of Sixty-Fifth Ross Conference on Pediatric Research, Columbus, Ohio, Ross Laboratories, 1973

Haesslein HC, Goodlin RC: Delivery of the tiny newborn. Am J Obstet Gynecol 134:192, 1979

Hatwick RE: Ethical Dilemmas in Current Obstetric and Newborn Care. Report of Sixty-Fifth

Ross Conference on Pediatric Research, Columbus, Ohio, Ross Laboratories, 1973

Haverkamp AD, Orleans M, Langendoerfer S, McFee J, Murphy J, Thompson HE: A controlled trial of the differential effects of intrapartum fetal monitoring. Am J Obstet Gynecol 134:399, 1979

Heinrichs WL, Storey CP: Fetal therapy: Glucocorticoids for respiratory maturation. Am J Obstet Gynecol 1980, In press

Hemminki E, Starfield B: Prevention and treatment of premature labor by drugs: Review of controlled clinical trials. Br J Obstet Gynaecol 85:411, 1978

Hesseldahl H: A Danish multicenter study of ritodrine in the treatment of pre-term labor. Danish Med Bull 26:116, 1979

Hobbins JC, Berkowitz RL, Grannum PAT: Diagnosis and antepartum management of intrauterine growth retardation. J Reprod Med 21:319, 1978

Hoffman HJ, Stark CR, Lunden FE Jr, Ashbrook JD: Analyses of birth weight, gestational age, and fetal viability, U.S. births, 1968. Obstet Gynecol Surv 29:651, 1974

Howie RN, Liggins GC: Clinical trial of antepartum betamethasone therapy for prevention of respiratory distress in pre-term infants. Proceedings of Fifth Study Group, Royal College of Obstetricians and Gynecologists. Oct., 1977, p. 281

Jimenez J, Tyson J, Santos-Ramos R, Duenhoelter J: Comparison of obstetric and pediatric evaluation of gestational age. Pediatr Res 14:497, 1979

Johnson JWC, Lee PA, Zachary AS, Calhoun S, Migeon CJ: High-risk prematurity-progestin treatment and steroid studies. Obstet Gynecol 54:412, 1979

Johnson JWC, Mitzner W, London WT, Palmer AE, Scott R: Betamethasone and the rhesus fetus. Multisystemic effects. Am J Obstet Gynecol 133:677, 1979

Jones MD Jr, Battaglia FC: Intrauterine growth retardation. Am J Obstet Gynecol 127:540, 1977

Jones MD Jr, Burd LI, Bowes WA Jr, Battaglia FC, Lubchenco LO: Failure of association of premature rupture of membranes with respiratory distress syndrome. N Engl J Med 292:1253, 1975

Jones RAK, Cummins M, Davies PA: Infants of very low birthweight. A 15-year analysis. Lancet 1:1332, 1979

Kirkpatrick SE, Pitlik PT, Hirschklau MJ, Friedman WF: Acute effects of maternal ethanol infusion on fetal cardiac performance. Am J Obstet Gynecol 126:1034, 1976

Kirschbaum TH: Discussion of paper by Knox GE, Huddleston JF, Flowers CE: Management of prolonged pregnancy: Result of a prospective randomized trial. Am J Obstet Gynecol 134:376, 1979

Knox GE, Huddleston JF, Flowers CE: Management of prolonged pregnancy: Result of a prospective randomized trial. Am J Obstet Gynecol 134:376, 1979

Kopelman AE: The smallest preterm infant. Am J Dis Child 132:461, 1978

Korda AR, Lyneham RC, Jones WR: The treatment of premature labour with intravenously administered salbutamol. Med J Austr I:744, 1974

Kristoffersen K, Hansen MK: The condition of the foetus and infant in cases treated with ritodrine. Danish Med Bull 26:121, 1979

Kubli F: In Anderson A, and others (eds): Preterm Labor. London, Royal College of Obstetricians and Gynaecologists, 1977, p. 218.

Landesman R: Premature labor: Its management and therapy. J Reprod Med 9:95, 106, 1972

Lauersen NH, Merkatz IR, Tejani N, Wilson KH, Roberson A, Mann LI, Fuchs F: Inhibition of premature labor: A multicenter comparison of ritodrine and ethanol. Am J Obstet Gynecol 127:837, 1977

Levin DL: Effects of inhibition of prostaglandin synthesis on fetal development, oxygenation, and the fetal circulation. Perinatal Seminars, in press

Liggins GC: The prevention of RDS by maternal betamethasone administration. In Lung Maturation and the Prevention of Hyaline Membrane Disease. Report of the Seventieth Ross Conference on Pediatric Research, Columbus, Ohio, Ross Laboratories, 1976

Liggins GC, Howie RN: The prevention of RDS by maternal steroid therapy. In Gluck 1 (ed): Modern Perinatal Medicine. Chicago, Year Book, 1974

Liggins GC, Vaughn GS: Intravenous infusion of salbutamol in the management of premature labour. J Obstet Gynaecol Br Commonw 80:29, 1973

Lubchenco LO: The High Risk Infant. Philadelphia, Saunders, 1976

Lubchenco LO, Hansman C, Dressler M, Boyd E: Intrauterine growth as estimated from liveborn birth weight data at 24 to 42 weeks of gestation. Pediatrics 32:793, 1963

Mann LI, Bhakthavathsalan A, Liu M, Makowski P: Placental transport of alcohol and its effects on maternal and fetal acid-base balance. Am J Obstet Gynecol 122:837, 1975

Mashiach S, Barkai G, Sack J, Stern E, Brish M, Goldman B, Serr DM: The effects of intraamniotic thyroxine administration on fetal lung maturity in man. J Perinat Med 7:161, 1979

Merkatz IR, Peter JB, Barden TP: Ritodrine hydrochloride: A betamimetic agent developed specifically for use in preterm labor. II. Evidence of efficacy. Am J Obstet Gynecol, in press

Morrison JC, Whybrew WD, Bucovaz ET, Schneider JM: Injection of corticosteroids into mother to prevent neonatal respiratory distress syndrome. Am J Obstet Gynecol 131:358, 1978

Mosier HD Jr, Dearden LC, Tanner SM, Jansons RA, Biggs CS: Disproportionate organ growth in the fetus after betamethasone administration. Pediatr Res 13:486, 1979

Naeye RL, Dixon JB: Distortions in fetal growth standards. Pediatr Res 12:987, 1978

Osler M: Side effects and metabolic changes during treatment with betamimetics (ritodrine). Danish Med Bull 26:119, 1979

Persson P-H, Grennert L, Gennser G: Impact of fetal and maternal factors on the normal growth of the biparietal diameter. Acta Obstet Gynecol Scand (Suppl) 78:21, 1978

Philip AGS: Fetal growth retardation: Femurs, fontanels, and follow-up. Pediatrics 62:446, 1978

Pomerance JJ, Ukrainski CT, Ukra T, Henderson DH, Nash AH, Meredith JL: Cost of living for infants weighing 1000 grams or less at birth. Pediatrics 61:908, 1978

Pritchard JA, Whalley PJ: High risk pregnancy and reproductive outcome. In Gluck L (ed): Modern Perinatal Medicine. Chicago, Year Book, 1974

Quirk JG, Raker RK, Petrie RH, Williams AM: The role of glucocorticoids, unstressful labor, and atraumatic delivery in the prevention of respiratory distress syndrome. Am J Obstet Gynecol 134:768, 1979

Reynolds JW: A comparison of salbutamol and ethanol in the treatment of premature labor. Aust NZ J Obstet Gynaecol 18:107, 1978

Ritchie K, McClure G: Prematurity. Lancet 2:1227, 1979

Rogge P, Young S, Goodlin R: Post-partum pulmonary oedema associated with preventive therapy for premature labour. Lancet 1:1026, 1979

Rydén G: The effect of salbutamol and terbutaline in the management of premature labour. Acta Obstet Gynecol Scand 56:293, 1977

Schifrin BS: The non-stress test. Presented at the Seventy-eighth Ross Conference on Pediatric Research (Obstetrical Decisions and Neonatal Outcome), San Diego, May 30, 1979

Schneider JM, Olson RW, Curet LB: Screening for fetal and neonatal risk in the postdate pregnancy. Am J Obstet Gynecol 131:473, 1978

Sell E, Harris TR: The influence of ruptured membranes (ROM) on fetal outcome. Pediatr Res 10:432, 1976

Sims CD, Chamberlain GVP, Boyd IE, Lewis PJ: A comparison of salbutamol and ethanol in the treatment of preterm labor. Brit J Obstet Gynaecol 85:761, 1978

Spellacy WN, Cruz AC, Birk SA, Buhi WC: Treatment of premature labor with ritodrine: A randomized controlled study. Obstet Gynecol 54:220, 1979

Steer CM, Petrie RH: A comparison of magnesium sulfate and alcohol for the prevention of premature labor. Am J Obstet Gynecol 129:1, 1977

Stewart AL, Turcan DM, Rawlings G, Reynolds EOR: Prognosis for infants weighing 1000g or less at birth. Arch Dis Child 52:97, 1977

Stubblefield RG: Pulmonary edema occurring after therapy with dexamethasone and terbutaline for premature labor: a case report. Am J Obstet Gynecol 132:341, 1978

Taeusch HW, Frigoletto F, Kitzmiller J, Avery ME, Hehre A, Fromm B, Lawson E, Neff RK: Risks of respiratory distress syndrome after prenatal dexamethasone treatment. Pediatrics 63:64, 1979

Tejani N, Mann LI: Diagnosis and management of the small-for-gestational age fetus. Clin Obstet Gynecol 20:943, 1977

Tinga DJ, Aarnoudse JG: Post-partum pulmonary oedema associated with preventive therapy for premature labour. Lancet 1:1026, 1979

Ulmsten U: Inhibition of myometrial hyperactivity by calcium antagonists. Danish Med Bull 26:125, 1979

Warshof SL, Gohari P, Berkowitz RL, Hobbins JC: The estimation of fetal weight by computer-assisted analysis. Am J Obstet Gynecol 128:881, 1977

Wright FH, Blough RR, Chamberlin A, Ernest T, Halstead WC, Meier P, Moore RY, Naunton RF, Newell FW: A controlled follow-up study of small prematures born from 1952 through 1956. Am J Dis Child 124:507, 1972

Yoon JJ, Harper RG: Observations on the relationship between duration of rupture of the membranes and the development of idiopathic respiratory distress syndrome. Pediatrics 52:161, 1973

Zlatnik FJ, Fuchs F: A controlled study of ethanol in threatened premature labor. Am J Obstet Gynecol 112:610, 1972

Zuckerman H, Reiss U, Robenstein I: Inhibition of human premature labor by indomethacin. Obstet Gynecol 44:787, 1974

Zuelzer WW: Ethical Dilemmas in Current Obstetric and Newborn Care. Report of the Sixty-fifth Ross Conference on Pediatric Research. Columbus, Ohio, Ross Laboratories, 1973

38

Other Diseases of the Fetus and Newborn Infant

The fetus and newborn infant are subject to a great variety of diseases, many of which are the direct consequence of maternal disease and have been considered along with the maternal disease, especially in Chapter 28. This chapter provides an introduction to other fetal and neonatal diseases of major clinical importance. Injuries and malformations of the fetus and newborn infants are considered in Chapter 39.

RESPIRATORY DISEASE

To provide prompt blood–gas exchange after birth, the infant must rapidly fill his lungs with air while clearing them of fluid, and he must simultaneously increase remarkably the volume of blood that perfuses his lungs. Some of the fluid is usually expressed as the chest is compressed during vaginal delivery; the remainder is absorbed especially through the lymphatics of the lungs. Of great importance is the presence of appropriate surfactant synthesized by the type II pneumocytes of the lungs to stabilize the air-expanded alveoli

by lowering surface tension and thereby preventing their collapse during expiration.

Idiopathic Respiratory Distress (Hyaline Membrane Disease). About two decades ago, the development of idiopathic respiratory distress-hyaline membrane disease was related to a deficiency of pulmonary surfactant. More recently, it has become apparent that the deficiency in surfactant may be qualitative as well as quantitative. Shelley and co-workers (1979), for example, found the amount of dipalmitoyl phosphatidylcholine, a major component of surfactant, to be lower and phosphatidylcholine containing unsaturated fatty acids to be higher in tracheal and pharyngeal aspirates from infants with respiratory distress than in aspirates from control infants. As the condition improved, the fatty contents of phosphatidylcholine became similar to that of the control group.

If the alveoli cannot be maintained in an expanded state because of inappropriate surfactant, obvious respiratory distress develops which is characterized by the formation of hyaline membrane in the distal bronchioles and alveoli, considerable cardiopulmonary shunting of blood, and the likelihood of death from hypoxia and acidosis unless treatment is prompt and appropriate.

DIAGNOSIS. The atelectatic lungs are stiff with very low compliance; thus the work of breathing is increased remarkably. Progressive shunting of blood through nonventilated areas of the lung contributes to the hypoxia and to both metabolic and respiratory acidosis. Clinically, the infants exhibit an increased respiratory rate accompanied by severe retraction. Expiration is often accompanied by a whimper and grunt; grunting is very common in the newborn whenever there is uneven expansion of the lungs or lower airway obstruction. Poor peripheral circulation and systemic hypotension may be evident.

A decade ago hyaline membrane disease accounted for one-fifth of all neonatal deaths (Farrell and Wood, 1976), but the actual number of deaths from respiratory distress-hyaline membrane disease undoubtedly has decreased since then (Table 38-1). Boys are more prone than girls to develop respiratory distress-hyaline membrane disease, and white infants appear to be more often affected than are black infants.

Other forms of respiratory insufficiency may be confused with idiopathic respiratory distress-hyaline membrane disease. These include respiratory insufficiency as the consequence of sepsis, pneumonia, aspiration, pneumothorax, diaphragmatic hernia, and heart failure. Common causes of cardiac decompensation in the early newborn period are patent ductus arteriosus and primary myocardial disease. The chest roentgenogram, coupled with a careful physical examination, is likely to be of considerable aid in differential diagnosis. In case of idiopathic respiratory distress, the chest roentgenogram reveals a diffuse reticulogranular infiltrate throughout the lung fields with an air-filled tracheobronchial tree (air bronchogram).

PATHOLOGY. In the fatal case, the atelectatic lungs on gross examination resemble liver. Histologically, many alveoli are collapsed while some are widely dilated; hyaline membranes of fibrin-rich protein and cellular debris line the dilated alveoli and the terminal bronchioles; and the epithelium underlying the membrane is necrotic.

TREATMENT. An arterial PO_2 below 40 mm Hg is indicative of need for effective oxygen therapy. Anaerobically collected blood is required to assess PO_2, PCO_2, and pH. The blood may be obtained from a peripheral artery but more easily from a catheter in an umbilical artery that may also be used for infusion of fluids. The concentration of oxygen administered to these infants should be sufficient to relieve hypoxia and acidosis but not higher. Arterial tensions of 50 to 70 mm Hg are adequate. Humidification of inspired air also is important in the management of these infants. During recovery, careful blood gas monitoring allows PO_2 to be maintained with lessening amounts of oxygen. The infant from the time of birth must be kept warm, since chilling increases oxygen consumption.

The use of oxygen-enriched air under pressure to prevent the collapse of unstable alveoli (continuous positive airway pressure) has brought about an appreciable reduction in the mortality rate from the respiratory distress syndrome. Chernik (1974), for example, reported a lowering of the fatality rate

TABLE 38-1.
IMPROVED SURVIVAL RATES (%) FOR
VERY SMALL INFANTS WITH RESPIRATORY
DISTRESS SYNDROME AT THE UNIVERSITY
OF CALIFORNIA AT SAN FRANCISCO

WEIGHT (kg)	1965–1968	1969–1973	1974–1978
<1.0	18	20	33
1–1.25	40	40	85
1.25–1.5	23	75	91
1.5–1.75	64	75	100
>1.75	64	94	99

From Creasy: Seventy-eighth Ross Conference on Pediatric Research, Obstetrical Decisions and Neonatal Outcome, San Diego, May 30, 1979.

with severe hyaline membrane disease from 72 percent to 28 percent. In order to be successful, any technic to augment ventilation requires continuous observation by skilled personnel in constant attendance. Successful ventilation usually reduces the high inspired oxygen concentrations that are otherwise required and thereby reduces oxygen toxicity to the lung. Disadvantages are that venous return to the heart may be impaired causing a fall in cardiac output, and there is always the possibility of rupture of the lung with interstitial emphysema and pneumothorax or pneumomediastinum. Moreover, vigorous mechanical ventilation is considered an important factor in the genesis of bronchopulmonary dysplasia as pointed out below.

The establishment of appropriately staffed and equipped neonatal intensive care units has served to reduce appreciably the number of deaths from idiopathic respiratory distress even in very small infants.

OTHER COMPLICATIONS. Oxygen therapy is not innocuous. Persistent hyperoxia is likely in itself to injure the lung, especially the alveoli and capillaries. If hyperoxemia is produced, the infant is at risk of developing *retrolental fibroplasia* (p. 960). Therefore, the concentration of oxygen administered must be reduced appropriately as the arterial PO_2 rises. Endotracheal tubes after prolonged use cause erosion and serious infection of the upper airway; thus, they must be removed as soon as possible. *Bronchopulmonary dysplasia* may develop in infants treated for severe respiratory distress (Workshop on Bronchopulmonary Dysplasia, 1979). Bronchopulmonary dysplasia is a chronic condition characterized by hypoxia, hypercarbia, and oxygen dependence as the consequence of alveolar and bronchiolar epithelial damage followed by peribronchial and interstitial fibrosis. Contributing to its development is the prolonged use of mechanical ventilators to deliver oxygen in high concentrations. Edwards and associates (1977) point out that large infants seldom develop the condition because of lack of need for such therapy and that neither do very small infants because

they are more likely to expire soon after birth. In one study the administration of vitamin E during the acute phase of the respiratory distress syndrome appeared to modify the development of bronchopulmonary dysplasia (Ehrenkranz et al., 1978).

SURVIVAL. Death from the respiratory distress syndrome formerly was quite common, especially among very small infants. In recent years, however, the mortality rate, even for very small infants, has decreased remarkably as borne out by data that are presented in Table 38-1.

Meconium Aspiration. The aspiration of normal amnionic fluid before birth is most likely a physiologic event (see Chap. 8, p. 198). Fetal distress, however, may lead to defecation of meconium into the amnionic fluid, and in more severe circumstances the meconium-contaminated fluid may become quite thick.

PATHOLOGY. Aspiration of meconium is likely to cause both mechanical obstruction of the airways and a chemical pneumonitis. Atelectasis, consolidation, and pneumothorax and pneumomediastinum may prove fatal unless vigorously treated. Yeh and co-workers (1979) have emphasized that the initial chest roentgenogram is useful for predicting outcome in infants with meconium aspiration. Consolidation or atelectasis, most commonly associated with aspiration of thick meconium, is indicative of a poor outcome.

Marshall and associates (1978) found no evidence of persistent chronic lung disease among survivors of meconium aspiration whom they followed. Two of three infants, however, who developed seizures while acutely ill subsequently demonstrated significant psychomotor retardation.

DIAGNOSIS AND MANAGEMENT. At Parkland Memorial Hospital, whenever meconium has been identified in amnionic fluid before or during delivery, someone especially skilled in resuscitative technics is present at the delivery. To prevent further aspiration, the mouth and nares are carefully suctioned by the obstetrician before the shoulders are delivered from the vagina, or as the mouth is visualized at cesarean section (see Chap. 20, p. 475). As soon as possible after delivery, all meconium-stained fluid that remains above the cords is aspirated and the vocal cords are visualized. Endotracheal intubation and suction are then applied and as much meconium as possible is aspirated from the trachea. It is essential to perform these procedures swiftly. The stomach is emptied to avoid the possibility of further meconium aspiration. *It is emphasized that ventilation of the lungs must not be delayed unduly while these procedures are carried out.* Subsequent treatment is generally similar to that described for respiratory distress. The value, if any, of corticosteroids, prophylactic antibiotics, and bronchodilators has not been established.

RETROLENTAL FIBROPLASIA

Retrolental fibroplasia had become by 1950 the largest single cause of blindness in this country. After the discovery that the etiology of the disease was hyperoxia, its frequency decreased remarkably.

Pathology. The retina of the eye vascularizes centrifugally from the optic nerve starting about the fourth month of gestation and continuing until shortly after birth. During the time of vascularization, the retinal vessels are very sensitive to and thus easily damaged by excess oxygen. The temporal portion of the retina, which is the last to be vascularized, is most vulnerable. Oxygen induces severe vasoconstriction, damage to the endothelium, and obliteration of the affected vessel. When the oxygen level is reduced, there is new vessel formation at the site of previous vasculature damage. The new vessels penetrate the retina and extend intravitreally where they are prone to leak proteinaceous material or actually burst and leak blood. Adhesions then form which detach the retina.

Prevention. The precise levels of hypoxemia that can be sustained without causing retrolental fibroplasia are not known. Unfortunately, a cooperative study that was carried out more recently did not provide answers to many difficult but important questions concerning arterial PO_2 levels and retrolental fibroplasia (Kinsey et al., 1977). It is felt by many pediatricians that the inhalation of air enriched with oxygen to no more than 40 percent will not cause retrolental fibroplasia. Some believe, however, that whenever oxygen-enriched air is provided the blood PO_2 must be monitored.

Preterm, small infants who develop respiratory distress are most likely to require ventilation with high concentrations of oxygen to maintain life until the respiratory distress clears. During this period, it is important that overzealous treatment does not lead to dangerous hyperoxia and, in turn, retrolental fibroplasia. Frequent measurements of PO_2, therefore, may be necessary first to assure adequate oxygen and then to prevent hypoxemia as the respiratory distress clears.

ANEMIA

Diagnosis. The diagnosis of anemia in the newborn infant is not always a simple process. After 35 weeks of gestation, the mean cord hemoglobin concentration is about 17.0 g per dl; values below 14.0 g may be regarded as pathologically low. During the first several hours of life, the hemoglobin value may rise by as much as 20 percent, especially when clamping of the cord was delayed. If, however, the placenta was cut or torn, a fetal vessel was perforated or lacerated, or the infant was held well above the level of the placenta for some time before cord-clamping, the hemoglobin concentration is more likely to fall during the hours after delivery.

FETAL TO MATERNAL HEMORRHAGE. The presence of fetal red cells in the maternal circulation may be identified by use of the acid elution principle described by Kleihauer, Brown, and Betke, or any of several modifications. Very small volumes of red cells commonly escape from the intravascular compartment of the fetus across the generally intact placental "barrier" into the maternal intervillous space. Although the bleed is usually small, it may incite maternal isoimmunization, as discussed below. Interestingly, evidence of maternal to fetal bleeding is very much less common (Bernard et al., 1977). Presumably a pressure gradient which is higher on the fetal than on the maternal side persists across the placenta.

Rarely, fetal to maternal hemorrhage may be so severe as to kill the fetus. The hypovolemic or severely anemic fetus-infant may be salvaged if the condition is recognized and treatment with blood, red cells, or both is promptly initiated. The fetus who is severely anemic is more likely to demonstrate one or more ominous heart rate patterns (see Chap. 14, p. 357). On occasion, the hemorrhage may have been chronic and so severe as to produce evidence of iron deficiency in the fetus (Pritchard and Cunningham, unpublished data). Maternal iron deficiency, however, even when severe, is not accompanied by anemia in the fetus; the same holds true for megaloblastic anemia due to folate deficiency (see Chap. 28, p. 720).

With large fetal to maternal hemorrhage there is most likely a placental lesion which fostered the leak. Chorioangiomas have been identified. Moreover, we know of two instances of severe fetal to maternal hemorrhage in which the mothers were later found to have choriocarcinoma. While neither placenta was studied, the subsequent recognition of choriocarcinoma in the mothers is suggestive that there was a placental lesion which was the site of transfer of blood from the fetus to the mother. Abruptio placentae, in our experience, does not appear to lead commonly to severe fetal to maternal hemorrhage.

At Parkland Memorial Hospital, for some time, maternal blood has been investigated for fetal red cells in each instance of stillbirth whenever a cause was not readily apparent. Massive fetal–maternal bleeds have been identified in a very small minority of stillbirths.

Large fetal to maternal hemorrhages may also prove dangerous to the mother. It is possible for up to 400 ml of fetal blood to be transferred from the fetal–placental circulation into the maternal circulation. A transfusion reaction may then develop in the mother whenever A or B antigen is present in fetal red cells but not the red cells of the mother. Bergin and associates (1978), for example, have described many of the characteristic features of a transfusion reaction developing in a mother who was blood type O immediately after delivery of an infant who was blood type B. The subject of fetal–maternal hemorrhage has been reviewed by Renaer and associates (1976).

HEMOLYSIS FROM MATERNAL Rho (D) ISOIMMUNIZATION

Ranking as major contributions to medicine are the delineation of the pathogenesis of most cases of hemolytic disease in the fetus and newborn infant by the observations especially of Levine and associates (1941), the related discovery of the Rh factor by Landsteiner and Wiener (1940), and the development of effective maternal prophylaxis by Freda, Gorman, and Pollack (1963) in the United States and Finn, Clarke, and associates in Great Britain (1961).

Blood Group Factors. Originally, the Rh concept was extremely simple, defined by one antiserum and two blood group factors, namely Rh positive and Rh negative. The Rh factors, however, have become increasingly complex, and a host of other red cell antigens have been identified. Although some of them are immunologically and genetically important, fortunately, many are so rare as to be of little clinical significance in the genesis of erythroblastosis fetalis.

Any person who lacks a specific red cell

antigen most likely will create an antibody when exposed to that antigen. The antibody may prove harmful to the individual in case of a blood transfusion or to her fetus when she conceives. The vast majority of human beings have at least one such factor inherited from their father and lacking in their mother. In these cases, the mother could be sensitized if enough erythrocytes from the fetus were to reach her circulation and an immune response were to be stimulated by the foreign antigen. In these terms, hemolytic disease is a possibility in nearly every pregnancy. That the disease occurs in very few pregnancies is a result of several circumstances. These include (1) the varying rates of occurrence of the offending red cell antigens, (2) their variable antigenicity, (3) insufficient transplacental crossing of antigen from fetus to mother, (4) the variability of maternal response to the antigen, and (5) lack of transfer of antibody across the placenta from mother to fetus in amounts sufficient to affect the fetus.

The Rh antigens are inherited independent of all other blood group antigens. There is apparently no difference in the distribution of the various Rh antigens with regard to sex. There are, however, important racial differences. American Indians and Chinese and other Asiatic peoples are almost all Rho (D) positive (99 percent). Among black Americans there is a lesser incidence of Rho negative individuals (7 to 8 percent) than among white Americans (13 percent). Of all racial and ethnic groups studied thus far, the Basques show the highest incidence of Rho negativity (34 percent).

At times, hemolysis in the fetus involves other antigen–antibody interactions, especially the ABO system. These are considered subsequently. *All pregnant women should be routinely tested for the presence or absence of Rho (D) antigen in their erythrocytes and for irregular antibodies in their serum, including anti-Rho.*

Mortality. The number of perinatal deaths from Rho hemolytic disease has dropped dramatically for the following reasons:

1. Pregnant women who are Rho negative and possess antibody to the Rho antigen can be readily identified.
2. Hemolysis in the fetus of the sensitized Rho negative woman can be predicted with considerable accuracy by the identification of abnormally high levels of bilirubin in the amnionic fluid.
3. The fetus who is most likely to be seriously affected can be treated by intraperitoneal transfusions of Rho negative red cells, or be delivered preterm before he expires in utero, or both.
4. Of greatest importance, the appropriate administration to the mother who is Rho negative of Rho immune globulin during or immediately after pregnancy has eradicated most, but not all, Rho isoimmunization among Rho negative women!

The favorable impact on reducing perinatal mortality as the consequence of these procedures is exemplified by the experiences in Manitoba. In that Canadian province, the number of perinatal deaths from hemolytic disease decreased from 29 in 1964 to zero in 1974 and one in 1975 (Bowman et al., 1977).

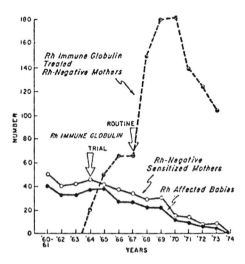

FIG. 38-1. Incidence of Rh disease correlated with Rh immune globulin treatment. (From Freda et al. *N Engl J Med* 292:1014, 1975)

Immune Globulin Prophylaxis for the Rho (D) Negative, Nonsensitized Mother.

Hemolytic disease of the fetus and newborn from Rho (D) isoimmunization has become a problem almost totally limited to Rho negative women who were sensitized before Rho (D) immune globulin* was available. Freda and co-workers (1975) summarized their 10 years of clinical experience with Rho immune globulin, confirming their original observations that such immune globulin given to the previously unsensitized Rho negative woman within 72 hours of delivery is highly protective, although not absolutely so (Figs. 38-1 and 38-2). There is good evidence to support the practice of giving the immune globulin promptly to previously unsensitized Rho negative women who have aborted including ectopic pregnancies and possibly hydatidiform moles, to women who undergo amniocentesis, and to those who bleed vaginally during pregnancy. The observation of Blajchman and co-workers (1974) of detectable fetal–maternal hemorrhage after at least 6 percent of amniocenteses has provided support for a policy that all unsensitized Rho negative women suspected of having an Rho positive fetus should receive Rho immune globulin following such a procedure. Freda (1973) has emphasized that when in doubt whether or not to give Rho immune globulin, the rule of thumb should be to give it.

While adherence to the above guidelines, including the administration of Rho immune globulin to the apparently nonsensitized mother within the first 72 hours after delivery of a Rho positive infant, has dramatically decreased the risk of maternal isoimmunization, the problem has not been eliminated. For example, Bowman and Pollock (1978) identified 1.8 percent of women to become isoimmunized in spite of adherence to the above recommendations for administering Rho immunoglobulin. He and his colleagues de-

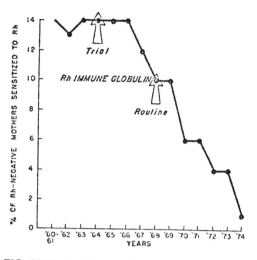

FIG. 38-2. Incidence of sensitization as a percentage of the total number of Rh-negative mothers seen per year. (From Freda et al. *N Engl J Med* 292:1014, 1975)

duced that most often the failures were the consequence of spontaneous silent fetal–maternal bleeds that occurred some time before delivery and therefore some time before the administration postpartum of Rho immune globulin. Therefore, to try to avoid isoimmunization from fetal–maternal bleeds that occurred remote from term, he administered routinely 300 μg intramuscularly to all nonsensitized Rho negative women at 28 weeks, and again at 34 weeks gestation, as well as at the time of amniocentesis or uterine bleeding. If the infant was Rho positive, a third dose of the immunoglobulin was administered to the mother after delivery. This program was followed by a reduction in the incidence of development of Rho isoimmunization during pregnancy from 1.8 percent to 0.07 percent. A single dose at about 28 weeks proved to be almost as effective as did the two doses antepartum; only 2 of 1799 Rho negative women showed evidence of Rho immunization, despite antenatal prophylaxis (Bowman and Pollock, 1978).

The small amount of antibody that crossed the placenta resulted at times in a weakly positive direct Coombs' test on cord and infant

---

* Rho (D) immune globulin is a 7S immune globulin (IgG) extracted by cold alcohol fractionation from plasma containing high titered Rho antibody. Each dose provides not less than 300 μg of Rho antibody as determined by radioimmunoassay.

blood. None of the infants, however, showed evidence of anemia or exaggerated hyperbilirubinemia.

RECOMMENDATIONS. A single intramuscular dose of 300 μg of Rho immunoglobulin is administered routinely to all Rho negative, *nonimmunized* women at 28 to 32 weeks of gestation and again within 72 hours of the birth of a Rho (D) positive infant. A similar dose is also given at the time of amniocentesis and whenever there is uterine bleeding, unless the routine dose at 28 to 32 weeks had been given very recently. If a massive fetal–maternal hemorrhage is recognized, more immune globulin should be given, as described below. One dose of 300 μg will protect the mother against a bleed of up to 15 ml of Rho positive red cells. Adoption of these dosage schedules should reduce the incidence of maternal isoimmunization to essentially zero.

ADVERSE MATERNAL REACTIONS. Only rarely do reactions occur after the intramuscular injection of commercially available Rho immunoglobulin. Usually the individual is IgA deficient and has previously developed an antibody to IgA. The Rho immune globulin that is currently available is likely to contain a small amount of IgA (Bowman, 1978). Rho immune globulin suitable for intravenous use very likely will become available.

MATERNAL–FETAL BLEED. Rarely, the Rho negative woman will have been exposed in utero to Rho antigen from her mother and become sensitized as the consequence. For this to occur, the woman's mother must have been Rho positive and a maternal–fetal bleed must have occurred sometime before the cord was severed. As with fetal–maternal bleeds, a major blood group (ABO) incompatibility most often appears to offer appreciable protection against Rho sensitization. Jen-

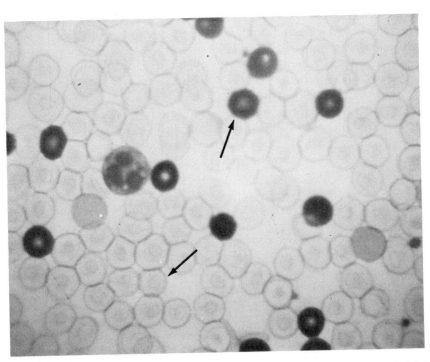

FIG. 38-3. Massive fetal to maternal hemorrhage. After acid elution treatment, fetal red cells rich in hemoglobin F stain darkly (upper arrow) whereas maternal red cells with only very small amounts of hemoglobin F (lower arrow) stain lightly.

nings and Clauss (1978) in a study of 105 Rho negative infants born to Rho positive mothers identified a maternal–fetal bleed in only two instances, or 1.9 percent, a value in very close agreement with that found by Cohen and Zuelzer (1965). Jennings and Clauss (1978) and Bowman (1978), on the basis of their extensive studies, do not believe that Rho immune globulin prophylaxis is warranted for Rho negative babies born to Rho positive mothers.

In case of larger fetal–maternal hemorrhage, the Rho positive erythrocytes may by careful examination be identified, at times, as clumps in the cross-match of the erythrocytes from maternal blood and the Rho immune globulin. The acid-elution technic, however, for identifying erythrocytes that contain appreciable alkaline-resistant (fetal) hemoglobin is best used to identify a major bleed and to approximate its magnitude.

When the acid-elution test is performed appropriately, red cells rich in fetal hemoglobin are easy to identify (Fig. 38-3). A careful differential count will serve to approximate closely the percentage of fetal cells in the maternal blood. From this value, coupled with the maternal hematocrit and an approximation of the maternal blood volume, an estimate of the volume of fetal red cells in the maternal circulation can be made. (Maternal blood volume will average about 5 liters before delivery and 4 liters shortly afterwards.) The volume of fetal red cells so calculated, then divided by 15 and multiplied by 300, provides a reasonable estimate for Rho immune globulin dosage in μg. If the estimate is doubled, almost certainly more than adequate protection would be afforded the mother.

Moreover, in cases of recognized major fetal–maternal hemorrhage, sensitization of the mother may be prevented by injecting sufficient immune globulin intramuscularly to maintain a demonstrable excess of antibody in the maternal serum.

In a case of massive fetal–maternal hemorrhage successfully treated at Parkland Memorial Hospital, 14 units of Rho immune globulin (4200 μg

at least) were injected intramuscularly over 48 hours to maintain a clearly demonstrable excess of antibody after delivery of a recently exsanguinated, very large infant. From the differential count of erythrocytes of maternal and fetal origin identified by acid-elution treatment of maternal blood and measurements of maternal hematocrit and blood volume, at least 150 ml of type O, Rho positive fetal erythrocytes were demonstrated to have entered the maternal circulation (Fig. 38-3). The mother did not become sensitized and subsequently gave birth to three unaffected type O, Rho positive infants, including twins. She remains free from evidence of Rho sensitization.

The Rho (D) Negative Sensitized Mother. The mother who is sufficiently immunized to produce enough antibody to cause overt hemolytic disease in the fetus and newborn infant will have demonstrable Rho antibody in her serum by the 36th week of gestation. Most often, if appropriate technics are used, the antibody will be demonstrable much earlier.

According to Freda (1973), if nothing is done in the way of interference in the pregnancy of a sensitized Rho negative woman with a Rho positive fetus, the perinatal mortality rate can be anticipated to be about 30 percent. With aggressive management, including diagnostic amniocenteses, intrauterine transfusions in selected cases, and early delivery in most cases, the perinatal mortality rate can be lowered to about 10 percent.

For optimal outcome, individualization of management should be practiced, aided by the following information:

1. Past obstetric history with emphasis on fetal outcome and how that outcome was achieved.
2. Accurate knowledge of fetal age.
3. The Rho zygosity of the father to identify those pregnancies in which the fetus has about a 50 percent chance of being Rho negative.
4. Maternal antibody measurements repeated throughout pregnancy.
5. Spectrophotometric analyses of amnionic fluid.

6. Identification of other maternal complications such as pregnancy-induced or -aggravated hypertension.

An antibody titer (indirect Coombs' test) that goes no higher than 1:16 almost always means that the fetus will not die in utero from hemolytic disease and that with appropriate care after birth he will survive. A titer higher than this indicates the *possibility* of severe hemolytic disease. It is emphasized that the titer in the previously sensitized woman may, during a subsequent pregnancy, rise infrequently to high levels even though her fetus is Rho negative.

A suspicious titer, i.e., 1:16 or higher, in most cases warrants appropriately timed amniocenteses and measurements of bilirubin pigment in amnionic fluid. The technic for amniocentesis is described in Chapter 14 (p. 330). If use of intrauterine transfusion is being considered, amniocentesis may be initiated at about 22 weeks' gestation.

The absorbence of the breakdown pigment, mostly bilirubin, in the supernatant of amnionic fluid, when measured in a continuously recording spectrophotometer, is demonstrable as a hump with maximum absorbence at 450 nm wavelength (ΔOD_{450}) as shown in Figure 38-4. The magnitude of the increase in optical density above baseline at 450 nm most often, but not always, correlates well, for any gestational age, with the intensity of the hemolytic disease.

Liley (1964) constructed a graph which provides for reasonably precise prediction of the severity of the hemolytic disease, a modification of which is demonstrated in Figure 38-5. His recommendations are as follows:

If the increase in optical density falls in Zone I at 28 to 31 weeks, the fetus will be unaffected or will have mild hemolytic disease. Repeat the amniocentesis in 2 or 3 weeks.

For Zone II, the prognosis is less accurate and may require repeated amniocenteses to indicate a trend. In lower Zone II, the infant's expected hemoglobin at birth will be between 11.0 and 13.9 g, whereas in upper Zone II, the infant's anticipated hemoglobin will range from 8.0 to 10.9 g. Trends and time of gestation will obviously indicate the necessity for early delivery or intrauterine transfusions.

Values in Zone III indicate a severely affected infant, and fetal death within 1 week to 10 days may be expected. The treatment—early delivery or intrauterine transfusion—will depend on the stage of gestation.

Pathologic Changes in Hemolytic Disease of the Fetus and Newborn.

Maternal antibodies gain access to the fetal circulation. In Rh positive infants, such antibodies are both adsorbed upon the Rho positive erythrocytes and exist in a free form in the infant's serum. The adsorbed antibodies act as hemolysins, leading to an accelerated rate of destruction of the red cells. The earlier this process begins in utero and the greater its intensity, the more severe will be the effect upon the fetus.

Maternal antibodies detectable at birth

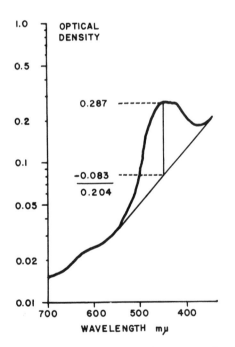

FIG. 38-4. Spectral absorption curve of amnionic fluid in hemolytic disease. (From Liley. In Greenhill L (ed.). *Yearbook of Obstetrics and Gynecology, 1964–1965* series, p 256. (Year Book)

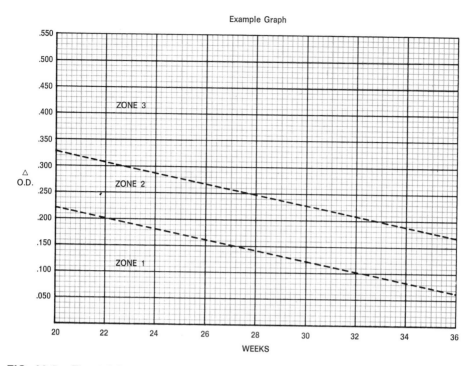

Example Graph

FIG. 38-5. The ΔO.D. value is plotted for the appropriate week of gestation. Zone 1 implies minimal hemolytic disease in the fetus, Zone 2 moderate to severe hemolytic disease, and Zone 3 impending fetal death. (From American College of Obstetricians and Gynecologists *Technical Bulletin No. 17,* July 1972)

gradually disappear from the infant's circulation over a period of 1 to 4 months. Their rate of disappearance is influenced to some extent by exchange transfusion. Detection of adsorbed antibodies is best accomplished by the direct Coombs' test. If Rho red cells coated with Rho antibody are typed with an anti-Rho saline agglutinin serum, they may be reported incorrectly as Rho negative because of the blocking effect produced by the adsorbed antibody. Therefore, erythrocytes reported to be Rho negative from an infant whose mother may be isoimmunized must always be checked by the direct Coombs' test.

The pathologic changes in the organs of the fetus and newborn infant vary with the severity of the process. The severely affected fetus or infant may show considerable subcutaneous edema as well as effusion into the serous cavities *(hydrops fetalis)*. At times, the edema is so severe that the diagnosis can be identified in the fetus by roentgenography (Fig. 38-6), or sonography (Fig. 38-7). In these cases, the *placenta* also is markedly edematous, appreciably enlarged and boggy, with large, prominent cotyledons and edematous villi. Excessive and prolonged hemolysis serves to stimulate marked erythroid hyperplasia of the bone marrow as well as large areas of *extramedullary hematopoiesis,* particularly in the spleen and liver. Histologic examination of the liver may serve to demonstrate, in addition, fatty degenerative parenchymal changes as well as deposition of hemosiderin and engorgement of the hepatic canaliculi with bile. There may be cardiac enlargement and pulmonary hemorrhages. Heart failure, however, at least at the outset, does not appear to play a prominent role in the development of ascites. Rather, portal hypertension and severe hypoalbuminemia are more likely the major factors in its develop-

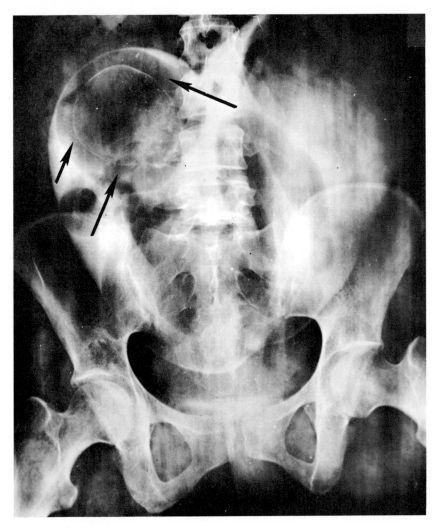

FIG. 38-6. Amniogram of a fetus with hydrops fetalis. *Arrows* point to severe edema of the scalp. (Courtesy of Dr. John T. Queenan)

ment. The ascites, and to a lesser degree hepatomegaly and splenomegaly, may be so massive as to lead to severe dystocia as the consequence of the greatly enlarged abdomen. Hydrothorax may be so severe as to compromise respirations after birth.

Fetuses with hydrops fetalis may die in utero from profound anemia and circulatory failure (Fig. 38-8). The liveborn hydropic infant appears pale, edematous, and limp at birth, often requiring resuscitation. The spleen and liver are enlarged, and there may be widespread ecchymoses or scattered petechiae. Dyspnea and circulatory collapse are common. Death may occur within a few hours in spite of transfusions.

Less severely affected infants may appear well at birth, only to become jaundiced within a few hours. Marked hyperbilirubinemia, if untreated, may lead to central nervous system damage, especially to the basal ganglia, which is characterized clinically by lethargy, stiffness of the extremities, retraction of the head, squinting, a high-pitched cry,

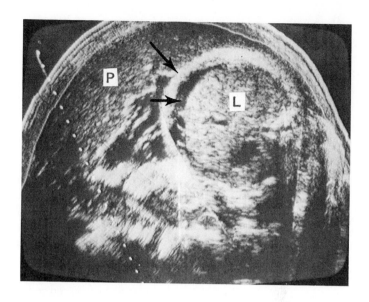

FIG. 38-7. Transverse sonogram of a hydropic fetus. Illustrated are fetal ascites (lower arrow), edema of fetal abdominal wall (upper arrow), liver (L), and large placenta (P). (Courtesy of Dr. R. Santos)

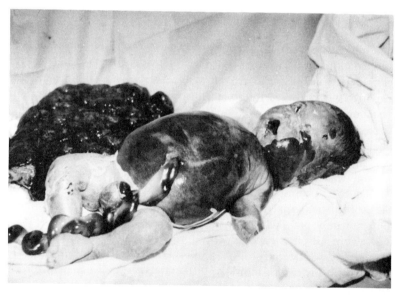

FIG. 38-8. Fatal erythroblastosis fetalis. Severely hydropic macerated stillborn infant and characteristically large placenta.

poor feeding, and convulsions. These signs are indicative of *kernicterus*. In such cases, death usually occurs within the first week of life. Surviving infants may be physically helpless, unable to support their heads or sit. Ability to walk is delayed or never acquired. In less severe forms, there may be varying degrees of motor incoordination, whereas some infants demonstrate residual nerve deafness as the only manifestation of neurologic injury.

Anemia, in part resulting from impaired erythropoiesis, may persist for many weeks to months in the infant who has demonstrated hemolytic disease at birth. In the absence of hypoxia, erythrocyte production normally falls after birth, especially in the premature infant. The observations of McIntosh (1975) serve to implicate low production of erythropoietin in this phenomenon.

Fetal Transfusions. The refinement in prognostic precision furnished by the analysis of amnionic fluid led Liley (1963) to try in apparently hopeless cases intrauterine transfusion of blood into the fetal peritoneal cavity. The procedure, in general, should be limited to cases in which, between 23 and 32 weeks, the spectrophotometric tracings and history forecast, in all likelihood, death of the fetus. Thirty-two weeks represents about the earliest gestational age at which the nontransfused affected fetus, if delivered, has a reasonable likelihood of surviving the adverse effects of prematurity, hemolytic disease, and exchange transfusion. For reasons that are not clear, the preterm infant with hemolytic disease from maternal Rh isoimmunization, unfortunately, is at increased risk of developing severe respiratory distresshyaline membrane disease. Bowman (1978) has emphasized that, in his hands, mortality following fetal transperitoneal transfusions at 32 weeks' gestation and delayed delivery is appreciably lower than with delivery at 32 weeks.

With intrauterine transfusion the overall survival rate in more recent years probably has been about 50 percent. Bowman reported

a survival rate of 70 percent if the initial transfusion was postponed to 26 weeks compared to 42 percent if the initial transfusion was required at 21½ to 23 weeks. Hamilton (1978) reported the survival of 76 percent of nonhydropic transfused fetuses. The results reported by some others have not been this good (Palmer and Gordon, 1976; Robertson et al., 1976).

Not only does fetal age and size at the time of the first transfusion affect the survival rate, the presence or absence of hydrops is of great importance. In Bowman's experience, the survival rate was only 21 percent if fetal ascites was encountered at the first transfusion, but 78 percent if no ascites was found at any time. In the presence of hydrops, absorption of the red cells from the peritoneal cavity appears to be markedly impaired. In the absence of hydrops, practically all of the erythrocytes are absorbed into the fetal circulation and survive there in normal fashion (Taylor et al., 1966).

The technic that has been used for fetal intraperitoneal transfusion at Parkland Memorial Hospital is very similar to that described in detail by Bowman (1978).

SUBSEQUENT CHILD DEVELOPMENT. Of 44 survivors of intrauterine transfusion followed by Holt and co-workers (1973), 43 were judged to be developing normally. Also, in Bowman's experience the great majority of fetal transfusion survivors developed normally; 74 of 89 tested when 18 months of age or older were completely normal and 4 were abnormal, while development in 11 appeared to be delayed somewhat perhaps because of preterm birth.

Delivery Before Term. In many circumstances, delivery before term is advantageous. Obviously, when it was considered necessary to utilize intrauterine transfusions, delivery, rather than further attempts at intrauterine transfusion, is desirable at the earliest date compatible with sufficient maturity to provide a good chance of survival. The exact timing of delivery in these cases depends on both clinical judgment and the results of the various laboratory tests. Delivery before the 32nd week in most instances is contraindicated by the extreme prematurity. Delivery may best be carried out at 34 weeks. At that time, the risk from prematurity probably is less than the risk of another intrauterine transfusion, at least at some institutions.

When intrauterine transfusion has not been performed, delivery before term may be considered for the following reasons: (1) previous history of an infant with unmistakable evidence of erythroblastosis, (2) a high titer of antibodies, (3) reasonable evidence of homozygosity of the father, and (4) evidence of potentially severe fetal disease from analysis of the amnionic fluid. The last is the most compelling reason for intervention, either delivery or an intrauterine transfusion.

Whenever a decision is reached to terminate pregnancy before term, adequate facilities for care of premature infants must be available, as well as the necessary equipment for carrying out exchange transfusion. The neonatologist should be advised of the situation well in advance of delivery, so that skilled personnel, blood, and equipment can be immediately available in or adjacent to the delivery room. The need for immediate transfusion is determined by the hemglobin concentration. Subsequently, the plasma bilirubin concentration is the important determinant.

METHOD OF DELIVERY. The fetus who is to be delivered remote from term because of evidence of hemolytic disease will sometimes benefit from cesarean section. By so doing, the time of birth is set and the "first team" of neonatologists and laboratory personnel can be assembled to provide for precise evaluation of the infant at birth and optimal treatment at that critical time, as well as subsequently. Moreover, the likelihood of a difficult, prolonged, or unsatisfactory induction of labor is avoided.

Exchange Transfusion for Hemolytic Disease of the Newborn. Examination of cord blood should be carried out immediately for any pregnancy in which the Rho negative mother is known to be sensitized. The cord blood hemoglobin concentration and the direct Coombs' test are of considerable importance when the infant is Rho positive. When the infant is overtly anemic, it is often best to carry out the initial exchange promptly to correct the anemia using recently collected packed type O, Rho negative red cells.

For infants who are not overtly anemic, exchange transfusion is determined by the rate of increase in bilirubin concentration, the maturity of the infant, and the presence or absence of other complications. While exchange transfusion is not an innocuous procedure, if moribund, hydropic, and kernicteric infants are excluded, the mortality rate is 1 percent or less.

Sensitization to Other Blood Group Factors. A variety of other fetal red cell antigens which are lacking in the mother may be involved in the genesis of hemolytic disease in the fetus and infant.

ABO INCOMPATIBILITY. The "major" blood group factors A and B are important causes of hemolytic disease. For example, group O women may from early life have anti-A and anti-B agglutinins, which may be augmented by pregnancy, particularly if the fetus is a secretor. Although about 20 percent of all infants have a "major" maternal blood group incompatibility, only 5 percent of them (1 percent of all babies) show overt signs of hemolytic disease. Moreover, when they do, the disease is usually much milder than that concerned with the Rho factor. Black infants are more likely to develop ABO disease than are white infants, according to Kirkman (1977). The disease does not appear to be any more severe, however, in black than in white infants (Peevy and Wiseman, 1978).

Desjardins and co-workers (1979) have intensively studied a large number of infants of blood group O mothers to try to identify a relationship between the degree of red cell sensitization by antibody and the cord blood hemoglobin and bilirubin concentrations. They found that when the infant blood type was A or B, the bilirubin was higher and hemoglobin was lower than in cord blood from blood group O infants even when no antibody was identified on the type A or B red cells. They concluded that ABO incompatibility represents a spectrum of hemolytic disease which ranges from those in which there is little laboratory evidence of red cell sensitization, but some evidence of hemolysis, to those with severe hemolytic disease in which red cell sensitization is readily demonstrable.

The usual criteria for diagnosis of hemolysis due to ABO incompatibility include the following: (1) The mother is group O, with anti-A and anti-B in her serum, while the fetus is A, B, or AB. (2) There is onset of jaundice within the first 24 hours. (3) There are varying degrees of anemia, reticulocytosis, and erythroblastosis. (4) There has been careful exclusion of other blood group sensitization. Unlike the result in Rh hemolytic disease, the Coombs' antiglobulin test in ABO incompatibility may be negative.

The principles of management of the newborn infant with Rh disease may be applied to ABO hemolytic disease, particularly with reference to the behavior of hemoglobin and bilirubin. For simple transfusion or exchange transfusion, group O blood is used. Quite dissimilar to Rh hemolytic disease, the incidence of stillbirths among ABO-incompatible pregnancies is not elevated (Freda, 1973). There is seldom justification for early induction of labor on this basis or for performing an amniocentesis.

Since there is no adequate method of antenatal diagnosis, careful observation is essential in the neonatal period if cases are to be detected. Although the infants with ABO hemolytic disease most often are less severely affected than are those with Rh hemolytic disease, they are equally incompetent in coping with excess bilirubin and its toxic effects on the central nervous system. Unlike Rh hemolytic disease, ABO disease frequently occurs in infants of primigravidas. It is likely but not certain to recur in subsequent pregnancies.

OTHER FETAL–MATERNAL BLOOD GROUP INCOMPATIBILITIES. Rho incompatibility and ABO heterospecificity account for approximately 98 percent of all cases of hemolytic disease. Instances of hemolytic disease resulting from rarer blood factors have been reported, but the detection of such cases requires extensive serologic study. The potential for hemolytic disease with rare blood groups may be suspected from the results of the screening test for abnormal antibodies in maternal serum. Summarized in Table 38-2 are various red cell antigens and their capacity for causing hemolytic disease when the fetus possesses the red cell antigen, and the mother is isoimmunized.

HYPERBILIRUBINEMIA

Bilirubin is formed from heme and transported in the circulation bound to albumin. In the sinusoidal circulation of the liver, a small fraction of bilirubin which dissociates from albumin enters hepatocytes where it attaches to receptor carrier proteins, the so-called Y and Z anion-binding proteins. Within hepatocytes, the bilirubin is conjugated with glucuronic acid.

Disposal of Bilirubin. Before birth, unconjugated, or free, bilirubin is readily transferred across the placenta from the fetal–maternal circulation (and vice versa, if the maternal plasma level is high). Unconjugated bilirubin is not excreted in the urine or to any extent in the bile, whereas the glucuronide of bilirubin is water-soluble and is normally excreted into the bile by the liver and when the plasma level is elevated by the kidney. Glucuronic acid is made available for this reaction by transfer from uridine diphosphoglucuronic acid catalyzed by the microsomal enzyme uridine diphosphoglucuronyl transferase. The conjugated bilirubin is secreted from the hepatocytes through the can-

TABLE 38-2.

OTHER RED CELL ANTIGENS AND THEIR PROPENSITY TO CAUSE HEMOLYTIC DISEASE IN
THE FETUS-INFANT WHOSE MOTHER IS ISOIMMUNIZED

BLOOD GROUP SYSTEM	ANTIGENS RELATED TO HEMOLYTIC DISEASE	SEVERITY OF HEMOLYTIC DISEASE	PROPOSED MANAGEMENT
Lewis*			
Kell	K	Mild to severe with hydrops fetalis	Amnionic fluid bilirubin studies
	k	Mild only	Expectant
	K_o	Mild only	Expectant
	Kp^a	Mild only	Expectant
	Kp^b	Mild only	Expectant
	Js^a	Mild only	Expectant
	Js^b	Mild only	Expectant
Duffy	Fy^a	Mild to severe with hydrops fetalis	Amnionic fluid bilirubin studies
	Fy^b†		
Kidd	Jk^a	Mild to severe	Amnionic fluid bilirubin studies
	Jk^b	Mild to severe	Amnionic fluid bilirubin studies
MNSs	M	Mild to severe	Amnionic fluid bilirubin studies
	N‡	Absent to moderate	Expectant
	S	Mild to severe	Amnionic fluid bilirubin studies
	s	Mild to severe	Amnionic fluid bilirubin studies
	U	Mild to severe	Amnionic fluid bilirubin studies
	Mi^a	Moderate	Amnionic fluid bilirubin studies
	Mt^a	Moderate	Amnionic fluid bilirubin studies
	Vw	Mild only	Expectant
Lutheran	Lu^a	Mild only	Expectant
	Lu^b	Mild only	Expectant
Diego	Di^a	Mild to severe	Amnionic fluid bilirubin studies
	Di^b	Mild only	Expectant
Xg	Xg^a	Mild only	Expectant
Public Antigens	Yt^a	Moderate to severe	Amnionic fluid bilirubin studies
	Lan	Mild only	Expectant
	Ge	Mild only	Expectant
	Co^a	Severe	Amnionic fluid bilirubin studies
Private antigens	Batty	Mild only	Expectant
	Becker	Mild only	Expectant
	Berrens	Mild only	Expectant
	Biles	Moderate	Amnionic fluid bilirubin studies
	Evans	Mild only	Expectant
	Gonzales	Mild only	Expectant
	Good	Severe	Amnionic fluid bilirubin studies
	Heibel	Moderate	Amnionic fluid bilirubin studies
	Hunt	Mild only	Expectant
	Jobbins	Mild only	Expectant
	Radin	Moderate	Amnionic fluid bilirubin studies
	Rm	Mild only	Expectant
	Ven	Mild only	Expectant
	Wright	Severe	Amnionic fluid bilirubin studies
	Zd	Moderate	Amnionic fluid bilirubin studies

* Not a proven cause of hemolytic disease.
† Not a cause of hemolytic disease.
‡ A rare cause of hemolytic disease
With slight modification from Weinstein: *Obstet Gynecol Surv* 31:581, 1976

alicular apparatus into the biliary tree and thus into the small intestine.

Kernicterus. The great concern over hyperbilirubinemia in the newborn infant is its association with *kernicterus.* This complication occurs with greater frequency in premature infants. The yellow staining of the basal ganglia and hippocampus is indicative of profound degeneration in these regions. If the infants survive, they show spasticity, muscular incoordination, and varying degrees of mental retardation. There is a positive correlation between kernicterus and unconjugated bilirubin levels above 18 to 20 mg per dl, although kernicterus may sometimes develop at levels lower than this, especially in very premature infants.

Factors other than the serum bilirubin concentration contribute to the development of kernicterus. Hypoxia and acidosis enhance bilirubin toxicity. Both hypothermia and hypoglycemia predispose the infant to kernicterus by raising the level of nonesterified fatty acids, which compete with bilirubin for the binding sites of albumin and inhibit bilirubin conjugation. Sepsis contributes to kernicterus too, although the mechanism of action is not altogether clear. Sulfonamides and salicylates such as aspirin may increase the incidence of kernicterus because they compete with unconjugated bilirubin for protein-binding sites. Sodium benzoate in injectable diazepam, as well as furosemide and gentamicin, also uncouple bilirubin from albumin. Excessive doses of vitamin K analogues may be associated with hyperbilirubinemia. The importance of the serum albumin concentration and the binding sites so provided is obvious.

OXYTOCIN AND HYPERBILIRUBINEMIA. It has been suggested that oxytocin administration to mothers during labor may in some way predispose to neonatal hyperbilirubinemia. Chalmers and associates (1975), in a retrospective study, found neonatal hyperbilirubinemia to be more common in infants born after oxytocin administration. Bearley

and Alderman (1975) identified a higher frequency of elevated bilirubin levels only when larger amounts of oxytocin were administered to the mothers. D'Souza and associates (1979) have also observed higher plasma levels of bilirubin after oxytocin. They attributed the hyperbilirubinemia, which appeared to be dose related, to increased breakdown of fetal red cells. Chew (1977) identified a higher bilirubin level in the neonate who was delivered after the administration of oxytocin to induce labor but not after prostaglandin E_2 given orally.

Friedman and Sachtleben (1976) considered the somewhat higher bilirubin levels in newborn infant plasma that has now been observed by several groups of investigators to be the consequence of fetal-neonatal bleeding induced by difficult deliveries associated with oxytocin stimulation. Singhi and Singh (1977) and Buchan (1979) have provided an intriguing explanation for the increase in bilirubin. They claim that cord blood erythrocytes are more fragile after oxytocin stimulation of labor because of a lowering of plasma osmolality as the consequence of water retention and hyponatremia. Water retention and hyponatremia are prevented by use of isotonic saline or lactated Ringer's solution as the vehicle for infusing oxytocin and by avoiding high infusion rates for oxytocin (see Chap. 17, p. 427).

There is no question that vigorous labor and traumatic delivery can cause hemorrhage in the fetus-infant, and thereby contribute to the development of hyperbilirubinemia. Stimulation of labor with oxytocin should never be so vigorous or carried out under circumstances so adverse as to incite such hemorrhages and, in turn, pathologic hyperbilirubinemia!

BREAST MILK JAUNDICE. Overt jaundice develops in approximately 1 percent of newborn infants as the consequence of breast feeding (Maisels, 1979). The jaundice has been attributed to the excretion of pregnane-3 (alpha), 20 (beta)-diol into the breast milk by some mothers. This steroid was reported by Arias and colleagues (1964) to block bilirubin conjugation by inhibiting glucuronyl transferase activity. These observations have not been confirmed, however. It now appears more likely that the milks which cause hyperbilirubinemia have an unusually high lipolytic activity and can liberate large quantities of fatty acids which can inhibit bilirubin conjugation (Foliot et al., 1976).

With breast milk jaundice the serum bilirubin level rises from about the fourth day after birth to a maximum by 15 days. If breastfeeding is continued, the high levels persist for another 10 to 14 days and decline slowly over the next several weeks.

No cases of overt bilirubin encephalopathy have been reported due to this phenomenon according to Maisels (1979), who also points out that there have been no prospective studies of the problem. The obvious solution to severe jaundice as the consequence of ingestion of breast milk is to discontinue breast feeding and substitute an appropriate formula.

"PHYSIOLOGIC" JAUNDICE.   By far the most common form of unconjugated nonhemolytic jaundice is so-called physiologic jaundice. In the mature infant, the jaundice increases for 3 or 4 days to achieve serum levels up to 10 mg per dl or so and then falls rapidly. In premature infants, the rise is more prolonged and may be more intense. The mechanisms involved in physiologic jaundice include, when compared to older children and adults: (1) normally increased rate of erythrocyte destruction, and, therefore, of bilirubin production; (2) probably a decreased rate of uptake of free bilirubin by hepatic cells because of lower levels of Y and Z anion-binding proteins; (3) decreased rate of conjugation of bilirubin in the liver; and (4) reduced conversion of bilirubin to urobilinogen by bacteria in the intestines, which, in turn, allows a greater fraction of excreted bilirubin to be reabsorbed (enterohepatic circulation). Thus, almost every phase of bilirubin metabolism has been implicated.

Jaundice in the newborn infant should not be ignored as being physiologic in the following circumstances:

1. The infant is visibly jaundiced in the first 24 hours after birth.
2. The total bilirubin concentration in serum is increasing daily by more than 5 mg per dl.
3. The total bilirubin concentration is above 15 mg per dl.
4. Jaundice is visible for more than 1 week in a term infant or 2 weeks in a preterm infant.

Long-term Effects of Hyperbilirubinemia.   The jaundiced infant who survives the neonatal period without neurologic evidence of involvement of the central nervous system has been thought most often to escape serious residual disease. Naeye (1979), however, on the basis of data obtained from the Cerebral Palsy Collaborative Study, has reported a significant increase in IQ scores below 90 at 4 years of age when the serum bilirubin concentration in the newborn period exceeded 8 mg per dl. This is worrisome. Previously, it had been generally accepted that there was usually no significant deficit in intellectual achievement in jaundiced infants who were neurologically normal even when bilirubin levels rose considerably above 8 mg per dl.

Treatments of Hyperbilirubinemia.   *Exchange transfusion* for hyperbilirubinemia is discussed earlier in this chapter. While exchange transfusion is not an innocuous procedure, the mortality rate is less than 1 percent if moribund, hydropic, and kernicteric infants are excluded.

Phototherapy is now widely used to treat hyperbilirubinemia. In most instances, its use leads to a lower bilirubin level from photooxidation of the compound. Light which penetrates the skin also increases peripheral blood flow which enhances photodestruction of bilirubin. By some unknown mechanism, light seems to promote excretion of unconjugated bilirubin by the liver. Moreover, intestinal transit time may be shortened thereby reducing reabsorption of bilirubin from the gut. A common situation in which phototherapy is justified, besides that of the infant with hemolytic disease, is the jaundiced infant of low birth weight who appears otherwise well.

As much of the infant's surface as possible should be exposed, and he should be turned every 2 hours. His eyelids should be closed and completely shielded from the light. The infant's temperature must be closely monitored and dehydration from the heat should be guarded against. Effective photodecomposition requires that the fluorescent bulbs be carefully selected and monitored for appropriate wavelength. The serum bilirubin concentration needs to be monitored for at least 24 hours after phototherapy has been stopped.

Phenobarbital has been shown to induce microsomal enzymes and thereby increase hepatic bilirubin conjugation and excretion. Halpin and associates (1972), beginning at 32 weeks' gestation, gave phenobarbital, 20 mg each night, to a general obstetric population and subsequently measured the bilirubin levels in the newborn infants. Fifteen percent of the infants demonstrated serum bilirubin levels above 10 mg per dl at 72 hours of age compared to 31 percent of their control group. McMullin and co-workers (1970) administered phenobarbital to Coombs'-positive newborn infants and reduced the number of exchange transfusions used by one-half. Possible adverse effects from such phenobarbital therapy must be considered, however. For example, phenobarbital inhibits fetal lung development in the rabbit fetus (Karotkin et al., 1976) and brain growth in newborn rats (Diaz et al., 1977).

HEMORRHAGIC DISEASE OF THE NEWBORN

Hemorrhagic disease of the newborn is a syndrome characterized by spontaneous internal or external bleeding accompanied by hypoprothrombinemia and very low levels of other vitamin-K-dependent coagulation factors (V, VII, IX, and X). Bleeding may begin any time after birth but typically is delayed for a day or two. The infant may be at term and healthy in appearance, although a greater incidence of the disease has been noted in preterm infants. The prothrombin time and partial thromboplastin time are greatly prolonged. The coagulation changes of vitamin K deficiency, especially if accompanied by a lowered platelet count, might lead to an erroneous diagnosis of disseminated intravascular coagulation, which has a much poorer prognosis (Hathaway et al., 1975). Moreover, the treatment of disseminated intravascular coagulation with anticoagulants, as recommended by some but not all, will intensify hemorrhagic disease of the newborn. In the differential diagnosis, hemophilia, congenital syphilis, sepsis of the newborn, thrombocytopenic purpura, erythroblastosis, and traumatic intracranial hemorrhage must also be considered.

As prophylaxis against hemorrhagic disease of the newborn, the intramuscular injection of 1 mg of vitamin K_1 has proved very efficacious. For treatment of active bleeding the vitamin is injected intravenously. Abnormalities in clotting are usually corrected over several hours.

The chief cause of hemorrhagic disease of the newborn from vitamin K deficiency appears to be a dietary deficiency of vitamin K resulting from the small amount of the vitamin in breast milk. The prothrombin time 24 hours after the start of feedings with cow's milk is comparable to that found 24 hours after vitamin K administration, whereas in infants receiving breast milk it remains prolonged (Keenan et al., 1971).

Serious reduction of vitamin-K-dependent clotting factors during the first week after birth in infants of women with epilepsy treated with anticonvulsant drugs has been described by Mountain and associates (1970).

The toxic effects of menadione, a synthetic vitamin K, and its derivatives in causing hyperbilirubinemia resulted from unnecessarily large doses, particularly to premature infants.

Allison's original report (1955), and the deluge of subsequent publications relating the administration of vitamin K to the development of hyperbilirubinemia and kernicterus, without exception, dealt with excessive doses of the drug. In short, there is no evidence that the small but effective dose of 1 mg of vitamin K_1 (phytonadione) to the infant, or 2.5 to 5 mg given to the mother in labor, is associated with significant hyperbilirubinemia or its sequelae.

Immune Thrombocytopenia. Antiplatelet IgG antibody transferred from the mother to the fetus and causing thrombocytopenia in the fetus-neonate can be suspected when the mother has thrombocytopenia from an autoimmune disease, especially immune ("idiopathic") thrombocytopenic purpura. Avoidance of traumatic delivery and appropriate corticosteroid therapy to try to improve hemostasis are important to a successful outcome (see Chap. 28, p. 728). The maternally produced antibody most often is directed against almost all platelets. Transfusion of donor platelets, therefore, is seldom of benefit. Corticosteroids given to the infant may be of benefit and, in desperation, exchange transfusion and platelet transfusion may be tried. Blood transfusion may be necessary to help combat hemorrhage.

Maternal isoimmunization against fetal platelet antigens is another mechanism by which thrombocytopenia may develop in the fetus-neonate. Even though diagnostic tests to type platelet antigens are not commonly available, the diagnosis can most often be made correctly on clinical grounds: The mother has a normal platelet count, and there is no history or evidence on physical examination of a disorder which causes autoimmune thrombocytopenia. The infant has thrombocytopenia without evidence of other disease. In case of active bleeding, treatment, ideally, should include transfusion with platelets compatible with those of the mother. Unfortunately, most of the donor population will have the platelet antigen to which the maternal antibody is directed. However, the mother's platelets are appropriate; therefore,

platelets collected from the mother by plasmapheresis and differential centrifugation are likely to be of greatest benefit. When one infant has been affected, there is appreciable likelihood that a subsequent one will also be affected. Cesarean section to minimize birth trauma is likely to be advantageous to the affected fetus-infant yet of little risk to the mother, since she is not thrombocytopenic.

Thrombocytopenia develops rather often in newborn infants who suffer a variety of illnesses, especially those sick infants who were born remote from term.

Polycythemia and Hyperviscosity. Several conditions predispose to polycythemia and hyperviscosity of the blood in the neonate. These include *transfusion* from the placenta, from a twin, or, much more rarely, from the mother, and *chronic hypoxia* in utero. As the hematocrit reading rises above 65, blood viscosity increases markedly. Signs and symptoms include plethora, cyanosis, and neurologic manifestations. Laboratory findings include hyperbilirubinemia, thrombocytopenia, fragmented erythrocytes, and hypoglycemia, as well as the high hematocrit reading. Treatment consists of prompt recognition and lowering of the hematocrit by partial exchange transfusion with plasma.

SOME INFECTIONS OF THE NEWBORN

While passive immunity is provided by the mother chiefly as IgG across the placenta, the immunologic capacity of the fetus and neonate is impaired, compared to that of older children and adults. Moreover, the degree of passive immunity is much lower in premature infants than in term infants.

Infection, especially in its early stages, may be difficult to diagnose because of the newborn infant's failure to respond in classic fashion. The signs of infection are frequently vague, nonspecific, and often not dramatic until the infant becomes moribund. If infected in utero, he may have had a poor

Apgar score for no other apparent reason. The infant may suck poorly, vomit, or develop abdominal distension. He may develop respiratory distress, which is quite similar in many ways to idiopathic respiratory distress. He may be lethargic or jittery. The response to sepsis may be hypothermia rather than hyperthermia, and the total leukocyte count in blood and the neutrophil count may not be influenced by sepsis, although the band count is likely to be increased (Akenzua et al., 1974).

Bacterial, viral, fungal, or parasitic disease may cross the placenta from the mother or, more commonly, after rupture of the membranes; the organisms may infect the fetus either in utero or during delivery. Thus, premature rupture of the membranes, prolonged labor, and excessive obstetric examinations and manipulations increase appreciably the risk of infection in the newborn infant. Sources of neonatal bacterial infections are as follows:

I. Intrauterine
  1. Transplacental
  2. Ascending amnionitis
    a. Premature rupture of membranes (common)
    b. Intact membranes (rare)
II. Intrapartum
  1. Maternal vaginal and cervical flora
  2. External contamination
III. Postnatal
  1. Transmission from handlers
  2. Equipment containing moisture
  3. Indwelling catheters

Infection at less than 72 hours of age is usually but not always caused by bacteria acquired in utero or during delivery, while infections after that time are most likely to have been acquired after birth.

A major mechanism for inducing infection in the newborn infant is transfer of pathogens from those caring for the infant; the handler may harbor the organisms or may passively transfer the organisms from another infected infant. The use of indwelling venous and arterial catheters in the umbilical vessels after delivery demands scrupulous care to prevent infection. Life-support systems that involve moisture easily become contaminated with bacteria and can be the source of a life-threatening infection.

Any infant who appears ill should be suspected of having an infection. If infection is suspected at vaginal delivery, cultures of a swabbing from the ear or of gastric aspirate may be made; at cesarean section, amnionic fluid can be collected from the sac and promptly cultured. Subsequently, cultures of blood and cerebrospinal fluid are essential for appropriate evaluation of such an infant.

Bacteria Responsible. The bacteria most often responsible for sepsis in the newborn infant have varied remarkably during the past several decades. In the 1930s and 1940s group A, β-hemolytic streptococci were principally involved. With the widespread use of penicillin, these streptococcal infections were reduced remarkably.

STAPHYLOCOCCI. In the 1950s, penicillin-resistant staphylococcal disease was observed in epidemic proportions. Reemphasis on hand washing, perhaps the use of hexachlorophene, screening for carriers of unusually virulent staphylococci, and newer antibiotics controlled the epidemics.

Colonization rates with *Staphylococcus aureus* have increased among newborn infants since 1973 when bathing with hexachlorophene was generally abandoned (Hargiss and Larson, 1978). Currently recommended procedures to control staphylococcal disease in newborn nurseries include the following: (1) Close attention is paid to each staff member's technic for handling infants; frequent, careful washing of the hands is important. (2) Routine umbilical care is performed, applying triple dye or bacitracin. (3) A program of continuous epidemiologic surveillance is essential.

GROUP B STREPTOCOCCI. Currently gram-negative organisms are the most common pathogens; however, group B, β-hemolytic streptococci also gives cause for concern.

It is clear that transmission to the fetus of group B streptococci from a colonized maternal genital tract can occur intrapartum, with the onset of severe sepsis in the infant soon after birth. Upwards to 40 percent of women during the third trimester of pregnancy harbor group B streptococci in the lower genital tract and up to 20 percent of newborn infants are colonized. Very few infants, perhaps 2 to 3 per thousand, develop clinical disease, however; for those who do demonstrate infection, unfortunately, the mortality rate is very high.

During the early 1970s, group B streptococcal infections increased remarkably in frequency, but then in many institutions the frequency decreased. The reasons for either the marked increase or the subsequent decrease are not clearly understood.

With the septicemia from group B streptococci that characterizes *early onset disease,* signs of serious illness develop within 48 hours of birth. Typically, membranes have been ruptured for some time before delivery. The preterm infant appears to be more prone to develop clinical infection. The signs of early onset infection include those of respiratory distress, apnea, and shock. At the outset, therefore, the physician must be astute to differentiate the illness from idiopathic respiratory distress or transient tachypnea of the newborn (Menke et al., 1979). Immediate treatment with antibiotics, as well as treatment of the respiratory problems, is mandatory if the infant is to survive. The mortality rate with early onset disease has varied from 30 percent to as high as 90 percent!

Late onset disease usually becomes evident as meningitis a week or more after birth. Whereas the serotype with early onset disease varies from infant to infant but most often is the same in the maternal vagina and in the infant, the serotype in cases of meningitis most often is serotype III. The mortality rate is appreciably less for late onset meningitis than for early onset sepsis.

Steigman and associates (1978) reported an absence of early onset group B streptococcal sepsis in 130,000 newborn infants who had received 50,000 units of aqueous penicillin G intramuscularly at birth as prophylaxis against ophthalmia neonatorum. This observation has not been confirmed at other institutions. For example, penicillin G, 100,000 units, given intramuscularly within 90 minutes of birth, did not eradicate group B streptococcal sepsis from the nursery at Cook County Hospital (Ramamurthy et al., 1979). An extensive study has also been carried out at Parkland Memorial Hospital. Aqueous procaine penicillin G, 50,000 units, was administered intramuscularly within 1 hour of birth to 7528 infants as prophylaxis against ophthalmia neonatorum and also to evaluate its impact on group B streptococcal infections. The incidence of group B streptococcal disease was less, but not absent, in those who received penicillin. There were 0.13 cases of early-onset of group B streptococcal disease per 1000 births compared to 1.2 cases per 1000 births among a similar number of infants who received tetracycline ointment applied to each eye for prophylaxis. Importantly, while the incidence of early-onset group B streptococcal disease was decreased in the penicillin treated infants, the incidence of infection caused by penicillin-resistant organisms and mortalities from these organisms were increased. On the basis of these observations the routine use of a single dose of penicillin is not recommended at this time (Siegel et al., 1979).

Prophylactic administration of penicillin or ampicillin to women who were demonstrated to harbor the organism in the vagina during the third trimester has not proved to be very effective. Recurrence was observed commonly (Hall et al., 1976; Gardner and associates, 1979). Moreover, an appreciable number of women whose cultures were negative when evaluated in the third trimester, subsequently before delivery, were demonstrated to harbor the organism.

A nosocomial source of infection has been suggested but not clearly established for some cases of group B infections in the newborn infant since (1) maternal vaginal cultures may be negative, (2) the cases at times occur in clusters, (3) the illness may have its onset many days after delivery, and (4) cultures of nursery personnel reveal a reservoir of group B streptococcus.

ANAEROBIC INFECTIONS. Infection with anaerobic pathogens also has been recognized more frequently, in part because of better culture technics and increased awareness of their importance. Chow and associates (1974) identified anaerobes in 26 percent of cases of neonatal bacteremia. In their experience, anaerobic bacteremia may be self-limited with a favorable prognosis, regardless of antimicrobial therapy, but more often, it is associated with serious perinatal morbidity or mortality.

Epidemic Diarrhea of the Newborn.
Outbreaks of epidemic diarrhea of the newborn may occur at any time, and many have been reported. Although it is unlikely that a single pathogen is responsible for all epidemics, certain pathogenic strains of *Escherichia coli* have been isolated in many outbreaks. It is probable that many of the epidemics are caused by these pathogenic colon bacilli and that the organism is brought into the nursery either by infected personnel, with or without symptomatic disease, or by an already infected infant.

The clinical symptoms are diarrhea with loose, watery, greenish stools, lethargy, dehydration, unstable temperature, and anorexia. The mortality rate varies, at times ranging as high as 6 percent in term infants and 35 percent in premature infants. No more infants should be admitted to the nursery; those affected should be isolated, and after the unit is evacuated, rigid cleansing of all equipment and of the nursery itself should be carried out. A stool culture should be obtained from all exposed infants to identify carriers and potentially ill babies.

Chlamydia.
The microbe *Chlamydia trachomatis* has been cultured from the cervix of upwards to 13 percent of pregnant women (Alexander, 1979; Frommell et al., 1979). The infants of infected women are at some risk of developing conjunctivitis and pneumonia. The pregnant woman who happens to be identified to have a chlamydial infection can be treated successfully with erythromycin as can an infected infant.

The absence of elevated IgM in the cord blood of infants whose mothers harbored *Chlamydia* in their cervices is evidence against intrauterine infection. Rather it is supportive of the infection being acquired during labor and delivery.

Necrotizing Enterocolitis.
This condition commonly presents with the clinical findings of abdominal distension, ileus, and bloody stools, and with radiologic evidence of pneumotosis intestinalis (gas in the intestinal wall as the consequence of invasion by gas-forming bacteria) and bowel perforation.

The disease is seen primarily in markedly preterm, low-birth-weight infants. Various causes have been suggested for necrotizing enterocolitis, including perinatal hypotension, perinatal hypoxia, sepsis, umbilical catheters, exchange transfusions, and the feeding of cow's milk and hypertonic solutions.

Suspicion of developing necrotizing enterocolitis is raised by the presence of abdominal distension or blood in the stools. Usually further oral feeding is withheld until these conditions clear. Although the prognosis appears to be improving with medical management and at times bowel resection, the etiology is not yet clear.

Syphilis.
In the past, syphilis accounted for nearly one-third of all fetal deaths. Indeed, delivery of a macerated fetus was considered diagnostic of syphilis. Today syphilis plays a smaller but persistent role in the causation of fetal death.

Syphilitic lesions in the internal organs comprise essentially interstitial changes in the lungs (pneumonia alba of Virchow), liver (hypertrophic cirrhosis), spleen, and pancreas, and osteochondritis in the long bones. Osteochondritis is most readily recognizable radiologically at the lower end of the femur and the lower ends of the tibia and radius.

Under the influence of syphilitic infection, the placenta becomes larger and paler and often dull and greasy. Microscopically, the villi appear to have lost their characteristic arborescent appearance and to have become thicker and more club-shaped. There is a marked decrease in the number of blood vessels, which in advanced cases almost entirely disappear as a result of endarteritis and proliferation of the stromal cells. Spirochetes are sparsely scattered through the placenta even when they are present in large numbers in the fetal organs. They may be demonstrated, however, by examination, under the dark-field microscope, of scrapings from the intima of the vessels of the fresh cord.

Syphilis is discussed further in Chapter 28, p. 752.

Drug   Addiction.   An   unfortunately large number of women use heroin and other "hard drugs" during pregnancy. These women and their offspring suffer not only from the direct effects of the drug or drugs but are at appreciably increased risk of coincidental infections and varying degrees of malnutrition. Pelosi and co-workers (1975) observed the risks of the following pregnancy complications to be increased 2 to 6 times among pregnant women who used heroin: low birth-weight (< 2500 g) from prematurity, growth retardation, or both; pregnancy-induced hypertension; late pregnancy bleeding; malpresentation; and puerperal morbidity. Interestingly, accelerated fetal lung maturation, manifested by a high L/S ratio in amnionic fluid and a low incidence of idiopathic respiratory distress in the newborn, is characteristic of pregnancies complicated by maternal heroin addition.

One-half or more of newborn infants of heroin addicts will develop withdrawal symptoms. Without treatment an appreciable number of these infants will die. The newborn infant must be closely watched during the first week of life for irritability, convulsions, nasal congestion, vomiting, diarrhea, tachypnea, and fever. Treatment has included paregoric, phenobarbital, chlorpromazine, and diazepam. Therapy is slowly withdrawn but reinstituted if the symptoms recur. Treatment may be required for many days to weeks.

Methadone treatment programs have commonly included pregnant women. Even though the drug is deleterious to the fetus-infant, it is probably less so than heroin. The newborn infant of the methadone-treated mother is also very likely to demonstrate withdrawal symptoms; Newman and co-workers (1975) reported an incidence of 80 percent and Harper and associates (1974) an incidence of 94 percent. Whereas withdrawal symptoms in the infant whose mother is addicted to heroin usually develop within 24 hours of delivery, the infant whose mother has been using methadone may not demonstrate signs of withdrawal for a week or so after birth.

A symposium has provided further insight into the many maternal and fetal-infant problems that arise as the consequence of pregnancy complicated by drug addiction (Zuspan, 1978).

REFERENCES

Akenzua GI, Hui YT, Milner R, Zipursky A: Neutrophil and band counts in the diagnosis of neonatal infections. Pediatrics 54:38, 1974

Alexander ER: Chlamydia: The organism and neonatal infection. Hosp Prac 14:63, July, 1979

Allison AC: Danger of vitamin K to newborn (Letters to the Editor). Lancet 1:669, 1955

Arias IM, Gartner LM, Seifter S, Furman M: Prolonged neonatal unconjugated hyperbilirubinemia associated with breast feeding and steroid, pregnane-3(alpha), 20(beta)-diol in maternal milk that inhibits glucuronide formation in vitro. J Clin Invest 43:2037, 1964

Bearley JM, Alderman B: Neonatal hyperbilirubinaemia following the use of oxytocin in labour. Br J Obstet Gynaecol 82:265, 1975

Bergin FT, Cefalo RC, Lewis PE: Self-limited hemolytic transfusion reaction in an ABO-incompatible maternal-fetal unit. Am J Obstet Gynecol 132:116, 1978

Bernard B, Presley M, Caudillo G, Clauss B, Rouault CL, McGregor J, Jennings ER: Maternal-fetal hemorrhage: Incidence and sensitization. Pediatr Res 11:467, 1977

Blajchman MA, Maudsley RF, Uchida I, Zipursky A: Diagnostic amniocentesis and fetal-maternal bleeding. Lancet 1:993, 1974

Bowman JM: The management of Rh-isoimmunization. Obstet Gynecol 52:1, 1978

Bowman JM: Suppression of Rh isoimmunization. A review. Obstet Gynecol 52:385, 1978

Bowman JM, Pollock JM: Antenatal Rh prophylaxis: 28 week gestation service program. Can Med Assoc J 118:622, 1978

Bowman JM, Chown B, Lewis M, Pollock J: Rh immunization, Manitoba, 1963–75. Can Med Assoc J 116:282, 1977

Buchan PC: Pathogenesis of neonatal hyperbilirubinemia after induction of labour with oxytocin. Brit Med J 2:1255, 1979

Chalmers I, Campbell H, Turnbull AC: Use of oxytocin and incidence of neonatal jaundice. Br Med J 2:116, 1975

Chernik V: Modern therapy of hyaline membrane disease by stabilization of alveoli. In Gluck L (ed): Modern Perinatal Medicine. Chicago, Year Book, 1974

Chew WC: Neonatal hyperbilirubinemia: a comparison between prostaglandin E_2 and oxytocin induction. Br Med J 2:679, 1977

Chow AW, Leake RD, Yamauchi T, Anthony BF, Guze LB: The significance of anaerobes in neonatal bacteremia: analysis of 23 cases and review of the literature. Pediatrics 54:736, 1974

Cohen F, Zuelzer WW: The transplacental passage of maternal erythrocytes into the fetus. Am J Obstet Gynecol 93:566, 1965

Desjardins L, Blajchman MA, Chintu C, Gent M, Zipursky A: The spectrum of ABO hemolytic disease of the newborn infant. J Pediatr 95:447, 1979

Diaz J, Schain RJ, Bailey BG: Phenobarbital-induced brain growth retardation in artifically reared rat pups. Biol Neonate 32:77, 1977

D'Souza SW, Black P, MacFarlane T, Richards B: The effect of oxytocin in induced labour on neonatal jaundice. Br J Obstet Gynecol 86:133, 1979

Edwards DK, Dyer WM, Northway WH Jr: Twelve years' experience with bronchopulmonary dysplasia. Pediatrics 59:839, 1977

Ehrenkranz RA, Bonta BW, Ablow RC, Warshaw JB: Amelioration of bronchopulmonary dysplasia after vitamin E administration. N Engl J Med 299:564, 1978

Farrell PM, Wood RE: Epidemiology of hyaline membrane disease in the United States: Analysis of national mortality statistics. Pediatrics 58:167, 1976

Finn R, Clarke CA, Donohoe W, McConnell RB, Sheppard PM, Lehane D, Kulke W: Experimental studies on the prevention of Rh haemolytic disease. Br Med J 1:1486, 1961

Foliot A, Ploussard JP, Housset E, Christoforov B: Breast milk jaundice: In vitro inhibition of rat liver bilirubin-uridine diphosphate glucuronyltransferase activity and Z protein—bromosulfonphtalein binding by human breast milk. Pediatr Res 10:594, 1976

Freda V: Hemolytic disease. Clin Obstet Gynecol 16:72, 1973

Freda VJ, Gorman JG, Pollack W: Successful prevention of sensitization to Rh with an experimental anti-Rh gamma₂ globulin antibody preparation. Fed Proc 22:374, 1963

Freda VJ, Gorman JG, Pollack W, Bowe E: Prevention of Rh hemolytic disease: ten years clinical experience with Rh immune globulin. N Engl J Med 292:1014, 1975

Friedman EA, Sachtleben MR: Neonatal jaundice in association with oxytocin stimulation of labour and operative delivery. Br Med J 1:198, 1976

Frommell GT, Rothenberg R, Wang S, McIntosh K: Chlamydial infections of mothers and their infants. J Pediatr 95:28, 1979

Gardner SE, Yow MD, Leeds LJ, Thompson PK, Mason EO Jr, Clark DJ: Failure of penicillin to eradicate group B streptococcal colonization in the pregnant woman. Am J Obstet Gynecol 135:1062, 1979

Hall RT, Barnes W, Krishnan L, Harris DJ, Rhodes PG, Fayez J, Miller GL: Am J Obstet Gynecol 124:630, 1976

Halpin TF, Jones AR, Bishop HL, Lerner S: Prophylaxis of neonatal hyperbilirubinemia with phenobarbital. Obstet Gynecol 40:85, 1972

Hamilton EG: Intrauterine transfusion for Rh disease: A status report. Hosp Prac 13:113, 1978

Hargiss C, Larson E: The epidemiology of staphylococcus aureus in a newborn nursery from 1970 through 1976. Pediatrics 61:348, 1978

Harper RG, Solish GI, Purow HM, Sang E, Panepinto WC: The effect of a methadone treatment program upon pregnant heroin addicts and their newborn infants. Pediatrics 54:300, 1974

Hathaway WE, Mahasandana C, Makowski EL: Cord blood coagulation studies in infants of high-risk pregnant women. Am J Obstet Gynecol 121:51, 1975

Holt EM, Boyd IE, Dewhurst CH, Murray J, Naylor CH, Smitham JH: Intrauterine transfusion: 101 consecutive cases treated at Queen Charlotte's Maternity Hospital. Br Med J 3:39, 1973

Jennings ER, Clauss B: Maternal-fetal hemorrhage: Its incidence and sensitizing effects. Am J Obstet Gynecol 131:725, 1978

Karotkin EH, Kido M, Redding R, Cashore WJ, Douglas W, Stern L, Oh W: The inhibition of pulmonary maturation in the fetal rabbit by maternal treatment with phenobarbital. Am J Obstet Gynecol 124:529, 1976

Keenan WJ, Jewitt T, Glueck HI: Role of feeding and vitamin K in hypoprothrombinemia of the newborn. Am J Dis Child 121:271, 1971

Kinsey VE, Arnold HJ, Kalina RE, Stern L, Stahlman M, Odell G, Driscoll J, Elliott J, Payne J, Patz A: PaO$_2$ levels and retrolental fibroplasia: A report of the cooperative study. Pediatrics 60:655, 1977

Kirkman HN Jr: Further evidence for a racial difference in frequency of ABO hemolytic disease. J Pediatr 90:717, 1977

Landsteiner K, Wiener AS: An agglutinable factor in human blood recognized by immune sera for Rhesus blood. Proc Soc Exp Biol NY 43:223, 1940

Levine P, Katzin E, Burnham L: Isoimmunization in pregnancy. JAMA 116:825, 1941

Liley AW: Intrauterine transfusion of foetus in hemolytic disease. Br Med J 2:1107, 1963

Liley, AW: Amniocentesis and amniography in hemolytic disease. In Greenhill JP (ed): Yearbook of Obstetrics & Gynecology, 1964–1965 series. Chicago, Year Book, 1964, p 256

McIntosh S: Erythropoietin excretion in the premature infant. J Pediatr 86:202, 1975

McMullin GP, Hayes MF, Arora SC: Phenobarbitone in rhesus haemolytic disease: a controlled trial. Lancet 2:949, 1970

Maisels MJ: Neonatal jaundice: III. Breast feeding and jaundice. Perinat Press 3:19, 1979

Marshall R, Tyrala E, McAlister W, Sheehan M: Meconium aspiration syndrome. Neonatal and follow-up study. Am J Obstet Gynecol 131:672, 1978

Menke JA, Giacoia GP, Jockin H: Group B beta hemolytic streptococcal sepsis and idiopathic respiratory distress syndrome: A comparison. J Pediatr 94:467, 1979

Mountain K, Hirsh J, Gallus AS: Neonatal coagulation defect and maternal anti-convulsant treatment. Lancet 1:265, 1970

Naeye RL: The role of congenital bacterial infections in low serum bilirubin brain damage, 1979, in press

Newman RG, Bashkow S, Calko D: Results of 313 consecutive live births of infants delivered to patients in the New York City methadone maintenance treatment program. Am J Obstet Gynecol 121:233, 1975

Palmer A, Gordon RR: A critical review of intrauterine fetal transfusion. Br J Obstet Gynaecol 83:688, 1976

Peevy KJ, Wiseman HJ: ABO hemolytic disease of the newborn: Evaluation of management and identification of racial and antigenic factors. Pediatrics 61:475, 1978

Pelosi MA, Frattarola M, Apuzzio J, Langer A, Hung CT, Oleske JM, Bai J, Harrigan JT: Pregnancy complicated by heroin addiction. Obstet Gynecol 45:512, 1975

Ramamurthy RS, Pyati SP, Pildes RS: Penicillin prophylaxis for neo-natal group-B streptococcal infection. Lancet 2:246, 1979

Renaer M, Van de Putte, Vermylen C: Massive feto-maternal hemorrhage as a cause of perinatal mortality and morbidity. Eur J Obstet Gynecol Reprod Biol 6:125, 1976

Robertson EG, Brown A, Ellis MI, Walker W: Intrauterine transfusion in the management of severe rhesus isoimmunization. Br J Obstet Gynaecol 83:694, 1976

Shelley SA, Kovacevic M, Paciga JE, Balis JU: Sequential changes of surfactant phosphatidylcholine in hyaline-membrane disease of the newborn. N Engl J Med 300:112, 1979

Siegel JD, McCracken GH Jr, Rosenfeld CR: Effects of a single intramuscular dose of penicillin on neonatal colonization and disease rates due to Group B and D streptococci. Presented at 11th International Congress of Chemotherapy—19th Interscience Conference on Antimicrobial Agents and Chemotherapy, Boston, Oct 1979

Singhi S, Singh M: Oxytocin induction and neonatal hyperbilirubinaemia. Br Med J 2:1028, 1977

Steigman AJ, Bottone EJ, Hanna BA: Control of perinatal group B streptococcal sepsis: Efficacy of single injection of aqueous penicillin at birth. Mount Sinai J Med 45:685, 1978

Taylor WW, Scott DE, Pritchard JA: Fate of compatible adult erythrocytes in the fetal peritoneal cavity. Obstet Gynecol 18:175, 1966

Workshop on Bronchopulmonary Dysplasia. J Pediatr 95:815, 1979

Yeh TF, Harris V, Srinvasin G, Lilien L, Pyati S, Pildes RS: Roentgenographic findings in infants with meconium aspiration syndrome. JAMA 242:60, 1979

Zuspan FP (ed): Drug addiction in pregnancy: An invitational symposium. J Reprod Med 20:301, 1978

Injuries and Malformations of the Fetus and Newborn Infant

Considered in this chapter are several varieties of birth injuries and malformation. Other birth injuries and malformations are described elsewhere in connection with the specific obstetric complication that led to or contributed to the injury or was created by the malformation. Hydrocephaly, for example, is considered under "Dystocia Caused by Abnormalities of the Fetus," (see Chap. 30, p. 822).

INJURIES

Intracranial Hemorrhage. The head of the fetus may undergo molding during passage through the birth canal. The skull bones, the dura mater, and the brain itself permit considerable alteration in the shape of the fetal head without untoward results. The dimensions of the head are changed, with lengthening especially of the occipitofrontal diameter of the skull (Fig. 39-1). Bridging veins from the cerebral cortex to the sagittal sinus may tear as the consequence of severe molding and marked overlap of the parietal bones or of difficult forceps delivery. Less

common are rupture of the internal cerebral veins, the vein of Galen at its junction with the straight sinus, or the tentorium itself. Compression of the skull can stretch the tentorium cerebelli and may tear the vein of Galen or its tributaries. The common types and locations of intracranial hemorrhages are illustrated in Figure 39-2.

Intracranial hemorrhages at one time were commonly encountered in newborn infants upon whom an autopsy was performed, but in recent years most obstetric services have shown a substantial reduction in the incidence of brain hemorrhage from trauma. Former studies, which demonstrated that one-third to one-half of all deaths within the first 2 weeks of life resulted from cerebral birth injuries, are no longer valid.

TRAUMA VS. HYPOXIA. Potter (1961) correctly distinguished between "birth injury" resulting from primary oxygen deficiencies and those resulting from mechanical injury. In accordance with that concept, intracranial hemorrhage can be divided into lesions initiated by hypoxia, which include ventricular and subarachnoid hemorrhages, subependymal hemorrhages, and isolated

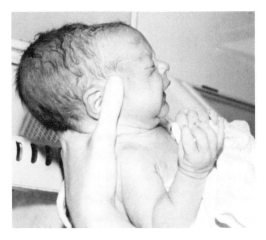

FIG. 39-1. Molding of head, newborn child.

hemorrhages in the pia mater, and those produced by mechanical trauma associated with subdural hematomas or dural tears.

Illingworth (1979), an English pediatrician, rightfully contended that, because of superficial thinking, obstetricians have been blamed unjustifiably for causing brain damage and other injuries, the genesis of which was not limited just to difficulties during labor and delivery, but involved prenatal factors, including those that were genetic and social in nature. Nonetheless, the elimination of difficult forceps operations, the use of cesarean section when there was cephalopelvic disproportion, the correct management of breech

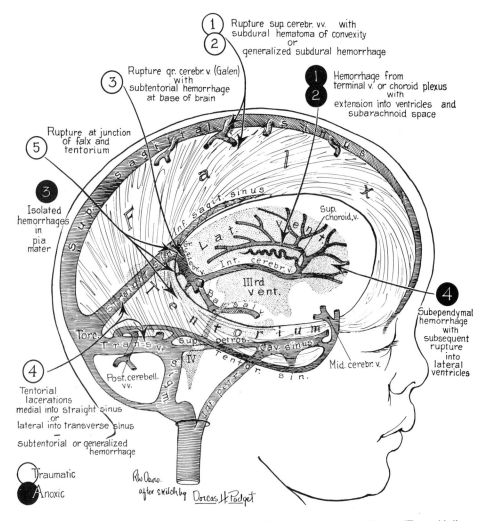

FIG. 39-2. The common types and locations of intracranial hemorrhage. (From Haller, Nesbitt, Anderson. *Obstet Gynecol Survey* 11:179, 1956)

delivery, and the virtual eradication of internal podalic version and extraction have all contributed significantly to the reduction in the incidence of all birth injuries, especially intracranial hemorrhage.

SIGNS AND SYMPTOMS. Commonly, the infants are born depressed but their conditions appear to improve until about 12 hours of age. Then drowsiness, apathy, feeble cry, pallor, failure to nurse, dyspnea, cyanosis, vomiting, and convulsions may become evident. Atelectasis, asphyxia neonatorum, meconium aspiration, and forceps trauma may be associated findings. To help rule out diaphragmatic hernia, congenital heart disease, atelectasis, idiopathic respiratory distress, and pneumonia, prompt roentgenologic examination of the chest is useful. In very recent years, scanning of the head using computerized axial tomography (CAT scan) has proved of diagnostic value.

TREATMENT. Therapy includes oxygen for the dyspnea and cyanosis, and sedation to control convulsions. The blood can be removed from some subdural hematomas by careful needle aspiration. In other instances surgical intervention is required. The value of administering clotting factors from plasma to infants with an intracranial hemorrhage is not clear. Prompt intramuscular administration of vitamin K to all newborn infants is indicated (p. 976).

The surviving infants may subsequently develop functional disturbances, including cerebral palsy and mental deficiency. Certain cases of idiopathic epilepsy may also be caused by intracranial injury sustained at birth.

Cerebral Palsy. Multiple definitions have been proposed for *cerebral palsy*. The term is probably most widely used to identify persons handicapped by motor disorders due to nonprogressive abnormalities of the brain which appeared early in life. Recognized patterns of motor disturbances include the spastic type, the athetoid type, the ataxic type, the atonic type, and mixed forms. Cerebral palsy may result from preterm birth

complicated by asphyxia in utero or in the newborn period, from severe hyperbilirubinemia, from cerebellar or cerebral malformations, and from infections acquired in utero, such as cytomegalovirus. Whenever possible, the specific brain lesion and its probable cause should be stated, rather than simply applying the term *cerebral palsy*.

Cephalhematoma. A cephalhematoma is caused by injury to the periosteum of the skull during labor or delivery (Fig. 39-3). Subperiosteal hemorrhages may develop over one or both parietal bones. The periosteal limitations with definite palpable edges differentiate the cephalhematoma from *caput succedaneum*. The latter lesion consists of a focal swelling of edema fluid that overlies the periosteum (Fig. 39-3). Furthermore, a cephalhematoma may not appear for hours after delivery, often growing larger and disappearing only after weeks or months (Fig. 39-4A, B). A caput succedaneum is present at birth, grows smaller, and disappears, if small, usually within a few hours and, even when very large, within a few days.

Increasing size of the hematoma and other evidence of extensive hemorrhage are indications for additional investigation, including x-ray films of the skull and assessment of coagulation factors, since the infant may have defective blood clotting, as exemplified by the infant with severe thrombocytopenia illustrated in Figure 28-4.

Spinal Injury. Overstretching of the spinal cord and associated hemorrhage may follow excessive traction during a breech delivery, and actual fracture or dislocation of the vertebrae may occur. Complete data on such lesions are lacking, since even the most careful autopsy does not always include thorough examination of the spinal column.

Brachial Plexus Palsy. As a result of a difficult delivery, and in rare cases after an apparently easy one, the infant is sometimes born with a paralyzed arm. Commonly known as *Duchenne's* or *Erb's paralysis,* this condition involves paralysis of the deltoid and infraspinatus muscles, as well as the flexor

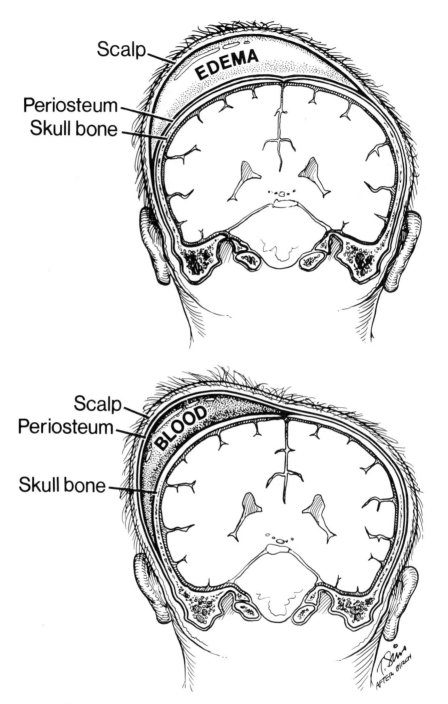

FIG. 39-3. Difference between a large caput succedaneum *(above)* and cephalhematoma *(below)*. In a caput succedaneum, the effusion overlies the periosteum and consists of edema fluid; in a cephalhematoma it lies under the periosteum and consists of blood.

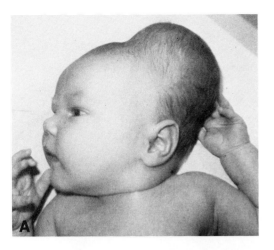

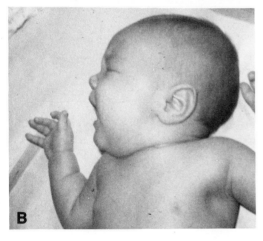

FIG. 39-4. **A.** A very large cephalhematoma photographed 2 weeks after delivery. **B.** The same infant 4 weeks later. (Courtesy of Dr. William Austin)

muscles of the forearm, causing the entire arm to fall limply close to the side of the body with the forearm extended and internally rotated. The function of the fingers is usually retained. The lesion results from stretching or tearing of the upper roots of the brachial plexus, which is readily subjected to extreme tension as a result of pulling laterally upon the head, sharply flexing it toward one of the shoulders. As traction in this direction is employed frequently to effect delivery of the shoulders in normal vertex presentations, Erb's paralysis may result without the

delivery appearing to be difficult. In extracting the shoulders, therefore, care should be taken not to bring about excessive lateral flexion of the neck. Most often, in case of cephalic presentations, the afflicted fetus is unusually large, typically weighing 4000 g or more.

In breech extractions, particular attention should be devoted to preventing the extension of the arms over the head. Extended arms not only materially delay breech delivery but also increase the risk of paralysis. The prognosis is usually good with prompt, appropriate physiotherapy (Bennet and Harrold, 1976). Occasionally, however, a case may resist all treatment, and the arm may remain permanently paralyzed. Less frequently, trauma only to the lower nerves of the brachial plexus leads to paralysis of the hand, or *Klumpke's paralysis.*

Occasionally, the child may be born with *facial paralysis,* a condition that may develop also shortly after birth (Fig. 39-5). It usually occurs in cases in which the head has been seized obliquely with forceps. It is caused by pressure exerted by the posterior blade of the forceps on the stylomastoid foramen, through which the facial nerve emerges. Very often, facial lacerations from the forceps are quite obvious. Not every case of facial paralysis following delivery by forceps should be attributed to the operation, however, since the condition is also encountered after spontaneous delivery. In fact, Hepner (1951) identified facial palsy to be as common following spontaneous delivery as after forceps delivery. Spontaneous recovery in a few days is the rule (Figs. 39-5, 39-6).

Skeletal Fractures. Fractures of the clavicle and the humerus are found with about the same frequency. Difficulty encountered in the delivery of the shoulders in vertex presentations and extended arms in breech are the main factors in the production of such fractures. A fractured femur is relatively uncommon and is usually associated with breech delivery. Fractures associated with delivery are often of the green-stick type, although complete fracture with overriding of the bones may occur. Palpation of

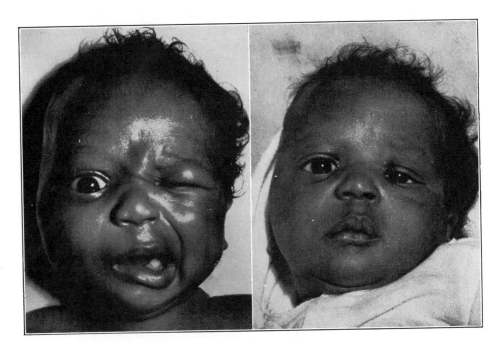

FIG. 39-5. Left, paralysis of right side of face 15 minutes after forceps delivery. Right, same infant 24 hours later. Recovery was complete in another 24 hours.

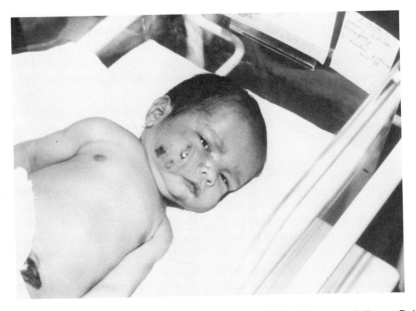

FIG. 39-6. Healing abrasions and lacerations from a difficult forceps delivery. Palsy of the right facial nerve has nearly cleared.

the clavicles and long bones should be performed on all newborn infants when a fracture is suspected, and any crepitation or unusual irregularity should be investigated by roentgenography. It is important to seek evidence of brachial palsy so that treatment for that condition can be instituted.

Fracture of the skull may occur, usually following forcible attempts at delivery, although it may follow spontaneous delivery (see Fig. 31-3, p. 835).

Muscular Injuries. Injury to the sternocleidomastoid muscle may occur, particularly during breech delivery. There may be a tear of the muscle or possibly of the fascial sheath, leading to a hematoma and gradual cicatricial contraction. As the neck lengthens in the process of normal growth, the child's head is gradually turned toward the side of injury, since the damaged muscle is less elastic and does not elongate at the same rate as its normal counterpart on the opposite side, thus producing the deformity of *torticollis.* Roemer (1954) reported that 27 of 44 infants showing this deformity in his series had been delivered by breech or internal podalic version. He postulates that lateral hyperextension sufficient to rupture the sternocleidomastoid may occur as the aftercoming head passes over the sacral promontory.

Congenital Amputations and Constricting Bands. Focal ring constrictions of the extremities and actual loss of a digit or a limb are rare complications. Their genesis is debated. Streeter (1930), and others since, have maintained that localized failure of germ plasm usually is responsible for the abnormalities. Torpin (1968), Higginbottom and coworkers (1979), and others have contended that the lesions are the consequence of early rupture of the amnion which then forms adherent tough bands that constrict and, at times, actually amputate an extremity of the fetus. Occasionally, the amputated part may be found within the uterus. A lesser constriction may result in considerable edema (Baker and Rudolph, 1971).

An unusual fatality from cord vessel occlusion by a "string" of amnion is demonstrated in Figure 39-7.

Congenital   Postural   Deformities. Mechanical factors arising from chronically low volumes of amnionic fluid and restrictions imposed by the small size and inappropriate shape of the uterine cavity may mold the growing fetus into distinct patterns of deformity, including talipes (clubfoot), sco-

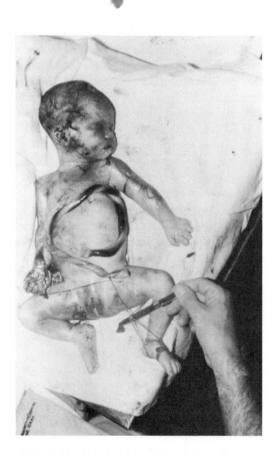

FIG. 39-7. Death of a fetus at term from an amnionic band that formed after premature rupture of the amnion. A tough string of rolled amnion was wrapped centrally around the cord and at each end was adherent to the right thigh and the left foot and ankle. Movements of these extremities tightened the amnionic string and constricted the cord. (Courtesy of Dr. Allan Dutton)

liosis, and hip dislocation. Hypoplastic lungs are also associated with oligohydramnios.

Coincidental Injuries. Experience at Parkland Memorial Hospital, with a very large trauma service, has been that severe trauma to the fetus inflicted at the time of severe trauma to the mother is less common than might be expected. As the fetus is floating in amnionic fluid he is likely to be effectively shielded from forces that cause serious injury to maternal structures close by.

Even so, the fetus is not completely immune to trauma from external forces, as emphasized by Buchsbaum (1979) in his book *Trauma In Pregnancy.* Moreover, fetal wellbeing may be indirectly jeopardized by injuries to the mother which lead to inadequate maternal oxygenation and, in turn, inadequate fetal oxygenation, or to maternal cardiac output insufficient for adequate perfusion of vital organs, including the placenta.

It is important that in case of accident the readily measurable vital sign of the fetus, i.e., the fetal heart rate, should be monitored, especially in the third trimester, when the fetus has achieved considerable potential for survival. At times, however, the fetus may expire before delivery can be safely accomplished. Such an instance is illustrated in Figures 21-5A and 5B (p. 499). The placenta was partially separated and grossly lacerated as the consequence of the mother's lower abdomen forcibly striking the steering wheel during an auto accident. The cause of fetal death was massive fetomaternal hemorrhage as the consequence of the gross laceration of the placenta. The fetus was not injured otherwise. The uterus was intact.

An unusual case was described by Buchsbaum and Caruso (1969) in which a pregnant woman was shot in the abdomen (Fig. 39-8). A roentgenogram showed that the bullet was most likely somewhere in the fetus, and at laparotomy an entrance wound was evident in the large pregnant uterus. However, a liveborn, apparently uninjured infant was delivered and no bullet was present in the uterus or elsewhere in the mother. It was then discovered that the rapidly decelerating bullet

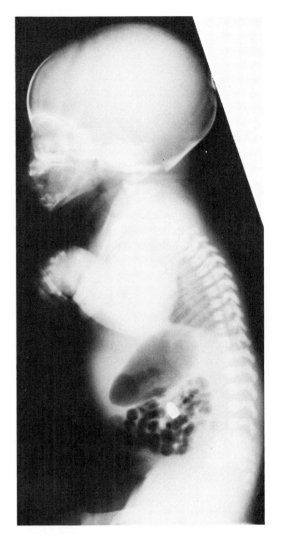

FIG. 39-8. A bullet in the stomach of a fetus following a gunshot wound to the mother's abdomen with penetration of the uterus. The fetus swallowed the bullet. (From Buchsbaum and Caruso. *Obstet Gynecol* 33:673, 1969)

had entered the mouth of the fetus and was swallowed; it was subsequently expelled per rectum.

MALFORMATIONS

Frequency. Congenital malformations are the third leading cause of deaths under

1 year of age, with 18 percent of deaths attributed to this underlying cause. Moreover, severe developmental defects are even more common among spontaneously aborted fetuses and stillbirths than among those who are liveborn.

Genetics and Environment. As was emphasized by Fraser (1959), a minority of congenital malformations appear to have a major environmental cause while a minority of congenital malformations have a major genetic cause. Most malformations probably result from complicated interactions between genetic predispositions and subtle factors in the intrauterine environment.

Perhaps the most familiar example of a major environmental cause of human malformation is maternal rubella during early pregnancy (see Chap. 28, p. 763). It produces congenital cataracts, cardiac defects, anomalies of the middle ear, microcephalus, and mental retardation.

In experimental animals, chiefly rodents, fetal malformations have been produced by withdrawing various vitamins from the maternal diet and adding their chemical analogues, by injecting certain chemicals at particular stages in pregnancy, by the administration of cortisone, by irradiation, and by other means. Although in many respects the results of these investigations may not be applicable to man, such research has brought out certain principles underlying induced malformations that bear on the etiology of many human deformities. They have been outlined by Wilson (1959) as follows:

1. The susceptibility of an embryo to a teratogen depends upon the developmental stage at which the agent is applied. The real determinant is the degree of differentiation within a susceptible tissue. Generally, all organs and systems seem to have a susceptible period early in the differentiation of their primordia. Susceptibility to teratogenic agents, in general, decreases as organ formation advances and usually becomes negligible after organogenesis is substantially completed.

2. Each teratogenic agent acts on a particular aspect of cellular metabolism. Different teratogenic agents, therefore, tend to produce different effects, although acting at the same period of embryonic development and on the same system. The same agent, moreover, may produce different effects when acting at different stages of embryonic development.

3. The genotype influences to a degree the animal's reaction to a teratogenic agent. In many malformations, therefore, both a genetic predisposition and a teratogenic agent are required to produce an anomaly.

4. An agent capable of causing malformations also causes an increase in embryonic mortality. This concept provides one explanation for early abortions.

5. A teratogenic agent need not be deleterious to the maternal organism. Subclinical maternal rubella, for instance, may lead to congenital malformations.

All the proven specific teratogens probably account for less than 5 percent of all anomalies of human development (Lowe, 1973).

The influence of purely genetic factors in the causation of congenital malformations is demonstrable in experimental animals and human beings. In certain strains of mice, for instance, about 15 percent of newborn young have cleft palate, but none has microphthalmia; in another strain, however, about 8 percent of the young have microphthalmia, but none has cleft palate (Fraser, 1959). These two examples indicate that the genes predispose one variety of embryo to cleft palate and the other to microphthalmia. In human beings, the high frequency of supernumerary digits in black infants, not only in this country but throughout the world, requires a genetic explanation.

Among the few drugs known to be definitely teratogenic in the human being are certain antifolic acid compounds and thalidomide. In addition, some progestational compounds masculinize the human fetus. A great many other drugs are suspect, either because they are teratogenic in animals or because there are clinical impressions of prev-

TABLE 39-1.

MAJOR FINDINGS IN ESTABLISHED CHROMOSOMAL ANOMALIES IN MAN
(FREQUENCY PER 1000)*

SYNDROME	CHROMOSOMAL COMPLEMENT	SEX CHROMATIN	NEWBORN BABIES	INSTITUTION POPULATIONS	SIGNS RECOGNIZABLE AT BIRTH	MEAN PARENTAL AGE†	
						Maternal	Paternal
Turner's	45/X	Negative‡	0.4		Lymphangiectatic edema of hands and feet Webbed neck	27.5	30.3
Klinefelter's	47/XXY	Positive	2.0	10–30	None	33.6	37.7
Triple X	47/XXX	Double	0.6	4–7	None	32.5	35.8
YY	47/XYY	Negative	1.4–4§	10–30‖	None		
Down's trisomy, 21	47	Depends on sex; ordinarily not abnormal	1.6	100	Mongoloid facies Simian line	36.7	
Translocation	46			Rare	Same		
Trisomy, 13–15	47			Rare	Cleft palate Harelip Eye defects Polydactyly		
Trisomy, 16–18	47			Rare	Finger flexion Low-set ears Digital arches	32.8	35.2
Cat cry	46 (Deletion B 5)			Rare	Cat cry Moon face		

* Data from Maclean and associates: *Lancet* 1:286, 1964
† Data from Hamerton JL (ed.): *Chromosomes in Medicine*, London, W. J. Heinemann Medical Books Ltd., and from Rohde RA, Hodgeman JE, Cleland RS: *Pediatrics* 33:258, 1964
‡ May be positive with iso-X complement
§ Ratcliffe and associates: *Lancet* 1:121, 1970; Sergovich and associates: *N Engl J Med* 280:851, 1969
‖ Court Brown WM: *J Med Genet* 5:341, 1968. Refers to penal institutions.

alence of congenital malformations associated with their use. Evidence from experimental animals can be misleading in support and elucidation of an etiologic relation between drugs and human congenital malformations. For example, on one hand, it was difficult to find an animal that demonstrates the teratogenic effect of thalidomide. On the other hand, some antihistaminic drugs are teratogenic in rodents but not in man (Yerushalmy and Milkovich, 1965). Although proof of these suspicions is virtually nonexistent and will be difficult to obtain, pregnant women should restrict the intake of all but essential drugs, especially during the early months of gestation.

Chromosomal Abnormalities.   The incidence of chromosome abnormalities in liveborn infants has been established by six studies to be between 1 in 150 and 1 in 200, and averaged 1 in 178, or 0.56 percent (Boué and Boué, 1978). The frequency among stillbirths and infants who died during the neonatal period was 6 to 7 percent. The incidence of various chromosome abnormalities among liveborn infants is presented in Table 39-1 and among stillbirths and neonatal deaths in Table 39-2. As pointed out in Chapter 24, chromosomal abnormalities occur in 60 percent or so of early spontaneous abortions.

Whether the involved chromosome is an autosome or a sex chromosome, the pathogenetic mechanism seems to be the same. During meiotic division in the gonad, a chromosome may "drop out" of the dividing cell (anaphase lagging) and thus be lost. Fertilization of such a gamete results in a zygote with one chromosome too few. In trisomies, one of the explanations of a chromosomal gain is *nondisjunction,* or failure of the gamete to split equally at meiotic division. If the cell with the extra chromosome if fertilized, the zygote becomes *trisomic.* These errors of meiotic division produce individuals whose cells are chromosomally equal but abnormal. If, however, nondisjunction occurs during mitosis after fertilization, the result is an individual with cells of two or rarely more different chromosomal constitutions, or a chromo-

TABLE 39-2.
INCIDENCE OF VARIOUS CHROMOSOMAL ABNORMALITIES AMONG STILLBIRTHS AND NEONATAL DEATHS

ABNORMALITY	PERCENT
Sex Chromosome	1.2
Autosomal Trisomies	
trisomy 21	0.7
trisomy 18	1.8
trisomy 13	0.5
Structural Anomalies	
balanced	0.35
unbalanced	0.5
Others	0.7
Triploidy	0.35
Total	6.1

Adapted from Boué and Boué. In *Towards the Prevention of Fetal Malformation.* Edinburgh, Edinburgh University Press, 1978

somal *mosaic.* In mosaicism, appraisal is more difficult, since the major phenotypic defects may be much less obvious, and karyotypes may be misleading unless many cells are examined.

DOWN   SYNDROME   (MONGOLISM). This is the most common chromosomal defect reliably detected by amniocentesis early in the second trimester (see Chap. 14, p. 338). Most cases of Down syndrome result from an extra chromosome (trisomy 21). Less common, is a chromosomal translocation defect. *Translocation* is the transfer of a segment of one chromosome to a different site on the same chromosome or to a different chromosome. In Down syndrome, such translocations are recognized by study of the karyotype. The important translocations in mongolism are 13–15/21, 21/21, and 21/22. A female carrier with a 13–15/21 translocation has about a 20 percent chance of producing a mongoloid infant. If either parent is a 21/21 carrier, 100 percent of the children will be affected; but if any normal children have been produced or if one of the carrier's parents has the same balanced translocation, the carrier almost certainly has a 21/22 defect. The rate of recurrence of this specific type of translocation is reported to be low. A 21/21 translocation cannot be distinguished from 21/22 except by the birth of a normal child, which rules out the 21/21 translocation.

This congenital malformation presents a striking clinical picture often recognizable at birth. The facies of the infants are mongoloid, with narrow, slanting, closely set palpebral fissures. The tongue is thick and fissured, and the palatal arch often high. Fingers are stubby and the hands present clearcut dermatoglyphic patterns, particularly a simian line. Mental retardation subsequently becomes apparent.

Whereas in mothers up to the age of 30 the risk of birth of a liveborn infant with Down syndrome is less than 1 in 800, this risk increases to about 1 in 100 by age 40, and to 1 in 32 by age 45 (Table 39-3). The frequency of Down syndrome among con-

ceptuses is higher than this but a sizable fraction, perhaps twice as many, are expelled from the uterus as abortuses or stillborn infants (Hook, 1978).

Often, but not always, an experienced individual can accurately diagnose Down syndrome from the general appearance of the newborn infant. Ideally, the capability for confirmation by chromosomal analysis should be immediately available for those instances in which other major complications are detected. Using bone marrow aspirate for culture, a karyotype can be obtained in a few hours. Thus, a decision as to the extent of treatment could be made promptly after *informed* consent for such treatment had been obtained from the parents (Francke et al., 1979).

Inborn Errors of Metabolism. There are several rare but heritable inborn errors of metabolism, most of which result from the absence of crucial enzymes, with resulting incomplete metabolism of proteins, sugars, or fats. In some cases, there are consequent high levels of toxic metabolites in the blood, causing mental retardation and other defects. These metabolic errors are true congenital defects, which are inherited most often as autosomol recessives (see Table 14-4, p. 340).

TABLE 39-3.
RISK OF GIVING BIRTH TO A DOWN SYNDROME INFANT BY MATERNAL AGE

MATERNAL AGE	FREQUENCY OF DOWN SYNDROME INFANTS AMONG BIRTHS
30	1/885
31	1/826
32	1/725
33	1/592
34	1/465
35	1/365
36	1/287
37	1/225
38	1/176
39	1/139
40	1/109
41	1/85
42	1/67
43	1/53
44	1/41
45	1/32
46	1/25
47	1/20
48	1/16
49	1/12

From Hook and Lindsjo: *Am J Hum Genet* 30:19, 1978

PHENYLKETONURIA. The inability to metabolize phenylalanine appropriately to tyrosine is an example of an inborn error of metabolism which is inherited in an autosomal recessive manner. Nationally, it is reported to occur about once in 10,000 to 15,000 white infants but only about once in 100,000 black infants. Because the associated mental retardation can often be prevented by a low phenylalanine diet, early diagnosis is important. Many states now require that some form of screening test for phenylketonuria be applied to all newborn infants. Screening before 4 days of age results in failure to recognize some cases of phenylketonuria whereas testing at 6 to 14 days is much more satisfactory (Starfield and Holtzman, 1975). The difficulties associated with obtaining blood or urine for screening after the 5th day are apparent.

Women with phenylketonuria adequately managed during childhood are likely to have poor pregnancy outcomes, including high frequencies of spontaneous abortion, microcephaly, and mental retardation. Women with phenylketonuria who wish to have children should be advised to switch to a strict diet low in phenylalanine before conception (Buist and co-workers, 1979). Even then, a normal outcome cannot be guaranteed (Smith et al., 1979).

Teratogenic Agents. Different teratogenic agents produce different effects. One that produced devastating effects on the human embryo in the form of phocomelia is thalidomide.

PHOCOMELIA. Phocomelia is a congenital malformation characterized by severe deformities of the long bones. Either the radius is absent or both radius and ulna are defective; in extreme cases, the radius, ulna, and humerus are lacking and the hand buds arise from the shoulders. The legs may be affected in the same manner. In extremely severe cases, both arms and legs are missing. The mental development of the vast majority of the children is normal, and about two-thirds of them survive (Taussig, 1962).

In 1961–1962, an outbreak of phocomelia occurred in West Germany and conclusive evidence indicated that it was attributable to the widespread use by pregnant women of a sedative and tranquilizing drug, thalidomide. In a large proportion of the cases, the drug was administered early in pregnancy for the treatment of nausea and vomiting. The fetus was most vulnerable to the teratogenic action when the drug was ingested by the mother between the 30th and 50th day of pregnancy. It has been estimated that the thalidomide tragedy involved at least 5,000 infants and possibly many more.

The most important practical lesson to be drawn from the experience with thalidomide is that no drug should be administered to pregnant women in the absence of a real therapeutic indication.

Genetic Predisposition and Environmental Factors. The genotype of the embryo may influence the response to environmental factors that otherwise would not be teratogenic. Possible examples follow:

ANENCEPHALY. Anencephaly is a malformation characterized by cerebral hemispheres that are either rudimentary or absent, and absence of the overlying skull (Fig. 39-9). Most often the pituitary gland also is either absent or very hypoplastic. The absence of the cranial vault renders the face very prominent and somewhat extended; the eyes often protrude markedly from their sockets, and the tongue hangs from the mouth. About 70 percent of anencephalic fetuses are females.

In addition to the virtual absence of brain tissue in anencephalic fetuses, typically there is extreme diminution in the size of the adrenal glands, the combined weight of which may be well under 1 g, in contrast to the usual weight of 5 g for the adrenals in normal term infants. The small size of the gland reflects the absence of the fetal, or provisional, cortex; it is commonly believed that the adrenal hypoplasia is secondary to the absence of the pituitary gland.

Nothing definite is known about the cause of anencephaly, but it again appears that both genetic and environmental factors are involved. A genetic factor is strongly suggested, of course, by the frequency with which this malformation recurs in subsequent pregnancies. Yen and MacMahon (1968) have pointed out, however, that the relatively small increase (about 5 percent) in sibship risk over the rate in the general population furnishes a strong argument against a single major-gene hypothesis. A polygenic predisposition is possible, but the very rare occurrence of concordance in twins is difficult to reconcile with either genetic or, for that matter, environmental causes.

Extreme examples of recurrence in siblings have been reported, in which women have produced four successive anencephalic infants (Horne, 1958). The reported geographic differences in the incidence of

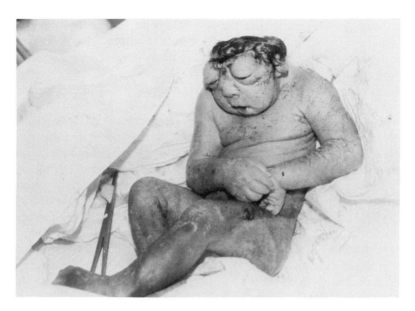

FIG. 39-9. Anencephalic monster.

anencephaly, however, have led to the belief that different environmental conditions in these several areas, notably differences in diets, predispose to the anomaly.

Inability to palpate a fetal head abdomi-

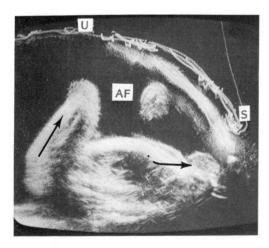

FIG. 39-10. Longitudinal sonogram that demonstrates an anencephalic fetus. The right arrow points to the rudimentary head without a calvarium. The left arrow overlies a lower extremity. Hydramnios is evident from the magnitude of the amnionic fluid (AF) between the fetus and the abdominal wall. (S = symphysis; U = umbilicus) (Courtesy of Dr. R. Santos)

nally is suggestive of anencephaly, but radiologic or sonographic examination provides for definitive diagnosis (Fig. 39-10). Since accompanying hydramnios occurs in the majority of cases, it too suggests anencephaly or, perhaps, another malformation. Anencephaly is probably the most common cause of gross hydramnios, which may occasionally be sufficiently massive to require amniocentesis. Because of the diminutive size and abnormal shape of the fetal head, breech and face presentations are frequent.

The most frequent practical question posed by pregnancies complicated by anencephaly is whether to initiate labor as soon as the diagnosis is confirmed. The uterus containing an anencephalic fetus may be refractory to oxytocin. Usually the slow aspiration of 2 to 3 liters of excess amnionic fluid transabdominally followed by the administration of oxytocin, at times repeatedly, accomplishes delivery.

Especially in the absence of hydramnios, the duration of anencephalic pregnancies may be remarkably long, exceeding that reported in any other form of gestation with a living fetus. In the well-authenticated case of Higgins (1954), for example, the duration of pregnancy was 1 year and 24 days after the last menstrual period, with fetal movements present until the moment of delivery.

Elevated levels of α-fetoprotein (see Chap. 14, p. 339) in amnionic fluid reliably predict the great majority of cases of larger open neural tube defects, including anencephaly. Knowledge of the duration of pregnancy is essential, however, since the level of α-fetoprotein normally varies remarkably with gestational age. Closed or very small open neural tube abnormalities may not be so detected. Lemire and co-workers (1978) have provided a book that deals specifically with anencephaly.

SPINA BIFIDA, MENINGOMYELOCELE. Spina bifida consists of a hiatus, usually in the lumbosacral vertebrae, through which a meningeal sac may protrude, forming a *meningocele* (Fig. 39-11). If the sac contains the spinal cord as well, the anomaly is called meningomyelocele. In the presence of complete rachischisis, the spinal cord is represented by a ribbon of spongy, red tissue lying in a deep groove. In these circumstances, the infant dies soon after birth. In other instances, the defect may be very slight, as in *spina bifida*

occulta. Associated malformations, particularly hydrocephaly, anencephaly, and clubfoot, are common. If part of the brain protrudes into the sac, a meningoencephalocele results (Fig. 39-12). In case of open neural tube defects, α-fetoprotein near midpregnancy is likely to be unusually high in both maternal plasma and in amnionic fluid (see Chap. 14, p. 343).

HYDROCEPHALY. Because of the clinical importance of hydrocephaly as a cause of dystocia and rupture of the uterus, this malformation is discussed in Chapter 30, (p. 822) together with other fetal causes of dystocia.

CONGENITAL HEART DISEASE. Because of the irregularity with which cases of congenital heart disease are reported, the frequency of this malformation cannot be stated precisely, but it is one of the more common abnormalities. The cardiac malformations include such conditions as patent ductus arteriosus, coarction of the aorta, septal defects, pulmonary stenosis, and tetralogy of Fallot. They

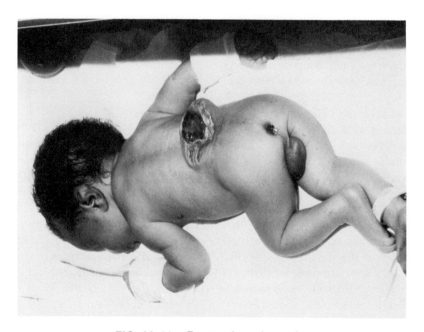

FIG. 39-11. Ruptured meningocele.

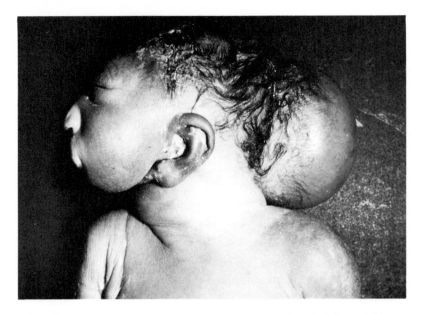

FIG. 39-12.   A large meningoencephalocele associated with agnathia.

commonly occur as part of a syndrome, such as Marfan's, Ellis-van Creveld's, Down, and other chromosomal disorders.

Infants with severe congenital heart disease may look and react quite normally at birth, only to deteriorate later. Therefore, one should consider the possibility of a cardiovascular defect in the mature infant who appears normal at birth and then develops tachypnea, cyanosis, marked tachycardia, and hepatomegaly in the early hours or days after birth. Arrhythmias are rare in the newborn.

RENAL AGENESIS. The incidence of complete absence of the kidneys is about 1 in 4000 births (Potter, 1965). The malformation occurs more frequently in male infants and is characteristically accompanied by oligohydramnios. The infant has prominent epicanthal folds, a flattened nose, and large, low-set ears. The skin is loose and the hands often seem large. A cardiac malformation is common. One-third of the infants are stillborn. The longest reported survival is 48 hours since pulmonary hypoplasia is found in practically all infants. Renal agenesis should be suspected when sonographic examination is indicative of scant to absent amnionic fluid and neither kidneys nor a filled bladder can be demonstrated. Renal agenesis and the associated changes are commonly referred to as Potter syndrome.

CLUBFEET (TALIPES EQUINOVARUS). The extremities are involved in a large number of congenital defects, most of which are rare. Clubfeet, however, are the most common, occurring about once in 1000 births. Since the borderline between the normal and the pathologic is not sharp in this malformation, early orthopedic consultation is essential.

CONGENITAL DISLOCATION OF THE HIP. This fairly common malformation is 6 times more frequent in girls than in boys (Record and McKeown, 1949), and more common in breech than in vertex deliveries. It shows geographic variations, having been noted with unusual frequency in northern Italy, for example. It is rarely seen in black infants. The cause is defective formation of the acetabulum, particularly its upper lip. As a result, the head of the femur may migrate upward and backward. In most cases, the displacement probably does not begin until after birth, developing gradually during the early weeks or months of life. From an obstetric point of view, the fact is worthy of note because it is sometimes alleged that these malformations were overlooked in the neonatal period. Carter (1963), reviewing the genetic aspects of the disease, found concordance in 40 percent of monozygous twins with congenital dislocation of the hip but in only 3 percent of dizygous twins. One percent of subsequent male siblings and 5 percent of later female siblings were affected.

POLYDACTYLISM. Supernumerary digits are occasionally seen, especially in black newborns. They usually consist of a small amount of skin and cartilage attached by a fine pedicle to the base of the fourth finger or toe. Simple ligation of the stalk with a silk thread is generally sufficient treatment. If the base is broad and the digit is well developed, however, surgical removal may be required.

CLEFT LIP AND CLEFT PALATE. A cleft in the lip, either unilateral or bilateral, may or may not be associated with a cleft in the alveolar arch or a cleft in the palate. It is one of the most frequent congenital deformities, with an incidence of approximately 1.3

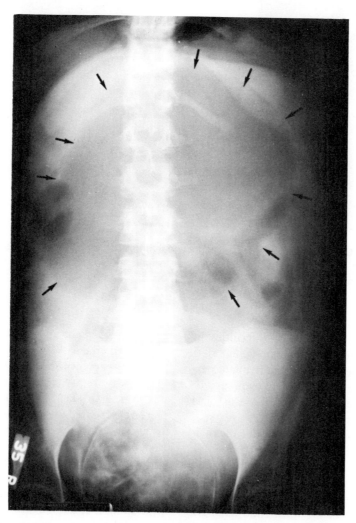

FIG. 39-13. **A.** Amniogram showing a large, relatively radioluscent area corresponding to the location of the sacrococcygeal tumor clearly outlined in the roentgenogram in B. *(Continued)*

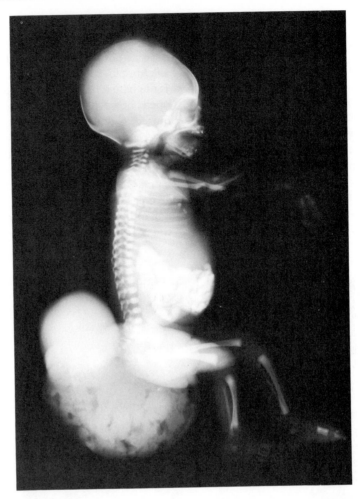

FIG. 39-13 (Cont.).   B. The large sacrococcygeal tumor contains air at the sites of rupture during labor and delivery. Note the outline of the intestinal tract from contrast material in the amnionic fluid swallowed in utero and concentrated in the intestine.

per 1000 births. Because of difficulties in feeding, it is advisable to operate upon a cleft lip as soon as the condition of the infant permits. Cleft palate may represent even greater difficulties in feeding, requiring use of a prosthesis until the age of 2 or 2½ years.

While the risk of the first child of unaffected parents having a cleft lip is about 1 per 1000, or 0.1 percent, the risk of cleft lip in the second child is about 40 times greater, or 4 percent. If both children are affected, the risk of the third child having a cleft lip is 10 percent. If a parent has a cleft lip, the risk of the first child being affected

is about 4 percent and when the first child is affected, the risk to the second child is about 10 percent (Habib, 1978).

OMPHALOCELE. The large circular defect left as the midgut returns to the abdomen at about 10 weeks gestation is normally closed by the rectus muscles and their interconnected fascial sheaths. At times, this closure fails to take place. An omphalocele results, consisting of a peritoneal sac covered with amnion and filled with intestines. Rupture of the sac, evisceration, and peritonitis are grave complications. Surgical correction may prove successful. An omphalocele is likely to be associated with elevated levels of α-fetoprotein in maternal serum and amnionic fluid (see Chap. 14, p. 343).

HERNIA: UMBILICAL AND INGUINAL. Umbilical hernias are common, especially in black infants. They are rarely serious, and strangulation of the bowel is almost unknown. Most small umbilical hernias disappear spontaneously within a few months, whereas the larger varieties are generally treated successfully by simple mechanical measures, such as strapping the surrounding skin with a band of adhesive tape. Inguinal hernias may correct themselves spontaneously during the first year of life. Inguinal hernias may undergo incarceration, especially in premature infants.

IMPERFORATE ANUS. In this abnormality, because of atresia of the anus, the rectum ends in a blind pouch. Examination of the newborn in the delivery room will usually reveal the condition. More commonly perhaps, it is discovered on the first attempt to record the infant's rectal temperature. Surgical intervention is, of course, imperative.

SACROCOCCYGEAL TERATOMA. These tumors are located over and under the coccyx; large ones fill the sacrum and buttocks. About 25 percent are malignant. An amniogram and a subsequent roentgenogram of a newborn infant with a very large sacrococcygeal tumor are shown in Figures 39-13. A and B. The mass ruptured during delivery with considerable bleeding; the infant expired. Especially with smaller lesions, resection may be accomplished successfully and the child not be incapacitated.

GENETIC COUNSELING

Genetic counseling supplies information to families with genetic problems, helping them to make intelligent decisions regarding future childbearing. A malformed child often precipitates the request for such guidance, although other problems leading to consultation include inheritable diseases in the family and consanguineous marriages. Human genetic counseling is by no means an exact science, but it becomes increasingly complex with the accumulation of additional information. Amateurish advice, particularly of the unjustifiably optimistic variety, may produce tragic results.

Forecasting the probability of an inherited disorder is an important step, but it requires a precise medical history. In addition to the routine history obtained on all women who are pregnant (see Chap. 13, p. 306), the specific questions listed in Figure 39-14 should be asked to help identify the expectant mother whose fetus is at unusual risk of having or subsequently acquiring a serious disability. The completed record also serves to document that the mother was informed of any unusual risk of the fetus being abnormal or that referral for further genetic counseling was advised.

Upon completion of the history, it is often possible to decide whether the disease follows an easily recognized pattern of inheritance or represents an isolated congenital defect. Most often, further steps to identify the fetus at risk of a serious disorder and to counsel the expectant parents are best handled through a specialized genetics center with established expertise in counseling and quality control over the variety of laboratory procedures that may be employed. The Council on Accreditation and Certification of the American Society of Human Genetics is now establishing standards of accreditation for genetic counselors. Technics for intrauterine diagnosis of fetal defects of genetic origin are considered especially in Chapter 14 (p. 338).

In addition to supplying positive information, appropriate genetic studies and subsequent counseling helps to dispel many misapprehensions and ill-founded rumors concerning congenital malformations. It also helps relieve the feeling of guilt after the birth of a defective child.

	Circle Appropriate Answer	
1. Will you be age 35 or older when the baby is due?	YES	NO
2. Have you or the baby's father or anyone in either of your families ever had:		
a. Down syndrome or mongolism?	YES	NO
b. Spina bifida or meningomyelocele (open spine)	YES	NO
c. Hemophilia (blood won't clot)?	YES	NO
d. Muscular dystrophy?	YES	NO
3. Have you or the baby's father had a child born dead or alive with a birth defect not listed in Question 2 above?	YES	NO

If Yes, describe: _____

4. Do you or the baby's father have any close relatives who are mentally retarded?	YES	NO

If Yes, list cause if known: _____

5. Do you or the baby's father or close relative in either of your families have any inherited genetic or chromosomal disease or disorder not listed above?	YES	NO
6. Have you, or the spouse of this baby's father in a previous marriage, had three or more spontaneous pregnancy losses?	YES	NO
7. Do you or the baby's father have any close relatives descended from Jewish people who lived in Eastern Europe (Ashkenazic Jews)	YES	NO
If Yes, have either you or the baby's father been screened for Tay-Sachs disease?	YES	NO

If Yes, indicate results and who screened: _____

_____

8. If patient or her spouse is black— Have you or the baby's father, or any close relative been screened for sickle cell trait and found to be positive?	YES	NO

I have discussed with my doctor the above questions which are answered "Yes" and
understand that I am at increased risk for _____
and that it is usually possible to diagnose an affected fetus by testing amniotic fluid
at about 16 weeks of pregnancy and I DO NOT want the test.

_____   _____
(PATIENT SIGNATURE)   (DATE)

Patient wants amniocentesis and fetal diagnoses for: _____

Patient referred for further testing or counseling concerning: _____

FIG. 39-14. Prenatal diagnosis screening questions. (From *Antenatal Diagnosis,* NIH Publication No. 79–1973, April, 1979)

Evaluation of Malformed Infants Who Die in the Perinatal Period.

A *detailed history* of events from before the time of conception through delivery should be obtained. Times of exposure to potential teratogens are especially important. *Photographs* should be made of the face, the body, and all anomalies. A *radiographic skeletal survey* may prove valuable. *Chromosomal analysis* is carried out either on 2 to 3 ml of blood collected aseptically from a large vessel or the heart, or on sterile skin, umbilical cord, amnion, or lung. A *complete autopsy* is performed and all malformations, both external and internal, should be described in detail. Histologic sections should be made of any tissue that appears abnormal.

Modes of Inheritance

DOMINANT INHERITANCE. A mutant gene producing its effects when present on one or both chromosomes of a given pair is referred to as a dominant gene. A recessive gene produces its effect only when present on both chromosomes. A dominantly inherited disease caused by a single dominant gene is transmitted from one generation to the next in a direct line so that each affected individual has an affected parent and there are no skipped generations. There is a 50 percent chance that the children of an affected parent married to an unaffected mate will inherit the condition. These affected children will in turn transmit the defect to half of their offspring.

A dominant trait may be sex-linked or autosomal. If the trait is dominant and linked to the X-sex chromosome, one-half of the daughters of an affected father whose wife is normal will inherit the gene, and none of the sons will be affected. If, however, the mother is heterozygous and affected and the father normal, she will transmit the condition to half of her daughters and half of her sons; but if the mother is homozygous and affected, she will transmit the condition to all her children.

Nongenetic factors may mimic inherited determinants in the production of disease, but these phenocopies can often be detected by adequate history, appropriate clinical examination, and studies in the laboratory. Familial recurrence is unlikely with phenocopies. Affected individuals are nearly always males in X-linked inheritance, for the female must have mutations in both her X chromosomes in order to manifest the disease. Red-green color blindness and hemophilia are well-known examples of sex-linked recessive inheritance.

PENETRANCE. A dominant gene with phenotypic expression in all individuals who carry the gene is said to be 100 percent penetrant. If not expressed in some individuals even though they have the gene, the gene is not completely penetrant. The degree of penetrance may be quantitatively expressed as the percentage ratio of carriers who show the trait to the total number of individuals who have the gene. A gene that is 80 percent penetrant is expressed in only 80 percent of the people who have that gene. The term *penetrance* is applicable not only to heterozygous dominant genes but also to homozygous genes, whether dominant or recessive.

The same gene may express itself in a variety of ways in different people. This characteristic is known as the *expressivity* of the condition. The expressivity of a gene varies from complete manifestation of the condition to complete absence.

RECESSIVE INHERITANCE. A child with an inherited disease that requires for its clinical expression the contribution of a duplicate mutant gene from each of its parents, as, for example, sickle cell anemia, is affected by a recessively inherited disease. Most all inherited enzyme defects are recessive disorders. The parents in these circumstances may be either heterozygous carriers of the mutant gene or homozygous and therefore affected.

If the recessively inherited disease is autosomal, either sex may be similarly affected, and the parents and more remote ancestors are usually unaffected. The probability of a subsequent child's being affected in such a family is one in four. The likelihood that a normal sibling of an affected child is a carrier of the defect is two chances out of three. The carrier child will not produce affected children, however, except by mating with another carrier or an affected individual. If a recessive gene is rare, there is, of course, only a remote chance that unrelated carriers will marry.

In sex-linked recessive inheritance, the affected individuals are nearly always males. The mothers of the affected males are the carriers, and, as with all sex-linked inheritance, male-to-male transmission does not occur. Positive information in this type of inheritance comes from the maternal side of the family pedigree, whereas the paternal history is of little consequence.

MULTIFACTORIAL OR POLYGENIC INHERITANCE. The largest source of genetic variability comes from the combined actions of a number of genes, each with a very small individual effect. The great range of effects so produced is thought to be responsible for the continuous variation seen in the vast majority of differences among normal human beings, as expressed in stature, intelligence, blood pressure, and quite likely in the susceptibility to a number of common diseases.

Many of the more common congenital malformations have a genetic factor in their causation. The increased incidence in relatives, compared with the incidence in the general population, is difficult to explain in terms of any known environmental factors and is much below that found in single-gene transmission. Common congenital malformations with an incidence at birth of at least 1 in 1000, such as cleft lip, pyloric stenosis, talipes equinovarus, congenital dislocations of the hip, spina bifida, anencephalus, and congenital heart defects, are polygenically inherited with varying degrees of environmental modification.

EMPIRIC RISKS. In the majority of cases, a simple pattern of inheritance cannot be demonstrated. In such patients, prognosis is derived from data on empiric risk, based on the pooled experience of many investigators. Such pooled data may be inapplicable to the individual case and occasionally misleading because they include "high-risk" and "low-risk" families. The average so obtained may thus either overestimate or underestimate the true risk. In many instances, however, such average data represent the only estimates available. As a rule of thumb, the risk of a significant malformation in any pregnancy is approximately 1 to 1.5 percent. The risk of a second malformed child is about 5 percent, increasing with subsequent malformed children.

CONSANGUINITY. The risks of recurrence of affected offspring is obviously greater for related than for not related parents, and the closer the relationship, the greater is the risk. Even for closely related couples, however, such as first cousins, the chance of having a significantly abnormal child, although twice that expected for children of nonrelatives, has been estimated by Motulsky and Hecht (1964) not to exceed 2 percent. Reed (1963) reported a risk of malformation of about 10 percent in a child resulting from a brother-sister union. Stevenson and colleagues (1966) indicate, from the 1958 WHO survey, that malformations of the neural tube occur in 1.42 percent of the offspring of first-cousin marriages, 0.8 percent of those from more remote cousin marriages, and 0.5 percent of the children from marriages of nonrelatives. These data suggest a relation between consanguinity and central nervous system malformations, but they are not conclusive. Because the likelihood of a normal child resulting from a cousin marriage is greater than that of an affected child, there is no compelling genetic reason to discourage cousin marriage unless there is familial evidence of recessive disease.

REFERENCES

Baker CJ, Rudolph AJ: Congenital ring constrictions and intrauterine amputations. Am J Dis Child 121:393, 1971

Bennett GC, Harrold AJ: Prognosis and early management of birth injuries to the brachial plexus. Br Med J 1:1520, 1976

Boué A, Boué J: Chromosomal abnormalities associated with fetal malformations. In Schrimgeour J (ed): Towards the Prevention of Fetal Malformation. Edinburgh, Edinburgh University Press, 1978

Buchsbaum HJ: Trauma In Pregnancy. Philadelphia, Saunders, 1979

Buchsbaum HJ, Caruso PA: Gunshot wound of the pregnant uterus. Obstet Gynecol 33:673, 1969

Buist NRM, Lis EW, Tuerck JM, Murphey WH: Maternal phenylketonuria. Lancet 2:589, 1979

Carter CO: Genetic factors in congenital dislocation of the hip. Proc R Soc Med 56:803, 1963

Francke U, Brown MG, Jones KL: Immediate chromosome diagnosis on bone marrow cells: An aid to management of the malformed newborn infant. J Pediatr 94:289, 1979

Fraser FC: Causes of congenital malformations in human beings. J Chron Dis 10:97, 1959

Habib Z: Genetic counselling and genetics of cleft lip and cleft palate. Obstet Gynecol Survey 33:441, 1978

Hepner WR Jr: Facial paresis in newborn infant. Pedatrics 8:494, 1951

Higgins LG: Prolonged pregnancy. Lancet 2:1154, 1954

Higginbottom MC, Jones KL, Hall BD, Smith DW: The amniotic band disruption complex: Timing of amniotic rupture and variable spectra of consequent defects. J Pediatr 95:544, 1979

Hook EB: Spontaneous deaths of fetuses with chromosomal abnormalities diagnosed prenatally. N Engl J Med 299:1036, 1978

Horne HW: Anencephaly in four consecutive pregnancies. Fertil Steril 9:67, 1958

Illingworth RS: Why blame the obstetrician? A review. Br Med J 1:797, 1979

Lemire RJ, Beckwith JB, Warkany J: Anencephaly. New York, Raven Press, 1978

Lowe CR: Congenital malformations and the problems of their control. Br Med J 3:515, 1973

Motulsky A, Hecht F: Genetic prognosis and counseling. Am J Obstet Gynecol 90:1227, 1964

Potter EL: Bilateral absence of ureters and kidneys: a report of 50 cases. Obstet Gynecol 25:3, 1965

Potter EL: Pathology of the Fetus and Infant, 2nd ed. Chicago, Year Book, 1961

Record RG, McKeown T: Congenital malformations of the central nervous system: I. A survey of 930 cases. Br J Soc Med 3:183, 1949

Reed SC: Counseling in Medical Genetics, 2nd ed. Philadelphia, Saunders, 1963

Roemer FJ: Relation of torticollis to breech delivery. Am J Obstet Gynecol 67:1146, 1954

Smith I, Erdohazi M, MacCartney FJ, Pincott JR,

Wolff OH, Brenton DP, Biddle SA, Fairweather DVI, Dobbing J: Fetal damage despite low-phenylalanine diet after conception in a phenylketonic woman. Lancet 1:17, 1979

Starfield B, Holtzman NA: A comparison of effectiveness of screening for phenylketonuria in the United States, United Kingdom and Ireland. N Engl J Med 293:118, 1975

Stevenson AC, Johnston HA, Stewart MIP, Golding DR: Congenital malformations. A report of a study of series of consecutive births in 24 centres. Bull WHO 34 (Suppl 9): 88, 1966

Streeter GL: Contrib Embryol 22:1, 1930

Taussig HB: A study of the German outbreak of phocomelia. JAMA 180:1106, 1962

Torpin R: Fetal malformations caused by amnion rupture during gestation. Springfield, Ill., Charles C Thomas, 1968

Wilson JG: Experimental studies on congenital malformations. J Chron Dis 10:111, 1959

Yen S, MacMahon B: Genetics of anencephaly and spina bifida. Lancet 2:623, 1968

Yerushalmy J, Milkovich L: Evaluation of the teratogenic effect of meclizine in man. Am J Obstet Gynecol 93:553, 1965

40

Family Planning

Justified alarm that the world was rapidly becoming overpopulated and recognition of the right of individuals to control their fertility have resulted in remarkable advances in the application of contraceptive technics. Indeed, governmental agencies—local, state, national, and international—are now obligated to try to provide family planning services for those individuals who desire them and cannot otherwise obtain them. This is a far cry from former years, when many public institutions, by inaction if not by proclamation, effectively impeded the application of family planning practices.

Population growth in the United States is now at replacement level, that is, essentially a 2-child family. Nonetheless, the momentum of previous growth will generate an increase in population for several decades (Fig. 40-1). Currently, the population of the United States is increasing at the rate of about 0.8 percent, or 1 million people per year.

The world's population now stands at 4 billion with a projection from the United States Bureau of the Census of 6.35 billion by the year 2000 (Fig. 40-2). Almost 80 million people are being added annually compared to but 10 million at the beginning of this century. If the population of the world continued to grow at its current rate, there would be at least 30 billion people 100 years from now! The predictable impact of population growth of this magnitude on food supply, natural resources, and political stability is ominous. It is imperative that all physicians be knowledgeable in the application of family planning technics.

WHO NEEDS CONTRACEPTION?

Sexually active couples both of whom are fertile but do not wish the woman to become pregnant need to use effective contraception. Young women who do not desire to be pregnant are best advised to use contraception whenever they become sexually active, no matter how young. At least some girls, and perhaps the majority, ovulate before their first menstrual period.

A much more difficult question to answer is, How late in life does a woman remain capable of becoming pregnant? Results of a recent study of women in the age range of 40 to 50 imply that ovulation is related more closely to the regularity of menstruation than to the age of the woman (Metcalf, 1979).

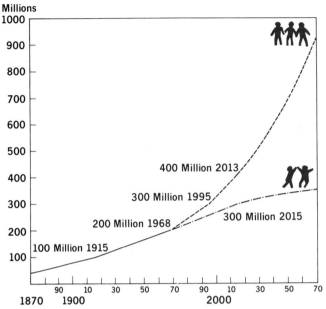

FIG. 40-1. U.S. population: 2-child versus 3-child family. (From *Population and the American Future, The Report of the Commission on Population Growth and the American Future*. Washington, D.C., US Gov Print Off, 1972, pp. 22–23)

Projections assume small future reductions in mortality and continuation of immigration at present levels . Population stabilizes at 350 million in 2070 with 2-child family.

When menstruation remained regular, there was evidence of ovulation in almost every cycle. A recent history of oligomenorrhea or of increasing cycle length was associated with a diminished frequency but not the complete absence of ovulation. Even the presence of hot flashes, amenorrhea, and elevated levels of follicle stimulating hormone in plasma or urine do not absolutely guarantee against subsequent ovulation (Metcalf and Donald, 1979). Primordial follicles with apparently normal oocytes have been observed in ovaries removed from women over 50 years of age and evidence of ovulation has been witnessed through the laparoscope.

On the other hand, pregnancies are rare

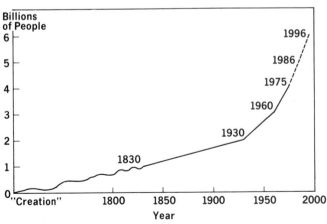

Years required to add one billion people : since creation to 1830; 100, 30, 15, 11, 10

FIG. 40-2. World population growth is exponential. (From The United Nations. Median variant projections, 1974)

TABLE 40-1.
CONTRACEPTIVE STATUS OF MARRIED WOMEN IN UNITED STATES

	AGE		
	15–44	15–29	30–44
Number of women	27,185,000	12,292,000	14,892,000
1. Fecund contraceptors (%)			
Oral contraceptive	22.3	35.1	11.8
Condom	7.1	6.5	7.7
Intrauterine device	6.1	6.9	5.4
Rhythm	3.4	2.6	4.0
Foam	3.0	3.3	2.8
Diaphragm	2.9	2.7	3.1
Withdrawal	2.0	1.7	2.3
Douche	0.7	0.4	0.9
Other	0.9	0.9	0.9
Total	48.6	60.2	39.1
2. Sterile couples (%)	30.2	11.6	45.7
3. Fecund noncontraceptors (%)			
(including pregnant)	21.1	28.2	15.2

From Advancedata. Vital and Health Statistics of the National Center for Health Statistics, No. 36, August 18, 1978.

in women over 50, and extremely rare after the age of 52 (Francis, 1970). Therefore, older women are probably best advised as follows: Regular menstrual periods imply recurrent ovulation irrespective of age; however, pregnancy is rare after the age of 50. A woman younger than this who has not menstruated for 2 years is very unlikely to ovulate spontaneously and to conceive, although there are reported instances in which conception occurred more than 2 years after the onset of documented hypergonadotropic, hypoestrogenic amenorrhea (Szlachter and co-workers, 1979).

COMMONLY EMPLOYED CONTRACEPTIVE TECHNICS

Methods of contraception of variable effectiveness currently employed include (1) oral steroidal contraceptives, (2) injected steroidal contraceptives, (3) intrauterine devices, (4) local physical or chemical barrier technics, (5) withdrawal before ejaculation, (6) sexual abstinence around the time of ovula-

tion, and (7) permanent sterilization. The results of a recent national survey of the contraceptive status and the various technics used by married women ages 15 through 44 are presented in Table 40-1. Estimates of the failure rate with each of these technics during the first year of use are presented in Table 40-2. It is emphasized that the rates of failure reflect patient misuse as well as method failure. Effective patient education, as well as

TABLE 40-2.
FIRST-YEAR CONTRACEPTIVE FAILURE RATES FOR WOMEN AGED 15–44 YEARS

TECHNIC	PERCENT
Sterilization	Rare
Oral contraceptives	2.0
Intrauterine devices	4.2
Condoms	10.1
Rhythm	19.1
Foam, cream, jelly	14.9
Diaphragm	13.1
All others	10.8

From Advancedata. Vital and Health Statistics of the National Center for Health Statistics, No. 26, April 6, 1978.

motivation, undoubtedly would have reduced the failure rate appreciably. Whereas the conception rates for the various technics range from rare after sterilization to nearly 20 percent for the rhythm method, *when no contraception is used about 80 percent of fertile women with fertile sex partners will conceive during one year.*

Abortion, strictly speaking, is not a contraceptive technic, although it serves at times as a less than ideal means for preventing unwanted children (see Chap. 24).

HORMONAL CONTRACEPTIVES

Nearly 6 million women in the United States use one of the variety of hormonal contraceptives available for fertility control. While hormonal contraceptives represented a dramatic departure from previous traditional methods, they also created a unique therapeutic dilemma. As stated in a report of an advisory committee to the Food and Drug Administration, "Never will so many people have taken such potent drugs voluntarily over such a protracted period for an objective other than for the control of disease." For some women, however, an unwanted pregnancy is in some ways a veneral disease. An account of the historical development of hormonal oral contraceptives has been provided by Goldzieher and Rudel (1974).

Estrogen plus Progestin Contraceptives. The oral contraceptives most often employed now consist of a combination of an estrogen and a progestational agent taken daily for 3 weeks and omitted for 1 week, during which time withdrawal uterine bleeding normally occurs. Usually the estrogen is ethinyl estradiol or its 3-methyl ether (mestranol). A greater variety of compounds with progestational activity is used, including norethindrone, norgestrel, ethynodiol diacetate, and norethynodrel. It is estimated that up to 40 percent of women aged 15 to 44 in the United States and Western Europe use oral contraceptives (Population Reports, January, 1979). Approximately 60 percent of women who intend to have more children use oral contraceptives.

MECHANISM OF ACTION. The contraceptive actions of the combined steroidal medication are mutiple. A most important effect is to prevent ovulation, almost certainly by suppression of hypothalamic releasing factors which, in turn, leads to inappropriate secretion by the pituitary of follicle-stimulating hormone and luteinizing hormone (Fig. 40-3). Other contraceptive effects induced by the combined steroids include altered maturation of the endometrium, rendering it inappropriate for successful implantation if a blastocyst were to develop, and the production of cervical mucus hostile to penetration by sperm. The possible role, if any, of altered tubal and uterine motility induced by the hormones is not clear. As the consequence of these actions, combined estrogen plus progestin oral contraceptives, *if taken daily for 3 weeks out of every 4,* provide virtually absolute protection against a conception. The failure rate, when taken appropriately, is less than 1 per 100 woman-years of use! An important exception, however, is the period of about a week immediately following initiation of use of an oral contraceptive. Indeed, in the woman with a maturing follicle who is soon to ovulate spontaneously, ovulation may actually be triggered by starting oral contraceptives in this circumstance.

The so-called *sequential oral contraceptive* was designed to provide estrogen alone for 2 weeks followed by estrogen plus a progestin for 1 week. The advantage originally claimed by commercial providers was that the sequential dosage scheme was more "physiologic." It does not take much thought to recognize the fallacy of implying that such potent medications to block ovulation, as well as induce a variety of other changes, are physiologic! The system of sequential dosage is little used because of the much higher pregnancy rates that result from its use. Moreover, Silverberg and Makowski (1975) and some others, in the course of investigating endometrial carcinoma among young women, noted that 13 of the 21 women had been using sequential oral contraceptives. This provided an additional reason for prohibiting further sale of sequential oral contraceptives.

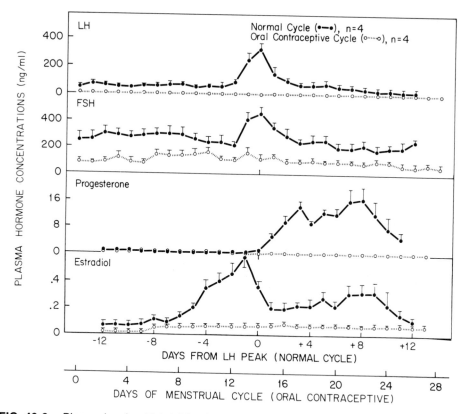

FIG. 40-3. Plasma levels of luteinizing hormone (LH), follicle stimulating hormone (FSH), progesterone, and 17-beta estradiol in 4 ovulatory women and in 4 women who were ingesting one tablet daily of an oral contraceptive that contained 80 μg of mestranol, and 1 mg of norethindrone. Note the suppression of all 4 hormones in the women taking the oral contraceptives. (From Carr, Parker, Madden, MacDonald, and Porter. *J Clin Endocrinol Metab* 49:346, 1979.)

DOSAGE. So as to prevent induction of ovulation, as well as to help recognize preexisting early pregnancy, it is generally recommended that women begin the use of oral contraceptives on the 5th day of the menstrual cycle. Many women, however, start their use after delivery or abortion, before the return of spontaneous menses. If their use is initiated at any time other than during or immediately after a normal menstrual cycle, or within 3 weeks of delivery, another means of birth control should be used throughout the first week to avoid the risk of induced ovulation.

To help achieve regular administration of the combined oral contraceptive, and thereby obtain maximum protection, several suppliers offer dispensers that provide sequentially 21 individually wrapped, identically colored tablets that contain the hormones, followed by seven inert tablets of another color (Fig. 40-4).

Since oral contraceptives have come into use, the amounts of estrogen and progestational agent contained in each tablet have been reduced considerably. It is now known that effective contraception can be achieved with doses of the steroids that are quite small compared to those originally used. This is of considerable importance, since adverse effects are to a degree dose-related. The lowest acceptable limit of dosage is set by the ability of the medication to prevent unacceptable breakthrough bleeding from the endometrium. The amount of estrogen most commonly administered daily probably is 50 μg

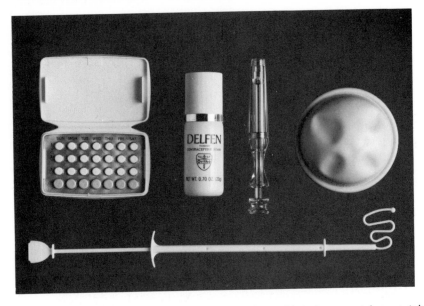

FIG. 40-4. Shown left to right are oral contraceptive tablets in a container, a tube of vaginal contraceptive cream plus applicator, a diaphragm, and, below, a Lippes Loop intrauterine device and inserter. Just before insertion, the rod is withdrawn until all of the device is pulled into the inserter tube.

of either mestranol or ethinyl estradiol. Oral contraceptive tablets that contain as little as 20 μg of ethinyl estradiol per tablet are commercially available. No tablet sold in the United States contains more than 100 μg. The amount of progestin varies, depending chiefly on the compound used.

Adverse Effects from Oral Contraceptives. Concern has been rightfully raised for the safety of users of oral contraceptives. Fortunately, no major disasters have occurred and, in general, the use of oral contraceptives, when appropriately monitored, has proved to be safe for the great majority of women.

METABOLIC CHANGES. A variety of metabolic changes, often qualitatively similar to those of pregnancy, have been identified in women taking oral contraceptives. For example, plasma thyroxine and thyroid binding proteins are elevated appreciably while triiodothyronine uptake by resin is lower than normal. Another change similar to that induced by normal pregnancy is elevation of plasma cortisol concentration with a compara-

ble increase in transcortin. It is extremely important, therefore, that evaluation of results of these laboratory tests and many others be considered in light of whether or not the woman is using oral contraceptives. Miale and Kent (1974) have provided a comprehensive review of the effects of oral contraceptives on various laboratory test values.

Most *plasma lipids* and *lipoproteins* usually are somewhat increased in women who use contraceptives that contain an estrogen and a progestin. Total cholesterol, triglycerides, low density lipoproteins, and very low density lipoproteins all have been found to be elevated compared to those of appropriate controls (Wallace et al., 1979). These changes are opposite to those that have been found in menopausal women who use estrogen alone. The importance of these changes in the genesis of vascular disease in users of oral contraceptives is not clear but, nonetheless, are cause for concern (p. 1017).

The contraceptive steroids may intensify preexisting *diabetes* or prove sufficiently diabetogenic to induce clinically apparent disease in women prone to develop diabetes.

In the great majority of women, however, the effect on carbohydrate metabolism is slight. Phillips and Duffy (1973), for example, identified 1-hour serum glucose levels after administration of 75 g of glucose orally to average 11 mg per dl more in users of oral contraceptives than in nonusers. As with pregnancy, diabetogenic effects most often appear to be reversible when use of the oral contraceptive is terminated (Wingrave et al., 1979).

Argument persists as to whether women with diabetes should use oral contraceptives. A general policy established early in the development of the Greater Dallas Family Planning Program operated by the Department of Obstetrics and Gynecology of the University of Texas Southwestern Medical School would preclude their use in this circumstance. The policy is as follows: *No women with systemic disease shall be given an oral contraceptive except in the infrequent circumstance where it can be verified that the merits from its use clearly outweigh any risks.*

Cholestasis and *cholestatic jaundice* are uncommon complications in users of oral contraceptives; the signs and symptoms clear when the medication is stopped. There appears to be no reason to withhold oral contraceptives from women fully recovered from viral hepatitis. A somewhat increased risk of surgically identified gallstones and *gallbladder disease* has been reported for users of oral contraceptives (Boston Collaborative Drug Surveillance Program, 1973). Interestingly, Javitt and co-workers (1975), using the baboon as an experimental model to study bile acid metabolism, reported that ethinyl estradiol caused a specific reduction in the proportion of chenodeoxycholate and thereby an increased risk of gallstone formation.

NEOPLASIA. Concern that the oral contraceptives might induce neoplasia appears, for the most part, to be unfounded. Case-control studies have not identified an increase of breast cancer in users of oral contraceptives, and the development of benign breast lesions appears actually to be reduced (Vessey et al., 1975, 1979). There is no evidence that use of oral contraceptives predisposes to invasive cervical malignancy and no convincing evidence of an increased risk of precancerous lesions.

Use of estrogen plus progestin contraceptives has been linked circumstantially with the development of hepatic focal nodular hyperplasia and actual tumor formation which most often, but not always, is benign. A prominent feature of the benign tumor nodules is increased vascularity with extensive proliferation of large and small thin-walled blood vessels. Therefore, the lesions, upon rupture, can be complicated by bleeding, hemoperitoneum, and shock which in 8 of 24 cases cited by Antoniades (1975) proved fatal. The liver may become enlarged to palpation, and by means of sonography, liver scans, and angiography, space-occupying lesion or lesions can be visualized. If identified before rupture, resection of the lesion, along with stopping the use of oral contraceptives, has been recommended. Some liver lesions appear to have disappeared after merely stopping the use of oral contraceptives. Increased growth and vascularity during pregnancy or the puerperium leading to rupture, and in one instance, causing death of the mother, have been described (Kent et al., 1978). Fortunately, such liver lesions associated with the use of oral contraceptives are rare.

NUTRITION. Aberrations in the levels of several *nutrients* have been described for women who use oral contraceptives and typically are similar to changes induced by normal pregnancy. Lower plasma or serum levels in users compared to nonusers have been described by some investigators, but not all, for ascorbic acid, folic acid, vitamin B_{12}, niacin, riboflavin, and zinc. Moreover, biochemical changes compatible with, but not necessarily proof of, vitamin B_6 deficiency have been documented repeatedly but do not differ from those that accompany normal pregnancy (Theur, 1972; Wynn, 1975).

The possibilities of folate deficiency and of vitamin B_6 deficiency as the consequence of oral contraceptives have received considerable attention. Folate deficiency developing from use of oral contraceptives was suggested by Streiff (1970), who described in women who were using oral contraceptives, severe megaloblastic anemia which responded to pteroylmonoglutamic acid but not to pteroylpolyglutamic acid unless the ingestion of the contraceptive was stopped. He believed that the estrogen of the contraceptive blocked intestinal conjugase (pteroylpolyglutamate hydrolase) and thereby prevented the cleavage of pteroylglutamate to an absorbable active form, a view not supported by the studies of Stephens and co-workers (1972). At about the same time, Shojania and associates (1968) reported serum folate levels of women who used oral contraceptives to be somewhat lower than those who did not. This triggered a chain reaction of reports that about equally confirmed and denied the findings of Shojania (1968).

The observations of Pritchard and associates (1971) may provide an explanation for the discrepancies. In our initial study, we compared plasma folate levels of socioeconomically somewhat privileged users and nonusers of oral contraceptives who were employed by the hospital or medical school or were wives of employees. No difference was found. We subsequently carried out similar studies in socioeconomically less privileged women who attended the free family planning clinics. Again we found no difference in plasma folate levels between users and nonusers, but their plasma folate levels were lower than those of the more affluent groups first studied. In other words, less affluent users and nonusers of oral contraceptives had lower folate levels than more affluent users.

Prasad and associates (1978) would appear to have utilized about all of the possible permutations for apparent effects of oral contraceptives on blood folate levels when they reported the following: For nonusers of oral contraceptives blood folate levels were higher in women of upper socioeconomic class. With use of oral contraceptives by women of upper socioeconomic class blood folate levels were lower than for nonusers in that class. In women of lower socioeconomic class, however, the blood folate levels were no lower in users than in nonusers.

A number of women with overt megaloblastic anemia resulting from folate deficiency during pregnancy have subsequently been followed by us, some of whom used an oral contraceptive beginning shortly after delivery (Scott and Pritchard, 1975). One relapsed remote from pregnancy while using an oral contraceptive, as did one who did not use an oral contraceptive. In both instances, relapse occurred while the women were consuming atrocious diets essentially devoid of any folate. We are therefore of the opinion that use of the typical estrogen–progestin oral contraceptive is rarely by itself a cause of clinically significant folate deficiency. This opinion is not shared by all.

Pyridoxine deficiency in women who use oral contraceptives has been implicated as a cause of mental depression, a phenomenon which is not a frequent complication of oral contraceptive use. Estrogens induce in the liver the rate-limiting enzyme, tryptophan oxygenase, which enhances tryptophan metabolism in a way that suggests pyridoxine deficiency (Wynn, 1975). To abolish these biochemical variations suggestive of pyridoxine deficiency, as much as 20 to 30 mg of pyridoxine, or 10 times the usual intake, need be ingested! Since altered tryptophan metabolism persists in contraceptive users even when other indices of vitamin B_6 nutrition are normal, Leklem and co-workers (1975) believe that oral contraceptives specifically affect tryptophan metabolism by some means other than through vitamin B_6 deficiency.

It has also been suggested that altered tryptophan metabolism, the consequence of oral contraceptives, may have a diabetogenic effect. For example, tryptophan has been reported to bind to insulin (Larrson-Cohn, 1975). Moreover, Spellacy and associates (1972) have claimed that women who were taking oral contraceptives and who experienced deterioration of glucose tolerance showed partial improvement in glucose tolerance after administration of pyridoxine. These observations have not been confirmed (see Chap. 13, p. 317).

The similarity of the changes in tryptophan and pyridoxine metabolism to those of normal pregnancy strongly implies that estrogen–progestin contraceptives do not induce significant pathologic changes as the consequence of pyridoxine deficiency any more than does normal pregnancy.

Combined estrogen–progestin oral contraceptives conserve iron by reducing blood loss from menstruation. Nilsson and Solvell (1967) compared hemoglobin shed by apparently normal women during spontaneous menses with hemoglobin of withdrawal bleeding following estrogen–progestin contraceptives and they noted that the contraceptives reduced the amount of hemoglobin shed by one-half. By quantitative measurements, we have demonstrated blood loss from spontaneous menses to decrease from as much as 400 ml per cycle to less than 30 ml when 100 μg of mestranol plus 2 mg of norethindrone was ingested daily by two young women with cyclic menorrhagia of unknown cause. The menorrhagia recurred when the oral contraceptive was stopped. It is apparent, therefore, that women who typically lose more than the average amount of blood with their periods may benefit from oral contraceptives by becoming iron sufficient. Moreover, women with *dysmenorrhea* from endometriosis or from idiopathic causes are likely to enjoy appreciable relief from pain while using combined oral contraceptives.

At times, while using the combined medication, the amount of blood and endometrium shed is so scant that the woman believes she is amenorrhic and concludes that she is pregnant, especially if she has missed a tablet or two. She then stops taking the medication and soon thereafter does conceive.

CARDIOVASCULAR EFFECTS. Certain vascular phenomena that are induced or enhanced by oral contraceptives, while rare, can be quite serious. In various studies, the risk of deep vein *thrombosis* and *pulmonary embolism* has been estimated to be 3 to 11 times greater in women who used oral contraceptives than in otherwise apparently similar women who did not. Vessey (1974) places the best estimate from pooled data at about 6 times greater. Kay (1975) has determined from the Royal College of General Practitioners Oral Contraceptive Study the likelihood of deep venous thrombosis among oral contraceptive users to be approximately 1 per 1000 woman-years of use, or nearly six times that of nonusers. Moreover, the use of oral contraceptives during the month before an operative procedure appears to increase the risk of postoperative thromboembolism significantly.

The mechanism by which estrogen plus progestin contraceptives enhance the risk of venous thrombosis and thromboembolism is not clear. Alterations in *blood coagulation factors,* including altered platelet function, and the development of distinctive vascular intimal and medial lesions with associated occlusive thrombi have been described (Irey et al., 1970). Alkjaersig and associates (1975) have identified high molecular weight fibrinogen complexes in plasma from 27 percent of women who use estrogen–progestin contraceptives compared to 6 percent in a control group. Thus, clinically silent circulating microthrombi were 4 times more common, a value similar to the probable degree of increased risk of clinically apparent thromboembolism induced by oral contraceptive use.

Almost certainly the estrogenic component is responsible for the risk of thromboembolism (Inman et al., 1970). This is but another reason to prescribe the smallest dose of estrogen that will prevent troublesome breakthrough bleeding. The enhanced risk of thromboembolism appears to decrease rapidly once the oral contraceptive is stopped. The woman who developed thromboembolism while taking estrogen-containing contraceptives, however, appears also to be at increased risk of thromboembolism during pregnancy and the early puerperium (Badaracco and Vessey, 1974).

Arterial thrombosis has also been attributed to the use of estrogen–progestin contraceptives. The relative risk of a cerebrovascular accident, or *stroke,* seems to be about 4 times greater than in women who do not use oral contraceptives (Collaborative Group for Study of Stroke, 1975). Again, the risk appears to correlate with the dose of estrogen (Inman et al., 1970).

An association between oral contraceptives and *hypertension* became apparent in the late 1960s, when several reports appeared of the occasional woman who, while using an estrogen–progestin contraceptive, became overtly hypertensive and usually, but not always, became normotensive when the medication was stopped (Weinberger, 1975). The oral contraceptives, presumably in response to the estrogen, were shown to increase markedly the plasma level of renin substrate and, to a lesser degree, renin to near the levels found in normal pregnancy. The great majority of women using oral contraceptives demonstrate these changes, as in pregnancy, yet do not become hypertensive. Fisch and Frank (1977), for example, have evaluated blood pressures of a large number of women who were using oral contraceptives and identified the mean systolic and diastolic blood pressures for the group to be 5 to 6 mm Hg and 1 to 2 mm Hg higher respectively than in the age-adjusted control group. Greenblatt and Koch-Wesser (1974), using case-control analysis, concluded that oral contraceptive-induced hypertension affects relatively few women and is usually mild in degree.

Unfortunately, normotensive women who are destined to become hypertensive in response to oral contraceptives usually cannot be identified in advance. The development of hypertension during pregnancy does not preclude subsequent use of oral contraceptives. Pritchard and Pritchard (1977) have evaluated the pressor response to oral contraceptives in young black women who had developed overt pregnancy-induced hypertension but subsequently had diastolic blood pressures of 90 mm Hg or less a few weeks later when oral contraceptives were started. The contraceptive dose most often used was 50 μg of mestranol and 1 mg of norethindrone daily. During an average of 1½ years, only 6 percent demonstrated a rise in diastolic pressure to above 90 mm Hg, a frequency not remarkably different from that observed in initially normotensive young nulligravid black women who used the same kind of oral contraceptive. Moreover, Fisch and Frank (1977) found no significant association between hypertension from use of oral contraceptives and previous hypertension during pregnancy.

The frequency and intensity of attacks of *migraine* may be enhanced appreciably by estrogen–progestin contraceptives. Therefore, this method of contraception is likely to be unacceptable to the woman who is prone to such attacks.

Several epidemiologic studies very strongly imply, at least, that use of estrogen plus progestin oral contraceptive increases the risk of *myocardial infarction.* Mann and Inman (1975) noted a significant association

which became stronger with increasing age. The relative risks for the groups 30 to 39 years and 40 to 44 years of age were 2.8 and 4.7 respectively. Use of oral contraceptives by women who were heavy smokers, were obese, were being treated for hypertension and diabetes, or who had type II hyperlipoproteinemia increased the risk of myocardial infarction remarkably, the effects being synergistic rather than merely additive.

In keeping with the policy of not giving estrogen–progestin contraceptives to women who demonstrate systemic disease, we do not give estrogen–progestin oral contraceptives to hypertensive women. Moreover, every woman's blood pressure is rechecked when contraceptive refills are provided 3 months and 6 months after starting the medication, and every 6 months thereafter. At each visit, usually a nurse or, at times, a physician also performs a brief but pertinent interrogation designed to uncover other possibly adverse effects from the use of oral contraceptives. Smoking is discouraged. Physical examination is repeated annually, or more often if an abnormality is suspected. Whenever hypertension is detected, the oral contraceptive is stopped and another form of contraception is substituted.

LETHALITY OF ORAL CONTRACEPTIVES. An increased risk of a number of adverse effects, some so serious as to cause death, has been identified for users of oral contraceptives. As borne out by the data in Table 40-3, fortunately, the risk of death from the use of an oral contraceptive is very low if the woman is under 35, has no systemic illness, and does not smoke. The risk of dying as the consequence of using an oral contraceptive certainly is less than that imposed by pregnancy and delivery, even though the risk with the latter is actually quite low.

Troublesome questions that persist are, Do the risks of death from circulatory disease related to use of the oral contraceptive increase with the number of years that it is used? To what degree do the risks persist after use of an oral contraceptive is stopped?

TABLE 40-3.

ESTIMATES OF MORTALITY RATES (PER 100,000) ASSOCIATED WITH PREGNANCY AND CHILDBIRTH, FIRST TRIMESTER LEGAL ABORTION, ORAL CONTRACEPTIVES, AND INTRAUTERINE DEVICES

AGE GROUP (YR)	PREGNANCY AND CHILDBIRTH	FIRST TRIMESTER LEGAL ABORTION	ORAL CONTRACEPTIVES		INTRAUTERINE DEVICES
			Nonsmokers	Smokers	
15–19	11.1	1.2	1.2	1.4	0.8
20–24	10.0	1.2	1.2	1.4	0.8
25–29	12.5	1.4	1.2	1.4	1.0
30–34	24.9	1.4	1.8	10.4	1.0
35–39	44.0	1.8	3.9	12.8	1.4
40–44	71.4	1.8	6.6	58.4	1.4

Adapted from Tietze. *Fam Plan Perspect* 9:74, 1977

It has been stated that women who use oral contraceptives for 5 or more years face a tenfold greater risk of death from circulatory disease than do women who have never used them (Population Reports, January, 1979).

EFFECTS ON REPRODUCTION. When the estrogen–progestin contraceptive is discontinued, ovulation usually, but not always, promptly resumes. Similar to the postpartum period, within 3 months at least 90 percent of women who previously ovulated regularly will have done so again. In the rare instance in which *anovulation* persists and is not caused by unrecognized early pregnancy or by premature menopause (in which case there would be high levels of follicle stimulating hormone in plasma and urine), ovulation may be induced with clomiphene or human menopausal gonadotropin. The possibility of a pregnancy with multiple fetuses must be kept in mind when either agent is administered.

Whether very recent use of oral contraceptives before a pregnancy or continued use during early unrecognized pregnancy might adversely affect the fetus has been the source of much concern. Even though an association between congenital defects and the use of oral contraceptives during early pregnancy has not been established conclusively, the woman who thinks that she may be pregnant might be best advised to stop the oral contraceptive *(but use another contraceptive technic)* until it can be established whether or not she is pregnant. Harlap and co-workers (1975) and others have reported a slight increase in both major and minor *fetal malformations* when the mother had recently used combined oral contraceptives. Teratogenic effects reported to date have included fetal limb-reduction deformities (Janevich et al., 1974; Nora and Nora, 1975). Rothman and Louik (1978), however, found no difference for major malformations between infants whose mothers had very recently used oral contraceptives and those whose mothers had not used them for at least 3 years prior to conception.

Use of contraceptive hormones by nursing mothers tends to reduce the amount of *breast milk;* moreover, the hormones are excreted in the milk.

OTHER EFFECTS. *Cervical mucorrhea* is fairly common in response to the estrogen contained, and the mucus at times may be irritating to the vagina and vulva. *Vaginitis* or *vulvovaginitis,* especially that caused by *Candida,* may develop. Antibiotic therapy increases the frequency of such an infection.

Hyperpigmentation of the face and forehead *(chloasma)* is more likely to occur in women who demonstrate such a change during pregnancy. *Acne* may improve or, at times, be aggravated.

Uterine *myomas* may increase in size more rapidly in response to the estrogen of oral contraceptives than they would otherwise but this is not a consistent phenomenon.

Weight gain has been a troublesome complaint from women who use oral contraceptives, although an increase in weight is far from a uniform phenomenon. Some of the weight may be caused by fluid retention, but it is likely to be a consequence of increased dietary intake.

In one case control study the risk of *ovarian carcinoma* was found to decrease as the number of pregnancies increased and to decrease with use of oral contraceptives. Casagrande and associates (1979) suggest that "incessant ovulation" may contribute to the development of ovarian cancer.

Oral contraceptives often ameliorate the dysmenorrhea associated with endometriosis. Their use may even reduce the risk of a woman developing severe endometriosis.

POSTPARTUM USE. Recently pregnant women who do not nurse their children, and especially those who have been aborted, may ovulate before 6 to 7 weeks after pregnancy termination (Ch. 19, p. 469; Ch. 24, p. 612). There is an advantage, therefore, to starting oral contraceptives before the traditional "6 weeks postpartum check." On the other hand, increased risks of adverse effects, especially venous thromboembolism, might be anticipated from use of estrogen–progestin contraceptives earlier in the puerperium. So far, in our now extensive experience in which oral contraceptives have been started typically during the third week postpartum, there has been no increased morbidity.

Oral Progestins Alone. The so-called mini-pill, consisting solely of 0.5 mg or less of a progestational agent daily, has not achieved widespread popularity because of the much higher incidence of irregular bleeding and a higher pregnancy rate. The progestational agent alone presumably impairs fertility without necessarily inhibiting ovulation by causing formation of cervical mucus that impedes sperm penetration and by altering endometrial maturation sufficiently to thwart successful implantation of a blastocyst.

Injectable Hormonal Contraceptives. Depot medroxyprogesterone acetate (Depo-Provera) has been widely used in several countries. It has been estimated that one million women throughout the world depend on an injectable progestin for contraception (Population Reports, March, 1975).

The advantages of depot medroxyprogesterone acetate are a contraceptive effectiveness comparable to the combined oral contraceptives, long-lasting action with injections required only 2 to 4 times a year, and lactation not likely to be impaired. The mechanisms of action appear to be multiple, and include inhibition of ovulation, increased viscosity of cervical mucus, and endometrium unfavorable for ovum implantation.

The disadvantages are prolonged amenorrhea or uterine bleeding or both, during and after its use, and prolonged anovulation after discontinuation (Cheng et al., 1974). The risk of venous thrombosis and thromboembolism appears to be increased, as with estrogen–progestin oral contraceptives (Schwallie, 1974). Obviously, these adverse effects must be explained to the woman and her consent obtained to use such a preparation for contraception. Unfortunately, the woman who may be best served by such a contraceptive agent may not be able to comprehend these potential problems. Currently, medroxyprogesterone acetate for injection is not marketed in the United States for contraceptive use, presumably because of the very unlikely possibility that the compound may cause breast cancer and fetal malformations if the fetus were exposed in utero.

Postcoital Contraception. Stilbestrol administered after intercourse to prevent unwanted pregnancy has come to be known as the "morning-after pill." Kuchara (1971) has reported no pregnancies in 1000 women who had inadequate contraceptive protection at the time of intercourse but within 3 days began to take stilbestrol, 25 mg twice daily for the next 5 days. The Food and Drug Administration has sanctioned the use of stilbestrol for this purpose. The mechanism of action is not fully understood but very likely implantation is interfered with in some way. Nausea and vomiting are common side effects.

Crist (1974) reported similar results for 194 women who, after sexual intercourse, ingested 10 mg of conjugated equine estrogens (Premarin) 3 times a day for 5 days. Presumably, other estrogens in comparable doses will prove to be effective.

Luteinizing Hormone Releasing Hormone.

The natural hormone and analogues of luteinizing hormone releasing hormone (LHRH) are being evaluated for contraceptive properties. LHRH administered daily as a nasal spray appears to inhibit ovulation without disrupting menstruation (Lambe and co-workers 1979). Further studies of the possible efficacy of LHRH as a contraceptive agent are awaited.

INTRAUTERINE CONTRACEPTIVE DEVICES

Since early in this century, attempts have been made, sporadic at the outset but very intense in recent years, to design a device which when inserted into the uterus would prevent pregnancy without causing adverse effects. It is estimated that in the United States 6 to 7 percent of married women of reproductive age use the intrauterine device for contraception. Some of the commonly used devices are demonstrated in Figures 40-4, 5, and 6. The pregnancy rates in larger studies generally vary from 2 to 5 per 100 woman-years, although rates as high as 10 and 15 per 100 woman-years have been reported (Perlmutter, 1974; Shine and Thompson, 1974).

One intriguing but unconfirmed story describes the first experience with an intrauterine device

to have been the insertion of a small stone into the uterus of the camel to prevent pregnancy during long caravans.

Theoretical Advantages.

An intrauterine device ideally would need to be inserted but once, would provide complete protection against pregnancy, would neither be expelled spontaneously nor have to be removed for adverse effects, and, after removal to allow a planned pregnancy, would have in no way induced changes detrimental to pregnancy. These objectives have not been fully achieved by any device so far.

Types of Intrauterine Devices.

In general, devices are of two varieties: (1) those that appear to be chemically inert, in that they are made of a nonabsorbable material, most often polyethylene impregnated with barium sulfate for radiopacity; (2) those in which there is more or less continuous elution from the device of a chemically active substance, such as copper or a progestational agent.

Of the chemically inert devices, the Lippes Loop, in various sizes, appears to be most popular. Of the chemically active devices, those whose surface is covered with metallic copper are being used extensively. The Copper T and Cu7 devices have been extensively evaluated in this country and elsewhere and have demonstrated desirable qualities. More recently, a T-shaped device (Progestasert) that releases progesterone, approximately 65 μg a day, through the wall of the vertical shaft of vinyl acetate copolymer has become popular, especially in the circumstance where use of another device had caused excessive bleeding or cramping.

Mechanisms of Action.

The mechanisms of action of the chemically inert device have not been precisely defined. Interference with successful implantation of the fertilized egg in the endometrium seems to be the most prominent contraceptive action. The interference may result from induction of a local nonspecific inflammatory response and lysosomal action on the blastocyst. Macrophages in the

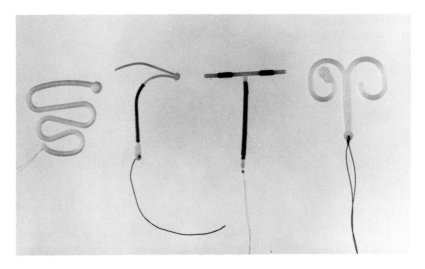

FIG. 40-5. Intrauterine contraceptive devices left to right are a Lippes Loop (size D), a Cu7, a Copper **T** (380 A), and a Safety-Coil.

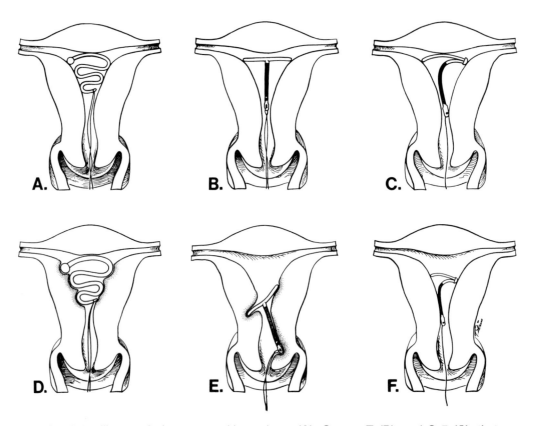

FIG. 40-6. Illustrated above are a Lippes Loop **(A)**, Copper **T (B)**, and Cu7 **(C)**, that are of appropriate size and are correctly positioned. Below are a Lippes Loop that is too large **(D)**, a prolapsed Copper **T** that has perforated the uterine isthmus and cervix **(E)**, and a Cu7 that is too small and has prolapsed into the uterine isthmus and cervical canal **(F)**.

vicinity of the device have been observed to phagocytize spermatozoa (Sagiroglu, 1974). Macrophages adherent to the device are also a source of prostaglandins (Myatt et al., 1975). Asynchronous development of the endometrium and increased uterine activity possibly from increased prostaglandin levels have been proposed to account for the antifertility effect (Wynn and Sawaragi, 1969). Impaired sperm transport to the oviducts in women who at midcycle underwent bilateral salpingectomy shortly after vaginal insemination has also been reported by Tredway and associates (1975). The experiences of Lippes and co-workers (1978) that insertion of a Copper T or Cu7 device up to 7 days after coitus effectively prevents pregnancy strongly support the concept that the intrauterine device does in some way compromise the blastocyst.

For the chemically inert devices, contraceptive effectiveness generally increases with size and extent of contact with the endometrium. For example, the small T-shaped polyethylene device designed by Tatum (1974) allowed a pregnancy rate of about 18 per 100 woman-years. However, with the addition of fine copper ribbon with a surface area of 200 sq mm, the pregnancy rate dropped to about 2 per 100 woman-years. A local, rather than systemic, action from copper must be of major importance, since metallic copper placed in one uterine horn of a rabbit prevents blastocyst implantation there but not in the adjacent horn. Zipper and co-workers (1969, 1971) have shown metallic copper in the uterine cavity to cause an infiltration of neutrophils and macrophages into the endometrium and uterine cavity.

The advantages to be gained from use of intrauterine devices that release locally a progestational agent do not appear to be as great as claimed at the time they were introduced. According to one report, 10 percent were removed within 1 year after insertion because of pain, bleeding, or both, a rate that is quite similar to that for most other devices (Population Reports, May, 1979).

Adverse Effects. A great variety of complications have been described during the use of various intrauterine devices but, for the most part, the common side effects have not been serious while the serious side effects have not been common. The earliest adverse effects are those associated with insertion. They include clinically apparent or silent *perforation of the uterus,* either while sounding the uterus or during insertion of the device, and *interruption of an unsuspected pregnancy.* The frequency of these complications will depend upon the skill of the operator and the precautions taken to avoid interrupting a pregnancy. Although devices may migrate spontaneously into and through the uterine wall at any time, most perforations occur, or at least begin, at the time of insertion.

Uterine *cramping* and some *bleeding* are likely to develop soon after insertion of an intrauterine device and to persist for variable periods of time. The smaller the device, the less the likelihood of cramping and bleeding but the greater the likelihood of a pregnancy either with the device in situ or after spontaneous expulsion. Conversely, the larger and more rigid the device, the lower the probability of expulsion and pregnancy but the greater the likelihood of troublesome cramping and bleeding.

Blood loss with menstruation commonly is increased by a factor of about 2 but may be so great as to cause severe iron deficiency anemia (Guttorm, 1971). Therefore, it is wise to make an annual check of the hemoglobin level or hematocrit reading of women with intrauterine devices as well as any time they complain of heavy periods.

As an aid for ascertaining appropriate placement in the uterine cavity, most devices have an attached synthetic filament, or tail, which protrudes through the external os and is cut off so that 2 to 3 cm are visible through the vagina. There has been concern from the outset that the tail might act as a wick and promote invasion of the uterine cavity by pathogenic bacteria. Purrier and co-workers (1979) have identified potentially pathogenic bacteria colonizing the mucus that coated the tails of more than half of intrauterine devices.

Pelvic infections, including septic abortion, have developed following the use of a variety of intrauterine devices. Tubo-ovarian abscess, usually unilateral, has been described by E. S. Taylor and co-workers (1975), Dawood and Birnbaum (1975), W. Taylor and associates (1973), and many others. When infection is suspected, the device should be removed and the woman, if not actively treated with effective antibiotics, must be observed very closely since there have been deaths from sepsis associated with use of an intrauterine device. Nonetheless, mortality attributable to such devices is lower than that attributed to estrogen–progestin oral contraceptives.

Locating a Lost Device. When the tail cannot be visualized protruding from the cervical canal, the possibilities of expulsion or of extrauterine location must be considered. In either event, pregnancy is likely to occur. The tail may, however, simply be located in the uterine cavity along with a normally positioned device. Often, gentle probing of the uterine cavity using a rod with a terminal

hook or with a Randall stone clamp will retrieve the device. The simple assumption that the device had been expelled and therefore another should be inserted was carried to the extreme in the case demonstrated in Figure 40-7. Adherent to the placenta at delivery were two Dalkon Shields and one Lippes Loop, each having been inserted because a tail was not visible through the vagina. Almost certainly, each tail was drawn into the uterine cavity by the rapidly growing pregnant uterus. The pregnancy, fortunately, was not otherwise complicated.

When the tail is not visible, sonography may be tried to identify a device that is in the uterine cavity. If a hysteroscope is available, this may also be used to identify a device in utero.

If not in the cavity, an extrauterine location may be confirmed by radiographic studies performed in the absence of pregnancy with either an opaque probe or another intrauterine device in the uterine cavity, or by

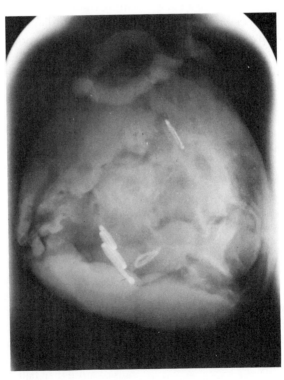

FIG. 40-7. A roentgenogram of a term placenta demonstrating two adherent Dalkon Shield intrauterine devices and one Lippes Loop.

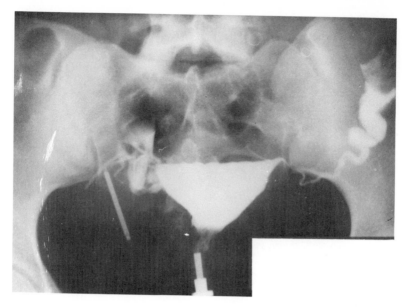

FIG. 40-8. Extrauterine location of a Copper T device is confirmed by hysterography.

filling the uterine cavity with appropriate radiocontrast material (hysterography) as shown in Figure 40-8.

An open device of an inert material, such as the Lippes Loop or Safety Coil, located outside the uterus may or may not do harm. Perforations of large and small bowel and bowel fistulas, with attendant morbidity, have developed remote from the time of insertion of the so-called inert devices. Closed devices, such as the Birnberg Bow, can cause *bowel obstruction* and for this reason are no longer used. A copper-bearing device in an extrauterine location is prone to induce a local inflammatory reaction and adhere to the inflamed structure. A Copper-T device firmly attached to the appendix is demonstrated in Figure 40-9. While chemically inert devices have been readily removed from the peritoneal cavity by laparoscopy or through a posterior colpotomy, the copper-bearing device is likely to be too firmly adherent for successful removal by these technics.

A device may penetrate the uterine wall in varying degrees. At times part of the device may extend into the peritoneal cavity while the remainder is firmly fixed in the myometrium (Fig. 40-10). In this case, at the time of repeat cesarean section, part of a Lip-pes Loop that was inserted 3 years before was found protruding from the fundus posteriorly. Omentum was firmly adherent to the uterus around the protruding loop. Oozing from the tract left after extracting the loop was controlled with deep mattress suture.

The intrauterine device can also penetrate into the cervix and actually protrude into the vagina (Fig. 40-5). This is more common with the Cu7 and Copper T device than with the Lippes Loop and Safety Coil. A more likely cause for pregnancy with a device in

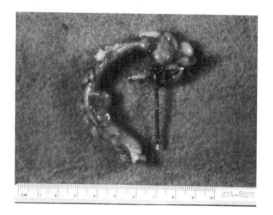

FIG. 40-9. Copper T device adherent to appendix.

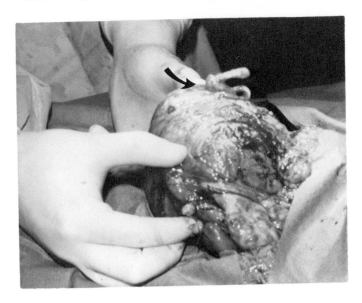

FIG. 40-10. Part of a Lippes Loop (arrow) covered by adhesions is protruding from the uterine fundus posteriorly. Repeat cesarean section has just been performed.

situ is displacement of the device into the uterine isthmus and cervix (Fig. 40-6), although successful nidation may occur with the device in the fundus of the uterus.

Pregnancy with a Device in Utero. When pregnancy is recognized and the tail is visible through the cervix, the device should be removed. This will reduce subsequent complications in the form of late abortion, sepsis, and prematurity. Tatum and co-workers (1976) observed the abortion rate to be 54 percent with the device left in compared to 25 percent if promptly removed. Moreover, with the device remaining in situ, the frequency of low birth weight was 20.3 percent, compared to 4.7 percent if the device was removed early. Vessey and associates (1979) have confirmed these observations. If the tail is not visible, attempts to locate and remove the device by instrumentation may lead to abortion. An increased incidence of malformation has not been noted with pregnancies complicated by the presence of an intrauterine device. Moreover, prior use of an intrauterine device does not have an adverse effect on pregnancies conceived subsequent to the removal of the device, according to Vessey and associates, 1979.

While most intrauterine pregnancies are prevented, the device provides no protection against nidation in other locations. There has been concern recently that use of an intrauterine device increases inordinately the risk of extrauterine pregnancy. Tatum and co-workers (1976) have noted a significant increase in ectopic pregnancies among women who have used intrauterine devices for more than 2 years compared to users for less than 2 years. However, Vessey and co-workers (1979) have found that the risk remains rather constant with duration of use at 1.2 per 1000 women per year.

Procedures for Insertion. The Food and Drug Administration requires that before an intrauterine device is inserted physicians must give women who request a device a detailed brochure spelling out the side effects and apparent risks from use of such a device.

Most devices have a special inserter, usually a sterile graduated plastic tube into which the device is withdrawn just before insertion (Fig. 40-4). Timing of the insertion of the device influences the ease of placement as well as the pregnancy and expulsion rates. Insertion near the end of a normal menstrual period when the cervix is usually softer and the canal somewhat more dilated may facilitate insertion and at the same time exclude an early pregnancy. However, insertion need not be limited only to this period. For the woman who is reasonably sure that she is not pregnant and she does not want to be pregnant, insertion may be carried out anytime during the menstrual cycle. Even though she has engaged in coitus during the previous week, she is unlikely to conceive if a Copper T or Cu7 device is used (Lippes et al., 1978).

Insertion at the time of delivery or very soon thereafter is followed by an unsatisfactorily high expulsion rate. The recommendation has been made, therefore, to withhold insertion for at least 8 weeks to reduce expulsions as well as to minimize the risk of perforation. The experience of the Greater Dallas Family Planning Program, however, has been that insertion during the 3rd week postpartum has not led to perforation or expulsion rates significantly higher than for insertion remote from pregnancy. In the absence of infection, the device may be inserted immediately after early abortion.

INSERTION AND FOLLOW-UP. Satisfactory technic for insertion and plan for follow-up are outlined below:

1. Obtain a careful gynecologic history. Contraindications to the use of an intrauterine device include the following: Untreated gonorrhea even though asymptomatic, a recent pelvic infection or a history of recurrent pelvic infections, severe dysmenorrhea, cervical stenosis, abnormalities of the uterine cavity, heavy menses, overt anemia, and abnormalities of blood coagulation. The woman who has had a previous ectopic pregnancy should be counseled against the use of an intrauterine device. She is already at considerable risk of another ectopic pregnancy but an intrauterine device does not prevent ectopic pregnancy.
2. Describe the various problems associated with use of an intrauterine device and obtain informed consent.
3. Perform a thorough pelvic examination to identify especially the position and size of the uterus and adnexa. If abnormalities are found, an intrauterine device often is contraindicated.
4. Visualize the cervix and grasp it with a tenaculum. Use sterile instruments and sterile intrauterine device. Wipe the cervix and the vaginal walls with an antiseptic solution. It is commonly recommended that the uterus first be sounded to help identify the direction and the depth of the uterine cavity. Before identifying the depth of the uterine cavity with a sound, the cervical canal and uterine cavity are first straightened by applying gentle traction on the tenaculum. A device of appropriate size is selected based on the length of the uterine cavity. The inserter (Fig. 40-3), with the device contained within its most distal portion, is gently inserted to the fundus of the uterus. After rotating the inserter so as to position the device in the transverse plane of the uterus (Fig. 40-5), the inserter is removed while the device is held in place in the fundus by the plastic rod within the inserter behind the device. Thus, the device is not pushed out of the tube, but rather it is held in place by the rod while the inserter tube is withdrawn.
5. Cut the marker tail 2 to 3 cm from the external os, remove the tenaculum, observe for bleeding from the tenaculum puncture sites, and if there is no bleeding, remove the speculum.
6. Provide analgesia with aspirin or codeine to allay cramps. Invite the woman to report promptly any apparent adverse effects.
7. Expulsion is most common during the first month of use. The recipient should be instructed on how to palpate the strings protruding from the cervix by either sitting on the edge of a chair or squatting down and then advancing the middle finger into the vagina until the cervix is reached. The woman should be checked in 1 month for appropriate placement of the device by identifying the tail protruding appropriately from the cervix. Barrier contraception may be desirable during this time, especially if a device has been expelled previously.

The chemically inert device may be left in the uterus indefinitely. The copper-bearing devices will have to be replaced periodically. For the Cu7 and Copper T devices, replacement every 3 years is recommended. The progesterone-bearing intrauterine device, Progestasert, should be replaced annually. (Many of the large number of publications dealing with intrauterine devices have been reviewed in Population Reports, May, 1979.)

LOCAL BARRIER METHODS

Condoms, vaginal diaphragms, and spermicidal agents placed in the vagina have long been used for contraception with variable success.

Condoms. To date, the condom represents in the United States the only reversible effective "male method" of contraception except for *coitus interruptus*. Condoms can provide effective contraception. Those currently on the market rarely contain holes or rupture during use. Their failure rate *when faithfully used* has been placed at less than 5 pregnancies per 100 couple-years of exposure (Population Report, Jan., 1976). As well as preventing pregnancy when used appropriately, the condom reduces significantly, but does not eliminate, the risk of acquiring a sexually transmitted disease (Barlow, 1977). It is estimated that up to 25 million couples in the world use condoms.

Historically, the original condoms were made of intestine and other materials, but with the introduction of rubber, the condom became much more effective, less expensive, and more widely available. The origin of the word "condom" is unknown. It has been stated that it refers to Dr. Condom, a physician who provided France's Charles II with a means of preventing more illegitimate offspring. Casanova (1725–1798) is said to have mentioned condoms several times in his exhaustive memoirs.

In Texas, and elsewhere, the earliest father-son discussion of sex and reproduction often has been stimulated by the presence of a number of condom-dispensing machines in the men's room of most service stations. It is of interest that condoms were widely available at a time when attempts to make other family planning technics more readily available were discouraged by much of society lest they promote sexual promiscuity or offend someone's religious beliefs. The condoms in the gas stations, allegedly, were provided to prevent veneral disease, which they do to a degree but not absolutely.

Intravaginal   Contraceptives. Such contraceptive agents are variously marketed as creams, jellies, suppositories, and in aerosol containers (Fig. 40-3). In this country, Delfen and Emko aerosol foams are widely used, especially by women who find the oral contraceptive or an intrauterine device unacceptable, or who need temporary protection, for example, during the first week after starting oral contraceptives or while nursing.

Most such intravaginal agents can be purchased "over-the-counter," i.e., a prescription is not needed. Typically, such preparations work by providing a physical barrier to sperm penetration as well as chemical spermicidal action. *To be highly effective, the agents must, shortly before intercourse, be deposited high in the vagina in contact with the cervix.* Their duration of maximal spermicidal effectiveness is usually no more than 1 hour and they therefore must be reinserted into the vagina before intercourse is repeated; douching should be avoided for at least 6 hours after intercourse.

Higher pregnancy rates are attributable chiefly to inconsistent use rather than to failure of the method during use. If inserted regularly and correctly, use of the foam preparations for contraception probably results in no more than 5 pregnancies per 100 woman-years of use.

DIAPHRAGM   PLUS   SPERMICIDAL AGENT. The vaginal diaphram (Fig. 40-3), consisting of a circular rubber dome of various diameters supported by a circumferentially placed metal spring, has long been used for contraception in combination with a spermicidal jelly or cream. The spermicidal agent is applied to the superior surface both along the rim and centrally. The device is then placed in the vagina so that the cervix, vaginal fornices, and anterior vaginal wall are effectively partitioned above the rest of the vagina and the penis. At the same time, the centrally placed spermicidal agent is held against the cervix by the diaphragm. When appropriately positioned in the vagina, the rim of the diaphragm is lodged superiorly deep in the posterior vaginal fornix and inferiorly the rim lies in close proximity to the inner surface of the symphysis immediately below the urethra (Fig. 40-11). If the diaphragm is too small, it will not remain in place. If too large, it will be uncomfortable when it is forced into position. A cystocele or uterine prolapse is very likely to result in instability of position and expulsion.

The diaphragm and spermicidal agent can be inserted even hours before intercourse and should be left for at least 6 hours afterward before removal.

An unacceptably high failure rate has been ascribed to the use of the diaphragm plus spermicidal agent in some reports (Peel and Potts, 1969). It is very likely, however, that failures most often occur in nonmotivated, inconstant users. The diaphragm requires a high level of motivation for proper use which, in turn, is accompanied by a quite low pregnancy rate. Vessey and Wiggins (1974) reported a pregnancy rate of only 2.4 per 100 woman-years for already established users of the diaphragm. They emphasized that established users need not be encouraged to change to a "more modern" method of birth control.

In prior centuries, a great variety of materials undoubtedly were inserted into the vagina by women who were desperately seeking an effective barrier that would prevent sperm from reaching the egg. Agents reported to have been used include oiled silk paper, sponges, gums, leaves, beeswax, or opium melted into discs. Casanova (apparently a very important figure historically in the design and the testing of a variety of barrier technics) allegedly recommended squeezing half a lemon and then inserting the rind into the vagina so as to cover the cervix. The lemon provided a barrier while the citric acid was spermicidal.

RHYTHMIC ABSTINENCE

The human ovum probably is susceptible to successful fertilization only for about 18 to 24 hours after ovulation. Motile sperm have been identified in oviducts of women undergoing laparotomy as long as 85 hours after coitus (Ahlgren, 1975). However, it is unlikely that sperm retain the capability for successful fertilization for this long a period. The "rhythm method" for preventing pregnancy is based on these considerations. Ovulation

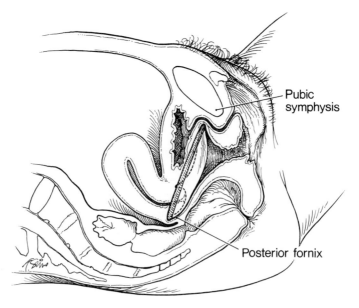

FIG. 40-11. A diaphragm in place creates a physical barrier between the vagina and cervix and, importantly, provides for intimate contact between the contraceptive jelly or cream and the cervix.

most often occurs about 14 days before the onset of the next menstrual period, but, unfortunately, not necessarily 14 days after the onset of the last menstrual period. Therefore, *calendar rhythm* is not always reliable.

Temperature rhythm relies on *slight* changes in basal body temperature which may occur just before ovulation. The temperature rhythm method is much more likely to be successful if during each cycle intercourse is restricted to well after the ovulatory temperature rise.

Cervical mucus rhythm depends upon awareness of "dryness" and "wetness" in the vagina as the consequence of changes in the amount and kind of cervical mucus formed at different times in the menstrual cycle. This approach has not achieved popularity.

The pregnancy rate with the rhythm methods has been placed as high as 21 to 38 per 100 woman-years (Mastroianni, 1974). Moreover, the possibility exists that rhythm methods may lead to fertilization involving overaged ova and yield pregnancies of inferior quality (Population Reports, 1974).

STERILIZATION

Prevalence.   According to the National Center for Health Statistics by 1976 at least one partner was sterile in nearly one-third of couples in which the wife was within the age limits of 15 to 44 years. By way of comparison, an oral contraceptive was being used by about 22 percent. More than 12 million Americans have already undergone voluntary sterilization and somewhat more than 1 million are being sterilized annually. Among white couples about an equal number of men and women have undergone sterilization. With the availability of new surgical methods and the increased use of those already established, estimates have been made that by 1985 more than 165 million couples throughout the world will choose sterilization.

Time of Tubal Sterilization.   The operation can be done at any time, but early in the puerperium is a particularly convenient

time. Because the fundus is near the umbilicus and the oviducts are readily accessible beneath the lower abdominal wall for several days after delivery, the operation is technically simple and hospitalization need not be prolonged.

It was recommended previously that puerperal sterilization by partial resection of the oviducts be accomplished before 72 hours postpartum so as to minimize infection from ascending bacterial invasion of the fallopian tubes. More recently, Laros and co-workers (1973), in a randomized prospective study, found no correlation between time interval and postoperative morbidity. At Parkland Memorial Hospital, the operation is performed in the obstetric surgical suite most often the morning after delivery to minimize hospital stay.

Sterilization at the time of vaginal delivery has some disadvantages. The likelihood of postpartum hemorrhage subsides remarkably during the first 12 hours after delivery and of especial importance, the status of the newborn infant can be much more accurately defined by that time.

Types of Operation.   A distinction can be made between *therapeutic* and *nontherapeutic sterilization.* Sterilization of a young healthy woman of low parity generally would fall into the nontherapeutic category. On the other hand, sterilization of the elderly woman, the woman of very high parity, or the woman with most chronic systemic diseases should be classified as therapeutic, since pregnancy is likely to be appreciably more hazardous in these latter groups.

A great variety of technics have been employed to try to disrupt tubal patency and thereby thwart union of sperm and egg. Some of these are considered below:

IRVING PROCEDURES.   This operation is least likely to fail. Briefly, as illustrated in Figure 40-12.A, the procedure involves severing the oviduct and separating it from the mesosalpinx sufficiently to create a medial segment, the end of which is buried within a tunnel into the myometrium posteriorly, and a short lateral segment, the proximal end

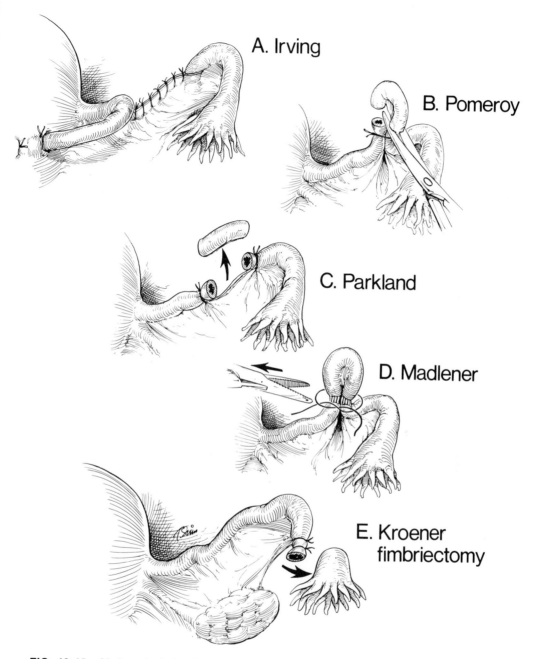

A. Irving

B. Pomeroy

C. Parkland

D. Madlener

E. Kroener
fimbriectomy

FIG. 40-12. Various technics for tubal sterilization. **A.** Irving procedure: The medial cut end of the oviduct is buried in the myometrium posteriorly and the distal cut end is buried in the mesosalpinx. **B.** Pomeroy procedure: A loop of oviduct is ligated and the knuckle of tube above the ligature is excised. **C.** Parkland procedure: A segment of tube is separated from the mesosalpinx at an avascular site, the separated tubal segment is ligated proximally and distally and then excised. **D.** Madlener procedure: A knuckle of oviduct is crushed and then ligated without resection. **E.** Kroener procedure: The distal portion of the ampulla, including all of the fimbriae, is resected.

of which is then buried within the mesosalpinx. The procedure requires considerably more exposure than do most other technics and the likelihood of hemorrhage is much greater.

POMEROY PROCEDURE. Of all the technics that divide the tube, the simplest, reasonably effective method of performing abdominal sterilization is the Pomeroy procedure (Fig. 40-12.B). It has generally been considered important that plain catgut be used to ligate the knuckle of tube, since the rationale of this procedure is based on absorption of the ligature and subsequent separation of the severed tubal ends, which most often become sealed over by fibrosis.

PARKLAND PROCEDURE. We avoid the initial intimate approximation of the cut ends of the oviduct which is inherent in the Pomeroy procedure (Fig. 40-12.C). Through an infraumbilical abdominal wall incision, typically just long enough to allow a small Richardson retractor to be inserted, the tube is

positively identified by grasping the midportion in a Babcock clamp and confirming by direct observation that indeed fimbriae are present on the distal end of the structure so held. Otherwise, it is easy to confuse the round ligament and the midportion of oviduct! Whenever the oviduct is inadvertently dropped, it is mandatory to repeat in toto the identification procedure. An avascular site (Fig. 40-13.A) in the mesosalpinx adjacent to the oviduct is perforated with a small hemostat and the jaws are opened to separate the oviduct from the adjacent mesosalpinx for about 2.5 cm (Fig. 40-13.B). The freed oviduct is ligated proximally and distally (Fig. 40-13.C) with 00 chromic suture and the intervening segment of about 2 cm is excised with sharp scissors (Fig. 40-13.D). After inspecting for hemostasis, the now discontinuous oviduct is dropped in place and the procedure is repeated on the other side. Both resected segments are labeled and submitted for histologic confirmation. Excluding instances in which an inexperienced operator failed to resect fallopian tube, which can be

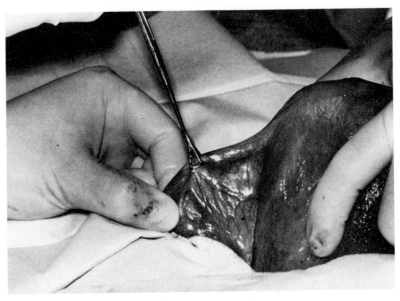

A

FIG. 40-13. Sterilization at cesarean section. **A.** An avascular site in the mesosalpinx adjacent to the midportion of the oviduct is looked for. On facing page: **B.** A small hemostat has been inserted through the avascular site and the jaws of the clamp opened to separate mesosalpinx from tube for about 2.5 cm. A ligature is being inserted. **C.** The segment of oviduct separated from mesosalpinx has been ligated. **D.** The ligated segment of oviduct has been resected. *(Continued)*

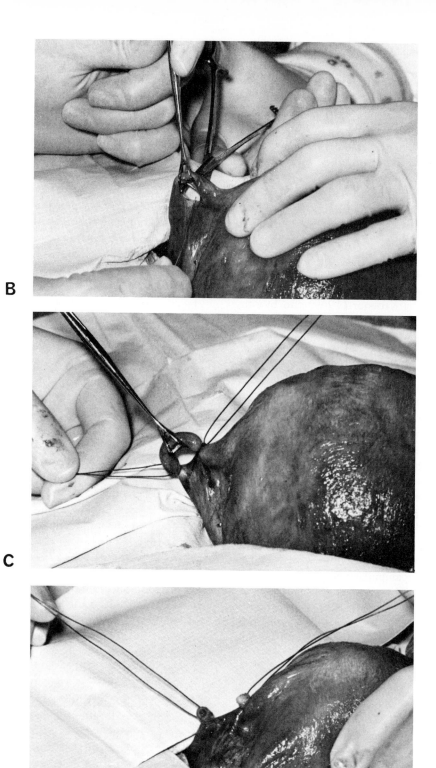

B

C

D

FIG. 40-13 (Cont.)

1033

confirmed promptly in the surgical pathology laboratory, the subsequent failure rate has been approximately 1 in 400 procedures.

MADLENER PROCEDURE. A knuckle of tube is crushed and ligated with nonabsorbable suture but not resected (Fig. 40-12.D). This procedure is mentioned only to discourage its use. Early experiences at Parkland Memorial Hospital indicated a failure rate of about 7 percent.

FIMBRIECTOMY. Removal of all of the fimbriae to effect sterilization has been recommended by Kroener (1969) and by others. Kroener doubly ligated the oviduct with silk suture and then excised the fimbriated end (Fig. 40-12.E). While Kroener reported no failures, others have, and in some instances the rate has been unacceptable. Taylor (1972), for example, observed 6 pregnancies among about 200 women who were subjected to fimbriectomy; usually when the tubes were examined, a small amount of fimbrial tissue had been left. Metz (1977) identified 7 failures among 388 women upon whom bilateral fimbriectomy was performed. Catgut suture had been used and the resected surface had been lightly electrocoagulated. In the cases that failed, tuboperitoneal fistulas lined with tubal endothelium were found in the remaining ampullary portion of the tube.

POSTOPERATIVE CARE. After puerperal sterilization, analgesia should be provided for abdominal soreness, which at times is aggravated in multiparous women by uterine "afterbirth pains." Meperidine, 75 mg intramuscularly, given intermittently as needed during the first 24 hours, provides excellent analgesia. Within 8 hours, most women can ambulate, eat a regular diet, and care for their babies. We have found discharge from the hospital on the second postoperative day to be satisfactory.

NONPUERPERAL TUBAL STERILIZATION. Laparotomy to perform sterilization can be a much more formidable procedure once the uterus has completely involuted and

returned to the true pelvis. However, much of the difficulty of obtaining exposure are removed if the uterus and adnexa are pushed out of the true pelvis to just beneath the abdominal wall just above the symphysis by means of a manipulator previously inserted into the uterus with the handle protruding from the vagina. Utilizing this technic, *"mini-laparotomies"* are being performed through a 3-cm incision made suprapubically. In most published reports, resection of the ampullary portion of the tube ("fimbriectomy") or a Pomeroy type sterilization usually has been performed.

Vaginal tubal sterilization may be performed after advanced pregnancy once the uterus has involuted and pregnancy-induced hyperemia has subsided. The peritoneal cavity is entered through the posterior vaginal fornix (colpotomy, culdotomy), the oviducts are grasped and drawn into view, and then, most often, either a Pomeroy type resection or fimbriectomy is performed. Yuzpe and associates (1974) described 700 such sterilizations, including 200 done at the time of curettage to terminate an *early* pregnancy. Cheng and co-workers (1975) reported a similar number of cases in which culdoscopy was used, often on an outpatient basis, to effect sterilization.

Veltman and Marshall (1973) analyzed the morbidity associated with various methods of sterilization, including vaginal tubal sterilization, carried out at the time of abortion. The results are presented in Table 40-4.

Great enthusiasm has been generated for interval as well as postabortal sterilizations using *laparoscopy*. An article in *Life* magazine (July 28, 1972) that referred to the technic as "Band-Aid" surgery undoubtedly brought the procedure to the attention of a great many women. Commonly, the woman is cared for in an ambulatory surgical setting. Anesthesia, either general usually with endotracheal intubation, or local, is induced, and after producing pneumoperitoneum with carbon dioxide, the sterilization procedure is accomplished. Most often a few hours later the woman can be discharged.

Typically, the midportion of the oviduct

TABLE 40-4.
MORBIDITY RATES FOR ABORTION/STERILIZATION PROCEDURES

OPERATION	OPERATIVE TIME (MIN)	ESTIMATED BLOOD LOSS (ml)	POST-OPERATIVE FEVER (%)	POST-OPERATIVE ANTIBIOTICS (%)	TRANSFUSION (%)
Hysterotomy therapeutic abortion-total abdominal hysterectomy	105*	500*	43.5†	40	8.3
Hysterotomy therapeutic abortion-bilateral tubal ligation	70	300	24.5	29	4.9
Vaginal hysterectomy	80	300	43	41	12
Vaginal tubal ligation	45	100	8	10	0

From Veltman and Marshall. *Am J Obstet Gynecol* 117:251, 1973
* Median values
† Temperature greater than 38C

is identified, grasped, and commonly has been electrocoagulated. Thompson and Wheeless (1975) reported a failure rate of 1 in every 60 cases with a previously used "one-burn" technic to disrupt tubal patency, but only one failure in every 220 when the electrocoagulation was repeated, usually 3 times, on each tube, along with complete transection of the tube. Specimens of electrocoagulated tissue provide little in the way of pertinent histologic information. Pregnancies after electroeoagulation are more likely to be ectopic (McCausland, 1980).

Damage to adjacent structures during electrocoagulation remains a problem. To avoid using cautery, occlusive devices, especially silicone-rubber bands such as the Yoon falope ring, are being used extensively. Yoon and Poliakoff (1979) report a known failure rate for interval sterilizations using the falope ring of 0.42 percent per 100 woman-years, excluding luteal phase pregnancies.

Hazards from Tubal Sterilization. The principal hazards associated with tubal sterilization are anesthetic complications, inadvertent coagulation of vital structures during laparoscopic sterilization, the rare occurrence of pulmonary embolism during the puerperium, and failure to produce sterility with an unrecognized and therefore inappro-

priately treated ectopic pregnancy as the result (see Chap. 22, p. 527).

The possibility has been raised of a "post-tubal ligation" syndrome variably characterized by pelvic discomfort, ovarian cyst formation, and especially menorrhagia. Stock (1978) identified the incidence of pelvic pain and of menorrhagia after tubal sterilization to be about 6 percent. Kasonde and Bonnar (1976) actually measured menstrual blood loss before and for 6 to 12 months after tubal sterilization and found that the operation made no significant difference in menstrual blood loss. They also noted that women who presented with menorrhagia soon after sterilization usually had the problem beforehand or had been using oral contraceptives which reduced blood loss and then reverted to spontaneous heavier periods when their use was stopped after sterilization.

The likelihood of tubal sterilization inducing any of these abnormalities remains to be established. While complete transection of the oviduct is mandatory, at the same time preservation of blood supply through the adjacent mesosalpinx is desirable to minimize the "post-ligation" abnormalities that have been attributed to tubal sterilization. The Parkland technic (Fig. 40-12.C) does not compromise blood supply to the ovary.

Women infrequently do request to have

their fallopian tubes reunited. Restitution of tubal continuity is technically feasible, but with an unknown success rate probably of less than 50 percent and appreciable risk of tubal pregnancy. Numerous gynecologists currently are enthusiastic about attempting to reestablish tubal function through the use of microsurgery. Hopefully, this enthusiasm, coupled at the outset with glowing reports of success, will not lead women who are considering tubal sterilization to believe anything other than that tubal sterilization must be considered permanent! If there is any doubt in the mind of the recipient, the sterilization should not be done rather than holding out hope that it can probably be reversed successfully.

Hysterectomy.   In the absence of uterine or other pelvic disease, hysterectomy for sterilization at the time of cesarean section, early in the puerperium, or remote from pregnancy, is difficult to justify statistically (Barclay et al., 1976; Laros and Work, 1975). Nonetheless, for the woman who desires no more children, hysterectomy has many theoretical advantages. The only known potential of the uterus, other than to house products of conception, is to harbor disease. Unfortunately, morbidity, mortality, and the cost of hysterectomy, compared to tubal sterilization, often preclude hysterectomy. With cesarean hysterectomy, blood loss is nearly always greater than with cesarean section plus tubal sterilization, leading to much more frequent use of blood transfusion and its sequelae. Injury to the urinary tract is also appreciably more common. For reasons that are hard to define, an increased failure rate for sterilization at the time of cesarean section has been observed by some. With the technic for tubal sterilization described above, however, no difference has been identified at Parkland Memorial Hospital (Husbands et al., 1970).

The extensive experiences of Barclay and associates (1976) should aid in the decision whether to perform a cesarean hysterectomy rather than a cesarean section and tubal sterilization:

Each surgeon, on the basis of his own surgical experience and these and other data, must decide in conjunction with each patient the best method of sterilization or treatment of uterine pathology at the time of elective cesarean section. Approximately 20 percent of patients undergoing cesarean hysterectomy will require one or more blood transfusions. Five to ten percent of patients will receive a unilateral oophorectomy for bleeding from the ovarian pedicle. A few patients will bleed excessively during the operative procedure and approximately 4 percent will develop a cuff hematoma or intraperitoneal bleeding although the latter will occur in only 2 percent of patients. The operating time will be increased by less than 30 minutes. The mean postoperative stay should not be prolonged beyond one day. Approximately one third of patients will develop postoperative febrile morbidity; however, this is also true after elective cesarean section. Perhaps 2 percent of patients will be readmitted to the hospital for treatment of a vaginal cuff infection or hematoma or for vaginal bleeding. An occasional vesicovaginal fistula is probably unavoidable. A ureteral injury should not occur; however, in instances of severe operative hemorrhage, damage is possible. The surgeon should be prepared to repair bladder lacerations which will occur in approximately 2 to 4 percent of patients, and to identify the ureter with certainty during the operation.

Hysteroscopy.   Sterilization   utilizing *hysteroscopy* to visualize the tubal ostia and somehow obliterate them is a worthy goal that has received considerable attention. To date, the failure rate and other problems limit the clinical utility of this approach.

Vasectomy.   Sterilization of the male has emerged as a popular form of family planning, especially among socioeconomically more priviledged, white couples. Through a small incision in the scrotum, the lumen of the vas deferens is disrupted in some way to block the passage of sperm from the testes (Fig. 40-14). The procedure is usually performed in 20 minutes or so on an outpatient

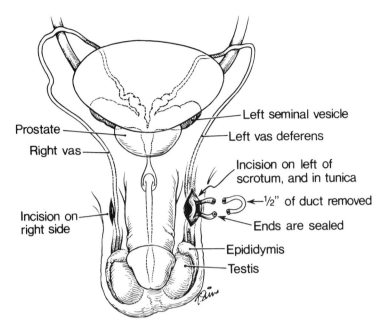

FIG. 40-14. Male reproductive system showing the site of vasectomy.

basis under local anesthesia. The procedure is less expensive than female sterilization.

A major disadvantage of vasectomy is that sterility is not immediate. Complete expulsion of sperm stored in the reproductive tract beyond the interrupted vas deferens may take a week to several months. The time appears to depend in part on the frequency of ejaculation. Semen should be checked until two consecutive sperm counts are negative. During this period, another form of contraception must be used. The failure rate for vasectomy is estimated to be about 1 in 100 (Population Reports, Jan., 1975).

Restoration of fertility after a successful vasectomy has been only partially successful. Even though the reappearance of sperm after reanastomoses has been described in from 40 to as high as 90 percent of men, functional success, i.e., the likelihood of a successful pregnancy, is appreciably lower. Three factors that appear to be important in restoration of fertility after previous vasectomy are: (1) the application of meticulous microsurgical technics for reanastomosis, (2) the length of time after vasectomy since chronic obstruc-

tion of the vas and possibly the development of sperm antibodies reduce progressively the capacity for spermatogenesis, and (3) the presence or absence of sperm granulomas (Silber, 1978).

Long-term storage of semen collected before vasectomy remains an experimental procedure. The cost of storing frozen semen is high, the availability of facilities is limited, and the results remain uncertain (Beck, 1978).

Sperm antibodies can be identified rather often after vasectomy. Concern remains over the possibility that the immune response may cause systemic changes of a harmful nature. To date, however, no such harm has been delineated (Lepow, Crozier, 1979).

REFERENCES

Ahlgren M: Sperm transport to and survival in the human fallopian tube. Gynecol Invest 6:206, 1975

Alkjaersig N, Fletcher A, Burstein R: Association between oral contraceptive use and thromboembolism: a new approach to its investigation based on plasma fibrinogen chromatography. Am J Obstet Gynecol 122:199, 1975

Antoniades K, Campbell WN, Hecksher RH, Kessler WB, McCarthy GE Jr: Liver cell adenoma and oral contraceptives. JAMA 234:628, 1975

Badaracco MA, Vessey MP: Recurrence of venous thromboembolic disease and use of oral contraceptives. Br Med J 1:215, 1974

Barclay DL, Hawks BL, Frueh DM, Power JD, Struble RH: Elective cesarean hysterectomy: a five year comparison with cesarean section. Am J Obstet Gynecol 124:900, 1976

Barlow D: The condom and gonorrhea. Lancet 2:811, 1977

Beck WW Jr: Artificial insemination and preservation of semen. Urol Clin North Am 5:593, 1978

Boston Collaborative Drug Surveillance Program. Oral contraceptives and venous thromboembolic disease, surgically confirmed gall bladder disease, and breast tumors. Lancet 1:399, 1973

Casagrande JT, Pike MC, Ross RK, Louie EW, Roy S, Henderson BE: "Incessant ovulation" and ovarian cancer. Lancet 2:170, 1979

Cheng MCE, Lim YC, Ng AYH, Ratnam SS: Six-monthly Depo-Provera injection as a contraceptive agent: its acceptability in Singapore. Aust NZ J Obstet Gynaecol 14:231, 1974

Cheng MCE, Khew KS, Chen C, Ratnam SS, Seng KM, Tarr WK: Culdoscopic ligation as an outpatient procedure. Am J Obstet Gynecol 122:109, 1975

Collaborative Group for Study of Stroke in Young Women: Oral contraceptives and stroke in young women. JAMA 231:718, 1975

Crist T: Post-coital estrogen. J Reprod Med 13:198, 1974

Dawood MY, Birnbaum SJ: Unilateral tubo-ovarian abscess and intrauterine contraceptive device. Obstet Gynecol 46:429, 1975

Fisch IR, Frank J: Oral contraceptives and blood pressure. JAMA 237:2499, 1977

Francis WJA: Reproduction at menarche and menopause in women. J Reprod Fertil suppl 12:89, 1970

Goldzieher JW, Rudel HW: How the oral contraceptives came to be developed. JAMA 230:421, 1974

Greenblatt DJ, Koch-Wesser J: Oral contraceptives and hypertension. Obstet Gynecol 44:412, 1974

Guttorm E: Menstrual bleeding with intrauterine contraceptive devices. Acta Obstet Gynecol Scand 50:9, 1971

Harlap S, Prywes R, Davies AM: Birth defects and oestrogens and progesterones in pregnancy. Lancet 1:682, 1975

Husbands ME Jr, Pritchard JA, Pritchard SA: Failure of tubal sterilization accompanying cesarean section. Am J Obstet Gynecol 107:966, 1970

Inman WHW, Vessey MP, Westerholm B, Engelund A: Thromboembolic disease and steroidal content of oral contraceptives. Br Med J 2:203, 1970

Irey NS, Nanion WC, Taylor HB: Vascular lesions in women taking oral contraceptives. Arch Pathol 89:1, 1970

Janevich DT, Piper JM, Glebatis DM: Oral contraceptives and congenital limb reduction defects. N Engl J Med 291:697, 1974

Javitt NB, Panveliwalla D, Morrissey K: Ethinyl estradiol: long term effects on bile acid metabolism in the baboon. Clin Res 23:439A, 1975

Kahn HS, Tyler CW Jr: Mortality associated with use of IUD's. JAMA 234:57, 1975

Kasonde JM, Bonnar J: Effect of sterilization on menstrual blood loss. Br J Obstet Gynaecol 83:572, 1976

Kay CR: Oral contraceptives and venous thrombosis. Lancet 1:1381, 1975

Kent DR, Nissen ED, Nissen SE, Ziehm DJ: Effect of pregnancy on liver tumor associated with oral contraceptives. Obstet Gynecol 51:148, 1978

Kroener WF Jr: Surgical sterilization by fimbriectomy. Am J Obstet Gynecol 104:247, 1969

Kuchara LK: Postcoital contraception with diethylstilbestrol. JAMA 218:562, 1971

Lambe RF, Werner-Zodrow I, Darragh A, Mall-Häfeli M: Contraceptive properties of luteinising hormone releasing hormone. Lancet 2:801, 1979

Laros RK Jr, Work BA Jr: Female sterilization. III. Vaginal hysterectomy. Am J Obstet Gynecol 122:693, 1975

Laros RK Jr, Zatuchni GI, Andros GJ: Puerperal tubal ligation morbidity, histology, and bacteriology. Obstet Gynecol 41:397, 1973

Larrson-Cohn U: Oral contraceptives and vitamins: a review. Am J Obstet Gynecol 121:84, 1975

Leklem JE, Brown RR, Rose DP, Linkswiler HM: Vitamin B$_6$ requirements of women using oral contraceptives. Am J Clin Nutrit 28:535, 1975

Lepow IH, Crozier R (eds): Summary and conclusions. In Vasectomy: Immunologic and Pathophysiologic Effects in Animals and man. New York, Academic, p. 581, 1979

Lippes J, Tatum HJ, Maulid D, Zielezny M: A continuation of the study of postcoital IUDs. Paper presented at the annual meeting of the Association of Planned Parenthood Physicians, San Diego, Oct. 25, 1978

Mann JI, Inman WHW: Oral contraceptives and death from myocardial infarction. Br Med J 2:245, 1975

Mastroianni L Jr: Rhythm: Systematized chance-taking. Fam Plann Perspect 6:209, 1974

McCausland A: High rate of ectopic pregnancy following laparoscopic tubal coagulation failures. Am J Obstet Gynecol 136:97, 1980

Metcalf MG: Incidence of ovulatory cycles in women approaching the menopause. J Biosoc Sci 11:39, 1979

Metcalf MG, Donald RA: Fluctuating ovarian function in a perimenopausal woman. Aust NZ Med J 89:45, 1979

Metz KGP: Failures following fimbriectomy. Fertil Steril 28:66, 1977

Miale JB, Kent JW: The effects of oral contraceptives on the results of laboratory tests. Am J Obstet Gynecol 120:264, 1974

Mishell DR Jr: Progress report: DMPA for contraception. Contemp Ob/Gyn 3:15, 1973

Myatt L, Bray MA, Gordon D, Morley J: Macrophages on intrauterine contraceptive devices produce prostaglandins. Nature 257:227, 1975

Nilsson L, Sölvell L: Clinical studies on oral contraceptives. Acta Obstet Gynecol Scand Suppl 8:46, 1967

Nora AH, Nora JJ: A syndrome of multiple congenital anomalies associated with teratogenic exposure. Arch Environ Health 30:17, 1975

Peel J, Potts M: Textbooks of Contraceptive Practice. New York, Cambridge University Press, 1969

Perlmutter JF: Experience with the Dalkon Shield as a contraceptive device. Obstet Gynecol 43:443, 1974

Phillips N, Duffy T: One-hour glucose tolerance in relation to the use of contraceptive drugs. Am J Obstet Gynecol 116:91, 1973

Population Reports. Periodic abstinence. Series I, No. 1, June 1974

Population Reports. Injectables and implants. Series K, No 1, March 1975

Population Reports. Vasectomy—What are the problems? Series D, No 1, Jan, 1975

Population Reports. Barrier Methods. Jan, 1976

Population Reports. OC's—Update on usage, safety, and side-effects. Jan, 1979, p A-133

Population Reports. IUD's—Update on safety, effectiveness, and research. May, 1979

Prasad AS, Lei KY, Moghissi KS: The effect of oral contraceptives on micronutrients. In Mosely WH (ed): Nutrition and Human Reproduction. New York, Plenum Press, 1978

Pritchard JA, Pritchard SA: Blood pressure response to estrogen-progestin oral contraceptive after pregnancy-induced hypertension. Am J Obstet Gynecol 129:733, 1977

Pritchard JA, Scott DE, Whalley PJ: Maternal folate deficiency and pregnancy wastage: IV. Effects of folic acid supplements, anticonvulsants, and oral contraceptives. Am J Obstet Gynecol 109:341, 1971

Purrier BGA, Sparks RA, Watt PJ, Elstein M: In vitro study of the possible role of the intrauterine contraceptive device tail in ascending infection of the genital tract. Br J Obstet Gynaecol 86:374, 1979

Rothman KJ, Louik C: Oral contraceptives and birth defects. N Engl J Med 299:522, 1978

Sagiroglu N: Local effects of polyethylene IUD's in women. Third International Conference on Intrauterine Contraception. Cairo, Egypt, Dec. 12–14, 1974

Schwallie PC: Experience with Depo-Provera as an injectable contraceptive. J Reprod Med 13:113, 1974

Scott DE, Pritchard JA: Hematologic effects of oral contraceptives after megaloblastic anemia in pregnancy. Gynecol Invest 6:40, 1975

Shine RM, Thompson JF: The in situ IUD and pregnancy outcome. Am J Obstet Gynecol 119:124, 1974

Shojania AM, Hornaday G, Barnes PH: Oral contraceptives and serum-folate levels. Lancet 1:1376, 1968

Silber SJ: Vasectomy and its microsurgical reversal. Urol Clin North Am 5:573, 1978

Silverberg SG, Makowski EL: Endometrial carcinoma in young women taking oral contraceptive agents. Obstet Gynecol 46:503, 1975

Spellacy WN, Buhi WC, Birk SA: The effects of vitamin B$_6$ on carbohydrate metabolism in women taking steroid contraceptives: preliminary report. Contraception 6:265, 1972

Stephens MEM, Craft I, Peters TJ, Hoffbrand AV: Oral contraceptives and folate metabolism. Clin Sci 42:405, 1972

Stock RJ: Evaluation of sequelae of tubal ligation. Fertil Steril 29:169, 1978

Streiff RR: Folate deficiency and oral contraceptives. JAMA 214:105, 1970

Szlachter BN, Nachtigall LE, Epstein J, Young BK, Weiss G: Premature menopause: a reversible entity? Obstet Gynecol 54:396, 1979

Tatum HJ: Copper-bearing intrauterine devices. Clin Obstet Gynecol 17:93, 1974a

Tatum HJ: Putting IUD's in perspective. Contemp Ob/Gyn 4:134, 1974b

Tatum HJ, Schmidt FH, Jain AK: Management and outcome of pregnancies associated with Copper-T intrauterine contraceptive device. Am J Obstet Gynecol 126:869, 1976

Taylor ES: Editorial comment. Obstet Gynecol Surv 27:168, 1972

Taylor ES, McMillan JH, Greer BE, Droegemueller W, Thompson HE: The intrauterine device and tubo-ovarian abscess. Am J Obstet Gynecol 123:338, 1975

Taylor WW, Martin FG, Pritchard SA, Pritchard JA: Complications from Majzlin spring intrauterine device. Obstet Gynecol 41:404, 1973

Theur RC: The effect of oral contraceptive agents on vitamin and mineral needs: a review. J Reprod Med 3:13, 1972

Thompson BH, Wheeless CR: Failures of laparoscopic sterilization. Obstet Gynecol 45:659, 1975

Tredway DR, Umezaki CU, Mishell DR Jr, Settlage DS: Effect of intrauterine devices on sperm transport in the human being: preliminary report. Am J Obstet Gynecol 123:734, 1975

Veltman LL, Marshall JR: Comparison of operative morbidity in abortion-sterilization procedures. Am J Obstet Gynecol 117:251, 1973

Vessey MP: Thromboembolism, cancer, and oral contraceptives. Clin Obstet Gynecol 17:65, 1974

Vessey MP, Doll R, Jones K: Oral contraceptives and breast cancer. Lancet 1:941, 1975

Vessey MP, Doll R, Jones K, McPherson K, Yeates D: An epidemiological study of oral contraceptives and breast cancer. Br Med J 1:1757, 1979

Vessey MP, Meisler L, Flavel R, Yeates D: Outcome of pregnancy in women using different methods of contraception. Br J Obstet Gynaecol 86:548, 1979

Vessey MP, Yeates D, Flavel R: Risk of ectopic pregnancy and duration of use of an intrauterine device. Lancet 2:501, 1979

Vessey MP, Wiggins P: Use-effectiveness of the diaphragm in a selected family planning clinic population in the United Kingdom. Contraception 9:15, 1974

Wallace RB, Hoover J, Barrett-Connor E, Rifkind BM, Hunninhake DB, Macenthun A, Heiss G: Altered plasma lipid and lipoprotein levels associated with oral contraceptive and oestrogen use. Lancet 2:111, 1979

Weinberger MH: Oral contraceptives and hypertension. Hosp Practice 10:65, 1975

Wingrave SJ, Kay CR, Vessey MP: Oral contraceptives and diabetes mellitus. Br Med J 1:23, 1979

Wynn R, Sawaragi I: Effects of intrauterine and oral contraceptives on the ultrastructure of human endometrium. J Reprod Fertil (Suppl) 8:45, 1969

Wynn V: Vitamins and oral contraceptive use. Lancet 1:561, 1975

Yoon IB, Poliakoff SR: Laparoscopic tubal ligation: A follow-up report on the Yoon falope ring methodology. J Reprod Med 23:76, 1979

Yuzpe AA, Anderson RJ, Cohen NP, West JL: A review of 1,035 tubal sterilizations by posterior colpotomy under local anesthesia or by laparoscopy. J Reprod Med 13:106, 1974

Zipper J, Medel M, Prager R: Suppression of fertility by intrauterine copper and zinc in rabbits. Am J Obstet Gynecol 105:529, 1969

Zipper JA, Tatum JH, Medel M, Pastene L, Rivera M: Contraception through the use of intrauterine metals: I. Copper as an adjunct to the T device. Am J Obstet Gynecol 109:771, 1971

41

Forceps Delivery and Related Technics

Obstetric forceps are designed for extraction of the fetus. The intriguing history of the early development and use of these instruments is presented at the end of this chapter.

GENERAL DESIGN

Forceps vary considerably in size and shape but consist basically of two crossing *branches* that are introduced separately into the vagina. Each branch is maneuvered into appropriate relationship with the fetal head and then articulated. Basically, each branch has four components. These are the *blade,* the *shank,* the *lock,* and the *handle.* Each blade has two curves, the *cephalic* and the *pelvic.* The cephalic curve conforms to the shape of the fetal head and the pelvic curve with that of the birth canal. The blades are oval to elliptical in outline and some varieties are fenestrated rather than solid to permit a more firm hold on the head.

The cephalic curve (Fig. 41-1) should be large enough to grasp the fetal head firmly without compression, but not so large that the instrument slips. The pelvic curve (Fig. 41-1) corresponds more or less to the axis of the birth canal, but varies considerably among different instruments. The blades are connected to the handles by the shanks, which give the requisite length to the instrument.

The kind of articulation, or *forceps lock,* varies among different instruments. The common method of articulation consists of a socket located on the shank at the junction with the handle and into which fits a socket similarly located on the opposite shank (Figs. 41-1, 41-2). This form of articulation is commonly referred to as the *English lock.* A *sliding lock* is used in some forceps, for example, Kielland forceps (Fig. 41-3) and Barton forceps in which a single U-shaped receptacle mounted midway on the left shank accepts the shank of the right branch. The sliding lock allows the shanks to move forward and backward independently. The components of a quite different type of lock, the *French lock,* are a threaded eye bolt screwed partway into a threaded hole in the left shank and a notch in the right shank that articulates with the eye bolt. After each branch has been applied to the fetal head, the notch is moved over the stem of the eye bolt and the eye bolt is tight-

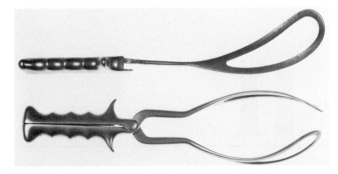

FIG. 41-1. Simpson forceps. Note the ample pelvic curve in the single blade above and cephalic curve evident in the articulated blades below. The fenestrated blade and the wide shank in front of the English style lock characterize the Simpson forceps.

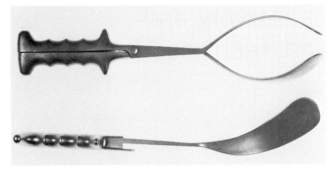

FIG. 41-2. Tucker-McLane forceps. The blade is solid and the shank is narrow.

ened to lock the branches firmly together. With one style, the Tarnier forceps (Fig. 41-4), there is included behind the French lock a hinged bolt with a wing nut mounted on one branch that, after the forceps are locked, is depressed medially into a U-shaped receiver mounted on the opposite shank. As the wing nut is tightened against the receiver, both blades of the forceps are forced against the fetal head. Use of Tarnier forceps was abandoned at Parkland Memorial Hospital long ago for obvious reasons.

DEFINITIONS AND CLASSIFICATION

Forceps operations on a fetus presenting by the vertex are classified as follows, according to the level and position of the head in the birth canal at the time the blades are applied:

Low forceps (outlet forceps) operations are those in which the instrument is applied after the fetal head has reached the perineal floor, the sagittal suture is in the anteroposterior diameter of the outlet, and scalp is visible at the vaginal introitus.

Midforceps operations are those in which forceps are applied before the criteria for low forceps are met but after engagement of the fetal head has taken place. Clinical evidence of engagement is usually afforded by the descent of the lowermost part of the skull to or below the level of the ischial spines, since the distance between the level of the ischial spines and the pelvic inlet ordinarily is greater than the distance from the biparietal diameter to the leading part of the fetal head (see Chap. 11, p. 282). Especially after vigorous labor, elongation of the fetal head from the combination of a marked degree of molding and caput formation will create the erroneous impression that the head is engaged even though the biparietal diameter has not passed through the pelvic inlet (see Chap. 31, p. 834).

The definition of midforceps as stated includes many levels of the fetal head and, therefore, a range of difficulty. For this reason, Dennen (1964) and some others subdivided midforceps operations as follows: A *midforceps delivery* is one performed when the leading bony portion of the head is at or just below the level of the ischial spines, with

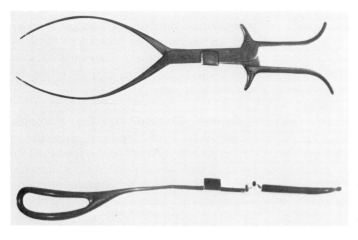

FIG. 41-3. Kielland forceps. The characteristic features are the sliding lock, a minimal pelvic curvature, and light weight.

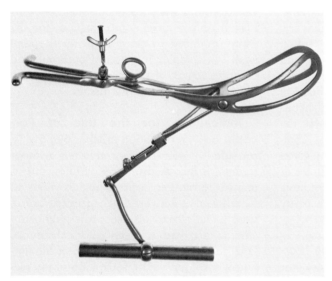

FIG. 41-4. Tarnier forceps and axis traction handle. The characteristic features are the French lock, the wing nut (which when dropped in place and tightened can apply excessive pressure against the fetal head), and the traction handle. These forceps have been used to effect vaginal delivery even in the presence of cephalopelvic disproportion. Trauma to fetus and mother, however, was a common result.

the biparietal diameter through the pelvic inlet; the head nearly fills the hollow of the sacrum. A *low midforceps delivery* is one performed when the biparietal diameter is at or below the level of the ischial spines and the leading part is within a finger's breadth of the perineum between contractions; the head fills the hollow of the sacrum.

The danger of trauma to the fetus and the mother from a so-called low midforceps delivery will vary remarkably depending upon circumstances that precede delivery. At times, the fetal head, as the consequence of appropriate uterine contractions and voluntary expulsive efforts of the mother, will descend to lie firmly against the perineum with the sagittal suture anteroposterior, yet subsequent to anesthesia for delivery, the fetal head recedes somewhat from the perineum and the sagittal suture reverts to an oblique position. Forceps delivery with episiotomy in this circumstance is very likely to be a benign procedure. On the other hand, if the fetal head has never reached the perineum and the sagittal suture has never achieved the anteroposterior position, so-called low midforceps delivery may prove traumatic to fetus, mother, or both. Forceps delivery in this latter situation should really be classified as a midforceps delivery.

High forceps operations are those in which forceps are applied before engagement has taken place. High forceps delivery has no place in modern obstetrics.

Incidence.   During much of the first half of this century, polarization of opinions over the use of forceps in obstetrics resulted in two very distinct schools of thought. One school vigorously maintained that forceps delivery should be accomplished as soon as the fetal head was engaged and the cervix fully dilated (or, at times, dilatable). The other contended with equal vigor that spontaneous delivery should be awaited. Subsequently, in objective analyses of outcomes it has been demonstrated repeatedly that increased perinatal morbidity and mortality and maternal morbidity result from midforceps delivery. Moreover, for reasons presented subsequently, there may be less perinatal and maternal morbidity with truly low forceps (outlet forceps) delivery and an adequate episiotomy compared to delayed spontaneous delivery without episiotomy. In general, the incidence of low forceps operations compared to spontaneous deliveries in any given institution will depend upon the attitude of the staff, the kinds of analgesia and anesthesia used for labor and delivery, and the parity of the obstetric population.

Functions and Choice of the Forceps.   The forceps may be used as a tractor or a rotator, or both. Its most important function is traction, although, particularly in transverse and posterior positions of the occiput, forceps may be employed successfully for rotation. Any properly shaped instrument will give satisfactory results, provided it is used intelligently. For general purposes, either Simpson or Tucker-McLane forceps are quite useful. In some circumstances, more specialized forceps may be preferable, for example, in some cases of *deep transverse arrest.* (When the progress of labor ceases with the fetal head in the transverse position, well down in the pelvis with the occiput below the spines, the situation is referred to as deep transverse arrest.) If there is no cephalopelvic disproportion, transverse arrest may be overcome with oxytocin stimulation, with resulting descent of the head to the perineum and

spontaneous anterior rotation. *If, however, there are indications for prompt delivery, as in instances of fetal distress, but easy vaginal delivery with no delay cannot be anticipated, cesarean section should be used.*

Forces Exerted by the Forceps. Obstetricians have long been interested in the forces extended by the forceps blades on the fetal skull and maternal tissues. If excessive, these forces can damage both the woman and her fetus. From experiments conducted on women in labor many years ago, Joulin (1867) estimated that a pull in excess of 60 kg might damage the fetal skull. These crude studies and subsequent ones have furnished only a gross approximation, for the force produced by the forceps on the fetal skull is a complex function of both pull and compression by the forceps and of friction produced by the maternal tissues.

Indications for the Use of Forceps.   The termination of labor by forceps, provided it can be accomplished without trauma, is indicated in any condition threatening the mother or fetus that is likely to be relieved by delivery. Such maternal indications include heart disease, acute pulmonary edema, intrapartum infection, or exhaustion. Fetal indications include prolapse of the umbilical cord, premature separation of the placenta, and abnormalities in fetal heart rate indicative of fetal distress.

Elective Low Forceps.   The vast majority of forceps operations performed in this country today are elective low forceps. One reason is that all methods of drug-induced analgesia, and especially conduction analgesia and anesthesia, often interfere with the woman's voluntary expulsive efforts, in which circumstances low forceps delivery becomes the most reasonable procedure.

The fact that the methods employed to relieve pain frequently necessitate forceps delivery is not an indictment of the procedures, provided the obstetrician adheres strictly to the definition of low forceps. The fetal head must be on the perineal floor with the sagittal suture anteroposterior. In these circumstances, forceps delivery preceded by episiotomy is a simple and safe operation requiring only gentle traction. By allowing the woman in labor ample time, the criteria for low forceps can usually be met despite the effects of analgesia. However, if the head does not descend and rotate, any forceps operations performed is not a low forceps but rather a midforceps operation. Although midforceps operations, especially those in which anterior rotation is the only criterion of low forceps not met, may occasionally be easy in expert hands, in general, the head is higher before rotation and more traction is usually required. For maximal safety of both mother and fetus, therefore, forceps should not be used *electively* until the criteria of a low forceps operation, as here defined, are fulfilled.

In a minority of nulliparous women, marked resistance of the perineum and the vaginal introitus may sometimes present a serious obstacle to the passage of the fetus, even when the expulsive forces are normal. In such cases, an episiotomy and outlet forceps delivery are beneficial to mother and fetus. Prolonged pressure of the fetal head against a rigid perineum sometimes results in injury to the brain. To prevent cerebral injury and to spare the mother the strain of the last minutes of the second stage, DeLee (1920) recommended the "prophylactic forceps operation," more commonly called "elective low forceps," on the grounds that the obstetrician elects to interfere knowing that it is not absolutely necessary, for spontaneous delivery may normally be expected within approximately 15 minutes.

PREREQUISITES FOR APPLICATION OF FORCEPS

1. *The head must be engaged and preferably deeply engaged.* Application of the blades before engagement, that is, high forceps, is an extremely difficult operation, often entailing brutal trauma to the maternal tissues and death of a large proportion of the babies. Many years ago, when cesarean section was also a highly dangerous operation, high forceps had a certain place in operative obstetrics. High forceps is rarely employed today, however, and is mentioned here only to condemn it. Even after engagement occurs, the higher the station of the fetal head, the more difficult and traumatic the forceps delivery becomes. Whenever the blades are applied before the head has reached the perineal floor, moreover, it is common to find the head decidedly higher than was believed to be the case from the findings of vaginal examination. This obtains because of extensive caput succedaneum formation and molding. These difficulties of midforceps operation obtain even in the presence of a valid maternal indication for forceps delivery. For instance, it is generally agreed that women with heart disease should be spared, as much as safely possible, the effort of bearing down during the second stage of labor. Such efforts, however, may be much less harmful than a difficult midforceps delivery. Therefore, forceps should not be used until the station of the head is low enough to assure a nontraumatic operative procedure. The same generalization applies to forceps for fetal distress when the head is not close to the perineal floor. Granted that the fetal heart rate in such a case may suggest that the infant is hypoxic, it may still be judicious to allow more time for the head to descend rather than to superimpose the trauma of a difficult midforceps operation on an already distressed infant. If delivery is mandatory, cesarean section is preferable to a difficult and damaging forceps operation.

2. *The fetus must present either by the vertex or by the face with the chin anterior.* The use of forceps is not applicable, of course, to transverse lies (shoulder presentation) nor is it intended for the breech.

3. *The position of the head must be precisely known so that the forceps can be appropriately applied to the fetal head.*

4. *The cervix must be completely dilated before the application of forceps.* Even a small rim of cervix may offer great resistance when traction is applied, causing extensive cervi-

cal lacerations that may reach the lower uterine segment. If prompt delivery becomes imperative before complete dilatation of the cervix, cesarean section is preferable.

5. *Before forceps application, the membranes must be ruptured to permit a firm grasp of the head by the blades of the forceps.*

6. *There should be no disproportion between the size of the head and that of the midpelvis or the outlet.* Since forceps should not be employed until after the head has passed through the pelvic inlet, contraction at the

pelvic inlet as a contraindication to forceps is not pertinent to present-day practices.

TECHNIC OF FORCEPS DELIVERY

Preparations for Operation. In the absence of previously instituted adequate continuous conduction anesthesia, a decision as to the type of anesthesia is made based on factors considered especially in Chapter 18. Pudendal block is not likely to provide sufficient anesthesia for forceps delivery. If spinal

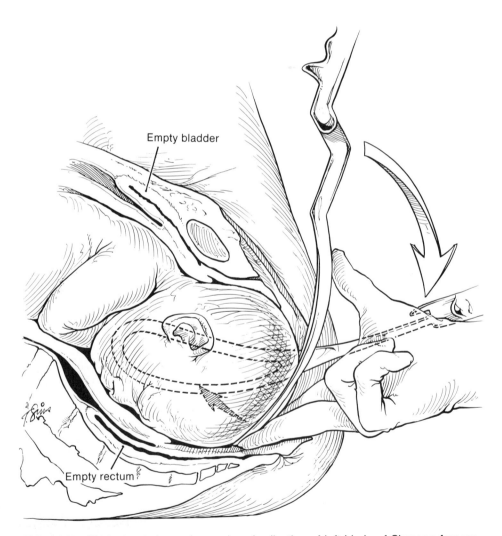

FIG. 41-5. Occiput anterior and crowning. Application of left blade of Simpson forceps. The right blade is next applied and the blades are articulated.

or epidural anesthesia is to be used, the anesthetic agent is introduced before placing the woman in the lithotomy position for delivery. If general anesthesia is to be used, the woman is placed in the lithotomy position, the pudenda are scrubbed and draped, and the obstetrician is ready to perform the forceps delivery before administering the anesthetic.

The woman's buttocks should be brought to the edge of the delivery table, and her legs held in position by appropriate stirrups. The woman is scrubbed and draped as described in Chapter 17, (p. 416). The bladder should be emptied by catheterization if a midforceps delivery is planned.

Application of Forceps.   Forceps are constructed so that their cephalic curve is closely adapted to the sides of the fetal head

(Fig. 41-5). The biparietal diameter of the fetal head corresponds to the greatest distance between the appropriately applied blades. Consequently, the head of the fetus is perfectly grasped only when the long axis of the blades corresponds to the occipitomental diameter, with the tips of the blades lying over the cheeks, while the concave margins of the blades are directed toward either the sagittal suture (occiput anterior position) or the face (occiput posterior position). Thus applied, the forceps should not slip, and traction may be applied most advantageously as illustrated in Figure 41-6. When forceps are applied obliquely, however, with one blade over the brow and the other over the opposite mastoid region, the grasp is less secure, and the fetal head is exposed to injurious pressure (Fig. 41-7). With most forceps, if

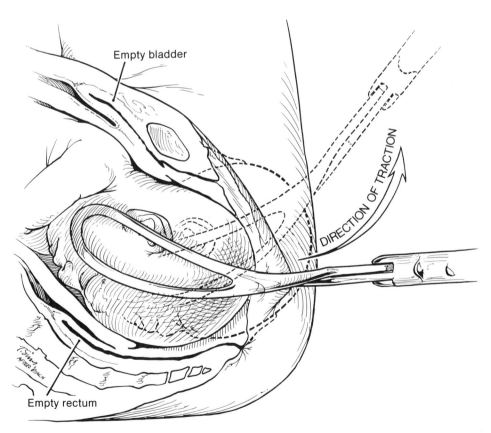

FIG. 41-6.   Occiput anterior. Delivery by low forceps (Simpson). The direction of gentle traction for delivering of the head is indicated.

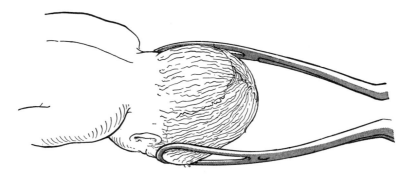

FIG. 41-7. INCORRECT application of forceps over brow and mastoid region.

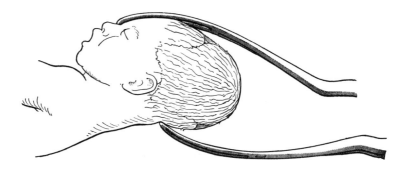

FIG. 41-8. INCORRECT application of forceps, one blade over occiput and the other over the brow. Note that the forceps cannot be locked.

one blade is applied over the brow and the other over the occiput, the instrument cannot be locked (Fig. 41-8), or, if locked, the blades slip off when traction is applied (Fig. 41-9) causing appreciable trauma. For these reasons, the forceps must be applied directly to the sides of the head along the *occipitomental diameter,* in what is termed the cephalic, biparietal, or bimalar application.

Identification of Position. Precise knowledge of the exact position of the fetal head is essential to a proper cephalic application. With the head low down in the pelvis, diagnosis of position is made by examination of the sagittal suture and the fontanels, but when it is at a higher station, an absolute diagnosis can be made by locating the posterior ear.

The term *pelvic application* is employed when the left blade is applied to the left and

right blade to the right side of the woman's pelvis, irrespective of the position of the fetal head. It follows that the head is grasped satisfactorily only when the sagittal suture happens to be directed anteroposteriorly. Pelvic application is likely to be injurious to the fetus and should not be practiced.

LOW FORCEPS. Delivery by low forceps is illustrated in Figures 41-10 through 41-18. With the head at the low station required in the definition of low forceps, the obstacle to delivery is usually insufficient expulsive forces, appreciable resistance of the perineum, or both. In such circumstances, the sagittal suture occupies the anteroposterior diameter of the pelvic outlet, with the small (posterior) fontanel directed toward either the symphysis pubis or the concavity of the sacrum. In either event, the forceps, if applied to the sides of the pelvis, grasps the head

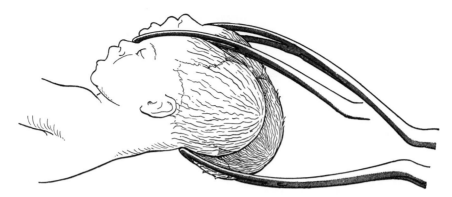

FIG. 41-9. Forceps applied INCORRECTLY as in Figure 41-8. Note extension of head and tendency of blades to slip off with traction.

ideally. The left blade is introduced into the left side of the pelvis and then the right blade into the right side of the pelvis, as follows: Two fingers of the right hand are introduced inside the left, posterior portion of the vulva into the vagina beside the fetal head. The handle of the left branch is then grasped between the thumb and two fingers of the left hand, as in holding a pen, and the tip of the blade is gently passed into the vagina between the fetal head and the palmar surface of the fingers of the right hand, which serve as a guide. The handle and branch are held at first almost vertically, but as the blade adapts itself to the fetal head, they are depressed, eventually to a horizontal position. The guiding fingers are then withdrawn, and the handle is left unsupported or held by an assistant. Similarly, two fingers of the left hand are then introduced into the right, posterior portion of the vagina to serve as a guide for the right blade, which is held in the right hand and introduced into the vagina. These guiding fingers are then withdrawn and the horizontally positioned branches are articulated, usually without difficulty. Otherwise, first one and then the other blade should be gently maneuvered until the handles are repositioned to effect easy articulation.

The application is now checked before any traction is applied. For the occiput anterior position, appropriately applied blades are equidistant from the sagittal suture. In the occiput posterior position the blades are equidistant from the midline of the face and brow. If cervical tissue has been grasped, the forceps should be loosened and, if possible, the incompletely retracted cervix pushed up over the head. When it is certain that the blades are placed satisfactorily and the cervix is not entrapped, gentle, intermittent, horizontal traction is exerted until the perineum begins to bulge. As the vulva is distended by the occiput, the handles are gradually elevated, eventually pointing almost directly upward as the parietal bones emerge. With the fetal head in the occiput anterior position, this maneuver takes advantage of the smallest diameters of the fetal head and brings the suboccipital region beneath the symphysis. As the handles are raised, the head is extended. Episiotomy is performed rarely just before application of the blades but most often when traction on the head begins to distend the perineum. During upward traction, the four fingers should grasp the upper surface of the handles and shanks, while the thumb exerts the necessary force upon their lower surface, as shown in Figure 41-17.

During birth of the head, spontaneous delivery should be simulated as closely as possible, employing minimal force. Traction should therefore be intermittent, and the head should be allowed to recede in intervals, as in spontaneous labor. Except when urgently indicated, as in fetal distress, delivery

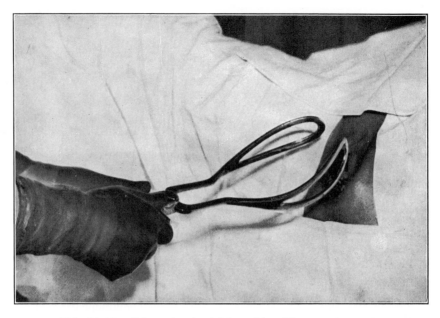

FIG. 41-10. Orientation for LOA position (Simpson forceps).

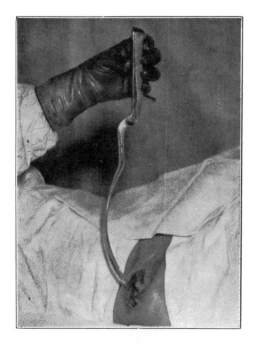

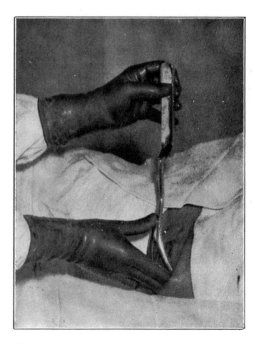

FIG. 41-11. The left handle held in the left hand. Simpson forceps.

FIG. 41-12. Introduction of left blade into left side of pelvis.

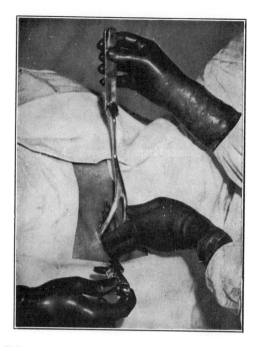

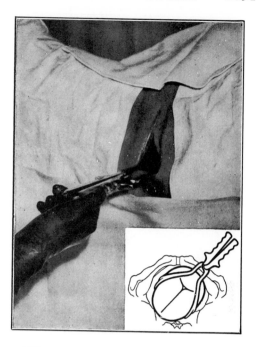

FIG. 41-13. Left blade in place; introduction of right blade by right hand.

FIG. 41-14. Forceps has been locked.

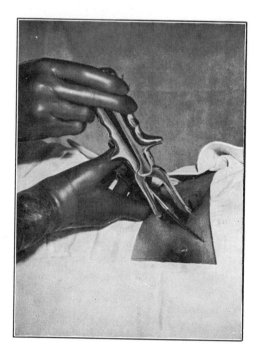

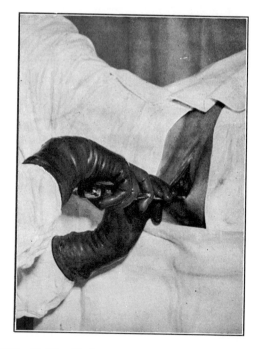

FIG. 41-15. Median or mediolateral episiotomy may be performed at this point. Left mediolateral episiotomy shown here.

FIG. 41-16. Horizontal traction; operator seated.

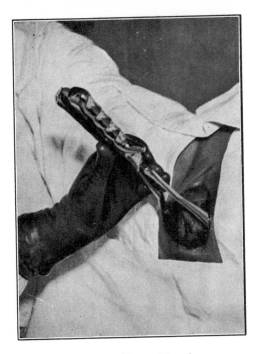

FIG. 41-17. Upward traction.

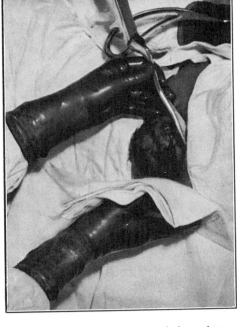

FIG. 41-18. Disarticulation of branches of forceps. Beginning modified Ritgen maneuver.

should be sufficiently slow, deliberate, and gentle to prevent undue compression of the fetal head.

After the vulva has been well distended by the head and the brow can be felt through the perineum, the delivery may be completed in several ways. Some obstetricians keep the forceps in place, in the belief that greatest control over the advance of the head is thus maintained. The thickness of the blades may at times add to the distension of the vulva, however, thus increasing the likelihood of laceration or necessitating a larger episiotomy. In such cases, the forceps are removed and delivery is completed by the modified Ritgen maneuver (Fig. 41-18), slowly expressing the head by using upward pressure upon the chin through the posterior portion of the perineum, while covering the anus with a towel to minimize contamination from the bowel. If the forceps is removed prematurely, the modified Ritgen maneuver may prove to be a tedious and inelegant procedure.

Midforceps Operations. When the head lies above the perineum, the sagittal suture usually occupies an oblique or transverse diameter of the pelvis. In such cases, the forceps should always be applied to the sides of the head. The application is best accomplished by introducing two or more fingers into the vagina to a sufficient depth to feel the posterior fetal ear, over which, whether right or left, the first blade should be applied.

Left Occiput Anterior Position. In left occiput anterior positions, the right hand, introduced into the left posterior segment of the vagina, should identify the posteriorly located left ear and at the same time serve as a guide for introduction of the left branch of the forceps, which is held in the left hand and applied over the left ear. The guiding hand is then withdrawn, and the handle is held by an assistant or left unsupported, the blade usually retaining its position without difficulty. Two fingers of the left hand are then introduced into the right posterior portion of the pelvis, but no attempt is yet made to reach the anteriorly located right ear, which lies near the right iliopectineal eminence. The right branch of the forceps, held in the right hand, is then introduced along the left hand as a guide. It must then be applied over the anterior ear of the fetus by gently sweeping the blade anteriorly until it lies directly opposite the blade that was introduced first. Of the two branches, when articulated, one occupies the posterior and the other the anterior extremity of the left oblique diameter.

Right Occiput Anterior Position.

In right positions, the blades are introduced similarly but in opposite directions, for in those cases the right ear of the fetus is the posterior ear, over which the first blade must be placed accordingly. After the blades have been applied to the sides of the head, the left handle and shank lie above the right. Consequently, the forceps does not immediately articulate. Locking of the branches is easily effected, however, by rotating the left around the right to bring the lock into proper position.

Occiput Transverse Positions.

If the occiput is in a transverse position, the forceps are introduced similarly, with the first blade applied over the posterior ear, and the second rotated anteriorly to a position opposite the first. In this case, one blade lies in front of the sacrum and the other behind the symphysis. The conventional Simpson or Tucker-McLane forceps (Figs. 41-1, 41-2) or the specialized Kielland (Fig. 41-3) or Barton forceps (Fig. 41-19) may be used.

ROTATION AND TRACTION. When the occiput is obliquely anterior, it gradually rotates spontaneously to the symphysis pubis as traction is exerted. When it is directed transversely, however, in order to bring it anteriorly a rotary motion of the forceps is required. The direction of rotation, of course, varies with the position of the occiput. Rotation from the left side toward the midline is required when the occiput is directed toward the left, and in the reverse direction when it is directed toward the right side of the pelvis. In infrequent circumstances, particularly when the Barton forceps is used in transverse positions in anteroposteriorly flattened (platypelloid) pelves, rotation should not be attempted until the fetal head has reached or approached the pelvic floor. Premature attempts at anterior rotation under such conditions may result in injury to the fetus and maternal soft parts. Regardless of the original position of the head, delivery is effected eventually by exerting traction downward until the occiput appears at the vulva; the rest of the operation is completed as described.

In exerting traction before the head appears at the vulva, one or both hands may be employed. To avoid excessive force, the operator should sit with his arms flexed and elbows held closely against the thorax, since the obstetrician's body weight must not be applied.

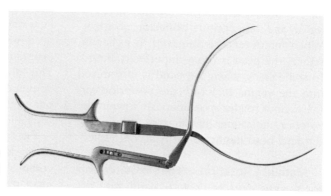

FIG. 41-19. Barton forceps. The characteristic features are the sliding lock and one hinged blade.

A

B

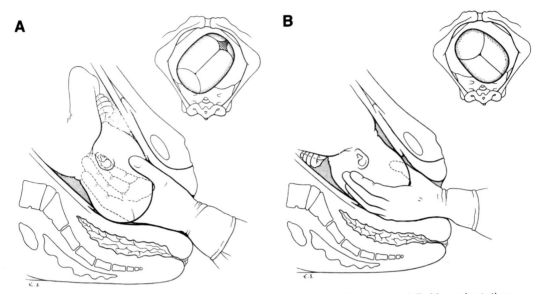

FIG. 41-20. **A.** Manual rotation; left hand in position grasping the head. **B.** Manual rotation accomplished to ROA. (Both A and B from Douglas and Stromme. Operative Obstetrics, 3rd ed., New York, Appleton, 1976.)

It is reemphasized that the possibility of serious trauma to the mother, and especially the fetus, must be kept in mind whenever midforceps delivery is considered. The remote fetal effects may be subtle. For example, Friedman and associates (1977) found that the mean IQ scores of 4-year old children who were delivered by midforceps was somewhat lower than the scores of those who were delivered spontaneously or by low forceps.

Use of Forceps in Obliquely Posterior Positions.   Prompt delivery may at times become necessary when the small (occipital) fontanel is directed toward one of the sacroiliac synchrondroses, i.e., in right occiput posterior and left occiput posterior positions. When interference is required in either instance, the head is often imperfectly flexed. In some cases, when the hand is introduced into the vagina to locate the posterior ear, the occiput rotates spontaneously toward the anterior indicating that manual rotation of the fetal head might be easily accomplished.

Manual Rotation.   The requirements for forceps must be met. A hand with the palm upward is inserted into the vagina and the fingers are brought in contact with that side of the fetal head which is to be pushed toward the anterior position while the thumb is placed over the opposite side of the head (Figs. 41-20. A, B). With the occiput in a right posterior position, the left hand is used to rotate the occiput anteriorly in a clockwise direction; the right hand is used for the left occiput posterior position. At the beginning of the rotation, it may be helpful to dislodge the head *slightly* upward in the birth canal but the head must not be disengaged. After the occiput has reached the anterior position, labor may be allowed to continue or, more commonly, forceps is used to effect delivery. First one blade is applied to that side of the head which is held by the fingers to help maintain the occiput in the anterior position. The other blade is immediately applied and delivery accomplished as described for occiput anterior forceps delivery.

Forceps Delivery as Occiput Posterior.   If manual rotation cannot be easily accomplished, application of the blades to the head in the posterior position and delivery from the occiput posterior position is the safest procedure. In many of these cases, the cause of the persistent occiput posterior position and of the difficulty in accomplishing rotation is an anthropoid pelvis, the architecture of which predisposes to posterior delivery and opposes rotation. When the occiput is directly posterior, horizontal traction should be applied until the root of the nose is under the symphysis. The handles should then be slowly elevated until the occiput gradually emerges over the anterior margin of the perineum. Then, by imparting a downward motion to the instrument, the forehead, nose, and chin successively emerge from the vulva. The extraction is more difficult than

when the occiput is anterior, and because of greater distension of the vulva, perineal lacerations are more common (Fig. 41-21).

Forceps Rotations. Tucker-McLane, Simpson, or Kielland forceps may be used to try to rotate the fetal head. The occiput may be rotated 45 degrees to the posterior position or 135 degrees to the anterior (Fig. 41-22). Except in the hands of experts with extensive experience in rotation, however, delivery of the head as an occiput posterior produces less maternal and fetal injury than does forceps rotation. In rotating the occiput anteriorly with forceps, the pelvic curvature, originally directed upward, at the completion

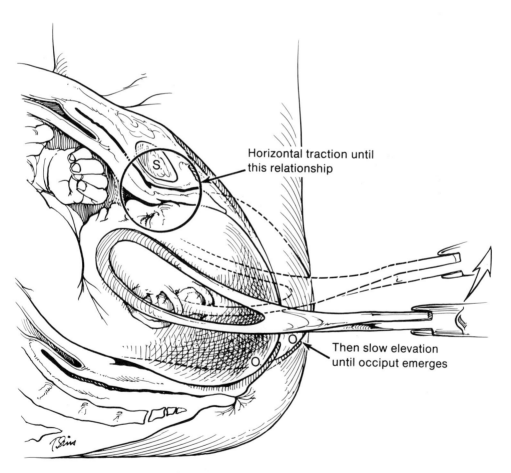

Horizontal traction until this relationship

Then slow elevation until occiput emerges

FIG. 41-21. Occiput directly posterior. Low forceps (Simpson) delivery as an occiput posterior.

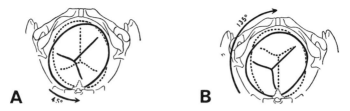

FIG. 41-22.   Rotation of obliquely posterior occiput to sacrum, **(A)** and symphysis pubis, **(B)**.

of rotation is inverted and directed posteriorly. Attempted delivery with the instrument in that position is likely to cause serious injury to maternal soft parts. To avoid such trauma, it is essential to remove and reapply the instrument as described in the following text.

TYPES OF SPECIAL MANEUVERS

Scanzoni-Smellie Maneuver.   The double application for forceps, which was first described by Smellie (1752) and rediscovered by Scanzoni (1853) about a century later, has given satisfactory results in some hands, but it is rarely necessary and is generally employed in only a small percentage of all obliquely posterior occipital positions. Since the right posterior variety is much more frequent, the steps of the operation in that case are here detailed:

In the first application, the blades of the forceps are applied to the sides of the head with the pelvic curve toward the face of the fetus, whereas in the second application the pelvic curve is directed toward the occiput. For the first application, the right hand is passed into the vagina posteriorly and the rear ear is located. The left blade is applied over the ear and held in position by an assistant, while the operator's left hand is passed into the right side of the vagina to control the introduction of the right blade, which is then rotated anteriorly until it lies over the left ear and opposite the first blade. The forceps is then locked and the handles elevated to flex the fetal head. Rotation may be facilitated by dislodging the fetal head

very slightly upward. *The head must not be disengaged from the pelvis.* To compensate for the pelvic curvature in Tucker-McLane forceps, or others with a pelvic curvature, the handles of the forceps are now gently rotated clockwise through an arc that extends well lateral to the circumference of the birth canal (Fig. 41-22). This serves to rotate the fetal head about the occipitomental diameter. With an appropriate initial forceps application, it is often possible to rotate the head completely to the occiput anterior position without undue force.

Once the occiput is rotated anteriorly, it is necessary to remove and reapply the forceps as described for an occiput anterior delivery. The forceps are unlocked and the branch on the left side of the pelvis (right branch) is removed by gently pulling the handle simultaneously downward and inward. During this maneuver, the other branch is held in position anteriorly by an assistant to help stabilize the occiput in an anterior position. The right branch is now inserted immediately after the remaining branch has been removed. During this time, the occiput typically will rotate back to a right occiput anterior position. After reapplication, some difficulty may arise in proper articulation, since the handle of the left branch lying above the right cannot be locked, but this can be readily overcome by rotating the handle of the left branch around the right to bring the lock into proper position. In left occiput posterior positions, the blades are applied similarly but in the reverse order.

Rotation   with   Kielland   Forceps. Kielland (1916) described a forceps with narrow, somewhat bayonet-shaped blades that he claimed could readily be applied to the sides of the head in the occiput transverse position and surpassed all other models as a rotator (Fig. 41-3). He held that his forceps was particularly useful when the station of the fetal head was high and when the sagittal suture was directed transversely. The Kielland forceps has almost no pelvic curve, but does have a sliding lock and is very light. On each handle is a small knob that indicates the direction of rotation.

There are two methods of applying the anterior blade. In one, *which may prove dangerous,* the anterior blade is introduced first with its cephalic curve directed upward and, after it has entered sufficiently far into the uterine cavity, it is turned through 180 degrees to adapt the cephalic curvature to the head. Kielland advised a more safe "wandering" or "gliding" method of application for the anterior blade when the uterus is tightly contracted about the head and the lower uterine segment is stretched and thin. In such cases, when the pelvis is slightly contracted, it is dangerous to introduce the anterior blade with its cephalic curvature directed upward to be followed by rotation of the blade. In the wandering or gliding method, the anterior blade is introduced at the side of the pelvis over the brow or face of the fetus. It is made to glide over the face to an anterior position, with the handle of the blade held close to the opposite maternal buttock throughout the maneuver. The second blade is introduced posteriorly and the branches are locked. Rotation is then accomplished at the station at which it may be most easily accomplished but not so high as to disengage the head from the pelvis.

With any forceps rotation, including Kielland, serious trauma may be induced unless considerable care is exercised. Pridmore and associates (1974) described laceration, hemorrhage, and edema of the cervical spinal cord following rotation of the fetal head from the posterior position with Kielland forceps. The problem appeared to have been tight encasement of the body of the fetus by a uterus that contained no amnionic fluid. Chis-

wick and James (1979) have looked carefully at neonatal morbidity and mortality following vaginal delivery with Kielland forceps or cesarean section after attempts at vaginal delivery with these forceps. Birth trauma was evident in 15 percent of infants so delivered. Neonatal mortality, most often from tentorial tears, was 3.5 percent. Factors significantly associated with the use of Kielland forceps were nulliparity, short maternal stature, induction of labor, late engagement of the fetal head, slow dilatation of the cervix, and epidural analgesia during labor (James, Chiswick, 1979).

Rubin and Coopland (1970) have summarized the experiences with Kielland's forceps rotation at Winnipeg General Hospital. Of the 1,000 consecutive cases surveyed, almost exactly one-half were occiput posterior and the remainder were occiput transverse. Rotation was accomplished successfully in 970. Practically always the same forceps were used for delivery following reapplication when necessary. There were eight perinatal deaths, including four with serious anomalies. Injuries to the infant were considered mostly minor. There were 27 injuries that were not minor, however, including seven fractured skulls.

Rotation with Barton Forceps. A forceps described by Barton and co-workers (1928) is illustrated in Figure 41-19. It differs from the usual types in that the anterior blade is hinged where it joins the shank. This forceps appears to be particularly useful when the sagittal suture occupies the transverse diameter of a platypelloid pelvis with a straight sacrum. For such cases, it has been used with presumably satisfactory results in several clinics in this country. The usual method of employing the Barton forceps involves wandering the hinged blade over the occiput or, less frequently, over the face. The posterior blade is then inserted directly into the hollow of the sacrum and the two branches of the forceps are articulated, adjusting the application, when necessary, by means of the sliding lock. Traction is applied in the transverse diameter of the pelvis, with rotation effected at or near the pelvic floor. Traction and rotation should not be performed simultaneously.

Application of Forceps in Face Presentations. In face presentations with the chin directed toward the symphysis, the application of forceps is used occasionally to effect vaginal delivery. The blades are applied to the sides of the head along the occipitomental diameter, with the pelvic curve directed toward the neck. Downward traction is exerted until the chin appears under the symphysis. Then, by an upward movement, the face is slowly extracted, the nose, eyes, brow, and occiput appearing in succession over the anterior margin of the perineum (Fig. 41-23).

Forceps should not be applied when the chin is directed toward the hollow of the sacrum, since delivery cannot be effected in that position.

Prognosis. The perinatal mortality rate associated with forceps deliveries depends on the condition of the fetus at the time the operation is undertaken, as well as the station of the head. Mortality should be zero when the head has reached the perineum. The application of forceps at higher stations, however, is attended by perinatal loss or damage in direct proportion to the height of the skull above the perineal floor. In such cases, the head may be subjected to injurious pressure

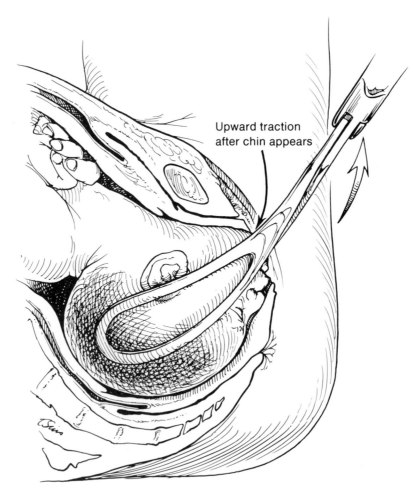

Upward traction after chin appears

FIG. 41-23. Face presentation, mentum (chin) anterior. Delivery with low forceps (Simpson).

that may lead to intracranial hemorrhage. Fortunately, the difficult forceps delivery has been largely supplanted by cesarean section.

Trial Forceps and Failed Forceps. In trial forceps, the operator attempts midforceps delivery with the full knowledge that a certain degree of disporportion at the midpelvis may make the procedure incompatible with safety for the fetus. With an operating room both equipped and staffed for immediate cesarean section, and after a good forceps application has been achieved, firm downward pulls on the instrument are made. If no descent occurs, the procedure is abandoned and cesarean section is performed (Douglass, Kaltreider, 1953).

The term *failed forceps* is applied to a case in which a forceps delivery was anticipated and a vigorous attempt was made to deliver with forceps but without success. The three fundamental factors responsible for such a failure are disproportion, incomplete cervical dilatation, and malposition of the fetal head. Most but not all such cases stem from inexperience and ignorance of obstetric fundamentals. In most areas of the United States, these cases are becoming much less frequent.

Since incomplete dilatation of the cervix is the cause of many cases of failed forceps, at times the problem can be solved by additional labor. Similarly, if the head does not rotate in occiput posterior positions, the case should be managed according to the principles set forth on page 1054. In the presence of overt disproportion, cesarean section is the only recourse with a living fetus. The prognosis for the infant is usually poor because of the trauma he has received. The outlook for the mother, however, is usually better, although it varies with the extent of trauma and infection.

VACUUM EXTRACTOR

There have been numerous attempts in the past to attach a tractor by suction to the fetal scalp. The theoretical advantages of the vacuum extractor over forceps include the avoidance of insertion of space-occupying steel blades within the vagina and of positioning the blades precisely over the fetal head as is necessary for safe forceps delivery, the ability to rotate the fetal head without the vacuum extractor impinging upon maternal soft tissues, and much less increase in intracranial pressure during traction with the vacuum extractor. All previously described instruments were unsuccessful until Malmström (1954) applied a new principle, namely, traction on a metal cap so designed that the suction creates an artificial caput within the cup that holds firmly and allows adequate traction.

In spite of some early enthusiasm for the instrument in the United States, the vacuum extractor is not used extensively now, partly because of reports of fetal damage, such as lacerations and abrasions of the scalp, cephalohematomas, intracranial hemorrhage, and death of infants. In contradistinction to the American hesitancy about the instrument, there has been an enthusiastic reception in many other parts of the world, although the enthusiasm has waned at least at some foreign institutions (Patel, 1979).

Use of the vacuum extractor has been reviewed by Sjösted (1967) and more recently by Plauché (1978), who emphasized the following basic requirements for its use:

1. The fetal membranes must be ruptured.
2. There must be no absolute cephalopelvic disproportion.
3. There must be a vertex presentation, preferably well flexed.
4. There must be cervical dilatation sufficient to apply the vacuum cup. Advanced dilatation allows the use of larger cups and results in safer, shorter procedures.
5. The cup should be placed as close to fetal occiput as possible.
6. Negative vacuum pressure should not exceed 0.7 to 0.8 kg/sq cm. Sufficient time (2 to 5 minutes) should be allowed for development of caput inside the cup.
7. The cup should not remain on the fetal scalp longer than a maximum of 45 minutes. Short application times reduce the incidence of damage to the fetal scalp.

8. Traction should be maintained at approximate right angles to the cup application. Diagonal, shearing forces and "rocking" motions increase the chances of scalp damage.
9. Traction should be applied concomitantly with uterine contractions and with the mother's voluntary expulsive efforts.
10. Traction should be perpendicular to the pelvic plane that the vertex is negotiating. This implies changing the direction of pull on high presentations from sharply downward, to parallel to the floor, to upward as the head advances. High applications thus require the operator to violate the principle of right angle traction and increase the likelihood of fetal scalp injury.
11. The cup should not be allowed to "pop off" thereby creating sudden pressure changes on the scalp. This usually occurs when insufficient time is allowed for the development of caput within the cup. The operator's nontraction hand can help by staying on the vertex, the index and middle fingers lifting the cervix up and over the vertex while the thumb maintains tight application of the cup and minimizes the shearing forces on the epicranial tissues.
12. Rotation of occiput transverse and posterior malpositions should be allowed to occur spontaneously with normal traction (autorotation) or should be performed manually prior to traction. The cup is a poor rotator and attempts to turn the cup itself when the fetal scalp is edematous and friable lead to "cookie cutter" avulsion injuries that can be severe.
13. If advancement is not evident after 3 or 4 pulls, the operator should stop, reevaluate the case, and consider the use of another mode of delivery. Vacuum extraction cannot safely overcome serious degrees of cephalopelvic disproportion.

CRANIOTOMY

The term *craniotomy,* as used in obstetrics, means an operation to collapse the fetal head for the purpose of facilitating its delivery. Widespread prenatal care, more astute management of pelvic contraction, antibiotics, and improvements in cesarean section have rendered craniotomy an exceedingly rare operation in modern obstetrics. As indicated in Chapter 30, page 824, cases of hydrocephalus are managed better by needle puncture and drainage than by craniotomy.

OPERATIONS PREPARATORY TO FORCEPS

Hysterostomatomy (Dührssen's Incisions). When immediate delivery is desirable before the cervix is fully dilated, multiple radial incisions may be made in the cervix and repaired immediately after delivery. These incisions are usually called Dührssen's incisions, after the German obstetrician who described them in 1890. While the complications may be formidable, the technic of the operation is simple: Three incisions, corresponding approximately to the hours of 2, 6, and 10 on the face of a clock, are made with scissors. Delivery is then effected by forceps or breech extraction, depending on the presentation. The operation should never be done unless the cervix is fully effaced and more than 7 cm dilated, lest profuse or even fatal hemorrhage result. The procedure is, of course, contraindicated in placenta previa.

Most obstetricians now consider the operation obsolete. It is included here only because of the rare possibility of its use in fetal distress when the cervix is almost fully dilated or the aftercoming head is trapped by the cervix.

Although the incisions themselves are simple to perform, the procedure involves major potential hazards, and cesarean section is most often preferable. For instance, in cases of uterine dysfunction in which the cervix is not yet fully dilated, the head is usually well above the pelvic floor, and a difficult midforceps operation, with its attendant trauma to mother and fetus, is often required. In such circumstances, severe maternal hemorrhage is common. Moreover, poor anatomic results, such as deep scars and adhesions between the cervix and the vaginal mucosa, are likely to be a result.

Manual Dilatation of the Cervix.

There is no such procedure as "manual dilatation of the cervix." What actually occurs when it is attempted is manual laceration of the cervix. The operation has no place in modern obstetrics.

Symphysiotomy and Pubiotomy.

Symphysiotomy is the division of the pubic symphysis with a wire saw or knife to effect an increase in the capacity of a contracted pelvis sufficient to permit the passage of a living child. In pubiotomy, the pubis is severed a few centimeters lateral to the symphysis. Because of interference with subsequent locomotion, bladder injuries, and hemorrhage, and because of the greater safety of cesarean section, these two operations have been abandoned in the United States. Symphysiotomy is still performed in parts of Africa and elsewhere, especially when it may be impossible to follow a patient in a subsequent pregnancy. Since, in these circumstances, a woman delivered by cesarean section for a mildly contracted pelvis might well die with a ruptured uterus in her next pregnancy, symphysiotomy may be indicated in such a case in an attempt to produce sufficient enlargement of the pelvis to allow vaginal delivery. Hartfield (1973) has provided a description of technic for subcutaneous symphysiotomy and summarized his experiences.

HISTORY OF FORCEPS

Crude forceps are an ancient invention, several varieties having been described by Albucasis, who died in 1112. Since their inner surfaces were provided with teeth to penetrate the head, however, it appears that they were intended for use only on dead fetuses.

The true obstetric forceps was devised in the latter part of the 16th or the beginning of the 17th century by a member of the Chamberlen family. The invention was not made public at the time, but was preserved as a family secret through four generations, not becoming generally known until the early part of the 18th century. Previously, version had been the only method that permitted the operative delivery of an unmutilated child. When that operation was impossible, imperative delivery was accomplished with hooks and crochets, which usually led to the destruction of the child. Thus, before the invention of forceps, the use of instruments was synonymous with the death of the child, and frequently of the mother as well.

William Chamberlen, the founder of the family, was a French physician who fled from France as a Huguenot refugee and landed at Southhampton in 1569. He died in 1596, leaving a large family. Two of his sons, both of whom were named Peter, and designated the elder and younger, respectively, studied medicine and settled in London. They soon became successful practitioners, devoting a large part of their attention to midwifery, in which they became very proficient. They attempted to control the instruction of midwives and, to justify their pretensions, claimed that they could successfully deliver patients when all others failed.

The younger Peter died in 1626 and the elder in 1631. The elder left no male children, but the younger was survived by several sons, one of whom, born in 1601, was likewise named Peter. To distinguish him from his father and uncle, he is usually spoken of as Dr. Peter, since the other two did not possess that title. He was well educated, having studied at Cambridge, Heidelberg, and Padua, and on his return to London was elected a Fellow of the Royal College of Physicians. He was most successful in the practice of his profession and counted among his clients many of the royal family and nobility. Like his father and uncle, he attempted to monopolize control of the midwives, but his pretensions were set aside by the authorities. These attempts gave rise to much discussion, and many pamphlets were written about the mortality of women in labor attended by men. He answered them in a pamphlet entitled "A Voice in Ramah, or the Cry of Women and Children as Echoed Forth in the Compassions of Peter Chamberlen." He was a man of considerable ability, combining some of the virtues of a religious enthusiast with many of the devious qualities of a pack. He died at Woodham Mortimer Hall, Moldon, Essex, in 1683, the place remaining in the possession of his family until well into the succeeding century. He was formerly considered the inventor of the forceps, a fact now known to be incorrect.

Chamberlen left a very large family, and three of his sons, Hugh, Paul, and John, became physicians who devoted special attention to the practice of midwifery. Of them Hugh (1630–?) was the most important and influential. Like his father, he was a man of considerable ability who took a practical interest in politics. Since some of his views were out of favor, he was forced to leave England for Paris, where in 1673 he attempted to sell the family's secret to Mauriceau for 10,000 livres, claiming that with forceps he could deliver in a very few minutes the most difficult case. Mauriceau placed at his disposal a rachitic dwarf whom he had been unable to deliver, and Chamberlen, after several futile hours of strenous effort, was obliged to acknowledge his inability to do so. Notwithstanding his failure, he maintained friendly relations with Mauriceau, whose book he translated into English. In his preface he refers to the forceps in the following words: "My father, brothers, and myself (though none else in Europe as I know) have by God's blessings and our own industry attained to and long practiced a way to deliver women in this case without prejudice to them or their infants."

Some years later he went to Holland and sold his secret to Roger Roonhuysen. Shortly afterward the Medico-Pharmaceutical College of Amsterdam was given the sole privilege of licensing physicians to practice in Holland, to each of whom, under the pledge of secrecy, was sold Chamberlen's invention for a large sum. The practice continued for a number of years until Vischer and Van de Poll purchased and made public the secret, whereupon it was discovered that the device consisted of only one blade of the forceps. Whether that was all Chamberlen sold to Roonhuysen, or whether the Medico-Pharmaceutical College had swindled the purchasers, is not known.

Hugh Chamberlen left a considerable family, and one of his sons, Hugh (1664–1728), practiced medicine. He was a highly educated, respected, and philanthropic physician, who numbered among his clients members of the best families in England. He was an intimate friend of the Duke of Buckingham, who had a statue erected in Chamberlen's honor in Westminster Abbey. During the later years of his life he allowed the family secret to leak out, and the instrument soon came into general use.

For more than 100 years Dr. Peter Chamberlen was considered the inventor of the forceps, but in 1813 Mrs. Kemball, the mother of Mrs. Codd, who was the occupant of Woodham Mortimer Hall at the time, found in the garret a trunk containing numerous letters and instruments, among

them four pairs of forceps together with several levers and fillets. As the drawings indicate (Fig. 41-24), the forceps were in different stages of development, one pair hardly applicable to the living woman, although the others were useful instruments. Aveling (1882), who carefully investigated the matter, believes that the three pairs of available forceps were used respectively by the three Peters, and that in all probability the first was devised by the elder Peter, son of the original William. The forceps came into general use in England during the lifetime of Hugh Chamberlen, the younger. The instrument was employed by Drinkwater, who died in 1728, and was well known to Chapman and Giffard.

In 1723, Palfyn, a physician of Ghent, exhibited before the Paris Academy of Medicine a forceps he designated *mains de fer*. It was crudely shaped and impossible to articulate. In the discussion following its presentation, De la Motte stated that it would be impossible to apply it to the living woman, and added that if by chance anyone should happen to invent an instrument that could be so used, and kept it secret for his own profit, he deserved to be exposed upon a barren rock and have his vitals plucked out by vultures. He had little knowledge that at the time he spoke such an instrument had been in the possession of the Chamberlen family for nearly 100 years.

The Chamberlen forceps, a short, straight instrument with only a cephalic curve, is perpetuated in the short forceps of today. It was used, with but little modification, until the middle of the 18th century, when Levret, in 1747, and Smellie, in 1751 independently added the pelvic curve and increased the length of the instrument. Levret's forceps was longer, with a more decided pelvic curve than that of Smellie. From these two instruments, the long forceps of the present day are descended.

As soon as forceps became public property, they were subjected to various modifications. As early as 1798, Mulder's atlas included illustrations of nearly 100 varieties. The modifications attempted in improving the instrument are pictured in Witkowski's *Obstetrical Arsenal*, illustrating several hundred forceps but representing only a small fraction of those devised. The monograph of Das contains excellent historical sketches of the development of the instrument. It is remarkable, however, that little advance was made over the instruments of Levret and Smellie until Tarnier, in 1877, clearly enunciated the principle of axis traction. These forceps were designed to cope with high

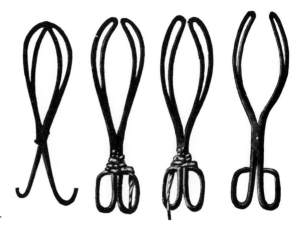

FIG. 41-24. Chamberlen forceps.

stations of the fetal head and contracted pelves. Such problems today, however, are generally solved by other means. Episiotomy, furthermore, has eliminated many of the difficulties stemming from the pelvic curve, and severe traction at the fenestra, as in the axis-traction forceps, is therefore unnecessary and probably undesirable (Rhodes, 1958).

Except for two specialized forceps, those of Barton and Kielland, very little that is both new and useful in modern obstetrics has been added to the development of the instrument in over 200 years.

REFERENCES

Aveling JH: The Chamberlens and the Midwifery Forceps. London, Churchill, 1882

Barton LG, Caldwell WE, Studdiford WE: A new obstetrical forceps. Am J Obstet Gynecol 15:16, 1928

Chiswick ML, James DK: Kielland's forceps: association with neonatal morbidity and mortality. Br Med J 1:7, 1979

DeLee JB: The prophylactic forceps operation. Am Obstet Gynecol 1:34, 1920

Dennen EH: Forceps Deliveries, 2d ed. Philadelphia, Davis, 1964

Douglas RG, Stromme WB: Operative Obstetrics, 3rd ed. New York, Appleton, 1976

Douglass LH, Kaltreider DF: Trial forceps. Am J Obstet Gynecol 65:889, 1953

Dührssen A: On the value of deep cervical incisions and episiotomy in obstetrics. Arch Gynaekol 37:27, 1890

Friedman EA, Sachtleben MR, Bresky PA: Dys-functional labor. XII. Long-term effects on the fetus. 127:779, 1977

Hartfield VJ: Subcutaneous symphysiotomy—time for a reappraisal? Aust NZ J Obstet Gynaecol 13:147, 1973

James DK, Chiswick ML: Kielland's forceps: role of antenatal factors in prediction of use. Br Med J 1:10, 1979

Joulin M: Study on the use of force in obstetrics. Arch Gen Med, 6th Series 9:149, 1867

Kielland C: On the application of forceps to the unrotated head, with description of a new model of forceps. Monatsschrift fur Geburtshilfe und Gynalkologie 43:48, 1916

Malmström T: The vacuum extractor, an obstetrical instrument. Acta Obstet Gynecol Scand (Suppl) 4:33, 1954

Patel N: Personal communication, 1980

Plauché WC: Vacuum extraction: Use in a community hospital setting. Obstet Gynecol 52:289, 1978

Pridmore BR, Hey EN, Aherne WA: Spinal cord injury of the fetus during delivery with Kielland's forceps. Br J Obstet Gynaecol 81:168, 1974

Rhodes P: A critical appraisal of the obstetric forceps. Br J Obstet Gynaecol 65:353, 1958

Rubin L, Coopland AT: Kielland's Forceps. Can Med Assoc J 103:505, 1970

Scanzoni FW: Lehrbuch der Geburtshülfe, 2nd ed. Vienna, Seidel, 1853, pp 838–840

Sjöstedt JE: The vacuum extractor and forceps in obstetrics: A clinical study. Acta Obstet Gynecol Scand 48: (Suppl 10):1, 1967 (360 references)

Smellie W: A Treatise on the Theory and Practice of Midwifery. London, Wilson & Durham, 1752

42

Technics for Breech Extraction and Version

The indications for vaginal delivery and cesarean section for breech presentations have been considered in Chapter 30, page 797.

There are three general methods of breech delivery through the vagina:

1. *Spontaneous breech delivery:* The infant is expelled entirely spontaneously without any traction or manipulation other than support of the infant. The mechanism of labor with spontaneous breech delivery is described elsewhere (see Chap. 30, p. 799). This form of delivery of mature infants is rare.
2. *Partial breech extraction:* The infant is delivered spontaneously as far as the umbilicus, but the remainder of the body is extracted.
3. *Total breech extraction:* The entire body of the infant is extracted by the obstetrician.

Since the technic of breech extraction differs in complete and incomplete breeches on the one hand, and frank breeches on the other, it is necessary to consider these conditions separately. (The varieties of breech presentation are illustrated in Chapter 30, Figs. 30-1, 2, and 3, p. 799.)

Timing of Delivery. In general, preparations for breech extraction should be initiated by the time that the buttocks or the feet appear at the vulva. It is essential that the delivery team include (1) an obstetrician skilled in the art of breech extraction, (2) an associate who is also scrubbed and gowned to assist with the delivery, (3) an anesthesiologist who can quickly induce appropriate general anesthesia when needed, (4) an individual trained to resuscitate the infant effectively, including endotracheal intubation, and (5) someone to provide general assistance.

Delivery is easier and, in turn, perinatal morbidity and mortality are lower when the breech of the fetus is allowed to deliver spontaneously. If fetal distress develops before this time, however, a decision must be made whether to perform a total breech extraction or, more likely, a cesarean section. It must be remembered that, for a favorable outcome with any breech delivery, at the very minimum the birth canal must be sufficiently large to allow passage of the fetus without trauma and the cervix must be effaced and fully dilated. If these conditions are lacking, cesarean section nearly always is the more appropriate method of delivery.

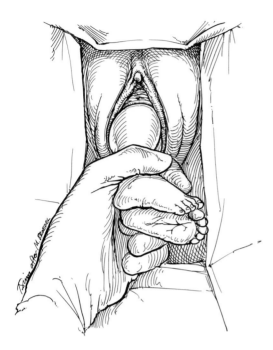

FIG. 42-1. Breech extraction. Traction on the feet and ankles.

EXTRACTION OF COMPLETE OR INCOMPLETE BREECH

Total Breech Extraction. During total breech extraction, the obstetrician's entire hand should be introduced through the vagina and both feet of the fetus grasped; the ankles are held with the second finger lying between them. The feet are then brought down the vagina, and gentle traction applied until they appear at the vulva. If difficulty is experienced in seizing both feet, first one foot should be drawn down the vagina to the introitus and then the other foot (Fig. 42-1).

Now both feet are grasped and pulled through the vulva simultaneously. Unless there is considerable relaxation of the perineum, an *episiotomy* is made. The episiotomy is an important adjunct to any type of breech delivery. A mediolateral episiotomy is usually preferred with a term-sized infant because it furnishes greater room and is less likely to extend into the rectum.

As the legs commence to emerge through

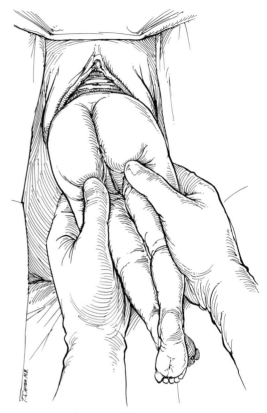

FIG. 42-2. Breech extraction. Traction on the thighs.

the vulva, they should be wrapped in a sterile towel to obtain a firmer grasp, for the vernix caseosa renders them slippery and difficult to hold. Many obstetricians prefer the towel to be moistened. The sterile water or normal saline used should be warm but not so hot as to burn the infant. Downward gentle traction is then continued.

As the legs emerge, successively higher portions are grasped, first the calves and later the thighs. When the breech appears at the vulva, gentle traction is applied until the hips are delivered. As the buttocks emerge, the back of the infant usually rotates to the anterior. The thumbs of the operator are then placed over the sacrum and the fingers over the hips, and gentle downward traction is continued until the costal margins, and then, the scapulas become visible (Figs. 42-2, 3). As traction is exerted and the scapulas be-

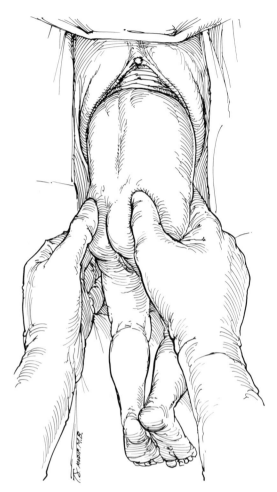

FIG. 42-3. Breech extraction. Extraction of the body. The obstetrician's hands are applied over, but not above, the infant's sacrum.

come visible, the back of the infant tends to turn spontaneously toward the side of the mother to which it was originally directed (Fig. 42-4). If turning does not occur, however, slight rotation should be added to the traction, with the object of bringing the bisacromial diameter of the fetus into the anteroposterior diameter of the pelvic outlet.

The cardinal rule in successful breech extraction is to employ steady, gentle, downward traction until the lower halves of the scapulas are delivered outside the vulva, making no attempt at delivery of the shoulders and arms until one axilla becomes visible. Frequently, failure to follow this rule will

cause an otherwise easy procedure to be difficult. The appearance of one axilla indicates that the time has arrived for delivery of the shoulders. Provided the arms are maintained in flexion, it makes little difference which shoulder is delivered first. Occasionally, while plans are made to deliver one shoulder, the other is born spontaneously.

There are two methods of delivery of the shoulders: (1) With the scapulas visible, the trunk is rotated in such a way that the anterior shoulder and arm appear at the vulva and can easily be released and delivered first. In Figure 42-2, the operator is shown rotating the trunk of the fetus counterclockwise to deliver the right shoulder and arm. The body of the fetus is then rotated in the reverse direction to deliver the other shoulder and arm. (2) If trunk rotation was unsuccessful, the posterior shoulder must be delivered first. The feet are grasped in one hand and drawn upward over the groin of the mother toward which the ventral surface of the fetus is directed; in this manner, leverage is exerted upon the posterior shoulder, which slides out over the perineal margin, usually followed by the arm and hand (Fig. 42-5). Then, by depressing the body of the fetus, the anterior shoulder emerges beneath the pubic arch, and the arm and hand usually follow spontaneously (Fig. 42-6). Thereafter, the back tends to rotate spontaneously in the direction of the mother's symphysis. If upward rotation fails to occur, it is effected by manual rotation of the body. Delivery of the head may then be accomplished.

Unfortunately, however, the process is not always so simple, and it is sometimes necessary first to free and deliver the arms. These maneuvers are much less frequently required today, presumably because of adherence to the principle of continuing traction without attention to the shoulders until an axilla becomes visible. Attempts to free the arms immediately after the costal margins emerge should be avoided.

Since there is more space available in the posterior and lateral segments of the normal pelvis than elsewhere, the posterior arm should be freed first. Since the corresponding

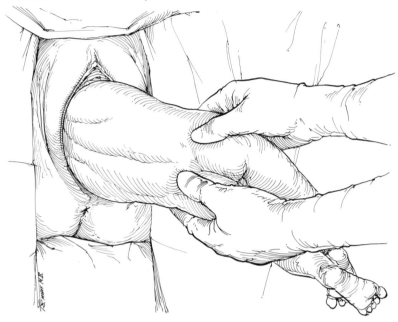

FIG. 42-4. Breech extraction. The scapulas are visible and the body is rotating.

axilla is already visible, upward traction upon the feet is continued, and two fingers of the obstetrician's other hand are passed along the humerus until the elbow is reached (Fig. 42-5). The fingers are now used to splint the arm, which is swept downward and delivered through the vulva. To deliver the anterior arm, depression of the fetal body of the infant is sometimes all that is required to allow the anterior arm to slip out spontaneously. In other instances, the anterior arm can be swept down over the thorax using two fingers as a splint. Occasionally, however, the body must be seized with the operator's thumbs over the scapulas and rotated to bring the undelivered shoulder near the closest sacro-sciatic notch. The legs are then carried upward to bring the ventral surface of the infant to the opposite groin of the mother; subsequently, the arm can be delivered as described previously.

If the arms have become extended over the head, their delivery, although more difficult, can usually be accomplished by the maneuvers just described. In so doing, particular care must be taken to carry the fingers up to the elbow and to use the fingers as a splint, for if the operator's fingers are merely hooked over the fetal arm, the humerus or clavicle is exposed to great danger of fracture. Infrequently, one or both fetal arms is found around the back of the neck *(nuchal arm),* and delivery is still more difficult. If the nuchal arm(s) cannot be freed in the manner described, extraction may be facilitated by rotating the fetus through half a circle in such a direction that the friction exerted by the birth canal will serve to draw the elbow toward the face. Should rotation of the fetus fail to free the nuchal arms, it may be necessary to push the fetus upward in an attempt to release them. If the rotation is still unsuccessful, the nuchal arm(s) is often forcibly extracted by hooking a finger over it. In that event, fracture of the humerus or clavicle is very common. Fortunately, good union almost always follows appropriate treatment.

After the shoulders are born, the head usually occupies an oblique diameter of the pelvis with the chin directed posteriorly. The fetal head may then be extracted either with

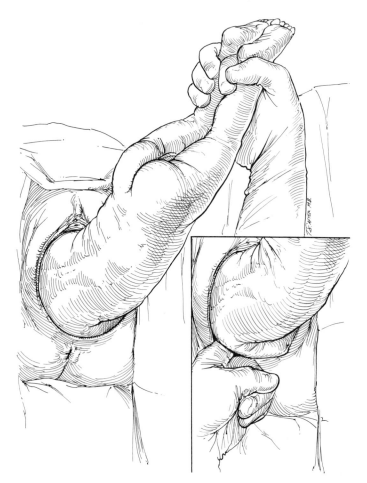

FIG. 42-5. Breech extraction. Upward traction to effect delivery of the posterior shoulder, followed by freeing the posterior arm (insert).

forceps, as illustrated in Figures 42-7 through 42-16, which is the method preferred by many obstetricians and is described subsequently, or by the so-called *Mauriceau maneuver* (Fig. 42-8B).

Employing the Mauriceau maneuver to help flex the head, the operator's index and middle finger of one hand are applied over the maxilla, while the fetal body rests upon the palm of the hand and forearm, which is straddled by the fetal legs. Two fingers of the operator's other hand are then hooked over the fetal neck, and grasping the shoulders, downward traction is applied until the suboccipital region appears under the symphysis. The body of the fetus is then elevated toward the mother's abdomen, and the mouth, nose, brow and eventually the occiput emerge successively over the perineum. Gentle traction should be exerted by the fingers over the shoulders. At the same time, suprapubic pressure, appropriately applied by an assistant, as shown in Figure 42-8B, is helpful in delivery of the head.

EXTRACTION IN FRANK BREECH PRESENTATIONS

At times, extraction of a frank breech may be accomplished by *moderate* traction exerted by a finger in each groin and facilitated by

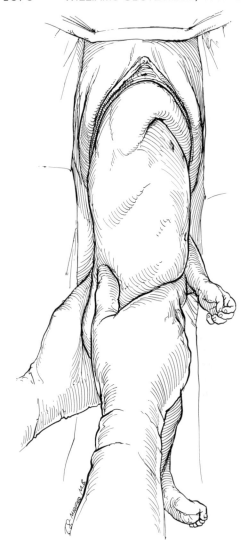

FIG. 42-6. Breech extraction. Delivery of the anterior shoulder by downward traction. The anterior arm may then be freed the same way as the posterior arm in Figure 42-5.

a generous episiotomy (Fig. 42-9). If moderate traction does not effect delivery of the breech, and cesarean section is not used, vaginal delivery can only be accomplished by *breech decomposition.* This procedure involves intrauterine manipulation to convert the frank breech into a footling breech by flexing both knees and extending the hips. The procedure is more readily accomplished if the membranes were ruptured recently but be-

comes extremely difficult if considerable time has elapsed after the escape of the amnionic fluid and if the uterus has become tightly contracted over the fetus.

In many cases, the *Pinard maneuver* aids materially in bringing down the feet. In that procedure, two fingers are carried up along one extremity to the knee to push it away from the midline. Spontaneous flexion usually follows, and the foot of the fetus is felt to impinge upon the back of the hand. The fetal foot may then be readily grasped and brought down (Fig. 42-10). As soon as the buttocks are born, first one leg and then the other are drawn out and extraction is accomplished as described under Extraction of Complete or Incomplete Breech, above.

FORCEPS TO THE AFTER-COMING HEAD

Piper forceps (Figs. 42-7–42-16) should be applied when the Mauriceau maneuver cannot be easily accomplished, or they may advantageously be applied electively instead of the Mauriceau procedure. The blades of the forceps should not be applied to the aftercoming head until it has been brought into the pelvis by gentle traction, combined with suprapubic pressure, and is engaged (Fig. 42-7). As shown in Figure 42-16, suspension of the body of the fetus in a towel keeps the arms out of the way and prevents excessive abduction of the trunk.

Entrapment of the Aftercoming Head. Occasionally, especially with small preterm fetuses, the incompletely dilated cervix will not allow delivery of the aftercoming head. Prompt action is necessary if the infant is to be delivered alive. With gentle traction on the fetal body, the cervix, at times, may be manually slipped over the occiput. If this maneuver is not readily successful, Dührssen's incisions can be made in the cervix. This is one of the few indications for this procedure in modern obstetrics (see Chap. 41, p. 1060).

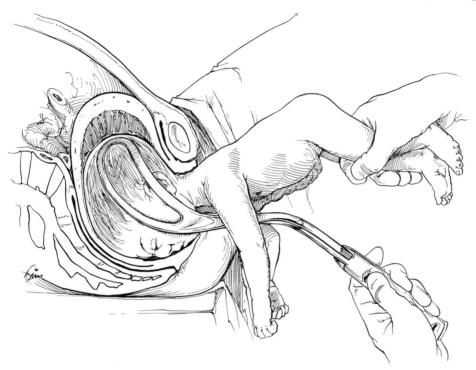

FIG. 42-7.   Forceps applied to after-coming head. The head has entered the pelvis and forceps have been applied (See Figs. 42-12–42-16.)

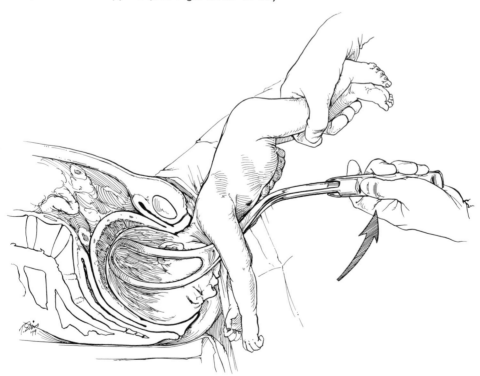

FIG. 42-8. A.   Forceps delivery of after-coming head *(Continued).*

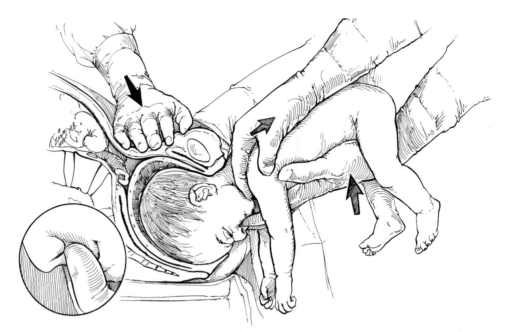

FIG. 42-8. B.   Delivery of after-coming head using the Mauriceau maneuver. Note that as the fetal head is being delivered, flexion of the head is maintained by suprapubic pressure provided by an assistant and simultaneously by pressure on the maxilla (insert) by the operator as traction is applied.

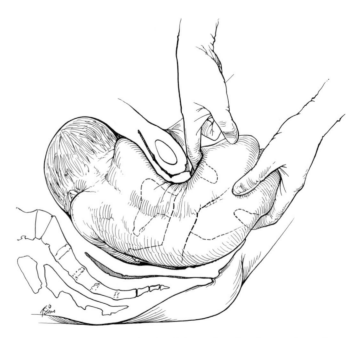

FIG. 42-9.   Extraction of a frank breech using fingers in groins.

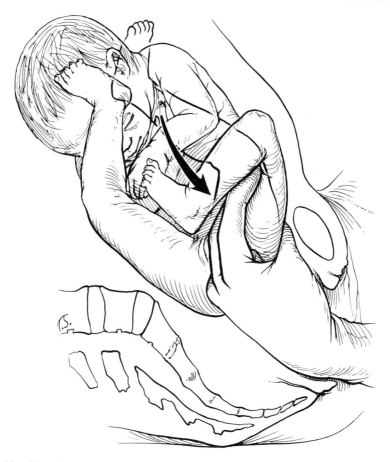

FIG. 42-10. Pinard maneuver sometimes used in case of a frank breech presentation to deliver a foot into the vagina.

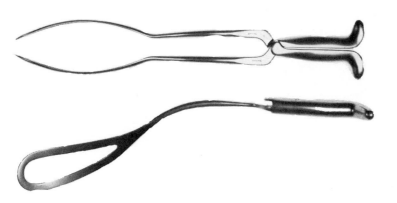

FIG. 42-11. Piper forceps.

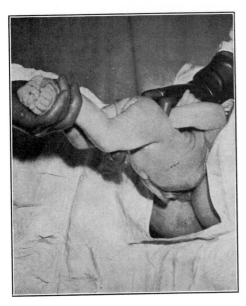

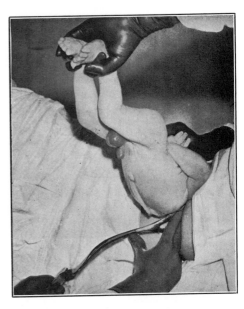

FIG. 42-12. Position of infant with head in pelvis prior to application of Piper forceps.

FIG. 42-13. Introduction of left blade to left side of pelvis. Note upward direction of forceps.

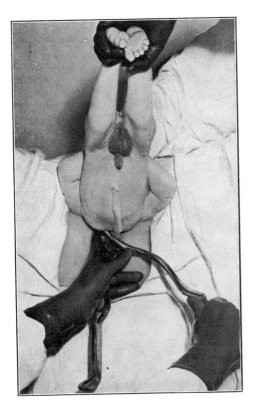

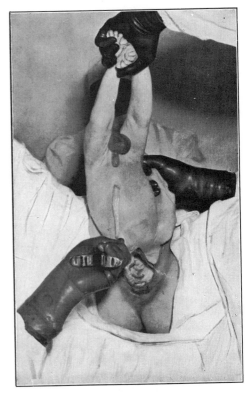

FIG. 42-14. Introduction of right blade, completing application.

FIG. 42-15. Forceps locked and traction applied; chin, mouth, and nose emerging over perineum.

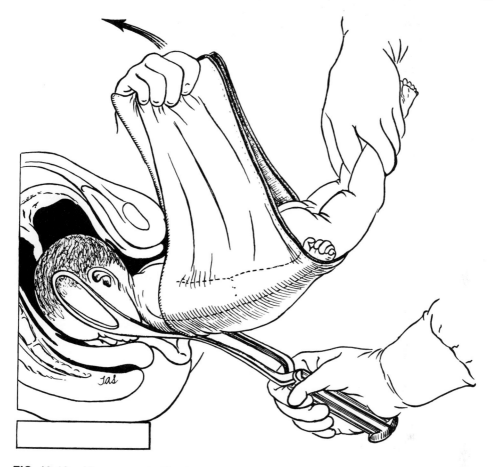

FIG. 42-16. Management of fetal arms in breech extraction. (From Savage. *Obstet Gynecol* 3:55, 1954)

PRAGUE AND BRACHT MANEUVERS

In the vast majority of cases, the back of the fetus eventually rotates toward the front, regardless of its original position, but when rotation fails to occur spontaneously, the movement may be initiated by applying stronger traction upon the leg. If even then the back remains posterior after birth of the shoulders, extraction must be begun with the occiput posterior. As a rule, rotation can still be effected by means of the finger in the mouth, and the head then extracted by the Mauriceau maneuver. When rotation is not possible, however, delivery of the head in its abnormal position must be attempted by the modified *Prague maneuver,* so called because it was strongly recommended by Kiwisch (1846) of that city. The Prague maneuver, as employed today with the fetal back down, is actually the reverse of the originally described

procedure, in which the fetal back was directed upward. In the procedure, two fingers of one hand grasp the shoulders from below, while the other hand draws the feet up over the abdomen of the mother. The Prague maneuver, as well as most breech extractions, is more easily performed after an adequate episiotomy is made.

In an effort to stimulate the forces of nature, Bracht (1936) employed a maneuver whereby the breech was allowed to deliver spontaneously to the umbilicus. The baby's body was then held, not pressed, against the mother's symphysis. The force applied in this procedure should be equivalent to that of gravity. The mere maintenance of this position, added to the effects of uterine contractions and moderate suprapubic pressure by an assistant, often suffices to complete the delivery spontaneously. The *Bracht maneuver* has been popular in Europe but has not gained wide acceptance in the United States. The procedure was thoroughly reviewed by Plentl and Stone (1953).

ANESTHESIA FOR BREECH DELIVERY

It is wise to allow the breech to deliver spontaneously to the umbilicus. Anesthesia for episiotomy and intravaginal manipulations that are needed for breech extraction usually can be accomplished with pudendal block and local infiltration of the perineum (see Chap. 18, p. 445). The inhalation of nitrous oxide plus oxygen provides further relief from pain. If for any reason general anesthesia is desired, it can be quickly induced with thiopental plus a muscle relaxant and maintained with nitrous oxide.

Anesthesia for decomposition and extraction must provide sufficient relaxation to allow intrauterine manipulation. Although successful decomposition has been accomplished using epidural, caudal, or spinal anesthesia, increased uterine tone may render the operation difficult. Then, preferably halothane can be used to relax the uterus, as well as provide pain relief.

PROGNOSIS

With complicated breech deliveries, there are increased maternal risks. Manual manipulations within the birth canal increase the risk of maternal infection. Intrauterine maneuvers, especially with a thinned-out lower uterine segment, or delivery of the after-coming head through an incompletely dilated cervix, may cause rupture of the uterus, lacerations of the cervix, or both. Such manipulations may also lead to extensions of the episiotomy or deep perineal tears. Anesthesia sufficient to induce appreciable uterine relaxation may cause uterine atony and, in turn, postpartum hemorrhage from the placental implantation site. Even so, the prognosis, in general, for *the mother* whose fetus is delivered by breech extraction is probably somewhat better than with cesarean section.

For *the fetus,* the outlook is less favorable and it becomes more serious the higher the presenting part is situated at the beginning of the breech extraction. In addition to the increased risk of tentorial tears and intracerebral hemorrhage, which are inherent in breech delivery, the perinatal mortality rate is augmented by the greater probability of other trauma during extraction. In incomplete breech presentations, moreover, prolapse of the umbilical cord is much more common than in vertex presentations and this complication further worsens the prognosis for the infant.

Fracture of the humerus and clavicle cannot always be avoided when freeing the arms, and fracture of the femur may occur during difficult frank breech extractions. Hematomas of the sternocleidomastoid muscles occasionally develop after the operation, though they usually disappear spontaneously. More serious problems, however, may follow separation of the epiphyses of the scapula, humerus, or femur. Exceptionally, paralysis of the arm follows pressure upon the brachial plexus by the fingers in exerting traction, but more frequently it is caused by overstretching the neck while freeing the arms. When the fetus is forcibly extracted through a contracted pelvis, spoonshaped depressions or actual fractures of the skull, generally fatal, may result. Occasionally, even the fetal neck may be broken when great force is employed. Perinatal morbidity and mortality are considered in greater detail in Chapter 30, page 802.

VERSION

Version, or turning, is an operation in which the presentation of the fetus is altered artificially, either substituting one pole of a longitudinal presentation for the other, or converting an oblique or transverse lie into a longitudinal presentation.

According to whether the head or breech is made the presenting part, the operation is designated cephalic or podalic version, respectively. It is also named according to the method by which it is accomplished. Thus, in *external version*, the manipulations are performed exclusively through the abdominal wall; in *internal version*, the entire hand is introduced into the uterine cavity.

External Cephalic Version. The object of the operation is to convert a less favorable presentation to that of a vertex.

INDICATIONS. If a breech or shoulder presentation (transverse lie) is diagnosed in the last weeks of pregnancy, its conversion into a vertex may be attempted by external maneuvers, provided there is no marked disproportion between the size of the fetus and the pelvis. Cephalic version is thought by some, but not most, obstetricians to be a frequently successful technic with little morbidity (see Chap. 30, p. 803), and therefore should be attempted in order to avoid the increased perinatal mortality that is attending breech delivery. If the fetus lies transversely, a change of presentation is usually the only alternative to cesarean section.

External cephalic version may be attempted only under the following conditions: (1) The presenting part must not be engaged. (2) The abdominal wall must be sufficiently thin to permit accurate palpation. (3) The abdominal and uterine walls must not be highly irritable. (4) The uterus must contain a sufficient quantity of amniotic fluid to permit easy movement of the fetus. Anesthesia should never be used, lest undue force be applied.

In the early stages of labor, before the membranes have ruptured, the same indications apply. They may then be extended to oblique presentations as well, although these unstable lies usually convert spontaneously to longitudinal lies as labor progresses. External cephalic version can rarely be effected, however, after the cervix has become fully dilated or the membranes have ruptured.

METHOD. Cephalic version is performed solely by *external manipulations* (Fig. 42-17). In the technic recommended, the

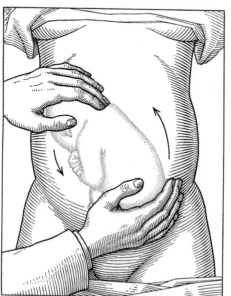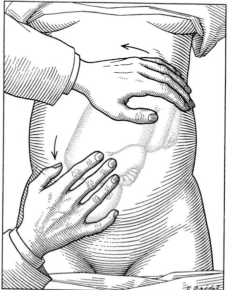

FIG. 42-17. External cephalic version.

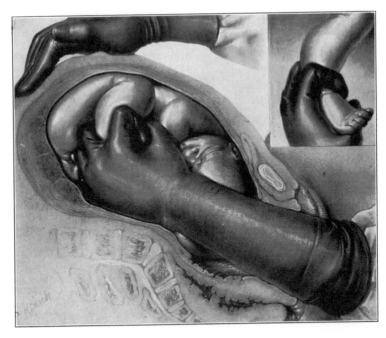

FIG. 42-18. Internal podalic version. Note use of long version gloves.

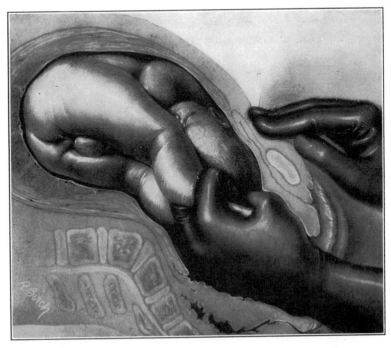

FIG. 42-19. Internal podalic version. Upward pressure on head is applied as downward traction is exerted on feet.

woman's abdomen is bared, and the presentation and position of the fetus are carefully ascertained. Each hand then grasps one of the fetal poles. The pole that is to be converted into the presenting part is then gently stroked toward the pelvic inlet while the other is moved in the opposite direction. After version has been completed, the fetus will tend to return to its original position unless the presenting part is fixed in the pelvis. During labor, however, the head may be pressed down into the pelvic inlet and held firmly in position until it becomes fixed under the influence of the uterine contractions.

Internal Podalic Version.   This maneuver consists of turning the fetus by the obstetrician inserting a hand into the uterine cavity, seizing one or both feet and drawing them through the cervix. The operation is followed by breech extraction.

INDICATIONS.   There are very few, if any, indications for internal podalic version other than for delivery of the second twin.

The technic for delivering the second twin has been described elsewhere (see Chap. 26, p. 661). Very occasionally, the procedure may be justified when the cervix is fully dilated, the membranes are intact, and the fetus in a transverse lie is either very small or dead. The possibility for serious trauma to the fetus and mother during internal podalic version from a cephalic presentation is apparent in Figures 42-18 and 42-19.

REFERENCES

Bracht E: Manual aid in breech presentation. Z. Geburtshilfe Gynaekol 112:271, 1936

Kiwisch FH: Beitrage zur Geburtskunde. Wurzburg, I Abth, 69, 1846

Mauriceau F: The method of delivering the woman when the infant presents one or two feet first. Traite des Maladies des Femmes Grosses, 6me ed, 1721, pp. 280–285

Pinard A: On version by external maneuvers. Paris, Traite de Palper abdominal, 1889

Plentl AA, Stone, RE: Bracht maneuver. Obstet Gynecol Survey 8:313, 1953

43

Cesarean Section and Cesarean Hysterectomy

CESAREAN SECTION

Definition. Cesarean section is defined as delivery of the fetus through incisions in the abdominal wall (laparotomy) and the uterine wall (hysterotomy). Therefore, it does not include removal of the fetus from the abdominal cavity in case of rupture of the uterus or abdominal pregnancy.

Indications. The indications for cesarean section are discussed in detail throughout the text wherever the fetal or maternal complications that might necessitate cesarean section are presented. The early history of cesarean section is considered at the end of this chapter. In general, cesarean section is used whenever it is believed that further delay in delivery would seriously compromise the fetus, the mother, or both, yet vaginal delivery cannot be safely accomplished. For reasons discussed in Chapter 33, once delivery has been effected by cesarean section, delivery in subsequent pregnancies is usually performed the same way, although some obstetricians contest this policy.

In recent years, the use of cesarean section has increased remarkably, in large measure because of the widespread emphasis that is directed toward recognition of impairment, actual or suspected, of fetal well-being if delivery were delayed or vaginal delivery were attempted. Moreover, with the prevailing enthusiasm for small families, many women whose first infants were delivered by cesarean section now wish sterilization after their second. In this circumstance, any slight advantage from vaginal delivery with the second pregnancy after initial cesarean section most often is offset by the need for laparotomy to accomplish sterilization subsequent to vaginal delivery.

The reduction in the parity of most women who now are being delivered, with up to to one-half of the population of pregnant women comprised of nulliparas, has led to cesarean section being done most often for those conditions that are especially common in nulliparous women. Delivery by cesarean section is most frequently performed in nulliparas for dystocia with suspected fetopelvic disproportion and for pregnancy-induced hypertension. At the same time, those abnormalities that are more common in multiparas, such as transverse lie of the fetus and placenta previa, are encountered less often than in former years. Also of importance is the fact that the opportunities for obstetricians-in-training to develop the skills required to accomplish successfully a potentially difficult breech delivery or to do an internal podalic version have diminished considerably, and for good reasons (see Chap. 30, p. 802). More and more, such problem cases are rightfully being managed by cesarean section.

The attitude of the past, that cesarean section was either an admission of lack of sophisticated obstetric skills or the coward's way to solve an obstetric problem, hopefully, has disappeared from the thinking of contemporary obstetrics in the United States. Nonetheless, the decision to perform, or not to perform, a cesarean section should be based on pertinent and precise medical observations rationally used to decide for that pregnancy the better method of delivery rather than be based on fear of legal repercussion if a cesarean section were not performed. Granted, it has long appeared that, if a cesarean section were performed, the woman and her family were usually convinced that all had been done that could have been done, irrespective of the outcome. For a variety of reasons, this attitude may not persist. Instead, the public's attitude is more likely to become one of suspicion that the obstetrician who performs a cesarean section may have interfered needlessly with a normal physiologic process, i.e., childbirth.

Frequency. The increase in cesarean section rate in California from 4.8 percent in 1960 to 12.7 percent in 1975 undoubtedly reflects the nationwide trend (Petitti et al., 1979). Recent cesarean section rates for several training institutions in the United States range from 10.1 percent to 22.0 percent, with a median value of 16 percent (Table 43-1).

At Parkland Memorial Hospital the frequency of cesarean section has increased progressively from 4.4 percent of deliveries in 1964 to 18.3 percent in 1979. A number of factors have contrib-

uted to this increase. For one, parity of the obstetric population has dropped appreciably. Thus the number of multiparous women who had previously been delivered vaginally and most likely would do so again has decreased. Only one-fourth of the women who were delivered in 1964 were having their first baby, compared to almost one-half in 1979. For another, the frequency of difficult or prolonged inductions of labor has diminished with the more frequent use of cesarean section. A third major factor has been a reduction in the number of potentially difficult vaginal deliveries, including the use of midforceps, the vaginal delivery of breeches, and the vaginal delivery of multiple fetuses.

Prognosis. Maternal and perinatal mortality and morbidity are typically higher with cesarean section than with vaginal delivery, in part because of the complication that led to the cesarean section and in part because of increased risks inherent in the abdominal route of delivery.

MATERNAL MORTALITY. In competent hands, maternal mortality from cesarean section is 2 per 1000 (0.2 percent) or less. At Parkland Memorial Hospital, from 1964 to 1978, cesarean section was performed 10,501 times with 9 fatalities (0.1 percent, or 1 in

TABLE 43-1.
FREQUENCY OF CESAREAN SECTION
DURING 1978 AT VARIOUS INSTITUTIONS

	PERCENT
University of Iowa Hospital	10.1
University of Southern California—Los Angeles County	12.0
University of Oklahoma Hospital	13.0
Harbor General Hospital	13.6
Ohio State University Hospital	14.0
University of Colorado Hospital	14.3
Grady Hospital	15.8
Wilford Hall Air Force Hospital	16.1
University of California at San Diego Hospital	16.8
Jackson Memorial Hospital	16.8
Washington University Hospital	16.9
Parkland Memorial Hospital	17.4
University of North Carolina Hospital	19.2
Boston Hospital for Women	22.0

1167 cesarean sections). Severe sepsis with multiple intra-abdominal abscesses and bowel fistulas proved fatal in one instance. Cardiac arrest near the completion of the operation caused another death; the mother was a 40-year-old gravida 15 who was markedly obese and diabetic; cesarean section was necessary to control active bleeding from placenta previa. One death occurred suddenly and unexpectedly following repeat cesarean section on a 16-year-old woman with twins; necropsy disclosed acute myocarditis and idiopathic cardiac hypertrophy. One woman discharged from the hospital after a benign postoperative course died two weeks later; idiopathic myocarditis was identified through autopsy. Death followed hysterotomy performed at midpregnancy on one woman with severe pulmonary hypertension. The rapid intravenous administration of 20 g of magnesium sulfate rather than 20 ml of a 20 percent solution as a loading dose proved fatal in a woman with eclampsia post-cesarean section. Aspiration pneumonitis killed 3 women; there have been no such maternal deaths however since the practice of ingesting 30 ml of milk of magnesia before induction of anesthesia was established.

Between 1968 and 1979, 10,231 cesarean sections were performed at Boston Hospital for women without a maternal death! (Frigoletto et al., 1980).

MATERNAL MORBIDITY. Even when morbidity from the problem that led to cesarean section is excluded, maternal morbidity is more frequent and likely to be more severe with cesarean section than with vaginal delivery. The common causes are infection, hemorrhage, and, less often, injury to the urinary tract.

PERINATAL MORTALITY. The frequency of stillbirth and neonatal death will depend, of course, on the underlying reason for the cesarean section and the gestational age of the fetus.

PERINATAL MORBIDITY. Birth trauma, in general, is much less likely with cesarean section than with vaginal delivery. Nonetheless, the fetus can be injured, especially if the uterine incision is inadequate for delivery of the fetus. For example, the head of the premature breech fetus may be entrapped because the incision through a thick uterine wall was too small, leading to serious trauma to the neck and spinal cord. There is always the risk of wounding the fetus during the course of making the uterine incision. A modicum of care, however, should minimize this risk.

Neonatal morbidity and mortality, primarily due to respiratory distress, has been claimed by some to be higher for repeat cesarean section than vaginal delivery. It is doubtful whether there is an appreciable difference, however, when the gestational ages of the fetuses are identical and fetal hypoxia and acidosis are avoided. To minimize the development of fetal hypoxia and acidosis, the woman before and during the operation should not be kept in the supine position, not be allowed to become hypoxic, and not be allowed to become hypotensive.

Timing of Repeat Cesarean Section. There are advantages to a predetermined time for carrying out repeat cesarean sections. For example, the family can better arrange for assistance in caring for other children while the mother is hospitalized and for the care of the mother and infant after leaving the hospital. Importantly, a competent team can be assembled more easily to provide optimal care, including anesthesia, infant resuscitation if needed, and subsequent care of the newborn. Conversely, with emergency repeat cesarean section, an operating room may not be immediately available, or the mother may have very recently eaten, which increases the anesthetic risk. Of considerable importance when dealing with a gravida with a previous cesarean section in which a vertical uterine incision was made is that the uterus may rupture with the onset of labor, resulting in death of the fetus and serious morbidity or even death of the mother. The likelihood before or during early labor of rupture of a scar from a transverse incision in the lower uterine segment with these disastrous consequences is very low.

Iatrogenic prematurity due to elective termination of pregnancy has been a major problem at some institutions. This unfortunate circumstance has led to the strong recommendation by some that amniocentesis with appropriate studies on the fluid obtained be performed before any elective delivery (Flaksman et al., 1978; Gluck, 1977). This approach is not without complications, however, for, at times, trauma to the placenta or fetus is caused by attempts to obtain amnionic fluid which may be of scant volume in pregnancies at or near term. Moreover, after an unsuccessful attempt at amniocentesis, the fetus has been known to succumb in utero awaiting a subsequent and hopefully successful attempt at aspiration of amnionic fluid and its analysis. Sonography at the time of amniocentesis dimishes the risk somewhat but adds further to the cost.

The guidelines for timing repeat cesarean section at Parkland Memorial Hospital do not include mandatory amniocentesis to measure the lecithin/sphingomyelin ratio. Instead, the following information is used to identify fetal maturity: (1) the date of onset of the last normal spontaneous menstrual period, (2) results of serial measurements of the height of the uterine fundus above the symphysis initiated in the first half of pregnancy, (3) the time when the fetal heart was first heard with a fetoscope, and (4) the estimated size of the fetus. Delivery is carried out after 38 completed weeks of gestation, based on the last normal menstrual period, without measuring the L/S ratio if the fetal heart was heard at a time when the fundal height was 18 to 20 cm; if the gestational age at that same time calculated from the normal last menstrual period was 18 to 20 weeks; and if the fetus is estimated by each of two experienced examiners to weigh as much as did the previous term infant, or more than 3000 g when the previous infant was premature or growth retarded. Delivery is postponed if there is discordance that implies a lower gestational age and there are no compelling reasons, maternal or fetal, to effect delivery before the onset of labor, such as a previous vertical incision in the uterus or strong suspicion of retarded fetal growth.

With this approach, about 60 percent of repeat cesarean sections are performed at Parkland Memorial Hospital at a scheduled time. The remainder are done during early labor. Respiratory distress has not been a problem in those pregnancies terminated by scheduled repeat cesarean section before the onset of labor.

A careful survey of the effectiveness of this policy in avoiding respiratory distress in the newborn infant was prompted by the widely publicized recommendation that before any elective cesarean section amniocentesis be performed to identify surfactant phospholipids in amounts sufficient to exclude the development of respiratory distress. Of 333 consecutive repeat cesarean sections at Parkland Memorial Hospital, reviewed recently, 58 percent were performed electively before the onset of labor or rupture of the membranes. Of the 191 infants delivered electively, one with congenital heart disease developed respiratory distress but survived. The infant weighed 2600 g, which was less than the birth weight of two siblings, but growth retardation rather than prematurity appeared to be the cause of the lower birth weight.

Toffle and associates (1978) analyzed their experiences with the management of elective, repeat cesarean section. They emphasize the following criteria pertaining to gestational age: (1) satisfactory menstrual history, (2) early bimanual examination, (3) fetal heart tones audible with fetoscope at 18 to 20 weeks, (4) appropriate uterine growth by fundal measurement, and (5) corroborative sonographic measurements of the biparietal diameter made at 28 weeks or before. In 60 percent of their patients these criteria were in good agreement, and cesarean section was repeated at 39 weeks' gestation. Otherwise, cesarean section was not performed electively until the amnionic fluid L/S ratio was demonstrated to be favorable. For further discussion of fetal maturity, see Chapters 12, 13, and 36.

Contraindications. In modern obstetric practice, there are virtually no contraindications to cesarean section. Cesarean section is seldom indicated, however, if the fetus is dead or too premature to survive. Exceptions to this generalization include pelvic contraction of such a degree that vaginal delivery by any means is impossible, most cases of placenta previa, and most cases of neglected transverse lie. Conversely, whenever the maternal coagulation mechanism is seriously impaired, delivery that minimizes incisions, i.e., vaginal delivery, is preferable in most instances (see Chap. 20).

TECHNIC OF CESAREAN SECTION

Type of Uterine Incision. A vertical incision made into the body of the uterus above the lower uterine segment and extending into the uterine fundus—the so-called classical cesarean section—is seldom used. Nearly always incision is initiated in the lower uterine segment either transversely ("Kerr technic") or less often vertically ("Krönig technic"). The lower segment transverse incision possesses the advantage of requiring only modest dissection of the bladder from the underlying myometrium. It has the disadvantage that, if the incision extends laterally, the lacerations may involve large branches of the uterine artery and veins. The low vertical incison has the advantage that in those circumstances where much more room is needed, the incision can be readily extended into the body of the uterus. Otherwise, it is a less desirable incision. More extensive dissection of the bladder is necessary to keep the vertical incision within the lower uterine segment. Moreover, if the vertical incision extends downward, it may tear through the cervix into the vagina and possibly involve the bladder. If, on the other hand, it is extended upwards, with incision into the body of the uterus, closure, including satisfactory reperitonealization, is more difficult and the likelihood of rupture in a subsequent pregnancy is increased. Importantly, it has been our experi-

ence that during the next pregnancy the vertical incision is much more prone to rupture, especially during labor, than is the lower segment transverse incision (see Chap. 33, p. 863).

Lower Segment Transverse Incision. For a cephalic presentation, most often a transverse incision through the lower uterine segment is the operation of choice. Generally, the transverse incision (1) results in less blood loss, (2) is easier to repair, (3) is located at a site least likely to rupture with extrusion of the fetus into the abdominal cavity during a subsequent pregnancy, and (4) does not promote adherence of bowel or omentum to the incisional site.

OPERATIVE TECHNIC. Hair is shaved from the abdominal wall from below the level of the mons pubis to somewhat above the umbilicus and laterally to about the level of the iliac crests. The bladder is emptied through an indwelling catheter and continuously drained during and after the procedure. The operative field is thoroughly scrubbed with a suitable detergent and then all of the abdomen is covered with sterile drapings, except for an area bounded by the mons pubis below to 4 cm or so above the umbilicus and for 2 cm to each side of the midline.

If general anesthesia is to be employed, all the above steps are carried out and the operating team is fully prepared to operate before induction of anesthesia. If continuous conduction anesthesia is to be used, it is necessary before scrubbing and draping the abdomen to insert the catheter into the epidural or caudal space. If single dose intrathecal (spinal) anesthesia is to be used, it is injected just before scrubbing and draping the abdomen.

An infraumbilical vertical incision is quickest to make. The abdominal wall is opened in layers from just above the upper margin of the symphysis to near the umbilicus. The incision should be long enough to allow the infant to be delivered without difficulty, but no longer. Therefore, its length should vary with the estimated size of the fetus. Sharp dissection is performed to the level of the anterior rectus sheath, which is freed of subcutaneous fat to expose a strip of fascia in the midline about 2 cm wide. Some operators prefer to incise the rectus sheath with the scalpel throughout the length of the fascial incision. Others prefer to make a small opening and then to incise the visualized fascial layer with scissors. There seems to be less bleeding with the latter approach, as well as reduced risk of inadvertently incising the structures, especially bowel, that might be lying beneath the peritoneum. The rectus and the pyramidalis muscles are separated in the midline by sharp and blunt dissection to expose the underlying transversalis fascia and peritoneum.

The transversalis fascia and properitoneal fat are carefully dissected beginning near the upper pole of the incision to reach the underlying peritoneum. The peritoneum near the upper end of the incision is elevated with two hemostats placed about 2 cm apart. The tented fold of peritoneum between the clamps is visualized and palpated to rule out the inclusion of omentum, bowel, or bladder, and only then is the peritoneum carefully opened. In women who have had previous intra-abdominal surgery, including cesarean section, omentum or even bowel may be adherent to the undersurface of the peritoneum. The peritoneum is incised superiorly to the upper pole of the incision and downward to just above the peritoneal reflection over the bladder.

Troublesome bleeding sites anywhere in the abdominal incision are clamped as encountered but are not ligated until later, unless the hemostats are in the way. Bleeding vessels should not be ignored, however, for it is essential that there be no active bleeding when the wound is closed.

The uterus is quickly but carefully palpated to identify the size and the presenting part of the fetus and to determine the direction and degree of rotation of the uterus. Commonly, the uterus is dextrorotated so that the left round ligament is more anterior and closer to the midline than the right. It may be levorotated, however. Some opera-

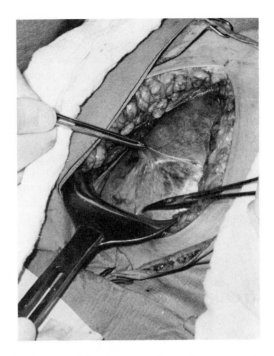

FIG. 43-1. The loose vesicouterine serosa is grasped in the forceps. The hemostat tip points to the upper margin of the bladder. The retractor is firm against the symphysis.

tors prefer to lay a moistened laparotomy pack in each lateral peritoneal gutter to absorb amnionic fluid and blood that escape from the opened uterus.

The typically rather loose reflection of peritoneum (serosa) above the upper margin of the bladder and overlying the anterior lower uterine segment is grasped in the midline with forceps (Fig. 43-1) and incised with a scalpel or scissors. Scissors, inserted between the serosa and myometrium of the lower uterine segment, are pushed laterally from the midline, while partially opening the blades, intermittently, to separate a 2 cm-wide strip of serosa which is then incised. As the lateral margin on each side is approached, the scissors are aimed somewhat more cephalad (Fig. 43-2). The lower flap of peritoneum is elevated and the bladder is gently separated by blunt dissection from the underlying myometrium (Fig. 43-3). In general, the separation of bladder should not exceed 5 cm in depth and is usually less. (It is possible, especially

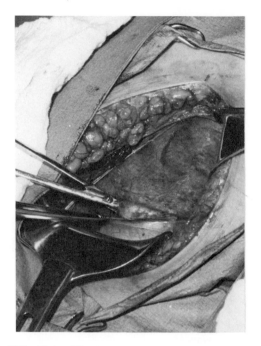

FIG. 43-2. The loose serosa above the upper margin of the bladder is being elevated and incised laterally.

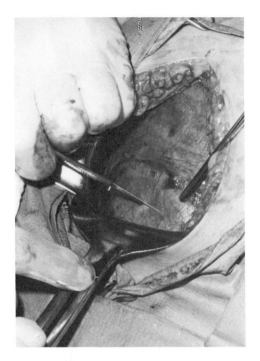

FIG. 43-4. The myometrium is being carefully incised to avoid cutting the fetal head.

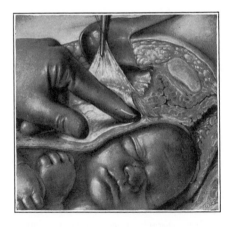

FIG. 43-3. Low segment cesarean section. Cross section showing dissection of bladder off uterus to expose lower uterine segment.

with an effaced, dilated cervix, to dissect downward so deeply as inadvertently to expose and then enter the underlying vagina rather than the lower uterine segment.) The developed bladder flap is held downward beneath the symphysis with a bladder retractor such as that used with a Balfour self-retaining retractor.

The uterus is opened through the lower uterine segment about 2 cm above the detached bladder. The uterine incision can be made by a variety of technics. Each is initiated by incising with a scalpel the exposed lower uterine segment transversely for 2 cm or so halfway between the lateral margins. This must be done carefully so as to cut completely through the uterine wall but not into the underlying fetus (Figs. 43-4, 43-5). Suctioning of the operative field by an assistant is especially important. Once the uterus is opened, the incision can be extended by cutting laterally and then slightly upward with bandage scissors; or when the lower segment is thin, the incision of entry can be extended by simply spreading the incision, using lateral pressure applied with each index finger (Fig. 43-6), or a combination of these technics can be used (Fig. 43-7). Exposure is aided by placement of a Richardson retractor into the wound and retracting the abdominal wall laterally as the incision is extended toward that

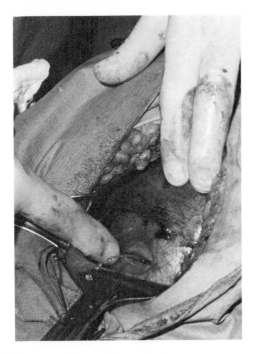

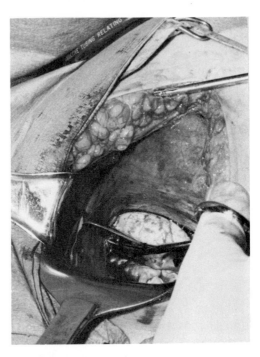

FIG. 43-5. The uterine cavity has been entered. Amnionic fluid is escaping through the incision.

FIG. 43-7. Bandage scissors are used to complete the transverse incision when resistance to spreading is encountered.

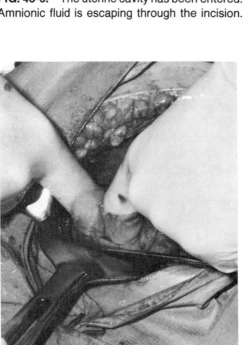

FIG. 43-6. The index fingers inserted through the incised lower uterine segment exert moderate pressure laterally to extend the opening in the uterus.

side. *It is very important to make the uterine incision large enough to allow delivery of the head and trunk of the fetus without either tearing into or having cut into the uterine arteries and veins that course through the lateral margins of the uterus.* If it appears that the uterine incision is going to be too small, some extra room may be obtained by curving the incision upward bilaterally to avoid the lateral uterine vessels. The membranes are incised if this was not done previously. If the placenta is encountered in the line of incision, it must be either detached or incised. Especially when incised, fetal hemorrhage may be severe. Therefore, the cord should be clamped as soon as possible.

DELIVERY OF INFANT. The retractors are removed, and if the vertex is presenting a hand is slipped into the uterine cavity between the symphysis and fetal head, and the head is gently elevated with the fingers and palm through the incision (Fig. 43-8.A, B) aided by modest transabdominal fundal pres-

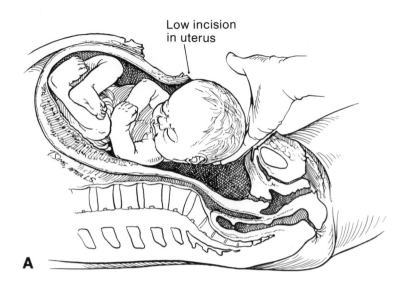

Low incision
in uterus

A

FIG. 43-8. A. Immediately after incising the uterus and fetal membranes, the operator's fingers are insinuated between the symphysis pubis and the fetal head until the posterior surface is reached. The head is carefully lifted anteriorly and, as necessary, superiorly to bring it from beneath the symphysis forward through the uterine and abdominal incisions. **B.** As the fetal head is lifted through the incision, pressure is usually applied to the uterine fundus through the abdominal wall to help expel the fetus.

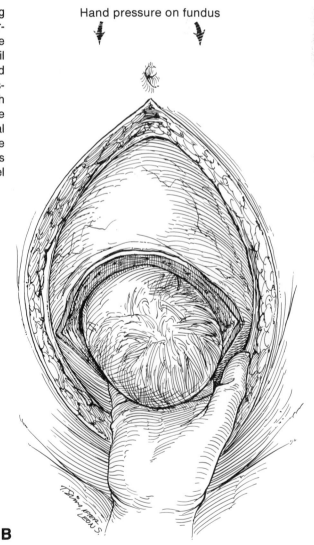

Hand pressure on fundus

B

sure. To minimize aspiration of amnionic fluid and its contents, the exposed nares and mouth are aspirated with a bulb syringe before the thorax is delivered. The shoulders are then delivered using gentle traction plus fundal pressure. The rest of the body readily follows.

Some operators favor delivery of the head with short-handled Simpson-type forceps. After a long labor with cephalopelvic disproportion, the fetal head may be rather tightly wedged in the birth canal. Upward pressure exerted through the vagina by the sterile-gloved hand of an associate will readily dislodge the head and allow its delivery above the symphysis pubis.

As soon as the shoulders are delivered (Fig. 43-9), an intravenous infusion containing about 20 units of oxytocin per liter is allowed to run in at the brisk rate of 10 ml per minute or so until the uterus contracts satisfactorily and then the rate is reduced to 2 to 4 ml per minute. The cord is promptly clamped with the infant at the level of the abdominal wall and the infant is given to the member of the team who will conduct resusci-

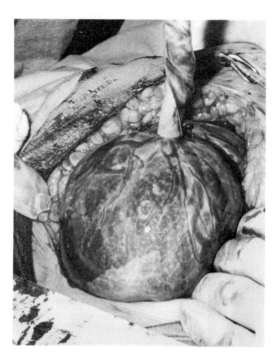

FIG. 43-10. Placenta bulging through uterine incision as uterus contracts.

tative efforts as they are needed. A sample of cord blood is obtained from the placental end of the cord.

If the fetus is not presenting as a vertex, or if there are multiple fetuses, a longitudinal incision through the lower segment may, at times, prove to be advantageous. The fetal legs must be carefully distinguished from the arms to avoid premature extraction of an arm and difficult delivery of the rest of the fetus.

The uterine incision is observed for any vigorously bleeding sites. These are promptly clamped, depending upon size and location, with Pean forceps, short-handled ring forceps, or similar instruments. The placenta is promptly removed manually, unless it is rapidly separating spontaneously (Fig. 43-10). Fundal massage, begun through the abdominal wall as soon as the fetus is delivered, reduces bleeding and hastens delivery of the placenta.

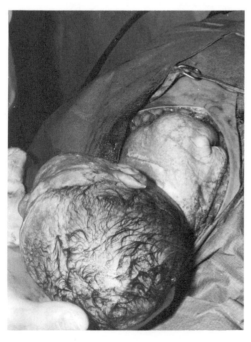

FIG. 43-9. Just as the shoulders are delivered, intravenous oxytocin infusion is started.

REPAIR OF UTERUS. After delivery of the placenta, the uterus may be lifted through the incision onto the draped abdominal wall and the fundus covered with a moistened laparotomy pack.*

Immediately after delivery and inspection of the placenta, the uterine cavity is inspected and may be wiped out with a gauze pack to remove shreds of membranes, vernix, clots, or other debris. If the cervical canal is not known to be patent, it should be probed with a Pean clamp to assure patency. The contaminated clamp is discarded from the field.

The upper and lower cut edges and each angle of the uterine incision are carefully examined for bleeding vessels. The lower margin of an incision made through a thinned-out lower uterine segment may be so thin as to be ignored inadvertently. At the same time, the posterior wall of the lower uterine segment may occasionally buckle anteriorly in such a way as to suggest that it is the lower margin of the incision. Incorporation of the posterior wall into the closure must be avoided.

The uterine incision may be closed with either one or the more traditional two layers of continuous chromic suture. Individually clamped large vessels are best ligated with a suture ligature. Concern has been expressed by some that sutures through the decidua may lead to endometriosis in the scar and a weak scar. In actuality, this is a rare complication. The initial stitch is placed just beyond one angle of the uterine incision. A running-lock

* Extra-abdominal exteriorization of the uterus immediately after delivery of the placenta often has advantages that outweigh the disadvantages. The relaxing uterus can be quickly recognized and fundal massage applied. The uterine incision and bleeding points along its cut margins are more easily visualized and sutured, especially when the incision extended during delivery of the fetus. There is also better exposure of the adnexa, especially the oviducts, which increases the ease and accuracy of tubal sterilization. The disadvantages are discomfort and, less often, vomiting during exteriorization or replacement when epidural or spinal anesthesia is used and possibly inadvertent displacement of a ligature from an oviduct at the site of discontinuity for sterilization. Hershey and Quilligan (1978), in the course of a study of the advantages and disadvantages of exteriorization of the uterus, did not find febrile morbidity to be more common in women whose uteri were exteriorized for closure.

suture is then carried out with each stitch penetrating the full thickness of the myometrium. It is important to select carefully the site of each stitch, and once the needle penetrates the myometrium, not to withdraw it. This minimizes the perforation of unligated vessels and subsequent bleeding from such. The running lock suture is continued just beyond the opposite angle of the incision.

Especially when the lower segment is thin, satisfactory approximation of the cut edges usually can be obtained with one layer of suture. When but one layer of suture is to be used, both hemostasis and closure may be better effected by tying the first running lock suture at about the middle of the incision, placing a new suture beyond the opposite angle in the same way as the first, and closing the remainder of the incision with a running lock stitch. If approximation is not satisfactory after a single-layer continuous closure, or if bleeding sites persist, either another layer of suture may be placed so as to achieve approximation and hemostasis, or sites of unsatisfactory approximation or lack of hemostasis can be treated with individual figure-of-eight or mattress sutures.

After making sure that there is no further bleeding after closure of the uterine incision, the cut edges of the serosa overlying the uterus and bladder are approximated with a continuous 00 chromic catgut suture (Figs. 43-11, 43-12). The lower edge of peritoneum should not be carried above the upper edge, since this tends to advance the bladder, especially if the procedure is repeated during subsequent cesarean sections. To do so may lead to bladder discomfort and undue urinary frequency during later pregnancies, as well as difficult dissection of an unusually adherent, overlapped peritoneum, with subsequent cesarean section or hysterectomy.

Tubal Sterilization.   If tubal sterilization is to be performed, it is done now. The failure rate after the following technic is low (Husbands et al., 1970):

1. Visualize the fallopian tube in its entirety.
2. Grasp the midportion in a Babcock clamp

at a site where the mesosalpinx is seen to be free of veins.

3. Perforate the mesosalpinx immediately beneath the fallopian tube with a fine hemostat and then open the jaws to separate the mesosalpinx from the tube for at least 2 cm.

4. Ligate the separated segment proximally and distally with individual pieces of 00 chromic suture so as to isolate a segment of at least 2 cm.

5. Excise the isolated segment, identify it, and submit it for histologic confirmation.

6. Observe sites of resection for bleeding and, if found, clamp and ligate with fine suture. This technic is described in Chapter 40, page 1032.

Abdominal Closure. Laparotomy packs, if used, are removed and the gutters and cul-de-sac emptied of blood and amnionic fluid by gentle suction. If general anesthesia is used, the interior of the abdominal cavity is systematically palpated as a rule, to evaluate the abdominal contents. With conduction anesthesia, however, this may produce considerable discomfort. The uterus is reexamined and compressed to express any blood within it.

As soon as the "sponge count" has been ascertained to be correct, the abdominal wall is closed. As each layer is closed, bleeding sites are searched for, clamped, and ligated. Continuous 00 chromic catgut suture is used to close the peritoneum, including the overlying transversalis fascia (Fig. 43-13). It is important to avoid leaving a defect at either end of the incision and to place each stitch far enough laterally to ensure a strong closure. The rectus muscles are allowed to fall into place and the overlying rectus fascia is closed with interrupted 00 silk or similar sutures that are placed well lateral to the cut fascial edges and no more than 1 cm apart. The subcutaneous tissue usually need not be closed separately if it is 2 cm or less in thickness, and the skin is closed with vertical mattress sutures of 000 or 0000 silk or equivalent

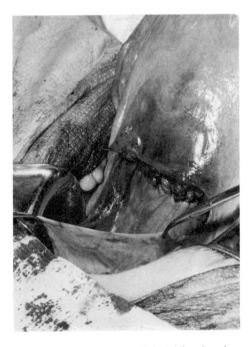

FIG. 43-11. The myometrial incision has been closed. The lower edge of the cut serosa is identified in the clamps.

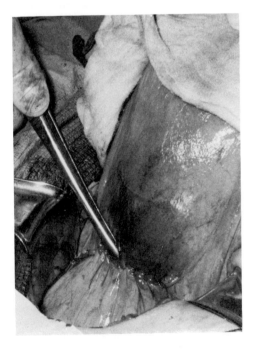

FIG. 43-12. The cut margins of the serosa have been approximated to reperitonealize the uterus.

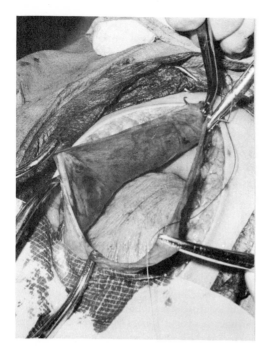

FIG. 43-13. The firmly contracted uterus is visible through the uterine incision. The cut margins of the parietal peritoneum are elevated and closure has been initiated.

suture. If there is more adipose tissue than this or if clips or subcuticular closure is to be used, a few interrupted 000 plain catgut sutures are used to obliterate dead space and reduce tension on the skin edges.

The abdominal wall in most circumstances need only be covered with a light dressing consisting of three 4 x 4 sponges unfolded once and fastened with three pieces of 1-inch tape.

Classical Cesarean Section. On occasion, it may be necessary to use a classical cesarean section to effect delivery, for example: (1) if the lower uterine segment cannot be exposed or entered safely because the bladder is densely adherent from previous surgery, or if a myoma occupies the lower uterine segment, or if there is invasive carcinoma of the cervix; (2) when there is a transverse lie of a large fetus, especially if the membranes are ruptured and the shoulder is impacted in the birth canal; (3) in some cases of placenta previa with anterior implantation of the placenta, especially if sterilization is to be performed (see Chap. 21, p. 508).

INCISIONS. The abdominal incision usually needs to extend somewhat higher than for a lower segment cesarean section. (Originally the classic incision extended to very near the top of the uterine fundus; therefore, to expose the uterus the vertical incision in the abdominal wall typically was made just below, lateral to, and above the umbilicus.) The vertical incision into the uterus is initiated with a scalpel beginning clearly above the level of the bladder. It is essential to incise through the uterine wall but not lacerate the fetus. Brisk bleeding during entry may make visualization difficult. Once sufficient room is made with the scalpel, the incision is extended cephalad with bandage scissors until sufficiently long to permit delivery of the fetus. Numerous large vessels that may bleed profusely are commonly encountered within the myometrium. As soon as the fetus has been removed, these vessels may best be clamped and eventually ligated with sutures of chromic catgut. As soon as the fetus has been delivered, oxytocin is administered and the placenta delivered as described above under "Lower Segment Transverse Incision."

REPAIR OF UTERUS. The uterus may be lifted through the incision and placed on the abdominal wall. The uterine incision is closed in such a manner that the cut edges are evenly and completely coapted and hemorrhage is controlled. One method employs a layer of continuous chromic catgut, size zero or one, to approximate the inner halves of the incision. The outer half of the uterine incision is then closed with similar chromic catgut suture, using either a continuous stitch or figure-of-eight sutures. Each stitch should be placed sufficiently deep into the myometrium that it will not pull out. No unnecessary needle tracts should be made lest myometrial vessels be perforated with hemorrhage or hematoma formation. To achieve good approximation and to prevent the suture from tearing through the myometrium, it is essential that an assistant compress the myometrium on each side of the wound medially as each suture is tied. The edges of the uterine serosa, if not already so, are approximated with continuous 00 chromic catgut. The operation is completed as described above under "Lower Segment Transverse Incision."

Extraperitoneal Cesarean Section. Early in this century, Frank (1907) and Latzko (1909) recommended extraperitoneal cesarean section rather than cesarean hysterectomy as a method of dealing with pregnancies with infected uterine contents. The goal of the operation was to open the uterus extraperitoneally by dissecting through the space of Retzius and then along one side and beneath the bladder to reach the lower uterine segment. The writings of Waters (1940) and Norton (1946) helped to popularize the operation in this country at midcentury. Enthusiasm for the procedure was transient, however, probably in large part because of the availability of a variety of effective antibacterial agents. The increased frequency in recent years of cesarean section, accompanied by either an actual increase in frequency and intensity of troublesome infections, or at least a reawareness of the problem, has rekindled interest in the use of extraperitoneal cesarean section. Perkins (1977), for example, has demonstrated some enthusiasm for the procedure, but, at the same time, has carefully pointed out the limitations of the procedure, as well as the benefits that might be derived from its use. He favors the technic described by Douglas and Stromme (1965), who have modified slightly those of Latzko and Norton.

Postmortem Cesarean Section. Both Weber (1970) and Arthur (1978) emphasize that a satisfactory outcome for the fetus is dependent upon (1) anticipation of death of the mother, (2) fetal age of more than 28 weeks, (3) personnel and appropriate equipment immediately available, (4) continued postmortem ventilation and cardiac massage for the mother, (5) prompt delivery, and (6) effective resuscitation of the infant. While a

few infants have survived with no apparent physical or intellectual compromise, others have not been so fortunate. In more recent years, the capability of life-support systems to maintain some level of vegetative function for long periods of time and the reluctance of physicians to pronounce a patient dead, have decreased further the likelihood of delivering an infant that will survive and thrive by postmortem cesarean section.

Choice of Abdominal Incisions. The most common abdominal incision for cesarean section or cesarean hysterectomy is the vertical incision described above under "Lower Segment Transverse Incision." With the alternative Pfannenstiel type of incision, the skin and subcutaneous tissue are incised transversely. Actually, a slightly curvilinear incision is made at the level of the pubic hairline to extend somewhat beyond the lateral borders of the rectus muscles. After the subcutaneous tissue has been separated from the underlying fascia for 1 cm or so on each side, the fascia is incised transversely the full length of the incision. The superior and inferior edges of the fascia are grasped with suitable clamps. First, the inferior margin is elevated by the assistant as the operator separates the fascial sheath from the underlying rectus muscles by blunt dissection with the scalpel handle. Then the superior fascial margin is elevated and the rectus sheath freed from the rectus muscles. Blood vessels coursing between the muscles and fascia are clamped, severed, and ligated. It is imperative that meticulous hemostasis be achieved. The separation is carried to near the umbilicus sufficient to permit an adequate midline longitudinal incision of the peritoneum. The rectus muscles are separated from each other and from the underlying transversalis fascia and peritoneum. The peritoneum is opened as described under "Lower Segment Transverse Incision." Closure in layers is carried out the same as with a vertical incision, except that many operators, in trying to prevent hematoma formation, place beneath the fascia small Penrose drains that exit from each angle of the fascial closure. The cosmetic advantage of the transverse skin incision is apparent. Moreover, the incision is said to be stronger with less likelihood of dehiscence or hernia formation. There are, nonetheless, disadvantages in use of the transverse incision. Exposure of the pregnant uterus and appendages is not as good. Whenever more room is needed, the vertical incision can be rapidly extended around and above the umbilicus, whereas the Pfannenstiel incision cannot. If the woman is obese, the operative field is even more restricted. Therefore, Pfannenstiel's incision tends to be used for thin women by operators who have achieved technical expertise while the vertical incision is used almost to the exclusion of the transverse incision whenever rapid delivery is indicated, or the woman is obese, or the operator is developing his skills. It is not appropriate to compare the vertical incision under these more adverse conditions to the transverse incision carried out under much more favorable circumstances. Finally, at the time of repeat cesarean section, reentry through Pfannenstiel's incision is likely to be more time consuming which, at times, can be detrimental to the fetus.

CESAREAN HYSTERECTOMY

Indications. The indications for cesarean hysterectomy have been discussed in connection with the various conditions that sometimes require the operation. In summary, intrauterine infection, a defective scar, a markedly hypotonic uterus that does not respond to oxytocics and massage, inadvertent laceration of major uterine vessels, significant myomas, severe dysplasia or carcinoma in situ, and placenta accreta or increta often may be best treated by immediate hysterectomy if cesarean section is being performed. The major deterrents to use of cesarean hysterectomy are increased blood loss and the frequency of damage to the urinary tract in the form of trauma to the ureters and more commonly to the bladder. The merits of cesarean hysterectomy for sterilization, rather than cesarean section plus partial tubal resection, remain the subject of much interest and are considered in Chapter 40, page 1036.

Technic. After delivery of the infant by either classical or lower segment cesarean section, supracervical or preferably total hysterectomy, usually with retention of the adnexa, can be carried out according to standard operative technics. Although *all vessels to the gravid uterus are appreciably larger than those of the*

nonpregnant organ, hysterectomy is usually facilitated by the ease of development of tissue planes. Blood loss commonly is appreciable, however. With cesarean hysterectomy performed primarily for sterilization, blood loss averages about 1500 ml, or about 500 ml more than with cesarean section (Pritchard, 1965).

As the infant's shoulders are delivered, oxytocin is infused intravenously until the uterus is removed. The major bleeding vessels are clamped and ligated quickly. The placenta is removed, and optionally to try to prevent excessive bleeding, a dry laparotomy pack is placed in the cavity over the implantation site before closing the uterine incision with either a continuous suture or a few interrupted sutures.

The uterus is elevated out of the abdominal cavity, and the round ligaments close to the uterus are divided between Heaney or Kocher clamps and doubly ligated. Either size 0 or 1 chromic catgut is used. The incision in the vesicouterine serosa, made to mobilize the bladder for cesarean section, is extended laterally and upward through the anterior leaf of the broad ligament to reach the incised round ligaments. Any actively bleeding vessels must be clamped and tied to minimize blood loss. The posterior leaf of the broad ligament adjacent to the uterus is perforated just beneath the fallopian tubes, utero-ovarian ligaments, and ovarian vessels, and these are then doubly clamped close to the uterus and severed; the lateral pedicle is doubly ligated. The pedicles adjacent to the uterus may be ligated and the clamps removed from the operative field. The posterior leaf of the broad ligament is next divided inferiorly toward the cardinal ligaments. Again, any bleeding vessels are discretely clamped and ligated. Next, the bladder and attached peritoneal flap are dissected from lower uterine segment and retracted out of the operative field. Usually this can be accomplished easily with gentle blunt dissection using gauze over the fingers. If the bladder flap is unusually adherent, as it may be after previous cesarean sections, careful sharp dissection with scissors is necessary.

Special care is necessary from this point on to avoid injury to the ureters, which pass beneath the uterine arteries. The ascending uterine artery and veins on either side are identified and near their origin are doubly clamped immediately adjacent to the uterus, and divided. The vascular pedicle is doubly ligated.

SUPRACERVICAL HYSTERECTOMY. To perform a subtotal hysterectomy, it is necessary only to amputate the body of the uterus at this level. The cervical stump may be closed with interrupted catgut sutures. If there is persistent oozing of blood or the likelihood of infection, the cervix may be dilated and a drain inserted into the vagina. Reperitonealization is performed as for total hysterectomy.

TOTAL HYSTERECTOMY. To perform a total hysterectomy, it is necessary to mobilize the bladder much more extensively in the midline and laterally. This will help carry the ureters inferiorly as the bladder is retracted beneath the symphysis and will also prevent cutting or suturing of the bladder during excision of the cervix and closure of the vagina. The bladder is dissected free for about 2 cm below the lowest margin of the cervix to expose the uppermost part of the vagina. If the cervix is no more than slightly effaced, it can be identified by palpation between the fingers with one hand in the cul-de-sac and the other anteriorly to identify the level at which the vagina can be entered yet remove all of the cervix. If the cervix is appreciably effaced and dilated, this maneuver usually cannot be performed satisfactorily. In this circumstance, the uterine cavity may be entered anteriorly in the midline either through the lower pole of the incision made for delivery of the fetus or through a stab wound made at the level of the ligated uterine vessels. A finger is directed inferiorly through the incision to identify the free margin of the dilated, effaced cervix and the anterior vaginal fornix.

The cardinal ligaments, the uterosacral ligaments, and the many large vessels the ligaments contain are systematically doubly clamped with Heaney-type curved clamps, Ochsner-type straight clamps, or similar instruments. The clamps are placed as close to the cervix as possible without including the cervix. It is imperative that not too large a volume of tissue be included in each clamp. The tissue between the pair of clamps is incised and the lateral pedicle, which invariably is vascular, is ligated appropriately. These steps are repeated until the level of the lateral vaginal fornix is reached. In this way, the descending branches of the uterine vessels are clamped, cut, and ligated as the cervix is dissected from the cardinal ligaments laterally and the uterosacral ligaments posteriorly.

Immediately below the level of the cervix, a curved clamp is swung in across the lateral vaginal fornix and the tissue is incised medially to the clamp. The excised lateral vaginal fornix commonly is simultaneously ligated and sutured to the stump of the cardinal ligament. The entire cervix is then excised from the vagina while an assistant systematically grasps the full thickness of the cut margins of the vagina with straight Ochsner or similar clamps.

The cervix is inspected to ascertain complete removal, and the vagina is repaired. Some operators prefer to close the vagina using figure-of-eight chromic catgut sutures. Perhaps the majority prefer to achieve hemostasis by using a running-lock stitch of chromic catgut suture placed through the mucosa and surrounding endopelvic fascia around the circumference of the vagina. The "open" vagina may promote drainage of fluids that would otherwise accumulate and contribute to abscess formation.

The peritoneal gutters and the cul-de-sac are emptied of blood and other debris. All sites of incision from the upper pedicle (fallopian tube and ovarian ligament) to the vaginal vault and bladder flap are carefully examined for bleeding. Any bleeding sites that are identified are clamped carefully and ligated appropriately. Care is necessary lest the ureter be compromised by such a hemostatic ligature.

The pelvis is reperitonealized. One method employs a continuous chromic suture starting with the tip of the ligated pedicle of fallopian tube and ovarian ligament which is inverted retroperitoneally. Sutures are then placed continuously so as to approximate the leaves of the broad ligament, to bury the stump of the round ligament, to approximate the cut edge of the vesicouterine peritoneum over the vaginal vault posteriorly to the cut edge of peritoneum above the cul-de-sac, to approximate the leaves of the broad ligament on the opposite side, and to bury the stump of the round ligament and finally the pedicle of the fallopian tube and ovarian ligament.

The abdominal wall normally is closed in layers as described under "Lower Segment Transverse Incision." In case of sepsis, the abdominal wound may be closed with permanent nonreactive sutures through the peritoneum and fascia while the subcutaneous tissue and skin are not closed until later.

Appendectomy and Oophorectomy.
The benefits compared to the risks from incidental appendectomy at the time of cesarean section or hysterectomy continue to be argued. Lacking are results of a study which demonstrate clearly that puerperal morbidity and mortality rates are not increased by appendectomy.

During cesarean hysterectomy, a decision as to the fate of the ovaries has to be made. Should the clamp be placed across the ovarian ligament and fallopian tube medial to the ovary or across the infundibulopelvic ligament just lateral to the ovary and tube? For women who are approaching menopause, the decision is not difficult, but few women who undergo cesarean hysterectomy are approaching the menopause. In general, preservation of the ovaries is favored by most obstetricians unless the ovaries are diseased.

PERIPARTAL MANAGEMENT

Preoperative Care. The woman scheduled for repeat cesarean section typically is admitted the day before surgery and evaluated by the obstetrician who will perform surgery and the anesthesiologist who will provide anesthesia. The hematocrit is rechecked and usually 1000 ml of compatible whole blood or its equivalent in blood fractions is reserved. A sedative such as secobarbital, 0.1 g, maybe given at bedtime the night before the operation. In general, no other sedatives, narcotics, or tranquilizers are administered until after the infant is born. Oral intake is stopped at least eight hours before surgery. An antacid such as a suspension of magnesium hydroxide (milk of magnesia), 30 ml, given shortly before the induction of a general anesthetic minimizes the risk of lung destruction from gastric hydrochloric acid should aspiration occur (see Chap. 18, p. 440). At Parkland Memorial Hospital, this is done routinely, even when regional conduction anesthesia will be used; at times it is necessary to switch to, or at least complement, the regional anesthesia with general anesthesia.

Intravenous Fluids. The requirements for intravenous fluids, including blood during and after cesarean section, can vary considerably. The woman of average size with a hematocrit of 33 or more and a normally expanded blood volume and extracellular fluid volume most often tolerates an actual blood loss of up to 1500 ml without difficulty. The concept that prevailed in some institutions not too long ago that blood loss should be matched milliliter for milliliter by blood transfusion is not tenable. Neither is disregard for excessive bleeding. Careful attention must be paid to blood loss so as to avoid both underestimation and overestimation. Unappreciated bleeding through the vagina during the procedure, or of bleeding concealed in the uterus after its closure, or both, commonly lead to underestimation. Blood loss averages about 1 liter but is quite variable (Wilcox et al., 1959; Pritchard, 1965).

Intravenously administered fluids consist of lactated Ringer's solution or similar solution and 5 percent dextrose in water. Typically, 1 to 2 liters that contain electrolyte are infused during and immediately after the operation. As the shoulders of the infant are delivered, oxytocin, 20 units per liter, is added to the infusion which is then infused for a few minutes at a brisk rate (5 to 10 ml per minute) until the uterus is well contracted. Throughout the procedure, and subsequently while in the postoperative recovery area, the blood pressure and urine flow are monitored closely to ascertain that perfusion of vital organs is satisfactory.

Recovery Suite. It is very important that the uterus remain firmly contracted. In the recovery suite, the amount of bleeding from the vagina must be closely monitored and the uterine fundus must be identified by palpation repeatedly to ascertain that the uterus is remaining firmly contracted. Unfortunately, as the patient awakens from general anesthesia or the conduction anesthesia dissipates, palpation of the abdomen is likely to produce considerable discomfort. This can be made much more tolerable by giving an effective analgesic intramuscularly such as meperidine (Demerol), 75 mg, or morphine, 10 mg. A thick dressing with an abundance of adhesive tape over the abdomen interferes with fundal palpation and massage and later causes discomfort as the tape and perhaps skin are removed. Deep breathing and coughing are encouraged.

Once the mother is fully awake, bleeding is minimal, the blood pressure is satisfactory, and urine flow is at least 30 ml per hour, she may be returned to her room.

Subsequent Care. Her subsequent care must include the following:

ANALGESIA. For the woman of average size, meperidine, 75 mg, is given intramuscularly as often as every three hours as needed for discomfort, or morphine, 10 mg, is similarly administered. If she is quite small, 50 mg, or if quite large, 100 mg of meperidine is more appropriate.

VITAL SIGNS. The patient is now evaluated at least hourly for four hours at the minimum, and blood pressure, pulse, urine flow, amount of bleeding, and status of the uterine fundus are checked at these times. Abnormal-

ities are reported immediately. Thereafter, for the first 24 hours, these are checked at intervals of four hours, along with the temperature.

FLUID THERAPY AND DIET. Unless there has been pathologic constriction of the extracellular fluid compartment (diuretics, sodium restriction, vomiting, high fever, prolonged labor without adequate fluid intake), the puerperium is characterized by the excretion of fluid that was retained during pregnancy and became superfluous once delivery was accomplished. Moreover, with the typical cesarean section or uncomplicated cesarean hysterectomy, significant sequestration of extracellular fluid in bowel wall and bowel lumen does not occur, unless it was necessary to pack the bowel away from the operative field or peritonitis develops. Thus the woman who undergoes cesarean section is rarely a candidate for the development, fluid compartment-wise, of a so-called third space. Quite the contrary, she normally begins surgery with a physiologic "third space" which she acquired during normal pregnancy, namely, the physiologic edema of pregnancy which after delivery she mobilizes and excretes. Therefore, large volumes of intravenous fluids during surgery and subsequently are not needed to replace sequestered extracellular fluid. As a generalization, three liters of fluid, including lactated Ringer's solution, should prove quite adequate during surgery and the first 24 hours thereafter. If urine output falls below 30 ml per hour, however, the patient should be reevaluated promptly. The cause of the oliguria may range from unrecognized blood loss to an antidiuretic effect from infused oxytocin (see Chap. 17, p. 427). In the absence of extensive intra-abdominal manipulation or sepsis, the woman nearly always should be able to tolerate oral fluids the day after surgery. If not, an intravenous infusion can be continued or restarted. By the second day after surgery, the great majority of women should tolerate a general diet.

BLADDER AND BOWELS. The catheter

most often can be removed from the bladder by 12 hours after the operation, or more conveniently, the morning after the operation. Subsequent ability to empty the bladder before overdistension develops must be monitored as with a vaginal delivery. Bowel sounds usually are not heard the first day after surgery, they are faint the second day, and they are active the third day. "Gas pains" from incoordinate bowel action may be troublesome the second and third days. Frequently, a rectal suppository followed by defecation, or, if that fails, an enema, provides appreciable relief.

AMBULATION. In most instances, on the first day after surgery the patient should, with assistance, get out of bed briefly at least twice. Ambulation can be timed so that a recently administered analgesic will minimize the discomfort. By the second day she may walk to the bathroom with assistance. With early ambulation, venous thrombosis and pulmonary embolism are extremely uncommon.

CARE OF WOUND. The incision is inspected each day. Thus a relatively light dressing without an abundance of tape is advantageous. Normally the skin sutures (or skin clips) are removed on the fourth day after surgery. By the third postpartum day, bathing, either by shower or by tub bath, is not harmful to the incision.

LABORATORY. The hematocrit is routinely measured the morning after surgery. It is checked sooner when there was unusual blood loss or when there is oliguria or other evidence to suggest hypovolemia. If the hematocrit is significantly decreased from the preoperative level, it is repeated and search instituted to identify the cause of the decrease. If the lower hematocrit is stable, the mother can ambulate without any difficulty, and if there is little likelihood of further blood loss, hematologic repair in response to iron therapy is preferred to transfusion.

BREAST CARE. Breast-feeding can be initiated the day after surgery. If the mother elects not to breast-feed, a breast binder that supports the breasts without marked compression will usually minimize discomfort.

DISCHARGE. Unless there are complications during the puerperium, the mother may be safely discharged from the hospital on the fifth postpartum day. The mother's activities during the following week should be restricted to self-care and care of her baby with assistance. It is advantageous to perform the initial postpartum evaluation during the third week after delivery rather than at the more traditional time of six weeks, for reason presented in Chapters 19 and 40.

Prophylactic Antibiotics. Febrile morbidity is not unusual in women who undergo cesarean section and, for reasons not altogether clear, it is more common in indigent, nonprivate patients than in socioeconomically more affluent private patients. Since the discovery of sulfonilamide and then penicillin, innumerable attempts have been made to quantify the value, if any, of antibacterial agents administered prophylactically to the patient who undergoes surgery. For prophylaxis, the sulfonamides were given at the time of cesarean section orally, or intravenously, or more or less randomly dumped into the uterine incision. For each route of administration, there were physicians who were favorably impressed. The results of somewhat more sophisticated studies on various antibiotics more recently suggest that, in general, morbidity can be reduced somewhat by administering them around the time of cesarean section but that antibiotics prophylactically are far from a panacea against sepsis. Gibbs, Hunt, and Schwarz (1973), for example, reported that the febrile morbidity rate was 25 percent in patients who had undergone cesarean section when antibiotics were given prophylactically, compared to 63 percent in those who received a placebo. Many others have reported similar results. Death from pseudomembranous enterocolitis has been reported following the prophylactic administration of antibiotics initiated during repeat cesarean section (Ledger, Puttler, 1975).

HISTORICAL

The origin of the term *cesarean section* is obscure. Three principal explanations have been suggested:

1. According to legend, Julius Caesar was born in this manner, with the result that the procedure became known as the "Caesarean operation." Several circumstances weaken this explanation, however. First, the mother of Julius Caesar lived for many years after his birth. Even as late as the 17th century, the operation was almost invariably fatal, according to the most dependable writers of that period. It is thus improbable that Caesar's mother could have survived the procedure in 100 B.C. Second, the operation, whether performed on the living or dead, is not mentioned by any medical writer before the Middle Ages. Historical details of the origin of the family name "Caesar" are found in Pickrell's monograph.

2. It has been widely believed that the name of the operation is derived from a Roman law, supposedly created by Numa Pompilius (eighth century, B.C.), ordering that the procedure be performed upon women dying in the last few weeks of pregnancy in the hope of saving the child. This explanation then holds that this *lex regia,* as it was called at first, became the *lex caesarea* under the emperors, and the operation itself became known as the *caesarean* operation. The German term *Kaiserschnitt* reflects this derivation.

Numa Pompilius, however, was said to be the successor to Romulus, the mythical "first king" of Rome. Any writings later attributed to Numa Pompilius are dismissed by modern historians as sheer forgeries. If, moreover, this operation had actually been a legal requirement in antiquity, it would certainly have been mentioned by medical writers of the period; but it was not.

3. The word *caesarean,* as applied to the operation, was derived sometime in the Middle Ages from the Latin verb *caedere,* "to cut." An obvious cognate is the word *caesura,* a "cutting," or pause, in a line of verse. This explanation of the term *caesarean* seems most logical, but exactly when it was first applied to the operation is uncertain. Since "section" is derived from the Latin verb "seco," which also means "cut," the term "caesarean section" seems tautological.

It is customary in the United States to replace the "ae" ligature in the first syllable of "caesarean" with the letter "e"; in Great Britain, however, the "ae" is still retained.

From the time of Virgil's Aeneas to Shakespeare's Macduff, poets have repeatedly referred to persons "untimely ripped" from their mother's womb. Ancient historians such as Pliny, moreover, say that Scipio Africanus (the conqueror of Hannibal), Martius, and Julius Caesar were all born thus. In regard to Julius Caesar, Pliny adds that it was from this circumstance that the surname arose by which the Roman emperors were known. Birth in this extraordinary manner, as described in ancient mythology and legend, was believed to confer supernatural powers and elevate the heroes so born above ordinary mortals.

In evaluating these references to abdominal delivery in antiquity, it is pertinent that no such operation is even mentioned by Hippocrates, Galen, Celsus, Paulus, Soranus, or any other medical writer of the period. If cesarean section were actually employed at that time, it is particularly surprising that Soranus, whose extensive work written in the second century A.D. covers all aspects of obstetrics, does not refer to it. In Genesis (II:21) it is written: "And the Lord God caused a deep sleep to fall upon Adam, and he slept: and he took one of his ribs, and closed up the flesh instead thereof." Are we to conclude from this statement that general anesthesia and thoracic surgery were known in pre-Mosaic times? It would probably be just as logical to draw comparable conclusions about the beginnings of cesarean section from the myths and fantasies that have come down to us.

Several references to abdominal delivery appear in the Talmud, compiled between the second and sixth centuries A.D., but whether they had any background in terms of clinical usage is conjectural. There can be no doubt, however, that cesarean section on the dead was first practiced soon after the Christian Church gained dominance, as a measure directed at baptism of the child. Faith in the validity of some of these early reports is rudely shaken, however, when they glibly state that a living, robust child was obtained 8 to 24 *hours* after the death of the mother.

Some of the early reports of cesarean section on the living excite similar skepticism. The case often cited as representing the first cesarean section performed on a living woman is that attributed to a German gelder named Jacob Nufer, who is said to have carried out the operation on his wife in the year 1500. Not only did his wife survive (a miracle in itself) but she lived to give birth to two subsequent children after normal labors, in a period when suturing of the uterine wound during cesarean section was unknown. The case was not reported until almost a hundred years later (1591), by an author who based his description on hearsay handed down through three generations.

Cesarean section on the living was first recommended, and the current name of the operation used, in the celebrated work of François Rousset entitled "Traité Nouveau de l'Hystérotomotokie ou l'Enfantement Césarien," published in 1581. Rousset had never performed or witnessed the operation, his information having been based chiefly on letters from friends. He reported 14 successful cesarean sections, a fact in itself difficult to accept. When it is further stated that 6 of the 14 operations were performed on the same woman, the credulity of the most gullible is exhausted.

The apocryphal nature of most early reports on cesarean section has been stressed because many of them have been accepted without question. Authoritative statements by dependable obstetricians about early use of the operation, however, did not appear in the literature until the mid-17th century, as for instance in the classic work of the great French obstetrician François Mauriceau, first published in 1668. These statements show without doubt that the operation was employed on the living in rare and desperate cases during the latter half of the 16th century, and that it was usually fatal. Details of the history of cesarean section are to be found in Fasbender's classic text (1906).

The appalling maternal mortality rate of cesarean section continued until the beginning of the 20th century. In Great Britain and Ireland, the maternal death rate from the operation had mounted in 1865 to 85 percent. In Paris, during the 90 years ending in 1876, not a single successful cesarean section had been performed. Harris noted that as late as 1887 cesarean section was actually more successful when performed by the patient herself, or when the abdomen was ripped open by the horn of a bull. He collected from the literature 9 such cases with 5 recoveries, and contrasted them with 12 cesarean sections performed in New York City during the same period, with only 1 recovery.

The turning point in the evolution of cesarean section came in 1882, when Max Sänger, then a 28-year-old assistant of Credé in the University Clinic at Leipzig, introduced suturing of the uterine wall. The long neglect of so simple an expedient as uterine suture was not the result of oversight, but stemmed from a deeply rooted belief that sutures in the uterus were superfluous as well as harmful. In meeting these objections Sänger, who had himself used sutures in only one case, documented their value, not from the sophisticated medical centers of Europe, but from frontier America. There, in outposts from Ohio to Louisiana, 17 cesarean sections had been reported in which silver wire sutures had been used with the survival of 8 mothers, an extraordinary record in those days. In a table included in his monograph, Sänger gives full credit to these frontier surgeons for providing the supporting data for his hypothesis. The problem of hemorrhage was the first and most serious problem to be solved. Details are found in Eastman's review (1932).

Although the introduction of uterine sutures reduced the mortality rate of the operation from hemorrhage, generalized peritonitis remained the dominant cause of death; hence, various types of operations were devised to meet this scourge. The earliest was the Porro procedure, in use before Sänger's time, which combined subtotal cesarean hysterectomy with marsupialization of the cervical stump. The first extraperitoneal operation was described by Frank in 1907 and with various modifications, as introduced by Latzko, Sellheim, and by Waters (1940), was employed until recent years.

In 1912, Krönig contended that the main advantage of the extraperitoneal technic consisted not so much in avoiding the peritoneal cavity as in opening the uterus through its thin lower segment and then covering the incision with peritoneum. To accomplish this end, he cut through the vesical reflection of the peritoneum from one round ligament to the other and separated it and the bladder from the lower uterine segment and cervix. The lower portion of the uterus was then opened through a vertical median incision and the child extracted by forceps. The uterine incision was then closed and buried under the vesical peritoneum. With minor modifications, this low-segment technic was introduced into the United States by Beck (1919) and popularized by DeLee (1922) and others. A particularly important modification was recommended by Kerr in 1926, who preferred a transverse rather than a longitudinal uterine incision. The Kerr technic is the most commonly employed type of cesarean section today.

REFERENCES

Arthur RK: Postmortem cesarean section. Am J Obstet Gynecol 132:175,1978

Beck AC: Observations on a series of cases of cesarean section done at the Long Island College Hospital during the past six years. Am J Obstet Gynecol 79:197, 1919

Cunningham FG: Personal communication, 1980

Cunningham FG, Hauth JC, Strong JD, Kappus SS: Infectious morbidity following cesarean section: Comparison of two treatment regimens. Obstet Gynecol 52:656, 1978

DeLee JB, Cornell EL: Low cervical cesarean section (laparotrachelotomy). JAMA 79:109, 1922

Douglas RG, Stromme WB: Operative Obstetrics, 2nd ed. New York, Appleton, 1965, pp 449–452

Eastman NJ: The role of Frontier America in the development of cesarean section. Am J Obstet Gynecol 24:919, 1932

Fasbender H: Geschichte der Geburlshufe. Jena, 1906, pp 979–1010

Flaksman RS, Vollman JH, Benfield DG: Iatrogenic prematurity due to elective termination of the uncomplicated pregnancy: A major perinatal health care problem. Am J Obstet Gynecol 132:885, 1978

Frank F: Suprasymphysial delivery and its relation to other operations in the presence of contracted pelvis. Arch Gynaekol 81:46, 1907

Frigoletto FD Jr, Ryan KJ, Phillippe M: Maternal mortality rate associated with cesarean section: An appraisal. Am J Obstet Gynecol 136:969, 1980

Gibbs RS, Hunt JE, Schwarz RH: A follow-up study on prophylactic antibiotics in cesarean section. Am J Obstet Gynecol 117:419, 1973

Gluck L: Iatrogenic RDS and amniocentesis. Hosp Prac 12:11, 1977

Harris RP: Lessons from a study of the caesarean operation in the City and State of New York. Am J Obstet 12:82, 1879

Hershey DW, Quilligan EJ: Extraabdominal uterine exteriorization at cesarean section. Obstet Gynecol 52:189, 1978

Husbands ME Jr, Pritchard JA, Pritchard SA: Failure of tubal sterilization accompanying cesarean section. Am J Obstet Gynecol 107:966, 1970

Kerr JMM: The technic of cesarean section with special reference to the lower uterine segment incision. Am J Obstet Gynecol 12:729, 1926

Krönig B: Transperitonealer Cervikaler Kaiserschnitt. In Doderlein A, Kronig B (eds): Operative Gynäkologie, 1912, p 879

Latzko W: Ueber den extraperitonealen Kaiserschnitt. Zentralbl Gynaekol 33:275, 1909

Ledger WJ, Puttler OL: Death from pseudomembranous entercolitis. Obstet Gynecol 45:609, 1975

Norton JF: A paravesical extraperitoneal cesarean section technique. Am J Obstet Gynecol 51:519, 1946

Perkins RP: Extraperitoneal section: a viable alternative. Contem Ob Gyn 9:55, 1977

Petitti D, Olson RO, Williams RL: Cesarean section in California—1960 through 1975. Am J Obstet Gynecol 133:391, 1979

Pickrell K: An inquiry into the history of cesarean section. Bull Soc Med Hist (Chicago) 4:414, 1935

Pliny the Elder, Natural History, Book VII, Chap IX. Cambridge, Mass, Harvard University Press, 1942. Translated by H. Rackham

Porro E: Della Amputazione Utero-ovarica. Milan, 1876

Pritchard JA: Changes in the blood volume during pregnancy and delivery. Anesthesiology 26:393, 1965

Rousset F: Traite Nouveau de l'Hysterotomotokie ou l'Enfantement Cesarien. Paris, Denys deVal, 1581

Sänger M: Der Kaiserschnitt bei Uterusfibromen. Leipzig, 1882

Toffle RC, MacFee MS, Porreco RP: The management of elective, repeat cesarean section. J Reprod Med 21:377, 1978

Waters EG: Supravesical extraperitoneal cesarean section: Presentation of a new techique. Am J Obstet Gynecol 39:423, 1940

Weber CE: Postmortem cesarean section: Review of the literature and case reports. Am J Obstet Gynecol 110:158, 1970

Wilcox CF, Hunt AB, Owen CA: The measurement of blood lost during cesarean section. Am J Obstet Gynecol 77:772, 1959

INDEX

(Italicized numbers refer to illustrations and tables.)

1103

Methylmalonic aciduria, fetal, disorder, *341*
Metritis
 abortion and, 613
 puerperal, 897
Metronidazole (Flagyl), 325
Miconazole, 325
Microangiopathic hemolysis, 720
Midforceps
 definition, 1042, 1052
 pelvic contraction and, 837, 838
Midpelvis
 contractions, 258, 836—38
 size estimation, 285, 836—37
Migraine, oral contraception and, 774, 1018
Milk, breast. *See also* Lactation
 antibodies in, 464—65
 bilirubin and, 974—75
 composition, human, *464*
 drugs secreted into, 465
 "drying up", 918—19
 ejection, or "letting down", 464
 fever, 465
 immunologic qualities, 464—65
 mammary development and, *461, 463*
 mastitis and, 919
 oral contraceptives and, 1019
Milk, cows', *464*
Milk-leg, 908
Minerals
 fetal, *204*
 maternal, 232, 234, 312
 prenatal dietary, *312*
"Mini-laparotomy" for sterilization, 1034
Miscarriage. *See* Abortion
Missed abortion, 596
Mitral valvotomy, 735
Mittelschmerz, 49
Molding of fetal head, 177, 403
 brow presentation, 812
 cerebral hemorrhage, 995
 pelvic contraction, 834
Mole
 blood (carneous), 591
 hydatidiform. *See* Hydatidiform mole
 invasive, 558, 571
 tuberous subchorial, 591
Morphine analgesia. *See* Analgesia, labor and delivery
Monad, 95
Mongolism. *See* Down's syndrome
Moniliasis, 325
Monitoring, 358. *See also specific technic*
 definition, 352
 fetal, intrapartum, 352—64,
Mons pubis, 11

Monsters. *See* Fetus, malformations
Mons veneris, 11
Montgomery, follicles of, 228
Morbidity, puerperal, definition, 893
"Morning-after pill", 1020—21
Morning sickness, 270, 322—23
Mortality fetal. *See* Mortality, perinatal
Mortality maternal, 3—5
 abdominal pregnancy, 545
 abortion, 611
 anesthesia as the cause, 1083
 breech presentation, 802
 carcinoma of cervix, 626
 causes, common, 4
 cesarean section, 1083
 compared to perinatal, 5
 decline, *4*
 definition, 3
 direct, 3
 diabetes, 740, 745
 eclampsia, 687, 1083
 hemorrhage, 4, 487
 hydatidiform mole, 565
 hypertension, 4
 indirect, 3
 infection, 4
 placenta previa, 514
 pregnancy-induced hypertension, 4, 687
 racial differences, 4
 sickle-cell diseases, 721, 723
Mortality, neonatal. *See also* Mortality, perinatal
 definition, 2
 rates, *5*
Mortality, perinatal, 5
 abdominal pregnancy, 545
 abnormal development, 545
 abortion, threatened and, 592
 after abortion, 612
 age, gestational, 587—88, 929—30, 949
 bacteriuria, 903—04
 breech presentation, 802—03
 black vs. white, 6
 causes, 5—6
 cerebral hemorrhage, 6, 985
 cesarean section, 1083
 compound presentation, 818
 definition, 2
 diabetes, 743, 745
 drug addiction, 981
 eclampsia, 687, 692
 fetal transfusion and, 970
 hemolytic disease, 962
 hyaline membrane disease, *958, 959*
 low birth weight and, 5—6, 923, 929